Atherosclerosis XI

Atherosclerosis XI

Proceedings of the XIth International Symposium on Atherosclerosis, held in Paris, France, on 5—9 October 1997

Editors:

B. Jacotot
Hôpital Henri Mondor
Créteil Cedex, France

D. Mathé
Institut de Protection et de Sûreté Nucléaire
Foutenay aux Roses Cedex, France

J.-C. Fruchart
Département d'Athérosclérose
INSERM
Institut Pasteur
Lille Cedex, France

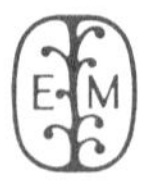

1998

ELSEVIER

Amsterdam – Lausanne – New York – Oxford – Shannon – Singapore – Tokyo

International Congress Series No. 1155
ISBN 0 444 82651 3

This book is printed on acid-free paper.

Published by:
Elsevier Science (Singapore) Pte Ltd.
No. 1 Temasek Ave.
#17-01 Millenia Tower
Singapore 039192

Printed in The Netherlands

Preface

This volume is the result of a fruitful experience, arising from the Eleventh International Symposium on Atherosclerosis, held in Paris on October 1997. As for the previous symposia of the International Atherosclerosis Society (IAS), every 3 years these proceedings will allow to widely spread the present situation of the research on Athero-thrombosis. Several hundred scientists have collaborated on the contribution to the proceedings. For their active participation in the conferences and their effort in the article writing, we express to all colleagues our warm gratitude.

The members of the French Atherosclerosis Society and ARCOL have joined their potentialities to make this symposium a privileged place of meetings and exchanges for thousands of participants coming from all over the world. We hope to have come up to their expectations.

The Paris meeting gave us the opportunity to express our admiration and our friendship to some colleagues, with honours being given in particular to: Daniel Steinberg, who received the 1997 Fredrickson Award; and Claude Lenfant and Philippe Douste-Blazy, who received the ARCOL Prizes.

The XIth Symposium on Atherosclerosis was also the occasion where homage could be paid to those colleagues who disappeared from the Montreal Symposium. We thank Daria Haust, historian of the International Atherosclerosis Society, who recalls in this book their outstanding careers and what they have brought to our branch of knowledge. Moreover, the memory of Gotthard Schettler, founder of the International Society and of the European Society of Atherosclerosis, was honoured by a memorial lecture given by the past president of the IAS, Antonio Gotto Jr. The memory of Schlomo Eisenberg, who tragically died near Paris 3 years ago, was honoured by a memorial lecture given by Jan Breslow.

Let me recall here the names of those IAS board members from previous years who trusted us with the organization of this symposium: Antonio M. Gotto Jr (President), Gotthard Schettler (Past-President), Rodolfo Paoletti (President-Elect), Maryvonne Rosseneu (Secretary), Daniel Pometta (Treasurer), Daria Haust (Historian), Jean Davignon, Yeckezkiel Stein and Akira Yamamoto (Members at large).

With Jean Charles Fruchart (Co-chairman), Denis Mathé (General Secretary), the Local Organizing Commitee members, the National Program Committee members and organizers of the Satellites Meetings, I would like to thank the generous sponsors who have allowed us to raise the welcome standard of the participants and the quality of the social program:
Major sponsors: Bristol Myers Squibb, Groupe Fournier, Merck & Co. Inc., Novartis, Parke Davis, Sanofi Recherche.

Main sponsors: Bayer AG, Pierre Fabre Santé.
Patron sponsors: Boehringer Mannheim, Rhone Poulenc Rorer.
Other sponsors: Otsuka Pharmaceutica, Daiichi Pharmaceutica, Laboratoires Servier.
Other contributors: AWD Arzneimittelwerk Dresden GmbH, Bristol Myers Squibb France, Fournier France, Gödecke AG Berlin, Immuno GmbH Heidelberg, Merckle GmbH Blauberen, MSD Sharp & Dohme GmbH Haar.
We look forward to meeting all of you again, in less than 3 years, on the occasion of the XIIth International Symposium on Atherosclerosis in Stockholm.

Bernard Jacotot

Committees

International Atherosclerosis Society

President:
A.M. Gotto Jr., USA
Past President:
G. Schettler, Germany
President Elect:
R. Paoletti, Italy
Secretary:
M. Rosseneu, Belgium
Treasurer:
D. Pometta, Switzerland
Historian:
D. Haust, Canada
Members at large:
Y. Stein, Israel
J. Davignon, Canada
A. Yamamoto, Japan

XIth International Symposium Organising Committee

B. Jacotot
J.C. Fruchart $\Big\}$ *Chairmen*
D. Mathé, *Secretary*
G. Ailhaud
F. Berthezène
B. Bihain
J. Bonnet
M.G. Bousser
L. Capron
M.J. Chapman
F. Delahaye
P. Douste Blazy
P. Ducimetière
I. Juhan-Vague
L. Robert
D. Thomas

Scientific Advisory Committee

N. Abdurhaman, Indonesia

P. Alaupovic, USA
G. Assmann, Germany
M. Aviram, Israel
G. Baggio, Italy
P. Barter, Australia
A. Bartomeo, Argentina
U. Beisiegel, Germany
D.J. Betteridge, UK
M. Bihari-Varga, Hungary
W.C. Breckenridge, Canada
J. Breslow, USA
H.B. Brewer, USA
G. Brook, Israel
M.S. Brown, USA
R. Carmena, Spain
A. Catapano, Italy
L. Chan, USA
B.N. Chiang, ROC Taiwan
G. Crepaldi, Italy
J. Davignon, Canada
G. De Baker, Belgium
D. De Bono, UK
M. De Oya Otera, Spain
D.W. Erkelens, The Netherlands
J. Fernadez-Britto, Cuba
V. Fuster, USA
J.L. Goldstein, USA
J. Gonzalez-Barranco, Mexico
Y. Goto, Japan
A.M. Gotto Jr., USA
S.M. Grundy, USA
Hai Jiang Cai, China
M.D. Haust, Canada
M. Hayden, Canada
S. Humphries, UK
H. Jellinek, Hungary
H. Kaffarnik, Germany
M.B. Katan, The Netherlands
N.M. Kipshidze, Georgia Rep.
T. Kita, Japan
G. Kostner, Austria
O. Kraupp, Austria
B. Lewis, UK

viii

R. Mahley, USA
M. Mancini, Italy
Y. Marcel, Canada
Y. Matsuzawa, Japan
T. Miettinen, Finland
S. Moncada, UK
N. Naruszewicz, Poland
P.J. Nestel, Australia
B.G. Nordestgaard, Denmark
O. Obregon, Venezuala
A.G. Olsson, Sweden
H. Orimo, Japan
R. Paoletti, Italy
J.R. Patsch, Austria
L. Pereira-Miguel, Portugal
D. Pometta, Switzerland
K. Pyorala, Finland
G. Ricci, Italy
W. Riesen, Switzerland
L. Robert, France
R. Ross, USA
M. Rosseneu, Belgium
E.M. Rubin, USA
E. Schaefer, USA
G. Schonfeld, USA
J. Scott, New Zealand
D. Seidel, Germany
J. Shepherd, UK
L. Simons, Australia
C.R. Sirtori, Italy
V.N. Smirnov, India
H.C. Stary, USA
O. Stein, Israel
Y. Stein, Israel
D. Steinberg, USA
G. Steiner, Canada
K, Steyn, South-Africa
F. Stoziky, Czech Rep.
A. Tall, USA
M.R. Taskinen, Finland
G. Thompson, UK
G. Utermann, Austria
A. Van Tol, The Netherlands
R.R. Williams, USA

A. Yamamoto, Japan
S. Young, USA

International Finance Committee

G. Campbell, Australia
H. Kritz, Austria
H. Dieplinger, Austria
L. Van Gaal, Belgium
T.C. Yang, China
O.S. Zakharova, CIS
J.A. Castillo, Cuba
E. Turzicka, Czech Rep.
M.C. Bourdillon, France
M.G. Kakaurize, Georgia Rep.
H. Heinle, Germany
A. Csaszar, Hungary
D.S. Gambhir, India
E. Leitersdorf, Israel
H. Tremoli, Italy
T. Takano, Japan
J. Scott, New Zealand
M. Naruszewicz, Poland
E. Castro, Portugal
S. Ylä-Herttuala, Scandinavia
M. de Oya Otero, Spain
T.A.B. Sanders, UK

National Program Committee

J.C. Fruchart, *Chairman*
J. Auwerx
B. Bihain
J. Bonnet
F. Cambien
M.J. Chapman
P. Denèfle
B. Jacotot
I. Juhan-Vague
Ph. Moulin
L. Robert
M. Rosseneu
B. Staels
P. Vanhoutte

Contents

Triglycerides are an independent risk factor for cornoary heart disease — a debate

Growth factors, cytokines and vasoactive peptides

Epidemiology: geographical variations of cardiovascular incidence and risk factors

Cellular and haemodynamic regulation of endothelial function

Immune and infectious factors in atherogenesis

New development in animal models for atherosclerosis

3

The apoE-deficient mouse model of atherosclerosis

Jan L. Breslow
Laboratory of Biochemical Genetics and Metabolism, New York, New York, USA

As a species the mouse is highly resistant to atherosclerosis. However, through induced mutations it has been possible to develop lines of mice that are susceptible to this disease. For example, mice that are deficient in apolipoprotein E, a ligand important in lipoprotein clearance, develop atherosclerotic lesions resembling those observed in humans. These lesions are exacerbated when the mice are fed a high-cholesterol, high-fat, Western-type diet. The apoE deficient mouse model is now being used to study the pathogenesis of atherosclerotic lesions, as well as the influence of genetics, environment, hormones, and drugs on lesion development.

Atherosclerotic cardiovascular disease is the major cause of morbidity and mortality in much of the world. Atherogenesis is a complex process in which the lumen of a blood vessel becomes narrowed by cellular and extracellular substances to the point of obstruction. Lesions tend to form at the branch points of arterial blood vessels and then progress through three stages. The first stage is the fatty streak lesion, which is characterized by the presence of lipid-filled macrophages (foam cells) in the subendothelial space. The second stage is the fibrous plaque, which consists of a central acellular area of lipid, derived from necrotic foam cells, covered by a fibrous cap containing smooth muscle cells and collagen. The final stage is the complex lesion, which shows evidence of thrombus formation with deposition of fibrin and platelets.

Researchers in vascular biology are working to identify the important cells and molecules involved in each stage of atherogenesis, as well as the environmental and genetic factors that promote lesion formation. These are complex questions that require in vivo models that mimic the human disease. Experimental approaches that deviate widely from the human disease or rely too heavily on in vitro systems could be misleading. Until recently, atherogenesis had been studied mainly in primates and in low-density lipoprotein (LDL) receptor-deficient rabbits. Unfortunately, these systems cannot provide sufficiently large numbers of animals, nor do they lend themselves to genetic analysis.

Address for correspondence: J.L. Breslow MD, Laboratory of Biochemical Genetics and Metabolism, The Rockefeller University, New York, NY 10021, USA.

4

Development of a mouse model

In 1992, two laboratories used gene knockout technology to generate mice deficient in apolipoprotein E (apoE) [1,2]. ApoE, which is made primarily in the liver, is a surface constituent of lipoprotein particles and a ligand for lipoprotein recognition and clearance by lipoprotein receptors. ApoE-deficient mice have delayed clearance of lipoproteins, and on a low-cholesterol, low-fat diet, their cholesterol levels reach 400–600 mg/dl as a result of accumulation of chylomicron and very low density lipoprotein (VLDL) remnants enriched in esterified and free cholesterol [3]. Notably, these mice develop not only fatty streaks but also widespread fibrous plaque lesions at vascular sites typically affected in human atherosclerosis [4,5]. Lesions form at the base of the aorta and the lesser curvature of the thoracic aorta; at the branch points of the carotid, intercostal, mesenteric, renal, and iliac arteries; and in the proximal coronary, carotid, femoral, subclavian, and brachycephalic arteries. Lesions begin at 5–6 weeks of age with monocyte attachment to the endothelium in lesion-prone areas and transendothelial migration. Fatty streak lesions begin to appear at 10 weeks, and intermediate lesions containing foam cells and spindle-shaped smooth muscle cells appear at 15 weeks. Fibrous plaques appear after 20 weeks; these consist of a necrotic core covered by a fibrous cap of smooth muscle cells surrounded by elastic fibers and collagen. In older mice, fibrous plaques progress. In some advanced lesions there is partial destruction of underlying medial cells with occasional aneurysm formation, and in others calcification occurs in the plaque. Extensive fibroproliferation can narrow the lumen, even to the point of occlusion of vessels. Complicated lesions characterized by thrombosis have not been found. One of the hallmarks of atherosclerosis is its exacerbation by high-cholesterol, high-fat diets. This effect is mimicked in apoE-deficient mice [4]. When these mice were fed a Western-type diet (containing 0.15% cholesterol and 21% fat, derived mainly from milk fat), their cholesterol levels rose to 3–4 times the levels on the low-cholesterol, low-fat diet, and their lesions increased in size and rate of progression.

Applications of the apo-E knockout models

The apoE knockout mouse model of atherosclerosis can provide insights into lesion pathogenesis, genetic modifiers, and the influence of environment, hormones, and drugs on the disease. With regard to lesion pathogenesis, it is now possible to study the molecular events involved in monocyte attachment to endothelium, monocyte transmigration to the subendothelial space, subintimal foam cell formation, foam cell necrosis and the ensuing fibroproliferative reaction, and the roles of immune cells, cytokines, and their receptors in lesion progression. These studies can be carried out by documenting the molecules and cell types present in the lesions, crossbreeding the atherosclerotic mice with other mutant mice harboring specific defects in the same molecules or cells, and then noting suppression or enhancement of the atherosclerosis phenotype.

The foam cell lesions of apoE-deficient mice contain oxidized epitopes of lipoprotein particles, accompanied by very high plasma levels of autoantibodies to oxidized lipoproteins [6]. On the basis of in vitro studies and lesion immunohistochemistry, lipoprotein oxidation in the subendothelium has been hypothesized to be necessary for foam cell formation. This mouse model can be used to test this hypothesis in vivo. Support for the hypothesis has come from a recent pharmacological study in which an antioxidant, N,N'-diphenyl-1, 4 phenylenediamine, was shown to decrease lesion area in apoE-deficient mice without affecting cholesterol levels [1]. The mouse atherosclerosis model can also be used to identify molecules involved in lipoprotein oxidation through crossbreeding with other appropriate mutant mice. Similarly, experiments could be designed to test whether autoantibodies to oxidized lipoproteins participate in lesion pathogenesis or are a response to lesion development.

In another study, the role of the macrophage in lesion development was tested by crossbreeding apoE-deficient mice with mice that have the op mutation, a mutation in the gene that codes for macrophage colony stimulating factor (MCSF). MCSF influences monocyte and macrophage development, and mice with the op mutation have reduced levels of blood monocytes and tissue macrophages [7]. Macrophages in the subendothelium have been hypothesized to protect against atherosclerosis by scavenging noxious materials such as oxidized lipoproteins, but they have also been hypothesized to contribute to foam cell formation and, by their death, to lesion progression. Lesions in mice that were doubly mutant (that is, apoE-deficient mice that also had the op mutation) were one-seventh the size of lesions in apoE-deficient mice, with almost no progression to the fibroproliferative stage, even though cholesterol levels in the doubly mutant mice were 2—3 times those in the apo-E deficient mice. These results strongly suggest that the net effect of the macrophage is proatherogenic. This hypothesis can be further tested by crossbreeding the apo-E deficient mice with mice that have mutations in other aspects of monocyte function.

The availability of mouse atherosclerosis models allows the use of a variety of techniques to identify genes that enhance or suppress the phenotype. Mice expressing the human apoA-I transgene were bred with apoE-deficient mice, and the offspring were fed a low-cholesterol, low-fat diet; at 4 months of age, fatty streak lesions were almost totally suppressed, whereas at 8 months some small fatty streaks had appeared but fibrous plaques were suppressed [8—10]. Thus, apoA-I expression led to decreased lesion area and inhibited lesion progression. These same mice showed a strong inverse correlation between HDL cholesterol levels and lesion size. This effect of HDL was independent of the effect of non-HDL cholesterol levels on lesion size. The relation between low HDL cholesterol levels and increased atherosclerosis observed in human epidemiological studies has been attributed largely to the association of low HDL cholesterol levels with high levels of atherogenic apoB-containing lipoproteins, such as VLDL, IDL, small dense LDL, and postprandial particles. These mouse studies suggest that

6

HDL has an additional independent protective effect, perhaps by accelerating reverse cholesterol transport or directly protecting the vessel wall against noxious atherogenic stimuli. Evidence for one or both of these proposed mechanisms of HDL action can now be sought in the mouse atherosclerosis models.

The mouse atherosclerosis models can also be used to test the effects of environment, hormones, and drugs on atherogenesis. In the apoE-deficient mouse, lesion size increases as the diet is changed from low-cholesterol low-fat to high-cholesterol high-fat [3]. Popular, but as yet unapproved, theories about the effects of various macro- and micronutrients on atherogenesis can also be tested. Finally, these mouse models can be used to test for drugs that inhibit atherogenesis. The availability of large numbers of atherosclerosis-prone mice will allow relatively inexpensive and thorough preclinical testing of new candidate drugs.

References

1. Plump AS, Smith JD, Hayek T, Aalto-Setälä K, Walsh A, Verstuyft JG, Rubin EM, Breslow JL. Severe hypercholesterolemia and atherosclerosis in apolipoprotein E-deficient mice created by homologous recombination in ES cells. Cell 1992;71:343–353.
2. Zhang SH, Hennessy DP, Cranwell PD, Noonan DE, Francis HJ. Physiological responses to exercise and hypoglycaemia stress in pigs of differing adrenal responsiveness. Comp Biochem Physiol Comp Physiol 1992;103(4):695–703.
3. Plump AS, Forte TM, Eisenberg S, Breslow JL. Atherogenic β-VLDL in the apo E-deficient mouse: composition, origin, and fate. AHA 66th Scientific Sessions 1993.
4. Nakashima Y, Plump AS, Raines EW, Breslow JL, Ross R. Apo E-deficient mice develop lesions of all phases of atherosclerosis throughout the arterial tree. Arterioscl Thromb 1994;14: 133–140.
5. Reddick RL, Zhang SH, Maeda N. Atherosclerosis in mice lacking apo E. Evaluation of lesional development and progression (published erratum appears in Arterioscl Thromb 1994;5:839) Arterioscl Thromb 1994;14(1):141–147.
6. Tangirala RK, Casanada F, Miller E, Witztum JL, Steinberg D, Palinski W. Effect of the antioxidant N,N′-diphenyl 1,4-phenylenediamine (DPPD) on atherosclerosis in apoE-deficient mice. Arterioscler Thromb Vasc Biol 1995;15(10):1625–1630.
7. Smith JD, Trogan E, Ginsberg M, Grigaux C, Tian J, Miyata M. Decreased atherosclerosis in mice deficient in both macrophage colony-stimulating factor (op) and apolipoprotein E. Proc Natl Acad Sci USA 1995;92(18):8264–8268.
8. Plump AS, Scott CJ, Breslow JL. Human apolipoprotein A-I gene expression raises HDL and suppresses atherosclerosis in the apo E-deficient mouse. Proc Natl Acad Sci USA 1994;91: 9607–9611.
9. Paszty C, Maeda N, Verstuyft J, Rubin EM. Apolipoprotein AI transgene corrects apolipoprotein E deficiency-induced atherosclerosis in mice. J Clin Invest 1994;94(2):899–903.
10. Palinski W, Ord VA, Plump AS, Breslow JL, Steinberg D, Witzum JL. Apoprotein E-deficient mice are a model of lipoprotein oxidation in atherogenesis: demonstration of oxidation-specific epitopes in lesions and high titers of autoantibodies to malondialdehyde-lysine in serum. Arterioscl Thromb 1994;14:605–616.

Increasing the throughput of mouse studies to search DNA sequence for function

Edward M. Rubin and Desmond J. Smith
Human Genome Center, University of California, Berkely, California, USA

Abstract. Nonvertebrate model organisms, despite their proven utility in deciphering gene function at the organismal level, are inadequate for modeling many complex mammalian physiological traits, such as heart disease. In contrast the mouse, as a mammal, has been used to successfully model many complex human conditions, although it classically has been used to look at one gene at a time. In order to increase the throughput of mouse studies for linking DNA sequence to function, we have developed a strategy to analyze several genes at a time in a single transgenic animal. This approach is based on the creation of panels of transgenics whose transgenes are derived from large insert clones (YAC or BACs) from a region of the genome where a particular phenotype has been mapped. These panels of transgenic mice, dubbed in vivo libraries, and their phenotypic analysis has enabled us to identify genes responsible for neurodegenerative and learning disorders in mice.

Keywords: functional assays, in vivo library, transgenic mice.

In vivo libraries: sifting through megabase regions of genomic sequence to link sequence to function

In general, transgenic approaches have largely analyzed the function of coding regions one at a time. The in vivo library approach [1] departs from these traditional strategies and involves making a series of large insert transgenic animals propagating DNA that covers a particular candidate region of the genome (Fig. 1). The region may be chosen based on the presence of a mapped genetic locus that plays a role in a disease or physiological process. As a result of the increased likelihood of including multiple genes as well as large genes, these large insert vectors (YACs or P1s) maximize the amount of information that can be derived from a relatively limited panel of founder transgenic animals. Furthermore, the use of genomic transgenes, because of the presence of normal cis regulatory elements, maximizes the likelihood of obtaining authentic patterns of expression and hence biological impact of the genes contained within the transgene.

Address for correspondence: E.M. Rubin, Human Genome Center, Lawrence Berkeley National Laboratory, One Cyclotron Road, 74–157, Berkeley, CA 94720, USA. E-mail: EMRubin@lbl.gov

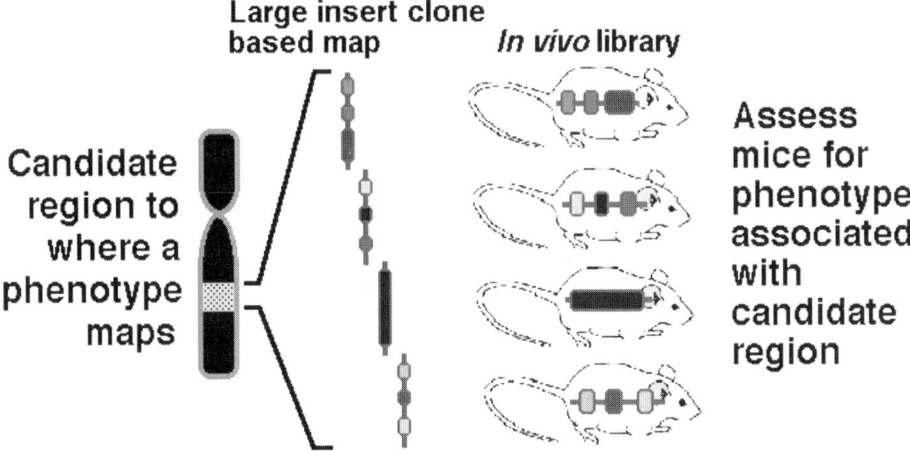

Fig. 1. In vivo library strategy: a chromosomal region to which a particular phenotype has been mapped is chosen for analysis. A large insert clone (YAC or BAC) contig is developed for the genetic interval and each clone is introduced individually into the mouse genome. The resulting panel of transgenic mice serve as an "in vivo" library of the candidate region. Members of the library are assessed for the phenotype mapped to the candidate region.

The use of in vivo libraries to identify a gene contributing to behavior

Studies of humans with partial trisomy of chromosome 21 [2], coupled with similar studies in mice trisomic for syntenic regions of mouse chromosome 16 [3–5], suggest that an extra dose of a limited region of these chromosomes, located at 21q22.2 in humans, may contribute to many of the phenotypic features associated with Down syndrome. The most variant of features observed in individuals trisomic for 21q22.2 are learning disorders. In order to identify the human sequences contributing to the learning defects, we created an in vivo library, based on the mapping studies, covering 2 Mb of 21q22.2 propagated as a panel of YAC transgenic mice [1]. Each member of the panel contains distinct 430–670 kb overlapping segments of the chromosome 21 region. Members of the library were subjected to detailed assays for learning and behavior in order to screen for genes which, when present at an extra dose, affect these phenotypes. From these screens, a 21q22.2 YAC was identified which caused distinct learning and behavioral deficits in several independent founder lines of mice. The gene on the YAC responsible for the defects was later identified by analyzing animals containing partial fragments of the initial 570 kb YAC [6]. This gene, DIRK, is of particular interest since mutations affecting the activity of the *Drosophila* homolog, minibrain, result in learning impairment in flies [7]. The parallel consequences of altering expression of minibrain in fruit flies and DIRK in mice support the role of this gene in learning/behavior and also the in vivo library approach as a strategy to identifying sequences impacting on behavior based on functional screens.

The use of in vivo libraries for cloning by complementation

Another application of the in vivo library approach for cloning genes based on their function, was the recent identification of the gene responsible for the murine neurodegenerative disorder, vibrator [8]. Using classical meiotic mapping, the responsible gene had been localized to a > 500 kb region. In order to narrow the interval containing the mutant gene, a library of transgenic animals was created with P1s spanning the critical region. Embryos were injected with two P1s at a time such that each transgenic mouse harbored two distinct but overlapping P1s, to maximize the information derived from each member of the library. Members of the library were then crossed with animals harboring the vibrator mutation. We eventually derived two separate lines of transgenic mice, each containing a common P1, that complemented the vibrator phenotype. The narrowing of the critical region from greater than half a megabase to a 70 kb region, based on functional complementation, dramatically reduced the number of genes requiring investigation. This led to the rapid identification of the mutation responsible for vibrator as being present in the pitpn gene which encodes the phosphatidylinositol transfer protein a isoform (PITPa).

Conclusions

The mouse, clearly the organism of choice for modeling human physiology, is encumbered by its small litter size, long reproductive cycle time, and its high cost, three features that appear to be recalcitrant to improvement. Where possible avenues of improvement do exist are in methods for multiplexing the amount of information derived from a single experiment. The approach described here consisted of screening in parallel the effect of many genes upon a single phenotype. The development of other novel higher "throughput" approaches employing the mouse are needed to ease the bottleneck of linking genotype/sequence information to function that has arisen as a result of the Human Genome Program.

Acknowledgements

This work was supported by National Institute of Health Grants to E.R., PPG HL18574. Research was conducted at the Lawrence Berkeley National Laboratory (Department of Energy Contract DE-AC0376SF00098), University of California, Berkeley.

References

1.   Smith DJ, Zhu Y, Zhang JL, Cheng JF, Rubin EM. Construction of a panel of transgenic mice containing a contiguous 2 Mb set of YAC/P1 clones from human chromosome 21q22.2. Genomics 1995;27:425—434.
2.   Rhamani Z, Blouin J, Creau-Goldgerg N et al. Critical role of the D21s55 region on chromo-

some 21 in the pathogenesis of Down syndrome. PNAS USA 1989;86:5958—5962.

3. Cox DR, Smith SA, Epstein LB, Epstein CJ. Mouse trisomy 16 as an animal model of human trisomy 21 (Down syndrome): production of viable trisomy 16 diploid mouse chimeras. Devel Biol 1984;101:416—424.

4. Gearhart JD, Davisson MT, Oster-Granite ML. Autosomal aneuploidy in mice: generation and developmental consequences. Brain Res Bull 1986;16:789—801.

5. Reeves RH, Irving NH, Moran TH et al. A mouse model for Down syndrome exhibits learning and behaviour deficits. Nature Genet 1995;11:177—184.

6. Smith DJ, Stevens ME, Sudanagunta SP et al. Functional screening of 2 Mb of human chromosome 21q22.2 in transgenic mice implicates *minibrain* in learning defects associated with Down syndrome. Nature Genet 1997;16:28—36.

7. Tejedor F, Zhu XR, Kaltenbach E et al. Minibrain: a new protein kinase family involved in post-embryonic neurogenesis in *Drosophila*. Neuron 1995;14:287—301.

8. Hamilton BA, Smith DJ, Mueller KL et al. The neurodegenitive vibrator mutation causes reduced expression of phosphatidylinositol transfer protein a: cloning by positional complementation in mice and mapping of an extragenic suppressor. Neuron 1997;18:711—712.

Use of transgenic animal models to study enzymes involved in lipoprotein metabolism and atherosclerosis

Silvia Santamarina-Fojo, Jeffrey M. Hoeg and H. Bryan Brewer Jr

Molecular Disease Branch, National Heart, Lung and Blood Institute, Bethesda, Maryland, USA

Abstract. Lecithin cholesteryl acyltransferase (LCAT) plays a major role in HDL metabolism by facilitating the esterification of free cholesterol present in circulating plasma lipoproteins. We have investigated the role that this enzyme plays in reverse cholesterol transport and the development of atherosclerosis by inducing the formation of aortic lesions using an atherogenic diet in transgenic mice and rabbits that overexpress human LCAT. Despite elevated plasma concentrations of HDL-cholesterol and apolipoprotein (apo) A-I, LCAT transgenic mice have enhanced diet-induced aortic atherosclerosis. In contrast, LCAT transgenic rabbits have increased plasma concentrations of HDL-cholesterol and apoA-I, reduced levels of apoB-containing lipoproteins and decreased aortic atherosclerosis. Reduced plasma concentrations of the proatherogenic apo-B-containing lipoproteins in rabbits but not in mice, as well as the presence of a "dysfunctional" HDL in LCAT transgenic mice may account for the differences in atherosclerosis between the two LCAT transgenic animal models. Our findings demonstrate the importance of LCAT in modulating the process of reverse cholesterol transport and atherosclerosis.

Keywords: atherosclerosis, high-density lipoproteins, lecithin cholesteryl acyltransferase, transgenic mice, transgenic rabbits.

Introduction

As the major enzyme responsible for the esterification of free cholesterol present in circulating plasma lipoproteins [1], lecithin cholesterol acyltransferase (LCAT) plays a major role in extracellular cholesterol metabolism. In plasma, LCAT is found to be primarily associated with HDL [2,3], where it promotes the synthesis of cholesteryl esters and lysolecithin from phosphatidylcholine and unesterified cholesterol [1,4]. The cholesteryl esters either become part of the lipoprotein core or are transferred by cholesteryl ester transfer protein (CETP) to other lipoproteins. LCAT function helps maintain a concentration gradient for the diffusion of free cholesterol from peripheral tissues to HDL [5]. Together with CETP, LCAT may not only modulate HDL concentrations in plasma but also play an important role in the processes of reverse cholesterol transport and atherosclerosis [6].

To examine this question, we induced the formation of aortic lesions in transgenic mice [7,8] and rabbits [9,10] overexpressing human LCAT, as well as age-

Address for correspondence: Silvia Santamarina-Fojo MD, PhD, Molecular Disease Branch, National Heart, Lung and Blood Institute, National Institutes of Health, Building 10, Room 7N115, 10 Center Drive MSC 1666, Bethesda, MD 20892-1666, USA.

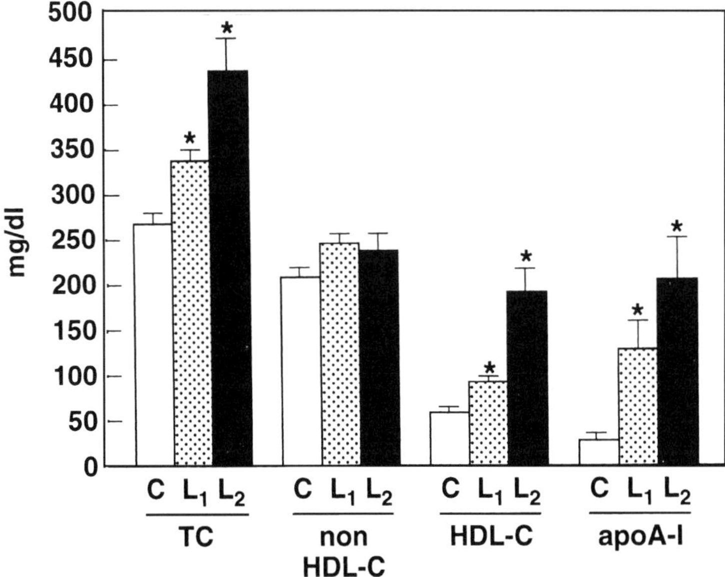

Fig. 1. Summary of the plasma lipid, lipoprotein and apolipoprotein concentrations in control (C), low expressor (L1) and high expressor (L2) LCAT transgenic mice after feeding a high-fat high-cholesterol diet.

and sex-matched control littermates, by feeding them an atherogenic diet. Overexpression of LCAT in rabbits results in increased plasma concentrations of

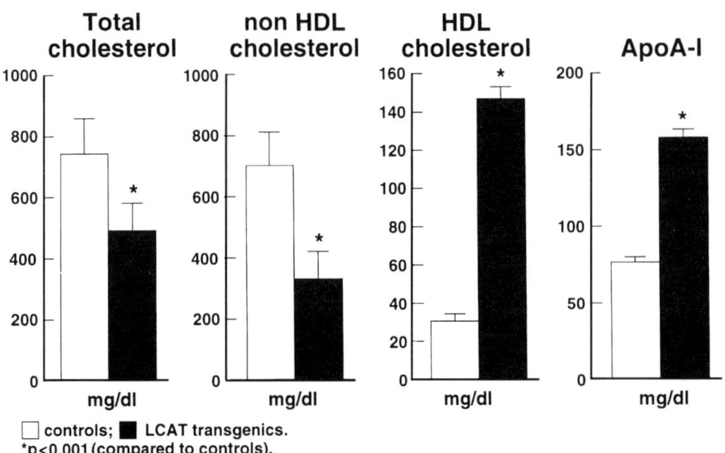

Fig. 2. Summary of the plasma lipid, lipoprotein and apolipoprotein concentrations in control (□) and LCAT transgenic (■) rabbits after feeding a high-cholesterol diet.

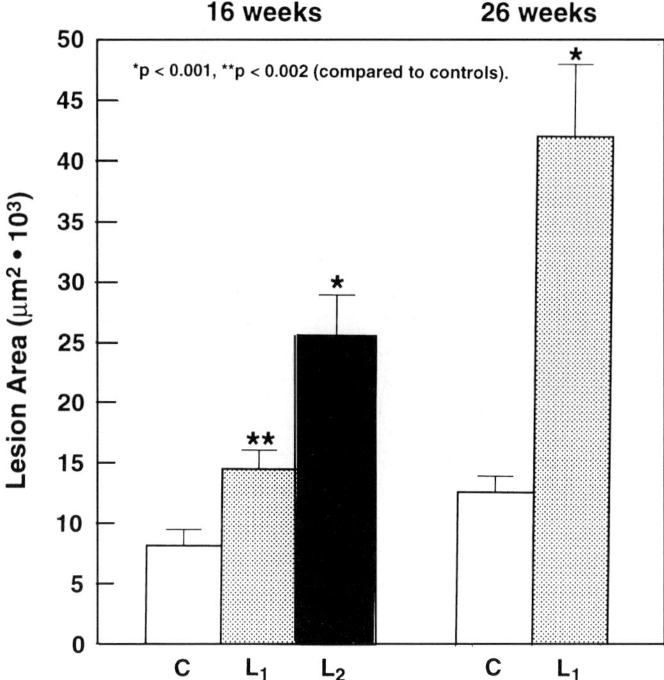

Fig. 3. Comparison of the mean aortic lesion area in control (C) and LCAT transgenic mice from the L1 and L2 lines, after being fed an antherogenic diet for 16 and 26 weeks.

HDL-cholesterol as well as reduced levels of the proatherogenic apoB-containing lipoproteins, [9] and marked reduction in the development of diet-induced aortic atherosclerosis [10]. In contrast, overexpression of human LCAT in mice leads to enhanced atherosclerosis, even though plasma HDL-cholesterol and apoA-I concentrations are significantly increased in these animals [8].

Results and Discussion

The plasma lipids, lipoproteins and apolipoproteins of control and LCAT transgenic mice and rabbits on a proatherogenic diet are summarized in Figs. 1 and 2. After being fed a high-fat, high-cholesterol diet [11] for 16 weeks, control (n = 14) as well as low expressor (n = 23) and high expressor (n = 7) LCAT transgenic mice [7] significantly increased their baseline plasma total cholesterol (p < 0.001), cholesteryl esters (p < 0.001) and non-HDL cholesterol (p < 0.001) concentrations (data not shown). However, compared to control animals (Fig. 1), LCAT transgenic mice had higher plasma levels of total (1.2- to 1.5-fold increase) and HDL-cholesterol (1.6- to 3.3-fold increase), as well as the major protein component of HDL, apoA-I (3.8- to 7.6-fold increase). Plasma non-HDL cholesterol levels were not significantly different (p > 0.05) among the three

14

study groups (Fig. 1). Consistent with these findings, immunoblot analysis of plasma apoB (the major apolipoprotein in non-HDL lipoproteins) demonstrated a similar increase in apoB in all three groups of mice (data not shown).

In contrast, in response to a high-cholesterol (0.3%) diet, control rabbits [10] had significantly higher plasma levels of total (1.5-fold) and non-HDL cholesterol (2.3-fold) concentrations than LCAT-transgenic rabbits ($p < 0.0001$; all). Like LCAT transgenic mice, the plasma HDL-cholesterol levels and apoA-I concentrations were higher in transgenic compared to control rabbits (4.7- and 2-fold, respectively).

Thus, in both mice and rabbits, LCAT modulates the lipoprotein response to an atherogenic diet, resulting in higher plasma concentrations of plasma HDL-cholesterol and apoA-I. However, the effect of LCAT expression on the plasma levels of the proatherogenic apoB-containing lipoproteins in mice and rabbits is different. Thus, LCAT transgenic rabbits had markedly decreased plasma concentrations of the apoB-containing lipoproteins compared to control, nontransgenic animals (Fig. 2) whereas no significant difference in these lipoproteins was observed between control and LCAT transgenic mice (Fig. 1).

Analysis of the aortic lesions in both control and LCAT transgenic mice was performed as described by Paigen et al. [11]. The mean aortic lesions of female transgenic mice containing either 100 (L1) or 240 (L2) copies of the human transgene were increased in size 1.8- to 3.5-fold compared with those of control animals (Fig. 3). LCAT overexpression increased the mean aortic lesion size from $12.63 \pm 0.66 \times 10^3$ μm^2 in controls to $42.7 \pm 5.2 \times 10^3$ μm^2 in L1 transgenic mice (26-week diet; $p < 0.001$). These findings demonstrate a dissociation between high plasma concentrations of the antiatherogenic lipoprotein HDL,

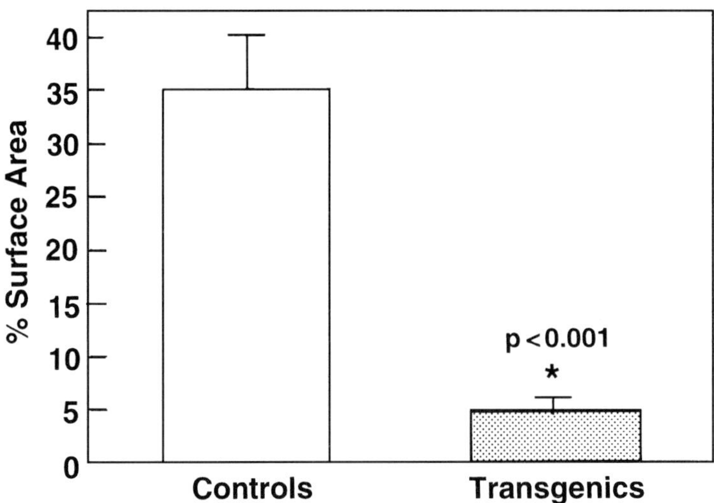

Fig. 4. Comparison of the atherosclerosis in control and transgenic rabbits overexpressing human LCAT after analysis by quantitative planimetry.

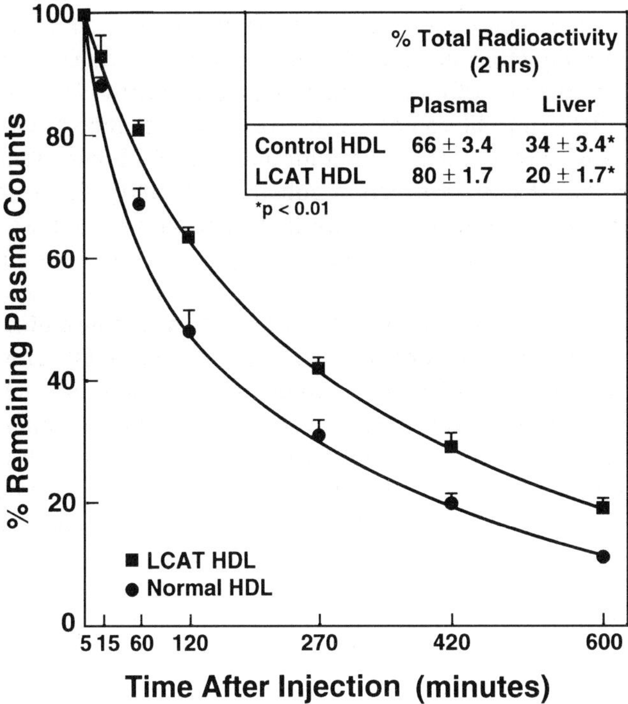

Fig. 5. Plasma decay curve of (^{3}H)cholesteryl ether HDL from control (●) and LCAT transgenic mouse (■) after injection of the radiolabelled lipoproteins in control C57Bl/6 mice. Inset, the percentage of total (^{3}H)cholesteryl ether counts present in the plasma and liver of C57Bl/6 mice 2 h after injection of (^{3}H)cholesteryl ether HDL isolated from control (n = 4) and LCAT transgenic (n = 5) mice; p < 0.01 is shown.

and the expected reduction in atherosclerosis in LCAT transgenic animals.

To evaluate the role of LCAT overexpression in the development of diet-induced athcrosclcrosis in rabbits, control and LCAT transgenic rabbits were placed on a 0.3% cholesterol diet. After 27 weeks, the aortas from control and LCAT transgenic animals were harvested and Sudan IV staining of the lipid droplets was used to quantify the percent of the surface area developing lesions [12]. The aortas of the control group (n = 9) had 35 ± 7% of the surface covered by plaque (Fig. 4). In marked contrast, only 5 ± 1% of the aortic surface was covered by plaque in the LCAT transgenic rabbits (n = 10; p < 0.009). Thus, opposite conclusions regarding the antiatherogenic potential of a candidate gene were obtained by expression of the same transgene in two different animal models.

In order to investigate potential mechanisms leading to differences in the role that LCAT plays in modulating diet-induced atherosclerosis in LCAT transgenic mice and rabbits, we evaluated the functional properties of transgenic mouse HDL using (^{3}H)cholesteryl ether-HDL. The plasma decay of (^{3}H)cholesteryl ether (Fig. 5) of transgenic HDL was significantly slower (fractional catabolic rate = 3.57 ± 0.34 units) than that of control HDL (FCR = 5.79 ± 0.18; $p < 0.002$). In addition, the accumulation of (^{3}H)cholesteryl ether (Fig. 5) derived from transgenic HDL in the liver (20% of total counts) was reduced by 41% compared with that of controls (34% of total counts; $p < 0.01$). These findings establish that the delivery of cholesterol from transgenic mouse HDL to the liver, and therefore the ability of this lipoprotein to function effectively in the process of reverse cholesterol transport, is significantly reduced compared with control mouse HDL.

Our findings emphasize the importance of evaluating the antiatherogenic potential of a candidate gene in different animal models. Key metabolic differences between rabbits and mice, including the presence of CETP-mediated transfer of cholesteryl esters from HDL to apoB-containing lipoproteins, as well as reduced plasma concentrations of the proatherogenic apo-B-containing lipoproteins in rabbits but not in mice, may account for the differences in atherosclerosis between the two LCAT transgenic animal models. Thus, although altered HDL composition and function in transgenic mouse HDL lead to impaired reverse cholesterol transport, this process appears to be normal in LCAT transgenic rabbits. Analysis of these two LCAT transgenic animal models provide in vivo evidence for dysfunctional HDL as a potential mechanism leading to increased atherosclerosis in the presence of high plasma HDL levels.

Acknowledgements

The authors would like to thank Ms Judith Burk for her excellent secretarial assistance.

References

1. Norum KR, Gjone E, Glomset JA. In: Scriver CR, Beaudet AL, Sly WS, Valle (eds) The Metabolic Basis of Inherited Disease. New York: McGraw-Hill Inc., 1989;1181–1194.
2. Francone OL, Gurakar A, Fielding C. Distribution and functions of lecithin:cholesterol acyltransferase and cholesteryl ester transfer protein in plasma lipoproteins. Evidence for a functional unit containing these activities together with apolipoproteins A-I and D that catalyzes the esterification and transfer of cell-derived cholesterol. J Biol Chem 1989;264:7066–7072.
3. Duverger N, Rader DJ, Duchateau P et al. Biochemical characterization of the three major subclasses of lipoprotein A-I (LpA-I) preparatively isolated from human plasma. Biochem 1993; 32:12373–12379.
4. Jonas A. Lecithin-cholesterol acyltransferase in the metabolism of high-density lipoproteins. Biochim Biophys Acta 1991;1084:205–220.
5. Glomset JA. The plasma lecithin:cholesterol acyltransferase reaction. J Lipid Res 1968;9: 155–167.
6. Glomset JA, Janssen ET, Kennedy R et al. Role of plasma lecithin:cholesterol acyltransferase in the metabolism of high-density lipoproteins. J Lipid Res 1966;7:638–648.
7. Vaisman BL, Klein H-G, Rouis M et al. Overexpression of human lecithin cholesterol acyltransferase leads to hyperalphalipoproteinemia in transgenic mice. J Biol Chem 1995;270: 12269–12275.
8. Berard AM, Foger B, Remaley AT et al. High plasma HDL concentrations associated with

enhanced atherosclerosis in transgenic mice overexpressing lecithin cholesteryl-acyl transferase. Nature Med 1997;3:744—749.

9. Hoeg JM, Vaisman BL, Demosky SJ Jr et al. Lecithin-cholesterol acyltransferase overexpression generates hyperalpha-lipoproteinemia and a nonatherogenic lipoprotein pattern in transgenic rabbits. J Biol Chem 1996;271:4396—4402.

10. Hoeg JM, Santamarina-Fojo S, Berard AM et al. Overexpression of lecithin: cholesterol acyltransferase in transgenic rabbits prevents diet-induced atherosclerosis. Proc Natl Acad Sci USA 1996;93:11448—11453.

11. Paigen B, Morrow A, Holmes PA et al. Quantitative assessment of atherosclerotic lesions in mice. Atherosclerosis 1987;68:231—240.

12. Kolodgie FD, Virmani R, Cornhill JF et al. Cocaine: an independent risk factor for aortic sudanophilia. A preliminary report. Atherosclerosis 1992;97:53—62.

Genetic dissection of high-density lipoprotein metabolism and reverse cholesterol transport

Gerd Assmann, Arnold von Eckardstein, Michael Walter and Paul Cullen
Institut für Arterioskleroseforschung an der Universität Münster, Münster; and Institut für Klinische Chemie und Laboratoriumsmedizin, Zentrallaboratorium, Westfälische Wilhelms-Universität Münster, Münster, Germany

Abstract. The reverse cholesterol transport model is widely used to explain the protective role of HDL in atherogenesis. HDL encompasses heterogeneous particles which are both structurally and functionally heterogeneous. Two-dimensional nondenaturing polyacrylamide gradient gel electrophoresis and subsequent immunoblotting differentiated minor HDL-subclasses from the bulk of HDL, which contains apoA-I and has electrophoretic α-mobility. Pulse-chase experiments have shown the minor HDL subclasses preβ$_1$-LpA-I, γ-LpE and LpA-IV to be initial and fast acceptors of cell-derived cholesterol while α-migrating HDL (i.e., α-LpA-I) is a late and slow acceptor. In plasmas of patients with certain forms of familial HDL-deficiency such as apoA-I deficiency and Tangier disease, preβ$_1$-LpA-I, γ-LpE and LpA-IV are the only HDL particles present and account for the significant residual cholesterol efflux capacity of these plasmas. These minor particles, however, also fulfil important roles in reverse cholesterol transport of normal plasma. Preβ$_1$-LpA-I, for example, is generated, during the interconversion of HDL by lipid transfer proteins. Thus incubation of plasma with phospholipid transfer protein increases the concentration of preβ$_1$-LpA-I and in parallel increases the cholesterol efflux capacity of plasma indicating that lipid transfer proteins modulate cholesterol efflux by modification of HDL subclass composition.

ApoE and γ-LpE are of special interest for reverse cholesterol transport since macrophages can produce apoE. We investigated the impact of apoE polymorphism on the ability of human macrophages to express apoE mRNA and secrete apoE. A reverse transcription-polymerase chain reaction assay with a competitive internal RNA standard did not identify genotype-related differences in apoE mRNA expression in non-cholesterol-loaded cells. Nevertheless, under these conditions apoE3/3 cells secreted approximately twice as much apoE than cells which did not express apoE3. Moreover, only the medium of apoE3-producing macrophages contained a particle with the mobility of γ-LpE. Loading with acetyl-LDL led to genotype-related increases in apoE mRNA in the order apoE4 → apoE3 → apoE2 and in apoE secretion in the order apoE4 → apoE2 → apoE3. Surprisingly, despite their increased secretion of apoE, E4 macrophages lacked effective net efflux of cholesterol.

Keywords: apoA-I, apoA-IV, apoE, HDL deficiency, HDL subclasses, macrophage, Tangier disease, transgenic mice.

Address for correspondence: Gerd Assmann, Institut für Klinische Chemie und Laboratoriumsmedizin, Zentrallaboratorium, Westfälische Wilhelms-Universität Münster, Albert-Schweitzer-Strasse 33, D-48149 Münster, Germany. Tel.: +49-251-83-56276. Fax: +49-251-83-56181.
E-mail: vonecka@uni-muenster.de

20

Introduction

High-density lipoproteins (HDLs) play an important role in the reverse transport of excess cholesterol from peripheral cells to the liver and steroidogenic organs [1−3]. HDL represents a very heterogeneous class of lipoproteins, most of which are lipid-rich, exhibit electrophoretic α-mobility and contain apolipoprotein (apo) A-I as the predominant protein constituent [1,4]. Quantitatively minor subgroups are lipid-poor or even lipid-free, exhibit electrophoretic preβ- or γ-mobilities, and contain apoA-I, apoA-IV, or apoE as the only protein constituents [1,4−8]. Lipid-rich and lipid-poor HDL-subclasses take up cholesterol from different cellular pools with different kinetics. A slow, unsaturable, and bidirectional flux of cholesterol takes place between all cell types investigated so far and lipid-rich HDLs but also between cells and LDL. Net cholesterol efflux from cells onto HDL depends on the esterification of cholesterol through lecithin:cholesterol acyltransferase (LCAT) [1−3,9−11]. By contrast, lipid-free apolipoproteins (e.g., apoA-I, apoA-IV, and ApoE) cause fast, saturable and unidirectional cholesterol efflux which is independent of LCAT [1−3,11−14]. This kind of efflux takes place, for example, in the presence of normal fibroblasts, macrophages, and smooth muscle cell-derived foam cells, but not in the presence of erythrocytes, native smooth muscle cells, and fibroblasts of Tangier disease (TD) patients [1−3,11−15]. Moreover, the fast and specific cholesterol efflux induced by lipid-free apoA-I is sensitive to the treatment of cells with proteases [9]. It is enhanced and suppressed by activation and inhibition of protein kinase C, respectively [16]. For these reasons and because apoA-I binds to cell membrane proteins, it has been hypothesized that apoA-I binds to a signal-transducing cell-surface receptor and that this binding facilitates the translocation of cholesterol from intracellular compartments to the plasma membrane [1−3].

This model of cholesterol efflux regulation is based mostly on experiments where cells were incubated with isolated lipoproteins or apolipoproteins. In vivo, however, the interaction between cells and extracellular acceptor particles is much more complex because both the quantity and quality of lipoproteins and apolipoproteins are modulated by lipid transfer proteins, because lipoproteins interact with one another, and because the plasma compartment may contain further as yet uncharacterized components which regulate cholesterol efflux. We have therefore investigated cholesterol efflux from cells into total plasma. Some rare inborn errors of HDL metabolism in man as well as gene-targeted defects in mice lead to the absence of all or some specific HDL particles from plasma. Plasmas of either patients or mice allowed us to investigate the contribution of various lipoproteins to cholesterol efflux from fibroblasts under more physiological conditions.

Lessons from Tangier disease and apoA-I(L141R)$_{Pisa}$

Plasmas of patients with Tangier Disease (TD) and of hemizygotes for apoA-

I(L141R)$_{Pisa}$ are characterized by the virtual absence of HDL and severely reduced levels of apoA-I. The residual apoA-I in plasmas of TD patients and of hemizygotes for apoA-I(L141R)$_{Pisa}$ resides in preβ$_1$-LpA-I [17—20]. In TD the presence of preβ$_1$-LpA-I but absence of α-LpA-I is associated with the absence of a plasma activity which normally converts preβ$_1$-LpA-I into α-LpA-I [21]. By contrast, the conversion activity is present in plasmas of hemizygotes for apoA-I(L141R)$_{Pisa}$ but the structurally defective apoA-I is resistant to preβ$_1$-LpA-I → α-LpA-I conversion [20].

Cholesterol efflux from fibroblasts into apoB-depleted plasma of TD patients and apoA-I(L141R)$_{Pisa}$ hemizygotes was saturated already after 1 min of incubation. At this time point, cholesterol efflux capacities of apoB-depleted plasmas from either normal donors or HDL-deficient patients did not differ significantly [20]. However, cholesterol efflux into apoB-depleted plasmas of normoalphalipoproteinemic donors slowly increased after this time and was not saturable. Thus, at later time points the capacity for cholesterol efflux was increased significantly relative to samples from HDL-deficient donors [20]. Cholesterol efflux from fibroblasts into apoB-free plasma clearly consists of two components. The fast and saturable component is observed in both HDL deficient and normoalphalipoproteinemic plasma samples. The slow and unsaturable component is only found in apoB-free plasmas of normoalphalipoproteinemic donors. Since plasmas of TD patients and hemizygotes for apoA-I(L141R)$_{Pisa}$ contain preβ$_1$-LpA-I but not α-LpA-I, this observation provides further evidence that preβ$_1$-LpA-I is responsible for fast and specific cholesterol efflux and that α-LpA-I causes slow and unspecific cholesterol efflux [20].

The contribution of lipid-poor HDL to cholesterol efflux is important not only in rare forms of HDL deficiency but also under normal circumstances. In the extravascular space, where cholesterol efflux from cells takes place in vivo, the concentration of lipid-poor HDL such as preβ$_1$-LpA-I relative to the concentration of lipid-rich alpha-migrating HDL is higher than in plasma [6,22,23]. Moreover, lipid poor preβ$_1$-LpA-I and lipid-rich HDL are part of a dynamic system, in which cholesteryl ester transfer protein (CETP) [24—26], phospholipid transfer protein (PLTP) [27,28], and hepatic lipase [29] produce, and LCAT and other factors consume, preβ$_1$-LpA-I [21,30—37]. Thus changes in the relative activities of preβ$_1$-LpA-I generating and converting enzymes should determine the cholesterol efflux capacity of plasma. In fact, supplementation of human plasma with exogenous PLTP or expression of CETP in transgenic mice have been shown to increase the concentration of preβ$_1$-LpA-I, cholesterol efflux into preβ$_1$-LpA-I, and total cholesterol efflux capacity of plasma [26,27].

Lessons from apoA-I-deficiency

Cholesterol efflux from fibroblasts into apoA-I-depleted plasmas or plasmas from apoA-I deficient patients is reduced by approximately 50% compared to normoalphalipoproteinemic plasmas [17,38]. This residual cholesterol efflux activity of plasma has formerly been attributed to albumin [38,39]. We searched for HDL-subclasses which are free of apoA-I but which fulfil important functions in reverse cholesterol transport. These experiments led to the identification of plasma lipoproteins which contain either apoE or apoA-IV as their only apolipoproteins and which have electrophoretic gamma-mobility (γ-LpE) or alpha-mobility (LpA-IV-1 and LpA-IV-2) [7,8,40,41]. Like preβ_1-LpA-I, both γ-LpE and LpA-IV-1 are relatively rich in sphingomyelin and phosphatidylcholine but poor in cholesterol [7,42]. After short pulse-incubations of plasma with ^{3}H-cholesterol labeled fibroblasts, significant amounts of radioactivity were detected in both γ-LpE and LpA-IV-1 [7,8,40]. During subsequent chase-incubations without cells the radiolabel disappeared from γ-LpE but not from LpA-IV-1 indicating that at least γ-LpE also serves as an initial acceptor of cell-derived cholesterol in the plasma compartment [7]. In contrast to both γ-LpE and preβ_1-LpA-I, cholesterol is esterified in LpA-IV-1 [8]. These observations indicate that γ-LpE and LpA-IV-1 are apoA-I-free lipoproteins which contribute to reverse cholesterol transport. We were also able to demonstrate that both γ-LpE and LpA-IV-1 are important contributors to the residual cholesterol efflux capacity of apoA-I-deficient plasma [17]. The contribution of apoE to cholesterol efflux capacity is also indicated by our observation that the cholesterol efflux capacity of plasma from an apoE-deficient patient is about 30% lower than that of normal control plasmas [43]. Moreover, cholesterol efflux capacity of plasmas from homozygotes for apoE4 who have either no or severely reduced levels of γ-LpE, was also reduced by about 30% compared to plasmas of apoE3 homozygotes [40].

Lessons from apoA-I- and apoE-deficient mice

We investigated the contribution of apoE to cholesterol efflux capacity of plasma also in the model of normal, apoA-I-, and apoE-deficient mice [44]. Plasmas of normal and apoA-I-deficient mice contain apoE in preβ-migrating VLDL as well as in HDL-like lipoproteins which have either electrophoretic α- or γ-mobilities. No apoE-containing lipoproteins were found in plasmas of apoE-deficient mice. Plasmas of apoA-I- and apoE-deficient mice released significantly less ^{3}H-cholesterol from radiolabeled fibroblasts than plasma of normal mice. Removal of apoE from plasmas of normal and apoA-I-deficient mice by anti-apoE-immunoaffinity chromatography decreased their cholesterol efflux capacities. In contrast anti-apoE-immunoaffinity chromatography of apoE-deficient plasma did not change its cholesterol efflux capacity. ApoE-deficient and apoE-depleted plasmas differ from normal plasmas in several respects. Not only apoE, but also other normal lipoproteins are absent, and abnormal remnant lipoproteins are present. Nevertheless, our data provide further evidence that apoE, in addition to apoA-I, determines the cholesterol efflux capacity of plasma. In agreement with this conclusion we have shown that low-dose expression of apoE in macrophages of apoE-deficient mice, which does not prevent remnant hyperlipidemia [45], corrects the defective cholesterol efflux capacity of apoE-deficient mouse plasma [46].

Some of the differences between cholesterol efflux into normal and apoE-deficient plasmas were attributable to the failure of apoE-deficient plasmas to take up cell-derived ^{3}H-cholesterol by γ-LpE and a reduced activity to take up cell-derived cholesterol by α-migrating HDL. Moreover, compared to normal plasma, both apoA-I-deficient and apoE-deficient plasmas were significantly decreased in their activity to esterify cell-derived ^{3}H-cholesterol. Anti-apoE-chromatography significantly decreased cholesterol esterification in normal plasma and apoA-I-deficient plasma, but not in apoE-deficient plasma. Taken together the data provide evidence that apoE is an important contributor to reverse cholesterol transport, partially due to uptake of cell-derived cholesterol by γ-LpE and apoE containing α-HDL, partially due to the contribution of apoE-containing lipoproteins to the esterification of cholesterol in plasma [44].

ApoE and macrophages

Three common isoforms of apoE exist in humans. These differ in only two amino acid positions and are designated E2, which contains cysteine at residues 112 and 158, E3 with cysteine at 112 and arginine at 158, and E4 with arginine at both 112 and 158 [47]. These isoforms are coded for by the respective alleles termed ε2, with a frequency in Caucasian populations of 8%, ε3 with a frequency of 77% and ε4 with a frequency of 15% [48]. This polymorphism has a significant effect on the risk of both coronary atherosclerosis (CHD) and Alzheimer's disease, both of which are more common in persons expressing the E4 isoform [49,50].

One reason for this difference in risk might lie in isoform-specific differences in the transcription, translation or posttranslational processing of apoE in macrophages. In order to investigate this, we used a reverse transcription-polymerase chain reaction assay with a competitive internal RNA standard to measure apoE mRNA levels in monocyte-derived macrophages from persons homozygous for each of the three apoE phenotypes, before and after cholesterol-loading of the cells by means of acetylated LDL. ApoE secretion was measured by ELISA and the cholesterol and cholesteryl ester concentration with an HPLC method developed in our laboratory [51]. Unloaded cells of all genotypes contained similar amounts of apoE mRNA. Despite this, E3/3 cells secreted 77 and 35% more apoE than E2/2 or E4/4 cells, respectively. Pulse-chase studies confirmed that the apoE secretion rate in unloaded cells was greatest in E3/3 and least in E2/2 cells. Moreover, a portion of the newly synthesized apoE2 and apoE4, but not apoE3, was degraded intracellularly. Nevertheless, all unloaded macrophages contained similar amounts of free cholesterol and cholesteryl ester. On cholesterol loading by means of acetylated LDL, apoE mRNA levels rose 2.2-fold in E3/3 and 4.5-fold in E4/4, but not in E2/2 cells. ApoE secretion also increased least in E2/2 and most in E4/4 cells. Intracellular cholesterol and cholesteryl ester content, however, rose most in E2/2 and least in E3/3 cells.

Incubations with 3H-cholesterol-AcLDL showed that E2/2 cells stored cholesterol most readily but were most efficient at secreting it. The greatest reuptake of ^{3}H-cholesterol-rich particles was observed from E4/4 macrophage-conditioned media. Thus it appears that E2/2 macrophages, despite a low apoE secretion rate, are protected from excessive cholesterol storage through apoE-mediated net cholesterol efflux. In E3/3 macrophages, cholesterol accumulation is lessened by a high basal apoE secretion rate. In E4/4 macrophages, despite the highest levels of apoE mRNA and protein secretion, effective net cholesterol efflux is lacking, probably due to enhanced reuptake of cholesterol-rich particles [52]. These findings may have implications for the isoform-specific differences in risk for both atherosclerosis and Alzheimer's disease.

Conclusions

In conclusion, lipid poor particles such as $pre\beta_1$-LpA-I, γ-LpE, and LpA-IV account for the significant residual cholesterol efflux capacity of HDL-deficient plasma but also fulfil important roles in reverse cholesterol transport of normal plasma. Cholesterol efflux by apoE-containing lipoproteins may play an important antiatherogenenic role since, although to a much lesser extent than by hepatocytes, apoE is also produced by macrophages [2,53]. Several lines of evidence indicate that macrophage-derived apoE contributes to reverse cholesterol transport. In vitro, lipid loading of macrophages stimulates synthesis and secretion of apoE, a process which was shown to facilitate cholesterol efflux from these cells [52,54—61]. In agreement with this, low dose expression of a human apoE transgene in macrophages of apoE-deficient mice did not correct remnant hyperlipidemia but significantly reduced the extent of atherosclerotic lesions [45] and transplantation of apoE-deficient bone marrow into apoE-deficient mice caused atherosclerosis [62].

Acknowledgements

The project was supported by grants from Deutsche Forschungsgemeinschaft (Ec116,2-2 and Ec116,3-2) to A. v. E. This manuscript summarizes previous work of the authors' laboratories most of which has been published in detail elsewhere. We thank all co-workers, especially our previous postdoctoral fellows Drs Yadong Huang, Andrea Cignarella, Roberto Miccoli, Shili Wu and Yenhong Zhu.

References

1. Fielding C, Fielding PE. Molecular physiology of reverse cholesterol transport. J Lipid Res 1995;36:211—228.
2. von Eckardstein A. Cholesterol efflux from macrophages and other cells. Curr Opin Lipid 1996;7:308—319.

3. Oram JF, Yokoyama S. Apolipoprotein-mediated removal of cellular cholesterol and phospholipids. J Lipid Res 1997;37:2473–2491.

4. von Eckardstein A, Huang Y, Assmann G. Physiological role and clinical relevance of high-density lipoprotein subclasses. Curr Opin Lipid 1994;5:404–416.

5. Barrans A, Jaspard B, Barbaras R, Chap H, Perret B, Collet X. Pre-β HDL: structure and metabolism. Biochim Biophys Acta 1996;1300:73–83.

6. Castro GR, Fielding CJ. Early incorporation of cell-derived cholesterol into pre-β-migrating high density lipoprotein. Biochemistry 1988;27:25–29.

7. Huang Y, von Eckardstein A, Wu S, Maeda N, Assmann G. A solely apolipoprotein E containing plasma lipoprotein with electrophoretic gamma-mobility takes up cellular cholesterol. Proc Natl Acad Sci USA 1994;91:1834–1838.

8. von Eckardstein A, Huang Y, Wu S, SaadatSarmadi A, Schwarz S, Steinmetz A, Assmann G. Lipoproteins containing apolipoprotein A-IV but not apolipoprotein A-I take up and esterify cell-derived cholesterol in plasma. Arterioscler Thromb Vasc Biol 1995;15:1755–1763.

9. Kawano M, Miida T, Fielding CJ, Fielding PE. Quantitation of preβ-HDL-dependent and nonspecific components of the total efflux of cellular cholesterol and phospholipid. Biochemistry 1993;32:5025–5028.

10. Czarnecka H, Yokoyama S. Regulation of cellular cholesterol efflux by lecithin:cholesterol acyltransferase reaction through nonspecific lipid exchange. J Biol Chem 1996;266:2023–2028.

11. Czarnecka H, Yokoyama S. Lecithin:cholesterol acyltransferase reaction on cellular lipid released by free apolipoprotein-mediated efflux. Biochemistry 1995;34:4385–4392.

12. Hara H, Yokoyama S. Interaction of free apolipoproteins with macrophages: formation of high density lipoprotein-like lipoproteins and reduction of cellular cholesterol. J Biol Chem 1991; 266:3080–3086.

13. Yancey PG, Bielicki JK, Johnson WJ, Lund-Katz S, Palgunachari MN, Anantharamaiah GM, Segrest JP, Phillips MC, Rothblat GH. Efflux of cellular cholesterol and phospholipid to lipid-free apolipoproteins and class A amphipathic peptides. Biochemistry 1995;34:7955–7965.

14. Li Q, Yokoyama S. Independent regulation of cholesterol incorporation into free apolipoprotein-mediated cellular lipid efflux in rat vascular smooth muscle cells. J Biol Chem 1995;269: 26216–26223.

15. Francis GA, Knopp RH, Oram JF. Defective removal of cellular cholesterol and phospholipids by apolipoprotein A-I in Tangier disease. J Clin Invest 1995;96:78–87.

16. Mendez AJ, Oram JF, Bierman EL. Protein kinase C as a mediator of high density lipoprotein dependent efflux of intracellular cholesterol. J Biol Chem 1991;266:10104–10111.

17. von Eckardstein A, Huang Y, Wu S, Noseda G, Assmann G. Reverse cholesterol transport in plasma of patients with different forms of familial high density lipoprotein deficiency. Arterioscler Thromb Vasc Biol 1995;15:690–701.

18. Assmann G, von Eckardstein A, Brewer HB Jr. Familial high density lipoprotein deficiency: Tangier disease. In: Scriver CR, Beaudet AL, Sly WS, Valle D (eds) The Metabolic Basis of Inherited Disease, 7th edn. New York: McGraw-Hill, 1995;2053–2072.

19. Miccoli R, Bertolotto A, Navalesi N, Odoguardi L, Boni A, Wessling J, Funke H, Wiebusch H, von Eckardstein A, Assmann G. Hemizygosity for a structural apolipoprotein A-I-variant — ApoA-I(L141R)$_{Pisa}$ — causes high density lipoprotein deficiency, corneal opacifications, and coronary heart disease. Circulation 1996;94:1622–1628.

20. Miccoli R, Zhu Y, Daum U, Wessling J, Huang Y, Navalesi R, Assmann G, von Eckardstein A. A natural apolipoprotein A-I variant — apoA-I(L141R)$_{Pisa}$ — interferes with the formation of alpha-high density lipoproteins (HDL) but not with the formation of prebeta$_1$-HDL: effects on cholesterol efflux into plasma. J Lipid Res 1997;38:1242–1253.

21. Huang Y, von Eckardstein A, Wu S, Assmann G. Generation of preβ$_1$-high density lipoprotein (HDL) and conversion into α-HDL: evidence for disturbed preβ$_1$-HDL conversion in Tangier disease. Arterioscler Thromb Vasc Biol 1995;15:1746–1754.

22. Asztalos BF, Sloop CH, Wong L, Roheim PS. Comparison of apo A-I-containing subpopula-

tions of dog plasma and prenodal peripheral lymph: evidence for alteration in subpopulations in the interstitial space. Biochim Biophys Acta 1993;1169:301–304.

23. Jaspard B, Collet X, Barbaras R, Manent J, Vieu C, Pontonnier G, Chap H, Perret B. Biochemical characterization of pre-β1- high-density lipoprotein from human ovarian follicular fluid: evidence for the presence of a lipd core. Biochemistry 1996;35:1352–1357.

24. Clay MA, Newnham HH, Forte TM, Barter PJ. Cholesteryl ester transfer protein and hepatic lipase activity promote shedding of apoA-I from HDL and susequent formation of discoidal HDL. Biochim Biophys Acta 1992;1124:52–58.

25. Hennessy LK, Kunitake ST, Kane JP. Apolipoprotein A-I-containing lipoproteins, with or without apolipoprotein A-II, as progenitors of preβ-high density lipoprotein particles. Biochemistry 1993;32:5759–5765.

26. Francone OL, Royer L, Haghpassand M. Increased preβ-HDL levels, cholesterol efflux, and LCAT mediated esterification in mice expressing the human cholesteryl ester transfer protein (CETP) and human apolipoprotein A-I (apoA-I) transgenes. J Lipid Res 1996;37:1268–1277.

27. von Eckardstein A, Jauhiainen M, Huang Y, Metso J, Langer C, Pussinen P, Wu S. Ehnholm C, Assmann G. Phospholipid transfer protein mediated conversion of high density lipoproteins (HDL) generates preβ₁-HDL. Biochim Biophys Acta 1996;1301:255–261.

28. Jiang X-J, Francone OL, Bruce C, Milne R, Mar J, Walsh A, Breslow JL, Tall AR. Increased preβ-high density lipoprotein, apolipoprotein AI, and phospholipid in mice expressing the human phospholipid transfer protein and human apolipoprotein AI transgenes. J Clin Invest 1996;98:2373–2380.

29. Barrans A, Collet X, Barbaras R, Jaspard B, Manent J, Vieu C, Chap H, Perret B. Hepatic lipase induces the formation of pre-beta 1 high density lipoprotein (HDL) from triacylglycerol-rich HDL2. A study comparing liver perfusion to in vitro incubation with lipases. J Biol Chem 1994;269:11572–11577.

30. Ishida BY, Albee D, Paigen B. Interconversion of prebeta migrating lipoproteins containing apoA-I and HDL. J Lipid Res 1990;31:227–236.

31. Neary R, Bhatnagar D, Durrington P, Ishola M, Arrol S, Mackness M. An investigation of the role of lecithin:cholesterol acyltransferase and triglyceride-rich lipoproteins in the metabolism of high density lipoproteins. Atherosclerosis 1991;89:35–48.

32. Miida T, Kawano M, Fielding CJ, Fielding PE. Regulation of the concentration of preβ high density lipoprotein in normal plasma by cell membranes and lecithin:cholesterol acyltransferase. Biochemistry 1992;31:11112–11117.

33. Liang H-Q, Rye K-A, Barter PJ. Remodelling of reconstituted high density lipoproteins by lecithin:cholesterol acyltransferase. J Lipid Res 1996;37:1962–1970.

34. Clay MA, Barter PJ. Formation of new HDL particles from lipid-free apolipoprotein A-I. J Lipid Res 1996;37:1722–1732.

35. Musliner TA, Long DL, Forte TM, Nichols AV, Gong EL, Blanche PJ, Krauss RM. Dissociation of high density lipoprotein precursors from apolipoprotein B-containing lipoproteins in the presence of unesterified fatty acids and a source of apolipoprotein A-I. J Lipid Res 1991;32:917–932.

36. Kunitake ST, Mendel CM, Hennessy LK. Interconversion between apolipoproteins of pre-beta and alpha electrophoretic mobilities. J Lipid Res 1992;33:1807–1816.

37. Liang H-Q, Rye K-A, Barter PJ. Cycling of apolipoprotein A-I between lipid-associated and lipid-free pools. Biochim Biophys Acta 1995;1257:31–37.

38. Fielding CJ, Moser K. Evidence for the separation of albumin- and apo A-I-dependent mechanisms of cholesterol efflux from cultured fibroblasts into human plasma. J Biol Chem 1982;257:10955–10960.

39. Zhao Y, Marcel YL. Serum albumin is a significant intermediate in cholesterol transfer between cells and lipoproteins. Biochemistry 1996;35:7174–7180.

40. Huang Y, von Eckardstein A, Wu S, Assmann G. Effects of the apolipoprotein E-polymorphism on uptake and transfer of cell-derived cholesterol in plasma. J Clin Invest 1995;96:2693–2701.

41. Krimbou JL, Tremblay M, Davignon J, Cohn JS. Characterization of human plasma apolipoprotein E containing lipoproteins in the high density lipoprotein size range: focus on prebeta1-LpE, prebeta2-LpE, and alpha-LpE. J Lipid Res 1997;38:35—48.

42. Duverger N, Ghalim N, Ailhaud G, Steinmetz A, Fruchart J-C, Castro G. Characterization of apo A-IV-containing lipoprotein particles isolated form human plasma and interstitial fluid. Arterioscler Thromb 1993;13:126—132.

43. von Eckardstein A, Zhu A, Bellosta S, Bernini F, Hoffmann M, März W, Assmann G. Defective cholesterol efflux into plasmas of apolipoprotein E-deficient men and mice. Eur J Clin Chem Clin Biochem (Abstract) 1997;(In press).

44. Huang Y, Langer C, Raabe M, Wiesenhütter B, Wu S, Seedorf U, Maeda N, Assmann G, von Eckardstein A. Effects of genotype and diet on cholesterol efflux into plasma and lipoproteins of normal, apolipoprotein A-I-, and apolipoprotein E-deficient mice. Arterioscler Thromb Vasc Biol 1997;17:2010—2019.

45. Bellosta S, Mahley RW, Sanan DA, Newland DL, Taylor JM, Pitas RE. Macrophage-specific expression of human apolipoprotein E reduces atherosclerosis in hypercholesterolemic apolipoprotein E-null mice. J Clin Invest 1995;96:2170—2179.

46. von Eckardstein A, Bellosta S, Zhu Y, Bernini F, Pitas RE, Assmann G. Macrophage specific expression of human apolipoprotein E in apolipoprotein E deficient mice increases cholesterol efflux and esterification capacities of plasma. Circulation (Abstract) 1997;(In press).

47. Utermann G, Langenbeck U, Beisiegel U et al. Genetics of the apolipoprotein E system in man. Am J Hum Genet 1980;32:339—347.

48. Davignon J, Gregg RE, Sing CF. Apolipoprotein E polymorphism and atherosclerosis. Arteriosclerosis 1988;8:1—21.

49. Ordovas JM, Schaefer MD. Apolipoprotein E polymorphisms and coronary heart disease risk. Cardiovasc Risk Fact 1994;4:103—107.

50. Corder EH, Saunders AM, Strittmatter WJ et al. Gene dose of apolipoprotein E type 4 allele and the risk of Alzheimer's disease in late onset families. Science 1993;261:921—923.

51. Cullen P, Fobker M, Tegelkamp K et al. An improved method for quantification of cholesterol and cholesteryl esters in human monocyte-derived macrophages by high performance liquid chromatography with identification of unassigned cholesteryl ester species by means of secondary ion mass spectrometry. J Lipid Res 1997;38:401—409.

52. Cullen P, Cignarella A, Brennhausen B, Mohr S, Assmann G. Phenotype-dependent differences in apoE metabolism and cholesterol homeostasis in human monocyte-derived macrophages. Atherosclerosis 1997;134:229.

53. Mazzone T. Apolipoprotein E secretion by macrophages: its potential functions. Curr Opin Lipidol 1996;7:303—310.

54. Cullen P, Cignarella A, von Eckardstein A, Mohr S, Assmann G. Phenotype-dependent differences in apolipoprotein E gene expression and protein secretion in human monocyte-derived macrophages. Circulation 1996;94:I-273.

55. Basu SK, Ho Y, Brown MS, Bilheimer DW, Anderson RGW, Goldstein J. Biochemical and genetic studies of the apoprotein E secreted by mouse macrophages and human monocytes. J Biol Chem 1982;257:9788—9795.

56. Basu S, Goldstein JL, Brown MS. Independent pathways for secretion of free cholesterol and apolipoprotein E by macrophages. Science 1983;219:871—873.

57. Dory L. Synthesis and secretion of apo E in thioglycolate-elicited mouse peritoneal macrophages: effect of cholesterol efflux. J Lipid Res 1989;30:809—816.

58. Mazzone T, Reardon C. Expression of heterologous human apolipoprotein E by J774 macrophages enhances cholesterol efflux to HDL$_3$. J Lipid Res 1994;35:1345—1353.

59. Kruth HS, Skarlatos SI, Gaynor PM, Gamble W. Production of cholesterol-enriched nascent high density lipoproteins by human monocyte-derived macrophages is a mechanism that contributes to macrophage cholesterol efflux. J Biol Chem 1994;269:24511—24518.

60. Hayek T, Oiknine J, Brook JG, Aviram M. Role of HDL apolipoprotein E in cellular cholesterol

efflux: studies in apoE knock out transgenic mice. Biochem Biophys Res Commun 1994;205: 1072–1078.

61. Zhang WY, Gaynor PM, Kruth HS. Apolipoprotein E produced by human monocyte-derived macrophages mediates cholesterol efflux that occurs in the absence of added cholesterol acceptors. J Biol Chem 1996;271:28641–28646.

62. Fazio S, Babaev VR, Murray AB, Hasty AH, Carter KJ, Gleaves LA, Atkinson JB, Linton MF. Increased atherosclerosis in mice reconstittued with apolipoprotein E null macrophages. Proc Natl Acad Sci USA 1997;94:4647–4652.

Leptin, leptin receptors and the regulation of body weight

Jeffrey M. Friedman
Howard Hughes Medical Institute, The Rockefeller University, New York, New York, USA

The molecular cloning of the mouse obesity (ob) and diabetic (db) genes has identified a new hormone, leptin, which plays an important role in regulating body weight. Recessive mutations in the mouse ob and db genes result in obesity and diabetes in a syndrome resembling morbid human obesity [1,2]. Affected ob and db mice have identical phenotypes, each mutant weighing 3 times that of normal mice with a 5-fold increase in body fat content. Coleman, using the method of parabiosis, predicted that the ob gene encoded a novel hormone and that the db gene encoded its receptor [1]. Available data are consistent with this hypothesis and suggest that body weight is regulated by a feedback loop integrated by the hypothalamus. Positional cloning was used to identify the ob and db genes [3,4]. The ob gene was localized to a 300 kB region on mouse chromosome 6. Exon trapping was employed to identify candidate genes from this interval. One exon detected a 4.5-kB fat-specific RNA which was shown to be allelic with ob [3,5—7]. The ob gene encodes a novel 167 amino acid protein. This protein sequence is novel and to date has no homologues in the public sequence database. The ob transcript is mutant in both of the available strains of ob mice. In ob^{2J} mice, a ~ 5 kB ETn transposon is inserted into the first intron (manuscript in preparation). This results in the synthesis of hybrid RNAs in which the splice donor of the noncoding ob first exon is spliced to splice acceptors in the transposon. Mature ob RNA is not synthesized in this mutant. In the original C57Bl/6J ob mutant, a nonsense mutation at codon 105 results in the synthesis of a truncated protein that is not detectable in mouse plasma. The ob protein has a functional signal sequence which initially suggested that the ob gene product was secreted [3]. In addition, the level of ob RNA was increased in ob mice suggesting that the ob gene is under feedback control. These data suggested that the protein product of the ob gene is an afferent signal in a negative feedback loop regulating the size of adipose tissue mass. However, this theory was unproven and required further experiments to establish the characteristics and function of the protein encoded by the ob gene. In order to establish that the ob gene product functions as a hormone controlling body fat content, the following criteria had to be satisfied:

Address for correspondence: Jeffrey M. Friedman, Howard Hughes Medical Institute, The Rockefeller University, New York, NY 10021, USA.

1) The ob gene should be expressed in adipocytes, the principle site of fat storage.
2) The ob protein should circulate in plasma.
3) The plasma level of the protein should increase in obese animals and decrease with weight loss.
4) Recombinant protein should reduce body fat content when injected into ob and wild-type, but not db mice.

In a collaborative study with the Ailhaud laboratory in Nice, France, in situ hybridization and cell fractionation were used to demonstrate that ob RNA is expressed only in adipocytes [7]. The ob gene product, known as LEPTIN, circulates as a 16 kDa protein in mouse and human plasma but is undetectable in plasma from C57BL/6J ob/ob mice [8]. Plasma levels of this protein are increased in diabetic mice, a mutant now confirmed to be resistant to the effects of ob [8]. The levels of protein are also increased in several other genetic and environmentally induced forms of rodent obesity including mice with lesions in the hypothalamus [7,9]. The plasma levels of leptin fall in both humans and mice after weight loss [9]. Daily intraperitoneal injections of recombinant mouse leptin, prepared in collaboration with the Burley laboratory at HHMI/Rockefeller, reduced body weight of ob/ob mice by 30% at 2 weeks and by 40% after 4 weeks but had no effect on db/db mice [8]. The protein reduced food intake and increased energy expenditure in ob/ob mice. Injections of wild-type mice twice daily with the mouse protein resulted in a sustained 12% weight loss, decreased food intake and a reduction of body fat from 12.2 to 0.7%. Recombinant human leptin reduced body weight with equivalent potency to mouse leptin when injected into ob mice [8]. These data suggested that leptin serves an endocrine function to regulate body fat stores. The data also suggested that the hypothalamus is an important target of leptin action [7].

Molecular cloning of the db gene: studies of leptin's site of action

The complete insensitivity of db mice to leptin and the identical phenotype of ob and db mice suggested that the db locus encoded the leptin receptor [1,8]. Additional experiments using mice with lesions of the hypothalamus led to the conclusion that leptin's effects were mediated via effects on the hypothalamus, a brain region known to control body weight [7]. Confirmation of this required the identification of the leptin receptor and/or the db mutation. The db gene was localized to a 300 kB interval on mouse chromosome 4 [4,10,11]. Exon trapping and cDNA selection from hypothalamus identified a candidate gene in this region. This candidate was found to be identical to a receptor (Ob-R) which was isolated by another group using expression cloning from choroid plexus [4,12]. However, the choroid plexus form of the receptor was normal in db mice. This suggested that the db mutation affected an alternatively spliced form of this receptor. The Ob-R gene was found to encode at least five alternatively spliced forms [4]. One of the splice variants, Ob-Rb,is expressed at a high level in the hypothalamus and at a lower level in other tissues. This transcript is mutant in C57BL/Ks db/db mice [4]. The mutation is the result of abnormal splicing leading to a 106 bp insertion into the 3' end of its RNA. The mutant protein is missing the cytoplasmic region and is likely to be defective in signal transduction (see [13]). A nonsense mutation in fa^{cp} rats, a rat equivalent of db, leads to premature termination NH2-terminal of the transmembrane domain (manuscript in preparation). In db^{3J} mice, a frame shift mutation in the extracellular region ablates expression of the wild-type receptor protein [4,13]. The phenotypes of C57BL/6J db/ob mice (mutant in Ob-Rb) and 129 db^{3J}/db^{3J} mice (mutant in all forms) are identical. These data suggest that the weight-reducing effects of leptin are mediated by signal transduction through a receptor, Ob-Rb, in the hypothalamus and perhaps elsewhere. Further evidence in support of a hypothalamic site of action was generated using in vivo assays of STAT activation in response to leptin [14]. Ob-R is a member of the cytokine family of receptors. These receptors regulate transcription via tyrosine phosphorylation of members of the STAT family of transcription factors. STAT activation was assayed in nuclear extracts from a number of mouse tissues after leptin treatment using gel shift assays. Dose-dependent activation of STAT3 is demonstrable in the hypothalamus of mice within 15 min of a single intravenous injection of leptin. This effect is not seen in C57Bl/KS db/db mice who have a defect in the Ob-Rb isoform of the leptin receptor. This work, which confirms a direct effect of leptin on hypothalamus, was a collaboration among the Friedman, Stoffel and the James Darnell laboratories at Rockefeller University. More recently, cells in hypothalamus that express leptin receptor in hypothalamus have been identified in the arcuate, VMH and LH nuclei [15]. These nuclei have all been shown to play a role in regulating food intake and weight. This knowledge sets the stage for further studies to establish the precise neuronal effects of leptin. These data do not exclude the possibility that leptin also acts on other tissues. Recently the effect of peripherally administered leptin has been compared to those of leptin administered directly into the mouse III ventricle using osmotic infusion pumps. Infusion of leptin ICV at a dose of 5 ng/h results in a more profound response (20% weight loss at 7 days) than that seen in response to a twice daily intraperitoneal dose of 250 μg (12% weight loss) [16]. The effect of the 5 ng/h ICV dose appears to be at the peak of the dose response curve as higher doses (50 and 500 ng/h) do not have a greater effect. Further studies are underway to establish the ED50 of ICV leptin. We have not yet identified any effects of peripheral leptin that are not reproduced by leptin infused into the ventricle. These data establish leptin as the most potent weight reducing peptide when delivered into the CSF and support the possibility that the CNS is a major site of leptin action.

Relevance of leptin to other forms of obesity

The relationship of leptin to other forms of obesity can be inferred by measurement of plasma leptin level [9]. An increase in plasma levels suggests that obesity is the result of an effect downstream of leptin. A low or normal plasma concentration of leptin in the context of obesity suggests a possible effect on leptin synthesis and/or secretion. An ELISA (developed in our laboratory in collaboration with Roger Lallone) has been used to measure plasma (leptin) in a number of animal obesities and in human (see below). In all forms of rodent obesity studied to date, the obese animals have a higher leptin level than controls (not including ob mice). The correlation between BMI (body mass index) and leptin concentration is 0.9 [9]. The animals studied included mutant A^y, fat and tub mice, diet-induced obese mice, New Zealand Obese mice (NZO), old mice and mice with hypothalamic lesions. These data suggest that these forms of animal obesity are the result of leptin resistance. Leptin infusion into obese animals has indicated that several obese rodents including diet induced obese (DIO), A^y and New Zealand Obese (NZO) mice are leptin-resistant [16]. DIO mice are partially resistant to peripheral leptin while A^y mice do not respond to subcutaneous leptin and respond poorly to ICV leptin (at 100-fold higher doses). NZO mice do not respond to peripheral leptin but respond normally to ICV leptin. The decreased potency of subcutaneous and ICV leptin in DIO, NZO and A^y mice indicate that obesity in these strains tested is likely to be the result of insensitivity to leptin. In NZO mice, leptin resistance may be the result of decreased transport of leptin into the CSF. In A^y mice, leptin resistance probably results from defects in the signaling pathway downstream of the leptin receptor in the hypothalamus. The basis for the partial leptin resistance of DIO mice is unknown. Further studies of the basis of leptin resistance in these and other obese strains may have important implications for understanding the pathogenesis of obesity and other mutational disorders. The apparent leptin resistance in other forms of rodent obesity suggests that, in many cases, the abnormality causing the obesity affects hypothalamic function. Indeed the A^y, fat and tub mutations all have been suggested, by others, to affect hypothalamic function. Ectopic expression of the agouti gene product in the hypothalamus has been suggested to affect activity of the Melanocortin 4 receptor, a receptor thought to regulate food intake in the paraventricular nucleus [17,18]. CPE, the gene product of the fat locus, alters posttranslational processing of many peptides including insulin and MCH, a hypothalamic peptide that increases food intake [19]. The tub gene product is expressed at high abundance in the paraventricular nucleus of the hypothalamus [20]. Further studies may reveal the link between these gene products and neurons expressing Ob-Rb.

Possible relevance of leptin to human physiology

The relationship of the ob gene to human obesity has been explored in several collaborative studies. In human subjects, a highly significant correlation between body fat content and plasma leptin concentration was observed. In general, obese humans have high leptin levels [9]. (This is also true, as mentioned, in obese rodents other than ob mice.) These data suggest that in most cases, human obesity is likely to be associated with insensitivity to leptin. However, some obese human subjects had low levels of leptin suggesting that, in a subset of cases, obesity results from a subnormal secretion rate of leptin from fat. Finally it was shown that weight loss by dieting results in a decrease in plasma leptin concentration [9]. This provides a possible explanation for the high failure rate of dieting, as a low leptin level is likely to be a potent stimulus to weight gain. In other studies to establish the relationship of leptin to other nutritional disorders, leptin levels were also measured in animals injected with endotoxin or in AIDS patients (submitted, 1996). Leptin levels increased in endotoxin-treated hamsters suggesting that some of the weight loss associated with LPS treatment is the result of increased plasma leptin [21]. In AIDS patients, leptin levels were not induced suggesting that weight loss is independent of leptin [22]. In almost all cases, obese subjects express at least some leptin, suggesting that human ob gene mutations are likely to be rare. This possibility is also suggested by the failure to find mutations in the human ob gene in more than 100 obese subjects [23]. However, two massively obese children with leptin mutations have recently been identified [24]. These findings confirm the importance of leptin in the regulation of body weight in human. The precise positioning of the human ob and db genes on the human genetic map will assist in further genetic studies to establish the genetic basis of human obesity [25,26]. Future research efforts will focus on several aspects of the physiology of leptin, its cellular effects on hypothalamic neurons and other possible targets, the regulation of the ob gene and the basis of leptin resistance. Other studies pertain to the genetic basis of obesity among the people of Kosrae, a South Pacific island.

References

1. Coleman DL. Obese and diabetes: two mutant genes causing diabetes-obesity syndromes in mice. Diabetologia 1978;14:141—148.
2. Friedman JM, Leibel RL. Tackling a weighty problem. Cell 1992;69:217—220.
3. Zhang Y, Proenca P, Maffei M, Barone M, Leopold L, Friedman JM. Positional cloning of the mouse obese gene and its human homologue. Nature 1994;372:425—432.
4. Lee GH, Proenca R, Montez JM, Carroll KM, Darvishzadeh JG, Lee JI, Friedman JM. Abnormal splicing of the leptin receptor in diabetic mice. Nature 1996;379:632—635.
5. Friedman JM, Leibel RL, Siegel DA, Walsh J, Bahary N. Molecular mapping of the mouse ob mutation. Genomics 1991;11:1054—1062.
6. Bahary N, Siegel DA, Walsh J, Zhang Y, Leopold L, Leibel R, Proenca P, Friedman JM. Microdissection of proximal mouse Chromosome 6: identification of RFLPs tightly linked to the ob mutation. Mammal Genome 1993;4:511—515.
7. Maffei M, Fei H, Lee GW, Dani C, Leroy P, Zhang Y, Proenca R, Negrel R, Ailhaud G, Friedman JM. Increased expression in adipocytes of ob RNA in mice with lesions of the hypothalamus and with mutations at the db locus. Proc Natl Acad Sci USA 1995;92:6957—6960.
8. Halaas JL, Gajiwala KS, Maffei M, Cohen SL, Chait BT, Rabinowitz D, Lallone RL, Burley SK, Friedman JM. Weight-reducing effects of the plasma protein encoded by the obese gene. Science 1995;269:543—546.
9. Maffei M, Halaas J, Ravussin E, Pratley RE, Lee GH, Zhang Y, Fei H, Kim S, Lallone R, Ranganathan S, Kern PA, Friedman JM. Leptin levels in human and rodent: measurement of plas-

ma leptin and ob RNA in obese and weight-reduced subjects. Nature Med 1995;1:1155−1161.

10. Bahary N, Leibel RL, Joseph L, Friedman JM. Molecular mapping of the mouse db mutation. Proc Natl Acad Sci USA 1990;87:8642−8646.

11. Bahary N, McGraw DE, Shilling R, Friedman JM. Microdissection and microcloning of mid-chromosome 4: genetic mapping of 41 microdissection clones. Genomics 1992;16:113−122.

12. Tartaglia LA, Dembski M, Weng X, Deng N, Culpepper J, Devos R, Richards GJ, Campfield LA, Clark FT, Deeds J, Muir C, Sanker S, Moriarty A, Moore KJ, Smutko JS, Mays GG, Woolf EA, Monroe CA, Tepper RI. Identification and expression cloning of a leptin receptor, OB-R. Cell 1995;83:1263−1271.

13. Lee GH, Li C, Montez J, Halaas J, Darvishzadeh J, Friedman JM. Leptin receptor mutations in 129 db^{3J}/db^{3J} mice and NIH fa^{cp}/fa^{cp} rats. Mammalian Genome 1997;8:445−447.

14. Vaisse C, Halaas JL, Horvath CM, Darnell JE Jr, Stoffel M, Friedman JM. Leptin activation of Stat3 in the hypothalamus of wild-type and ob/ob mice but not db/db mice. Nature Genet 1996;14:95−97.

15. Fei H, Okano HJ, Li C, Lee G-H, Zhao C, Darnell R, Friedman JM. Anatomic localization of alternatively spliced leptin receptors (Ob-R) in mouse brain and other tissues. Proc Natl Acad Sci USA 1997;94:7001−7005.

16. Halaas JL, Boozer C, Blair-West J, Fidahusein N, Denton D, Friedman JM. Physiological response to long-term peripheral and central leptin infusion in lean and obese mice. Proc Natl Acad Sci USA 1997;94:8878−8883.

17. Fan W, Boston BA, Kesterson RA, Hruby VJ, Cone RD. Role of melanocortinergic neurons in feeding and the agoutiobesity syndrome. Nature 1997;385:165−168.

18. Huszar D, Lynch CA, Fairchild-Huntress V, Dunmore JH, Fang Q, Berkemeier LR, Gu W, Kesterson RA, Boston BA, Cone RD, Smith FJ, Campfied LA, Burnt P, Lee F. Targeted disruption of the melanocortin-4 receptor results in obesity in mice. Cell 1997;88:131−141.

19. Naggert JK, Fricker LD, Varlamov O, Nishina PM, Rouille Y, Steiner DF, Carroll RJ, Paigen BJ, Leiter EH. Hyperproinsulinaemia in obese fat/fat mice associated with a carboxy peptidase E mutation which reduces enzyme activity. Nature Genet 1995;10:135−142.

20. Kleyn PW, Fan W, Kovatas SG, Lee JJ, Pulido JC, Wu Y, Berkemeir LR, Misumi DJ, Holmgren L, Charlat O, Woolf EA, Tayber O, Brody T, Shu P, Hawkins F, Kennedy B, Baldini L, Ebeling C, Alperin GD, Deeds J, Lakey ND, Culpepper J, Chen H, Glucksmann-Kuis MA, Carlson GA, Duyk GM, Moore KJ. Identification and characterization of the mouse obesity gene tubby: a member of a novel gene family. Cell 1996;85:281−290.

21. Grunfeld C, Zhao C, Fuller J, Pollock A, Moser A, Friedman JM, Feingold KR. Endotoxin and cytokines induce expression of leptin, the ob gene product, in hamsters: a role for leptin in the anorexia of infection. J Clin Invest 1996;97:2152−2157.

22. Yarasheski KE, Zachwieja JJ, Horgan MM, Powderly WG, Santiago JV, Landt M. Serum leptin concentrations in human immunodeficiency virus-infected men with low adiposity metabolism. Clin Experiment 1997;46:303−305.

23. Maffei M, Stoffel M, Barone M, Moon B, Dammerman M, Ravussin E, Bogardus C, Ludwig DS, Flier JS, Talley M, Auerbach S, Friedman JM. Absence of mutations in the human ob gene in obese/diabetic subjects. Diabetes 1996;45:679−682.

24. Montaque CT, Farooqi IS, Whitehead JP, Soos MA, Rau H, Wareham NJ, Sewter CP, Digby JE, Mohammed SN, Hurst JA, Cheetham CH, Early AR, Barnett AH, Prins JB, O'Rahilly S. Congenital leptin deficiency is associated with severe early-onset obesity in humans. Nature 1997;387:903−908.

25. Green ED, Maffei M, Braden VV, Proenca R, DeSilva U, Zhang Y, Chua SC, Leibel RL, Weissenbach J, Friedman JM. The human obese (OB) gene: RNA expression pattern and mapping on the physical, cytogenetic, and genetic maps of chromosome 7. Genome Res 1995;5:5−12.

26. Winick JD, Stoffel M, Friedman JM. Identification of microsatellite markers linked to the human leptin receptor gene on chromosome 1. Genomics 1996;36:221−222.

PPAR activators improve glucose homeostasis by changing fatty acid partitioning

Geneviève Martin, Kristina Schoonjans, Bart Staels and Johan Auwerx

U.325 INSERM, Département d'Athérosclérose, Institut Pasteur, Lille, France

Keywords: fatty acids, gene expression, lipid metabolism, nuclear receptors, peroxisomes, transcription factors.

Non-insulin-dependent diabetes mellitus (NIDDM) and obesity

Non-insulin-dependent diabetes mellitus (NIDDM) affects approximately 10 million people in the USA and many more millions around the world. A reduced ability of tissues to respond to insulin (insulin resistance (IR)) and a relative insulin deficiency seem to be the hallmarks of this disorder. Studies in families and in twins [1] have shown that genetic factors contribute in a major way to the development of NIDDM [2], although the genes that determine susceptibility to its development have not yet been identified. Its inheritance does not follow a simple mendelian inheritance pattern suggesting that it is an oligogenic disorder. Superimposed on the complex genetic factors underlying this disorder, it is known that IR and the subsequent development of NIDDM are influenced by environmental factors, such as diet and lack of exercise. Often one of the earliest abnormalities seen in subjects predisposed to NIDDM is the accumulation of intra-abdominal fat leading to subsequent insulin resistance. This visceral obesity/insulin resistance syndrome is almost invariably accompanied by the occurrence of a subtle dyslipidemia, characterized by high triglyceride levels, low HDL cholesterol levels and the occurrence of small dense LDL. This lipid pattern is a major risk factor in the development of premature atherosclerosis, the most important cause of mortality in NIDDM patients [3–7].

These observations clearly underscore the importance of adipose tissue and visceral obesity in the pathogenesis of NIDDM. Obesity is a widespread disorder affecting approximately 30% of the USA population, and is a major risk factor for developing IR, hyperlipidemia and NIDDM [8–10]. More than 80% of subjects with NIDDM are also obese. In fact, reduction of obesity by diet and exercise is a commonly employed strategy in combating obesity-linked diabetes. This strongly suggests that the formation and metabolic activities of adipose tissue play an important role in the effect of insulin on other tissues and point to the

Address for correspondence: Dr J. Auwerx MD, PhD, U.325 INSERM, Institut Pasteur, 1 Rue Calmette, 59019 Lille Cedex, France. Fax: +33-20-877360. E-mail: Johan.Auwerx@pasteur-lille.fr

importance of adipose tissue and lipids in the pathogenesis of insulin resistance, NIDDM and associated disorders. Although IR-NIDDM affects a large number of subjects, its pathogenesis remains ill understood. In view of the hypothesis that variation in the function or synthesis of key adipocyte proteins contributes to IR-NIDDM, we will outline in this review our current views about how alterations in fatty acid metabolism induced by activation of PPARγ impede the development of this syndrome.

Key target genes controlling triglyceride and fatty acid metabolism

Several highly specialized proteins are involved in triglyceride and fatty acid homeostasis and in the next section we will briefly review them. One of them is lipoprotein lipase (LPL) which catalyzes the hydrolysis of triacylglycerols of lipoprotein particles [11]. LPL is synthesized by many cell types including macrophages, neonatal liver, skeletal and cardiac muscle but its expression is highest in adipose tissue. All these tissues have a high demand for fatty acids [12]. After secretion LPL becomes bound to glycosaminoglycans on the luminal surface of the capillary endothelium, where it hydrolyzes core triglycerides in triglyceride-rich lipoproteins, such as chylomicrons and very low density lipoproteins [13] (reviewed in [11]). The released free fatty acids (FFAs) are either oxidized to generate ATP in muscle, re-esterified and stored in adipose tissue, or secreted in milk by the mammary gland. LPL therefore occupies a pivotal position in both lipoprotein and energy metabolism. In fact, the activity of this enzyme regulates in part the flux of free fatty acids towards the different tissues. LPL activity furthermore shows an interesting tissue-specific regulation. This differential regulation may explain how fat calories and lipids are partitioned between storage or energy production [14]. For instance, LPL activity in adipose tissue is high during feeding and the immediate postprandial period but is downregulated during fasting, probably to direct the flux of FFAs towards tissues which need energy. In addition to the prandial state, FFA and a long list of hormones affecting FFA flux regulate LPL in a tissue-specific manner. In the absence of LPL, adipose tissue and muscle are essentially unable to absorb FFA from plasma.

Although the FFAs generated by LPL can be taken up by diffusion through the plasma membrane [15], the recently identified fatty acid transport protein (FATP) can facilitate rapid uptake and coordinate the import of FFA in harmony with metabolic demands [16]. FATP is a 63 kDa protein with six predicted membrane-spanning regions, and which is integrally associated with the plasma membrane. Expression of FATP stimulates FFA uptake by adipocytes in a concerted action with acyl-CoA synthetase (ACS) [17], the latter enzyme preventing afflux of fatty acids from the cell by generating acyl-CoA derivatives from them and effectively rendering the FFA uptake unidirectional [16]. Furthermore, fatty acid-binding proteins (FABPs), such as liver FABP or the adipocyte-specific aP2 protein, can act as cytoplasmic sink for these incorporated fatty acids. High level of expression of LPL, FATP, ACS, and FABPs is characteristic of tissues utilizing

FFA such as adipose tissue and/or cardiac and skeletal muscle.

In the adipocytes intracellular triglycerides can again be hydrolysed by a fine-tuned lipolytic pathway [7], liberating FFAs from the fat cell to the bloodstream, where they bind to albumin and are transported to other organs for utilization. This intracellular lipolysis is stimulated by another lipase, hormone-sensitive lipase (HSL), which is exclusively localized within the adipocyte. Insulin has an important function as the hormone responsible for suppressing plasma free fatty acid levels, a function often impaired in the plurimetabolic syndrome [18]. The adipocyte hence stores an important pool of releasable fatty acids which can interfere with metabolic functions.

In addition to these proteins produced mainly in the peripheral tissues (adipose tissue and muscle), which affect triglyceride and fatty acid metabolism, several other liver proteins also affect these parameters. Apo C-III is an apolipoprotein secreted by the liver and intestine, which is involved in the determination of serum triglycerides levels. This apolipoprotein limits the clearance of triglyceride-rich lipoproteins [12,19]. In transgenic animals, overexpressing apo C-III gene, plasma triglycerides levels are proportional to plasma apo C-III concentration [20−22], providing evidence for the causal relationship between increased apo C-III levels and hypertriglyceridemia. In addition to apo C-III, stimulation of oxidative metabolism of fatty acids either by peroxisomal or mitochondrial enzymes also affects the capacity of the liver to produce and secrete FFAs and triglycerides (reviewed in [23−25]). Hence the rate-limiting enzymes involved in these metabolic pathways, such as acyl-CoA oxidase (ACO; peroxisomes) [26,27] and medium chain acyl-CoA dehydrogenase (MCAD; mitochondria) [28] are important control elements in FFA homeostasis.

PPARs, a finely tuned control mechanism of fatty acid metabolism

The expression and activity of the above-mentioned genes is under the control of a group of transcription factors called peroxisome proliferator-activated receptors (PPARs), which hence play an integrative role in the control of fatty acid metabolism (reviewed in [23−25]). Three mammalian PPAR subtypes α, γ and the ubiquitously expressed PPARβ/δ have been described. PPARγ is found predominantly in adipose tissue [29−31], where it plays a crucial role in adipocyte differentiation and fat storage, whereas PPARα, the main PPAR subtype in liver, plays an important role in lipid oxidation [32,33]. PPARs play an integrative role in the control of gene expression by nutritional factors. Following heterodimerization with the retinoid X receptor (RXR) [34], the receptor for 9-*cis*-retinoic acid, PPAR transcription factors bind to PPAR response elements (PPRE) in the DNA. The PPRE consensus sequence is composed of two direct repeats separated by one nucleotide. The PPAR-RXR heterodimer governs the expression of many genes involved in lipid metabolism (reviewed in [24,25]). However, not only are genes involved in lipid metabolism regulated by PPARs, but conversely, lipids are also shown to regulate PPAR activity. This idea first arose from the

38

observation that a wide variety of compounds such as fibrates, other peroxisome proliferators and thiazolidinediones affect PPAR activity (reviewed in [23–25]). The only thing these compounds have in common are that they affect the metabolism of fatty acids, hence the hypothesis that fatty-acid-derived metabolites were the endogeneous PPAR ligands and activators. In fact, both PPARα and PPARγ are activated by naturally occurring arachidonic acid metabolites, prostaglandin J2 [35,36] being a ligand for PPARγ, and eicosanoids, such as 8-S-hydroxyeicosa-tetranoic [37,38] and pentanoic [38] acid and leukotriene B4 [39] being described as a ligand for PPARα. In addition, synthetic ligands and activators for these PPARs are described and it is now well-established that antidiabetic thiazolidinediones are ligands for PPARγ [40], whereas fibrates appear to be ligands for PPARα [37–39]. The main characteristics of the two most important PPARs in this context, PPARα and γ, are shown in Table 1.

PPARγ in adipose tissue

The PPARγ gene gives rise to three distinct mRNAs, i.e., PPARγ1, PPARγ2, and PPARγ3, each differing in their 5′ ends and each under control of their own promoter [30,31,41] (Fajas, unpublished data). All three PPARγ subtypes contain the common exons 1–6. Human PPARγ1 contains in addition the exons A1 and A2 at its 5′ end. PPARγ2 contains the B exon, whereas PPARγ3 contains only the A2 exon. PPARγ1 and 3 give rise to the same protein encoded by exons 1 to 6, since neither the A1 nor the A2 exon are translated. In PPARγ2 the B exon is translated producing a protein with an additional 28 amino acids at its NH2 terminus. In man, PPARγ1 and 3 expression has been found to be highest in large intestine and adipose tissue although measurable expression was also found in kidney, liver, and small intestine [31,33] (L. Fajas, G. Martin, L. Gelman and J. Auwerx, unpublished data). PPARγ2 expression was highest in adipose tissue, with minimal expression in liver, but no expression at any other site [31,33,42]. Perhaps surprisingly, expression of PPARγ in muscle, which is classically thought to be involved in glucose disposal, was very low [31,33]. These mRNA expression studies have also been confirmed by immunocytochemistry, showing that transcription and translation coincide. The high level expression of PPARγ in adipose tissue points to the important function of this transcription

Table 1. Main characteristics of PPARα and PPARγ.

PPARα	PPARγ
Mainly liver (also present in other tissues)	Mainly adipose tissue and colon
Stimulation of β-oxidation	Stimulation of fat storage
Lipid metabolism	Glucose and lipid metabolism
Inflammation (stimulates breakdown of inflammatory fatty acids)	Fat formation
Leukotriene B4, 8-S-HETE, and fibrates	Prostaglandin J2 and thiazolidinediones

factor in adipogenesis and adipocyte gene expression.

Adipogenesis involves multiple transcription factors (reviewed in [10,43]). Adipogenic stimuli such as insulin, dexamethasone, or cAMP are known to activate the transcription factors C/EBPβ and δ. Both these transcription factors directly induce the expression of PPARγ [44,45] which subsequently stimulates the expression of adipocyte-specific genes such as aP2, LPL, and ACS, both alone and in cooperation with two other transcription factors, C/EBPα and adipocyte differentiation and determination factor 1 (ADD-1)/sterol response element binding protein 1 (SREBP-1) [46,47]. This is highly remarkable, because both the activity of PPARγ-RXR (fatty acids, vitamin A) and the ADD-1/SREBP-1 (cholesterol) transcription factors are regulated by different nutrients and both are involved in adipocyte differentiation [10,25,48].

PPARγ activation and insulin sensitivity

The clinical importance of the above findings concerning PPARγ mRNA expression is that the antidiabetic thiazolidinediones, potent PPARγ ligands, are very unlikely to have an important direct transcriptional effect on glucose metabolism in the muscle because there is very little PPARγ expressed there. This implicates that the effect of thiazolidinediones on insulin sensitivity must be due to an indirect effect most likely mediated due to their actions on PPARγ in adipose tissue. The crucial role of adipose tissue in glucose homeostasis was supported by the clinical observation that both lipatrophy [49,50] and obesity are accompanied by insulin resistance [10], which indicates that an approximately "normal" amount of adipose tissue is required for normal insulin sensitivity. The currently favored hypothesis suggests that the beneficial effects of PPARγ on glucose homeostasis are caused by the induction of signalling molecules in adipose tissue, which indirectly would cause an improvement in muscle glucose disposal.

Two groups of mediators generated in adipose tissue might influence glucose metabolism in the muscle. On the one hand, adipocyte-derived protein-based mediators such as tumor necrosis factor α [51,52], plasminogen activator inhibitor-1 [53—55], and leptin [56] interact with insulin signalling pathways and affect muscle glucose disposal. On the other hand, lipid-derived mediators such as free fatty acids (FFAs) are at least equally important determinants of muscle insulin sensitivity [57,58] (reviewed in [25]). Fatty acids are released from adipocytes on activation of hormone sensitive lipase and are also generated during the lipolysis of triglyceride-rich lipoproteins by LPL. The fatty acids are taken up by the cells via a specific fatty acid transporter protein. In the cells fatty acids are converted into metabolic active acyl-CoA derivatives by the action of ACS. Fatty acids are usually equally distributed between adipose tissue and muscle because both tissue express roughly equivalent amounts of the above-mentioned proteins involved in the generation and uptake of fatty acids.

Studies with PPARγ activators suggested that the expression of all of these genes involved in fatty acid metabolism, i.e., LPL, FATP, and ACS are affected

40

in such a way as to improve muscle glucose disposal (Fig. 1). In fact, in adipose
tissue, in 3T3/L1 and Ob1771 adipocyte-like cell lines, activation of PPARγ
induces the above-mentioned genes leading to an enhancement of FFA uptake
into this tissue. Hence treatment with PPARγ activators shifts FFAs into fat cells,
an effect corroborated by the observation that PPARγ agonists induce both adipocyte hypertrophy and hyperplasia and weight gain in rodents [59]. This change
is usually associated with an increased insulin sensitivity of the adipocyte and
will hence also result in a decrease in HSL activity [18]. Since extremely low levels
of PPARγ are expressed in muscle, treatment with a PPARγ agonist does not
affect expression of any of the above-mentioned genes in this tissue. Therefore
FFA uptake is decreased in the muscle in favor of an uptake in the adipocyte.
This decreased availability of FFAs in muscle produced by this adipocyte "FFA
steal" results, via the Randle cycle [57], in an improvement muscle insulin sensitivity.

It is interesting to note that the increase in adipose tissue mass following therapy with PPARγ agonists is not only explained by the selective redistribution of
FFA to this tissue. In fact, food consumption in animals also increases after treatment with the PPARγ agonist, BRL49653 [59]. This effect was caused by a reduction of ob gene expression and leptin production, resulting in enhanced food
consumption [59–61].

A role for PPARα activation in glucose homeostasis?

An additional improvement in insulin sensitivity could perhaps be obtained by
further reducing triglyceride levels (FFA precursors) by treatment with PPARα

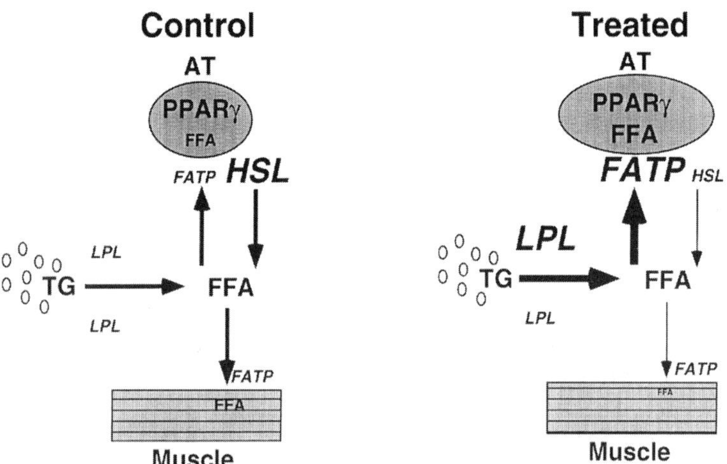

Fig. 1. Scheme representing the effect of treatment with PPARγ activators on key genes involved in
FFA metabolism and FFA partitioning between muscle and adipose tissue. The size of the lettering,
arrows, and symbols corresponds with the relative activity of the various proteins and pathways.

agonists, such as the fibrate hypolipidemic drugs (Fig. 2). In liver and in liver cell lines, activation of PPARα by fibrates enhances fatty acid β-oxidation, decreases apo C-III production, and lowers triglyceride and VLDL secretion, ultimately resulting in a substantial reduction in circulating triglyceride levels [23,24,62]. Such a decrease in triglyceride and FFA supply would, in the same context as discussed above for PPARγ activators, lead to an improvement in glucose homeostasis. Evidence of such a beneficial effect is found in both human and animal studies summarized below [63–65], although not all studies have confirmed this beneficial effect [66,67]. Bezafibrate treatment of rats leads to an improvement in insulin sensitivity [63]. Another fibrate, clofibrate, has also been shown to increase insulin sensitivity in NIDDM subjects independently of insulin-receptor and postreceptor functions [64,65]. Altogether these studies suggest that the combination of a PPARα and a PPARγ agonist might have an additive effect on circulating triglycerides levels, improving insulin sensitivity and glucose homeostasis.

Mechanisms of fatty acid interference with glucose homeostasis

The hypothesis of a redistribution of fatty acid, with a pivotal role for adipose tissue in the control of glucose homeostasis, is in apparent contrast with current opinions concerning insulin-stimulated glucose disposal. Normally, liver and adipose tissue only contribute minimally (< 10%) to glucose disposal, whereas muscle is responsible for most of the glucose uptake. Fatty acid partitioning, linked to the relative expression levels of PPARγ among the different tissues, however, provides an attractive hypothesis to explain the multiple abnormalities seen in

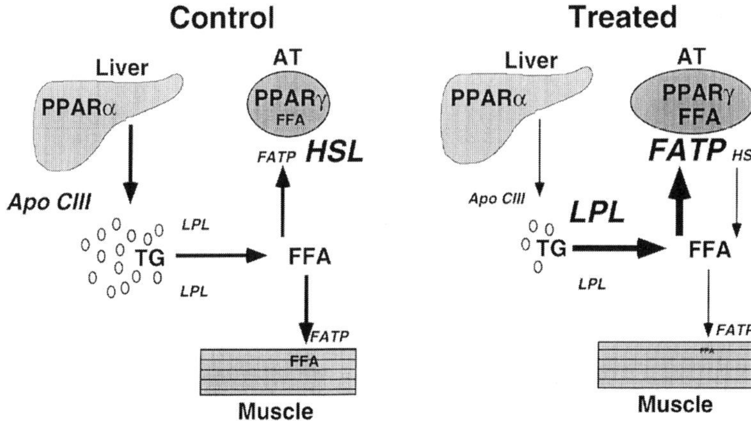

Fig. 2. Scheme representing the effect of combination treatment with PPARγ and PPARα activators on key genes involved in FFA metabolism and FFA partitioning between muscle and adipose tissue. The size of the lettering and arrows corresponds with the relative activity of the various proteins and pathways.

the IR-NIDDM syndrome as well as the beneficial effects of PPAR agonists on this syndrome [68]. This becomes especially evident when one considers the interference between muscle fatty acid and glucose metabolism.

Glucose and long chain fatty acids are known to be competitive substrates in insulin-dependent tissues [57,69]. Free fatty acids greatly interfere with glucose utilization. Lipid infusion was followed by a reversible increase in fat oxidation and decrease in insulin stimulated total body carbohydrate oxidation [70]. This inhibition may be due to different steps in glucose utilization: glucose transport, glucose phosphorylation, glucose oxidation and glycogen synthesis.

The GLUT-4 transporter is mainly expressed in insulin-sensitive tissues and its function depends on insulin which enhances its translocation towards the membrane. Randle showed in the 1960s that increased availability of fatty acid enhanced fat oxidation and decreased carbohydrate oxidation and glucose uptake in perfused rat heart and to a lesser extent in rat diaphragm [57]. He suggested that alteration of rat intramuscular free fatty acid metabolism plays an important role in the pathogenesis of the insulin resistance observed in patients with NIDDM. Although several groups have tried unsuccessfully to reproduce this inhibition of glucose metabolism [71,72], several subsequent studies firmly demonstrated an inhibitory effect of free fatty acids on glucose uptake and metabolism [58,73]. In 1994 Boden et al. demonstrated a dose-dependent negative relationship between plasma free fatty acid concentrations and glucose uptake [58]. Moreover, fat infusion in patients with NIDDM did not affect basal postabsorptive glucose uptake, but selectively inhibited insulin-stimulated glucose uptake [74]. Proportional inhibition of glucose uptake, glycogen synthase, and glycolysis suggested that fat caused a major defect involving glucose transport and or phosphorylation and subsequent metabolism.

Once glucose enters the cell, it is phosphorylated to glucose 6 phosphate (G6P) to avoid accumulation of free glucose, which would inhibit further glucose uptake. Insulin regulates this phosphorylation by controlling hexokinase II activity. Fatty acid utilization consumes NAD and generates NADH. The depletion of NAD, induced by fatty acid utilization, will impair the citric acid or Krebs cycle leading indirectly to an accumulation of citrate which on its turn will inhibit of glucose and fructose phosphorylation.

Once phosphorylated in the cell, glucose can either be converted in glycogen or enter the glycolytic pathway. In fact, Roden et al. [75] explained that free fatty acid concentration causes insulin resistance not only by inhibition of glucose transport or phosphorylation but also through a subsequent reduction in the rates of glucose oxidation and muscle glycogen synthesis. When fatty acid accumulates intracellularly, enhanced β-oxidation leads to an accumulation of acetyl-CoA, a powerful inhibitor of pyruvate dehydrogenase activity [57], resulting in a decrease in glucose oxidation via the Krebs cycle. In the liver, fatty acyl CoA derivatives also directly inhibit glycogen synthase [76,77]. In addition, glycogen synthase activity can also be indirectly inhibited by citrate accumulation. In fact, glycogen synthesis depends not only on the activity of the rate limiting enzyme glycogen synthetase but also on the availability of its main substrate G-6-P/UDP Glucose, which becomes limiting in view of the citrate inhibition of glucose phosphorylation [58].

Free fatty acid has also a positive relationship with insulin level. The ability of the pancreatic β-cell to secrete insulin is absolutely dependent upon the elevated level of circulating FFAs, characteristic of the fasted state. The action of nicotinic acid, a powerful antilipolytic agent, abolishes in fact the glucose-stimulated insulin secretion [78].

Conclusions

PPARs are fine-tuned transcription factors involved in many aspects of metabolic control. PPARα plays a prime role in the control of lipid metabolism in the liver, whereas PPARγ has a pivotal role in the control of glucose homeostasis. The activity of both these transcription factors is strongly influenced by their natural fatty-acid-derived ligands. In addition, these receptors constitute excellent targets for pharmacological intervention since highly selective and potent synthetic ligands (such as the thiazolidinediones and fibrates) can control their activity. In the present manuscript we review the evidence supporting a role for PPARγ and to a lesser extent for PPARα in glucose homeostasis. Activation of these nuclear receptors will selectively induce the expression of several genes involved in fatty acid uptake, such as lipoprotein lipase, fatty acid transport protein and acyl-CoA synthetase, in adipose tissue without changing their expression in muscle tissue. This coordinate regulation of fatty acid partitioning by these two nuclear receptors results in an adipocyte "FFA steal", causing a relative depletion of fatty acids in the muscle. Based on the well-established interference of muscle fatty acid and glucose metabolism it is hypothesized that reversal of muscle fatty acid accumulation will improve whole body glucose homeostasis.

Acknowledgements

We acknowledge discussions with Drs Samir Deeb, Hubert Vidal, Mike Briggs, Rich Heyman, Jim Paterniti, Mark Leibowitz, David Moller, and Didier De Chaffoy. Research in the laboratory of the authors is supported by INSERM, CNRS, Institut Pasteur, Association pour la Recherche contre le Cancer, Fondation pour la Recherche Medicale, and grants from Ligand Pharmaceuticals, Merck Research Laboratories, and the Janssen Research Foundation.

References

1. Barnett AH, Eff C, Leslie RDG, Pyke DA. Diabetes in identical twins: a study of 200 pairs. Diabetologia 1981;20:600—609.
2. Granner DK, O'Brien RM. Molecular physiology and genetics of NIDDM; importance of metabolic staging. Diabet Care 1992;15:369—395.

3. Brunzell JD, Albers JJ, Chait A, Grundy SM, Groszek E, McDonald GB. Plasma lipoproteins in familial combined hyperlipidemia and monogenic familial hypertriglyceridemia. J Lipid Res 1983;24:147—156.

4. Sniderman AD, Wolfson C, Teng B, Franklin F, Bachorik PS, Kwiterovich PO. Association of hyperapobetalipoproteinemia with endogeneous hypertriglyceridemia and atherosclerosis. Ann Int Med 1982;97:833—839.

5. DeFronzo RA, Ferrannini E. Insulin resistance: a multifacetted syndrome responsible for NIDDM, obesity, hypertension, dyslipidemia and atherosclerotic vascular disease. Diabet Care 1991;14:173—194.

6. Cabezas MC, de Bruin TWA, de Valk HW, Shoulders CC, Jansen H, Erkelens DW. Impaired fatty acid metabolism in familial combined hyperlipidemia. A mechanism associating hepatic apolipoprotein B overproduction and insulin resistance. J Clin Invest 1993;92:160—168.

7. Arner P. Is familial combined hyperlipidaemia a genetic disorder of adipose tissue? Curr Opin Lipid 1997;8:89—94.

8. Howard BH, Howard WJ. Dyslipidemia in non-insulin-dependent diabetes mellitus. Endocrine Rev 1994;15:205—216.

9. Flier JS. The adipocyte: storage depot or node on the energy information superhighway. Cell 1995;80:15—18.

10. Spiegelman BM, Flier JS. Adipogenesis and obesity: rounding out the big picture. Cell 1996;87:377—389.

11. Auwerx J, Leroy P, Schoonjans K. Lipoprotein lipase: recent contributions from molecular biology. Crit Rev Clin Lab Sci 1992;29:243—268.

12. Wang C-S, McConathy WJ, Kloer HU, Alaupovic P. Modulation of lipoprotein lipase activity by apolipoproteins. Effect of apolipoprotein C-III. J Clin Invest 1985;75:384—390.

13. Olivecrona G, Olivecrona T. Triglyceride lipases and atherosclerosis. Curr Opin Lipid 1995;6: 291—305.

14. Zechner R. The tissue-specific expression of lipoprotein lipase: implications for energy and lipoprotein metabolism. Curr Opin Lipid 1997;8:77—88.

15. Kamp F, Hamilton JE, Westerhoff HV. Movement of fatty acids, fatty acid analogues, and bile acids accross lipid bilayers. Biochemistry 1993;32:11074—11086.

16. Schaffer JE, Lodish HF. Expression cloning and characterization of a novel long chain fatty acid transport protein. Cell 1994;79:427—436.

17. Suzuki H, Kawarabayasi Y, Kondo J et al. Structure and regulation of rat long-chain acyl-CoA synthetase. J Biol Chem 1990;265:8681—8685.

18. Groop LC, Bonadonna RC, Del Prato S. Glucose and free fatty acid metabolism in non-insulin-dependent diabetes mellitus: evidence for multiple sites of insulin resistance. J Clin Invest 1989;84:205—213.

19. Ginsberg HN, Le N-A, Goldberg IJ et al. Apolipoprotein B metabolism in subjects with deficiency of apolipoproteins CIII and AI: evidence that apolipoprotein CIII inhibits catabolism of triglyceride-rich lipoproteins by lipoprotein lipase in vivo. J Clin Invest 1986;78:1287—1295.

20. Ito Y, Azrolan N, O'Connell A, Walsh A, Breslow JL. Hypertriglyceridemia as a result of human apo CIII gene expression in transgenic mice. Science 1990;249:790—793.

21. de Silva HV, Lauer SJ, Wang J et al. Overexpression of human apolipoprotein C-III in transgenic mice results in an accumulation of apolipoprotein B48 remnants that is corrected by excess apolipoprotein E. J Biol Chem 1994;269:2324—2335.

22. Maeda N, Li H, Lee D, Oliver P, Quarfordt SH, Osada J. Targetted disruption of the apolipoprotein C-III gene in mice results in hypertriglyceridemia and protection from postprandial hypertriglyceridemia. J Biol Chem 1994;269:23610—23616.

23. Schoonjans K, Staels B, Auwerx J. Role of the peroxisome proliferator activated receptor (PPAR) in mediating effects of fibrates and fatty acids on gene expression. J Lipid Res 1996; 37:907—925.

24. Schoonjans K, Staels B, Auwerx J. The peroxisome proliferator activated receptors (PPARs) and

their effects on lipid metabolism and adipocyte differentiation. Biochim Biophys Acta 1996; 1302:93–109.

25. Schoonjans K, Martin G, Staels B, Auwerx J. Peroxisome proliferator-activated receptors, orphans with ligands and functions. Curr Opin Lipid 1997;8:159–166.

26. Osumi T, Wen JK, Hashimoto T. Two cis-acting regulatory elements in the peroxisome proliferator-responsive element enhancer region of rat acyl-CoA oxidase gene. Biochem Biophys Res Commun 1991;175:866–871.

27. Tugwood JD, Isseman I, Anderson RG, Bundell KR, McPheat WL, Green S. The mouse peroxisome proliferator activated receptor recognizes a response element in the 5′ flanking sequence of the rat acyl CoA oxidase gene. EMBO J 1992;11:433–439.

28. Gulick T, Cresci S, Caira T, Moore DD, Kelly DP. The peroxisome proliferator-activated receptor regulates mitochondrial fatty acid oxidative enzyme gene expression. Proc Natl Acad Sci USA 1994;91:11012–11016.

29. Tontonoz P, Hu E, Spiegelman BM. Stimulation of adipogenesis in fibroblasts by PPARγ2, a lipid-activated transcription factor. Cell 1994;79:1147–1156.

30. Tontonoz P, Hu E, Graves RA, Budavari AI, Spiegelman BM. mPPARγ2: tissue-specific regulator of an adipocyte enhancer. Genes Devel 1994;8:1224–1234.

31. Fajas L, Auboeuf D, Raspe E et al. Organization, promoter analysis and expression of the human PPARγ gene. J Biol Chem 1997;272:18779–18789.

32. Braissant O, Foufelle F, Scotto C, Dauca M, Wahli W. Differential expression of peroxisome proliferator-activated receptors: tissue distribution of PPARα, β and γ in the adult rat. Endocrinology 1995;137:354–366.

33. Auboeuf D, Rieusset J, Fajas L et al. Tissue distribution and quantification of the expression of PPARs and LXRa in humans: no alterations in adipose tissue of obese and NIDDM patients. Diabetes 1997;48:1319–1327.

34. Kliewer SA, Umesono K, Noonan DJ, Heyman RA, Evans RM. Convergence of 9-cis retinoic acid and peroxisome proliferator signalling pathways through heterodimer formation of their receptors. Nature 1992;358:771–774.

35. Forman BM, Tontonoz P, Chen J, Brun RP, Spiegelman BM, Evans RM. 15-Deoxy-D12,14 prostaglandin J2 is a ligand for the adipocyte determination factor PPARγ. Cell 1995;83:803–812.

36. Kliewer SA, Lenhard JM, Willson TM, Patel I, Morris DC, Lehman JM. A prostaglandin J2 metabolite binds peroxisome proliferator-activated receptor γ and promotes adipocyte differentiation. Cell 1995;83:813–819.

37. Kliewer SA, Sundseth SS, Jones SA et al. Fatty acids and eicosanoids regulate gene expression through direct interactions with peroxisome proliferator-activated receptors α and γ. Proc Natl Acad Sci USA 1997;94:4318–4323.

38. Forman BM, Chen J, Evans RM. Hypolipidemic drugs, polyunsaturated fatty acids, and eicosanoids are ligands for peroxisome proliferator-activated receptors α and δ. Proc Natl Acad Sci USA 1997;94:4312–4317.

39. Devchand PR, Keller H, Peters JM, Vazquez M, Gonzalez FJ, Wahli W. The PPARα-leukotriene B4 pathway to inflammation control. Nature 1996;384:39–43.

40. Lehmann JM, Moore LB, Smith-Oliver TA, Wilkison WO, Willson TM, Kliewer SA. An antidiabetic thiazolidinedione is a high affinity ligand for Peroxisome Proliferator-Activated Receptor γ. J Biol Chem 1995;270:12953–12956.

41. Zhu Y, Qi C, Korenberg JR et al. Structural organization of mouse peroxisome proliferator activated receptor γ gene: alternative promoter use and different splicing yield two mPPARg isoforms. Proc Natl Acad Sci USA 1995;92:7921–7925.

42. Vidal-Puig A, Jimenez-Linan M, Lowell BB et al. Regulation of PPARgamma gene expression by nutrition and obesity in rodents. J Clin Invest 1996;97:2553–2561.

43. Auwerx J, Martin G, Guerre-Millo M, Staels B. Transcription, adipocyte differentiation, and obesity. J Molec Med 1996;74:347–352.

44. Wu Z, Bucher NLR, Farmer SR. Induction of peroxisome proliferator-activated receptor γ dur-

ing the conversion of 3T3 fibroblasts into adipocytes is mediated by C/EBPγ, C/EBPδ, and glucocorticoids. Molec Cell Biol 1996;16:4128−4136.

45. Wu S, Xie Y, Bucher NLR, Farmer SR. Conditional ectopic expression of C/EBPb in NIH-3T3 cells induces PPARγ and stimulates adipogenesis. Genes Devel 1995;9:2350−2363.

46. Tontonoz P, Kim JB, Graves RA, Spiegelman BM. ADD1: a novel helix-loop-helix transcription factor associated with adipocyte determination and differentiation. Molec Cell Biol 1993;13:4753−4759.

47. Kim JB, Spiegelman BM. ADD1/SREBP1 promotes adipocyte differentiation and gene expression linked to fatty acid metabolism. Genes Devel 1996;10:1096−1107.

48. Brown MS, Goldstein JL. The SREBP pathway: regulation of cholesterol metabolism by proteolysis of a membrane-bound transcription factor. Cell 1997;89:331−340.

49. Moller DE, Flier JS. Insulin resistance-mechanisms, syndromes, and implications. N Engl J Med 1991;325:938−948.

50. Flier JS. Syndromes of insulin resistance and mutant insulin. In: De Groot LJ (ed) Endocrinology, vol 2. Philadelphia: W.B. Saunders, 1995;1592−1604.

51. Hotamisligil GS, Shargill NS, Spiegelman BM. Adipose expression of tumor necrosis factor-α: direct role in obesity-linked insulin resistance. Science 1993;259:87−91.

52. Hotamisligil GS, Peraldi P, Budavari A, Ellis R, White MF, Spiegelman BM. IRS-I-mediated inhibition of insulin receptor tyrosine kinase activity in TNF-α- and obesity induced insulin resistance. Science 1996;271:665−668.

53. Auwerx J, Bouillon R, Collen D, Geboers J. Tissue-type plasminogen activator antigen and plasminogen activator inhibitor in diabetes mellitus. Arteriosclerosis 1988;8:68−72.

54. Shimomura I, Funahashi T, Takahashi M et al. Enhanced expression of PAl-I in visceral fat: possible contributor to vascular disease in obesity. Nature Med 1996;2:800−803.

55. Landin K, Stigendal L, Eriksson E et al. Abdominal obesity is associated with an impaired fibrinolytic activity and elevated plasminogen activator inhibitor-1. Metabolism 1990;39:1044−1048.

56. Cohen B, Novick D, Rubinstein M. Modulation of insulin activities by leptin. Science 1996;274:1185−1188.

57. Randle PJ, Garland PB, Hales CN, Newsholme EA. The glucose-fatty acid cycle; its role in insulin sensitivity and metabolic disturbances of diabetes mellitus. Lancet 1961;I:785−789.

58. Boden G, Chen X, Ruiz J, White JV, Rossetti L. Mechanisms of fatty acid-induced inhibition of glucose uptake. J Clin Invest 1994;93:2438−2446.

59. De Vos P, Lefebvre AM, Miller SG et al. Thiazolidinediones repress ob gene expression via activation of PPARγ. J Clin Invest 1996;98:1004−1009.

60. Zhang B, Graziano MP, Doebber TW et al. Down-regulation of the expression of the *obese* gene by antidiabetic thiazolidinedione in Zucker diabetic fatty rats and *db/db* mice. J Biol Chem 1996;271:9455−9459.

61. Kallen CB, Lazar MA. Antidiabetic thiazolidinediones inhibit leptin (ob) gene expression in 3T3-L1 adipocytes. Proc Natl Acad Sci USA 1996;93:5793−5796.

62. Auwerx J, Schoonjans K, Fruchart JC, Staels B. Transcriptional control of triglyceride metabolism; fibrates change the expression of the LPL and apo C-III genes by activating the nuclear receptor PPAR. Atherosclerosis 1996;124(Suppl):S29−S37.

63. Matsui H, Okumura K, Kawakami K, Hibino M, Toki Y, Ito T. Improved insulin sensitivity by bezafibrate in rats; relationship to fatty acid composition of skeletal muscle triglycerides. Diabetes 1997;46:348−353.

64. Kobayashi J, Shigeta Y, Hirata Y et al. Improvement of glucose tolerance in NIDDM by clofibrate: randomized double-blind study. Diabe Care 1988;11:195−499.

65. Daubresse JC, Daigneux D, Bruwier M, Luyckx A, Lefebvre PJ. Clofibrate and diabetes control in patients treated with oral hypoglycemic agents. Br J Clin Pharmac 1979;7:599−603.

66. Karhapaa P, Uusitupa M, Voutilainen E, Laakso M. Effect of bezafibrate on insulin sensitivity and glucose tolerance in subjects with combined hyperlipidemia. Clin Pharmacol Ther 1992;

52:620—626.
67. Riccardi G, Genovese S, Saldamacchia G et al. Effects of bezafibrate on insulin secretion and peripheral insulin sensitivity in hyperlipidemic patients with and without diabetes. Atherosclerosis 1989;75:175—181.
68. Saltiel AR, Olefsky JM. Thiazolidinediones in the treatment of insulin resistance and type R diabetes. Diabetes 1996;45:1661—1669.
69. Ferrannini E, Barrett EJ, Bevilacqua S, DeFronzo RA. Effect of fatty acids on glucose production and utilization in man. J Clin Invest 1983;72:1737—1747.
70. Boden G, Jadali F, White J et al. Effects of fat on insulin-stimulated carbohydrate metabolism in normal men. J Clin Invest 1991;88:960—966.
71. Bonadonna RC, Zych K, Boni C, Ferrannini E, De Fronzo RA. Time dependence of the interaction between lipid and glucose in humans. Am J Physiol 1989;257:E49—E56.
72. Bevilacqua S, Buzzigoli G, Bonadonna R et al. Operation of Randle's cycle in patients with NIDDM. Diabetes 1990;39:383—389.
73. Felley CP, Felley EM, van Melle GD, Frascarolo P, Jequier E, Felber J-P. Impairment of glucose disposal by infusion of triglycerides in humans: role of glycemia. Am J Physiol 1989;256:E747—E752.
74. Boden G, Chen X. Effects of fat on glucose uptake and utilization in patients with non-insulin-dependent diabetes. J Clin Invest 1995;96:1261—1268.
75. Roden M, Price TB, Perseghin G et al. Mechanism of free fatty acid-induced insulin resistance in humans. J Clin Invest 1996;97:2859—2865.
76. Wititsuwannakul D, Kim K. Mechanism of palmityl coenzyme A inhibition of liver glycogen synthase. J Biol Chem 1977;252:7812—7817.
77. Thiebaud D, DeFronzo RA, Jacot E. Effect of long chain triglyceride infusion on glucose metabolism in man. Metabolism 1982;31:1128—1136.
78. Stein DT, Esser V, Stevenson BE et al. Essentiality of circulating fatty acids for glucose-stimulated insulin secretion in the fasted rat. J Clin Invest 1996;97:2728—2735.

The WHO MONICA project: changes in coronary risk in the 1980s

A. Evans[1], A. Dobson[2], M. Ferrario[3], K. Kuulasmaa[4], V. Moltchanov[4], S. Sans[5], H. Tunstall-Pedoe[6], J. Tuomilehto[4], H. Wedel[7] and J. Yarnell[1] for the WHO MONICA project

[1] *The Queen's University of Belfast, Belfast, UK;* [2] *University of Newcastle, Newcastle, NSW, Australia;* [3] *University of Milan, Milan, Italy;* [4] *National Public Health Institute, Helsinki, Finland;* [5] *Institut d'Estudis de la Salut, Barcelona, Spain;* [6] *University of Dundee, Dundee, UK; and* [7] *Nordic School of Public Health, Sweden*

Abstract. *Background.* The WHO MONICA project is a 10-year study monitoring trends and determinants of cardiovascular disease in geographically defined populations.

Methods and Results. Data were collected from randomly selected participants in two risk factor surveys conducted approximately 5 years apart. The net effects of changes in the risk-factor levels were estimated using risk scores derived from longitudinal studies in the Nordic countries. Prevalence of cigarette smoking decreased among men in most populations, but trends for women varied. Prevalence of hypertension declined in two-thirds of the populations. Changes in prevalence of raised total cholesterol were small. Prevalence of obesity increased in about three-quarters of the populations for both men and women. In almost half the populations there were statistically significant declines in estimated coronary risk for both men and women, although for Beijing the risk score increased significantly for both genders.

Conclusions. The net effect of changes in risk-factor levels in the 1980s in the study populations of the WHO MONICA project is that rates of coronary disease are predicted to decline in the 1990s.

Keywords: coronary heart disease, epidemiology, risk factors.

Introduction

The multifactorial origin of coronary heart disease (CHD) is now well-established. Levels of the major risk factors are changing in many countries [1—4]. Understanding the joint effect of these changes on possible future trends in CHD is vital for combating the disease.

The World Health Organization (WHO) MONICA project was established to MONItor trends and determinants of CArdiovascular disease [5]. Trends in risk-factor levels were measured in independent, periodic community surveys conducted in geographically defined areas starting in the 1980s. The study centres cover many differing populations in Europe as well as a few in North America, Asia and Australasia. The objectives of this paper are to report changes in the

Address for correspondence: Prof Alun Evans, Division of Epidemiology, The Queen's University of Belfast, Mulhouse Building, Grosvenor Road, Belfast BT12 6BJ, Northern Ireland. Tel.: +44-1232-240503 (Ext. 2717). Fax: +44-1232-236298. E-mail: belfastmon@qub.ac.uk

major risk factors which occurred during the 1980s and to estimate the changes in overall risk for coronary events.

Methods

Risk-factor surveys

The study populations of the WHO MONICA project are residents of well-defined geopolitical areas [6]. In each population, smoking habits, blood pressure, serum total cholesterol, weight and height were measured using standardised methods in independent, random samples in the early and late 1980s [7]. Surveys in the same populations were conducted at the same time of year to avoid seasonal variation. Details of the survey periods, sampling schemes and response rates have been given elsewhere [8].

The age of a subject at the last birthday on or before participation in the survey was classified by 10-year age group; data for the age groups 35—64 years are considered in this paper. Information on smoking was obtained by self-completed questionnaires or by interview. A current cigarette smoker was defined as a person who reported smoking cigarettes regularly at the time of the survey [8]. Blood pressure was measured on the right arm, with the subject in the sitting position after at least 5 min rest. Two consecutive measurements were taken, to the nearest 2 mmHg, and the mean value was used in the present analysis [9]. A person was defined as hypertensive if he or she had systolic blood pressure greater than or equal to 160 mmHg and/or diastolic blood pressure greater than or equal to 95 mmHg and/or was known to be on antihypertensives. A venous blood sample was drawn from the antecubital vein with the subject in the sitting position and with minimal use of a tourniquet [10]. Fasting was not required. Raised cholesterol was defined as greater than or equal to 6.5 mmol/l. Height and weight were measured in light clothing without shoes and outer garments. Body mass index (BMI) was calculated as the weight (kg) divided by the square of height (m). Obesity was defined as BMI greater than or equal to 30 kg/m^2 in both genders.

Results for study populations are included in the analyses reported here if data for all four major risk factors at both surveys met the quality control requirements of the WHO MONICA project.

Risk scores

In order to estimate the combined effects of these four major risk factors, prediction equations were obtained from the NOrdic Risk Assessment (NORA) study using pooled data from longitudinal studies in the Nordic countries with CHD death as an outcome variable (unpublished data from H. Wedel).

The NORA study involves data for over 100,000 men and women, and more than 1,500 deaths from CHD. For each survey participant a risk score was calcu-

lated using smoking status (SMOKE 1 for a current regular smoker or 0 otherwise), systolic blood pressure (SBP mmHg), total blood cholesterol (CHOL mmol/l) and BMI (kg/m^2). The equations are:
1) For men, $0.818 \times$ SMOKE $+ 0.015 \times$ SBP $+ 0.286 \times$ CHOL $+ 0.049 \times$ BMI.
2) For women, $1.000 \times$ SMOKE $+ 0.021 \times$ SBP $+ 0.225 \times$ CHOL $+ 0.002 \times$ BMI.

Estimation of trends

Trends over time in levels of each risk factor and in risk scores were estimated by fitting simple linear-regression models calculated separately for each sex and 10-year age group within each population. The response variable was the measurement for each subject (in either survey) and the explanatory variable was the calender year of measurement. The average change over 5 years was estimated by 5 times the regression slope coefficient.

Age-standardized mean levels and changes in risk factors were calculated from the age-specific estimates by direct standardization using the world standard population weights of 12/31, 11/31 and 8/31 for the 10-year age groups 35—44, 45—54 and 55—64 years, respectively.

Associations between changes in risk-factor levels or risk scores among men and women in the same population were assessed using Pearson correlation coefficients.

Results

Risk factor changes

The age-standardized 5-year changes in prevalence for each of the major risk factors are shown in Table 1. The prevalence of cigarette smoking among men decreased in most populations but in Beijing it increased significantly. Among women, there were decreases in prevalence of cigarette smoking in some populations and increases in others. The decreases among men and women were greatest in Stanford. The prevalence of hypertension declined in about two-thirds of the populations for both men and women. The prevalence of raised total blood cholesterol varied less than for the other risk factors. Prevalence of obesity increased in almost three-quarters of the populations for men and women.

The changes in risk scores are shown in Table 2. For almost half of the populations there were statistically significant declines in estimated risk for both men and women. For Beijing the risk score increased significantly for both sexes. The decreases in systolic blood pressure contributed consistently to the decrease in estimated overall risk. For men, the decrease in smoking was also important, increases in cholesterol contributed to increased risk while BMI had little effect. For women, cigarette smoking and cholesterol contributed toward increases in estimated risk in some populations and decreases in others while changes in BMI made no important contribution. In several populations decreases in two

52

Table 1. Changes in prevalence of major risk factors: age-standardised average 5 year absolute changes (ages 35–64 years).

Population	Men				Women			
	Cigarette smoking[a]	Hypertension[b]	Cholesterol ≥ 6.5 mmol/l[c]	BMI ≥ 30[d]	Cigarette smoking[a]	Hypertension[b]	Cholesterol ≥ 6.5 mmol/l[c]	BMI ≥ 30[d]
Australia - Newcastle	− −	−	−	++	− −	−	−	++
Australia - Perth	− −	−	+	++	+	− −	+	+
China - Beijing	++	+	+	+	−	+	++	−
Denmark - Glostrup	−	−	++	−	−	−	++	−
Finland - Kuopio Province	−	−	+	−	+	− −	−	++
Finland - North Karelia	−	+	−	++	++	−	− −	+
Finland - Turku/ Loimaa	−	−	+	+	−	+	−	++
Germany - Augsburg (rural)	−	++	+	+	+	−	+	+
Germany - Augsburg (urban)	−	−	+	−	++	−	+	+
Germany - Berlin - Lichtenberg	−	−	−	*	*	−	−	−
Iceland	−	+	++	+	−	− −	−	+
Italy - Area Brianza	−	−	−	+	−	+	+	+
Italy - Friuli	−	+	− −	+	−	−	− −	−
Lithuania - Kaunas	−	+	+	+	+	−	++	−
Poland - Warsaw	−	− −	+	+	++	−	++	+
Spain - Catalonia	−	*	− −	++	++	+	− −	++
Switzerland - Vaud/ Fribourg	+	−	+	−	+	+	+	−
UK - Belfast	+	−	++	+	− −	−	++	+
UK - Glasgow	− −	− −	− −	++	− −	− −	− −	++
USA - Stanford	− −	−	− −	++	− −	+	+	+

++ indicates an increase with statistical significance level $p < 0.05$; + indicates an increase with $p > 0.05$; * indicates no change; − indicates a decrease with $p > 0.05$; − − indicates a decrease with $p < 0.05$. [a]Prevalence of regular smoking of cigarettes; [b]prevalence of hypertension; [c]prevalence of hypercholesterolaemia: total; [d]prevalence of obesity: body mass index 30 kg/m^2.

or three of the risk factors contributed to the overall decline in estimated risk. In contrast, in Beijing all four risk factors contributed to increased estimated risk.

Discussion

In most of the study populations the prevalence of cigarette smoking and hypertension clearly decreased during the 1980s. Changes in cholesterol were smaller and less consistent. The prevalence of obesity increased, especially among men.

Table 2. Age-standardized 5-year changes in coronary risk score (age 35—64).

| | Change (95% CI) | |
Population	Men	Women
ITA—FRI	−0.21 (−0.33, −0.10)	−0.21 (−0.31, −0.10)
GER—BER	−0.14 (−0.25, −0.04)	−0.14 (−0.24, −0.04)
POL—WAR	−0.14 (−0.21, −0.07)	−0.04 (−0.11, 0.04)
UNK—GLA	−0.14 (−0.20, −0.07)	−0.20 (−0.27, −0.12)
ITA—BRI	−0.13 (−0.24, −0.03)	−0.05 (−0.14, 0.04)
USA—STA	−0.13 (−0.20, −0.06)	−0.17 (−0.23, −0.11)
AUS—PER	−0.09 (−0.16, −0.02)	−0.09 (−0.16, −0.02)
FIN—KUO	−0.09 (−0.16, −0.02)	−0.11 (−0.17, −0.05)
SPA—CAT	−0.07 (−0.12, −0.01)	−0.06 (−0.11, −0.00)
FIN—TUL	−0.05 (−0.11, 0.01)	−0.05 (−0.11, 0.01)
AUS—NEW	−0.04 (−0.09, 0.01)	−0.07 (−0.12, −0.02)
DEN—GLO	−0.04 (−0.12, 0.05)	−0.09 (−0.18, −0.01)
FIN—NKA	−0.04 (−0.09, 0.02)	−0.06 (−0.11, −0.02)
GER—AUU	−0.03 (−0.10, 0.04)	0.08 (0.01, 0.14)
LTU—KAU	−0.01 (−0.10, 0.07)	−0.01 (−0.08, 0.07)
GER—AUR	0.00 (−0.06, 0.07)	−0.00 (−0.06, 0.05)
UNK—BEL	0.02 (−0.08, 0.12)	−0.10 (−0.20, 0.00)
SWI—VAF	0.03 (−0.06, 0.12)	−0.07 (−0.02, 0.16)
ICE—ICE	0.05 (−0.00, 0.11)	−0.03 (−0.09, 0.02)
CHN—BEI	0.26 (0.18, 0.35)	0.13 (0.06, 0.21)

The net effects appear to be declines in overall estimated risk of CHD in most but not all of the populations, with Beijing being an obvious exception.

The net reductions in estimated risk were mainly due to reductions in prevalence of cigarette smoking and blood-pressure levels.

The increase in prevalence of obesity, especially among men is of public health concern. Overweight is associated with increased levels of blood pressure and cholesterol and incidence of diabetes which, in turn, lead to increased risk of CHD [11]. The long-term effects of increasing BMI could negate some of the gains from reductions in other risk factors.

In the WHO MONICA project, changes in rates of CHD events during the same study period are currently being analysed. The original design of the WHO MONICA project anticipated that a minimum 10-year period is needed to test the hypothesis relating trends in CHD risk factors and event rates. The present findings show that it is possible to monitor cardiovascular risk factors in populations in a standardized way over time in numerous different settings. The trends in risk factors are important for evaluating preventive activities in addition to predicting future patterns of CHD and other noncommunicable diseases.

Acknowledgements

MONICA Centres are funded predominantly by regional and national governments, research councils and research charities. The study is coordinated by the World Health Organization (WHO). The MONICA Data Centre (MDC) in Helsinki is supported by the National Public Health Institute of Finland and a contribution to WHO from the National Heart, Lung and Blood Institute, National Institute of Health, Bethesda, Maryland, USA. Grants from ASTRA Hässle AB, Sweden; Hoechst AG, Germany; Hoffmann-La Roche AG, Switzerland; and the Institut de Recherches Internationales Servier, France, help to support data analysis and preparation of publications.

References

1. Beaglehole R. International trends in coronary heart disease mortality, morbidity and risk factors. Epidemiol Rev 1990;12:1–15.
2. McGovern PG et al. for the Minnesota Heart Survey Investigators. Recent trends in acute coronary heart disease: mortality, morbidity, medical care, and risk factors. N Engl J Med 1996; 334:884–890.
3. Sigfusson N et al. Decline in ischaemic heart disease in Iceland and change in risk factor levels. Br Med J 1991;302:1371–1375.
4. Vartiainen E et al. Twenty-year trends in coronary risk factors in North Karelia and in other areas of Finland. Int J Epidemiol 1994;23:495–504.
5. Tunstall-Pedoe H et al. for the WHO MONICA project. The World Health Organization MONICA project (MONItoring trends and determinants in CArdiovascular disease): a major international collaboration. J Clin Epidemiol 1988;41:105–113.
6. Tunstall-Pedoe H et al. for the WHO MONICA project. Myocardial infarction and coronary deaths in the World Health Organization MONICA project: registration procedures, event rates, and case-fatality rates in 38 populations from 21 countries in four continents. Circulation 1994;90:583–612.
7. Keil U, Kuulasmaa K for the WHO MONICA project. WHO MONICA project: risk factors. Int J Epidemiol 1989;18(Suppl 1):546–555.
8. Dobson A et al. for the WHO MONICA project. Changes in cigarette smoking among adults in 35 populations in the mid 1980s (Submitted).
9. Hense H-W et al., for the WHO MONICA project. Assessment of blood pressure measurement quality in the baseline surveys of the WHO MONICA project. J Hum Hypertens 1995;9: 935–949.
10. Döring A et al. for the WHO MONICA project. Method of total cholesterol measurement in the baseline survey of the WHO MONICA project. Rev Epidem et Sante Publ 1990;38:455–461.
11. Pi-Sunyer FX. Health implications of obesity. Am J Clin Nutr 1991;53(Suppl):51595–51603.

Appendix

Key personnel: sites, principal investigators (PI) and key personnel of contributing MONICA centres.
Australia: University of Western Australia, Perth; M.S.T. Hobbs (PI), K. Jamrozik (PI), P.L. Thompson; and University of Newcastle; A. Dobson (PI), H. Alexander, R. Heller.
China: Beijing Heart, Lung and Blood Vessel Research Institute, Beijing; Wu Zhaosu (PI), Yao Chonghua, Zhang Ruisong.
Denmark: Centre of Preventive Medicine (The Glostrup Population Studies), Copenhagen University; M. Schroll (PI), M. Kirchhoff, A. Sjøl, S. Quitsau-Lund.
Finland: National Public Health Institute, Helsinki; J. Tuomilehto (PI), H. Korhonen, M. Jauhiainen, A. Nissinen, E. Vartiainen, P. Pietinen.

Germany: GSF-Institute of Epidemiology, Neuherberg/Munich; U. Keil (PI), J. Stieber, A. Döring, B. Filipiak, U. Härtel, H.W. Hense; and Centre for Epidemiology & Health Research, Berlin (from October 1990, previously German Democratic Republic); W. Barth (PI), L. Heinemann (PI), A. Assmann, S. Böthig, G. Voigt, S. Brasche, D. Quietsch, E. Classen.

Iceland: Heart Preventive Clinic, Reykjavik; N. Sigfússon (PI), I.I. Gudmundsdóttir, I. Stefánsdóttir, Th. Thorsteinsson, H. Sigvaldason.

Italy: Institute of Cardiology, Regional Hospital, Udine; G.A. Feruglio (PI), D. Vanuzzo, M. Palmieri, M. Spanghero, M. Scarpa, L. Pilotto, G. Cignacco, R. Marini, G. Zilio; and University of Milan, Research Center for Chronic Degenerative Diseases, Monza; G.C. Cesana (PI), M. Ferrario (PI), R. Sega, P. Mocarelli, G. DeVito, F. Valagussa.

Lithuania: Kaunas Medical Academy Institute of Cardiology; J. Bluzhas (PI), S. Domarkiene, A. Tamosiunas, R. Reklaitiene.

Poland: National Institute of Cardiology, Warsaw, Department of Cardiovascular Epidemiology and Prevention; S.L. Rywik (PI), G. Broda, M. Polakowska, P. Kurjata.

Spain: Institute of Health Studies, Department of Health and Social Security, Barcelona; S. Sans (PI), I. Balaguer-Vintro (PI), Ll. Balanà, G. Paluzie, T. Puig.

Switzerland: University Institute of Social and Preventive Medicine, Lausanne; F. Gutzwiller (PI), M. Rickenbach, V. Wietlisbach, F. Barazzoni, F. Mainieri, B. Tullen.

UK: The Queen's University of Belfast, Northern Ireland; A. Evans (PI), E. McCrum, T. Falconer, S. Cashman, C. Patterson, M. Kerr, D. O'Reilly, A. Scott, M. McConville, I. McMillan; and University of Dundee, Scotland; H. Tunstall-Pedoe (PI), C. Morrison (PI), R. Tavendale, K. Barrett, C. Brown, M. Shewry. Former key personnel: W.C.S. Smith, I. Crombie, M. Kenicer.

USA: Stanford Center for Research in Disease Prevention, California; S.P. Fortmann (PI), A. Varady, M. Hull.

MONICA Management Centre: World Health Organization, Geneva. Responsible officer: I. Martin. Former responsible officers: I. Gyarfas, Z. Pisa, S.R.A. Dodu, S. Böthig. Key personnel: M.J. Watson, M. Hill.

MONICA Data Centre: National Public Health Institute, Helsinki, Finland. Responsible officer: K. Kuulasmaa. Former responsible officer: J. Tuomilehto. Key personnel: V. Moltchanov, A. Molarius, E. Ruokokoski.

MONICA Steering Committee: M. Hobbs (Chair), M. Ferrario (Publications Coordinator), A. Evans, H. Tunstall-Pedoe (Rapporteur), I. Martin, K. Kuulasmaa, A. Shatchkute (WHO, Copenhagen). Consultant: A. Dobson. Previous Steering Committee Members: S. Sans, F. Gutzwiller, S.P. Fortmann, A. Menotti, P. Puska, S.L. Rywik, U. Keil, R. Beaglehole, and former chiefs of CVD/HQ, Geneva (listed above), V. Zaitsev, J. Tuomilehto, I Gyarfas. Former Consultants: Z. Pisa, O.D. Williams, M.J. Karvonen, R.J. Prineas, M. Feinleib, F.H. Epstein.

Recent progress in the epidemiology of haemostatic factors

Gordon D.O. Lowe
University Department of Medicine, Royal Infirmary, Glasgow, UK

Abstract. Plasma fibrinogen is consistently associated with both incident and prevalent cardiovascular disease (CVD): there is a 2-fold increased risk in the highest third of the population. Standardisation of methods is progressing. While proof as a causal risk factor awaits the results of large trials of fibrates which lower fibrinogen by about 20%, causality is suggested by a consistent, dose-dependent association with CVD, associations of the "high-fibrinogen" BclI genotype with CVD and plausible mechanisms for promoting ischaemia (including atherogenesis, thrombogenesis and increased blood viscosity). Other variables increasing viscosity include haematocrit, white cell count, and lipoproteins: reductions in lipoproteins (but not fibrinogen) by pravastatin significantly reduced viscosity in the West of Scotland Coronary Prevention Study.

Other coagulation factors (VII, VIII, IX) increase with conventional risk factors, but so do coagulation inhibitors (antithrombin, proteins C and S) and hence coagulation balance (plasma activation markers) is little changed. Increased plasminogen activator inhibitor (PAI) and tissue plasminogen activator (tPA) antigen are associated with triglyceride and insulin: the latter may also reflect endothelial disturbance, as does von Willebrand factor (vWF). These variables are associated with incident and prevalent CVD (as is fibrin D-dimer, a marker of fibrin turnover) and merit assessment for both risk stratification and antithrombotic prophylaxis.

Keywords: coagulation, fibrinogen, fibrinolysis, viscosity.

Introduction

In recent years evidence has accumulated that thrombosis plays an important role in common cardiovascular diseases such as ischaemic heart disease (IHD), stroke and peripheral arterial disease. Thrombosis plays an important role in atherogenesis and also precipitates clinical episodes of ischaemia and infarction following rupture of an atherosclerotic plaque. Thromboembolism from the heart (e.g., due to atrial fibrillation) remains an important cause of stroke.

Thrombosis has been called "haemostasis in the wrong place" [1]. Following traumatic rupture of blood vessels, activation of the haemostatic system results in a platelet-fibrin plug, which is subsequently lysed by the fibrinolytic system in parallel with tissue repair processes. Following rupture of an atherosclerotic plaque, a similar local activation of the haemostatic system results in a platelet-fibrin thrombus, which may either develop into an occlusive thrombus, embolise to cause distal occlusion, be incorporated into the plaque causing increased ste-

---

Address for correspondence: Prof G.D.O. Lowe, University Department of Medicine, Royal Infirmary, 10 Alexandra Parade, Glasgow G31 2ER, UK.

nosis, or be entirely cleared by thrombolysis and/or microembolisation. The importance of the platelet, coagulation and fibrinolytic systems in acute IHD has been clearly demonstrated by the efficacy of antiplatelet, anticoagulant and thrombolytic drugs [2].

It seems reasonable to hypothesise that blood levels of haemostatic factors may be related to cardiovascular risk and to prevalent cardiovascular (or arterial) disease, and that these factors may be mechanisms through which conventional risk factors might promote ischaemic events. The present review briefly summarises recent progress in testing these hypotheses through epidemiological studies, but more detailed reviews have been published recently [3–6].

Fibrinogen

Of all haemostatic variables, plasma fibrinogen is the best established predictor of IHD, stroke and peripheral arterial disease. At least 10 prospective studies of cohorts who were mostly free of clinically detectable cardiovascular disease have shown consistently that risk increases with increasing fibrinogen level. A meta-analyses of the first seven reported studies (Gothenburg, Leigh, Northwick Park (London), Framingham, Caerphilly-Speedwell, Münster (PROCAM) and Göttingen (GRIPS)) showed a relative risk of 2.45 (95% CI 2.05–2.93) in the highest third of the population [7]. We have recently confirmed these results in three large Scottish prospective studies: the Edinburgh Artery Study [8], Scottish Heart Health Study [9] and West of Scotland Coronary Prevention Study (WOSCOPS) [10].

The Scottish Heart Health Study [9] is worth emphasising. It was a large, random sample of both men and women from the middle-aged Scottish population. Fibrinogen was associated with a similar relative risk of incident IHD in men and in women, and in those with baseline evidence of IHD and in those without. The strength of association was similar to that of the three major conventional risk factors (smoking, blood pressure and cholesterol), and fibrinogen added to risk prediction with any combination of these three conventional factors. Fibrinogen was also a strong predictor of both cardiovascular and total mortality. These results support the case for adding fibrinogen to the IHD risk profile, as recently suggested for the American Heart Association profile, based on the Framingham data [11].

However, before fibrinogen is adopted in clinical practice as a risk predictor, two practical problems have to be addressed: biological variability and laboratory standardisation. Fibrinogen varies with time in individuals, for example, due to "acute phase" reactions to various stresses (physical, mental, infections) and to seasonal variation [4]. This biological variability appears intermediate between that of cholesterol and that of triglyceride. As with other risk predictors (blood pressure, cholesterol) up to three measurements may be required to identify "hyperfibrinogenaemia" for risk stratification.

Interlaboratory variation depends partly on methodology (assays of "total" fibrinogen, e.g., by precipitation or immunological nephelometry, give higher readings than assays of "clottable" fibrinogen) and partly on the historical lack of international standards. An international standard for clottable fibrinogen was introduced in 1992 [12]. Only one prospective study (Caerphilly-Speedwell) has prospectively compared two types of fibrinogen assay: heat-precipitation nephelometry showed a significantly higher predictive value than the von Clauss assay of clottable fibrinogen (Sweetnam et al., submitted). Further collaborative studies are required to define the optimum assay for risk prediction and the relative risks associated with standardised unit increase in plasma fibrinogen.

Evidence for a pathological role for fibrinogen in cardiovascular disease consists not only of these consistent associations with incident disease (in different cohorts of varying age, country and assay methods), but also of:
— its consistent relationships to prevalent clinical IHD, stroke, peripheral arterial disease; and to the extent of coronary, cerebral and peripheral arterial disease [4];
— the associations of high-fibrinogen genotypes (e.g., Bcl1) with peripheral and coronary arterial disease [4], which suggest that fibrinogen elevation may precede disease;
— the associations of fibrinogen with many risk factors, both positive (Caucasian race, age, winter season, smoking, infections, diabetes, obesity, lack of exercise, oral contraceptives, menopause, trauma and surgery), and inverse (alcohol, hormone replacement therapy) [4]; and
— the benefits of fibrinogen reduction in controlled trials: of thrombolysis in acute IHD [2]; of defibrination with ancrod in acute stroke [4]; of bezafibrate (which lowers fibrinogen by about 20%) after premature myocardial infarction [4].

Larger, ongoing trials of ancrod in acute stroke and of fibrates in secondary prevention of IHD, should provide further evidence as to whether or not fibrinogen is a causal risk factor.

Four plausible mechanisms through which increasing fibrinogen may promote ischaemic events have been suggested [3—5]:
1) arterial wall infiltration and atherogenesis;
2) increased platelet aggregation (fibrinogen is a key ligand in platelet aggregation);
3) increased fibrin thrombus formation and persistence (due to formation of dense fibrin strands which reduces thrombus deformability and lysability); and
4) increased blood viscosity (due to increased plasma viscosity and increased red cell aggregation), which may have atherogenic and thrombogenic effects and which may reduce blood flow distal to atherothrombotic stenoses. About 50% of the predictive value of fibrinogen for IHD events in the Caerphilly-Speedwell study could be attributed to its effects on plasma viscosity, and vice versa [13].

Blood viscosity

The possibility that increasing fibrinogen levels might promote ischaemic events partly through increasing plasma and blood viscosity is consistent with the predictive value of viscosity for IHD and stroke in three prospective studies [8,10,13]. Lipoproteins (as well as fibrinogen) increase plasma and blood viscosity. In the West of Scotland Coronary Prevention Study, we observed that pravastatin significantly lowered plasma and blood viscosity [10]. This appeared due to reductions in plasma LDL and VLDL, because pravastatin had no significant effect on fibrinogen levels. We have suggested that this early reduction in viscosity may be one mechanism for the early reduction in risk of IHD by statins in clinical trials, which cannot be explained by regression of atherosclerosis [10].

Blood viscosity is influenced by haematocrit as well as plasma viscosity. Haematocrit is a risk predictor for IHD and stroke, partly due to its effects on blood viscosity [8,10]. The blood white cell count is also a risk predictor for IHD and stroke [10,14] which may again be a rheological effect: increased numbers of leucocytes rarely increase bulk blood viscosity, but markedly reduce the filterability of blood through microvessels, which may potentially affect microcirculatory flow in ischaemic organs.

Other coagulation factors

Factor VII

Factor VII plays a key role in activation of the extrinsic pathway of coagulation, interacting with tissue factor. Plasma factor VII activity levels were associated with incident IHD in the Northwick Park Study [15] and PROCAM Study [16], although this association appeared confined to fatal events [15] and may be partly due to its strong association with triglyceride levels [16]. No association was apparent in the Caerphilly Study [17] or Edinburgh Artery Study [18]. The potential risk factor role of factor VII will be illuminated by the results of ongoing studies of primary IHD prevention by low-dose warfarin, which lowers high factor VII levels.

Factor VIII/von Willebrand factor

Coagulation factor VIII circulates bound to von Willebrand factor (vWF), which is released from endothelial cells and which plays an important role in platelet adhesion and aggregation. Both factor VIII and vWF were associated with incident IHD in both the Northwick Park Study [19] and Caerphilly Study [17].

Coagulation inhibitors and activation markers

Increases in coagulation factors VII, VIII and IX within the general population are associated with increased thrombin generation, as measured by plasma levels of the coagulation activation markers, prothrombin fragment F1+2 and thrombin-antithrombin complexes [20]. Conversely, increases in the coagulation inhibitors, antithrombin, protein C and protein S are associated with decreased levels of these activation markers [20]. Most conventional cardiovascular risk factors are associated with increases in both coagulation factors and inhibitors, resulting in no overall increase in coagulation activation [21], although a trend is observed in older men [19]. These associations may explain why neither of these two coagulation activation markers was associated with incident IHD in the Caerphilly Study [17].

Fibrinolytic factors

Increased plasma levels of both tissue plasminogen activator (tPA) antigen, and its major inhibitor, plasminogen activator inhibitor type I (PAI-1) are associated with incident IHD and stroke, probably reflecting tPA-PAI-1 complexes [5,6]. As with factor VII, these relationships are partly explained by their strong associations with triglyceride levels [5,6]. Furthermore, tPA antigen may (like vWF antigen) be a marker of endothelial disturbance [5, 6]. The potential risk factor role of PAI-1 may be illuminated by future studies of specific inhibitors [7].

Increased plasma levels of fibrin D-dimer, a marker of increased fibrin turnover (formation, followed by plasmin-mediated fibrinolysis) have also been associated with incident IHD and stroke [5,17,18,22]. This is not due to associations with fibrinogen, tPA or PAI-1 [22]. Increased plasma levels also occur in patients with atrial fibrillation, and may be relevant to the increased risk of stroke in this disorder [23]. These increased levels may be normalised by either cardioversion or full-dose warfarin [23]. We have suggested that D-dimer levels merit evaluation both in identifying persons at high risk of fibrin-rich thrombosis who may benefit from prophylactic anticoagulation, and also in monitoring the antithrombin effects of anticoagulants [23].

References

1. Macfarlane RG. Introduction. Br Med Bull 1977;33:183—185.
2. Collins R, Peto R, Baigent C, Sleight P. Aspirin, heparin and fibrinolytic therapy in suspected acute myocardial infarction. N Engl J Med 1997;336:847—860.
3. Meade TW. Haemostatic function and arterial disease. Br Med Bull 1994;50:755—775.
4. Lowe GDO, Fowkes FGR, Koenig W, Mannucci PM (eds). Fibrinogen and cardiovascular disease. Eur Heart J 1995;16(Suppl A):1—63.
5. Lowe GDO. Haemostatic risk factors for arterial and venous thrombosis. In: Poller L, Ludlam CA (eds) Recent Advances in Blood Coagulation 7. Edinburgh: Churchill Livingstone, 1997; 69—96.
6. Juhan-Vague I, Alessi MC. PAI-1, obesity, insulin resistance and risk of cardiovascular events. Thromb Haemost 1997;78:656—660.
7. Resch KL, Ernst E. The complex impact of fibrinogen on atherosclerosis-related disease. In: Koenig W, Hombach V, Bond MG, Kramsch DM (eds) Progression and Regression of Athero-

sclerosis. Vienna: Blackwell MZV, 1995;36–40.

8. Lowe GDO, Lee AJ, Rumley A, Price JF, Fowkes FGR. Blood viscosity and risk of cardiovascular events: the Edinburgh Artery Study. Br J Haematol 1997;96:168–173.

9. Woodward M, Lowe GDO, Rumley A, Tunstall-Pedoe H. Fibrinogen as a risk factor for coronary heart disease and mortality in middle-aged men and women — The Scottish Heart Health Study. Eur Heart J 1997;(In press).

10. Rumley A, Lowe GDO, Norrie J, Ford I, Shepherd J, Cobbe SM, for the West of Scotland Coronary Prevention Study Group. Blood rheology and outcome in the West of Scotland Coronary Prevention Study: is the benefit of lipoprotein reduction partly due to lower viscosity? Br J Haematol 1997;97(Suppl 1):78.

11. Kannel WB. Influence of fibrinogen on cardiovascular disease. Drugs 1997;54(Suppl 3):32–40.

12. Gaffney PJ, Wong MT. Collaborative study of a proposed international standard for plasma fibrinogen measurement. Thromb Haemost 1992;68:428–432.

13. Sweetnam PM, Thomas HF, Yarnell JWG et al. Fibrinogen, viscosity and the 10-year incidence of ischaemic heart disease. The Caerphilly and Speedwell Studies. Eur Heart J 1996;17: 1814–1820.

14. Yarnell JWG, Baker IA, Sweetnam PM et al. Fibrinogen, viscosity and white blood cell count are major risk factors for ischaemic heart disease. The Caerphilly and Speedwell Studies. Circulation 1991;83:836–844.

15. Ruddock V, Meade TW. Factor VII activity and ischaemic heart disease: fatal and nonfatal events. Quart J Med 1994;87:403–406.

16. Junker R, Heinrich J, Schulte H, van de Loo J, Assmann G. Coagulation factor VII and the risk of coronary heart disease in healthy men. Arterioscl Thromb Vasc Biol 1997;17:1539–1544.

17. Lowe GDO, Rumley A, Sweetnam PM, Yarnell JWG, Thomas HF, Ford RP. Coagulation factors, activation markers and risk of ischaemic heart disease in the Caerphilly Study. Br J Haematol 1997;97(Suppl 1):49.

18. Smith FB, Lee AJ, Fowkes FGR, Price JF, Rumley A, Lowe GDO. Haemostatic factors as predictors of ischaemic heart disease and stroke in the Edinburgh Artery Study. Arterioscl Thromb Vasc Biol 1997;(In press).

19. Meade TW, Cooper J, Stirling Y et al. Factor VIII, ABO blood group and the incidence of ischaemic heart disease. Br J Haematol 1994;88:601–607.

20. Lowe GDO, Rumley A, Woodward M et al. Epidemiology of coagulation factors, inhibitors and activation markers: the Third Glasgow MONICA Survey. I. Illustrative reference ranges by age, sex and hormone use. Br J Haematol 1997;97:775–784.

21. Woodward M, Lowe GDO, Rumley A et al. Epidemiology of coagulation factors, inhibitors and activation markers: the Third Glasgow MONICA Survey. II. Relationships to cardiovascular risk factors and prevalent cardiovascular disease. Br J Haematol 1997;97:785–797.

22. Lowe GDO, Yarnell JWG, Sweetnam PM, Rumley A, Thomas HF, Elwood PC. Fibrin D-dimer, tissue plasminogen activator, plasminogen activator inhibitor, and the risk of major ischaemic heart disease in the Caerphilly Study. Thromb Haemost 1997;(In press).

23. Lip GYH, Lowe GDO. Fibrin D-dimer: a useful clinical marker of thrombogenesis? Clin Sci 1995;89:205–214.

63

The pleiotropic effects of drugs affecting lipid metabolism

Jean Davignon
Hyperlipidemia and Atherosclerosis Research Group, Clinical Research Institute of Montreal; and Department of Medicine, University of Montreal, Montreal, Quebec, Canada

Abstract. A drug impacting on different systems or metabolic processes is said to have pleiotropic effects. Whether discovered a posteriori or obtained by design, these properties may enhance the cardiovascular benefit of a lipid-lowering agent, lead to new indications or be at the origin of a new class of drugs. The lipid-lowering effect of niacin is an example of a new indication derived from the pleiotropic effect of a vitamin given at high doses. The antioxidant properties of probucol, its ability to improve endothelial dysfunction or increase CETP mass and activity were found a posteriori and contributed to the design of new antiatherogenic drugs. Fibrates have ubiquitous effects on lipoprotein metabolism, many of which are mediated via the PPAR system. They lower fibrinogen, blood viscosity and PAI-1; these and many other pleiotropic effects were not anticipated when their prototype clofibrate was developed. Similarly, statins have a plethora of pleiotropic effects including class effects such as improvement of endothelial dysfunction. They also have effects that are not necessarily shared by all members of the class on heart transplant rejection, oxidative processes, ex vivo platelet aggregation, cell proliferation and migration, adhesion molecules, tissue factor expression, etc. These may account for their impressive ability to lower CAD events with evidence of early benefit in clinical trials. Pleiotropic effects should be given more attention in clinical practice for a better understanding of drug actions, interactions and indications. Industry takes advantage of their existence and is currently developing drugs with multiple effects.

Keywords: atherosclerosis, dyslipidemia, fibrates, lipoproteins, probucol, vastatins.

Definition and scope

Drugs usually have multiple effects, through an analogy with single genes which affect more than one system or determine more than one phenotype, they are currently referred to as "pleiotropic effects" (from the Greek πλειων for "more" and τροπος for "direction or turn"). These may be related or unrelated to the primary mode of action of the drug. Pleiotropic effects may emerge during preclinical and clinical studies in drug development but, more often than not, they are discovered a posteriori long after the therapeutic agent is marketed. They may be undesirable and recognized as adverse side effects, they may be neutral, or they may be beneficial, enhancing the desirable effect of a drug. Over the years, the discovery of such effects has expanded the spectrum of action of drugs (i.e., enhancing the primary effect or adding a new property), led to new indications or contributed to the creation of a new class of therapeutic agents. In the hyper-

---

Address for correspondence: Jean Davignon MD, Director, Hyperlipidemia and Atherosclerosis Research Group, IRCM, 110 Pine Avenue West, Montreal, QC, Canada H2W 1R7.

tension field, for instance, minoxidil, an arteriolar vasodilator with potent anti-hypertensive properties was found to cause hypertrichosis [1]. This property was exploited in the development of a 2% topical spray for the treatment of baldness under the trade name rogaine®. Therefore, an unanticipated side effect created a new indication. Similarly, the use of niacin as a lipid-modulating agent results from the discovery by Altschul et al. [2] in 1955 that a vitamin which prevents the development of pellagra, was endowed with the ability to lower plasma cholesterol and triglycerides when given in very large doses. When using niacin for the treatment of dyslipidemia, one is in fact taking advantage of the pleiotropic effect of a vitamin which has found a new indication at large doses. Further development led to the formulation of slow-release preparations and analogues [3]. Recognition of the importance of pleiotropic effects has influenced industry in designing a priori molecules with multiple effects. The fact that drugs affecting lipid metabolism have pleiotropic effects has far-reaching implications for the practice of medicine as well as for drug discovery and development. In recent years, there has been growing evidence from major clinical trials and ancillary studies that part of the impressive effects of lipid-lowering drugs on the occurrence or recurrence of coronary events could be ascribed to their pleiotropic effects [4,5]. This review will briefly consider the pleiotropic effects of probucol and fibrates and more extensively those of HMG CoA reductase inhibitors (HCRIs) with particular attention to their potential clinical relevance. Negative pleiotropic effects of these drugs will not be discussed in this review.

Probucol

Probucol, developed as a cholesterol-lowering agent, was found to be a potent antioxidant with antiatherogenic properties in rabbits and monkeys (reviewed in [6]). This discovery had major repercussions on the oxidation theory of atherosclerosis [7] and resulted in the development of a new class of antioxidant drugs for their potential antiatherogenic effects [8]. A major free radical scavenger, probucol was found to protect low-density lipoproteins (LDL) and lipoprotein(a) (Lp(a)) against oxidative modifications [9] and to prevent the inhibition of endothelium-dependent relaxation by LDL in vitro [10]. The demonstration that a combination of probucol and lovastatin can improve endothelium-dependent vasodilator responses to acetylcholine in coronary artery disease (CAD) patients [11], and that the vasodilator response to acetylcholine was directly related to the resistance of LDL to oxidation [12] have emphasized the clinical relevance of these experimental findings. New drugs such as ACA-147 [13] have been designed a priori with multiple effects including an antioxidant component to enhance the antiatherogenic potential of another action, the inhibition of ACAT activity. Although probucol was withdrawn after the negative results of the PQRS trial (Probucol Quantitative Regression Swedish Trial) [14,15], there has been a renewed interest in this drug following the demonstration [16] that it improves the restenosis rate after coronary angioplasty if given 4 weeks prior to the intervention, confirming and expanding previous findings [17–19]. Among the many other pleiotropic effects of probucol, its ability to increase CETP activity and mass [20,21], to inhibit IL-1 secretion in vivo [22] and its gene expression in vitro [23] by THP-1 macrophages, to inhibit neointimal cell proliferation in balloon-injured rat carotid artery [24], and to block copper-induced tissue factor expression in macrophages [25], should be mentioned. The premature withdrawal of probucol ignored these and other beneficial effects [6,26] which have not been fully tested for their clinical relevance.

Fibrates

Clofibrate, the prototype of fibrates was developed to lower plasma lipids and was found to lower plasma triglycerides and raise high-density lipoproteins efficiently [27,28]. Several unanticipated pleiotropic effects seemingly unrelated to the primary mode of action of the drug have since been discovered including an insect repellent activity [29], an antiviral effect [30], a stimulatory effect on antidiuretic hormone secretion [31] and the ability to protect experimental animals against the hepatotoxicity of acetaminophen [32]. With the development and clinical use of several new class analogues (with animal experimentation and metabolic studies in humans) fibrates were found to have a multiplicity of effects on plasma lipoproteins and ubiquitous sites of action [33,34]. A paradoxical increase in LDL-C in some patients and a lithogenic potential were among the negative findings. Their ability to shift the atherogenic small dense LDL towards more buoyant LDL particles of larger size, to reduce postprandial lipemia and lower Lp(a) to a modest extent, stood among added pleiotropic advantages. The recent discovery that many of their effects on plasma lipoproteins were exerted via the peroxisome proliferator activated receptor (PPAR) pathway constitutes a major breakthrough in our understanding of their mode of action [35]. Unknowingly, when giving fibrates, physicians have been directly modulating gene expression, inhibiting the transcription of apo CIII [36,37] and enhancing that of apo AI [38–40], apo AII [41] and lipoprotein lipase [42].

Beneficial effects of fibrates on fibrinolysis and thrombosis have emerged over the years adding to their cardiovascular pleiotropic effect profile [34]. High-plasma fibrinogen [43] and plasminogen activator inhibitor-1 (PAI-1) [44,45] levels, which are associated with impaired fibrinolysis, constitute established CAD risk factors. Most fibrates lower plasma fibrinogen concentrations [46] and as a consequence decrease blood viscosity [47]. This has been shown for clofibrate [27], bezafibrate [48–51], fenofibrate [47,52] and ciprofibrate [53–56]. Gemfibrozil does not seem to share this effect to the same extent. Except for one study reporting a decrease in plasma fibrinogen [57], it has been shown either to increase [46,54,58], or to have little or no effect [56,59,60] on fibrinogen in dyslipidemic patients. On the other hand, there is evidence that gemfibrozil [61] and bezafibrate [51] may lower plasma PAI-1. Although PAI-1 is associated with triglyceride-rich lipoproteins and should be expected to be decreased by any measure lowering plasma TG [62], there is evidence that fibrates may exert a more direct action. Gemfibrozil inhibits basal and EGF- or TGFβ-stimulated PAI-1 synthesis in HepG2 cells [44] as well as PAI-1 synthesis induced by insulin and its precursors in noninsulin-dependent diabetes mellitus (NIDDM) [63]. It also suppresses PAI-1 synthesis and gene expression in cultured cynomolgus monkey primary hepatocytes, an effect that is independent of TG concentration in the culture medium, is not shared to the same extent by other fibrates and could be mediated by the PPAR pathway [64]. The issue is still controversial, as two studies reported no effect of gemfibrozil on plasma PAI-1 levels [60,65] while another showed that gemfibrozil had an effect on PAI-1 only when TG were reduced maximally to $\leqslant 2.8$ mmol/l in hypertriglyceridemic patients [45]. Furthermore, very low density lipoprotein (VLDL) were shown to regulate PAI-1 gene expression in HepG2 cells [66]. One report showed that gemfibrozil increases platelet count, in vivo platelet aggregability and urinary excretion of thromboxane B2 [67]. Because of this potentially prothrombotic negative pleiotropic effect, the authors proposed that gemfibrozil administration should be combined with aspirin for maximal benefit. This is in contrast with studies showing that gemfibrozil decreases factor VII-phospholipid complex with no effect on platelet count in myocardial infarction patients [68], decreases prothrombin fragment F_{1+2} [58] and platelet activity [69,70].

The beneficial multifunctional effects of fibrates acting in synergy to improve cardiovascular endpoints may account in part for the positive results of clinical trials such as the Helsinki Heart Study (HHS), a primary prevention trial [71], and the Bezafibrate Coronary Artery Intervention Trial (BECAIT), an angiographic study [72]. The latter, carried out in young male hyperlipidemic myocardial infarction survivors ($\leqslant 45$ years of age) showed a marked decrease in myocardial infarction recurrence associated with a significant decrease in triglycerides (-36%) and fibrinogen (-12%), a significant increase in HDL-C ($+9\%$) but no significant effect on LDL-C (-2%) over a period of 5 years.

HMG CoA reductase inhibitors

Compactin, the first of the HMG CoA reductase inhibitors (HCRIs) was designed to lower plasma LDL-C by inhibiting cholesterol synthesis. With the development of new analogues (either fungal metabolites (lovastatin, simvastatin, pravastatin) or synthetic compounds (fluvastatin, atorvastatin and cerivastatin)) a large number of new properties became apparent a posteriori [4,73,74]. These include the ability to raise plasma HDL-C, to lower plasma β-VLDL and TG-rich lipoproteins and to inhibit VLDL production. In addition, studies in cell cultures, experimental animals and humans carried out over the past few years have provided strong evidence that HCRIs have major unanticipated pleiotropic effects which are beneficial to the cardiovascular system. It has been proposed that these may have contributed in part to the impressive success of the major clinical trials (conducted with HCRIs) at reducing the number of CAD events and lowering total mortality. Several compelling arguments support this hypothesis, the major one being that a cardiovascular benefit was observed too early to be accounted for by atherosclerosis regression which is a slow process. In the West of Scotland Coronary Prevention (WOSCOP) Study [75], for instance, the pravastatin treatment curve separates early from the placebo curve so that by 18 months the cumulative CAD events (fatal and nonfatal MI) are significantly different between the two groups (Ian Ford, personal communication). Similarly, in the PLAC-II (Pravastatin, Lipids and Atherosclerosis in the Carotids) trial, a reduction in fatal and nonfatal coronary events occurred in as little as 36 months of follow-up [76]. In contrast, in the POSCH (Program on the Surgical Control of the Hyperlipidemias) trial, where the major impact of treatment was on LDL-C (-33%), with little HDL-C raising effect ($+4\%$) and no TG-lowering effect ($+19\%$), it took 5 years for the treatment curve (i.e., patients having had partial ileal bypass surgery) to separate from the nonintervention curve [77]. An extended analysis of the results of the WOSCOP Study by Packard et al. [78] shows that more benefit for cardiovascular risk was obtained from the treatment of patients with pravastatin than would have been anticipated according to the Framingham model (a 35% underestimation), whereas this model predicted with accuracy what was observed in the placebo group. Gould and co-workers [79], using positron emission tomography (PET) imaging, were able to show that intensive cholesterol-lowering with diet, lovastatin and cholestyramine could markedly improve myocardial perfusion in CAD patients in only 90 days of therapy, too short a period of time for anatomic regression to have occurred. Such findings strongly support the view that pleiotropic effects of HRCIs are involved in the seemingly disproportionate cardiovascular benefits observed with HCRIs. Some of these may be related to inhibition of cholesterol synthesis, the primary pharmacological action of HCRIs; in this instance the effect can be inhibited or reversed by mevalonate. Others may be unrelated to this primary mechanism and provide a benefit beyond that attributable to LDL-C reduction.

Three pleiotropic effects may be considered to have major clinical significance. The first is the ability of HCRIs to improve endothelial dysfunction in hypercholesterolemic and CAD patients. This has been studied in different vascular beds with a variety of techniques and appears to be a class effect, as it is shared among all HCRIs which were tested, whether lipophilic or hydrophilic. It has been demonstrated with pravastatin [80], lovastatin [11,81], fluvastatin [82] and simvastatin [83,84]. A combination of lovastatin and probucol was particularly effective at improving coronary blood flow after acetylcholine infusion [11], an effect which was correlated with the ability of LDL to resist oxidation by copper in vitro [12]. The role of enhanced oxidative processes and reduced nitric oxide production in the pathogenesis of the endothelial dysfunction associated with hypercholesterolemia and CAD is strongly supported by animal experimentation [85,86]. That HCRIs may exert an antioxidant activity is also borne out from the observation that simvastatin and pravastatin [87] as well as fluvastatin [88] reduce LDL susceptibility to oxidation in vitro, that fluvastatin reduces plasma lipid peroxides induced by cholesterol feeding in rabbits [89] and that simvastatin inhibits the ability of human monocyte-derived macrophages to oxidize LDL in vitro [90]. The latter is prevented by mevalonate indicating that the effect is linked to the primary mode of action of the drug. The demonstration that pravastatin can reduce transient myocardial ischemia in a 2-year randomized prospective study in patients with stable angina pectoris may be related to improvement in myocardial perfusion, and demonstrates further the clinical relevance of improving endothelial dysfunction [91]. The second pleiotropic effect of major clinical relevance is the capacity of HCRIs to improve survival and reduce graft rejection in immunosuppressed patients after cardiac transplantation. This was shown with the administration of pravastatin [92] and simvastatin [93]. Pravastatin prevented the rise in cholesterol which follows transplantation, markedly decreased the number of rejections with hemodynamic compromise and significantly improved 1-year survival as compared to a control group [92]. A similar effect was observed over 4 years by maintaining posttransplantation plasma LDL-C concentration at < 120 mg/dl (3.1 mmol/l) with simvastatin [93]. In this study, a reduction of intimal thickening assessed by intracoronary ultrasonography was documented in a subset of patients with LDL-C < 110 mg/dl (2.84 mmol/l). Several pleiotropic effects of HCRIs have been considered to account for this beneficial result: decreased natural killer cells cytotoxicity [92,94,95], inhibition of monocyte chemotaxis [96], inhibition of smooth muscle cell proliferation [97] (see below), interference with cell cycling [98] and a putative potentiation of the immunosuppressive effect of cyclosporin A [93]. A third property which could have clinical relevance is the recent observation that pravastatin improves ex vivo platelet aggregation in hypercholesterolemic patients [99] (an effect not shared with simvastatin [22a]) that would be additive to the effect of aspirin. Similarly, a recent study in a rabbit model has shown that atorvastatin (but not simvastatin) reduces platelet aggregation in a superfusion chamber lined with a mildly injured, but not with a severely injured, rabbit artery [100]. Since similar cholesterol reductions are achieved in both cases, the difference in responses may not be simply attributed to the LDL-C lowering effect of the drugs.

Inhibition of cell proliferation is another consistent pleiotropic effect of HCRIs, with suggestive but not conclusive evidence that the degree of lipophilicity may be involved in determining the magnitude of the effect. Interference with cell proliferation has been shown with smooth muscle cells (SMC) (all except pravastatin) [101−103], fibroblasts (all except pravastatin) [103], endothelial cells (all except pravastatin) [103], mesangial cells (lovastatin) [104], striated myoblasts (lovastatin, simvastatin, not pravastatin) [105], pancreatic cancer cells (lovastatin) [106], neuroblastoma cells (lovastatin) [107], glioma cells (simvastatin) [108,109], malignant B lymphocytes (simvastatin) [110], leukemic progenitor cells (simvastatin) [111], and breast cancer cells (lovastatin, simvastatin) [112]. Simvastatin ($IC_{50} = 0.1\mu M$) and pravastatin ($IC_{50} = 80\ \mu M$) also interfere with macrophage growth induced by oxidized LDL in vitro [113]. The findings on SMC in vitro have been complemented by studies in vivo demonstrating inhibition of neointimal cell proliferation in the carotid artery of rabbits by fluvastatin, lovastatin and simvastatin, but not pravastatin [101], and by cerivastatin [114]. The action appears to be mediated by interference with cholesterol synthesis, the primary mechanism, since it is abolished by mevalonate and partially prevented by farnesol or geranyl-geraniol [102]. In addition, simvastatin was shown to interfere with smooth muscle cell migration [115]. Six HCRIs have been compared head-to-head recently for their ability to inhibit in vitro the proliferation of human SMC, fibroblasts and endothelial cells [103]. The magnitude of the effect was consistent for each HCRI across the three cell types, pravastatin being the least effective (IC_{25} 37.6 ± 6.8 µM on SMC) and cerivastatin the most effective (IC_{25} 0.02 ± 0.01 µM on SMC). Unexpectedly, although atorvastatin was the most potent HCRI after cerivastatin at reducing LDL-C, it was the least effective after pravastatin (IC_{25} 1.0 ± 0.6 µM on SMC). The biological significance of the interference of HCRIs with cell proliferation remains to be established, especially as far as its antiatherogenic influence is concerned. It shows promise in oncology, however, as HCRIs may eventually be used as adjuvants to chemotherapy [109,116—118]. Other pleiotropic effects which may become clinically relevant include the ability of HCRIs to lower plasma soluble E selectin (an adhesion molecule) in hypercholesterolemic patients [119], to inhibit the transcription of tissue factor [120] (a major thrombogenic determinant in plaque rupture by macrophages in vitro), to lower the concentration of PAI-1 antigen levels in hyperlipidemic patients [121] (a known risk factor for recurrent myocardial infarction [122]), to reduce the overproduction of thromboxane A2 [123] and to lower blood viscosity [124] in hyperlipidemic patients.

The range of HCRI pleiotropic effects has increased considerably over the last few years to encompass many properties that could not have been predicted at the outset. These include effects as diverse as the ability to protect rat neonatal cardiomyocytes against hypoxic injury in vitro [125], to lower angiotensin converting enzyme activity in aorta of cholesterol fed rabbits [89], to inhibit SMC calcium mobilization by angiotensin II, platelet-derived growth factor and vasopressin [126,127], and to induce apoptosis in a variety of cells [128—130]. More and more attention is being given today to the growing list of unanticipated pleiotropic effects of HCRIs [4,5,118,131—133]. It is likely that they have contributed to the inhibition of atherothrombosis and to the reduction in total mortality reported in several major clinical trials.

Conclusion

Pleiotropic effects of drugs affecting lipid metabolism are numerous and varied, they may add to the desirable effect of a drug or be undesirable and interfere with the benefit of treatment. They have led to new indications, expanded the spectrum of action of existing drugs and they may create new classes of drugs. As the list of pleiotropic effects of lipid-lowering agents is expanding rapidly, it will become essential to establish their relative biological significance and clinical relevance. It will be important to take action on the new indications which have emerged from consideration of these effects, the most obvious being the use of HCRI in improving graft rejection and survival of immunosuppressed subjects submitted to organ transplantation. An effort will be needed to separate the effects resulting from the lipid-lowering properties from those due to the primary mode of action of the drug or to a new unrelated effect of the molecule. The place of pleiotropic effects in current medical practice, in drug development and in drug licensing will have to be reappraised. A full pleiotropic effect profile will have to be established for each agent of a class to take full advantage of the nonlipid beneficial properties in clinical practice and determine whether the observed differences among agents of a class may refine their respective indications. Pleiotropic effects will continue to be exploited for the benefit of patients and for marketing advantages while opening new avenues of research. They will provide a better understanding of drug action, help explain certain drug interactions and side effects, and facilitate the choice of a drug for combination therapy. The trend of developing molecules with multiple effects by design will persist and new therapeutic options for cardiovascular diseases as well as for cancer will emerge.

References

1. Burton JL, Marshall A. Hypertrichosis due to minoxidil. Br J Dermatol 1979;101:593—595.
2. Altschul R, Hoffer A, Stephen MJ. Influence of nicotinic acid on serum cholesterol in man. Arch Biochem Biophys 1955;54:558—559.
3. Efthymiopoulos C, Edwards DMF, Strolin-Benedetti M, Ruff F, Advenier C, Bianchini R et al. Pharmacokinetics of acipimox and of its N-deoxy metabolite following single and repeated oral administration of a sustained release formulation to healthy volunteers. Int J Pharm 1993;95:127—133.
4. Davignon J, Montigny M. The future of drug therapy for the treatment of dyslipoproteinemia. Acta Angiol 1996;2:11—26.
5. Vaughan CJ, Murphy MB, Buckley BM. Statins do more than just lower cholesterol. Lancet 1996;348:1079—1082.
6. Davignon J. Probucol. In: Schettler G (ed) Handbook of Experimental Pharmacology. Vol. 109 — Principles and Treatment of Lipoprotein Disorders. Berlin: Springer-Verlag, 1994:429—469.
7. Steinberg D, Witztum JL. Lipoproteins and atherogenesis. Current concepts. JAMA 1990;264: 3047—3052.
8. McCarthy PA. New approaches to atherosclerosis. An overview. Med Res Rev 1993;13: 139—159.
9. Naruszewicz M, Selinger E, Dufour R, Davignon J. Probucol protects lipoprotein(a) against oxidative modification. Metabolism 1992;41:1225—1228.
10. Plane F, Jacobs M, McManus D, Bruckdorfer KR. Probucol and other antioxidants prevent the inhibition of endothelium-dependent relaxation by low-density lipoproteins. Atherosclerosis 1993;103:73—79.
11. Anderson TJ, Meredith IT, Yeung AC, Frei B, Selwyn AP, Ganz P. The effect of cholesterol-lowering and antioxidant therapy on endothelium-dependent coronary vasomotion. N Engl J Med 1995;332:488—493.
12. Anderson TJ, Meredith IT, Charbonneau F, Yeung AC, Frei B, Selwyn AP et al. Endothelium-dependent coronary vasomotion relates to the susceptibility of LDL to oxidation in humans.

Circulation 1996;93:1647—1650.

13. Adelman SJ, McKean M, Prozialeck DH, Clark DE, Fobare WF. ACA-147: an inhibitor of ACAT and of the oxidative modification of LDL. In: Woodford FP, Davignon J, Sniderman A (eds) Atherosclerosis X. Amsterdam: Elsevier Science B.V., 1995:316—320.

14. Walldius G, Erikson U, Olsson AG, Bergstrand L, Hadell K, Johansson J et al. The effect of probucol on femoral atherosclerosis — The Probucol Quantitative Regression Swedish Trial (PQRST). Am J Cardiol 1994;74:875—883.

15. Steinberg D. Clinical trials of antioxidants in atherosclerosis: are we doing the right thing? Lancet 1995;346:36—38.

16. Tardif JC, Côté G, Lespérance J, Bourassa M, Lambert J, Doucet S et al. Probucol and multivitamins in the prevention of restenosis after coronary angioplasty. N Engl J Med 1997;337: 365—372.

17. Lee YJ, Yamaguchi H, Daida H, Yokoi H, Miyano H, Takaya J et al. Pharmacological intervention to modify restenosis. Circulation 1991;84:II—299

18. Setsuda M, Inden M, Hiraoka N, Okamoto S, Tanaka H, Okinaka T et al. Probucol therapy in the prevention of restenosis after successful percutaneous transluminal coronary angioplasty. Clin Ther 1993;15:374—382.

19. Watanabe K, Sekiya M, Ikeda S, Miyagawa M, Hashida K. Preventive effects of probucol on restenosis after percutaneous transluminal coronary angioplasty. Am Heart J 1996;132:23—29.

20. Franceschini G, Chiesa G, Sirtori CR. Probucol increases cholesteryl ester transfer protein activity in hypercholesterolaemic patients. Eur J Clin Invest 1991;21:384—388.

21. McPherson R, Hogue M, Milne RW, Tall AR, Marcel YL. Increase in plasma cholesteryl ester transfer protein during probucol treatment: relation to changes in high-density lipoprotein composition. Arterioscl Thromb 1991;11:476—481.

22. Ku G, Doherty NS, Schmidt LF, Jackson RL, Dinerstein RJ. Ex vivo lipopolysaccharide-induced interleukin-1 secretion from murine peritoneal macrophages inhibited by probucol, a hypocholesterolemic agent with antioxidant properties. FASEB J 1990;4:1645—1653.

22a. Lacoste L, Lam JYT. Comparative effect of pravastatin and simvastatin on platelet-thrombus formation in hypercholesterolemic coronary patients. J Am Coll Cardiol 1996;27:413A (Abstract).

23. Akeson AL, Woods CW, Mosher LB, Thomas CE, Jackson RL. Inhibition of IL-1β expression in THP-1 cells by probucol and tocopherol. Atherosclerosis 1991;86:261—270.

24. Ishizaka N, Kurokawa K, Taguchi J, Miki K, Ohno M. Inhibitory effect of a single local probucol administration on neointimal formation in balloon-injured rat carotid artery. Atherosclerosis 1995;118:53—56.

25. Crutchley DJ, Que BG. Copper-induced tissue factor expression in human monocytic THP-1 cells and its inhibition by antioxidants. Circulation 1995;92:238—243.

26. Kaul N, Siveski-Iliskovic N, Hill M, Khaper N, Seneviratne C, Singal PK. Probucol treatment reverses antioxidant and functional deficit in diabetic cardiomyopathy. Molec Cell Biochem 1996;161:283—288.

27. Hunninghake DB, Probstfield JL. Drug treatment of hyperlipoproteinemia. In: Rifkind BM, Levy RI (eds) Hyperlipidemia, Diagnosis and Therapy. New York: Grune & Stratton, 1977: 327—362.

28. Hunninghake DB, Peters JR. Effect of fibric acid derivatives on blood lipid and lipoprotein levels. Am J Med 1987;83(Suppl 5B):44—49.

29. Levinson HZ, Levinson AR. Insectistatic action of the lipid antagonist ethyl-p-chlorophenoxyisobutyrate. Naturwissenschaften 1973;60:1—3.

30. Steinhart WL, Hogeman CS, Powanda MC. Inhibition of the production of infectious herpes simplex virus by clofibrate. Virology 1976;70:241—243.

31. De Gennes JL, Bertrand C, Bigorie B, Truffert J. Première démonstration de l'activité antidiurétique, pharmacologique et thérapeutique du clofibrate (atromid-S) dans le diabète insipide. C R Acad Sci Paris 1969;269:2607—2610.

32. Manautou JE, Hart SGE, Khairallah EA, Cohen SD. Protection against acetaminophen hepatotoxicity by a single dose of clofibrate: Effects on selective protein arylation and glutathione depletion. Fundam Appl Toxicol 1996;29:229–237.

33. Davignon J. Fibrates: a review of important issues and recent findings. Can J Cardiol 1994; 10:61B–71B.

34. Schonfeld G. The effects of fibrates on lipoprotein and hemostatic coronary risk factors. Atherosclerosis 1994;111:161–174.

35. Schoonjans K, Staels B, Auwerx J. Role of the peroxisome proliferator-activated receptor (PPAR) in mediating the effects of fibrates and fatty acids on gene expression. (Review) (193 refs). J Lipid Res 1996;37:907–925.

36. Staels B, Vu-Dac N, Kosykh VA, Saladin R, Fruchart J-C, Dallongeville J et al. Fibrates downregulate apolipoprotein C-III expression independent of induction of peroxisomal acyl coenzyme A oxidase. A potential mechanism for the hypolipidemic action of fibrates. J Clin Invest 1995;95:705–712.

37. Hertz R, Bishara-Shieban J, Bar-Tana J. Mode of action of peroxisome proliferators as hypolipidemic drugs. Suppression of apolipoprotein C-III. J Biol Chem 1995;270:13470–13475.

38. Vu-Dac N, Schoonjans K, Laine B, Fruchart J-C, Auwerx J, Staels B. Negative regulation of the human apolipoprotein A-I promoter by fibrates can be attenuated by the interaction of the peroxisome proliferator-activated receptor with its response element. J Biol Chem 1994;269: 31012–31018.

39. Berthou L, Duverger N, Emmanuel F, Langouët S, Auwerx J, Guillouzo A et al. Opposite regulation of human vs. mouse apolipoprotein A-I by fibrates in human apolipoprotein A-I transgenic mice. J Clin Invest 1996;97:2408–2416.

40. Kockx M, Princen HMG, Kooistra T. Studies on the role of PPAR in the fibrate-modulated gene expression of apolipoprotein A-I, plasminogen activator inhibitor 1, and fibrinogen in primary hepatocyte cultures from cynomolgus monkey. Ann NY Acad Sci 1996;804:711–712.

41. Berthou L, Saladin R, Yaqoob P, Branellec D, Calder P, Fluchart JC et al. Regulation of rat liver apolipoprotein A-I, apolipoprotein A-II and acyl-coenzyme A oxidase gene expression by fibrates and dietary fatty acids. Eur J Biochem 1995;232:179–187.

42. Staels B, Schoonjans K, Fruchart JC, Auwerx J. The effects of fibrates and thiazolidinediones on plasma triglyceride metabolism are mediated by distinct peroxisome proliferator activated receptors (PPARs). Biochimie 1997;79:95–99.

43. Ernst E, Resch KL. Fibrinogen as a cardiovascular risk factor: a meta-analysis and review of the literature. Ann Int Med 1993;118:956–963.

44. Fujii S, Sobel BE. Direct effects of gemfibrozil on the fibrinolytic system. Diminution of synthesis of plasminogen activator inhibitor type I. Circulation 1992;85:1888–1893.

45. Keber I, Lavre J, Suc S, Keber D. The decrease of plasminogen activator inhibitor after normalization of triglycerides during treatment with fibrates. Fibrinolysis 1994;8(Suppl 2):57–59.

46. Branchi A, Rovellini A, Sommariva D, Gugliandolo AG, Fasoli A. Effect of three fibrate derivatives and of two HMG-CoA reductase inhibitors on plasma fibrinogen levels in patients with primary hypercholesterolemia. Thromb Haemost 1993;70:241–243.

47. Leschke M, Höffken H, Schmidtsdorff A, Blanke H, Egbrink R, Joseph K et al. The effect of fenofibrate on fibrinogen concentration and blood viscosity: its possible consequence for myocardial microcirculation in coronary heart disease. Dtsch Med Wochenschr 1989;114:939–944.

48. Niort G, Bulgarelli A, Cassader M, Pagano G. Effect of short term treatment with bezafibrate on plasma fibrinogen, fibrinopeptide A, platelet activation and blood filterability in atherosclerotic hyperfibrinogenemic patients. Atherosclerosis 1988;71:113–119.

49. Pazzucconi F, Mannucci L, Mussoni L, Gianfranceschi G, Maderna P, Werba P et al. Bezafibrate lowers plasma lipids, fibrinogen and platelet aggregability in hypertriglyceridaemia. Eur J Clin Pharmacol 1992;43:219–223.

50. De Faire U, Ericsson CG, Grip L, Nilsson J, Svane B, Hamsten A. Retardation of coronary atherosclerosis: the bezafibrate coronary atherosclerosis intervention trial (BECAIT) and other

angiographic trials. Cardiovasc Drugs Ther 1997;11:257–263.

51. Ishiwata S, Nakanishi S, Nishiyama S, Seki A. Prevention of restenosis by bezafibrate after successful coronary angioplasty. Coronary Artery Dis 1995;6:883–889.

52. Farnier M, Bonnefous F, Debbas N, Irvine A. Comparative efficacy and safety of micronized fenofibrate and simvastatin in patients with primary type IIa or IIb hyperlipidemia. Arch Int Med 1994;154:441–449.

53. Simpson IA, Lorimer AR, Walker ID, Davidson JF. Effect of ciprofibrate on platelet aggregation and fibrinolysis in patients with hypercholesterolaemia. Thromb Haemost 1985;54:442–444.

54. Knipscheer HC, De Valois J, Van den Ende B, Ten Cate JW, Kastelein JJP. Ciprofibrate vs. gemfibrozil in the treatment of primary hyperlipidaemia. Atherosclerosis 1996;124:S75–S81.

55. Kontopoulos AG, Athyros VG, Papageorgiou AA, Hatzikonstandinou HA, Mayroudi MC, Boudoulas H. Effects of simvastatin and ciprofibrate alone and in combination on lipid profile, plasma fibrinogen and low-density lipoprotein particle structure and distribution in patients with familial combined hyperlipidaemia and coronary artery disease. Coronary Artery Dis 1996;7:843–850.

56. De Maat MPM, Knipscheer HC, Kastelein JJP, Kluft C. Modulation of plasma fibrinogen levels by ciprofibrate and gemfibrozil in primary hyperlipidaemia. Thromb Haemost 1997;77:75–79.

57. Athyros VG, Papageorgiou AA, Avramidis MJ, Kontopoulos AG. Long-term effect of gemfibrozil on coronary heart disease risk profile of patients with primary combined hyperlipidaemia. Coronary Artery Dis 1995;6:251–256.

58. Wilkes HC, Meade TW, Barzegar S, Foley AJ, Hughes LO, Bauer KA et al. Gemfibrozil reduces plasma prothrombin fragment F1+2 concentration, a marker of coagulability, in patients with coronary heart disease. Thromb Haemost 1992;67:503–506.

59. Bröijersén A, Hamsten A, Silveira A, Fatah K, Goodall AH, Eriksson M et al. Gemfibrozil reduces thrombin generation in patients with combined hyperlipidaemia, without influencing plasma fibrinogen, fibrin gel structure or coagulation factor VII. Thromb Haemost 1996;76:171–176.

60. Bröijersén A, Eriksson M, Wiman B, Angelin B, Hjemdahl P. Gemfibrozil treatment of combined hyperlipoproteinemia – No improvement of fibrinolysis despite marked reduction of plasma triglyceride levels. Arterioscl Thromb Vasc Biol 1996;16:511–516.

61. Cimminiello C, Vigorelli P, Piliego T, Soncini M, Toschi V, Arpaia G et al. Fibrinolytic response in subjects with hypertriglyceridemia and low HDL cholesterol. Biomed Pharmacother 1997;51:164–169.

62. Mussoni L, Mannucci L, Sirtori M, Camera M, Maderna P, Sironi L et al. Hypertriglyceridemia and regulation of fibrinolytic activity. Arterioscl Thromb 1992;12:19–27.

63. Nordt TK, Kornas K, Peter K, Fujii S, Sobel BE, Kübler W et al. Attenuation by gemfibrozil of expression of plasminogen activator inhibitor type 1 induced by insulin and its precursors. Circulation 1997;95:677–683.

64. Arts J, Kockx M, Princen HMG, Kooistra T. Studies on the mechanism of fibrate-inhibited expression of plasminogen activator inhibitor-1 in cultured hepatocytes from cynomolgus monkey. Arterioscl Thromb Vasc Biol 1997;17:26–32.

65. Haire WD. Gemfibrozil predictably lowers triglycerides but does not significantly change plasminogen activator inhibitor activity in hypertriglyceridemic patients with a history of thrombosis. Thromb Res 1991;64:493–501.

66. Sironi L, Mussoni L, Prati L, Baldassarre D, Camera M, Banfi C et al. Plasminogen activator inhibitor type-1 synthesis and mRNA expression in HepG2 cells are regulated by VLDL. Arterioscl Thromb Vasc Biol 1996;16:89–96.

67. Bröijersén A, Eriksson M, Angelin B, Hjemdahl P. Gemfibrozil enhances platelet activity in patients with combined hyperlipoproteinemia. Arterioscl Thromb 1995;15:121–127.

68. Andersen P, Smith P, Seljeflot I, Brataker S, Arnesen H. Effects of gemfibrozil on lipids and

haemostasis after myocardial infarction. Thromb Haemost 1990;63:174—177.

69. Avellone G, Di GV, Panno AV, Cordova R, Lepore R, Strano A. Changes induced by gemfibrozil on lipidic, coagulative and fibrinolytic pattern in patients with type IV hyperlipoproteinemia. Int Angiol 1988;7:270—277.

70. Sirtori CR, Franceschini G, Gianfranceschi G, Sirtori M, Montanari G, Tremoli E et al. Effects of gemfibrozil on plasma lipoprotein-apolipoprotein distribution and platelet reactivity in patients with hypertriglyceridemia. J Lab Clin Med 1987;110:279—286.

71. Frick MH, Elo O, Haapa K, Heinonen O, Heinsalmi P, Helo P et al. Helsinki Heart Study: primary-prevention trial with gemfibrozil in middle-aged men with dyslipidemia. Safety of treatment, changes in risk factors and incidence of coronary heart disease. N Engl J Med 1987; 317:1237—1245.

72. Ericsson C-G, Hamsten A, Nilsson J, Grip L, Svane B, De Faire U. Angiographic assessment of effects of bezafibrate on progression of coronary artery disease in young male postinfarction patients. Lancet 1996;347:849—853.

73. Davignon J, Montigny M, Dufour R. HMG-CoA reductase inhibitors: a look back and a look ahead. Can J Cardiol 1992;8:843—864.

74. Davignon J. Atorvastatin: a statin with a large spectrum of action. Atherosclerosis ID research alert 1997;2:233—252.

75. Shepherd J, Cobbe SM, Ford I, Isles CG, Lorimer AR, Macfarlane PW et al. Prevention of coronary heart disease with pravastatin in men with hypercholesterolemia. N Engl J Med 1995; 333:1301—1307.

76. Furberg CD, Byington RP, Crouse JR, Espeland MA. Pravastatin, lipids, and major coronary events. Am J Cardiol 1994;73:1133—1134.

77. Buchwald H, Varco RL, Matts JP, Long JM, Fitch LL, Campbell GS et al. Effect of partial ileal bypass surgery on mortality and morbidity from coronary heart disease in patients with hypercholesterolemia — Report of the Program on the Surgical Control of the Hyperlipidemias (POSCH). N Engl J Med 1990;323:946—955.

78. Packard CJ, Norrie J, Cobbe SM, Shepherd J. Influence of pravastatin and plasma lipids on clinical events in the West of Scotland Coronary prevention Study (WOSCOPS). Atherosclerosis 1997;134:49 (Abstract).

79. Gould KL, Martucci JP, Goldberg DI, Hess MJ, Edens RP, Latifi R et al. Short term cholesterol lowering decreases size and severity of perfusion abnormalities by positron emission tomography after dipyridamole in patients with coronary artery disease: a potential noninvasive marker of healing coronary endothelium. Circulation 1994;89:1530—1538.

80. Egashira K, Hirooka Y, Kai H, Sugimachi M, Suzuki S, Inou T et al. Reduction in serum cholesterol with pravastatin improves endothelium-dependent coronary vasomotion in patients with hypercholesterolemia. Circulation 1994;89:2519—2524.

81. Treasure CB, Klein JL, Weintraub WS, Talley JD, Stillabower ME, Kosinski AS et al. Beneficial effects of cholesterol-lowering therapy on the coronary endothelium in patients with coronary artery disease. N Engl J Med 1995;332:481—487.

82. Eichstädt HW, Eskötter H, Hoffmann I, Amthauer HW, Weidinger G. Improvement of myocardial perfusion by short-term fluvastatin therapy in coronary artery disease. Am J Cardiol 1995;76(Suppl):122A—125A.

83. Vogel RA, Corretti MC, Plotnick GD. Changes in flow-mediated brachial artery vasoactivity with lowering of desirable cholesterol levels in healthy middle-aged men. Am J Cardiol 1996; 77:37—40.

84. O'Driscoll G, Green D, Taylor RR. Simvastatin, an HMG-coenzyme A reductase inhibitor, improves endothelial function within 1 month. Circulation 1997;95:1126—1131.

85. Osborne JA, Lento PH, Siegfried MR, Stahl GL, Fusman B, Lefer AM. Cardiovascular effects of acute hypercholesterolemia in rabbits: reversal with lovastatin treatment. J Clin Invest 1989; 83:465—473.

86. Lefer AM, Ma X. Decreased basal nitric oxide release in hypercholesterolemia increases neu-

trophil adherence to rabbit coronary artery endothelium. Arterioscl Thromb 1993;13: 771–776.

87. Kleinveld HA, Demacker PN, De Haan AF, Stalenhoef AF. Decreased in vitro oxidizability of low-density lipoprotein in hypercholesterolaemic patients treated with 3-hydroxy-3-methylglutaryl-CoA reductase inhibitors. Eur J Clin Invest 1993;23:289–295.

88. Hussein O, Schlezinger S, Rosenblat M, Keidar S, Aviram M. Reduced susceptibility of low-density lipoprotein (LDL) to lipid peroxidation after fluvastatin therapy is associated with the hypocholesterolemic effect of the drug and its binding to the LDL. Atherosclerosis 1997; 128:11–18.

89. Mitani H, Bandoh T, Ishikawa J, Kimura M, Totsuka T, Hayashi S. Inhibitory effects of fluvastatin, a new HMG-CoA reductase inhibitor, on the increase in vascular ACE activity in cholesterol-fed rabbits. Br J Pharmacol 1996;119:1269–1275.

90. Giroux LM, Davignon J, Naruszewicz M. Simvastatin inhibits the oxidation of low-density lipoproteins by activated human monocyte-derived macrophages. Biochim Biophys Acta 1993;1165:335–338.

91. Van Boven AJ, Jukema JW, Zwinderman AH, Crijns HJGM, Lie KI, Bruschke AVG. Reduction of transient myocardial ischemia with pravastatin in addition to the conventional treatment in patients with angina pectoris. Circulation 1996;94:1503–1505.

92. Kobashigawa JA, Katznelson S, Laks H, Johnson JA, Yeatman L, Wang XM et al. Effect of pravastatin on outcomes after cardiac transplantation. N Engl J Med 1995;333:621–627.

93. Wenke K, Meiser, Thiery J, Nagel D, Von Scheidt W, Steinbeck G et al. Simvastatin reduces graft vessel disease and mortality after heart transplantation, a 4 year randomized trial. Circulation 1997;96:1398–1402.

94. Cutts JL, Bankhurst AD. Reversal of lovastatin-mediated inhibition of natural killer cell cytotoxicity by interleukin 2. J Cell Physiol 1990;145:244–252.

95. Katznelson S, Wilkinson AH, Kobashigawa JA, Wang XM, Chia D, Ozawa M et al. The effect of pravastatin on acute rejection after kidney transplantation — A pilot study. Transplantation 1996;61:1469–1474.

96. Kreuzer J, Bader J, Jahn L, Hautmann M, Kübler W, Von Hodenberg E. Chemotaxis of the monocyte cell line U937: dependence on cholesterol and early mevalonate pathway products. Atherosclerosis 1991;90:203–209.

97. Corsini A, Raiteri M, Soma MR, Gabbiani G, Paoletti R. Simvastatin but not pravastatin has a direct inhibitory effect on rat and human myocyte proliferation. Clin Biochem 1992;25: 399–400.

98. Doyle JW, Kandutsch AA. Requirement for mevalonate in cycling cells: quantitative and temporal aspects. J Cell Physiol 1988;137:133–140.

99. Lacoste L, Lam JYT, Hung J, Letchacovski G, Solymoss CB, Waters D. Hyperlipidemia and coronary disease — Correction of the increased thrombogenic potential with cholesterol reduction. Circulation 1995;92:3172–3177.

100. Alfon J, Pueyo AF, Badimon L. Regulation by atorvastatin, a novel HMG-CoA reductase inhibitor, of plasma lipids and thrombotic risk in atherosclerotic rabbits. 66th Congress of the European Atherosclerosis Society, Florence 1996;201.

101. Soma MR, Donetti E, Parolini C, Mazzini G, Ferrari C, Fumagalli R et al. HMG CoA reductase inhibitors: in vivo effects on carotid intimal thickening in normocholesterolemic rabbits. Arterioscl Thromb 1993;13:571–578.

102. Corsini A, Raiteri M, Soma MR, Bernini F, Fumagalli R, Paoletti R. Pathogenesis of atherosclerosis and the role of 3-hydroxy-3-methylglutaryl coenzyme A reductase inhibitors. Am J Cardiol 1995;76(Suppl):21A–28A.

103. Nègre-Aminou P, Van Vliet AK, Van Erck M, Van Thiel GCF, Van Leeuwen REW, Cohen LH. Inhibition of proliferation of human smooth muscle cells by various HMG-CoA reductase inhibitors: comparison with other human cell types. Biochim Biophys Acta 1997;1345: 259–268.

104. O'Donnell MP, Kasiske BL, Kim Y, Atluru D, Keane WF. Lovastatin inhibits proliferation of rat mesangial cells. J Clin Invest 1993;91:83–87.

105. Van Vliet AK, Nègre-Aminou P, Van Thiel GCF, Bolhuis PA, Cohen LH. Action of lovastatin, simvastatin, and pravastatin on sterol synthesis and their antiproliferative effect in cultured myoblasts from human striated muscle. Biochem Pharmacol 1996;52:1387–1392.

106. Sumi S, Beauchamp RD, Townsend CM Jr, Pour PM, Ishizuka J, Thompson JC. Lovastatin inhibits pancreatic cancer growth regardless of RAS mutation. Pancreas 1994;9:657–661.

107. Maltese WA, Defendini R, Green RA, Sheridan KM, Donley DK. Suppression of murine neuroblastoma growth in vivo by mevinolin, a competitive inhibitor of 3-hydroxy-3-methylglutaryl-coenzyme A reductase. J Clin Invest 1985;76:1748–1754.

108. Soma MR, Pagliarini P, Butti G, Paoletti R, Paoletti P, Fumagalli R. Simvastatin, an inhibitor of cholesterol biosynthesis, shows a synergistic effect with N,N'-bis(2-chloroethyl)-N-nitrosourea and β-interferon on human glioma cells. Cancer Res 1992;52:4348–4355.

109. Kikuchi T, Nagata Y, Abe T. In vitro and in vivo antiproliferative effects of simvastatin, an HMG-CoA reductase inhibitor, on human glioma cells. J Neurol 1997;34:233–239.

110. Vitols S, Angelin B, Juliusson GJ. Simvastatin impairs mitogen-induced proliferation of malignant B-lymphocytes from humans – In vitro and in vivo studies. Lipids 1997;32:255–262.

111. Newman A, Clutterbuck RD, DeLord C, Powles RL, Catovsky D, Millar JL. The sensitivity of leukemic bone marrow to simvastatin is lost at remission: a potential purging agent for autologous bone marrow transplantation. J Invest Med 1995;43:269–274.

112. Addeo R, Altucci L, Battista T, Bonapace IM, Cancemi M, Cicatiello L et al. Stimulation of human breast cancer MCF-7 cells with estrogen prevents cell cycle arrest by HMG-CoA reductase inhibitors. Biochem Biophys Res Commun 1996;220:864–870.

113. Sakai M, Kobori S, Matsumura T, Biwa T, Sato Y, Takemura T et al. HMG-CoA reductase inhibitors suppress macrophage growth induced by oxidized low-density lipoprotein. Atherosclerosis 1997;133:51–59.

114. Igarashi M, Takeda Y, Mori S, Ishibashi N, Komatsu E, Takahashi K et al. Suppression of neointimal thickening by a newly developed HMG-CoA reductase inhibitor, BAYw6228 and its inhibitory effect on vascular smooth muscle cell growth. Br J Pharmacol 1997;120:1172–1178.

115. Hidaka Y, Eda T, Yonemoto M, Kamei T. Inhibition of cultured vascular smooth muscle cell migration by simvastatin (MK-733). Atherosclerosis 1992;95:87–94.

116. Buchwald H. Cholesterol inhibition, cancer, and chemotherapy. Lancet 1992;339:1154–1156.

117. Soma MR, Baetta R, De Renzis MR, Mazzini G, Davegna C, Magrassi L et al. In vivo enhanced antitumor activity of carmustine (N, N'-bis(2-chloroethyl)-N-nitrosourea) by simvastatin. Cancer Res 1995;55:597–602.

118. Massy ZA, Keane WF, Kasiske BL. Inhibition of the mevalonate pathway: Benefits beyond cholesterol reduction. Lancet 1996;347:102–103.

119. Hackman A, Abe Y, Insull W Jr, Pownall H, Smith L, Dunn K et al. Levels of soluble cell adhesion molecules in patients with dyslipidemia. Circulation 1996;93:1334–1338.

120. Colli S, Eligini S, Lalli M, Camera M, Paoletti R, Tremoli E. Vastatins inhibit tissue factor in cultured human macrophages – a novel mechanism of protection against atherothrombosis. Arterioscl Thromb Vasc Biol 1997;17:265–272.

121. Isaacsohn JL, Setaro JF, Nicholas C, Davey JA, Diotalevi LJ, Christianson DS et al. Effects of lovastatin therapy on plasminogen activator inhibitor-1 antigen levels. Am J Cardiol 1994; 74:735–737.

122. Hamsten A, Walldius G, Szamosi A, Blombäck M, De Faire U, Dahlén G et al. Plasminogen activator inhibitor in plasma: risk factor for recurrent myocardial infarction. Lancet 1987;2: 3–9.

123. Notarbartolo A, Davì G, Averna M, Barbagallo CM, Ganci A, Giammarresi C et al. Inhibition of thromboxane biosynthesis and platelet function by simvastatin in type IIa hypercholesterolemia. Arterioscl Thromb 1995;15:247–251.

124. Tsuda Y, Satoh K, Kitadai M, Takahashi T, Izumi Y, Hosomi N. Effects of pravastatin sodium

and simvastatin on plasma fibrinogen level and blood rheology in type II hyperlipoproteinemia. Atherosclerosis 1996;122:225—233.

125. Bastiaanse EML, Atsma DE, Kuijpers MMC,Van der Laarse A. Simvastatin-sodium delays cell death of anoxic cardiomyocytes by inhibition of the Na^+/Ca^{2+} exchanger. FEBS Lett 1994;343:151—154.

126. Escobales N, Castro M, Altieri PI, Sanabria P. Simvastatin releases Ca^{2+} from a thapsigargin-sensitive pool and inhibits $InsP_3$-dependent Ca^{2+} mobilization in vascular smooth muscle cells. J Cardiovasc Pharmacol 1996;27:383—391.

127. Escobales N, Crespo MJ, Altieri PI, Furilla RA. Inhibition of smooth muscle cell calcium mobilization and aortic ring contraction by lactone vastatins. J Hypertens 1996;14:115—121.

128. Jones KD, Couldwell WT, Hinton DR, Su Y, He S, Anker L et al. Lovastatin induces growth inhibition and apoptosis in human malignant glioma cells. Biochem Biophys Res Commun 1994;205:1681—1687.

129. Reedquist KA, Pope TK, Roess DA. Lovastatin inhibits proliferation and differentiation and causes apoptosis in lipopolysaccharide-stimulated murine B cells. Biochem Biophys Res Commun 1995;211:665—670.

130. Satoh T, Isobe H, Ayukawa K, Sakai H, Nawata H. The effects of pravastatin, an HMG-CoA reductase inhibitor, on cell viability and DNA production of rat hepatocytes. Life Sci 1996; 59:1103—1108.

131. Gaw A. Can the clinical efficacy of the HMG CoA reductase inhibitors be explained solely by their effects on LDL-cholesterol? Atherosclerosis 1996;125:267—269.

132. Corsini A, Bernini F, Quarato P, Donetti E, Bellosta S, Fumagalli R et al. Nonlipid-related effects of 3-hydroxy-3-methylglutaryl coenzyme A reductase inhibitors. Cardiology 1996;87: 458—468.

133. Davignon J. Lipid lowering in patients with coronary artery disease: low-density lipoprotein cholesterol and beyond. Evidence-based Cardiovasc Dis 1997;1:34—35.

Interaction of oxidized LDL with arterial proteoglycans

Alan Chait, Mary Y. Chang, Katherine Olin, Kevin O'Brien and Thomas Wight
University of Washington, Seattle, Washington, USA

The retention of lipoproteins by extracellular matrix molecules is believed to be a critical step in the pathogenesis of atherosclerosis [1]. The major extracellular-matrix molecules with which lipoproteins interact are proteoglycans, which are secreted by smooth muscle cells and other cells of the artery wall. Positively charged residues on lipoproteins such as low-density lipoprotein (LDL) undergo ionic interactions with negatively charged sulfate and carboxylic acid residues on the glycosaminoglycan chains of proteoglycans, resulting in retention of the lipoproteins in the arterial intima. These retained lipoproteins are highly susceptible to subsequent oxidation modification. Oxidized LDL can influence many of the biological processes that are involved in atherogenesis and, therefore, is an important factor in the pathogenesis of atherosclerosis [2].

There are several ways in which oxidized LDL can influence lipoprotein-proteoglycan interactions. Firstly, oxidized LDL can influence the amount of proteoglycan synthesis by arterial smooth muscle cells. Oxidized LDL selectively stimulates the expression of biglycan (a small dermatan sulfate-rich proteoglycan) by arterial smooth muscle cells [3]. The expression of versican and decorin, two other proteoglycans produced by vascular smooth muscle cells, is not increased. Secondly, oxidized LDL also has a more generalized effect on elongation of glycosaminoglycan chains on all of the proteoglycans secreted by arterial smooth muscle cells [3], which tends to favor further retention of lipoproteins in the arterial intima. Thirdly, the extent of oxidation can influence the binding of LDL to proteoglycans and other matrix molecules.

The binding of lipoproteins to purified arterial smooth muscle cell proteoglycans can be assessed in vitro using a gel-shift assay performed under nondenaturing conditions [4]. Using this assay, LDL binding to either biglycan or versican (a chondroitin sulfate-rich proteoglycan that is a major component of atherosclerotic lesions) is reduced as the LDL becomes progressively oxidized. Extensively oxidized LDL does not bind to these proteoglycans to any significant extent. These observations are what would be predicted as a result of the reduction in the positive charge of LDL that occurs during its oxidation. These findings also are consistent with the possibility that LDL might be released from its pro-

---

Address for correspondence: Alan Chait MD, Professor of Medicine, Department of Medicine, P.O. Box 356426, University of Washington, Seattle, WA 98195-6426, USA.

teoglycan-binding sites after becoming oxidized [5]. However, oxidized LDL can be bound to proteoglycans if lipoprotein lipase, a secretory product of macrophages in atherosclerotic lesions [6] is present [7]. This ability of lipoprotein lipase to act as a bridging molecule for the binding of oxidized lipoproteins to smooth muscle cell proteoglycans is similar to that demonstrated for the binding of lipoproteins to endothelial cell-derived matrix molecules [8]. Thus, this macrophage secretory product may facilitate retention of LDL by arterial wall proteoglycans even after the lipoprotein becomes oxidized.

Retention of lipoproteins by arterial smooth muscle cell matrix also can be evaluated in vitro by measurement of binding to a complex matrix secreted by arterial smooth muscle cells under physiological conditions. In addition to proteoglycans, this matrix contains molecules such as collagen, fibronectin and elastin [9]. LDL that has been oxidized by several different mechanisms is retained by this complex matrix to a much greater extent than is native LDL, although the affinity of binding is somewhat reduced. These findings are in marked contrast to that observed for the binding of oxidized LDL to purified proteoglycans, in which oxidized LDL binds less well than native LDL. The binding of oxidized LDL to this complex matrix was also not proportional to changes in the charge of the lipoprotein that occurred as result of its oxidation. These observations suggest that oxidized LDL can bind to matrix molecules other than proteoglycans. Consistent with this hypothesis, the binding of oxidized LDL to the arterial smooth muscle cell-derived matrix was not reduced by digestion of the matrix by either chondroitinase ABC or heparitinase, nor was it reduced by digestion of collagen molecules with collagenase. These in vitro findings support the following schema depicting the initiating role of lipoprotein-proteoglycan interaction

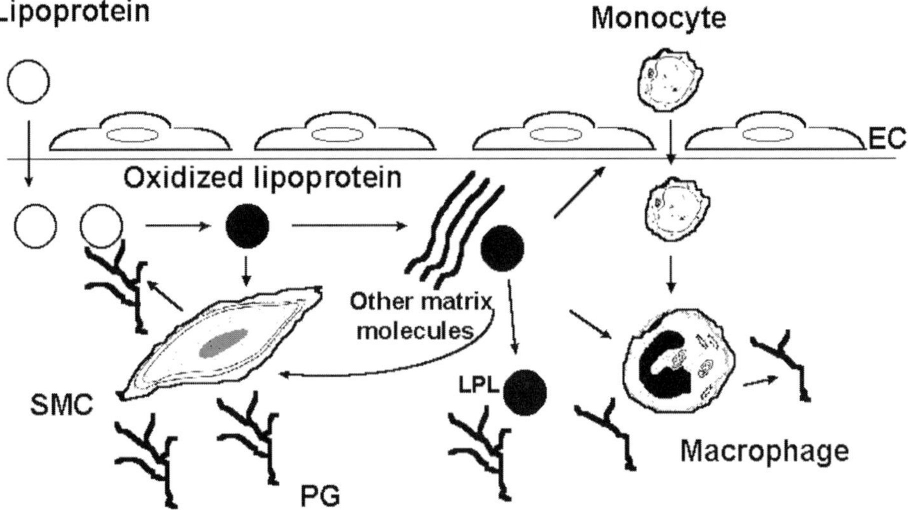

Fig. 1. Retention and oxidation of lipoproteins by arterial wall matrix molecules. PG = proteoglycans; SMC = smooth muscle cells; EC = endothelial cells; and LPL = lipoprotein lipase.

in the pathogenesis of atherosclerosis (Fig. 1). LDL enters the arterial wall where it initially binds to smooth muscle cell-derived proteoglycans and becomes oxidized. This oxidized LDL can stimulate further synthesis of proteoglycans with enhanced lipoprotein trapping capability. While oxidized LDL is not retained by proteoglycans, it can bind to other matrix molecules and can then influence the various biological processes involved in atherogenesis.

To determine the relationship between lipoproteins and proteoglycans in vivo, studies have commenced in which these molecules have been evaluated by immunohistochemistry in human coronary arteries obtained from individuals undergoing cardiac transplantation. Oxidation-specific epitopes occur in two major distributions. While a small amount of oxidation-specific epitopes are seen in the matrix colocalized with apolipoprotein B, most of the oxidation-specific epitopes occur intracellularly in areas that are not stained for apolipoprotein B. In addition, the extent of extracellular apolipoprotein B deposition was far greater than that of the oxidation-specific epitopes, suggesting that most of the apolipoprotein B seen in human atherosclerotic lesions is not present in oxidized lipoproteins. The proteoglycan, versican, was present in virtually all coronary artery segments, independent of whether they showed diffuse intimal thickening (which is the normal appearance in adult humans) or were affected by atherosclerosis. In contrast, extensive deposits of biglycan were seen commonly only in atherosclerotic segments. A surprising observation was that there was a striking colocalization of biglycan and apolipoprotein E [10], an apolipoprotein that is present in the remnants of the triglyceride-rich lipoproteins and in a small subset of high-density lipoprotein particles. Apolipoproteins B and A-I also were detected in regions with biglycan and apolipoprotein E deposits, as well as in regions adjacent to plaque neovasculature. Deposits of apolipoproteins E and B were much less prevalent in nonatherosclerotic intima. In vitro experiments show that biglycan binds with high affinity to HDL that contains apolipoprotein E, but does not bind to HDL that is devoid of apolipoprotein E, indicating that apolipoproteins A-I and A-II do not bind biglycan. Thus, biglycan in the artery wall may be trapping apolipoprotein E- and B-containing remnants of the triglyceride-rich lipoproteins, thereby facilitating their oxidation or uptake by cells. Biglycan also may be acting as a bridging molecule to trap certain HDL particles in the atherosclerotic intima, thereby potentially interfering with reverse cholesterol transport. Thus, there appears to be a complex interplay between lipoproteins and proteoglycans of the artery wall, in which lipoproteins that are trapped might undergo oxidation, which in turn can influence a myriad of biological processes involved in atherosclerosis, including the regulation of expression of proteoglycans, which may in turn lead to further retention of lipoproteins.

References

1. Williams KJ, Tabas I. The response-to-retention hypothesis of early atherogenesis. Arterioscl Thromb 1995;15:551–561.

2. Young SG, Parthasarathy S. Why are low-density lipoproteins atherogenic? West J Med 1994; 160:183–184.

3. Chang MY, Perigo S, Chait A, Wight TN. Regulation of vascular smooth muscle cell proteoglycan genes by oxidized low-density lipoproteins. J Vasc Res 1996;33:S1–49.

4. Camejo G, Fager G, Rosengren B, Hurt-Camejo E, Bondjers G. Binding of low-density lipoproteins by proteoglycans synthesized by proliferating and quiescent human arterial smooth muscle cells. J Biol Chem 1993;268:14131–14137.

5. Hurt-Camejo E, Camejo G, Rosengren B, Lopez F, Ahlstrom C, Fager G, Bondjers G. Effect of arterial proteoglycans and glycosaminoglycans on low-density lipoprotein oxidation and its uptake by human macrophages and arterial smooth muscle cells. Arterioscl Thromb 1992;12: 569–583.

6. O'Brien K, Gordon DS, Deeb S, Ferguson M, Chait A. Lipoprotein lipase is synthesized by macrophage-derived foam cells in human coronary atherosclerotic plaques. J Clin Invest 1992; 89:1544–1550.

7. Olin KL, Wight TN, Chait A. Lipoprotein lipase enhances the binding of native and oxidized low-density lipoproteins to biglycan and versican. Circulation (In press).

8. Saxena U, Klein MG, Vanni TM, Goldberg IJ. Lipoprotein lipase increases low-density lipoprotein retention by subendothelial cell matrix. J Clin Invest 1992;89:373–380.

9. Schonherr E, Jarvelainen HT, Kinsella MG, Sandell LJ, Wight TN. Platelet-derived growth factor and transforming growth factor-βI differentially affect the synthesis of biglycan and decorin by monkey arterial smooth muscle cells. Arterioscl Thromb 1993;13:1026–1036.

10. O'Brien KD, Alpers CE, Ferguson M, Wight T, Chait A. Colocalization of apolipoprotein E and biglycan in human atherosclerotic plaques. Circulation 1994;90:I–403.

The increasing significance of the unstable atheroma

Richard T. Lee and Peter Libby
Vascular Medicine and Atherosclerosis Unit, Brigham and Women's Hospital, Harvard Medical School, Boston, Massachusetts, USA

As we move into the next millennium, it is interesting to consider the increasing contribution of unstable vascular syndromes to the global burden of disease. As cardiovascular disease emerged as the leading cause of death in developed countries, we have also made great strides in treating and preventing these diseases. In the USA, age-adjusted rates of stroke and coronary death have steadily declined, the result of both intensive public education measures and treatment advances [1]. With the recent success of cholesterol-lowering therapy, some investigators have even speculated that cardiovascular disease may no longer be a major problem for future generations [2].

However, careful studies of patterns of disease in the world indicate that cardiovascular disease will in fact be the dominant health problem of the next century. By the year 2020, cardiovascular disease will be the leading cause of global disease burden, as infectious disease mortality continues to decline throughout the world and people live longer [3]. Therefore, it is critical for us to continue to develop preventive strategies and therapies for vascular disease, particularly the unstable vascular syndromes. We have learned a great deal about the natural history of atherosclerosis in the past decade, and it is now widely accepted that unstable atheroma and subsequent plaque rupture is a leading cause of acute myocardial infarction. However, recent studies indicate that plaque rupture may be a common and important cause of many cardiovascular diseases in addition to acute myocardial infarction. Here we will briefly review the pathophysiology of plaque rupture in causing myocardial infarction. We will also discuss recent exciting data that suggest that prevention of plaque rupture may have dramatic and unforeseen clinical benefits.

The mechanism of plaque rupture

The pathologic features of the unstable lesion have been well-described by Davies, Falk and others [4—6]. The unstable lesion has an eccentric and often large lipid pool beneath a thin fibrous cap. Davies et al. studied 100 consecutive cases of acute coronary thrombosis with careful histopathology [7]. They found

---

Address for correspondence: Richard T. Lee MD, Cardiovascular Division, Brigham and Women's Hospital, 75 Francis Street, Boston, MA 02115, USA. Tel.: +1-617-732-7146. Fax: +1-617-277-4981. E-mail: RTLEE@BICS.BWH.HARVARD.EDU

that the vast majority of these lesions had this particular geometrical configuration, with only a minority having calcification or concentric atherosclerotic lesions without lipid pools. These observations led to the hypothesis that a specific mechanical process caused tearing of the fibrous cap. Structures of human atheroma were subsequently studied with modern powerful computer techniques for analyzing complex structures [7,8]. These studies confirmed that the unstable atherosclerotic lesion has enormous stresses in the fibrous cap, particularly when the fibrous cap thickness is less than 200 microns. In these lesions, the peak stresses can reach many thousands of millimeters of mercury, greater than the fracture stress of the fibrous cap tissue (that is, the maximum stress the tissue can bear without fracturing). Therefore, geometrical and structural considerations are important components of plaque stability. These findings provide further incentive for the development of high-resolution imaging techniques such as intravascular ultrasound and optical coherence tomography for defining lesion structure in vivo; if we could image beneath the lumen, we could identify some unstable lesions before they rupture.

However, it is also quite clear that mechanical forces do not alone determine plaque stability. Fibrous cap strength varies widely, and some fibrous caps have sufficient intact fibrillar collagen to withstand thousands of mmHg [9,10]. Other fibrous caps have much less strength, particularly when infiltrated by inflammatory cells. How might leukocyte infiltration influence the strength of the atherosclerotic lesion? Leukocytes, and particularly activated macrophages, are potent promoters and mediators of extracellular matrix degradation; degradation of matrix then causes mechanical weakening of the tissue.

There are several major classes of enzymes that degrade and weaken extracellular matrix [11]. One class includes the serine proteases, most commonly known in cardiovascular diseases as enzymes in the blood that can degrade fibrin such as plasmin and urokinase. These enzymes also exist in the extracellular space and are capable of degrading matrix components. A second class of enzymes is the cysteine proteases, such as cathepsin B and D. These proteases have a wide range of substrates and generally act within the cytosol itself, although cathepsin S also has extracellular activity. A third class of enzymes is the family of matrix metalloproteinases. These enzymes include at least 12 members that are active in the extracellular space at neutral pH. The matrix metalloproteinases have broad specificities and some can degrade fibrillar collagen, the major structural backbone of the fibrous cap.

Many members of the metalloproteinase family (including the enzymes that degrade collagen) are overexpressed in the atherosclerotic lesion. Galis et al. demonstrated that both smooth muscle cells and macrophages in the human atheroma overexpressed these enzymes [12]. In addition, zymographic techniques showed that these enzymes are active and are likely to promote matrix degradation in the human atheroma.

One fascinating and unexplained feature of metalloproteinase overexpression in the human atheroma is that expression occurs at specific critical locations [13].

For example, matrix metalloproteinase-1 is commonly found at the "shoulder" regions of the fibrous cap. These shoulder regions are the same locations as the high mechanical stress areas; therefore, it appears that the excess matrix degradation activity is occurring at the same locations where the highest forces are borne by the plaque. This suggests that plaque rupture is the interaction between the mechanical forces and matrix degradation at these locations (Fig. 1).

This proposed pathophysiology of plaque rupture, the intersection of high mechanical stresses and matrix degradation at rupture locations, agrees well with clinical data. Angiography cannot determine the instability of atherosclerotic lesion, and indeed the greatest information regarding lesion stability is in fact beneath the surface of the lumen and not related to stenosis severity itself [14]. In addition, these data suggest that lesion stability can be improved without dramatic changes in the degree that the lumen is compromised, either by altering the stress distribution beneath the surface of the lesion or by decreasing the inflammatory activity. This scenario may explain the dramatic benefits of cholesterol-lowering therapy despite rather modest changes in the angiographic appearance of the lesion [15].

Although we have learned a great deal about how plaques rupture and why, many additional questions have arisen. These issues, which we will discuss below, suggest that prevention of plaque rupture may have very broad benefits in preventing many acute vascular syndromes (Table 1).

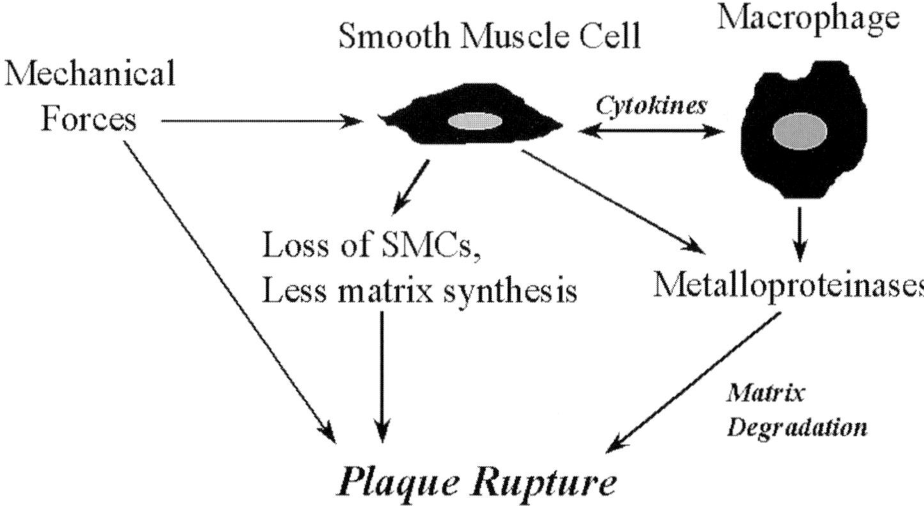

Fig. 1. Pathophysiology of plaque rupture. Plaque stability is determined by several parameters, including mechanical forces and the mechanical strength of the fibrous cap. High mechanical forces develop in lesions with thin fibrous caps overlying large lipid pools. Smooth muscle cells (which normally secrete extracellular matrix molecules such as fibrillar collagen) may decrease in number or synthetic activity, leading to less matrix. Both smooth muscle cells and macrophages can secrete metalloproteinases, enzymes that degrade the extracellular matrix. The weakened matrix is particularly susceptible to the high mechanical forces, leading to plaque rupture.

86

Table 1. Potential benefits of improving plaque stability.

Decrease in myocardial infarction; allowing collateral vessels to develop in ischemic territory.
Decrease in asymptomatic lesion growth; decrease in chronic stable angina.
Decrease in aortic atheroemboli, a potentially major cause of cardiogenic stroke.
Decrease in carotid artery stroke.
Decrease in peripheral artery symptomatic disease.
Decrease in congestive heart failure due to coronary artery disease.

Asymptomatic plaque rupture

Asymptomatic plaque rupture occasionally occurs in the coronary artery. Davies et al. observed asymptomatic plaque rupture in approximately 9% of coronary disease patients, and up to 22% in patients who had multiple coronary risk factors including hypertension and diabetes [16]. Other investigators have not found asymptomatic plaque ruptures at this high frequency. It does certainly appear, however, that asymptomatic plaque rupture can occur in the coronary artery, and occurs in other larger arteries as well. Even angiographic data (which is insensitive for determining plaque stability) suggests that asymptomatic coronary plaque disruption can occur. Chester et al. studied the natural history of complex coronary plaques [17]. In their study, 222 patients with chronic stable angina underwent cardiac catheterization and then waited an average of 7 months to have an intervention, usually an angioplasty. In this study, 4% of smooth lesions progressed more than 15% by quantitative angiography. However, 14% of lesions that appeared complex at the first angiogram progressed in these patients, despite clinical stability. This information suggests that the unstable atheroma can grow in a stepwise process with plaque rupture and subsequent healing, even in the absence of symptoms. This scenario can certainly be seen in some patients with unstable angina who have complex lesions, but with anticoagulation and conservative therapy, they then become stable for long periods without requiring revascularization procedures. Thus, prevention of asymptomatic rupture events could decrease lesion growth and decrease the prevalence of chronic stable angina. Slower growth of the lesion could also allow the development of collateral vessel supply.

Plaque rupture in noncoronary beds

An additional major question concerns the role of plaque rupture in noncoronary beds. For example, in the abdominal aorta, ruptured plaques with small overlying thrombi are frequently found, without apparent clinical significance given the size of the aorta. Recently, thoracic aortic arch complicated plaques with thrombi have been recognized as a potential major cause of cardiogenic emboli [18]. These lesions can often be seen by transesophageal ultrasound. The role of plaque rupture in carotid artery disease is incompletely defined but also possibly very important. Carr et al. studied plaque rupture and other morphologic features of the unstable atheroma in patients who had symptomatic and asymptomatic carotid artery disease [19]. In endarterectomy specimens, asymptomatic plaque rupture occurred in 32% of patients compared with 74% of patients who had symptomatic carotid lesions. These data strongly suggest that plaque rupture is an important step in the natural history of the carotid atheroma. In the case of the carotid artery, it may not be acute occlusion overlying the thrombus, but subtotal thrombosis with embolization that causes the transition from asymptomatic to symptomatic. Plaque rupture may also be a precipitant of symptomatic peripheral artery disease as well [20].

Prevention of congestive heart failure

Ischemic cardiomyopathy is a rapidly growing problem worldwide. Successful therapies such as pharmacologic therapy, transplantation, and artificial devices are improving the outlook for these patients, but attempts at regenerating viable and functional myocardium are far from the clinical arena. The optimal strategy, therefore, is prevention of loss of myocardial tissue. We have made progress in preserving myocardium after patients present with acute ischemia, but the greatest potential for limiting myocardial damage lies in preventing the acute event. For this reason, prevention of plaque rupture should be considered a major therapeutic target for heart failure.

Plaque rupture as a key therapeutic target

Despite the benefits of proven therapies such as aspirin and cholesterol reduction agents, acute vascular syndromes will become an even greater medical and economic global burden. Improving lesion stability will not only reduce the incidence of acute myocardial infarction, but will also most likely have broad benefits for patients with atherosclerosis.

Acknowledgements

Supported in part by a Grant-in-Aid from the American Heart Association and grants from the National Heart Lung and Blood Institute (HL-47840, HL-48743, HL-54759).

References

1. Goldman L, Cook EF. The decline in ischemic heart disease mortality rates. An analysis of the comparative effects of medical interventions and changes in lifestyle. Ann Int Med 1984;101: 825–836.
2. Brown MS, Goldstein JL. Heart attacks: gone with the century. Science 1996;272:629.
3. Murray CJL, Lopez AD. The Gobal Burden of Disease. Global Burden of Disease and Injury Series. The Harvard School of Public Health/Harvard University Press, 1996;1–34.

4. Davies MJ. Stability and instability: two faces of coronary atherosclerosis. Circulation 1996;94: 2013—2020.

5. Falk E. Progressive atherogenesis: why do plaques rupture. Circulation 1992;86(Suppl III): III30—III42.

6. MacIsaac AI, Thomas JD, Topol EJ. Toward the quiescent coronary plaque. J Am Coll Cardiol 1993;22:1228—1241.

7. Richardson PD, Davies MJ, Born GVR. Influence of plaque configuration and stress distribution on fissuring of coronary atherosclerotic plaques. Lancet 1989;2:941—944.

8. Loree HM, Kamm RD, Stringfellow RG, Lee RT. Effects of fibrous cap thickness on peak circumferential stress in model atherosclerotic vessels. Circ Res 1929;71:850—858.

9. Lendon CL, Davies MJ, Born GVR, Richardson PD. Atherosclerotic plaque caps are locally weakened when macrophage density is increased. Atherosclerosis 1991;87:87—90.

10. Loree HM, Grodzinsky AJ, Park SY, Gibson LJ, Lee RT. Static circumferential tangential modulus of human atherosclerotic tissue. J Biomech 1994;27:195—204.

11. Lee RT, Libby P. The unstable atheroma. Arterioscl Thromb Vasc Biol (In press).

12. Galis ZS, Muszynski M, Sukhova GK, Simon-Morrissey E, Unemori EN, Lark MW, Amento E, Libby P. Cytokine-stimulated human vascular smooth muscle cells synthesize a complement of enzymes required for extracellular matrix digestion. Circ Res 1994;75:181—189.

13. Lee RT, Schoen FJ, Loree HM, Lark MW, Libby P. Circumferential stress and matrix metalloproteinase 1 in human coronary atherosclerosis: implications for plaque rupture. Arterioscl Thromb Vasc Biol 1996;16:1070—1073.

14. Ambrose JA, Tannenbaum MA, Alexopoulos D, Monsen CS, Weiss M, Borriw S, Gorlin R, Fuster V. Angiographic progression of coronary artery disease and the development of myocardial infarction. J Am Coll Cardiol 1988;12:56—62.

15. Topol EJ, Nissen SE. Our preoccupation with coronary luminology: the dissociation between clinical and angiographic findings in ischemic heart disease. Circulation 1995;92:2333—2342.

16. Davies MJ, Bland JM, Hangartner JRW, Angelini A, Thomas AC. Factors influencing the presence or absence of acute coronary artery thrombi in sudden ischaemic death. Eur Heart J 1989;10:203—208.

17. Chester MR, Chen L, Kaski JC. The natural history of unheralded complex coronary plaques. J Am Coll Cardiol 1996;28:604—608.

18. Amarenco P, Cohen A, Tzourio C, Bertrand B, Hommel M, Besson G, Chauvel C, Touboul P, Bousser M. Atherosclerotic disease of the aortic arch and the risk of ischemic stroke. N Engl J Med 1994;331:1474—1479.

19. Carr S, Farb A, Pearce WH, Virmani R, Yao JST. Atherosclerotic plaque rupture in symptomatic carotid artery stenosis. J Vasc Surg 1996;23:755—766.

20. Mecley M, Rosenfield K, Kaufman J, Langevin RE, Razvi S, Isner JM. Atherosclerotic plaque hemorrhage and rupture associated with crescendo claudication. Ann Int Med 1929;117: 663—666.

Atherosclerosis XI.
B. Jacotot, D. Mathé and J.-C. Fruchart, editors.

Probing the etiology of elevated plasma levels of Lp(a) in African-Americans

Vincent Mooser[1], Jonathan Cohen[2] and Helen H. Hobbs[2]
[1]*Department of Internal Medicine, University Hospital, Lausanne, Switzerland; and* [2]*Departments of Molecular Genetics and Internal Medicine, University of Texas Southwestern Medical Center at Dallas, Dallas, Texas, USA*

Abstract. Plasma levels of lipoprotein(a) (Lp(a)) are 2- to 3-fold higher in Africans and their descendants than Caucasians. In Caucasians, the interindividual variation in plasma levels of Lp(a) is determined largely by sequences linked to the gene encoding apo(a), the highly polymorphic glycoprotein which distinguishes Lp(a) from low-density lipoprotein (LDL). To elucidate the genetic architecture of plasma levels of Lp(a) in African-Americans, we examined the segregation of apo(a) alleles and plasma levels of Lp(a) in 52 African-American families. Comparison of the mean sibling and mid-parental levels of plasma Lp(a) disclosed a relatively high heritability ($H^2 = 0.77$). Sibling pair analysis indicated that polymorphism in the apo(a) gene accounts for $\sim 85\%$ of the variation in plasma Lp(a) levels. We found no evidence for an African-specific sequence variant in the apo(a) gene accounting for the higher plasma Lp(a) levels. To determine if the higher plasma levels of Lp(a) in Africans were due to reduced proteolytic cleavage of apo(a) into fragments, we compared the relationship between plasma levels of apo(a) fragments and Lp(a) in African-Americans and Caucasians; no differences were observed between the two groups. We conclude that the genetic architecture of plasma levels of Lp(a) in African-Americans is similar, although not identical, to Caucasians and the higher plasma levels in this population are not due to a difference in the proteolysis of apo(a). The factor(s) responsible for the higher levels of plasma Lp(a) in individuals of African descent remain to be determined.

Keywords: apo(a) fragments, apolipoprotein(a), genetics, heritability, sib-pair analysis.

Introduction

Lipoprotein(a) or Lp(a) is a lipoprotein made up of a low-density lipoprotein (LDL) particle to which a highly polymorphic glycoprotein, apolipoprotein(a) (apo(a)), is covalently linked [1]. In all ethnic group studies to date, plasma levels of Lp(a) vary widely between individuals [2,3]. Africans as well as their descendants have 2- to 3-fold higher median plasma Lp(a) levels than Caucasians [4,5]. In Caucasians, plasma levels of Lp(a) are highly heritable and are largely determined by sequences at the apo(a) locus [6]. The genetic architecture of plasma Lp(a) levels in African-Americans and the reason(s) why they have higher levels of Lp(a) than Caucasians have been recently investigated [7].

Address for correspondence: Helen H. Hobbs, Department of Molecular Genetics, UT Southwestern Medical Center, 5323 Harry Hines Blvd, Dallas, TX 75235, USA. Tel.: +1-214-648-6724. Fax: +1-214-648-7539. E-mail: Hhobbs@mednet.swmed.edu

Materials and Methods

A total of 52 families of African ascendance were recruited from Dallas, Texas and New Orleans, Louisiana [7]. Plasma levels of Lp(a) were quantitated by enzyme-linked immunoabsorbent assay (ELISA) using antiapo(a) mouse monoclonal antibodies of well-characterized specificity [8]. The heritability of plasma Lp(a) levels was estimated by comparing the mid-parental and the mean offspring plasma levels of Lp(a). The contribution of the apo(a) gene to plasma levels of Lp(a) was examined in the families using a sibling (sib) pair method [6]. In this analysis, the highly polymorphic size of the apo(a) gene was used to identify pairs of sibs who inherited one, two or no apo(a) alleles identical by descent (ibd) from their parents. The number of kringle 4 repeats in the apo(a) gene, which varies from $12-51$, was assessed by Southern blot analysis of Hpal-digested high molecular weight genomic DNA after size fractionation of the digested fragments by pulsed-filed gel electrophoresis (PFGE) [9]. Two apo(a) alleles of different sizes on PFGE analysis were identified in all but three parents; a total of 49 families, including 257 sib-pairs, were included in the analysis.

To determine if higher plasma levels of Lp(a) in African-Americans were due to a reduced proteolysis of plasma apo(a) into fragments, plasma levels of Lp(a) and apo(a) fragments were quantitated as described [8,10] in 26 African-Americans and 26 Caucasians with normal renal function, and in 52 individuals on hemodialysis for end stage renal disease (ESRD). The two groups were matched for ethnicity, sex and size of apo(a) isoforms. Apo(a) fragments in plasma were assayed by ELISA after precipitation of Lp(a) using heparin-chromotography [10].

Results

The heritability of plasma level of Lp(a) was determined in 307 individuals from 52 unrelated African-American families [7] by comparing mid-parental and mean plasma concentrations of Lp(a) in the offspring. The heritability was relatively high ($H^2 = 0.77$). Removal of a single outlying family resulted in an even higher heritability ($H^2 = 0.96$). The heritability of plasma levels of Lp(a) in these 52 African-American families was similar to the estimate obtained previously in a sample of Caucasian families [6].

Sibling-pair analysis was performed to estimate the contribution of the apo(a) gene to the interindividual variation in plasma levels of Lp(a). The results of this analysis are summarized in Fig. 1. Parental apo(a) alleles were arbitrarily designated 1 and 2 for the father and 3 and 4 for the mother. In the example given in Fig. 1, the first child inherited apo(a) allele 1 from her father and apo(a) allele 3 from her mother. The second child inherited alleles 2 and 4. Accordingly, these two sibs share no apo(a) alleles in common. The second and third sibling share one apo(a) allele in common (apo(a) allele 2). Finally, the third and fourth siblings share both apo(a) alleles in common (alleles 2 and 3). In 49 families, 70

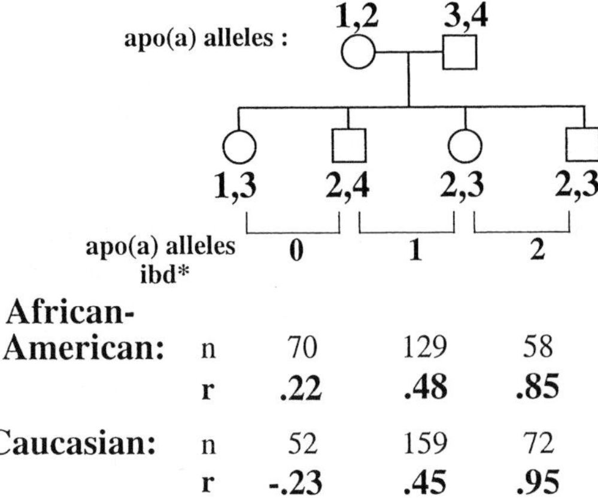

		0	1	2
African-American:	n	70	129	58
	r	.22	.48	.85
Caucasian:	n	52	159	72
	r	-.23	.45	.95

* identical by descent

Fig. 1. Sibling-pair analysis of plasma Lp(a) levels in 49 African-American and 43 Caucasian families. PFGE analysis of the apo(a) gene was used to differentiate parental apo(a) alleles of different sizes [9]. Segregation analysis of the apo(a) gene and plasma Lp(a) levels was performed and plasma levels of Lp(a) were compared in siblings who inherited one, two or no apo(a) alleles identical by descent (ibd) [6,7].

pairs of the African-American sib-pairs shared no apo(a) alleles in common and only a weak correlation of plasma Lp(a) levels were found in this subgroup (r = 0.22). The correlation coefficient increased progressively to 0.48 in the sib-pairs that shared one apo(a) allele in common (n = 129), to finally 0.85 in the 58 sib-pairs who inherited both apo(a) alleles ibd.

Comparison of the results of the sibling-pair analysis to that previously obtained in a sample of 48 Caucasian families [6] is shown in Fig. 1. In general, the correlation coefficients were somewhat higher in the Caucasian sibling pairs than in the African-Americans and the contribution of the apo(a) gene to plasma levels of Lp(a) were estimated at ~85% in the African-Americans compared with ~91% in the Caucasians. Taken together, these results indicated the apo(a) gene is a major contributor to the interindividual variation in plasma Lp(a) levels in both African-Americans and Caucasians.

Apo(a) alleles of smaller sizes are usually associated with higher plasma levels of Lp(a) [11]. To determine if the higher plasma levels of Lp(a) in African-Americans were due to a greater proportion of apo(a) alleles in this ethnic group being of smaller size, the distribution of apo(a) alleles in our sample was compared to that previously found in a Caucasian sample of similar size [6]. The distribution of apo(a) alleles appeared similar in the two groups [7]. The results of the analysis of the kringle 4-encoding region of the apo(a) gene, as assessed by PFGE analysis, were compared to immunoblot analysis of apo(a) in plasma. Within the intermediate-size category of apo(a) alleles, fewer alleles were associated with very low plasma levels of Lp(a) in the African-American sample than in the Caucasian, which is similar to previous observations by Marcovina and her colleagues [4].

We used two-length polymorphisms in the apo(a) gene, the K4 repeat polymorphism and a pentanucleotide TTTTA tandem repeat in the 5′ flanking region of the apo(a) gene [12] to construct apo(a) haplotypes [13]. We reasoned that if an African-specific sequence variation in the apo(a) gene is responsible for the higher plasma levels of Lp(a), there may be a common haplotype associated with higher levels of plasma Lp(a) in this population. No such haplotype at the apo(a) locus sequence variant was identified. In general, the plasma levels of Lp(a) associated with specific apo(a) haplotypes were higher in African-Americans than Caucasians over the entire size spectrum of apo(a) alleles. The lack of a common African-specific haplotype suggests the elevated levels of Lp(a) are not due to a common sequence difference in the apo(a) gene, unless the sequence variant is ancient and predates the generation of the kringle 4 length polymorphism.

The apo(a) that circulates in plasma is synthesized in the liver and secreted from hepatocyte where it joins LDL to form Lp(a). The fate of the Lp(a) that circulates in plasma is largely unknown. Some of the apo(a) is proteolytically processed to generate apo(a) fragments that circulate in plasma (Fig. 2) [10]. Previously, we provided evidence that the apo(a) fragments in plasma are the source of the apo(a) fragments in human urine [14]. As a first step in determining whether higher plasma levels of Lp(a) in African Americans are due to reduced activity of this catabolic pathway, we compared plasma concentrations of apo(a)

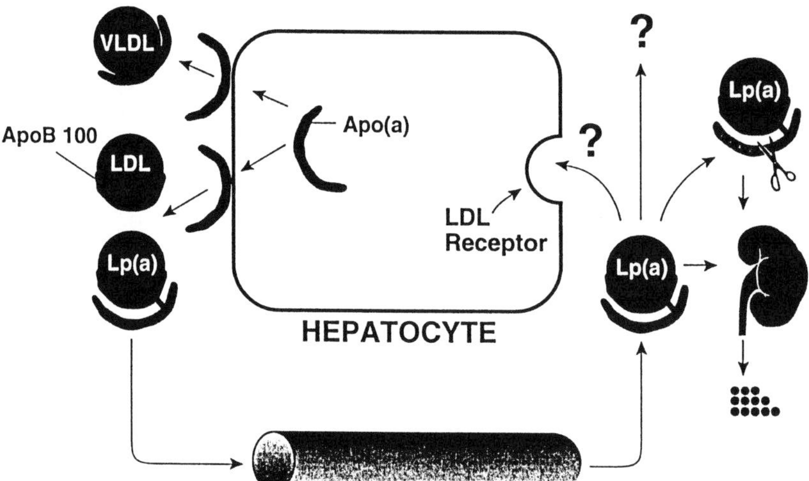

Fig. 2. The metabolism of apo(a) and Lp(a). Apo(a) is synthesized and secreted by the liver. The apo(a) a covalent attaches to the apoB-100 of LDL to form Lp(a). The Lp(a) circulates but its eventual fate is uncertain. Some apo(a) undergoes proteolytic cleavage into fragments [10] that are excreted by the kidney and appear in urine [14].

fragments and Lp(a) in 26 Caucasian and 26 African-American individuals [15]. The relationship between the plasma levels of apo(a) fragments and plasma levels of Lp(a) was similar in both groups (Fig. 3). We also examined the relationship between plasma levels of Lp(a) and apo(a) fragments in 26 African-Americans and 26 Caucasians on hemodialysis for end stage renal disease (ESRD). In this case, the apo(a) fragments cannot be excreted into the urine. In both the African-Americans and Caucasians, plasma levels of apo(a) fragments were higher in hemodialysis subjects than in controls [15], but the relationship between the plasma levels of apo(a) fragment and Lp(a) were comparable in the two groups. Taken together, these data are consistent with the higher plasma Lp(a) levels in African-Americans not being due to reduced proteolysis of circulating apo(a).

Discussion

In this paper we have reviewed our studies exploring why plasma levels of Lp(a) are higher in African Americans than in Caucasians. We have found that the overall genetic architecture in African-Americans is similar, although not identical, to that of Caucasians. In both groups, the heritability of plasma Lp(a) levels is high. Heritability is composed of two components, shared genes and shared environment. It is unlikely that the high heritability of plasma Lp(a) in African-Americans is due to shared environmental factors since plasma levels of Lp(a) are higher in all individuals of African descent, irrespective of geographic region.

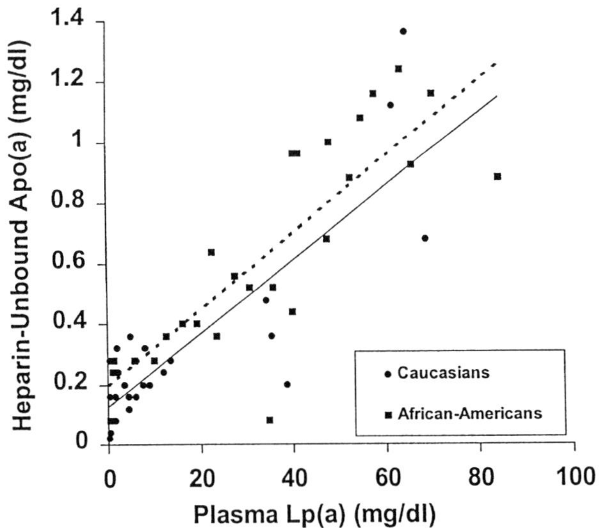

Fig. 3. Relationship between plasma levels of Lp(a) and heparin-unbound apo(a) in 26 African-American and 26 Caucasian apparently healthy individuals. The plasma was subjected to heparin-chromatography to remove Lp(a) and heparin-unbound apo(a) was quantitated by ELISA exactly as described [14].

We have shown that a major factor contributing to the high heritability plasma Lp(a) levels in Africans, as well as Caucasians, are sequence differences in the apo(a) locus. We have found no evidence supporting the existence of an African-specific Lp(a)-elevating sequence variant(s) in the apo(a) gene, although this has not been formally excluded. Our data are most consistent with the higher plasma levels of Lp(a) in African-Americans being due to a transacting factor(s). Studies to examine and compare the metabolism of Lp(a) in African-Americans to that of Caucasians are needed to determine if the higher plasma levels of Lp(a) in individuals of African descent are due to an increase in Lp(a) synthesis or a decrease in its catabolism.

Acknowledgements

Rudy Guerra, Santica Marcovina, Douglas Sheer and Jinping Wang contributed to the studies on the genetic architecture of plasma Lp(a) levels in African-Americans. This work was in part supported by the Swiss National Foundation (SCORE A grant no 32-44471.95 to VM), NIH-HL47619 and the Perot Family Fund.

References

1. Utermann G. The mysteries of lipoprotein(a). Science 1989;246:904–910.
2. Albers JJ, Marcovina SM, Lodge MS. The unique lipoprotein(a): properties and immunochemical measurement. Clin Chem 1990;36:2019–2026.
3. Sandholzer C, Hallman DM, Saha N, Sigurdsson G, Lackner C, Csaszar A, Boerwinkle E, Utermann G. Effects of the apolipoprotein(a) size polymorphism on the lipoprotein(a) concentration in 7 ethnic groups. Hum Genet 1991;86:607–614.
4. Marcovina SM, Albers JJ, Wijsman, Zhang Y, Chapman NH, Kennedy H. Differences in Lp(a) concentrations and apo(a) polymorphs between black and white populations. J Lipid Res 1996; 37:2569–2585.
5. Gaw A, Boerwinkle E, Cohen J, Hobbs HH. Comparative analysis of the apo(a) gene, apo(a) glycoprotein and plasma concentrations of Lp(a) in three ethnic groups. J Clin Invest 1994; 93:2526–2534.
6. Boerwinkle E, Leffert CC, Lin J, Lackner C, Chiese G, Hobbs HH. Apoliprotein(a) gene accounts for greater than 90% of the variation in plasma lipoprotein(a) concentrations. J Clin Invest 1992;90:52–60.
7. Mooser V, Sheer D, Marcovina SM, Wang J, Guerra R, Cohen J, Hobbs HH. The apo(a) gene is the major determinant of variation in plasma Lp(a) levels in African Americans. Am J Hum Genet 1997;61:402–417.
8. Marcovina SM, Albers JJ, Gabel B, Koschinsky ML, Gaur VP. Effect of the number of apolipoprotein(a) kringle 4 domains on immunochemical measurements of lipoprotein(a). Clin Chem 1995;4:246–255.
9. Lackner C, Cohen JC, Hobbs HH. Molecular basis of apolipoprotein(a) isoform size heterogeneity as revealed by pulsed-filed gel electrophoresis. J Clin Invest 1991;87:2077–2086.
10. Mooser V, Marcovina SM, White AL, Hobbs HH. Kringle-containing fragments of apolipoprotein(a) circulate in human plasma and are excreted into the urine. J Clin Invest 1996;98: 2414–2424.
11. Utermann GH, Menzel HJ, Kraft HG, Duba HC, Kemmler HG, Seitz C. Lp(a) glycoprotein

phenotypes. Inheritance and relation to Lp(a)-lipoprotein concentrations in plasma. J Clin Invest 1987;80:458—465.

12. Wade DP, Glarke JG, Lindahl GE, Liu AC, Zysow BR, Meer K, Schwartz K, Lawn RM. 5′ control regions of the apolipoprotein(a) gene and members of the related plasminogen gene family. Proc Nat Acad Sci USA 1993;90:1369—1373.

13. Mooser V, Mancini FP, Bopp S, Pethö-Schramm A, Guerra R, Boerwinkle E, Muller HR, Hobbs HH. Sequence polymorphism in the apo(a) gene associated with specific levels of Lp(a) in plasma. Hum Mol Genet 1995;4:173—181.

14. Mooser V, Seabra MC, Abedin M, Landschulz KT, Marcovina SM, Hobbs HH. Apo(a) kringle-4 containing fragments in human urine — relationship to plasma levels of lipoprotein(a). J Clin Invest 1996:97:858—864.

15. Mooser V, Marcovina SM, Wang J, Hobbs HH. High plasma levels of apo(a) fragments in Caucasians and African-Americans with end stage renal disease: implications for plasma Lp(a) assay. Clin Genet 1997;(In press).

Advanced glycoxidation: a vascular enemy with many faces

Helen Vlassara
The Picower Institute for Medical Research, New York, New York, USA

Introduction

It is estimated that more than 50% of all deaths in the adult population are due to vascular causes, most frequently manifested as hypertension (HTN) or arterio-/ atherosclerotic heart disease (ASCHD) [1]. Such incremental mortality late in adulthood suggests multiple pathogenic influences in this population. Among these, hyperglycemia, obesity, smoking and hyperlipidemia have been proven as major risk factors [2,3] which might be present in young adulthood, and together with genetic factors, (e.g., diabetes, apoprotein isoform E4, race (African American, American Indian)) may determine cardiovascular disease in the third and fourth decades of life [4,5].

In the midst of a plethora of pathogenic mechanisms that contribute to eventual vascular decline (which present investigators with a daunting challenge) a unifying systemic, as well as local "triggering" process, termed glycation has begun to emerge [6,7].

It is now confirmed that glycation is a ubiquitous biochemical process, which together with the interrelated processes of free radical generation and oxidative tissue damage, is believed to account for many of the typical features of cardiovascular disease [8,9]. The narrowing of vascular lumen, resulting from abnormal basement membrane and subintimal thickening, focal proliferation of vascular cells, loss of elasticity, thrombotic diathesis, abnormal deposition of cholesterol esters and fibrinin all lead to an increase in peripheral resistance and hydrostatic pressure [10,11]. Since diabetes frequently accompanies normal aging (sharing many of the typical features of aging vasculopathy) it is now accepted that hyperglycemia compounds the effects of aging alone [12].

Ambient blood glucose concentrations inevitably lead to nonenzymatic glycosylation reactions on proteins, lipids and nucleic acids [6,7,13]. Work from our and other laboratories has demonstrated that the aldehyde or keto groups of reducing sugars are capable of reacting with amino groups of amino acids or nucleic acids to form Schiff bases, which can rearrange to become irreversible, highly cross-linking advanced glycation endproducts (AGEs). These late rearrangements of the covalent modification of proteins and lipids by glucose have been shown to slowly accumulate in vascular, renal and other tissues with aging [14,15] and at a more rapid rate in diabetes [6,7] exerting considerable damage.

In the following update we will provide a general overview and recent evidence of the pathogenetic pluripotential of these ubiquitous substances.

Receptor-mediated AGE turnover and toxicity

Numerous studies have indicated that reactive AGEs can directly alter physical and structural properties of the endothelial and subendothelial components, for instance, by inducing collagen cross-linking, basement membrane thickening and covalent trapping of plasma proteins and lipids [7,16,17], or by directly reacting with nitric oxide thus negatively impairing vascular dilatory capacity [18,19]. In addition, AGEs are known to elicit a wide range of cell-mediated responses, thereby "indirectly" mediating phenotypic changes that can lead to vascular cell adhesion molecule expression [20,21] — with their attendant cascade of leucocyte adhesion, infiltration and activation [19], increased permeability and thrombotic diathesis [22], which could be responsible for some of the pathologic features characteristically observed in the subendothelium of vasculature in the aged.

A number of these cellular responses are thought to be induced through an AGE-specific cell-surface receptor system which has now been identified on many cell types, among which the monocyte/macrophage receptors were the first to be identified as mediating AGE uptake and degradation [23,24]. Investigation in our and other laboratories has revealed that the interaction of AGE-modified proteins with these well conserved among species receptors not only serves toward the catabolism and elimination of AGEs, but also toward the initiation of tissue repair and protein turnover, via the coordinate synthesis and release of cytokines and growth factors [25—27]. The AGE-receptor system (AGEr) comprises several components, including a 50 kD or OST-48 AGE-binding protein, a 80—90 kD or 80 K-H, a protein substrate for kinase C, and a 30—35 kD AGE-binding protein known as galectin-3, found on endothelial cells as well as on other systems, including hemopoetic, renal and neural cell membranes [28]. Other investigators have reported additional AGE-binding proteins including: a 35-kD peptide termed RAGE [29,30], lactoferin [29] and lysozyme [31], further expanding the known cell-associated or soluble polypeptides with AGE-binding capacity. These observations point to the existence of a heterogeneous and complex system of natural AGE-binding or AGE-transporter molecules, some of which may contribute to their catabolism, while others may participate in their transportation across plasma membranes, or tissues or may initiate cellular activation with tissue-specific secondary responses. In addition, it is important to point out that the catabolic byproducts of AGEs are in large part excreted by the kidney [32]. In fact, tissue and serum AGE levels correlate inversely with renal function and are markedly elevated in patients with end stage renal disease (ESRD) with or without diabetes [33,34] thus placing the kidney among the major distal regulators of AGE metabolism.

As anticipated, the interaction of AGEs with cell-specific AGE-receptor gene products and alterations in these genes have emerged as a mechanism of primary importance in atherosclerosis, hypertension, as well as renal disease. Preliminary support to this notion was obtained indirectly from studies on nondiabetic NOD mice, known for a genetic predisposition to nephropathy independent of diabetes. While kidney tissue and serum AGEs were surprisingly elevated more than 2-fold in the absence of diabetes, AGE-R1 expression at the mRNA and peptide levels were significantly reduced, as was AGE-binding activity, compared to normal controls [35]. Although preliminary, the findings have prompted the speculation that low AGE-R1 expression and function may enhance early accumulation of glycotoxins in tissues, promoting early tissue injury.

Plasma AGE-modified ApoB levels correlate with carotid artery AGEs in nondiabetic patients

Using carotid artery tissue and plasma samples obtained from nondiabetic patients undergoing endarterectomy, we have compared circulating AGE-modified ApoB and tissue AGE levels and the cellular distribution of AGE receptor, and using antibodies to AGEs, to the recently characterized AGE receptor proteins (AGE-R1 and AGE-R2) and to cell-specific leukocyte markers [36] (Fig. 1). Importantly, although none of the patients were hyperlipidemic nor diabetic, arterial tissue AGE levels correlated with plasma AGE-ApoB levels (r = 0.7) (Fig. 2) and with the severity of atheromatous lesions (graded 0−3+). In early lesions, AGE-immunoreactivity occurred mostly extracellularly in the thickened intima, and in more advanced lesions within lipid-containing macrophages and smooth muscle cells in fatty streaks and atheromatous plaques. Extracellular

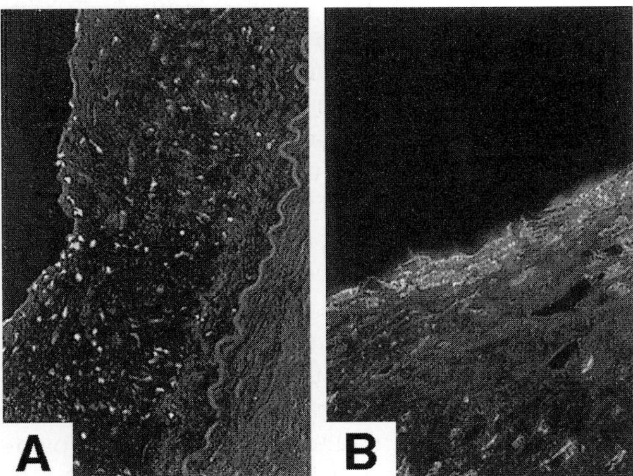

Fig. 1. AGE-receptor localization in atheromatous human artery. **A**: AGE-R1 staining prominently mononuclear cells infiltrating through endothelium and thickened intima (mag × 100). **B**: AGE-R2 staining of adjacent area of section shown in **A**; endothelium is stained more intensely and diffusely than migrating mononuclear cells (mag × 200) [55].

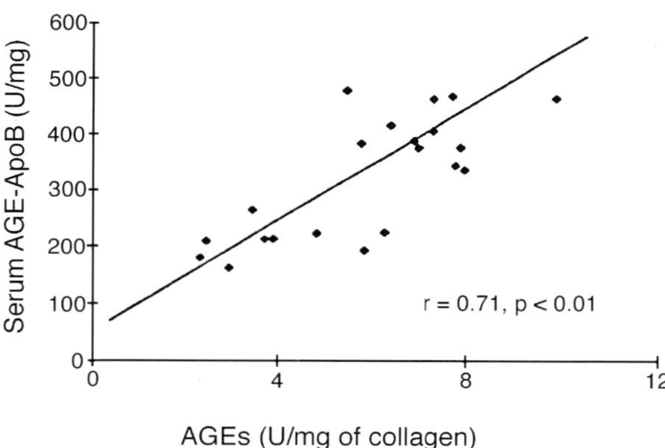

AGEs (U/mg of collagen)

Fig. 2. Correlation of circulating serum AGE-ApoB levels with arterial tissue AGE-collagen levels in nondiabetic patients with occlussive atherosclerosis [55].

AGE staining was also intense in late stage and acellular plaques. AGE receptors colocalized with infiltrating monocytes, endothelial and smooth muscle cells in early stage lesions, while in later stage plaques they colocalized with foam cells and macrophages [36]. These data point to a link between plasma AGE-ApoB levels and severity of vascular disease in nondiabetic, nonuremic patients.

In vivo AGE-mediated acceleration of atherosclerosis

To evaluate the atherogenic potential of exogenous AGEs, low doses of in vitro prepared AGE-modified rabbit serum albumin were administered to normal rabbits for 4 months either alone (AGE) or in combination with a 2-week period of a cholesterol-rich diet (AGE + CRD). The AGE content of aortic tissue increased by 2.2-fold in AGE-infused rabbits and by 3.2-fold in AGE+CRD-fed rabbits compared to normal saline-treated (CL) rabbits ($p < 0.025$ and 0.001, respectively) [20]. Serum AGE levels in the AGE and AGE+CRD groups rose up to 3-fold above CL ($p < 0.025$ and $p < 0.01$). Ascending aortic sections from AGE-treated rabbits showed significant focal intimal proliferation, enhanced endothelial cell adhesion with infrequent intimal macrophages, oil-red-O-staining lipid deposits and positive focal expression of vascular cell adhesion molecule-1 (VCAM-1), and intercellular adhesion molecule-1 (ICAM-1), a pattern not observed in the CL group. These AGE-induced changes were markedly enhanced in animals placed on CRD, consisting of multifocal atheromas containing foam-like cells, massive lipid droplets and strong endothelial expression of VCAM-1 and ICAM-1 restricted to the lesions. This study provided further in vivo support for a causal relationship between glycated substance accumulation and athero-sclerosis.

Cerebral neurotoxicity of exogenous AGEs in a stroke model

Given the increasing incidence and severity of stroke in aging individuals, we investigated the potential neurotoxicity of AGEs to rats by systemic administration of in vitro prepared AGE-proteins, with or without aminoguanidine, just prior to inducing a middle cerebral artery infarction. Glycotoxin infusion significantly increased cerebral infarct size even when applied transiently [37]. This was attenuated in animals that also received aminoguanidine. These data suggest that elevated levels of glycotoxins and their derivatives, as they may occur with age, diabetes, or renal insufficiency may potentiate neurotoxicity secondary to ischemic stroke.

Aging-related cardiovascular and renal disease; prevention by AGE-inhibition

Based on recent animal data indicating that AGE-inhibitors, such as aminoguanidine can to a large extent prevent exogenous AGE-mediated damage, we examined the effects of aminoguanidine (AG) (0.1% in drinking water) on vascular/ renal changes attributed to normal aging, during a 2-year study in normal Sprague-Dawley (SD) and F344 rats (n = 10/group) [38]. Blood pressure studies of both rat strains revealed markedly defective vasodilatory responses (to acetylcholine and nitroglycerine) with advancing age, accountable for the cardiomegaly found in these animals; aminoguanidine treatment prevented this defect, as well as the age-linked cardiomegaly. In both untreated strains of old rats (SD more than F344), marked albuminuria and proteinuria developed as a function of time. In contrast, AG-treated rats (SD more than F344) retained significantly lower levels of urinary albumin:creatinine ratio ($p < 0.05$) and proteinuria ($p < 0.02$; F344, $p < 0.02$). Thus, in spite of the genetic variability, the AGE-inhibitor aminoguanidine, while maintaining reduced tissue glycotoxin levels, preserved normal blood pressure responses, and cardiac size and protected renal function, pointing to the importance of glycotoxin metabolism and turnover in the natural history of these disorders.

Lipid/lipoprotein modification by glycation enhances oxidation and atherogenesis

Recent studies have identified a new endogenous mechanism for the formation of proatherogenic, oxidized LDL, namely advanced glycation. AGE modification has been found on both the phospholipid and apolipoprotein components of LDL, based on an AGE-ELISA [39,40], together with increased lipid oxidation products, measured as MDA equivalents. More recently, GC-MS analyses have led to the identification of the specific fatty acid oxidation products 4-hydroxynonenal and 4-hydroxyhexenal as consequences of this reaction [41]. The inclusion of the advanced glycation inhibitor aminoguanidine blocked the increases in fluorescence, AGE formation and lipid oxidation products. Incubating purified

LDL with glucose also resulted in a time-dependent increase in LDL oxidation, which also was blocked by aminoguanidine. These observations recently led to the structural elucidation of a dideoxyosone as an AGE reactive intermediate [42,43] which has provided a potential conceptual framework for investigating the direct contribution of AGEs to oxidative chemistry. Lipid-linked dideoxyosones may rearrange to an electron accepting "piperidine dione" directly within the hydrophobic micro environment of phospholipids. Taken together, these observations provide important clues for beginning to understand how lipid-linked AGEs may play a role in the propagation of oxidative reactions in vivo, found markedly enhanced in senescence.

An important source for the latter — overlooked until now — has turned out to be the influx of exogenous, food-derived glycotoxins, present in Western diet, consumed by the general population [44] and in cigarette smoke [45,46]. These may well be found to represent a key mechanism accelerating age-related tissue damage and organ failure.

Anti-AGE strategies

Pharmacologic intervention of the glycoxidation pathway has been under evaluation. An important inhibitor of this process has been the nucleophilic compound aminoguanidine (Fig. 3). Known to be a potent and specific inhibitor of glucose-mediated cross-linking and tissue damage in vitro and in vivo [47]. The terminal amino group of aminoguanidine, by virtue of its low pKa, reacts specifically with glucose-derived reactive intermediates and prevents protein-protein or protein-lipid AGE cross-links from forming. This mechanism of action of aminoguanidine has now been confirmed in a number of studies, in which aminoguanidine was shown to prevent diabetes-related vascular complications in experimental animals [40,48—53]. From these extensive studies, it is apparent that aminoguanidine can be used to prevent advanced glycosylation and the AGE-mediated tissue in animal models of diabetes and aging. Of direct relevance to atherosclerosis, in a clinical study aminoguanidine caused a 28% decrease in LDL-cholesterol, a 20% decrease in total cholesterol and a 20% decrease in triglycerides [39]. Aminoguanidine and related advanced glycosylation inhibitors may eventually find widespread use in diabetics or in individuals at risk of age-

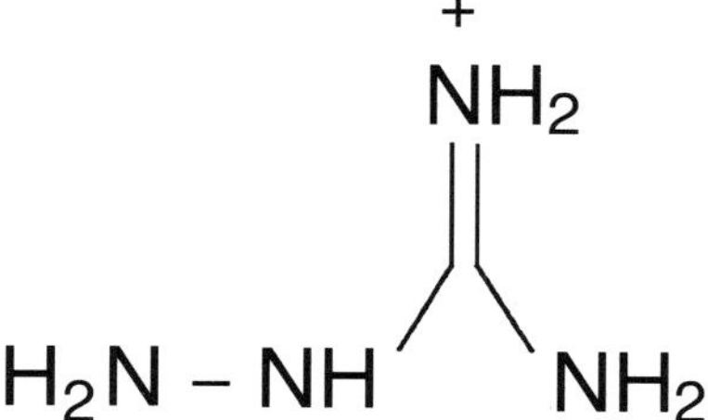

Fig. 3. The chemical structure of the AGE-inhibitor aminoguanidine.

related vascular sequelae. Development of aminoguanidine is now at phase II/III efficacy trials. A subsequently discovered agent, effective at "breaking" AGE cross-links is under intense investigation as it offers the promise of reversing a number of AGE-mediated adverse effects [54].

It has been recently suggested that individuals with high levels of AGE-LDL in serum may actually show enhanced AGE deposition in their vessel walls and are, therefore, at increased risk of atheroma formation [36]. High levels of circulating AGEs in nondiabetic and otherwise healthy adults may be a reflection of a dysfunction in AGE-receptor-mediated clearance mechanisms since receptor expression is likely to be highly variable. Therefore, early testing for AGE-related metabolic markers, such as AGE-ApoB [40,46] may prove prudent as an early warning to those persons that are especially at risk to complications, enabling timely adjustments in dietary and lifestyle prior to pharmacologic/invasive interventions.

References

1. Goldstein RS, Tarloff JB, Hook JB. Age-related nephropathy in laboratory rats. FASEB J 1988; 2:2241—2251.
2. McGill HC Jr, McMahan CA, Malcom GT, Oalmann C, Strong JP. Relation of glycohemoglobin and adiposity to atherosclerosis in youth: pathobiological determinants of atherosclerosis in youth (pday) research group. Arterioscl Thromb Vasc Biol 1995;15:431—440.
3. Strong JP, Malcom GT, Oalmann MC. Environmental and genetic risk factors in early human atherogenesis: lessons from the pday study, pathobiological determinants of atherosclerosis in youth. Pathol Int 1995;45:403—408.
4. Solberg LA, Ishii T, Strong JP, Guzman MA, Hosoda Y, Tsugane S, Newman WP III, Tracy RE. Comparison of coronary atherosclerosis in middle-aged Norwegian and Japanese men: an autopsy study. Lab Invest 1987;56:451—456.
5. Hornick CA, Baker HN, Malcom GT, Newman WP, Roheim PS, Strong JP. Lipoproteins and apolipoproteins in postmortem serum. Mod Pathol 1988;1:480—484.
6. Brownlee M, Cerami A, Vlassara H. Advanced glycosylation end products in tissue and the biochemical basis of diabetic complications. N Engl J Med 1988;318:1315—1321.
7. Vlassara H, Bucala R, Striker L. Pathogenic effects of advanced glycosylation: biochemical, biologic, and clinical implications for diabetes and aging. Lab Invest 1994;70:138—151.
8. Davies KJA, Weise AG, Sevanian A, Kim EH. Repair systems in oxidative stress. In: Finch CE, Johnson TE (eds) Molecular Biology of Aging. New York: Wiley-Liss, 1990;123—141.
9. Mackay W, Orr WC, Bewley GC. Genetic and molecular analysis of antioxidant enzymes in *Drosophila* melanogaster: A correlation between catalase activity levels, life span, and spontaneous mutation rate. In: Finch CE, Johnson TE (eds) Molecular Biology of Aging. New York: Wiley-Liss, 1990;157—170.
10. Lakatta EG, Cohen JD, Fleg JL, Frohlich ED, Gradman AH. Hypertension in the elderly: age- and disease-related complications and therapeutic implications. Cardiovasc Drug Ther 1993;7: 643—653.
11. Belz GG. Elastic properties and windkessel function of the human aorta. Cardiovasc Drug Ther 1995;9:73—83.
12. Rowe JW, Resnick NM. Disorders of the kidney and urinary tract. In: Andres R, Bierman EL, Hazzard WR (eds) Principles of Geriatric Medicine. New York: McGraw-Hill, 1995;614—628.
13. Bucala R, Vlassara H, Cerami A. Advanced glycosylation endproducts. In: Harding JJ, Crabbe MJC (eds) Post-Translational Modifications of Proteins. Boca Raton, Florida: CRC Press Inc.,

1992;53—59.

14. Lindeman RD, Tobin J, Shock NW. Longitudinal studies on the rate of decline in renal function with age. J Am Geriatr Soc 1985;33:278—285.

15. Sell DR, Monnier VM. Structure elucidation of a senescence crosslink from human extracellular matrix: implication of pentoses in the aging process. J Biol Chem 1989;264:21597—21602.

16. Eble AS, Thorpe SR, Baynes JW. Nonenzymatic glycosylation and glucose-dependent crosslinking of proteins. J Biol Chem 1983;258:9406—9412.

17. Brownlee M, Ponger S, Cerami A. Covalent attachment of soluble proteins by nonenzymatically glycosylated collagen: role in the in situ formation of immune complexes. J Exp Med 1983; 158:1739—1744.

18. Bucala R, Tracey KJ, Cerami A. Advanced glycosylation products quench nitric oxide and mediate defective endothelium-dependent vasodilatation in experimental diabetes. J Clin Invest 1991;87:432—438.

19. Vlassara H, Fuh H, Makita Z, Krungkrai S, Cerami A, Bucala R. Exogenous advanced glycosylation end products induce complex vascular dysfunction in normal animals: a model for diabetic and aging complications. Proc Natl Acad Sci USA 1992;89:12043—12047.

20. Vlassara H, Fuh H, Donnelly T, Cybulsky M. Advanced glycation endproducts promote adhesion molecule (vcam-1, icam-1) expression and atheroma formation in normal rabbits. Molec Med 1995;1:447—456.

21. Schmidt AM, Hori O, Chen JX, Li JF, Crandall J, Zhang J, Cao R, Yan SD, Brett J, Stern D. Advanced glycation endproducts interacting with their endothelial receptor induce expression of vascular cell adhesion molecule-1 (vcam-1) in cultured human endothelial cells and in mice: a potential mechanism for the accelerated vasculopathy of diabetes. J Clin Invest 1995; 96:1395—1403.

22. Esposito C, Gerlach H, Brett J, Stern D, Vlassara H. Endothelial receptor-mediated binding of glucose-modified albumin is associated with increased monolayer permeability and modulation of cell surface coagulant properties. J Exp Med 1989;170:1387—1407.

23. Vlassara H, Brownlee M, Cerami A. High-affinity receptor-mediated uptake and degradation of glucose-modified proteins: a potential mechanism for the removal of senescent macromolecules. Proc Natl Acad Sci USA 1985;82:5588—5592.

24. Vlassara H, Brownlee M, Cerami A. Novel macrophage receptor for glucose-modified proteins is distinct from previously described scavenger receptors. J Exp Med 1986;164:1301—1309.

25. Vlassara H, Brownlee M, Manogue KR, Dinarello CA, Pasagian A. Cachectin/tnf and il-1 induced by glucose-modified proteins: role in normal tissue remodeling. Science 1988;240: 1546—1548.

26. Kirstein M, Brett J, Radoff S, Ogawa S, Stern S, Vlassara H. Advanced protein glycosylation induces transendothelial human monocyte chemotaxis and secretion of platelet-derived growth factor: role in vascular disease of diabetes and aging. Proc Natl Acad Sci USA 1990;87: 9010—9014.

27. Kirstein M, Aston C, Hintz R, Vlassara H. Receptor-specific induction of insulin-like growth factor i in human monocytes by advanced glycosylation end product-modified proteins. J Clin Invest 1992;90:439—446.

28. Li YM, Mitsuhashi T, Wojciechowicz D, Shimizu N, Li J, Stitt A, He C, Banerjee D, Vlassara H. Molecular identity and cellular distribution of advanced glycation endproduct receptors: relationship of p60 to ost-48 and p90 to 80k-h membrane proteins. Proc Natl Acad Sci USA 1996; 93:11047—11052.

29. Schmidt AM, Vianna M, Gerlach M, Brett J, Ryan J, Kao J, Esposito C, Hegarty H, Hurley W, Clauss M et al. Isolation and characterization of two binding proteins for advanced glycosylation end products from bovine lung which are present on the endothelial cell surface. J Biol Chem 1992;267:14987—14997.

30. Neeper M, Schmidt AM, Brett J, Yan SD, Wang F, Pan YC, Elliston K, Stern D, Shaw A. Cloning and expression of a cell surface receptor for advanced glycosylation end products of proteins. J

Biol Chem 1992;267:14998—15004.
31. Li YM, Tan AX, Vlassara H. Antibacterial activity of lysozyme and lactoferrin is inhibited by binding of advanced glycation-modified proteins to a conserved motif (see comments). Nat Med 1995;1:1057—1061.
32. Makita Z, Radoff S, Rayfield EJ, Yang Z, Skolnik E, Friedman EA, Cerami A, Vlassara H. Advanced glycation endproducts in patients with diabetic nephropathy. N Engl J Med 1991; 325:836—842.
33. Makita Z, Bucala R, Rayfield EJ, Friedman EA, Kaufman AM, Korbet SM, Barth RH, Winston JA, Fuh H, Manogue KR et al. Reactive glycosylation endproducts in diabetic uraemia and treatment of renal failure. Lancet 1994;343:1519—1522.
34. Gugliucci A, Bendayan M. Renal fate of circulating advanced glycated end products (AGE): evidence for reabsorption and catabolism of AGE-peptides by renal proximal tubular cells. Diabetologica 1996;39:149—160.
35. He CJ, Li YM, Liu C, Mitsuhashi T, Vlassara H. Oral absorption, turnover and renal clearance of dietary glycotixins (reactive AGEs) in the rat. J Am Soc Nephrol 1996;7:1870—1871 (Abstract).
36. Stitt AW, Friedman S, Scher L, Rossi P, Ong H, Founds H, Bucala R, Vlassara H. Carotid artery advanced glycation endproducts and their receptors correlate with severity of lesion and with plasma AGE-ApoB levels in nondiabetic patients. 1996 FASEB Meeting (Abstract).
37. Zimmerman GA, Meistrell M III, Bloom O, Cockroft KM, Bianchi M, Risucci D, Broome J, Farmer P, Cerami A, Vlassara H et al. Neurotoxicity of advanced glycation endproducts during focal stroke and neuroprotective effects of aminoguanidine. Proc Natl Acad Sci USA 1995; 92:3744—3748.
38. Li YM, Steffes M, Donnelly T, Liu C, Fuh H, Basgen J, Bucala R, Vlassara H. Prevention of cardiovascular and renal pathology of aging by the advanced glycation inhibitor aminoguanidine. Proc Natl Acad Sci USA 1996;93:3902—3907.
39. Bucala R, Makita Z, Vega G, Grundy S, Koschinsky T, Cerami A, Vlassara H. Modification of low-density lipoprotein by advanced glycation end products contributes to the dyslipidemia of diabetes and renal insufficiency. Proc Natl Acad Sci USA 1994;91:9441—9445.
40. Bucala R, Makita Z, Koschinsky T, Cerami A, Vlassara H. Lipid advanced glycosylation: pathway for lipid oxidation in vivo. Proc Natl Acad Sci USA 1993;90:6434—6438.
41. Al-Abed Y, Liebich H, Voelter W, Bucala R. Hydroxyalkenal formation induced by advanced glycosylation of low-density lipoprotein. J Biol Chem 1996;271:2892—2896.
42. Pokorny J. Browning from lipid-protein interactions. Prog Ed Nutr Sci 1981;5:421—428.
43. Zhang X, Ulrich P. Directed approached to reactive Maillard intermediates: Formation of a novel 3-alkylamino-2-hydroxy-4 hydroxymethyl-2-cyclopenten-1-one ("cypentodine"). Tetrahedron Lett 1996;7:4667—4670.
44. Koschinsky T, He C, Mitsuhashi T, Bucala R, Liu C, Buenting C, Heitmann K, Vlassara H. Orally absorbed reactive glycation products (glycotoxins)-A potential risk factor in diabetic nephropathy. PNAS 1997;94:6474—6479.
45. Founds HW, Giordano D, Mitsuhashi T, Stitt AW, Finch G, Cerami A, Vlassara H, Bucala R. Tobacco smoke is a source of advanced glycation endproducts (AGEs): possible role in the accelerated vascular disease of smokers. J Clin Invest 1996;44:200A (Abstract).
46. Cerami C, Founds H, Nicholl I, Mitsuhashi T, Giordano D, VanPatten S, Lee A, Al-Abed Y, Vlassara H, Bucala R, Cerami A. Tobacco smoke is a source of toxic reactive glycation products. PNAS 1998;(In press).
47. Brownlee M, Vlassara H, Cerami A. Nonenzymatic glycosylation products on collagen covalently trap low-density lipoprotein. Diabetes 1985;34:938—941.
48. Nicholls K, Mandel TE. Advanced glycosylation end-products in experimental murine diabetic nephropathy: effect of islet isografting and of aminoguanidine. Lab Invest 1989;60:486—491.
49. Ellis EN, Good BH. Prevention of glomerular basement membrane thickening by aminoguanidine in experimental diabetes mellitus. Metabolism 1991;40:1016—1019.

50. Soulis-Liparota T, Cooper M, Papazoglou D, Clarke B, Jerums G. Retardation by aminoguanidine of development of albuminuria, mesangial expansion, and tissue fluorescence in streptozocin-induced diabetic rat. Diabetes 1991;40:1328—1334.
51. Edelstein D, Brownlee M. Mechanistic studies of advanced glycosylation end product inhibition by aminoguanidine. Diabetes 1992;41:26—29.
52. Cho HK, Kozu H, Peyman GA, Parry GJ, Khoobehi B. The effect of aminoguanidine on the blood-retinal barrier in streptozotocin-induced diabetic rats. Ophthalmic Surg 1991;22:44—47.
53. Hammes HP, Martin S, Federlin K, Geisen K, Brownlee M. Aminoguanidine treatment inhibits the development of experimental diabetic retinopathy (published erratum appears in Proc Natl Acad Sci USA 1992;89(19):9364). Proc Natl Acad Sci USA 1991;88:11555—11558.
54. Vasan S, Zhang X, Zhang X, Kapurniotu A, Bernhagen J, Teichberg S, Basgen J, Wagle D, Shih D, Terlecky I, Bucala R, Cerami A, Egan J, Ulrich P. An agent cleaving glucose-derived protein crosslinks in vitro and in vivo. Nature 1996;382:275—278.
55. Stitt AW, He C, Friedman S, Scher L, Rossi P, Ong L, Founds H, Li YM, Bucala R, Vlassara H. Elevated AGE-modified ApoB in sera of euglycemic, normolipidemic patients with atherosclerosis: relationship to tissue AGEs. Molec Med 1997;3:617—627.

Receptor-dependent interaction of native and modified lipoproteins with liver: a concerted action of various cell types

Theo J.C. van Berkel, Johan K. Kruijt, Patrick C.N. Rensen, Kees Fluiter, Agnes van Velzen, Carla J.M. Vogelezang and Bertjan Ziere
Division of Biopharmaceutics, Leiden/Amsterdam Center for Drug Research, Sylvius Laboratories, Leiden, The Netherlands

Abstract. Apolipoprotein E (apoE) is an important determinant for the liver uptake of triglyceride-rich lipoproteins and exerts affinity for both the low-density lipoprotein (LDL) receptor and a liver-specific non-LDL-receptor recognition system. The mechanism underlying the receptor-specificity of apoE-carrying lipoproteins was investigated in wild-type vs. LDL-receptor knock-out mice by using human recombinant apoE and triglyceride-rich emulsions of 50, 80 and 150 nm. The serum decay, tissue distribution and the intrahepatic processing of the large emulsion were independent of the LDL-receptor, while the serum decay and liver uptake of the small emulsion was 6- to 8-fold retarded in the knock-out mice. It is concluded that particle size determines the metabolic behaviour and the receptor-specificity of chylomicrons. HDL cholesteryl esters (HDL-CE) are selectively taken up by liver parenchymal cells without parallel apolipoprotein uptake. In vitro competition experiments with isolated liver parenchymal cells show that acetylated LDL (Ac-LDL) and oxidized LDL (OxLDL) did inhibit HDL-CE uptake by 35 and 80%, respectively. The inhibition profile of the selective uptake of HDL-CE in liver parenchymal cells suggests that in the liver scavenger receptor B1 is responsible for the efficient uptake of HDL-CE.

Introduction

Apolipoprotein E (apoE), a 34-kDa glycoprotein, plays a key role in the hepatic metabolism of triglyceride-rich lipoproteins such as chylomicrons, very low density lipoproteins (VLDL) [1], and emulsions [2]. Within the blood compartment, triglyceride-rich lipoproteins are converted into remnants through the hydrolysis of core triglycerides by lipoprotein lipase (LPL) [3] and the concomitant enrichment with apoE. These remnants are subsequently taken up by the liver, but the precise mechanism of recognition is still unclear. Various apoE-recognizing systems have been proposed to participate in remnant removal, including the LDL (apoB, E) receptor (LDLr) [4], a distinct specific apoE receptor [5], the low-density receptor-related protein/α_2-macroglobulin receptor (LRP) [6], heparan sulfate proteoglycans (HSPG) [7], as well as LPL [8] and hepatic lipase (HL) [9] in concert with proteoglycans and/or LRP. Whereas the lipases (LPL and HL) and proteoglycans may be involved in the initial low-affinity binding of remnants to the liver, the dominant role of both the LDLr and a distinct receptor (possibly LRP) in endocytosis of remnants has been clearly demonstrated [10].

Address for correspondence: Theo van Berkel, Division of Biopharmaceutics, Leiden/Amsterdam Center for Drug Research, Sylvius Laboratories, P.O. Box 9503, 2300 RA Leiden, The Netherlands.

The existence of an apoE-recognizing receptor in addition to the LDLr has been suggested by several independent lines of evidence [11]. Chylomicron remnants appeared not to accumulate in Watanabe heritable hyperlipidemic (WHHL) rabbits [11], LDLr knockout mice or human familial hypercholesterolemia homozygotes [12].

At present, it is still unclear which factor(s) determine(s) the specificity of remnants for the different receptor systems in vivo. Recently, we described a triglyceride-rich apolipoprotein-free emulsion model of native chylomicrons with well-defined physicochemical characteristics [2]. Upon intravenous injection into rats, the emulsion was extensively processed by LPL [13], acquired apolipoproteins (e.g., apoE and apoCs) and was subsequently taken up by liver parenchymal cells via lactoferrin-sensitive apoE-specific receptors, similar to endogenous chylomicrons. The rate of liver uptake was greatly increased by preloading the emulsion with recombinant (rec-) apoE. We fractionated this emulsion into well-defined size populations in order to evaluate the effects of emulsion size vs. composition on the relative roles of the LDLr and the distinct apoE-specific receptor in the hepatic clearance. We used wild-type vs. LDLr knockout mice, allowing unequivocal evaluation of the role of the LDLr.

The mechanism of selective uptake of cholesteryl esters from HNL (HDL-CE) is largely unestablished. It is restricted to the adrenals, ovary and liver [14], while within the liver the parenchymal cells are solely responsible for the selective uptake of HDL-CE [15,16]. Rinninger et al. [17] showed that there are distinct sites on liver parenchymal cells for the binding of the protein moiety of HDL and selective CE uptake.

Recently, Acton et al. [18] provided evidence that scavenger receptor class B (SR-B1) (a member of the CD 36 family) not only mediates HDL binding but also selective CE uptake in vitro with murine-SR-B1 transfected CHO cells. SR-B1 was found to bind a broad spectrum of ligands, including modified lipoproteins, native lipoproteins and anionic phospholipids [18]. However, scavenger class B receptors do not bind the broad array of polyanions (e.g., fucoidin, polyinosinic acid) which are classical ligands for scavenger class A receptors. In vivo, SR-B1 is expressed mainly in the adrenals, ovary and to a much lesser extent in the liver of rats and mice [19]. In the present work we also studied the potential role of SR-B1 in the selective uptake of HDL-CE by rat liver parenchymal.

Results and Discussion

Effect of particle size on the interaction with the LDL receptor vs. the remnant receptor

The differential ultracentrifugation procedure from Redgrave and Maranhao [20] was used to divide the initial emulsion into three populations, based on their particle-size-dependent flotation properties. The size and composition of the emulsion fractions are summarized in Table 1. The average particle size of the emul-

Table 1. Size, electrophoretic mobility and lipid composition of emulsion fractions.

	Emulsion fraction		
	1	2	3
Mean diameter (nm)	152.3 ± 7.0	80.0 ± 2.4	47.8 ± 1.7
R_f on agarose	0.09 ± 0.01	0.16 ± 0.01	0.14 ± 0.01
Composition (%w/w)			
Triolein	84.1 ± 0.8	78.1 ± 0.6	67.7 ± 2.4
Phosphatidylcholine	10.5 ± 0.6	15.4 ± 0.7	26.9 ± 2.2
Cholesteryl oleate	2.8 ± 0.3	4.2 ± 0.3	2.6 ± 0.3
Cholesterol	2.6 ± 0.4	2.4 ± 0.1	2.8 ± 0.1

Emulsions were obtained by sonication of a lipid mixture (triolein: egg yolk phosphatidylcholine: lysophosphatidylcholine: cholesteryl oleate: cholesterol = 70: 22.7: 2.3: 3.0: 2.0, w/w), subdivided into three fractions by differential ultracentrifugation, the mean particle size (mean ± SE; n = 11), electrophoretic mobility (R_f) on agarose (mean ± SD; n = 3), and composition (mean ± SE; n = 4—6) of the fractions were determined.

sion fractions decreased with increasing fraction number.

In order to assess the relative contribution of the LDLr to the in vivo clearance of the three emulsion fractions, the kinetics of the emulsions were determined in both LDLr (+/+) and LDLr (−/−) mice (Fig. 1). The absence of the LDLr in LDLr (−/−) mice was functionally verified by the 2.6-fold increased serum half-life of human ^{125}I-LDL (9.1 ± 0.6 h) as compared to that in wild-type mice (3.5 ± 0.3 h).

Upon injection of the emulsions into LDLr (+/+) mice, the in vivo kinetics were again highly size-dependent, with the serum half-lives being <2 min (fraction 1), 32.0 ± 2.0 min (2), and 47.6 ± 7.6 min (3). Accordingly, 64 ± 7% (fraction 1), 52 ± 2% (2), and 41 ± 3% (3) of the injected doses were taken up by the liver at 30 min after injection (Fig. 1). The effects of the particle size on the serum clearance and liver uptake are clearly expressed within LDLr (−/−) mice. Whereas the serum half-life of the large emulsion (<2 min) did not differ from that observed in LDLr (+/+) mice, 3.1- and 7.8-fold increased half-lives were observed for the medium-sized (97.5 ± 7.8 min) and small (371.2 ± 42.7 min) emulsion, respectively. Accordingly, the liver uptake of the large emulsion (69 ± 2%) was not altered, but was reduced by 1.7- and 5.9-fold for the medium-sized (30 ± 8%) and small emulsion (7 ± 1%), respectively, at 30 min after injection.

At present, the mechanism for the hepatic uptake of triglyceride-rich lipoprotein remnants is still under active discussion. It is now generally accepted that the LDLr can contribute to the clearance of both VLDL (remnants) and chylomicrons in animals. However, its relative importance as compared to uptake systems that are not related to the LDLr, and the mechanism that determines LDLr vs. non-LDLr (remnant receptor) mediated uptake are unclear.

In this study we investigated the factor(s) that determine(s) the specificity of triglyceride-rich lipoproteins (remnants) for both the LDLr and non-LDLr uptake

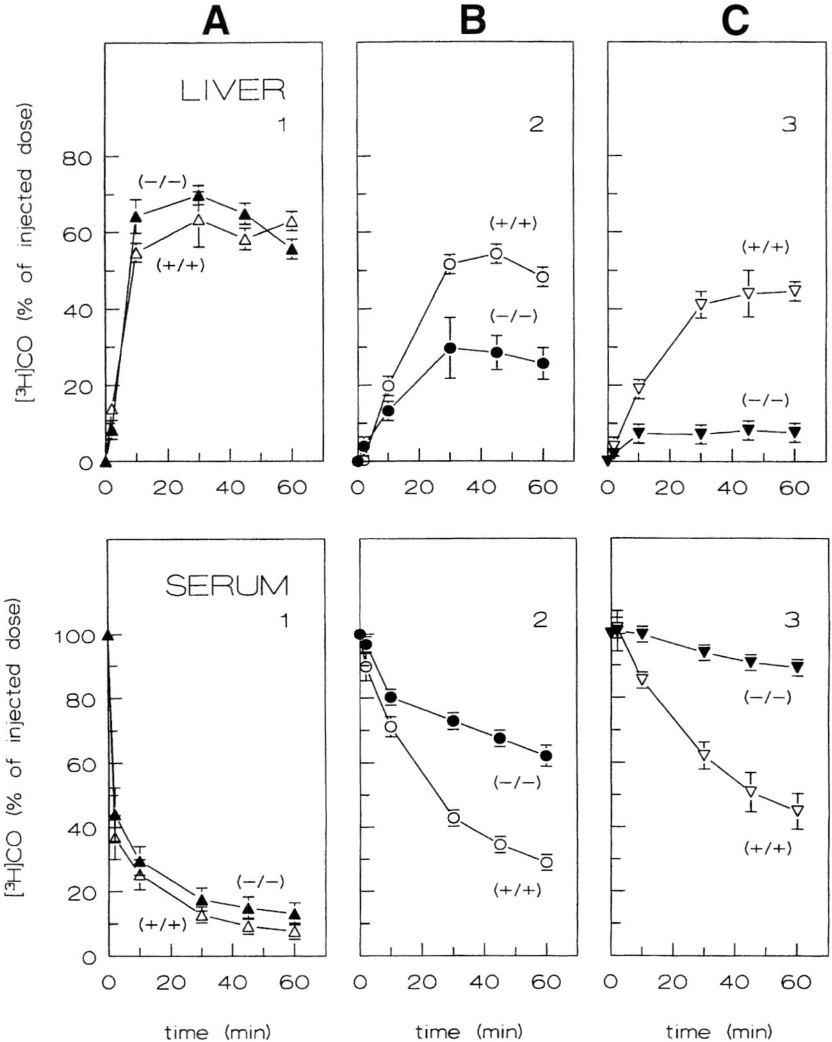

Fig. 1. Liver uptake and serum decay of the emulsion fractions in mice. [³H]Cholesteryl oleate labeled emulsion fraction 1 (**A**), 2 (**B**) and 3 (**C**) (150 μg of emulsion-triglyceride) were injected into fasted anesthetized wild-type (+/+) (open symbols) and LDLr (−/−) (closed symbols) mice. At the indicated times, the liver uptake (top) and serum decay (bottom) were determined. Liver values are corrected for serum radioactivity. Values are means ± variation (fraction 2; n = 2) or SE (fraction 1 and 3; n = 3−6).

site(s) in vivo using a defined emulsion model of chylomicrons, which was fractionated into homogeneous size populations with mean diameters of about 50, 80, and 150 nm. Taken together with the size-dependent liver uptake patterns and serum kinetics, it is clear that the affinity of emulsions for this recognition site (termed the remnant receptor) decreases as the particle size decreases without induction of extrahepatic uptake. Using both wild-type and LDLr $(-/-)$ mice, we demonstrate that the contribution of the LDLr to emulsion clearance increases with decreasing particle size, as is evident from the association of emulsions with the liver. In fact, whereas the in vivo behaviour of the large emulsion is virtually independent of the LDLr, the behaviour of the small emulsion appeared almost completely dependent on the presence of the LDLr.

Elucidation of the nature of the (non-LDLr) initial recognition system, which is responsible for the high liver association rate of the large emulsion, was not primarily aimed at by our present experiments. Possible sites include:
1) the LRP,
2) proteoglycans,
3) lipases such as LPL and HL in concert with proteoglycans and/or LRP, and
4) a remnant receptor of an unidentified nature.

In conclusion, the present data can explain the long-term discrepancy between various research groups with respect to the appreciation of the relative role of the LDLr in the clearance of triglyceride-rich lipoproteins, as these groups used a wide variety of substrates mostly with a heterogenous size distribution. Our data demonstrate unambiguously that the particle size of triglyceride-rich emulsions determines receptor specificity. Whereas small emulsions directly interact with the LDLr, possibly dependent on a favourable apoE conformation and/or apoE:C ratio, the hepatic uptake of the large emulsion is not dependent on this receptor. The concerted action of apoE and lipases (i.e., LPL and HL) may result in the initial association of large emulsions to hepatic HSPG, which is coupled to endocytosis as mediated by LRP and/or an as yet unidentified remnant receptor.

Role of SR-B1 in the selective uptake of HDL-cholesteryl esters

As mentioned in the introduction, the mechanism of selective uptake of HDL-CE in liver is largely unestablished. We studied the ability of (modified) lipoproteins to inhibit the selective cholesteryl ester uptake, while also the effect on ^{125}I-HDL association was studied.

The ability of (modified) lipoproteins to compete for [^{125}I]-HDL and [^{3}H]2CE-HDL association was tested by coincubation with either 100 µg of protein/ml unlabeled HDL, LDL, AcLDL or OxLDL (Fig. 2). Both HDL particle association, as measured by [^{125}I]-HDL association, and [^{3}H]-CE HDL association were inhibited for approximately 50% when 100 µg/ml unlabeled apoE-free HDL protein was added. Further inhibition of both [^{125}I]-HDL association and [^{3}H]CE-HDL association up to 75% could be achieved by increasing the excess of unlabeled HDL to 500 µg/ml (data not shown). In contrast to HDL, addition of either 100 µg of /ml LDL protein or modified LDL protein did only marginally ($<10\%$) decrease the cell association of [^{125}I]-HDL. [^{3}H]CE-HDL association was approximately 20% decreased by addition of LDL. However, addition

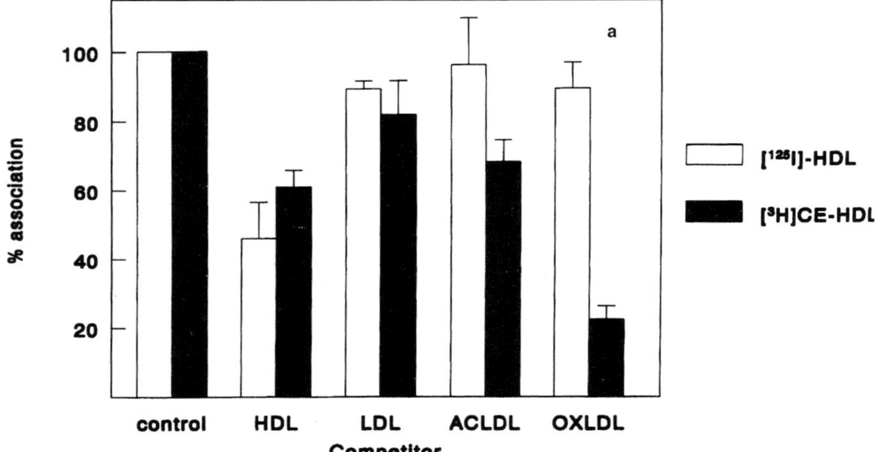

Fig. 2. Effect of native and modified lipoproteins on the parenchymal cell association of [^{125}I]- or [^{3}H]-Ch18:1 labeled HDL. Rat liver parenchymal cells were incubated for 3 h at 37°C with 10 μg/ml labeled HDL in the absence or presence of 100 μg protein/ml of unlabeled competing lipoproteins in DMEM with 2% BSA. The 100% value for association of [^{3}H]-Ch18:1 labeled HDL was 202 ± 14 ng HDL/mg cell protein and for [^{125}I]-HDL association was 36 ± 3 ng HDL/mg cell protein. The association is expressed as the percentage of the radioactivity obtained in the absence of competitor. The results are given as means ± SEM (of three separate cell isolations). [a]Indicates significant difference between the value and the control; p < 0.005 (unpaired Student's t test).

of AcLDL led to a significant inhibition of 35% (p < 0.005) while OxLDL decreased [^{3}H]CE-HDL association up to 80%.

Effect of OxLDL on selective HDL-CE uptake

The inhibitory effect of OxLDL on the the selective uptake of HDL-CE was further analyzed with respect to efficiency of competition. Increasing concentrations of OxLDL were added to freshly isolated parenchymal cells in the presence of [^{3}H]Ch18:1 labeled HDL. Already at 20 μg/ml OxLDL protein the association of HDL-CE was inhibited for more than 50% (Fig. 3). Poly I, an established inhibitor of scavenger receptor class A, did not lower the cell association of [^{125}I]-HDL or [^{3}H]Ch18:1 HDL, but instead increased both particle association and CE association. The simultaneous presence of increasing concentrations of OxLDL and 100 μg/ml poly I did not influence the inhibitory action of OxLDL, indicating that the effect of OxLDL was not due to interaction with a poly I sensitive site.

Apparently, scavenger-receptor class A is not involved, since the OxLDL mediated inhibition of HDL-CE uptake by rat liver parenchymal cells was not dependent on a poly I sensitive site. Therefore, we specifically studied the role of the scavenger class B receptors by analysing the effect of anionic phospholipid

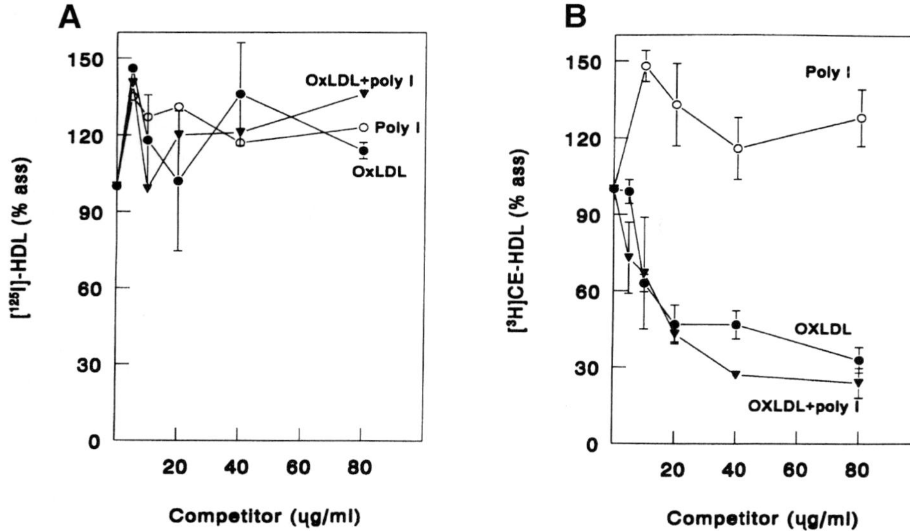

Fig. 3. Effect of increasing concentrations of OxLDL and poly I on the parenchymal cell association of (**A**) [^{125}I] or (**B**) [^{3}H]-Ch18:1 labeled HDL. Rat liver parenchymal cells were incubated for 3 h at 37°C with 10 µg/ml labeled HDL in the presence of the indicated amounts of OxLDL and when indicated poly I (100 µg/ml). The association is expressed as the percentage of the radioactivity obtained in the absence of competitor. The 100% value for association of [^{3}H]-Ch18:1 labeled HDL without competitor was 202 ± 14 ng HDL/mg cell protein and for [^{125}I]-HDL without competitor, association was 36 ± 3 ng HDL/mg cell protein. The results are given as means ± SEM (of three separate cell isolations).

liposomes. These liposomes do effectively interact with scavenger class B receptors. Liposomes consisting of phosphatidylcholine, cholesterol and the anionic phospholipid phosphatidylserine inhibited HDL-CE association for 40% (Table 2) while [^{125}I]-HDL association was increased. Neutral liposomes, consisting

Table 2. Effect of phosphatidyl serine liposomes and neutral liposomes on the cell association of ^{125}I or [^{3}H]-Ch18:1 labeled HDL.

	^{125}I-HDL	[^{3}H]Ch18:1-HDL
Control	100	100
N-lipo	105 ± 4	100 ± 20
PS-lipo	150 ± 30	58.3 ± 7[a]

Rat liver parenchymal cells were incubated for 3 h at 37°C with 10 µg/ml labeled HDL in the absence or presence of liposomes (100 µg phospholipid/ml) in DMEM with 2% BSA. The 100% value for association of [^{3}H]Ch18:1 labeled HDL was 202 ± 14 ng HDL/mg cell protein and for [^{125}I] − HDL association was 36 ± 3 ng HDL/mg cell protein. The association is expressed as the percentage of the radioactivity obtained in the absence of competitor. The results are given as mean ± SEM (of three separate cell isolations). [a]Indicates significant difference between the value and the control; p < 0.005 (unpaired Student's t test).

only of phosphatidylcholine and cholesterol, did not influence HDL-CE association.

Selective delivery of CE from HDL to the liver is an important direct route for reverse cholesterol transport. The precise mechanism of this selective uptake and the cellular mediators is not known. SR-B1 might be involved in this process, but until now direct involvement of SR-B1 in reverse cholesterol transport has not been shown. Unlike scavenger class A receptors, SR-B1 is insensitive for polyanions like poly I. The selective uptake of HDL-CE by liver parenchymal cells is completely blocked by the presence of OxLDL, while also anionic phospholipids and to a lesser extent AcLDL are effective inhibitors. It can be calculated that OxLDL inhibits the selective uptake of HDL-CE nearly completely, as the residual association of HDL-CE equals particle association as measured with $[^{125}I]$-HDL. It thus appears that the selective HDL-CE uptake by rat liver parenchymal cells is mediated by a recognition site which possesses recognition properties characteristic for SR-B1. The finding that the inhibitory effect of OxLDL on HDL-CE uptake was not influenced by the simultaneous presence of poly I is consistent with the characteristic property of SR-B1, which unlike the other scavenger receptor classes is insensitive to poly I.

In conclusion, our present data provide the first evidence that the selective uptake route of HDL-CE in rat parenchymal cells can be inhibited by competitors of SR-B1. Although SR-B1 is expressed in liver at a lower concentration than in the adrenals or ovary, the relatively high amount of liver mass and its high efficiency, suggests an important function in the liver uptake of HDL-CE and thus in reverse cholesterol transport.

References

1. Weisgraber KH. Apolipoprotein E: structure-function relationships. Adv Protein Chem 1994; 45:249–302.
2. Rensen PCN, Van Dijk MCM, Havenaar EC, Bijsterbosch MK, Kruijt JK, van Berkel ThJC. Selective liver targeting of antivirals by recombinant chylomicrons — a new therapeutic approach to hepatitis B. Nat Med 1995;1:221–225.
3. Osborne JC, Bengtsson-Olivecrona Jrg, Lee NS, Olivecrona T. Studies on inactivation of lipoprotein lipase: role of the dimer to monomer dissociation. Biochemistry 1985;24:5606–5611.
4. Windler EET, Greeve J, Daerr WH, Greten H. Binding of rat chylomicrons and their remnants to the hepatic low-density-lipoprotein receptor and its role in remnant removal. Biochem J 1988;252:553–561.
5. Herz J, Qiu SQ, Oesterle A, DeSilva HV, Shafi S, Havel RJ. Initial hepatic removal of chylomicron remnants is unaffected but endocytosis is delayed in mice lacking the low density lipoprotein receptor. Proc Natl Acad Sci USA 1995;92:4611–4615.
6. Ziere GJ, van der Kaaden ME, Vogelezang CJM, Boers W, Bihain BE, Kuiper J, Kruijt JK, van Berkel ThJC. Blockade of the α_2-macroglobulin receptor/low-density-lipoprotein-receptor-related protein on rat liver parenchymal cells by the 39-kDa receptor-associated protein leaves the interaction of β-migrating very-low-density lipoprotein with the lipoprotein remnant receptor unaffected. Eur J Biochem 1996;242:703–711.
7. Herz J, Hamann U, Rogne S, Myklebost O, Gausepohl H, Stanley KK. Surface location and high affinity for calcium of a 500-kd liver membrane protein closely related to the LDL-receptor

suggest a physiological role as lipoprotein receptor. EMBO J 1988; 7:4119—4127.

8. Beisiegel U, Weber W, Bengtsson-Olivecrona G. Lipoprotein lipase enhances the binding of chylomicrons to low density lipoprotein receptor-related protein. Proc Natl Acad Sci USA 1991; 88:8342—8346.

9. Shafi S, Brady SE, Bensadoun A, Havel RJ. Role of hepatic lipase in the uptake and processing of chylomicron remnants in rat liver. J Lipid Res 1994;35:709—720.

10. De Faria E, Fong LG, Komaromy M, Cooper AD. Relative roles of the LDL receptor, the LDL receptor-like protein, and hepatic lipase in chylomicron remnant removal by the liver. J Lipid Res 1996;37:197—209.

11. Kita T, Goldstein JL, Brown MS, Watanabe Y, Hornick CA, Havel RJ. Hepatic uptake of chylomicron remnants in WHHL rabbits: a mechanism genetically distinct from the low density lipoprotein receptor. Proc Natl Acad Sci USA 1982;79:3623—3627.

12. Goldstein JL, Brown MS. Familial hypercholesterolemia. In: Scriver CR, Beaudet AL, Sly WS, Valle D (eds) The Metabolic Basis of Inherited Disease. New York: McGraw-Hill, 1989; 1215—1250.

13. Rensen PCN, van Berkel ThJC. Apolipoprotein E effectively inhibits lipoprotein lipase-mediated lipolysis of chylomicron-like triglyceride-rich lipid emulsions in vitro and in vivo. J Biol Chem 1996;271:14791—14799.

14. Pittman RCC, Knecht TP, Rosenbaum MS, Taylor CI Jr. A nonendocytotic mechanism for the selective uptake of high density lipoprotein-associated cholesterol esters. J Biol Chem 1987; 262:2443—2450.

15. Fluiter K, Vietsch H, Biessen EAL, Kostner GM, van Berkel ThJC, Sattler W. Increased selective uptake in vivo and in vitro of oxidised cholesteryl esters from high density lipoprotein by rat liver parenchymal cells. Biochem J 1996;319:471—476.

16. Pieters MN, Schouten D, Bakkeren HF, Esbach B, Brouwer A, Knook DL, van Berkel ThJC. Selective uptake of cholesteryl esters from apolipoprotein-E-free high-density lipoproteins by rat parenchymal cells in vivo is efficiently coupled to bile acid synthesis. Biochem J 1991;280: 359—365.

17. Rinninger F, Jaeckle S, Greten H, Windler E. Selective association of lipoprotein cholesteryl esters with liver plasma membranes. Biochim Biophys Acta 1993;1166:284—299.

18. Acton S, Rigotti A, Landschulz KT, Xu S, Hobbs HH, Krieger M. Identification of scavenger receptor SR-BI as a high density lipoprotein receptor. Science 1996;271:518—520.

19. Landschulz KT, Pathak RK, Rigotti A, Krieger M, Hobbs HH. Regulation of scavenger receptor, class B, type I, a high density lipoprotein receptor, in liver and steroidogenic tissues of the rat. J Clin Invest 1996;98:984—995.

20. Redgrave TG, Maranhao RC. Metabolism of protein-free lipid emulsion models of chylomicrons in rats. Biochim Biophys Acta 1985;835:104—112.

Atherosclerosis XI.
B. Jacotot, D. Mathé and J.-C. Fruchart, editors.

Expanding roles for apolipoprotein E in health and disease

Robert W. Mahley
Departments of Pathology and Medicine, Cardiovascular Research Institute, Gladstone Institute of Cardiovascular Disease, San Francisco, California, USA

Abstract. Apolipoprotein E is a major component of plasma lipid metabolism. Recent studies have also identified a significant role for apolipoprotein E in neurobiology. This review summarizes the structural and functional studies that have provided considerable insight into the involvement of this protein in neurobiology and Alzheimer's disease, as well as lipid metabolism.

Keywords: Alzheimer's disease, lipoproteins, neurobiology.

Introduction

Apolipoprotein (apo-) E, a key component of lipid metabolism, has been the subject of considerable research for its role in cardiovascular disease. Recent discoveries have revealed an additional role for apo-E in neurobiology and Alzheimer's disease (AD). An understanding of the structure and function of this important protein is likely to be valuable in order to progress against these two major diseases.

Apolipoprotein E occurs as three major allelic forms with differences at only two amino acid positions. The most common isoform, apo-E3, contains cysteine and arginine at positions 112 and 158, respectively. Apolipoprotein E2 has cysteine at both sites, and apo-E4 has arginine at both sites (for review [1—3]). Each isoform has its own physical and physiological characteristics and each is associated with different human disorders. Apolipoprotein E2 preferentially binds to small, phospholipid-rich high-density lipoproteins (HDL), has defective receptor binding and is associated with type III hyperlipoproteinemia. Apolipoprotein E4 interacts preferentially with large, triglyceride-rich very low density lipoproteins (VLDL) and has normal receptor binding compared to apo-E3. More recently, apo-E4 has been identified as a risk factor for AD [4—6].

Cellular uptake of lipoproteins

As one of several apolipoproteins associated with VLDL, intermediate density lipoproteins (IDL), chylomicron remnants and certain subclasses of HDL, apo-E participates in the clearance of these lipoproteins from the plasma by mediat-

---

Address for correspondence: Robert W. Mahley MD, PhD, Gladstone Institute of Cardiovascular Disease, P.O. Box 419100, San Francisco, CA 94141-9100, USA. Tel.: +1-415-826-7500. Fax: +1-415-285-5632.

ing their binding to specific cell-surface receptors (including the low-density lipoprotein (LDL) receptor related protein (LRP), cell-surface heparan sulfate proteoglycans (HSPG), and the newly described VLDL receptor) [1]. Cellular uptake of lipoproteins containing apo-E occurs by one of two pathways. The first pathway involves a direct interaction of apo-E with the LDL receptor. The second is a two-step process involving the LRP and HSPG. The HSPG-LRP pathway is initiated by the interaction of the apo-E-containing lipoproteins with cell-surface HSPG. The HSPG-bound lipoproteins are then transferred to the LRP. The LRP-HSPG-lipoprotein complex is internalized by the cell. Alternatively, but less likely, the LRP may initiate the uptake without the HSPG involvement. Under certain conditions, it seems that the HSPG can mediate lipoprotein uptake alone.

Apolipoprotein E structure and domain interaction

The structure of apo-E is intimately involved with its function (for review [3]). Apolipoprotein E has two structural domains which are joined by a short hinge region of about 20–30 amino acids. The amino-terminal domain (residues 1–191, 22 kDa) accounts for about two-thirds of the molecule and contains the receptor-binding region. Six to eight critical arginine and lysine residues and a histidine residue in the region of amino acids 136–150 mediate the interaction with the ligand-binding domain of the LDL receptor. Most likely, the same residues also mediate binding to the LRP and the VLDL receptors, since regions in these receptors are highly homologous with the ligand-binding domains of the LDL receptor. As determined by X-ray crystallography, the amino-terminal domain contains five α-helices, four of which are arranged in an antiparallel four-helix bundle. The carboxyl-terminal domain (residues 216–299, 10 kDa) accounts for the remaining one-third of the molecule and contains the major lipid-binding region (residues 244–272). The structure of the carboxyl-terminal domain is less clear but is predicted to contain primarily α-helices.

The great differences in the structural and physiological characteristics of apo-E3 and apo-E4 seem incongruous with the single amino acid difference between them. It is even more remarkable that the amino acid difference occurs in the amino-terminal domain, whereas the major lipid-binding region where the difference is manifested, is in the carboxyl-terminal domain. Early clues to this apparent mystery came from comparative studies of the apo-E from various species. Arginine at position 61 is a distinguishing feature of human apo-E. The apo-Es of other species have threonine at position 61 and preferentially associate with HDL. This suggested that arginine-61 preferentially directs apo-E to the large VLDL particles [7,8].

Recent studies by Dong and Weisgraber [9] support a model in which arginine-61 is implicated as a key residue in a domain-domain interaction that alters lipoprotein-binding preference. They constructed internal deletion mutants of apo-E4 that eliminated increasing portions of the hinge region. While deletion of the residues 186—202 or 186—223 had no effect, deletion of residues 186—244 resulted in a loss of VLDL binding. They further hypothesized that a specific acidic residue in the carboxyl terminus interacts with arginine-61. To identify that residue, they substituted alanine for each of the six acidic residues in that region and tested the mutants for their lipid-binding preferences. Only substitution of glutamic acid 255 changed the preference of apo-E4 from VLDL to HDL. The arginine at position 112 causes a conformational change in the protein so that arginine-61 forms a salt bridge with glutamic acid 255 and results in domain interaction. In contrast, apo-E3 with cysteine in position 112 lacks that interdomain salt bridge. The conformation of the carboxyl-terminal lipid-binding region may allow apo-E4 to interact with lipoproteins (VLDL) with a greater radius of curvature. Alternatively, apo-E3 interacts with HDL, suggesting a different conformation of the lipid-binding region.

Residue 158, which lies outside this highly basic region, has an indirect influence on receptor binding. Although the crystallographic backbone structures of apo-E3 and apo-E2 [10] are essentially identical, there are differences in side chain conformations in the region of residue 158. In apo-E3, arginine-158 is involved in two salt bridges: one to glutamic acid 96 in helix 3 and one to aspartic acid 154 in helix 4. In apo-E2, with cysteine-158, the salt bridges are different. Aspartic acid 154 in apo-E2 interacts with arginine-150, causing the side chain of arginine-150 to swing into a new plane. The substitution of cysteine for arginine at residue 158 alters the conformation of the receptor-binding region (residues 136—150) and indirectly disrupts receptor binding.

Therefore, in summary, residues 136—150 are directly involved in receptor-binding activity, whereas residue 158 modulates receptor-binding indirectly. The significance of the domain interaction extends beyond its implications for lipid binding. The isoform-specific roles of apo-E in AD which will be discussed below may be another manifestation of this phenomenon.

Metabolism of apo-E-containing lipoproteins by neurons: relationship of apolipoprotein E4 to Alzheimer's disease

A role for apo-E in neurobiology is not surprising. The brain is second only to the liver in production of apo-E [11]. Apolipoproteins E, C-I, and C-III are found in human cerebrospinal fluid [12]. Neurons in the central and peripheral nervous systems express the LDL receptor and the LRP in vivo and in cultured cells [13—19]. The HSPG/LRP pathway is active in neurons, and the VLDL receptor is present in the brain [20—24].

Alzheimer's disease (AD) is a neurodegenerative disorder associated with progressive memory loss and dementia. The link between apo-E and AD was established by an exciting and intriguing report from Dr Allen Roses and his colleagues at Duke University. They noted a marked overrepresentation of the apo-E4 allele in AD patients [1—3]. Both late-onset familial and sporadic AD have been correlated to the apo-E locus on chromosome 19. Based on Dr Roses' work, apo-E4 is a major risk factor for about 50% on the late-onset form of the disease. These observations have stimulated numerous studies attempting to define the involvement of apo-E4 in this disorder.

There are two characteristic neuropathologic lesions seen in AD (for review [25,26]). Various schools of thought ascribe cause and effect to one or the other of these lesions. Whatever the case, apo-E is associated with both types. Amyloid plaques are extracellular deposits of the amyloid β (Aβ) peptide; apo-E, along with numerous other proteins is localized in the plaques. Apolipoprotein E4 has been linked to the formation of the amyloid plaques. In vitro studies demonstrated that apo-E4 forms a very stable complex with the Aβ peptide, whereas apo-E3 interacts less avidly [27]. Incubation of the Aβ peptide with apo-E4 results in a much more complex, dense network of fibers compared to that formed with apo-E3 [28]. This electron microscopic observation has been confirmed by other studies [29,30].

The second AD lesion is the neurofibrillary tangle which consists of paired helical filaments of a microtubule-associated protein called tau [25]. Apolipoprotein E is colocalized with hyperphosphorylated tau in these intracellular deposits [28]. Because tau normally participates in microtubule assembly and stability, the occurrence of neurofibrillary tangles suggests that the cytoskeleton is involved in the disease process. We have focused our attention on the effects of apo-E on the cytoskeleton. This hypothesis is supported by results from the laboratory of Dr Eliezer Masliah [31]. By immunolocalization of the microtubule-associated protein that functions in stabilizing the cytoskeleton of neurons, they have demonstrated a 15—40% loss of synapto-dendritic connections in the cortex of apo-E null mice and an abundant vacuolization and distortion of dendrites.

We have developed a model to explain the involvement of apo-E4 in the development of AD. Our working hypothesis is that apo-E modulates neuronal repair and/or remodeling. We have used various neurons in culture to determine the apo-E isoform-specific effects on neurite remodeling [16,32—34]. We believe that one or more injurious agents could cause neuronal damage which would require neuronal repair or neurite remodeling. Our model postulates that apo-E3 is a neurotrophic/neuroprotective agent, crucial to neurite remodeling and cytoskeleton maintenance. It further postulates that apo-E4 is deficient in these functions.

In our initial studies, we used rabbit dorsal root ganglia and Neuro-2a cells in culture to show that apo-E alone without added lipid had no effect on neurite outgrowth. Adding lipid (e.g., β-VLDL) caused increased branching of the neurite but had little effect on neurite extension. However, when rabbit apo-E was added along with a source of lipid, there was marked neurite extension and a reduction in branches [16].

When the effects of human apo-E3 and apo-E4 were compared, a distinct isoform-specific effect was revealed [32]. Addition of β-VLDL plus apo-E3 to the dorsal root ganglion cells in culture resulted in a significant increase in neurite extension. In contrast, addition of β-VLDL plus apo-E4 in a similar experiment resulted in little neurite extension. Thus the two isoforms displayed differential effects on the cytoskeleton.

Based on these preliminary results, we have attempted to answer two questions. First, what types of lipids or lipoproteins can serve as a carrier or vehicle to transport apo-E into the neurons? Second, which receptors or processes are involved in the uptake of apo-E?

To answer the first question, we have extended our studies on neurite extension to other cell types and other lipid sources. In our initial experiments, cholesterol-rich lipoprotein from cholesterol-fed rabbits (β-VLDL) were used as a model lipoprotein to serve as a transport vehicle for apo-E. We have also examined other triglyceride-rich VLDL and various lipid emulsions, including significantly, apo-E-containing lipoproteins in the cerebrospinal fluid. All yielded similar isoform-specific effects [16,32–34].

Several lines of evidence suggest that the isoform-specific effects may be mediated by lipoprotein receptor pathways [32,34]. Reductive methylation of apo-E, which blocks receptor- and heparin-binding activity, prevents the apo-E3-induced stimulation or the apo-E4-induced inhibition of neurite outgrowth. Furthermore, addition of the monoclonal antibody 1D7, which binds to the receptor-binding region of apo-E and prevents it from interacting with receptors and HSPG, blocks the apo-E isoform-specific effects on neurite outgrowth. When we inhibited the HSPG/LRP pathway in our cultured cells, we abolished the isoform-specific effects on neurite outgrowth [32]. Heparinase or chlorate treatment were used to interfere with the sulfated HSPG on the cell surface [34]. In addition, various inhibitors of the LRP receptor (such as the 39-kDa protein) were used to block the receptor-ligand interactions. Inhibition of the HSPG/LRP pathway prevents apo-E3 maximal stimulation and apo-E4 inhibition of neurite extension. We have also undertaken to find out if there was a direct effect of apo-E on the cytoskeleton by looking a the effect of apo-E on tubulin in the neuroblastoma cells [33]. The cells were incubated with a source of lipid plus apo-E3 or apo-E4. The microtubules were observed by immunolocalization using an antibody to β-tubulin and visualized using confocal microscopy. In these cases, the microtubules of neurons incubated with β-VLDL and apo-E3 are well-formed and extend throughout the cells. This observation has been confirmed by electron microscopy and is consistent with the polymerization of a large amount of tubulin. In contrast, cells incubated with apo-E4 and β-VLDL show dispersed tubulin. There were no well-formed microtubules. Electron microscopic examination showed only a few short microtubules, and biochemical tests found mostly monomers of tubulin [33].

Immunofluorescent localization of apo-E in neurons and skin fibroblasts revealed that apo-E3, incubated with β-VLDL, accumulated in cell bodies and neurites and was widespread throughout. In contrast, apo-E4 showed little accumulation. In skin fibroblasts, we have determined that apo-E3 accumulated to levels 3- to 6-fold over those of apo-E4.

We have used similar experiments to determine the pathways that are used in the uptake of apo-E. In tests to determine the amounts of iodinated apo-E3 and apo-E4 that accumulate in fibroblasts that lack LDL receptors, we found a 3-fold greater accumulation of apo-E3 than apo-E4, thus showing that the differential accumulation is unrelated to the activity of the LDL receptor. Tests of apo-E accumulation in fibroblasts lacking the LRP (generously provided by Dr Joachim Herz) gave similar results, indicating that the LRP is not directly involved in apo-E accumulation. However, when the fibroblasts lacking the LDL receptors were treated with heparinase to remove the sulfates from the HSPG, the differential uptake was eliminated and the accumulations of both apo-E3 and apo-E4 were very low. Thus, the differential accumulation somehow relates to a difference in the way that apo-E3 and apo-E4 interact with cell surface HSPG.

From these results, we have two primary hypothesis that form our working model. The first suggests that there may be a specific HSPG that has a somewhat greater affinity for apo-E3 than for apo-E4. Alternatively, the internalized HSPG apo-E complexes may be treated differently. More apo-E3 may be retained in the cell, whereas apo-E4 may undergo a process called retroendocytosis and be expelled from the cell. We are pursuing additional studies to resolve this question.

Conclusion

In summary, our model predicts that apo-E is involved in neuronal repair and remodeling. The effects of both isoforms are mediated by the HSPG-LRP pathway. Apolipoprotein E3 with an appropriate lipid transport vehicle is internalized by the neurons and facilitates cytoskeletal or microtubular assembly. A variety of injurious agents may cause the initial insult to the neurons. Depending on the severity of the stress, apo-E3 (and apo-E2) may be able to effect some repair. In contrast, apo-E4 may not support the repair process and may actually block cytoskeletal assembly and impair neurite extension. As a result, apo-E4 is a significant risk factor for the development of AD. Even though individuals with apo-E4 have normal neuronal development, the impact of apo-E4 may be on selected types of neurons during remodeling that occurs later in life or following central nervous system injury.

Acknowledgements

This work was funded in part by National Institutes of Health Program Project Grants HL41633 and HL47660.

References

1. Mahley RW. Apolipoprotein E: cholesterol transport protein with expanding role in cell biology. Science 1988;240:622–630.
2. Mahley RW, Rall SC Jr. Type III hyperlipoproteinemia (dysbetalipoproteinemia): the role of

apolipoprotein E in normal and abnormal lipoprotein metabolism. In: Scriver CR, Beaudet AL, Sly WS, Valle D (eds) The Metabolic and Molecular Bases of Inherited Disease, 7th edn. New York: McGraw-Hill, 1995;1953—1980.

3. Weisgraber KH. Apolipoprotein E: structure—function relationships. Adv Protein Chem 1994; 45:249—302.

4. Corder EH, Saunders AM, Strittmatter WJ, Schmechel DE, Gaskell PC, Small GW, Roses AD, Haines JL, Pericak-Vance MA. Gene dose of apolipoprotein E type 4 allele and the risk of Alzheimer's disease in late onset families. Science 1993;261:921—923.

5. Saunders AM, Strittmatter WJ, Schmechel D, St George-Hyslop PH, Pericak-Vance MA, Joo SH, Rosi BL, Gusella JF, Crapper-MacLachlan DR, Alberts MJ, Hulette C, Crain B, Goldgaber D, Roses AD. Association of apolipoprotein E allele ε4 with late-onset familial and sporadic Alzheimer's disease. Neurology 1993;43:1467—1472.

6. Mayeux R, Stern Y, Ottman R, Tatemichi TK, Tang M-X, Maestre G, Ngai C, Tycko B, Ginsberg H. The apolipoprotein ε4 allele in patients with Alzheimer's disease. Ann Neurol 1993;34: 752—754.

7. Dong L-M, Wilson C, Wardell MR, Simmons T, Mahley RW, Weisgraber KH, Agard DA. Human apolipoprotein E. Role of arginine 61 in mediating the lipoprotein preferences of the E3 and E4 isoforms. J Biol Chem 1994;269:22358—22365.

8. Dong L-M, Weisgraber KH. Apolipoprotein E4 preference for very low density lipoproteins results from domain interaction mediated by glutamic acid 255 and arginine-61. Circulation 1995;92:I427—I428 (Abstract).

9. Dong L-M, Weisgraber KH. Human apolipoprotein E4 domain interaction. Arginine 61 and glutamic acid 255 interact to direct the preference for very low density lipoproteins. J Biol Chem 1996;271:19053—19057.

10. Wilson C, Mau T, Weisgraber KH, Wardell MR, Mahley RW, Agard DA. Salt bridge relay triggers defective LDL receptor binding by a mutant apolipoprotein. Structure 1994;2:713—718.

11. Elshourbagy NA, Liao WS, Mahley RW, Taylor JM. Apolipoprotein E mRNA is abundant in the brain and adrenals, as well as in the liver, and is present in other peripheral tissues of rats and marmosets. Proc Natl Acad Sci USA 1985;82:203—207.

12. Roheim PS, Carey M, Forte T, Vega GL. Apolipoproteins in human cerebrospinal fluid. Proc Natl Acad Sci USA 1979;76:4646—4649.

13. Hofmann SL, Russell DW, Goldstein JL, Brown MS. mRNA for low-density lipoprotein receptor in brain and spinal cord of immature and mature rabbits. Proc Natl Acad Sci USA 1987; 84:6312—6316.

14. Swanson LW, Simmons DM, Hofmann SL, Goldstein JL, Brown MS. Localization of mRNA for low-density lipoprotein receptor and a cholesterol synthetic enzyme in rabbit nervous system by in situ hybridization. Proc Natl Acad Sci USA 1988;85:9821—9825.

15. Boyles JK, Zoellner CD, Anderson LJ, Kosik LM, Pitas RE, Weisgraber KH, Hui DY, Mahley RW, Gebicke-Haerter PJ, Ignatius MJ, Shooter EM. A role for apolipoprotein E, apolipoprotein A-I, and low-density lipoprotein receptors in cholesterol transport during regeneration and remyelination of the rat sciatic nerve. J Clin Invest 1989;83:1015—1031.

16. Handelmann GE, Boyles JK, Weisgraber KH, Mahley RW, Pitas RE. Effects of apolipoprotein E, β-very low density lipoproteins, and cholesterol on the extension of neurites by rabbit dorsal root ganglion neurons in vitro. J Lipid Res 1992;33:1677—1688.

17. Moestrup SK, Gliemann J, Pallesen G. Distribution of the α_2-macroglobulin receptor/low-density lipoprotein receptor-related protein in human tissues. Cell Tissue Res 1992;269:375—382.

18. Rebeck GW, Reiter JS, Strickland DK, Hyman BT. Apolipoprotein E in sporadic Alzheimer's disease: allelic variation and receptor interactions. Neuron 1993;11:575—580.

19. Rebeck GW, Harr SD, Strickland DK, Hyman BT. Multiple, diverse senile plaque—associated proteins are ligands of an apolipoprotein E receptor, the α_2-macroglobulin receptor/low-density lipoprotein receptor—related protein. Ann Neurol 1995;37:211—217.

20. Takahashi S, Kawarabayasi Y, Nakai T, Sakai J, Yamamoto T. Rabbit very low density lipoprotein

receptor: a low-density lipoprotein receptor-like protein with distinct ligand specificity. Proc Natl Acad Sci USA 1992;89:9252—9256.

21. Jokinen EV, Landschulz KT, Wyne KL, Ho YK, Frykman PK, Hobbs HH. Regulation of the very low density lipoprotein receptor by thyroid hormone in rat skeletal muscle. J Biol Chem 1994;269:26411—26418.

22. Gåfvels ME, Paavola LG, Boyd CO, Nolan PM, Wittmaack F, Chawla A, Lazar MA, Bucan M, Angelin B, Strauss JF III. Cloning of a complementary deoxyribonucleic acid encoding the murine homolog of the very low density lipoprotein/apolipoprotein-E receptor: expression pattern and assignment of the gene to mouse chromosome 19. Endocrinology 1994;135:387—394.

23. Webb JC, Patel DD, Jones MD, Knight BL, Soutar AK. Characterization and tissue-specific expression of the human "very low density lipoprotein (VLDL) receptor" mRNA. Hum Mol Genet 1994;3:531—537.

24. Oka K, Ishimura-Oka K, Chu M-J, Sullivan M, Krushkal J, Li W-H, Chan L. Mouse very low density lipoprotein receptor (VLDLR) cDNA cloning, tissue-specific expression and evolutionary relationship with the low-density lipoprotein receptor. Eur J Biochem 1994;224:975—982.

25. Roses AD. The Alzheimer diseases. Curr Neurol 1994;14:111—141.

26. Selkoe DJ. The molecular pathology of Alzheimer's disease. Neuron 1991;6:487—498.

27. Strittmatter WJ, Weisgraber KH, Huang DY, Dong L-M, Salvesen GS, Pericak-Vance M, Schmechel D, Saunders AM, Goldgaber D, Roses AD. Binding of human apolipoprotein E to synthetic amyloid β peptide: isoform-specific effects and implications for late-onset Alzheimer disease. Proc Natl Acad Sci USA 1993;90:8098—8102.

28. Sanan DA, Weisgraber KH, Russell SJ, Mahley RW, Huang D, Saunders A, Schmechel D, Wisniewski T, Frangione B, Roses AD, Strittmatter WJ. Apolipoprotein E associates with β amyloid peptide of Alzheimer's disease to form novel monofibrils. Isoform apoE4 associates more efficiently than apoE3. J Clin Invest 1994;94:860—869.

29. Ma J, Yee A, Brewer HB Jr, Das S, Potter H. Amyloid-associated proteins α_1-antichymotrypsin and apolipoprotein E promote assembly of Alzheimer β-protein into filaments. Nature 1994; 372:92—94.

30. Wisniewski T, Castaño EM, Golabek A, Vogel T, Frangione B. Acceleration of Alzheimer's fibril formation by apolipoprotein E in vitro. Am J Pathol 1994;145:1030—1035.

31. Masliah E, Mallory M, Ge N, Alford M, Veinbergs I, Roses AD. Neurodegeneration in the central nervous system of apoE-deficient mice. Exp Neurol 1995;136:107—122.

32. Nathan BP, Bellosta S, Sanan DA, Weisgraber KH, Mahley RW, Pitas RE. Differential effects of apolipoproteins E3 and E4 on neuronal growth in vitro. Science 1994;264:850—852.

33. Nathan BP, Chang K-C, Bellosta S, Brisch E, Ge N, Mahley RW, Pitas RE. The inhibitory effect of apolipoprotein E4 on neurite outgrowth is associated with microtubule depolymerization. J Biol Chem 1995;270:19791—19799.

34. Bellosta S, Nathan BP, Orth M, Dong L-M, Mahley RW, Pitas RE. Stable expression and secretion of apolipoproteins E3 and E4 in mouse neuroblastoma cells produces differential effects on neurite outgrowth. J Biol Chem 1995;270:27063—27071.

Atherosclerosis XI.
B. Jacotot, D. Mathé and J.-C. Fruchart, editors.

125

Antiatherogenic effects of high-density lipoproteins: mechanisms

Philip J. Barter[1−3], Kerry-Anne Rye[2,3], Moira A. Clay[1,3], Dale Ashby[1,3], Paul W. Baker[1,3], Pu Xia[3], Jenny R. Gamble[3] and Mathew A. Vadas[3]

[1] *University of Adelaide Department of Medicine;* [2] *Royal Adelaide Hospital Cardiovascular Investigation Unit; and* [3] *Hanson Centre for Cancer Research, Adelaide, South Australia, Australia*

Abstract. An inverse relationship between the concentration of high-density lipoprotein (HDL) cholesterol and the development of coronary heart disease (CHD) in humans is well-established. Furthermore, studies of transgenic mice indicate that HDLs are directly antiatherogenic. The mechanism by which HDLs inhibit atherosclerosis remains unclear, but may be secondary to several known functions of these lipoproteins. Such functions include the capacity of HDLs to promote the efflux of cholesterol from cells, the antioxidant properties of HDLs and the ability of HDLs to inhibit the expression of adhesion molecules on the surface of endothelial cells. This report is concerned mainly with the effects of HDLs on endothelial cell adhesion molecule expression.

Keywords: atherosclerosis, cell adhesion molecules, coronary heart disease.

Introduction

The concentration of high-density lipoprotein (HDL) cholesterol is a powerful and independent inverse predictor of premature coronary heart disease (CHD) in humans [1]. While this relationship may be one of cause and effect, the possibility has also been raised that a low HDL concentration in patients with CHD may be an epiphenomenon, with the low HDL being a marker of some other factor which is the true cause of the CHD. However, recent studies of transgenic animals engineered to overexpress HDL apolipoproteins have tipped the balance in favour of the view that a high concentration of HDLs is directly protective against atherosclerosis and CHD.

Evidence that HDLs protect against CHD

To date there have been no reports of human intervention studies designed specifically to determine whether raising the level of HDLs translates into a reduced incidence of CHD. There are, however, intervention studies designed primarily to determine the effects of lowering low-density lipoprotein (LDL) cholesterol and plasma triglyceride in which treatment-induced elevations of HDL cholesterol are independently predictive of both a reduction in CHD events [2] and a

---

Address for correspondence: Prof P.J. Barter, University of Adelaide Department of Medicine, Royal Adelaide Hospital, North Terrace, Adelaide, SA 5000, Australia.

126

reduced progression of coronary atherosclerosis [3]. Direct evidence that HDLs are atheroprotective is provided by studies of transgenic animals. Overexpression of the human apo A-I gene in transgenic mice results in an increase in the concentration of HDL cholesterol which is accompanied by a dramatic protection against both diet-induced atherosclerosis [4] and the spontaneous atherosclerosis which develops in apo E-deficient mice [5]. A direct protective role of HDLs has also been demonstrated in studies of cholesterol-fed rabbits in which a regression of atherosclerosis accompanies prolonged intravenous infusions of HDLs [6].

HDL subpopulations and atherosclerosis

Human case control studies have suggested that the inverse relationship between HDL cholesterol and the development of premature CHD is a function mainly of the concentration of the HDL_2 subfraction [7]. In other studies, however, the development of CHD has been reported to correlate significantly and inversely with the concentrations of both HDL_2 and HDL_3 [8].

In terms of apolipoprotein-specific subpopulations of HDLs, studies of transgenic animals suggest that A-I HDLs may be superior to both A-I/A-II HDLs and A-II HDLs in their ability to protect against atherosclerosis. Mice overexpressing the combination of human apoA-I and apoA-II [9] or human apo A-II alone [10] are partly protected but not to the same extent as is observed in the apo A-I transgenic animals, even when levels of HDL cholesterol are comparable. Mice engineered to overexpress murine apo A-II appear to have an increased susceptibility and develop spontaneous atherosclerosis [11].

The situation in humans is uncertain. There have been no prospective studies of the relationship between apolipoprotein-specific subpopulations of HDLs and CHD. Nor are there any intervention studies assessing the impact of changing apolipoprotein-specific subpopulations of HDLs in human subjects.

Potential antiatherogenic properties of HDLs

The most widely documented function of HDLs relates to their ability to promote the efflux of cholesterol from cells in the first step of the pathway of reverse cholesterol transport. As outlined below, this function is clearly one possible mechanism through which HDLs protect against atherosclerosis. However, HDLs have a number of other functions that appear to be unrelated to their role in plasma cholesterol transport but which may contribute to a protection against atherosclerosis [12]. HDLs have been reported to be mitogenic, to bind lipopolysaccharide, to protect erythrocytes against the generation of procoagulant activity, to ameliorate the abnormal vasoconstriction which is a feature of early atherosclerosis, to reduce epidermal growth-factor-induced DNA synthesis in vascular smooth muscle cells, to stimulate endothelial cell prostacyclin synthesis, to bind prostacyclin and thus prolong its half-life, to inhibit the transmigration of monocytes induced by oxidised LDLs, to inhibit the oxidative modification of LDLs and to inhibit the adhesion of monocytes to endothelial cells.

All of these functions of HDLs may contribute in some way to their ability to inhibit the development of atherosclerosis. Their functions as mediators of cholesterol efflux, as antioxidants and as inhibitors of endothelial cell adhesion molecule expression have major antiatherogenic potential as shown schematically in Fig. 1.

HDL-mediated cell cholesterol efflux as an antiatherogenic process

It is commonly believed that HDLs protect against the development of atherosclerosis by virtue of their ability to extract cholesterol from cells. This view holds that HDLs counteract the effects of LDLs by removing cholesterol from cells in the arterial intima, thus preventing the formation of foam cells. In support of this view, the ability of HDLs to promote the efflux of cholesterol from cells is well known. Furthermore, the ability of serum to promote cholesterol efflux from a rat hepatoma cell line has been shown to correlate significantly with the serum HDL cholesterol concentration [13].

Virtually all HDL subpopulations are able to accept cholesterol from cells [14]. However, the preferred initial acceptor of cell cholesterol is a minor subpopulation of small, pre-β-migrating, apo A-I-containing particles [15]. These particles have been designated pre-β_1 HDLs and have been identified in plasma [15] and interstitial fluid [16]. It is not known, however, what regulates their concentration in plasma, let alone in extravascular compartments. In vivo, the concentration of pre-β HDLs in plasma is elevated in subjects with hypertriglyceridemia [17];

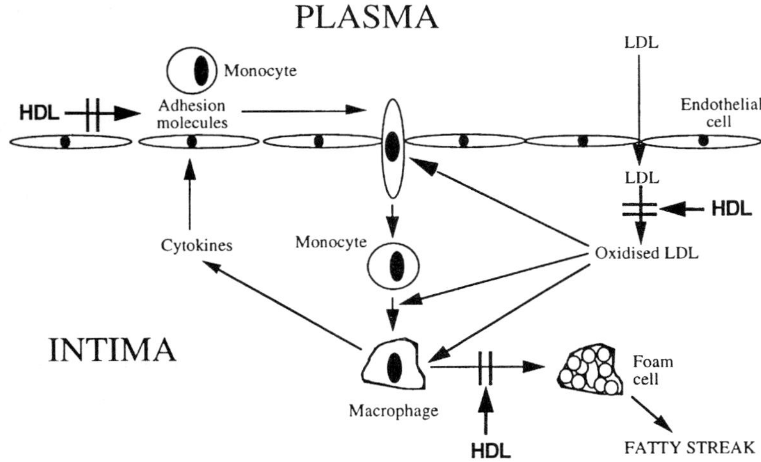

Fig. 1. Schematic design of three points at which HDLs may inhibit the development of atherosclerosis. They may inhibit the formation of foam cells by promoting the efflux of cholesterol from macrophages. They may inhibit the oxidative modification of LDLs. They may inhibit the adhesion of monocytes to endothelial cells.

128

it should be noted that the concentration of the total HDL fraction tends to be low in such subjects. In vitro, small, pre-β-migrating HDLs are generated by the interaction of HDLs with CETP [18], activity of which also tends to reduce the concentration of HDLs [19]. Thus, circumstances favouring high levels of pre-β HDLs are those in which the concentration of the total HDL fraction is low rather than high. Therefore, it follows that an increased rate of reverse cholesterol transport that may be associated with an increased concentration of pre-β HDLs will also tend to be associated with a low rather than a high total HDL level. Such a scenario is not consistent with the view that a high level of HDLs protects against atherosclerosis by enhancing the rate of reverse cholesterol transport.

The second main step in reverse cholesterol transport is the esterification of cholesterol on the surface of HDLs in a reaction catalysed by LCAT [20]. This reaction depletes the HDL surface of unesterified cholesterol and thus generates a concentration gradient which promotes the transfer of cholesterol from cell membranes to HDLs. An increased rate of LCAT-catalysed cholesterol esterification would, therefore, be predicted to enhance the rate of reverse cholesterol transport. It is known that the rate of the LCAT reaction in plasma correlates negatively rather than positively with the concentration of HDL cholesterol [21]. Thus, subjects with low concentrations of HDL cholesterol, especially if they also have elevated levels of plasma triglyceride [22], tend to have high rather than low rates of plasma cholesterol esterification, and by inference, high rather than low rates of reverse cholesterol transport. Again, this is not consistent with the view that the increased coronary risk in subjects with low levels of HDL cholesterol is secondary to a reduced rate of reverse cholesterol transport. This raises the possibility that the inverse relationship between HDL concentration and the development of CHD may be mediated by a mechanism which is independent of the involvement of HDLs in reverse cholesterol transport.

Antioxidant property of HDLs as an antiatherogenic process

It is widely believed that oxidative modification of LDLs within the arterial intima is a key early event in atherogenesis. HDLs are known to inhibit the oxidation of LDLs [23]. This may reflect the activity of paraoxonase which is known to be a component of HDLs and which has been shown to prevent the accumulation of lipoperoxides in LDLs [24].

HDL-mediated inhibition of endothelial cell adhesion molecules as an antiatherogenic process

Adhesion molecules and atherosclerosis

It is generally accepted that the adhesion of monocytes to the vascular endothelium is an early event in atherogenesis. This adhesion is mediated by endothelial cell adhesion molecules which include vascular cell adhesion molecule

(VCAM)-1, intercellular adhesion molecule (ICAM)-1 and E-selectin, all of which are rapidly synthesised in response to the inflammatory cytokines, tumour necrosis factor-α (TNFα) and interleukin-1 (IL-1). VCAM-1 is a member of the immunoglobulin-like superfamily and is primarily involved in the adhesion of mononuclear leukocytes to the endothelium. ICAM-1 (another member of the immunoglobulin-like superfamily) is expressed on many cell types and is involved in both monocyte and lymphocyte adhesion to activated endothelium. E-selectin, a member of the selectin family of molecules, is an endothelial specific adhesion molecule which is important in the adhesion of polymorphonuclear leukocytes, monocytes and lymphocytes to cytokine-stimulated endothelial cells. E-selectin has also been shown to play a role in capturing leukocytes from the axial stream so as to enable them to roll along the endothelium. These adhesion molecules appear to be involved both in early atherogenesis [25] and in the progression of mature atherosclerotic plaques [26].

Effects of HDLs on expression of adhesion molecules in endothelial cells

We have shown that HDLs have the capacity to inhibit by 65—90% the cytokine-induced (both TNFα and IL-I) expression of VCAM-1, ICAM-1 and E-selectin in endothelial cells grown in tissue culture [27]. This inhibition is concentration-dependent over the physiological range of HDL concentrations and is paralleled by significant reductions in the steady-state mRNA levels of these adhesion molecules [27].

We have excluded the possibility that the inhibiting properties of HDLs are mediated by contaminating plasma components which coisolate with the HDLs by using reconstituted HDLs (rHDLs) containing purified apo A-I (the main HDL apolipoprotein) as their sole protein component and phosphatidylcholine as their sole lipid. When these rHDLs are presented to monolayers of human umbilical vein endothelial cells (HUVECs), the TNF-induced expression of endothelial cell VCAM-1 is inhibited in a concentration-dependent manner comparable to that observed with native HDLs isolated from plasma.

Results comparable to those with HUVECs have also been obtained with human umbilical artery endothelial cells and the HUVEC-derived transformed cell line, C11STH [27].

Effects of HDL subpopulations on endothelial cell adhesion molecule expression

In studies designed to compare the effectiveness of various HDL subpopulations as inhibitors of endothelial cell adhesion molecule expression, we have found that HDL$_2$ and HDL$_3$ as well as HDLs with markedly different apolipoprotein composition all have the capacity to inhibit cytokine-induced VCAM-1 expression in HUVECs. However, at equivalent concentrations of either apo A-I or cholesterol, the HDL$_3$ subfraction is clearly superior to HDL$_2$ in terms of inhibiting the cytokine-induced expression of VCAM-1 in HUVECs. In other studies designed to investigate the influence of apolipoprotein composition on the ability of HDLs to inhibit adhesion molecule expression, preparations of HDL_3 were incubated in vitro with apo A-II which displaced all of the apo A-I from the particles to produce a population of particles containing apo A-II without apo A-I. These modified A-II HDLs were identical in terms of their ability to inhibit endothelial cell adhesion molecule expression to the unmodified HDL_3 which contained a mixture of A-I HDLs and A-I/A-II HDLs.

To the extent that an inhibition of VCAM-1 by HDLs contributes to the anti-atherogenic properties of this lipoprotein fraction, the results of these studies suggest that the ability of HDLs to protect against CHD may be independent of apolipoprotein composition. They also raise the possibility that it may be the HDL_3 rather than HDL_2 subfraction that protects against CHD in most subjects. This would account for the persistence of an inverse relationship between HDL levels and CHD even when the HDL cholesterol concentration is below 1.0 mmol/l [28] and there is no longer any measurable HDL_2.

Mechanism by which HDLs inhibit endothelial cell adhesion molecule expression

The mechanism by which HDLs inhibit endothelial cell adhesion molecule expression has been investigated. It has been found that exposure of HUVECs to HDLs prior to the addition of TNFα has the capacity to inhibit VCAM-1 expression even if the HDLs are removed before adding the cytokine. Exposure of the cells to HDLs for only 2–4 h is sufficient to achieve maximum inhibition of cytokine-induced VCAM-1 expression; furthermore, we have found that the inhibition persists for 8–12 h after the HDLs have been removed from the cells.

Coincident with their effects on endothelial cell adhesion molecule expression, we have found that HDLs inhibit the TNFα-induced translocation of NF-κB, the transcription factor essential for the expression of VCAM-1, ICAM-1 and E-selectin. We have found that HDLs also inhibit the TNFα-induced activation of sphingosine kinase and, as a consequence, markedly reduce the accumulation of sphingosine-1-phosphate (Sph-1-P) in HUVECs. We have subsequently found that Sph-1-P induces both NF-κB translocation and VCAM-1 expression in HUVECs in a manner comparable to TNFα and that the inhibitor of sphingosine kinase, dimethyl sphingosine, mimics HDLs in terms of inhibiting the effects of TNFα on NF-κB and VCAM-1 expression. These results suggest that Sph-1-P may be an important component of a signalling pathway by which cytokines induce inflammatory responses and that HDLs act by inhibiting their formation (Fig. 2).

Conclusion

Much is known about the relationship between HDLs and CHD, but there is still

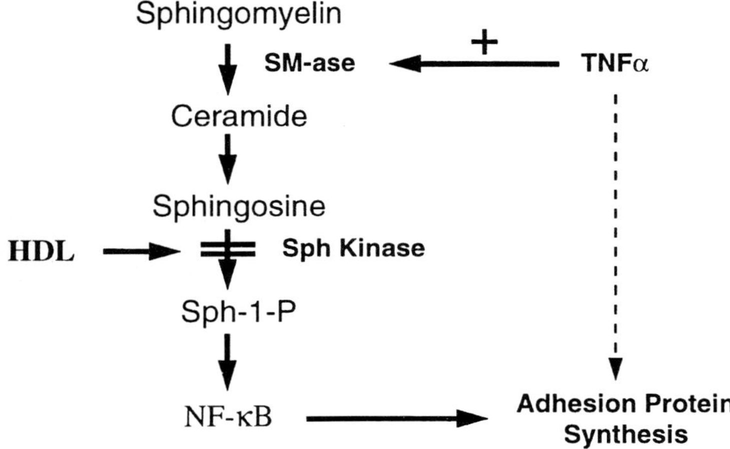

Fig. 2. Proposed mechanism by which HDLs inhibit the cytokine-induced expression of adhesion molecules in endothelial cells.

a lot that is not yet understood. The fact that the concentration of HDL cholesterol correlates inversely with the development of premature CHD has been well-established, as has the demonstration that the relationship is at least partly cause and effect. However, the mechanism by which HDLs protect against CHD remains to be established with certainty. The capacity of HDLs to promote the efflux of cholesterol from cells is viewed most widely as the mechanism by which HDLs inhibit the development of atherosclerosis. However, there is growing evidence that the atheroprotective effects of HDLs may relate to other functions of these lipoproteins such as their possible role in preventing the oxidative modification of LDLs or their ability to inhibit the cytokine-induced expression of adhesion molecules in endothelial cells. We suggest that this latter function may be an important mechanism by which HDLs inhibit the development of premature CHD.

References

1. Gordon DJ, Probstfield JL, Garrison RJ, Neaton JD, Castelli WP, Knoke JD, Jacobs DR, Bangdiwala S, Tyroler HA. High-density lipoprotein cholesterol and cardiovascular disease. Four prospective American studies. Circulation 1989;79:8—15.
2. Manninen V, Elo O, Frick MH, Haapa K. Heinonen OP, Heinsalmi P, Helo P, Huttunen JK, Kaitaniemi P, Koskinen P, Maenpaa H, Malkonen M, Manttari M, Norola S, Pasternack A, Pikkarainen J, Romo M, Sjoblom T, Nikkila EA. Lipid alterations and decline in the incidence of coronary heart disease in the Helsinki Heart Study. JAMA 1988;260:641—651.
3. Brown G, Albers JJ, Fisher LD, Schaefer SM, Lin JT, Kaplan C, Zhao XQ, Bisson BD, Fitzpatrick VF, Dodge HT. Regression of coronary artery disease as a result of intensive lipid-lowering therapy in men with high levels of apolipoprotein B. N Engl J Med 1990;323:1289—1298.
4. Rubin EM, Krauss RM, Spangler EA, Verstuyft JG, Clift SM. Inhibition of early atherogenesis in transgenic mice by human apolipoprotein AI. Nature 1991;353:265—267.

132

5. Paszty C, Maeda N, Verstuyft J, Rubin EM. Apolipoprotein AI transgene corrects apolipoprotein E deficiency-induced atherosclerosis in mice. J Clin Invest 1994;94:899—903.

6. Badimon JJ, Badimon L, Fuster V. Regression of atherosclerotic lesions by high-density lipoprotein plasma fraction in the cholesterol-fed rabbit. J Clin Invest 1990;85:1234—1241.

7. Robinson D, Ferns GA, Bevan EA, Stocks J, Williams PT, Galton DJ. High-density lipoprotein subfractions and coronary risk factors in normal men. Arteriosclerosis 1987;7:341—346.

8. Stamper MJ, Sacks FM, Salvini S, Willett WC, Hennekens CH. A prospective study of cholesterol, apolipoproteins and the risk of myocardial infarction. N Engl J Med 1991;325:373—381.

9. Schultz JR, Verstuyft JG, Gong E, Nichols AV, Rubin EM. Protein composition determines the antiatherogenic properties of HDL in transgenic mice. Nature 1993;365:762—764.

10. Schultz JR, Rubin EM. The properties of HDL in genetically engineered mice. Curr Opin Lipid 1994;5:126—137.

11. Warden CH, Hedrick CC, Qiao J-H, Castellani LW, Lusis AJ. Atherosclerosis in transgenic mice overexpressing apolipoprotein A-II. Science 1993;261:469—472.

12. Barter PJ, Rye K-A. High-density lipoproteins and coronary heart disease. Atherosclerosis 1996;121:1—12.

13. de la Llera Moya M, Atger V, Paul JL, Fournier N, Maotti N, Giral P, Friday KE, Rothblat G. A cell culture system for screening human serum for ability to promote cellular cholesterol efflux. Relations between serum components and efflux, esterification, and transfer. Arterioscl Thromb 1994;14:1056—1065.

14. Barter PJ. High-density lipoproteins and reverse cholesterol transport. Curr Opin Lipid 1993;4:210—17.

15. Castro GR, Fielding CJ. Early incorporation of cell-derived cholesterol into preβ-migrating high-density lipoprotein. Biochemistry 1988;27:25—29.

16. Asztalos BF, Sloop CH, Wong L, Roheim PS. Comparison of apo A-I-containing subpopulations of dog plasma and prenodal peripheral lymph: evidence for alteration in subpopulations in the interstitial size. Biochim Biophys Acta 1993;1169:301—304.

17. Ishida BY, Frolich J, Fielding CJ. Prebeta migrating high-density lipoproteins: quantitation in normal and hyperlipidemic plasma by solid phase radioimmunoassay following electrophoretic transfer. J Lipid Res 1987;28:778—786.

18. Kunitake ST, Mendel CM, Hennessy LK. Interconversion between apolipoprotein A-I-containing lipoproteins of prebeta and alpha electrophoretic mobilities. J Lipid Res 1992;33:1807—1816.

19. Marotti KR, Castle CK, Murray RW, Rehberg EF, Polites HG, Melchior GW. The role of cholesteryl ester transfer protein in primate apolipoprotein A-I metabolism. Insights from studies with transgenic mice. Arterioscl Thromb 1992;12:736—744.

20. Glomset JA. The plasma lecithin:cholesterol acyltransferase reaction. J Lipid Res 1968;9:155—167.

21. Wallentin L, Vikrot O. Lecithin:cholesterol acyl transfer in plasma of normal persons in relation to lipid and lipoprotein concentration. Scand J Clin Lab Invest 1975;35:669—676.

22. Nestel PJ, Monger EA. Turnover of plasma esterified cholesterol in normocholesterolemic and hypercholesterolemic subjects and its relation to body build. J Clin Invest 1967;46:967—974.

23. Parthasarathy S, Barnett J, Fong LG. High-density lipoprotein inhibits the oxidative modification of low-density lipoprotein. Biochim Biophys Acta 1990;1044:275—283.

24. Mackness MI, Arrol S, Abbott CA, Durrington PN. Protection of low-density lipoprotein against oxidative by high-density lipoprotein associated paraoxonase. Atherosclerosis 1993;104:129—135.

25. Cybulsky MI, Gimbrone MA Jr. Endothelial expression of a monocyte leukocyte adhesion molecule during atherogenesis. Science 1991;251:788—791.

26. Wood KM, Cadogan MD, Ranshaw AL, Parums DV. The distribution of adhesion molecules in human atherosclerosis. Histopathology 1993;22:437—444.

27. Cockerill GW, Rye K-A, Gamble JR, Vadas MA, Barter PJ. High-density lipoproteins inhibit

cytokine-induced expression of endothelial cell adhesion molecules. Arterioscl Thromb Vasc Biol 1995;15:1987—1994.
28. Gordon T, Castelli WP, Hjortland MC, Kannel WB, Dawber TR. High-density lipoprotein as a protective factor against coronary artery disease. The Framingham study. Am J Med 1977; 62:707—714.

Atherosclerosis XI.
B. Jacotot, D. Mathé and J.-C. Fruchart, editors.

Cholesteryl ester transfer protein deficiency: virtue or vice?

Yuji Matsuzawa, Shizuya Yamashita, Naohiko Sakai, Ken-ichi Hirano and Takao Maruyama
Second Department of Internal Medicine, Osaka University Medical School, Osaka, Japan

Serum high-density lipoprotein (HDL) has been widely recognized as an anti-atherogenic lipoprotein and the reduction of plasma HDL-cholesterol level is related to the occurrence of atherosclerotic cardiovascular diseases. Therefore, the increase in serum HDL-cholesterol has been considered to protect against the development of atherosclerosis. Since the early 1980s, several groups reported cases with marked elevation of serum HDL-cholesterol, which is a clinical marker of serum HDL level. By analyzing the biochemical basis of hyperalphalipo-proteinemia in these cases, the deficiency of plasma cholesteryl ester transfer protein (CETP) was identified.

Plasma CETP is a 74 kDa glycoprotein which facilitates the transfer of cholesteryl ester from HDL to apolipoprotein (apo) B-containing lipoproteins such as very low density lipoprotein (VLDL), intermediate-density lipoprotein (IDL) and low-density lipoprotein (LDL). However, most of these reporters discussed CETP deficiency from the standpoint that these cases are in an antiatherogenic state because of the increase in HDL [1], and in some cases hyper-HDL-choles-terolemia was called "longevity syndrome" without clear evidence. Among these reports, the hyper-HDL-cholesterolemic case that we reported in 1983 had a peculiar corneal opacity, a typical expression of lipid depositions in tissues [2]. Thereafter, we identified an additional case with hyper-HDL-cholesterolemia who was accompanied by massive corneal opacity and angina pectoris. Therefore, we have been working on HDL metabolism from the viewpoint that the marked elevation of HDL-cholesterol caused by CETP deficiency does not always show a protective ability against lipid accumulation in human tissues including athero-sclerotic lesions. In the current report, the molecular defects of CETP genes and lipoprotein abnormalities in these CETP-deficient cases are presented. Further-more, the atherogenicity of CETP deficiency is discussed, especially from the observations in a peculiar area of Japan where genetic CETP deficiency is ex-tremely frequent.

Address for correspondence: Yuji Matsuzawa, Second Department of Internal Medicine, Osaka University Medical School, 2-2 Yamadaoka, Suita, Osaka 553, Japan.

Molecular defect of plasma cholesteryl ester transfer protein

Two common mutations have been identified from the Japanese subjects with deficiency of CETP activity. One is a G-to-A mutation in the 5′-splice donor site of intron 14, which results in an impaired splicing of pre-mRNA. The other is a missense mutation (442D:G) in the exon 15. Both mutations are reportedly common in the Japanese cases with hyper-HDL-cholesterolemia, and the prevalence of the heterozygotes of intron 14 mutation is estimated to be about 1–2% in the Japanese general population. Moreover, nonsense CETP mutations in exon 6 and exon 10 have recently been identified. An additional defect in the intron 10 splice donor site has been identified, which causes exon 10 skipping, resulting in abnormal downstream splice site selection. All mutations induce a marked increase in serum HDL-cholesterol in homozygotes and less markedly in heterozygotes. However, in the case of missense mutation of exon 15 even heterozygotes sometimes show the phenotype of homozygotes, such as total deficiency of CETP activity with marked hyperalphalipoproteinemia. This evidence suggests that the mutation may have dominant negative effects on CETP activity in vivo. This was confirmed by in vitro study by the expression of wild-type and mutant protein in COS cells [3].

Lipoprotein abnormalities in the subjects with CETP deficiency

Serum-cholesterol levels of the CETP-deficient patients are moderately elevated and serum HDL-cholesterol is remarkably increased 3- to 6-fold (110–280 mg/dl) in homozygotes [4]. Serum apo A-I, C-III and E are also markedly increased in CETP-deficient patients, while apo B is normal or slightly decreased on average. The increase in HDL-cholesterol is attributed solely to the increase in HDL_2-cholesterol. The HDL particles of the patients are markedly rich in cholesteryl ester and poor in triglycerides compared with normal HDL particles. On the contrary, the content of cholesteryl ester is decreased and that of triglycerides is increased in the VLDL and LDL particles of the patients. In the ultracentrifugally isolated LDL fraction (d = 1.019–1.063 g/ml), apo E-rich HDLs which migrate with a slow α-mobility in agarose gel electrophoresis are detected in addition to apo B-containing LDL. These HDLc-like particles have a higher affinity than normal LDL to the LDL receptors of fibroblasts.

The particle size of HDL_2 of the CETP-deficient patients is remarkably enlarged while HDL_3 particles keep a normal size. In addition to the abnormalities of HDL particles, apo B-containing LDL particles in CETP deficiency show peculiar abnormalities. Polyacrylamide gradient gel electrophoresis demonstrated that LDL particles are small in the average size and show marked polydispersity. Equilibrium density gradient ultracentrifugation revealed that the LDLs of CETP-deficient patients comprised a group of heterogeneous lipoprotein particles distributed in a wide density range, without a prominent peak like normal LDLs. The LDL in each subfraction from the patients is poor in cholesteryl ester and rich in triglycerides. By native polyacrylamide gradient gel electrophoresis, each subfraction of normal control LDL contains only one species of homogeneous LDL particles, which progressively decrease in size with an increase in the density. In contrast, each subfraction of the patients' LDL contains two species of LDL particles; smaller LDL particles are found in addition to those which are identical to the normal control LDL. The IDLs of the patients are also composed of two species of lipoproteins. These data suggest that two metabolic pathways might exist in the process of mature LDL formation. VLDL is secreted by the liver as two species of lipoprotein particles different in size, and the VLDL is successively metabolized to LDL through IDL by a separate pathway [5]. Various modulations might be involved in producing homogeneous cholesterol-rich LDL particles which may possess a high affinity to LDL receptors. The hydrolysis of triglycerides by lipoprotein lipase (LPL) and hepatic triglyceride lipase (HTGL) may be important for this process. In addition, CETP plays a crucial role in converting small cholesteryl ester-poor LDL particles to large homogeneous and cholesterol-rich LDL particles by transferring cholesteryl ester from HDL particles.

HDL has been shown to protect macrophages from cholesterol accumulation when incubated with acetylated LDL, and also to enhance cholesterol efflux from lipid-laden macrophages. Cholesteryl ester-rich large HDL_2 from CETP-deficient subjects have been shown to be abnormal in these functions. Namely, the HDL_2 particles from the subjects show a reduced ability to inhibit acetyl LDL-induced accumulation of cholesteryl ester in mouse peritoneal macrophages [6]. Furthermore, these HDL_2 particles have less capacity than normal HDL_2 for cholesterol efflux from macrophages preloaded with cholesteryl ester by acetylated LDL. These data indicate that large HDL_2 particles enriched with cholesteryl ester in CETP deficiency may not have antiatherogenic function. In addition to the functional abnormalities of HDL_2 particles, small and polydisperse LDLs observed in homozygous patients, have a reduced-binding affinity for LDL receptors, which also induces a delayed catabolism of LDL and may finally cause susceptibility to various modifications of LDLs.

Is CETP deficiency atherogenic or antiatherogenic?

Species with high or moderate levels of CETP activity are susceptible to atherosclerosis, while species with low levels of CETP activity are resistant to atherosclerosis. In addition, a CETP transgenic mouse line developed aortic atherosclerosis after cholesterol feeding. From these observations, CETP was hypothesized to be proatherogenic and its deficiency might be antiatherogenic. However, the atherogenicity of CETP even in animal models has recently become controversial since Hayek et al. [7] reported that atherosclerosis was inhibited by co-overexpressing CETP in the transgenic mice overexpressing apo CIII to induce hyperlipidemia.

Although we have documented that the lipoprotein abnormalities observed in

138

CETP-deficient patients do not seem to be antiatherogenic but rather atherogenic, the demonstration of atherogenicity of CETP deficiency was not successful in clinical studies. This was probably because the number of CETP-deficient subjects was not enough for statistical analysis and the prevalence of atherosclerotic diseases is basically extremely low in the Japanese general population. However, we have recently identified a unique area in the northern part of Japan, Omagari in the Akita prefecture, where the prevalence of the intron 14 splice defect is enormously high, reaching 28 times that in the other parts of Japan such as Osaka or Tokyo [8]. In the Omagari area, the prevalence of hyper-HDL-cholesterolemic individuals with serum HDL-cholesterol more than 100 mg/dl was much lower in individuals over 80 years of age than in those under 80 years. Moreover, the frequency of CETP gene mutation was also reduced in individuals over 80 years of age compared with those under 80 years, suggesting that CETP deficiency is never a longevity syndrome, but may be related to rather short life.

In the Omagari study, the prevalence of ischemic changes in electrocardiogram was increased in individuals whose serum HDL-cholesterol was more than 90 mg/dl compared with those whose serum HDL-cholesterol was 50—70 mg/dl. It is speculated that hyper-HDL-cholesterolemia caused by CETP deficiency might be accompanied by atherosclerotic cardiovascular diseases. More recently, Zhong et al. [9] reported that in the Japanese-American men living in Hawaii, the incidence of coronary heart disease was higher in individuals with CETP gene mutations than in those without mutations. Hirano of our group investigated the clinical and metabolic characteristics of hyper-HDL-cholesterolemic subjects with coronary artery disease (CAD) and demonstrated that the reduction of both CETP and HTGL activities relates to the occurrence of atherosclerosis [10]. The accumulation of large cholesteryl ester-rich HDL particles in CETP-deficient individuals have a reduced capacity for cholesterol efflux from vascular wall cells such as macrophages. However, the addition of CETP alone or together with HTGL transforms large HDL particles of CETP-deficient subjects into small ones such as pre-β HDLs, which have a potent antiatherogenic function [11]. Thus, our clinical and in vitro studies on CETP-deficient subjects strongly suggest that CETP may have an antiatherogenic function as an enhancer of the reverse cholesterol system in humans.

References

1. Tall AR. Plasma cholesteryl ester transfer protein. J Lipid Res 1993;34:1255—1274.
2. Matsuzawa Y, Yamashita S, Kameda K, Kubo M, Tarui S, Hara I. Marked hyper-HDL$_2$-cholesterolemia associated with premature corneal opacity; a case report. Atherosclerosis 1984;53: 207—212.
3. Takahashi K, Jiang X-C, Sakai N, Yamashita S, Hirano K, Bujo H, Yamazaki H, Kusunoki J, Miura T, Kussie P, Matsuzawa Y, Saito Y, Tall AR. A missense mutation in the cholesteryl ester transfer protein gene with dominant effects on plasma high-density lipoproteins. J Clin Invest 1993;92:2060—2064.
4. Yamashita S, Sakai N, Hirano K, Arai T, Ishigami M, Maruyama T, Matsuzawa Y. Molecular

genetics of plasma cholesteryl ester transfer protein. Curr Opin Lipid 1997;8:101–110.
5. Sakai N, Matsuzawa Y, Hirano K, Yamashita S, Nozaki S, Ueyama Y, Kubo M, Tarui S. Detection of two species of low-density lipoprotein particles in cholesteryl ester transfer protein deficiency. Arterioscl Thromb 1991;11:71–79.
6. Ishigami M, Yamashita S, Sakai N, Arai T, Hirano K, Hiraoka H, Takemura K, Matsuzawa Y. Large and cholesteryl ester-rich high-density lipoproteins in cholesteryl ester transfer protein deficiency cannot protect macrophages from cholesterol accumulation induced by acetylated low-density lipoproteins. J Biochem 1994;116:257–262.
7. Hayek T, Masucci-Magoulas L, Jiang X, Walsh A, Rubin E, Breslow JL, Tall AR. Decreased early atherosclerotic lesions in hypertriglyceridemic mice expressing cholesteryl ester transfer protein transgene. J Clin Invest 1995;96:2071–2074.
8. Hirano K, Yamashita S, Nakajima N, Arai T, Maruyama T, Yoshida Y, Ishigami M, Sakai N, Kameda-Tekemura K, Matsuzawa Y. Genetic cholesteryl ester transfer protein deficiency is extremely frequent in the Omagari area of Japan; marked hyperalphalipoproteinemia caused by CETP gene mutation is not associated with longevity. Arterioscl Thromb Vasc Biol 1997;17: 1053–1059.
9. Zhong S, Sharp DS, Grove JS, Bruce C, Yano K, Curb JD, Tall AR. Increased coronary heart disease in Japanese-American men with mutations in the cholesteryl ester protein gene despite increased HDL levels. J Clin Invest 1996;97:2917–2923.
10. Hirano K, Yamashita S, Kuga Y, Sakai N, Nozaki S, Kihara S, Arai T, Yanagi K, Takami S, Menju M, Ishigami M, Yoshida Y, Kameda-Tekemura K, Hayashi K, Matsuzawa Y. Atherosclerotic disease in marked hyperalphalipoproteinemia; combined reduction of cholesteryl ester transfer protein and hepatic triglyceride lipase. Arterioscl Thromb Vasc Biol 1995;15:1849–1856.
11. Yamashita S, Ishigami M, Arai T, Sakai N, Hirano K, Kameda-Tekemura, Tokunaga K, Matsuzawa Y. Very high density lipoprotein (VHDL) induced by plasma cholesteryl ester transfer protein (CETP) have a potent antiatherogenic function. Ann NY Acad Sci 1995;748:606–608.

Postprandial lipaemia and coronary heart disease

Anders Hamsten, Johan Björkegren, Susanna Boquist, Lennart Nilsson, Giacomo Ruotolo, Per Eriksson, Angela Silveira and Fredrik Karpe
Atherosclerosis Research Unit, King Gustaf V Research Institute, Karolinska Hospital, Stockholm, Sweden

Background

Most of our lives are spent in the postprandial state. Postprandial triglyceride-rich lipoproteins (chylomicrons, very low density lipoproteins (VLDL) and their remnants) are a heterogeneous population of particles varying in origin, structure and interactions with cellular receptors. Differences in atherogenic properties may well exist between the various subclasses. The fact that epidemiological studies have not included determinations of postprandial lipoproteins might have contributed to the persisting confusion concerning the role of triglycerides as a risk factor for coronary heart disease (CHD).

The liver secretes apolipoprotein (apo) B-100 into a wide spectrum of VLDL particles. Normal metabolic conditions favour the production of smaller particle species. These appear to be precursors of low-density lipoprotein (LDL). The presence of an excess of substrate for triglycerides promotes the formation of larger triglyceride-loaded VLDLs. These are cleared from the circulation without being converted to LDL [1]. Dietary fats are to a major extent incorporated into chylomicrons containing apo B-48 and then secreted into the circulation. Chylomicron metabolism is thought to take place in two stages, involving hydrolysis of triglycerides by lipoprotein lipase (LPL) with subsequent removal of resulting remnant particles mainly by specific receptors in the liver. Throughout this process apo B-48 remains an integral part of the chylomicron particle and its remnants. Like large VLDL, there is no significant conversion of chylomicrons to intermediate density lipoprotein (IDL) or LDL [2]. Triglyceride-rich lipoproteins from both the liver and the intestine make a significant contribution to the normal postprandial triglyceridemia found in humans fed a fat-rich meal [3].

Insulin resistance appears to play a major role in the perturbed metabolism of postprandial triglyceride-rich lipoproteins underlying a prolonged and enhanced alimentary lipaemia (reviewed in [4]). Increased flux of free fatty acids (FFA) to the liver, secondary to a failure of insulin to suppress FFA release from adipose tissue is an important factor leading to elevation of circulating triglyceride-rich

---

Address for correspondence: Prof Anders Hamsten, King Gustaf V Research Institute, Karolinska Hospital, S-171 76 Stockholm, Sweden. Tel.: +46-8-517-73201. Fax: +46-8-311298.

lipoproteins. The normal effect of insulin is most pronounced in the postprandial period and is mediated both through inhibition of the intracellular hormone-sensitive lipase and through an increase in the re-esterification of fatty acids within adipose tissue. The mechanism linking increased flux of FFA to the liver to increased secretion of VLDL is probably an increase in the amount of lipoproteins directed to the secretory pathway and protection of apo B-100 from post-translational degradation. Furthermore, the insulin activation of adipose tissue LPL is blunted in the insulin-resistance syndrome, which impedes the clearance of VLDL particles and lowers HDL. Thus, disruption of the normal precise coordination of postprandial lipid metabolism by insulin can be envisaged to account for the elevated postprandial triglyceride and low HDL cholesterol concentrations seen in insulin-resistant subjects.

VLDL and chylomicron remnants are considerably larger than LDL, and it has, therefore, been argued that they cannot readily penetrate the endothelium. However, the smaller (Sf 12–60) cholesteryl ester enriched particles — chylomicron remnants and small VLDL — share with LDL the ability to mediate cholesterol influx into the arterial wall intima in humans [5]. Intact triglyceride-rich lipoproteins have also recently been isolated from the plaque tissue [6]. These lipoproteins resembled the triglyceride-rich lipoproteins encountered in plasma, except for a slightly larger particle size and enrichment in apolipoprotein E. Interestingly, plasma contained apo B-48, whereas the plaques did not. This could be interpreted as meaning that chylomicron remnants are not directly implicated in atherogenesis.

The clinical evidence

A relationship between postprandial lipaemia and CHD was also established already in the 1950s. However, it was only recently that Patsch and colleagues provided evidence that the postprandial triglyceride concentration is an independent predictor of coronary artery disease [7]. Postprandial triglyceridaemia has also been independently associated with the presence of carotid atherosclerosis as determined by B-mode ultrasound measurement of intima-media thickness [8]. It could, therefore, now be argued that hypertriglyceridaemia at late time points after a standardized oral fat load might reflect a kind of fat intolerance that is of clinical importance. Simple measurements such as postprandial triglycerides, in particular late (6–8 h) after oral fat intake, might serve as a good indicator of an atherogenic lipoprotein pattern which is not detectable in fasting plasma.

Almost two decades ago, Zilversmit advanced the hypothesis that chylomicron remnants are important in atherogenesis in humans [9]. However, the evidence was indirect and this hypothesis has not yet been definitely confirmed or refuted, since epidemiological and clinical studies including specific determinations of subfractions of triglyceride-rich lipoproteins are still sparse. Recent studies of coronary patients using retinyl palmitate as a marker for the intestinally derived triglyceride-rich lipoprotein lipid have demonstrated the persistence of elevated plasma levels of chylomicron remnants for up to 24 h after ingestion of a fat meal [10—12]. Importantly, this also pertains to normolipidaemic patients [11,12]. Another study using the ratio of apo B-48 to apo B-100 in plasma as a measure of chylomicronaemia also proposed that this parameter was an independent metabolic risk factor for CHD [13]. However, that study did not aim at absolute quantification of apo B-48 and B-100.

In the one study published so far in which a specific method was used to quantify postprandial lipoproteins in patients with CHD, apo's B-48 and B-100 were measured in fractions of postprandial triglyceride-rich lipoproteins from patients with premature coronary artery disease who had previously undergone two coronary angiographies with an intervening time period of more than 5 years [14]. This study suggested that the different subclasses of triglyceride-rich lipoproteins vary considerably in their association with the development of coronary atherosclerosis and that alimentary lipaemia is likely to represent an important atherogenic mechanism. Importantly, only the postprandial plasma levels of small chylomicron remnants (Sf 20—60 lipoproteins containing apolipoprotein B-48) appeared to be distinctly associated with the rate of progression of coronary atherosclerosis. However, the interpretation of these data is not entirely straightforward. The concentrations of apo B-48 are very low in the fraction containing small chylomicron remnants and also correlate significantly with the plasma levels of small dense LDL [15], which have been linked to CAD in many other studies.

Atherogenic mechanisms

Molecular mechanisms have been described whereby chylomicron remnants might be directly involved in atherogenesis. Several experimental studies have demonstrated that uptake of chylomicron remnants by macrophages may lead to intracellular accumulation of cholesteryl esters and conversion into foam cells [16—18]. Studies in hypertriglyceridaemic subjects have subsequently indicated that postprandial triglyceride-rich lipoproteins in the S_f 100—400 and $S_f > 400$ ranges have enhanced ability to cause lipid loading of macrophages compared with the same postprandial lipoproteins from normolipidaemic individuals [19]. Thus, chylomicrons and large VLDL from hypertriglyceridaemic patients are the only native plasma lipoproteins that, without prior modification in vitro, can cause receptor-mediated lipid uptake into monocytes-macrophages in vitro, converting them to foam cells.

Generation of postprandial lipoproteins directly involved in atherogenesis is not the only mechanism by which alimentary lipaemia may contribute to premature coronary atherosclerosis. Associated alterations in the metabolism and composition of the other major lipoproteins, IDL, LDL and high-density lipoprotein (HDL), which influence the roles of these lipoproteins in atherogenesis have to be considered. During alimentary lipaemia there is a very active exchange of lipids and apolipoproteins between plasma lipoproteins. HDL is thought to undergo triglyceride and phospholipid enrichment through transfer of triglycerides from apo B-containing lipoproteins in exchange for cholesteryl ester. Subsequently, triglyceride-enriched, large HDL particles are converted to smaller ones by the action of hepatic lipase (HL). In this scenario, cholesterol initially contained in HDL is misdirected by the triglyceride exchange mechanism from its centripetal path, from tissues to the liver into triglyceride-rich lipoproteins which may end up in the arterial wall. The work of Patsch and his colleagues [20] has particularly linked the chylomicron remnant hypothesis to the known inverse relationship between HDL cholesterol and CHD. According to their concept, individuals with normal fasting plasma lipids and high levels of HDL_2 cholesterol catabolize chylomicrons and chylomicron remnants at a faster rate than do individuals with normal fasting lipids and low HDL_2 cholesterol. High plasma concentrations of HDL_2 are consequently considered as a result rather than a cause of processes which protect against atherosclerosis. The hypothesis advanced by these authors states that LPL activity limits the magnitude of postprandial lipaemia, which determines the triglyceride content of HDL_2 that, in turn, influences the levels of HDL_2 through the action of HL [21,22]. Low HDL cholesterol concentrations may thus reflect a proneness to coronary atherosclerosis because of diminished capacity to eliminate possibly atherogenic postprandial triglyceride-rich lipoproteins from plasma, and not because of a deficiency of HDL per se.

LDL (the true remnant particle of endogenous triglyceride-rich lipoproteins), has been assumed to be a passive bystander unaffected by the rapid events of triglyceride metabolism. However, LDL metabolism now seems to be influenced by alimentary lipaemia [23]. Incubation of a macrophage-like cell line (P388) with postprandial LDL-induced enhanced cholesteryl ester accumulation compared with LDL isolated from fasting plasma. The postprandial LDL also produced far more thiobarbituric acid substances after incubation with either $CuSO_4$ or P388 cells. These results imply that the postprandial LDL might be more atherogenic due to enhanced susceptibility to oxidative modification.

Recent metabolic findings: focus on the postprandial VLDL particle

The advent of methods to quantify chylomicrons, VLDL and their remnants by means of their specific apo B species (apo B-48 or apo B-100) and to separate the postprandial VLDL from chylomicron remnants have opened up a new window on the study of postprandial lipoprotein metabolism and its clinical consequences. Based on these techniques, a slightly revised concept for the clinical implications of postprandial lipoprotein metabolism is beginning to emerge. Recent studies have shown that most of the cholesterol contained in triglyceride-rich lipoproteins or transferred to triglyceride-rich lipoproteins during alimentary lipaemia is bound to endogenous VLDL containing apo B-100, whereas chylomicron remnants containing apo B-48 are consistently present at very low concentrations in both fasting and postprandial plasma [24–27]. Furthermore, chylomicron remnants seem to leave the circulation long before they reach the particle size, which is likely to allow them to be deposited in the arterial wall [27,28]. Around 80% of the postprandial increase in apo B-containing lipoproteins is accounted for by VLDL [24–26]. Whereas the bulk of the postprandial triglyceride increase is carried by chylomicron remnants [26], only about 20% of the increment in postprandial lipoprotein particle number is thus accounted for by these particles. It is, therefore, speculated that the metabolism of chylomicrons and chylomicron remnants represents a repeated daily atherogenic influence on other lipoprotein species in plasma rather than inducing atherosclerosis per se. Accordingly, recent studies conducted in our laboratory, both on rats [29] and humans [30], have shown that reduced lipolysis of VLDL (secondary to competition from chylomicrons) is the main cause of the postprandial accumulation of VLDL particles, a physiological phenomenon first suggested by Brunzell [31]. VLDL isolated from postprandial plasma shows significant compositional alterations, such as enrichment with apo E, apo C-I and cholesterol, and depletion of apo C-II [32]. These compositional perturbations are likely to account for the association between small cholesterol ester-enriched VLDL and precocious coronary atherosclerosis [33,34] and could be of importance for the implication of large VLDL in thrombosis [35].

Alimentary lipaemia is a hypercoagulable state

Triglyceride-rich lipoproteins appear to be involved in determining coagulation factor VII (FVII) mass and activity. Activation of FVII was recently demonstrated during alimentary lipaemia [36–38] and shown to relate to lipolysis of triglyceride-rich lipoproteins and generation of FFA from intestinal lipoproteins [37]. Furthermore, long-term increase in FVII coagulant activity (FVIIc) such as in hypertriglyceridaemia, appears to be associated with a rise in factor FVII protein concentration [39]. Based on in vitro experiments and studies of the hypercholesterolaemic rabbit it has earlier been hypothesized that large triglyceride-rich lipoprotein particles, such as chylomicrons, VLDL and their remnants, carrying the appropriate FFA at a sufficient density of negative charge, activate FVII through the intrinsic coagulation pathway and activated factor XII [40–43]. The generation and subsequent transfer of FFA from the triglyceride core to the phospholipid surfaces of large triglyceride-rich lipoproteins through the action of LPL plays an important role in this sequence of events [44]. In this way, the contact system would serve an important function in priming the extrinsic pathway of blood coagulation by increasing the levels of circulating activated FVII molecules (FVIIa), and contributing to the basal rate of thrombin generation. This could be particularly important in individuals with manifest atherosclerosis in whom increased plasma concentrations of FVIIa would be expected to generate thrombin at a higher rate at sites where tissue factor is expressed.

Another striking feature of VLDL is its positive association with plasma plasminogen activator inhibitor-1 (PAI-1) activity [45]. PAI-1 is the major determinant of the fibrinolytic activity in plasma. Elevated PAI-1 activity may be of particular importance for myocardial infarction in young patients, particularly in subjects with hypertriglyceridaemia [45,46]. Furthermore, most clinical studies performed so far have shown an association of elevated plasma PAI-1 activity with manifest CHD [47] and with increased risk of major cardiovascular events in patients with a history of cardiovascular disorders [46,48,49].

In vitro, VLDL induces a dose-dependent increase in PAI-1 secretion from endothelial cells [50,51] and liver cells [51]. In addition to VLDL, LDL oxidized by ultraviolet light stimulates the synthesis and secretion of PAI-1 from cultured endothelial cells [52]. The molecular mechanism/s by which VLDL and modified LDL initiate secretion of PAI-1 from endothelial and liver cells need/s further clarification. Recently, a VLDL-response element in the promoter region of the PAI-1 gene locus has been identified that mediates a VLDL-induced increase in PAI-1 transcription in endothelial cells [53]. In HepG2 cells, on the other hand, VLDL does not primarily increase PAI-1 gene transcription but instead stabilizes the two PAI-1 mRNA transcripts [54]. The VLDL-response element shows homology with a peroxisomal proliferator response element (PPRE) [53]. This finding, along with the responsiveness of a VLDL-induced transcription factor to clofibric acid and to polyclonal antibodies directed against peroxisome proliferator activator receptor (PPAR), suggests that the VLDL-induction of PAI-1 could be mediated by a member of the PPAR family. PPAR belongs to the steroid hormone receptor superfamily. The members of this family are ligand-dependent transcription factors that bind their cognate ligand with high affinity and specificity and then activate gene transcription through binding to a specific hormone response element in the promoter region of the target gene. Fatty acids are natural ligands of PPAR. This argues for a nutritional regulation of PAI-1 secretion from endothelial cells by fatty acids derived from VLDL triglycerides.

Conclusions

The corollary of the current data is that repeated episodes of exaggerated or perturbed alimentary lipaemia are linked to multiple disturbances of lipoprotein metabolism, which are related to precocious coronary atherosclerosis. These include abnormal cholesteryl ester enrichment of VLDL, abnormal LDL composition reflected by a predominance of small dense LDL or triglyceride accumulation in the dense LDL fraction, and an increased propensity of LDL to undergo oxidative modification. Postprandial lipaemia is likely to represent an important atherogenic and prothrombotic state.

References

1. Packard CJ, Munro A, Lorimer AR, Gotto AM Jr, Shepherd J. Metabolism of apolipoprotein B in large triglyceride-rich very low density lipoproteins of normal and hypertriglyceridemic sub-

jects. J Clin Invest 1984;74:2178—2193.

2. Stalenhoef AFH, Malloy MJ, Kane J, Havel RJ. Metabolism of apo B-48 and B-100 of triglyceride-rich lipoproteins in normal and lipoprotein lipase-deficient humans. Proc Natl Acad Sci USA 1984;81:1839—1843.

3. Cohn JS, McNamara JR, Cohn SD, Ordovas JM, Schaefer EJ. Plasma apolipoprotein changes in the triglyceride-rich lipoprotein fraction of human subjects fed a fat-rich meal. J Lipid Res 1988;29:925—936.

4. Frayn KN. Insulin resistance and lipid metabolism. Curr Opin Lipid 1993;4:197—204.

5. Shaikh M, Wootton R, Nordestgaard BG, Baskerville P, Stuart-Lumley J, La Ville AE, Quiney J, Lewis B. Quantitative studies of transfer in vivo of low density, Sf 12—60, and Sf 60—400 lipoproteins between plasma and arterial intima in humans. Arterioscl Thromb 1991;11:569—577.

6. Rapp JH, Lespine A, Hamilton RL, Colyvas N, Chaumeton AH, Tweedie-Hardman J, Kotite L, Kunitake ST, Havel RJ, Kane JP. Triglyceride-rich lipoproteins isolated by selected-affinity anti-apolipoprotein B immunosorbtion from human atherosclerotic plaque. Arterioscl Thromb 1994;14:1767—1774.

7. Patsch JR, Miesenböck G, Hopferwieser T, Mühlberger V, Knapp E, Dunn JK, Gotto AM Jr, Patsch W. The relationship of triglyceride metabolism and coronary artery disease. Studies in the postprandial state. Arterioscl Thromb 1992;12:1336—1345.

8. Ryu JE, Howard G, Craven TE, Bond MG, Hagaman AP, Crouse J III. Postprandial triglyceridemia and crotid atherosclerosis in middle-aged subjects. Stroke 1992;23:823—828.

9. Zilversmit DB. Atherogenesis: a postprandial phenomenon. Circulation 1979;60:473—485.

10. Simpson HS, Williamson CM, Olivecrona T, Pringle S, Maclean J, Lorimer AR, Bonnefous F, Bogaievsky Y, Packard CJ, Shepherd J. Postprandial lipemia, fenofibrate and coronary artery disease. Atherosclerosis 1990;85:193—202.

11. Groot PHE, van Stiphout WAHJ, Krauss XH, Jansen H, van Tol A, van Ramshorst E, Chin-On S, Hofman A, Cresswell SR, Havekes L. Postprandial lipoprotein metabolism in normolipidemic men with and without coronary artery disease. Arterioscl Thromb 1991;11:653—662.

12. Weintraub MS, Grosskopf I, Rassin T, Miller H, Charach G, Rotmensch HH, Liron M, Rubinstein A, Iaina A. Clearance of chylomicron remnants in normolipidemic patients with coronary heart disease: case control study over three years. Br Med J 1996;312:935—939.

13. Simons LA, Dwyer T, Simons J, Bernstein L, Mock P, Poonia NS, Balasubramaniam S, Baron D, Branson J, Morgan J, Roy P. Chylomicrons and chylomicron remnants in coronary artery disease: a case-control study. Atherosclerosis 1987;65:181—189.

14. Karpe F, Steiner G, Uffelman K, Olivecrona T, Hamsten A. Postprandial lipoproteins and progression of coronary atherosclerosis. Atherosclerosis 1994;106:83—97.

15. Karpe F, Tornvall P, Olivecrona T, Steiner G, Carlson LA, Hamsten A. Composition of human low density lipoproteins; effects of postprandial triglyceride-rich lipoproteins, lipoprotein lipase, hepatic lipase and cholesteryl ester transfer protein. Atherosclerosis 1993;98:33—49.

16. Goldstein JL, Yo YK, Brown MS, Innerarity TL, Mahley RW. Cholesteryl ester accumulation in macrophages resulting from receptor-mediated uptake and degradation of hypercholesterolaemic canine beta-very low density lipoproteins. J Biol Chem 1980;255:1839—1848.

17. Mahley RW, Innerarity TL, Brown MS, Ho YK, Goldstein JL. Cholesteryl ester synthesis in macrophages: stimulation by beta-very low density lipoproteins from cholesterol-fed animals of several species. J Lipid Res 1980;21:970—980.

18. Van Lenten BJ, Fogelman AM, Jackson RJ et al. Receptor-mediated uptake of remnant lipoproteins by cholesterol-laden human monocyte-macrophages. J Biol Chem 1985;260:8783—8788.

19. Gianturco S, Bradley WA, Nozaki S, Vega GL, Grundy SM. Effects of lovastatin on the levels, structure, and atherogenicity of LDL in patients with moderate hypertriglyceridemia. Arterioscl Thromb 1993;13:472—481.

20. Patsch JR, Karlin JB, Scott LW, Smith LC, Gotto AM Jr. Inverse relationship between blood levels of high-density lipoprotein subfraction 2 and magnitude of postprandial lipemia. Proc Natl Acad Sci USA 1983;80:1449—1453.

21. Patsch JR, Prasad S, Gotto Jr AM, Bengtsson-Olivecrona G. Postprandial lipemia. A key for the conversion of high-density lipoprotein2 into high-density lipoprotein3 by hepatic lipase. J Clin Invest 1984;74:2017−2023.
22. Patsch JR, Prasad S, Gotto AM Jr, Patsch W. High-density lipoprotein2. Relationship of the plasma levels of this lipoprotein species to its composition, to the magnitude of postprandial lipemia, and to the activities of lipoprotein lipase and hepatic lipase. J Clin Invest 1987;80: 341−347.
23. Lechleitner M, Hoppichler F, Föger B, Patsch JR. Low-density lipoproteins of the postprandial state induce cellular cholesteryl ester accumulation in macrophages. Arterioscl Thromb 1994; 14:1799−1807.
24. Karpe F, Steiner G, Olivecrona T, Carlson LA, Hamsten A. Metabolism of postprandial triglyceride-rich lipoproteins. J Clin Invest 1993;91:748−759.
25. Schneeman BO, Kotite L, Todd KM, Havel RJ. Relationships between the responses of triglyceride-rich lipoproteins in blood plasma containing apolipoproteins B-48 and B-100 to a fat-containing meal in normolipidemic humans. Proc Natl Acad Sci USA 1993;90:2069−2073.
26. Cohn JS, Johnson EJ, Millar JS, Cohn SD, Milne RW, Marcel YL, Russell RM, Schaefer EJ. Contribution of apoB-48 and apoB-100 triglyceride-rich ripoproteins (TRL) to postprandial increases in the plasma concentration of TRL triglycerides and retinyl esters. J Lipid Res 1993; 34:2033−2040.
27. Karpe F, Bell M, Björkegren J, Hamsten A. Quantification of postprandial triglyceride-rich lipoproteins in healthy men by retinyl ester labelling and simultaneous measurement of apolipoproteins B-48 and B-100. Arterioscl Thromb Vasc Biol 1995;15:199−207.
28. Karpe F, Hultin M. Endogenous triglyceride-rich lipoproteins accumulate in rat plasma when competing with a chylomicron-like triglyceride emulsion for a common lipolytic pathway. J Lipid Res 1995;36:1557−1566.
29. Karpe F, Olivecrona T, Hamsten A, Hultin M. Chylomicron/chylomicron remnant turnover in man. Evidence for argination of chylomicrons and poor conversion of larger to smaller chylomicron remnants. J Lipid Res 1997;38:949−961.
30. Björkegren J, Packard C, Hamsten A, Bedford D, Caslake M, Foster L, Shepherd J, Stewart P, Karpe F. Accumulation of large very low density lipoprotein in plasma during intravenous infusion of a chylomicron-like emulsion reflects competition for a common lipolytic pathway. J Lipid Res 1996;37:76−86.
31. Brunzell JD, Hazzard WR, Porte DJ, Bierman EL. Evidence for a common, saturable, triglyceride removal mechanism for chylomicrons and very low density lipoprotein in man. J Clin Invest 1973;52:1578−1585.
32. Björkegren J, Hamsten A, Milne RW, Karpe F. Compositional changes of VLDL during alimentary lipemia. J Lipid Res 1997;38:301−314.
33. Tornvall P, Båvenholm P, Landou C, de Faire U, Hamsten A. Relationship of angiographically defined coronary artery disease to plasma levels and composition of apolipoprotein B-containing lipoproteins in patients with myocardial infarction at young age. Circulation 1993;88(Part 1):2180−2189.
34. Phillips NR, Waters D, Havel RJ. Plasma lipoproteins and progression of coronary artery disease evaluated by angiography and clinical events. Circulation 1993;88:2762−2770.
35. Hamsten A, Eriksson P, Karpe F, Silveira A. Relationships of thrombosis and fibrinolysis to atherosclerosis. Curr Opin Lipid 1994;5:382−389.
36. Salomaa V, Rasi V, Pekkanen J, Jauhiainen M, Vahtera E, Pietinen P, Korhonen H, Kuulasmaa K, Ehnholm C. The effects of saturated fat and n-6 polyunsaturated fat on postprandial lipemia and hemostatic activity. Atherosclerosis 1993;103:1−11.
37. Silveira A, Karpe F, Blombäck M, Steiner G, Walldius G, Hamsten A. Activation of coagulation factor VII during alimentary lipemia. Arterioscl Thromb 1994;14:60−69.
38. Silveira A, Karpe F, Johnsson H, Bauer K, Hamsten A. In vivo demonstration in humans that large postprandial triglyceride-rich lipoproteins activate coagulation factor VII through the

intrinsic coagulation pathway. Arterioscl Thromb Vasc Biol 1996;16:1333—1339.

39. Scarabin PY, Bara L, Samama M, Orssaud G. Further evidence that activated factor VII is related to plasma lipids. Br J Haematol 1985;61:186—187.

40. Mitropoulos KA, Esnouf MP, Meade TW. Increased factor VII coagulant activity in the rabbit following diet-induced hypercholesterolaemia. Evidence for increased conversion of VII to VIIa and higher flux within the coagulation pathway. Atherosclerosis 1987;63:43—52.

41. Mitropoulos KA, Esnouf MP. Turnover of factor X and of prothrombin in rabbits fed on a standard or cholesterol-supplemented diet. Biochem J 1987;244:263—269.

42. Mitropoulos KA, Martin JC, Reeves BEA, Esnouf MP. The activation of the contact phase of coagulation by physiological surfaces in plasma: the effect of large negatively charged liposomal vesicles. Blood 1989;73:1525—1533.

43. Mitropoulos KA, Reeves BEA, O'Brien DP, Cooper JA, Martin JC. The relationship between factor VII coagulant activity and factor XII activation induced in plasma by endogenous or exogenously added contact surface. Blood Coag Fibrinol 1993;4:223—234.

44. Mitropoulos KA, Miller GJ, Watts GF, Durrington PN. Lipolysis of triglyceride-rich lipoproteins activates coagulant factor XII: a study in familial lipoprotein-lipase deficiency. Atherosclerosis 1992;95:119—125.

45. Hamsten A, Wiman B, de Faire U, Blombäck M. Increased plasma levels of a rapid inhibitor of tissue plasminogen activator in young survivors of myocardial infarction. N Engl J Med 1985; 313:1557—1563.

46. Hamsten A, de Faire U, Walldius G, Dahlén G, Szamosi A, Landou C, Blombäck M, Wiman B. Plasminogen activator inhibitor in plasma: risk factor for recurrent myocardial infarction. Lancet 1987;II:3—9.

47. Wiman B, Hamsten A. Impaired fibrinolysis and risk of thromboembolism. Prog Cardiovasc Dis 1991;34:179—192.

48. Cortellaro M, Cofrancesco E, Boschetti C et al., for the PLAT Group. Increased fibrin turnover and high PAI-1 activity as predictors of ischemic events in atherosclerotic patients. A case-control study. Arterioscl Thromb 1993;13:1412—1417.

49. Juhan-Vague I, Pyke SDM, Alessi MC, Jespersen J, Haverkate F, Thompson SG, on behalf of the ECAT Study Group. Fibrinolytic factors and the risk of myocardial infarction or sudden death in patients with angina pectoris. ECAT Study Group. European Concerted Action on Thrombosis and Disabilities. Circulation 1996;94:2057—2063.

50. Stiko-Rahm A, Wiman B, Hamsten A, Nilsson J. Secretion of plasminogen activator inhibitor-1 from cultured human umbilical vein endothelial cells is induced by very low density lipoprotein. Arteriosclerosis 1990;10:1067—1073.

51. Mussoni L, Mannucci L, Sirtori M, Camera M, Maderna P, Sironi L, Tremoli E. Hypertriglyceridemia and regulation of fibrinolytic activity. Arterioscl Thromb 1992;12:19—25.

52. Latron Y, Chautan M, Anfosso F, Alessi MC, Nalbone G, Lafont H, Juhan-Vague I. Stimulating effect of oxidized low density lipoproteins on plasminogen activator inhibitor-1 synthesis by endothelial cells. Arterioscl Thromb 1991;11:1821—1829.

53. Eriksson P, Nilsson L, Karpe F, Hamsten A. A very low density lipoprotein response element in the promoter region of the human plasminogen activator inhibitor-1 gene implicated in the impaired fibrinolysis of hypertriglyceridaemia. Arterioscl Thromb Vasc Biol (In press).

54. Sironi L, Mussoni L, Prati L, Baldassarre D, Camera M, Banfi C, Tremoli E. Plasminogen activator inhibitor type-1 synthesis and RNA expression in HepG2 cells are regulated by VLDL. Arterioscl Thromb Vasc Biol 1996;16:89—96.

History of International Atherosclerosis Society — a personal journey*

M. Daria Haust

Department of Pathology, The University of Western Ontario, London, Ontario, Canada

Keywords: International Program Committee (IPC), International Symposia on Atherosclerosis.

Introduction

Inherent in the definition of any history is the premise that accounts be provided accurately. Historians who research their subjects of history attempt to arrive at accurate accounts by studying the available information (be it archival or contemporary) from various and contradictory sources. The aim has always been to present the history as objectively as possible.

It has been customary and an accepted practice in scientific writings in English not to write in the narrative, the first person, but rather the third person, avoiding the "I" and the "we" (and their possessive forms) at all costs. This format is believed to enhance the credibility of objectivity (of scientific writings), and precludes a personal element. On the other hand, the scientific reporting in other languages (e.g., German, French) had always expressed linguistically a very personal involvement ("I found"; "our results showed"; "we decided to proceed", etc.).

The above comments are intended to explain that a decision had to be made prior to the present writing: should it be in the accepted English format, in a more personal style, or could one use a "mixed" form and narrate in a personal form whenever one's own involvement is recounted? The decision was made in favour of the last, perhaps in part because having been with the IAS for the past 20 years and from its very "birth", the Society became almost a second family for this writer. How then can one write about one's own (quasi) family in an impersonal language only? Thus, instead of referring to oneself in the text as "the writer" or per initials ("MDH") it seems so much more natural and personal to use the more direct format (I, my, we, our, etc.). The readers may be assured that by the usage of a more personal style, neither the objectivity nor the accuracy of this reporting will be affected.

Address for correspondence: Prof M. Daria Haust MD, FRCP(C), Department of Pathology, The University of Western Ontario, London, Ontario, Canada, N6A 5C1.
*Dedicated to the memory of my departed friends who accompanied me on this journey.

152

Background

The idea of "creating" the IAS was conceived at the meeting of the International Program Committee held in Tokyo, August 1976, on the occasion of the IVth International Symposium on Atherosclerosis. At this meeting Dr Antonio M. Gotto Jr, the designated Chairman of the next, i.e., the Vth International Symposium scheduled for 1979 in Houston, reported that he encountered difficulties in obtaining funds in support of the Symposium, in part because no definable Society sponsored these Symposia. Moreover, it was learned that the Tokyo hosts experienced similar difficulties in preparation for their 1976 Symposium. Since the number of scientists in attendance (approximately 100 at their inception in Athens) grew steadily through subsequent Symposia in Chicago and Berlin, to some 800 in Tokyo, and it was anticipated that the registration in Houston may approach 1,000, the costs with each consecutive Symposium also increased (with the number of participants).

Perhaps it is appropriate while writing on the topic of the history of the IAS, to digress to earlier beginnings, including those of the International Program Committee (IPC).

It all began when the idea of organizing an International Symposium on Atherosclerosis in 1966 in Athens was conceived and executed largely by three colleagues who were actively engaged in the field: Dr N. Miras (Athens; host), Dr R. Paoletti (Milan), and Dr A. Howard (Cambridge). Whereas, until that time, several excellent Symposia with international "flavour" took place on both sides of the Atlantic prior to the above Athens gathering (Toronto, 1961; Chicago, 1962), there was never a very concerted effort to seek out participating scientists from as many countries as possible, or to consult with a designated body representing the diverse national or regional communities of scientists in the field of atherosclerosis. Thus, the IPC was "born" in 1966.

The 1966 Symposium in Athens was a resounding success. In many instances one could put for the first time a name known from the literature to a face. In the small group of participants (approximately 100) that stayed together for almost 1 week in the lecture room and for the scheduled social events, close contacts and even friendships developed, as well as a desire to seize the momentum, and establish such meetings on a more regular and permanent basis; the IPC retaining the "core" scientific and organizational role for that purpose. Thus, it was with much enthusiasm that at the parting address given on behalf of the North American Participants by Dr Robert Wissler, the group endorsed unanimously his suggestion that the next gathering be in Chicago, 3 years hence. Dr Robert Furman (one of the past Presidents of the AHA-Council on Arteriosclerosis present in Athens) reinforced the invitation for the group to come to the USA. Parenthetically, in view of the novelty of the undertaking of such an international task, Dr Wissler required a little longer than 3 years to organize and host in Chicago the next International Symposium (November, 1969).

The proceedings of the Athens' first Symposium were published by Karger, and thus, too, initiated another tradition, as Proceedings of all subsequent Symposia (Chicago, 1969; Berlin, 1973; Tokyo, 1976; Houston, 1979; Berlin, 1982; Melbourne, 1985; Rome 1988; (Jerusalem) Rosemont-Chicago, 1991; and Montreal, 1994) appeared in print. Subsequently, other publishers were given this task (Springer-Verlag for Symposia II—VI; R & L Creative Communication, Tel-Aviv for Symposium IX, and Excerpta Medica (Elsevier), Amsterdam for Symposia: VIII, X and XI.

I wish to express (again) on behalf of the scientists in the field of atherosclerosis throughout the world, a renewed gratitude to the three colleagues who, over 30 years ago, conceived the idea of getting us together across the lands and oceans, i.e., Drs Miras, Paoletti and Howard. No doubt they must have received many expressions of appreciation in the past. However, their contribution to the initiation of the International Symposia on Atherosclerosis and the establishment of the IPC as a "standing" body (that later constituted the Charter Membership of the IAS), should be documented in print and be part of the permanent record of our Society. It is also quite befitting that one of these three "visionary" colleagues, Dr Rodolfo Paoletti, is assuming the Office of the IAS-President at this Symposium.

Foundation of the society; the initial period

The First Chapter in the IAS-history began with the Tokyo (IV)-Symposium. It was decided there at the meeting of the IPC that a Task Force, consisting of Drs William Holmes (USA), Roldolfo Paoletti (Italy) and M. Daria Haust (Canada; the recording secretary), explore the "pros and cons" of establishing an international society[1]. The Task Force was instructed to consult with as many colleagues at the international level as possible including all the members of the IPC, and report back to that Committee.

The IPC constituted in Athens in 1965 was largely responsible for the programs of the Symposia that followed (those of Chicago, 1969; Berlin, 1973 and Tokyo, 1976), i.e., until the "take over" by the IAS. Of the members to whom the voting ballot was sent (along with the minutes of both meetings) by the Task Force, 32 members replied (and became later Charter Members of the IAS) and no answer

---

[1] It is most regrettable that under the time constraints to reply to the Editorial comments made about the IAS in the Newsletter (SC-83-A) [1] of the AHA-Council on Arteriosclerosis, I failed to check the minutes of the Task Force prior to my replying in the next Newsletter [2] and reported erroneously that Dr Antonio M. Gotto was also elected to the Task Force. In fact, the Task Force consisted of only three (remaining) members. However, Dr David Kritchevsky was invited to attend the first Task Force meeting as an advisor, and Dr Gotto was invited to the second meeting (as the Chairman of the forthcoming V. International Symposium, communications with him deemed desirable). Regrettable is moreover, that the above error was perpetuated by myself when — again in a great hurry to "pacify" the disquiescent IAS-membership by any news after the long absence (1985—1988) of written or printed reports the same misinformation appeared in a widely read Journal [3]. Trusting that my statements were correct, Dr Gotto repeated this misinformation also in print [4], but this is solely my responsibility ("mea maxima culpa").

was received from five. Thus, the charter members of the (later) IAS were: Drs C. Adams (UK), J.-L. Beaumont (France), H. Buchwald (USA), W. Connor (USA), A. Day (Australia), F. Epstein (Switzerland), S. Gerö (Hungary), Y. Goto (Japan), A. Gotto (USA), M.D. Haust (Canada), W. Holmes (USA), A. Klimov (former USSR), D. Kritchevsky (USA), K.T. Lee (USA), R. Lovell (Australia), H. McGill (USA), C. Miras (Greece), E. Nikkilä (Finland), M. Oliver (UK), R. Paoletti (Italy), G. Rothblatt (USA), G. Schettler (Germany), G. Schlierf (Germany), D. Seidel (Germany), T. Shimamoto (Japan), E. Smith (UK), Y. Stein (Israel), D. Steinberg (USA), N. Werthessen (USA), R. Wissler (USA) and S. Wolf (USA).

The members of the Task Force consulted extensively with colleagues of their own groups, and this included consultations with the members of the Council on Arteriosclerosis of the American Heart Association (AHA). The Task Force met on three different occasions to discuss their findings and to formulate recommendations. At its first meeting (August 1976, Tokyo) the agenda consisted of exploring the feasibility of the IPC-members becoming the Charter Members of an International Atherosclerosis Society, the choice of incorporation site, considering all the pros and cons for creation of the society, and finally formulating the recommendations. Dr Holmes was assigned the function of working with a lawyer on the matters of incorporation technicalities (what is needed in terms of by-laws, constitution, committees, executive board, finances and the most suitable state in USA). The long discussion regarding the pros and cons yielded only two serious disadvantages vs. nine advantages in proceeding with the creation of the IAS. Of interest is that one of the two reservations were summarized as follows: "Apprehension, that the happy atmosphere of the voluntary association between colleagues and friends from various countries will suffer within the structured formal framework of an organized society". But even to this reservation a good-will answer was found: "The congenial atmosphere prevailing at present does not have to change because the more structured format is only an *external* factor, whereas the people will remain the same! As long as the members *themselves* don't change (and human nature is, indeed, at times unpredictable) the warm and congenial atmosphere will retain all the basis necessary for its maintenance and survival".

The second gathering of the Task Force took place at the time of the AHA-meeting in Miami, Florida, November 1976. Dr Paoletti could not attend, but we invited Dr Gotto as a guest. Since the last meeting, Dr Holmes worked on the incorporation with a lawyer; it seemed that the most suitable state was Pennsylvania, but for incorporation, bylaws of the proposed Society had to be drawn up and an Executive Board constituted (it had to include at least three members residing in Pennsylvania). Thus, in addition to Dr Holmes, Drs Kritchevsky and Rothblatt were invited to serve. The Board was thus to consist of all five Chairmen of Symposia to date (Drs Miras, Wissler, Schettler, Goto and Gotto), members of the Task Force (Holmes, Paoletti and Haust) and the two additional residents of Pennsylvania (Kritchevsky and Rothblatt). After the second meeting a ballot vote was sent out (with the minutes) to all the members of the IPC. Two questions were to be answered:

1. Do you accept the recommendations of the Task Force for incorporating the group (IPC) as the International Atherosclerosis Society — with terms and goals outlined in the accompanying minutes?
2. Do you empower the Proposed Executive Board to proceed with steps necessary for the implementation of the Task Force recommendations?

All the ballots returned were in the affirmative on both questions. The comments included on one return are of interest. Dr F. Epstein wrote: "Weighing pros and cons I still have considerable misgiving about creating a new society, especially if Gotthard Schettler puts life into the ISC-Council on Arteriosclerosis. All the same, one could not in good conscience vote "no". There are too many "pros"!".

There was some misconception in certain quarters about the aims and objectives of the IAS (that were as yet not known widely). I remember making a journey from a meeting in Vienna to a conference in Budapest in mid-April of 1977 in a car driven by a friend. Travelling with us was also a colleague from the USA who learned from someone about the efforts to establish the IAS. He was quite negative in his attitude. "Well, I hear you are establishing a new international society. I expect that it will be quite an exclusive club! But after all it may not survive for long." My attempts at explaining that the aims of the society were intended to bring all the scientists of the world closer, rather than creating an exclusive club, met with a disbelieving (and maybe even contemptuous) smile and silence. This was quite a sad experience. In the end there are some good news to report today, as this very colleague is co-chairing a Workshop at the present Symposium, precisely 20 years later. Alas, our IAS proved not to be an Exclusive Club, nor has it been short-lived.

Other opposition was of a more serious nature and was damaging to our goals because it came from a rather respected person and by its nature, was widely disseminated. Moreover, it occurred after the IAS had been in existence for a few years and proved its viability. I wish to quote one example. In January, 1983, an editorial carried in the Newsletter of the Council on Arteriosclerosis, AHA [1] discussed the IAS in particular (probably) as a nondemocratic entity, because: "With no discussion, the IAS decided that there would be an annual fee". Just how anyone arrived at the conclusion that the IAS-Executive and Council decided such a matter with no discussion was puzzling, as was the fact that anyone would expect an International Society to function without annual membership fees. The damage control was undertaken swiftly and my reply (instead of a rebuke) published in the next issue of the same Newsletter [2] took advantage to inform the readers of all the important developments of the IAS to that date as well as explain in detail our aims and goals. My reply ended with the statement: "These and other developments relating to the IAS support the contention of many good-will people that a benevolent and cooperative spirit rather than restrictive measures and limitation will contribute to the progress and to an understanding not only amongst scientists, but between all peoples of the world".

There was an overwhelming support for the creation of an International Atherosclerosis Society and the recommendation by the Task Force to this effect was presented to and endorsed by the IPC early during the course of the International Conference on Atherosclerosis in Milan (November, 1977). Later in the week the IPC met again and elected a slate of officers and the Council from its membership, and appointed a small committee to formulate the Constitution and Bylaws of the IAS. Since some members of the IPC were not present in Milan, it was also decided that all members should be asked to vote on the ratification of the elected Officers and Council as well as approve later the Constitution and Bylaws written by myself with Dr Schlief's assistance. The voting ballot was unanimously favourable on all three accounts. Thus, the IAS had its First Execu-

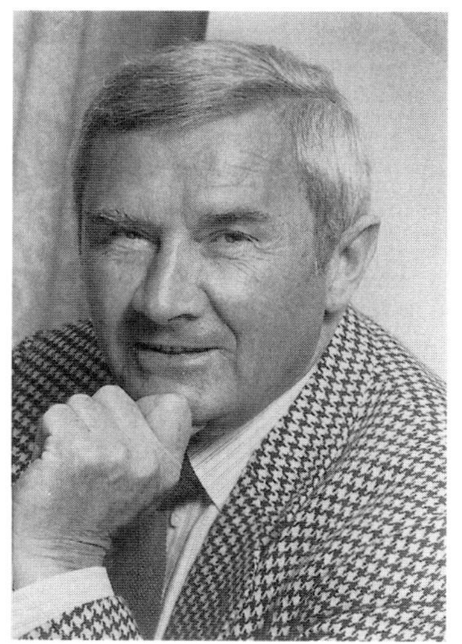

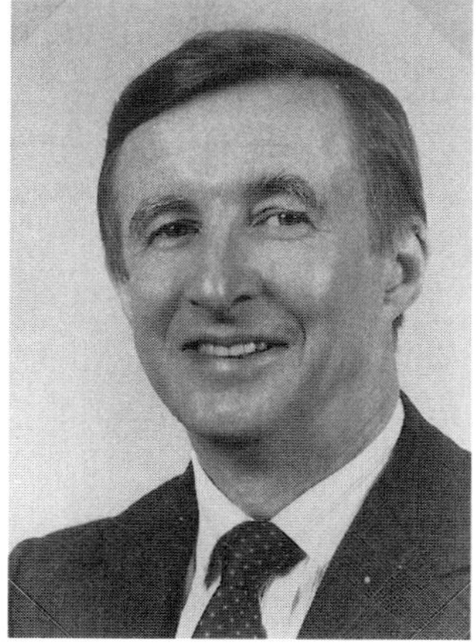

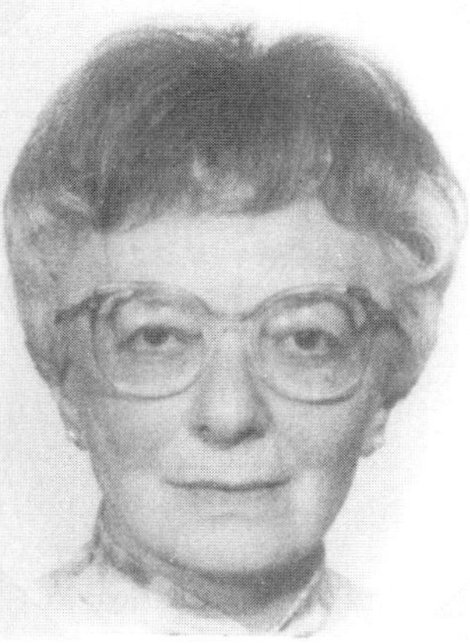

Fig. 1. The Founding Executive Committee of the International Atherosclerosis Society. Top: Dr Gotthard Schettler (dec): President. Bottom left: Dr Antonio Gotto Jr: Vice-President. Bottom right: Dr M. Daria Haust: Secretary-Treasurer.

tive Committee, i.e., President: Dr Gotthard Schettler (Germany), Vice-President: Dr Antonio Gotto Jr (USA) and Secretary-Treasurer: Dr M. Daria Haust (Canada), elected in Milan (November, 1977) and ratified by voting per mail ballot (in early 1978) (Fig. 1).

In the meantime Dr Holmes completed the necessary procedures for the IAS to become incorporated in the Commonwealth of Pennsylvania, Department of State (3-1-78: 521, 1705) on 29 November 1978. We were now in the possession of our own corporate seal (Fig. 2), able to apply (Fig. 3) to the Department of Treasury, Internal Revenue Service of the USA-Government for Federal Tax exemption, and obtained this status on 5 September 1980 (Fig. 4). This opened the door for collection of membership dues and for soliciting corporate support.

Shortly before the Houston Symposium (1979), a letter was received from Dr Harry Jellinek of Hungary, regarding the fact that no potential members from the countries of Eastern Europe would be able to join the IAS because of state regulations. It suggested, at least on behalf of the Hungarian Atherosclerosis Society, that the only avenue for them to join would be via en bloc membership. In order to allow for en bloc membership, the newly written Constitution would have to be rewritten; prior to such (considerable) undertaking, it seemed advisable to explore with the other existing national or regional societies whether

Fig. 2. IAS-Corporate Seal (1978).

law to be filed in any state, territory, or dependency of the United States, or in any foreign country, in which said officers shall find it necessary or expedient to file the same to authorize the corporation, to transact business in such state, territory, dependency or foreign country.

    RESOLVED, That the proper officers of the corporation are hereby authorized and directed to make application for exemption from income tax under the appropriate section of the United States Internal Revenue Code and to file all necessary documents and forms in connection therewith.

Dated: November 29, 1978

DR. COLIN ADAMS	DR. S. GERO
DR. Y. GOTO	DR. A. GOTTO
DR. M.D. HAUST	DR. W. L. HOLMES
DR. D. KRITCHEVSKY	DR. C. MIRAS
DR. R. PAOLETTI	DR. G. ROTHBLAT
DR. G. SCHETTLER	DR. C. SCHLIERF
	DR. R. WISSLER

Fig. 3. Signatures of the majority of Members of the Executive Council on the document empowering the IAS to seek the Federal Tax exemption.

158

Internal Revenue Service
District Director

Department of the Treasury

Date: SEP 05 1980

RECEIVED
SEP 8 1980
DEPT. OF RESEARCH

Employer Identification Number:
23-2099003
Accounting Period Ending:
November
Form 990 Required: ☒ Yes ☐ No

International Atherosclerosis
Society, Dept. of Research
Lankenau Hospital
Lancaster and City Line Aves.
Phila., PA 19151

Person to Contact:
Mrs. S. Pratt
Contact Telephone Number:
(215) 597-4168

Dear Applicant:

   Based on information supplied, and assuming your operations will be as stated
in your application for recognition of exemption, we have determined you are exempt
from Federal income tax under section 501(c)(3) of the Internal Revenue Code.

   We have further determined that you are not a private foundation within the
meaning of section 509(a) of the Code, because you are an organization described
in section 509(a)(1) & 170(b)(1)(A)(vi).

Fig. 4. The document from the US-Government Treasury Department re: Federal Tax exemption status of the IAS (1980).

they, too, would envisage joining en bloc. For that purpose, the representatives of the known existing Societies for the study of Atherosclerosis were invited to meet with the Executive Committee of the IAS on the occasion of the Houston Symposium. After discussion in depth, all representatives of the various Societies expressed the desire to join the IAS en bloc as Constituent Societies; they took this matter to their respective Societies for ratification. The representatives present at the above meeting reported shortly thereafter of the desire of their Societies to join as Constituent-Societies, although officially only five were able to complete this step immediately (French, Italian, Japanese, Scandinavian and the European Atherosclerosis Groups).

   Subsequently, other Societies also applied for a similar status. At the time of the Rome Symposium (1988) there were 18 Constituent Societies in the IAS in addition to numerous individual and Corporate Members (vide infra). Upon our initiative several Societies were constituted de novo and at least one, that was dormant, was reactivated.

   To allow the Societies to join en bloc, the Constitution had to be rewritten (by myself) and approved by the now existing members of the IAS. Moreover, to reflect the new membership-structure of the IAS, the originally constituted Council had to be replaced by representatives of all Constituent Societies — a task completed only in the early spring of 1983. These representatives were nominated now by the Constituent Societies as were those serving on the Program and International Finance Committees (for the Symposia).

It is reasonable to assume that the Constituent Societies opted for an "en bloc" membership because of the US$2.00 dues for a Society member/per annum instead of US$10.00 required for the Individual Membership, the representation on the Council, the input into the programs of the International Symposia, the interaction between the various Constituent Societies, and the eligibility to apply on behalf of any member for the Fellowships and Scholarships (that were established later; vide infra), to name only a few.

As in all existing societies, the membership fee (whether for individual members or through the Constituent Societies) was calculated on an annual basis. Compared with the fees in other societies the US$2.00 per annum per member (of the Constituent Society) was quite a bargain, particularly if one added to it the privilege of subscribing (as a member of the IAS), at a considerably reduced price, to "Atherosclerosis", the leading international journal in the field, and published "in affiliation with" the IAS.

Returning to the goals of the IAS: these have been, of course, much broader than only the organization of the triennial International Symposia on Atherosclerosis. These goals were stated in general terms in Article III of the Constitution and were excerpted in part in the President's Message (then Dr Schettler) published in the October 1980 issue of the Newsletter (IAS) as well as in the first 1981 issue of "Atherosclerosis".

Already, with the second (1982) Berlin Symposium, steps were undertaken to facilitate the participation of young investigators from underprivileged or monetarily restricted countries; our International Finance Committee helped finance the attendance of several young colleagues as well as of some colleagues from various Constituent Societies who needed assistance. It was envisaged from the beginning that the Fellowships for young investigators in support of travel to various centers for a time of study will be established as soon as the accumulated funds will permit it.

Some other goals mentioned in the President's Message were also achieved in a short time of the IAS existence. For example two of the oldest existing Societies that were rather exclusive and restrictive, increased their membership to almost twice their former number and admitted quite a few young investigators — a feature hardly thinkable even a few years prior to the IAS' existence. There is little doubt that the presence and the activities of the IAS contributed substantially to the changing attitudes of the "old guard".

Financial matters

Throughout the almost 5 years (1976—1980) since the creation of the Task Force (Tokyo) to late 1980 when the Internal Revenue Service of the Department of Treasury of the USA-Government granted the IAS a Federal income tax exempt status (Fig. 4), there were no financial resources to support the activities of the IAS developing on several fronts. The funds needed for the purpose of the incorporation (the fees of incorporation in Pennsylvania and those of the lawyer)

160

were provided to the IAS by the Executive Committee (Dr Schettler: US$400.00 borrowed from and later reimbursed to The (German) Association for Advancement of Investigations in Myocardial Infarction; Dr Gotto: US$400.00 from Baylor College of Medicine (return not requested) and Dr Haust: US$100.00 — personal donation (return not requested). Upon designing our IAS-logo Dr Schettler made available to the Executive Committee members printed IAS stationary — at no expense.

All the remaining ongoing expenses (secretarial work, innumerable long-distance telephone calls, postage, xeroxing and travel, see below) were in part carried by my office at the University of Western Ontario; London, Canada, but largely on my research grants. These considerable expenses extending over almost 5 years were never reimbursed to my grants or my University office. It was therefore a great relief to begin receiving the US$2.00/person/year for members in the Constituent-Societies and US$10.00 per Individual Member as of 1980. Moreover, Dr Schettler almost single handedly succeeded in obtaining support from 18 corporations (largely placed in Germany). The contributions were modest, ranging from US$100.00 to 500.00 per annum; some were only a one-time donation, some limited their support for 5 to 7 years but, two (ASTRA Chemicals and Pfizer Gmbh) continue supporting the IAS to this very day, i.e., annually, since 1980).

I wish to express our sincere appreciation to these small and not-so-small corporations without whose help in those initial months and years of establishing the IAS the task would have been so much more difficult.

Newsletter; Journal affiliation

It was considered essential that two avenues of communications between the Executive Committee and the membership; as well as between the various groups and individuals of the IAS be established as soon as possible. Anxious to establish the two avenues, the Secretary-Treasurer (MDH) "produced" the first Newsletter of the Society in October 1980, i.e., shortly after the tax exemption document (Fig. 4) was received from the USA-Federal Government. The Newsletter was produced in a rather modest form (but proudly exhibited the already acquired IAS-logo) with her own laboratory and secretarial staff; 200 copies of it were taken kindly by one of her colleagues to the annual meeting of the Council on Arteriosclerosis of the AHA for distribution (as she was unable to attend herself). The plan was that someone else would continue with the editing of the Newsletter, as it was humanly impossible for the Secretary-Treasurer to assume also this (important!) job. As no volunteers were found, this remained the only issue until the Newsletter was "revived" years later.

The matter of Journal affiliation faired better. At the time of the IAS development, three journals were published that potentially would have been suitable for publications of the members of the IAS but were not already associated or "bound" to other scientific bodies: "Artery" — a new small size journal of yet not established reputation; "Paroi Arterielle" ("Arterial Wall") published in Paris by Centre National de la Recherche Scientifique (carrying publications in both English and French since the mid-60s), and "Atherosclerosis" published in English by Elsevier Science, being the oldest in existence (on whose Editorial Board served in earlier years colleagues of outstanding reputation). "Artery" was soon ruled out as a suitable vehicle. In view of the strong desire of my respected colleague and Editor-in-Chief of the "Paroi Arterielle", Dr L. Scebat, to "win" our favour, I travelled to Paris (on the occasion of one of my journeys to Europe) to discuss with him this matter in person. I left without any commitment and subsequently met with the Editor-in-Chief of "Atherosclerosis", Dr Colin Adams, a trusted and respected colleague and friend; he brought along to our meeting Mrs Judith Taylor from the representative publishers, Elsevier Science.

It soon became apparent that both journals were in a somewhat difficult phase of their operations, but the status of the "Paroi Arterielle" seemed to me more precarious. To associate ourselves with a Journal that had little prospect of surviving (and perhaps therefore saw in our joining or affiliation a form of rescue) would have been a folly, as we would have gone "down" with that Journal in our then difficult financial status. Whereas the motives of "Atherosclerosis" may have been similar to those of the "Paroi Arterielle", at least I was able to negotiate with Dr Adams an association that would give the IAS the needed exposure, a forum, advantages of special subscription for members, but no obligations whatsoever, as we would be: "affiliated" with the Journal rather than "associated" or sponsoring it. And finally, I believed that this Journal had a better chance of survival than the "Paroi Arterielle".

Thus, after communicating the results of my explorations to Dr Schettler by telephone and his agreement, this matter was discussed and approved officially by the Executive and Council, and "Atherosclerosis" was chosen as the "home" Journal for the IAS. The terms of reference of the Affiliation were meticulously defined in a document signed by the three representatives: Dr Adams, Mrs Taylor and myself. Amongst the terms: "Printing of announcements of meetings, Conferences, and other important news of the IAS in "Atherosclerosis" without charge; a 50% reduction of the Journal's subscription cost to *every* member of the IAS, and the representation of the IAS on the policy making body of the Journal". The concessions to the Journal from the IAS: the Editor-in-Chief to be an ex-Officio member on the IAS-Council, "Affiliated with the IAS" to be printed on the front page of the Journal, and an agreement that Elsevier Science would be given *a chance* to compete for publishing any or all Supplements, as well as books, and Proceedings of Symposia and meetings compiled or written by the IAS-members. It is fair to state that the choice of this Journal was the right one and we have been existing in a satisfactory "symbiosis" ever since. (Parenthetically, the "Paroi Arterielle" (Arterial Wall) ceased its publication in 1983.)

The logo (reproduced in green on the stationary and Program of this Symposium) represents an arterial cross-section with a prominent atherosclerotic plaque protruding into and narrowing the lumen. In its original format it is bright red on a white background; as such it appears on all official IAS-stationary and the Newsletter (vide infra) and was adopted in other colours for the stationeries and programmes of the more recent International Symposia on Atherosclerosis (blue — Montreal, 1994; green — Paris, 1997).

There is a personal touch to the story under which conditions the logo (Fig. 5) was "born". It was a beautiful afternoon one summer day in 1979 in Heidelberg when Dr Schettler and I sat on the balcony off his imposing office at the Ludolf-Krehl Clinic, discussing, as we ceasingly did in those days, "our" IAS and all the outstanding matters that required action. And the matter of a logo came up (I believe that in Germany in those days a logo was of little importance). We both embarked upon the drawings of various shapes and nature aiming at simplicity and easy reproducibility. The logo as we know it was accepted. Dr Schlettler summoned immediately his secretary advising that several sheets with this logo be printed prior to my departure for Canada! What a feeling of "security" it was to carry the stationary along with me home! Whenever I see the logo today — I see also the lovely scene on a balcony and feel that in each of our logos there is a grain of Dr Schettler and of myself.

The period of transition

There was a "change of guards" at the VII International Symposium in Melbourne (1985), and a new Executive Committee took over: Dr Antonio Gotto Jr — President; Dr Gotthard Schettler — Past President, Dr Louis Smith — Secretary and Dr M. Daria Haust — Treasurer. (Later, when the decision was made that the next, i.e., Symposium VIII would take place in Rome, Dr Gaetano Crepaldi, the host of that Symposium became Vice-President.)

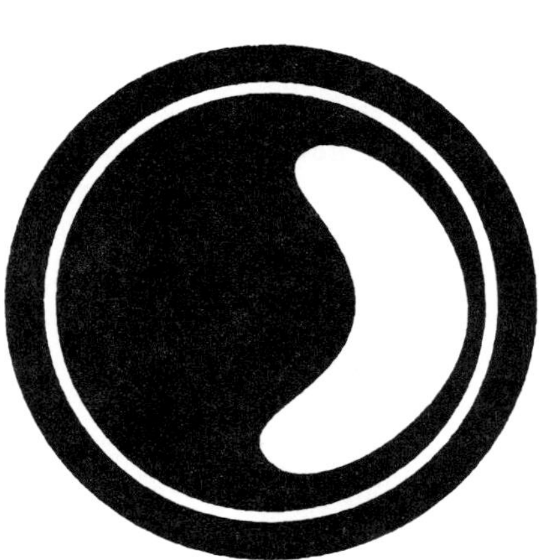

Fig. 5. IAS-logo.

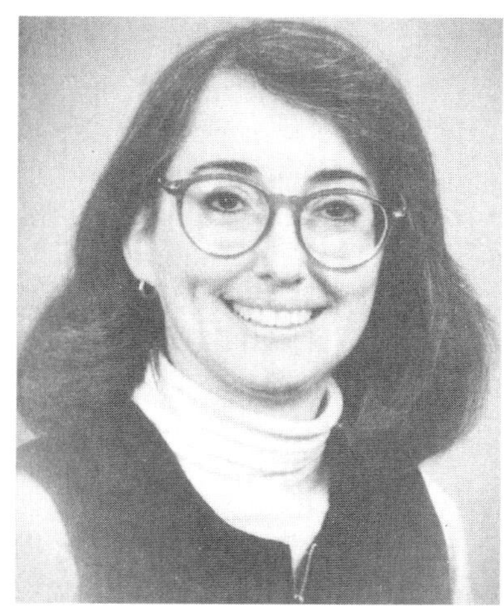

Fig. 6. Ms Barbara Gordin, Executive Director, IAS.

The reasons for the change in the leadership have never been articulated in the open, and even the most strongly argued argument did not quite hold true: "The Constitution & By-laws provide that the President holds his office for six years and thus we need to comply. Moreover, six years is much too long for a term and the Constitution and By-laws need to be rewritten reducing the term to three years only". The first part of this argument did not reflect the actual facts because our Constitution and Bylaws as written by me in the final version was endorsed by members only in 1980, thus the term of President's Office was 1 year short of the 6 years. Moreover, one could hardly count as an actual term of office the initial years of "building" the IAS. In that initial period not only the President but we all in the Executive Committee tried to find our ways through totally unknown territory; and such time of uncertainties, trials and tribulations can hardly be considered a "time in office". Finally, the explanation that the term of Office needed to be reduced to 3 years (and therefore the Constitution & By-laws be once again rewritten) appears in retrospect surprising.

As the IAS-Secretary, I wrote my last Minutes of the Executive Committee and Council Meetings as well as of the General Business Meeting in Melbourne, and as in the years before, the copies were mailed individually to all in attendance.

In January, 1986, Dr Louis Smith, the new Secretary of the IAS, came to London, Ontario (he must have been very cold arriving from sunny Houston) to take over this part of my Office (I continued as the Treasurer). We spent 3 days in which we made strenuous attempts of "indoctrinating" him with his duties. But it was difficult for both of us to work in an organized fashion, because the different working routes and patterns since my days on the Task Force were so intertwined with each other! The many boxes (prepared by my secretary with files on IAS) seemed like mountains that could not be conquered, ever. I myself had not realized until then how much material had accumulated since the idea of the IAS was conceived. I have always been in the habit of providing the Executive Members and other concerned parties with copies of the pertinent correspondence; the bulk of the latter seemed to be never-ending in the course of our review and work. The kind and gentle Dr Smith never lost his patience, but after the 3 days it was decided to ship to him (in Houston) all materials concerning the Secretary's job for his further study, along with important documents and items (the Society's seal; documents of Incorporation; originals of the various Constitutions and Bylaws, etc.). I also provided him with a set of all minutes of all meetings written and sent out by me, and all the ballots ever sent out for voting by mail. Of all that material the only items kept by myself were personal letters written often in confidence to me by my colleagues and friends while we were "building" the IAS. In April of the same year I travelled to Houston, to complete with Dr Smith his takeover of the Secretary's duties and much was accomplished on that visit.

It seems that a certain "hiatus" set in during the period between the Melbourne (1985) and the Rome (1988) Symposia, as neither Executive Committee meetings nor any regular kind of communication between the IAS-office and the IAS-membership occurred in that period. Expressions of concern at this turn of events were conveyed to me from time to time and I was alarmed by the possibility that all the years of effort put into the project of the IAS may prove futile. To prevent any real or perceived disaster ("revolution"?) a quick remedy was advisable prior to the Rome Symposium (1988). I therefore proposed to furnish a (quickly written) brief history of the IAS for publication in "Atherosclerosis" prior to the Rome Symposium. The strategy worked but the hurried time and deadline were responsible for a grave mistake committed by me (I included, incorrectly, Dr Gotto with those who were elected in Tokyo to serve on the Task Force).

I believe that as of the Rome Symposium "life began slowly returning to the IAS". The Constitution and Bylaws commissioned by Dr Gotto from someone who was apparently very experienced in writing such documents, proved totally unsuitable for our purposes, and the work of rewriting had to begin again. On this occasion of rewriting the Constitution and Bylaws I was assisted quite energetically by Dr Louis Smith. We first spent a couple of days working on this project in Houston, and later he joined me in London, Ontario, for completing this work. The new version was circulated to all members on the Executive Committee and at a special meeting, section by section was discussed in detail.

During this period of transition some inconsistencies appeared imperceptibly in the "structuring" of the Executive Committee. For example, with no appropriate provision in the Bylaws, for the first time and without any discussion, the Chairman of the forthcoming Symposium in Melbourne (Dr P. Nestel) became the Vice-Chairman of the Executive Committee. Amazed by this development and anxious not to see the legitimate Vice-President (Dr A. Gotto) "dislodged" I proposed that he should remain on the Executive Committee as Vice-President II, and retain his rightful function. Subsequently, this matter became even more complex with a real "crowding" around the Vice-Presidency. Prior to the X. Symposium in Montreal in 1994, there was Vice-President I (Dr J. Davignon; Chairman of the X. Symposium), Vice-President II (Dr Y. Stein; Chairman of the past IX. Symposium) and Vice-President III (Dr G. Crepaldi; Chairman of the past VIII. Symposium). It was unknown, however, who of the three gentlemen was the holder of the actual (legitimate) Office of the Vice-Presidency of the IAS. Indeed, it was high time to complete the rewriting of the Constitution and Bylaws, a process intended since the VII. Symposium in Melbourne (1985).

A revised version of the Constitution and Bylaws was finally ratified by all Constituent Societies at the Council Meeting in Rosemount-Chicago (1991) at the IX. Symposium, but it was presented to the membership at the General Business Meeting 3 years later (1994) at the X. Symposium in Montreal. The other changes voted upon the recommendation of the Executive Committee and Council at the IX. Symposium were the increases in annual dues: from US$2.00 to 3.00 for each member of a Constituent Society and from US$10.00 to 15.00 for Individual Members.

As the Individual Members (formerly a large group) in time joined their newly established national and regional (Constituent) Societies, their number in the IAS diminished progressively to only a few. Conversely, the Constituent Societies grew in number steadily (see infra).

Present status

As the IAS grew in size and stature it was becoming increasingly apparent that even with separation of the previous duties of a Secretary-Treasurer into two posts (Secretary and Treasurer) it would be impossible to attend to all existing needs and to develop programs as set out in our goals and objectives without securing an assistance in carrying out certain tasks. This became particularly acute in the face of the many obligations and increasing workload of our President, Dr Gotto. Thus, with the generous sponsorship of four large pharmaceutical companies, a permanent office of the IAS was established at the Baylor Medical College in Houston, TX, and Ms Barbara Gordin (Fig. 6) was appointed as the part-time Executive Director and supported by part-time secretarial help. The work of Ms Gordin and her staff contributed enormously to the streamlining of the IAS activities. Amongst other functions Ms Gordin undertook to handle almost all correspondence with the growing members of the IAS as well as concerning herself with the dues, and other communications relating to the IAS. Conscientious, dependable, tactful and always pleasant, Ms Gordin has been a soothing element that added the human touch to the IAS. One of the early tasks of her office was to assemble a database of all members of the IAS. It is largely owing to her presence and work that the IAS-Newsletter (issued only once in 1980) was reinstituted biannually and sent individually to every IAS-member. There is little doubt that many other activities of the IAS were enabled by the help provided by Ms Gordin.

In addition to issuing regularly the biannual newsletter, the IAS was able to realize in the past few years one of its most important and ambitious goals: it instituted two Visiting Fellowships with the objectives of improving the awardee's skills and knowledge, learning new research techniques and entering new fields of scientific areas. The first of these Fellowships (not intended for trainees or postgraduate fellows) is for a period of 3 months; the second (established at the X. Symposium in Montreal, 1994), i.e., the "M. Daria Haust-Award", is for a period of 6 months and intended explicitly for young investigators (under the age of 35 years). Thus, the Fellowship Program (of which we dreamed so longingly in those early days of the IAS) became a reality, and to date allowed 38 fellows to spend several months in a host laboratory. This program is a truly international endeavour, with 34 of the fellows living in Europe, the Middle East, Asia and the Pacific Region, and four being from North America. A number of the fellows reside in the Eastern European Countries; without the IAS-funding, their travel abroad would be impossible considering the economic conditions of their homelands. In 1995, the IAS was honoured by the American Society of Association Executives; our Fellowship Program was added to their Association's Advance America Honor Roll.

In addition to the Fellowship Program the Donald S. Frederickson Award was established in 1991 to honour a senior investigator at the time of the IAS-International Symposia. The (third) recipient of this prestigious Award at the forthcoming XI. Symposium in Paris will be Dr Daniel Steinberg of San Diego, California.

We have been fortunate, too, to receive several bequests, but it has been largely the continuous generous support from our main corporate sponsors (at present: Merck Sharp & Dohme, Parke-Davis, Division of Warner-Lambert Co. and Novartis Pharmaceuticals Corp.; for a number of previous years also: the Bristol-Myers Squibb Co.) that enabled the IAS to advance and fulfill its goals.

As indicated above the ratified latest "edition" of the revised Constitution and Bylaws went into effect at the X. Symposium in Montreal (1994). Its aim has been to streamline and clarify the governance of today's IAS, whose operations and activities became increasingly complex with its growth. Today the IAS "embraces" 36 national or regional Societies from around the world and from all continents (including one of Africa), with a total membership amounting to almost 7,000. The last (X) International Symposium in Montreal in 1994 was attended by 3,100 people. This indicates that we have achieved a considerable prominence in the world of science.

The new Constitution and Bylaws formalize the relation of the IAS to the IAS-International Symposia and to their sponsoring (host) societies, specify procedures for elections of the governing body, terms of Office and succession of Officers. The previously governing Executive Committee consisting of five Officers has been replaced by a larger Executive Board. It consists of the President (Dr A. Gotto), Past President (Dr G. Schettler — dec), President-Elect (Dr R. Paoletti), Secretary (Dr M. Rosseneu), Treasurer (Dr D. Pometta), and three Members-at-Large (Drs J. Davignon, Y. Stein, A. Yamamato); it includes the Historian (Dr M. Daria Haust). The Executive Board meets at least once per year.

"Epilogue"

Since this writing aspires to "live-up" to its title ("IAS — a personal journey"), how would I view my own role or place in that 20-year-long journey? I believe my role has been largely that of a "facilitator". This may be best illustrated by activities "behind the scenes". In particular, countless colleagues were assisted in their quest of joining the IAS as individual members in those years when no societies existed in Central and Eastern Europe, and in other politically restrictive countries. Similarly, persistent (even if at times years-long) efforts were made to assist groups of colleagues in similar regions to obtain the permission of their governments to constitute themselves into Societies that could "en bloc" join the IAS. Such permissions were not easily obtained, but it was even more difficult, if not impossible, to be provided with the means of paying the necessary annual membership dues in foreign currency (US$). In several instances, the initial dues for such societies were possible by a private loan by this writer — a loan that was always returned later with gratitude.

In other instances, particularly in the early phases of our development, it was essential to attend the scientific (and thus the Business) Meetings of well-established Societies to speak on behalf of the IAS and convince the members of the advantages in joining the IAS. Other colleagues, especially those from previously politically constrained countries required the advice and the "know how" in their preparations for a Constituent Society status in the IAS.

Looking back on that time (that continued until as late as last year), one remembers vividly every instance with pleasure, and every travel related to these activities as a true adventure, as well as a privilege. These travels took me to Sweden (April, 1977) where in Stockholm, consulted by Dr Sören Björkerud about the advisability of creating the Scandinavian Atherosclerosis Society despite a very strong opposition by most prominent Swedish scientists, I not only encouraged him to proceed, but was able to secure for him support from other prominent Swedish scientists (while in Malmö). When the Hungarian Society tried in vain to obtain permission to join us, I traveled to attend the 6th Hungarian Arteriosclerosis Conference in Dobogokö (September, 1981) where (I knew from Prof Gerö's communication) I would meet their guest, the Minister of Health. There was no problem to convince the charming gracious Minister how important for Hungary's population it would be if the Society were in the mainstream of the current scientific knowledge on the "killer disease". The Hungarians quickly obtained the permission to join the IAS and paid their dues in US$! Some such efforts took a much longer time, but were equally successful in the end. After some 6 years of writing to the various authorities in the (then) USSR (without receiving any reply), I finally traveled to (then) Leningrad upon Prof A. Klimov's invitation (seemingly to participate in a special scientific Conference) in the main because I was informed that Prof Chazov, the powerful Minister of Health, would be attending too, as would Prof V. Smirnov (who was on "our" side and anxious to join the IAS). It so happened that Prof Chazov received a while earlier an honorary degree from Queen's University, here in Canada, and Queen's is my Alma Mater. This common bond facilitated greatly our conversation in Leningrad, and shortly thereafter the "Atherosclerosis Group" of the Soviet Society of Cardiology, was permitted to join the IAS. Space does not permit for more anecdotal accounts in such detail, but it may be of interest that my travels (for the same purposes) to China, Tbilisi (Georgia), Cuba, the Czech Republic and Slovakia, all culminated in the creation of respective National Societies for the purpose of joining the IAS as Constituent Societies. In still other instances my travels were timed to allow me to speak to (and "convert") membership of a Society not inclined to join the IAS (then: British Atherosclerosis Discussion Group; Cambridge, 1980), or to members of a newly constituted Society, explaining the advantages of the IAS-membership (Spanish Society; Valencia, 1987). One had also the pleasure and privilege to assist colleagues who on their own wished to create national Societies but required information or guidance (the Polish, Argentinean, Indian, Portuguese, New Zealand and Austrian Societies). And naturally, to keep step with other groups we have constituted ourselves in Canada into a Society, too (only in 1983).

It may not seem modest but it is correct to state that of today's 36 Constituent Societies of the IAS, the role of a "facilitator" was played by me in half (18) of these. In all, but one, instances (Stockholm, Sweden) the travel expenses for the above purposes were carried only by myself, and there never was any financial contribution to these "escapades" from the meager coffers of the IAS.

Prior to closing that journey, let me review objectives and goals of the IAS set out in our first Constitution and Bylaws, and assess how far we have gone in the past 20 years in reaching these goals.

"The International Atherosclerosis Society (IAS) was incorporated in 1978 and obtained a tax-free status in 1980. It promotes, at an international level, the advancement of science, research, and teaching in the field of atherosclerosis. It endeavours to achieve these objectives by promoting the exchange of existing knowledge; encouraging new research ventures and interdisciplinary approaches; establishing visiting fellowships for investigators; fostering the dissemination of knowledge by organizing international symposia and interim meetings; and through affiliation with a scientific journal. Membership is open to active researchers who join one of the 36 IAS national or regional Constituent Societies, as individual members from countries which do not have an IAS-affiliated society; and to corporate organizations facilitating the objective of the IAS."

The above citation, concurs, indeed, that our goals and objectives are being met, almost beyond any ambitious expectations.

The history of our (compassionate) Society would be incomplete were we not to pay tribute to those colleagues and friends who departed since the last International Symposium (Montreal, 1994). Their scientific contributions and human attributes could be summarized only briefly; our Society is much indebted to the eight outstanding people whom we shall miss very much.

In memoriam (1995—1997) (in alphabetical order)

Pietro Avogaro

Pietro Avogaro was born in Venice, Italy, on 20 March 1923 and died there on 12 June 1995 after a long distressing illness which he faced with dignity and a rare courage.

Avogaro (known to his friends as Piero) received his medical degree in 1947 from the University of Padova. Continuing his postgraduate studies he became a "specialist" in Physiology (1950; University of Napoli), Hematology (1956; University of Padova) and Gerentology (1967; University of Cagliari, Sardinia). His academic career began in 1958 under the direction of Prof Gino Patrassi, Department of Medicine, the University of Padova, culminating with the rank of

Professor in the School of Cardiology at the same University (1982—1992).

Avogaro began working in the field of metabolic disorders in the late 50s. While at the University of Padova he published with Gaetano Crepaldi the first account and delineation of the "plurimetabolic syndrome" (later renamed: "syndrome X"). His main contributions to atherosclerosis and related fields were made after his return to Venice (1967), where he established and directed (1968—1995) a large, well-organized clinical centre and supporting laboratories for lipid research.

With his large staff and many collaborators Avogaro was very prolific. Of his 356 publications most are concerned with the results of research carried out at that centre (Ospedale Regionale Generale di Venezia) where he served as the Physician-in-Chief (1967—1988). He was also the Director of the Section on Clinical Epidemiology at the Specialized Regional Centre (in Venice) for the Study of Atherosclerosis (1970—1988), and since 1988 until his death, its Primario Emeritus and Scientific Director.

Important of the "Venice period" are the studies on: apoproteins as predictors of cardiovascular risk, familial hyper-α-lipoproteinemia and the significance of Lp(a). In the last years of his life, Avogaro concerned himself with the mechanisms of LDL-oxidation and the identification of in vivo markers of LDL-oxidation.

Avogaro was a member of many national and international scientific societies and of several editorial boards of scientific publications. As an invited speaker he lectured often at international scientific gatherings. He received a number of awards in recognition for his scientific contributions. One of the latest ("Andreas Vesalius Medal") was awarded to him in Padua from his Alma Mater (University of Padova) (25 May 1993).

Whereas in his work Piero — a very disciplined man — was demanding of and strict with himself and his co-workers, he knew also the pleasurable side of life. He has been missed not only by his beloved wife Bruna and his son and daughter, but also by his many friends at home and abroad.

Edwin L. Bierman

Edwin L. Bierman was born in Far Rockaway, New York, USA on 17 September 1930 and died in Seattle, Washington, on 5 July 1995 after a long but courageous battle with cancer.

After receiving his MD-degree from Medical College, Cornell University (1955), Bierman (known to his colleagues and friends as Ed) spent in New York a year (1955—1956) of internship at the New York Hospital, another at the Rockefeller Institute of Medical Research (1956—1957) and moved to Denver, Colorado, working as an Assistant Chief and Chief of Metabolic Research Division, US-Army Medical Research & Nutrition Lab (1957—1959). He returned to New York to complete his residency (1959—1960) in Medicine and began his academic career as an Assistant Professor at Rockeffeler Institute (1960—1962).

170

He left for the University of Washington School of Medicine, Seattle, WA, where after a year as an Assistant Professor (1962–1963) he was promoted quickly (1963–1968: Associate Professor) to full Professor in Medicine (1968). he also served as Director of the Northwest Lipid Research Clinic (1971–1973), and was Head of the Division of Metabolism, Endocrinology and Gerentology (1975–1994) and Co-Director, Clinical Nutrition Research Unit at the University of Washington. He remained and continued working at this University virtually until his death.

Bierman has a long record of research accomplishments in fields of diabetes, obesity, hyperlipidemia and atherosclerosis. The prevailing theme in his studies was an attempt at elucidating abnormalities of processing and transport of energy-rich metabolites in human disease and their relation to atherosclerosis. His investigations included: insulin's role in lowering plasma free fatty acids in diabetes mellitus by limiting their outflow from adipose tissues; abnormalities of triglyceride transport in pathogenesis of hyperlipidemias in man; the role of diet in regulating the plasma glucose homeostasis and lipid metabolism; and many others. It was also he who first utilized cultured arterial smooth muscle cells in the study of LDL-metabolism, thus opening the door for future evaluations (by others) of the role of the LDL-receptor and cholesterol metabolism in smooth muscle cells. In midcareer, Bierman became a major figure in the development of medical and health policies. His clinical research led to changes in managing diabetic patients; this he championed within the American Diabetes Association as Chair of its Food and Nutrition Committee, as Chair of the Nutrition Committee of the American Heart Association (AHA), and in several similar bodies.

Bierman was a member of 20 professional and scientific USA-societies, numerous national scientific and academic Committees, Boards, Task Forces, Study Sections (NIH) and Councils, and was elected Chairman, Co-Chairman or President of a number of scientific Societies (Western Association of Physicians; AHA-Council on Arteriosclerosis; American Society of Clinical Nutrition, and Food and Nutrition Board, National Academy of Sciences). He served on eight Editorial Boards of Scientific Journals, and in 1980 became the Founding Editor of "Arteriosclerosis" (now: "Arteriosclerosis, Thrombosis and Vascular Biology") of the AHA; he was Chief Editor for a decade. He was a prolific writer with over 250 publications and six books to his name.

Bierman was a dedicated educator and a true mentor. His role in the development and promoting of young colleagues was well known; many of his "disciples" went on to distinguished careers in biomedical sciences.

In recognition for his numerous contributions to science, academia and public life he received (some) 15 Awards or Honours. He was the Lyman Duff Lecturer (AHA, 1991) and obtained from the AHA the Merit, Gold Heart, Special Recognition (Council on Arteriosclerosis) and Scientific Councils Distinguished Achievement Awards. He was elected to the Institute of Medicine of the National Academy of Sciences, USA in 1988, and was invited as a Visiting Professor to Hebrew University, Hadassah Medical School (1972–1973), Jerusalem, Israel.

As a man Ed will be remembered for his warmth, grace, great sense of humour and work ethic, and for his dedication and commitment to his family. He left his beloved wife Marilyn and his two loving children in deep mourning. To young academicians for whom he was a role model and to colleagues for whom he was a mentor, a counselor or a friend, his loss left an irreplaceable void.

Meier Burstein

Meier Burstein was born in Pinsk (at that time: Russia) in 1908 and died in Paris, France on March 22, 1995.

Burstein studied medicine at the University in Paris, receiving his MD-degree in 1935. His postgraduate studies, upon which he embarked subsequently, were interrupted by the invasion of France in the WWII, and his deportation to Auschwitz (1943). Surviving the latter ordeal, he returned to Paris after the war. Here he was appointed to the staff of the National Centre for Blood Transfusion.

At the National Centre Burstein became engaged in investigations of blood coagulation and the role of heparin. His work culminated in the findings that heparin could precipitate lipoproteins. He utilized this knowledge in developing a simple precipitation method that allowed for the separation of various plasma lipoproteins. In 1955 he published the method for the separation of HDL from LDL and VLDL using heparin and manganese. This (relatively easily carried out) method was suitable for adoption by clinical laboratories throughout the world for the measurements of lipoproteins. It was utilized in epidemiological studies concerned (amongst others) with the HDL-cholesterol concentration in relation to the cardiovascular risk.

Following his initial publication in 1955, Burstein, using combinations of polyanions and divalent cations, developed methods for the separation of individual lipoprotein classes. In 1977 he isolated β 2-glycoprotein-II which interacted with triglyceride-rich lipoproteins; he designated it as apoprotein H.

Burstein was known for his unusual kind of humour. Shortly before his death he requested that the level of his cholesterol be determined. He explained to the surprised bystanders that he required this information in order to inform the devil whether to fry him in saturated or unsaturated oil. He continued working in his laboratory almost until the end of his life.

By the scientific community, Burstein will be remembered for his valuable contributions to the methodology of separating and determining the various classes of plasma lipids and their relevance to atherosclerosis. However, his intellect, spirit and determination that were not broken by his horrifying personal experiences in the WWII, deserve an admiration by all mankind.

Francisco Grande-Covián

Francisco Grande-Covián was born in Colunga (Asturias), Spain on 29 June 1909 and died in Madrid, Spain, on 26 June 1995.

Grande-Covián (to his friends: Paco Grande) obtained his medical license in 1931 and his MD-degree in 1932 from the Faculty of Medicine, University of Madrid. His postdoctoral studies in Physiology and Biochemistry took him to the Universities of Copenhagen (Denmark), Lund (Sweden) and London (UK) (1932–1934). He began his independent research as the Chief of Physiology and Vice-Director of the National Institute of Alimentation (1937–1939) in Madrid, moving (1940) to the Institute of Medical Investigations to chair the Department of Physiology. He became full Professor of Physiology and Biochemistry, Faculty of Medicine at the University of Zaragoza in 1950, and after 3 years (1953) left for the University of Minnesota, Minneapolis, USA. He worked here with Ancel Keys in the Laboratory of Physiological Hygiene (until 1974) and held the appointment of Professor of Physiology (of Hygiene and Nutrition) at the Graduate School (1958–1974). He was also the Director of the Jay Phillips Institute of Investigation at Mount Sinai Hospital of Minneapolis. During his USA stay he was a Visiting Professor in Physiology, Faculty of Medicine at the University of California. Upon returning to Spain (1975) he embarked on yet another academic career: Honorary Professor of Biochemistry, Faculty of Sciences at the University of Zaragoza.

Nutrition, and the impact of diet and lipid metabolism on atherosclerosis and cardiovascular risk were the main interests of Grande-Covián. He published with Keys and Anderson in the mid-60s a seminal series of articles including that on the famous formula for predicting the serum cholesterol changes in relation to the dietary fatty acids composition. His 300 original publications, four books and several chapters contributed to other books, attest to many areas of his expertise (biochemistry and physiology of muscle; cardiac metabolism; vitamins; and others). He was an active member of four scientific societies abroad and served on the editorial board of the Am J Clin Nutr.

In recognition of his many contributions to science he was awarded an honorary membership in a number of Academies of Medicine in Spain and in scientific societies in foreign countries and Spain; made an academician of the Academy of (Exacting) Sciences in Zaragoza; received the Rodriguez Pascual Medical Prize (1972), honorary degrees from three universities (Santiago de Compostela, 1970; Oviedo, 1981; Madrid, 1984), and the Great Crosses of Public Health and "El Sabio" of Alfonso X. He was the Honorary President of the Spanish Society for Atherosclerosis.

Raphael Carmena, his first "disciple" in Minneapolis (1965–1971) wrote: "I loved him dearly. He was a very charming and generous person, and we all miss him enormously".

Shlomo Eisenberg

Shlomo Eisenberg was born in Tel-Aviv, Israel in 1935 and died suddenly (while attending a scientific meeting) in France on 17 February 1995.

Eisenberg obtained his MD-degree in 1965 from the Hebrew University —

Hadassah Medical School in Jerusalem. Here he did his residency and later joined the staff. In 1975 he became the Physician-in-Chief of the Department of Medicine B, directing eventually the Unit for Diagnosis and Treatment of Hyperlipidemias. He was promoted to full Professor in 1979 and later served as the Vice-Dean of Medicine (1988—1992). In 1993 he became the Chairman of the Department of Medicine C and the director of a new Institute for Lipid and Atherosclerosis Research at the Sheba Medical Centre and Professor of Medicine in Sackler School of Medicine at Tel-Aviv University.

Eisenberg began his research in lipid, and phospholipid metabolism of arterial wall in 1965 with Olga and Yechezkiel Stein. He spent a postdoctoral year (1970—1971) in NIH, Bethesda, USA, with the Fredrickson-Levy group, and was involved there in early studies on lipoprotein and apoprotein kinetics which defined the major pathways of lipoprotein catabolism and interconversion. Upon his return to Jerusalem he continued animal experimentations and in vitro studies on lipoprotein and apoprotein turnover. He demonstrated that during in vitro lipolysis of VLDL, two major types of particles were formed: "surface remants" and "core remnants". He defined how these components were lost sequentially from the VLDL-particles in the course of lipolysis: the "surface components" were shed as apoprotein-phospholipid-cholesterol discs which fused with pre-existing HDL-particles, whereas apolipoprotein B consistently remained on the "core remnant". Amongst other contributions he presented solid evidence that one VLDL-particle yields one LDL-particle.

In recent years Eisenberg studied the metabolism of postprandial lipoproteins. He established fruitful international collaborations while on sabbatical visits to Sweden (University of Umea) and the USA (Baylor College of Medicine, Houston; University of Washington, Seattle; Rockefeller University, New York City — where he was an Adjunct Professor since 1988).

Eisenberg's seminal contributions to the understanding of lipoprotein metabolism and effects of diet and drugs upon it, and to the insight into the pathophysiology of dyslipoproteinemias earned him an international reputation. In 1993 (May) he was awarded the prestigious Morgani Prize from the University of Padova, Padua, Italy. He served on several Editorial Boards of scientific journals and was a member of a number of international scientific Societies.

Eisenberg's attributes as a scientist were matched by his human characteristics: his warmth; generosity of spirit; infectious vitality; exuberance; keen sense of humour and zest of life. With his untimely death, the scientific world lost an outstanding physician and investigator, his wife Aviva a loving husband, and his four children a caring father. His many colleagues and friends have been missing a special human being. "Let his memory be blessed" said his friend Yechezkiel Stein in Shlomo's native language.

Frederick H. Epstein

Frederick H. Epstein was born in Frankfurt, Germany on 24 July 1916 and died suddenly in Zürich, Switzerland on 23 May 1995.

Epstein (to his friends: Fred) studied Biochemistry at the University of Zürich (1936—1937) but continued at Cambridge University (UK). With the beginning of the WWII he switched to medicine, taking his clinical training at University College Hospital, London (UK) from which he graduated in 1944. After the war he moved to the USA and worked in renal physiology at the New York University College of Medicine, New York. In 1951 he undertook (with Ernst Boas — a known investigator of cholesterol and coronary disease) to study why the rates of atherosclerosis were different in Italian and Jewish descendants. This "Italian and Jewish Garment Workers Study" was a landmark in the emerging field of Epidemiology, and one of the first conducted in the new research department of the Sidney Hillman Health Centre which Epstein directed (1951—1956). It was also decisive in his embarking upon a distinguished, lifelong career in Epidemiology. In 1956 he moved to the Department of Epidemiology, School of Public Health at the University of Michigan, Ann Arbor (1956—1959, Assistant Professor; 1959—1963, Associate Professor; 1963—1973, Full Professor). Here he headed the famous "Tecumseh Study" designed to assess the health and disease of an entire community, to determine common causes of the latter and provide strategies for prevention in youth. This was one of the first studies of risks in cardiovascular (and other) diseases.

In 1973 Epstein joined the Institute of Social and Preventative Medicine of the University of Zürich, serving also as a Scientific Consultant to the Swiss National Science Foundation's program on Prevention of Cardiovascular Disease. Here he remained active until his death.

Epstein's pioneering work in Epidemiology of cardiovascular diseases gained early an international reputation. In 1959 he participated in the first WHO-Conference on Methods in Cardiovascular Epidemiology and throughout his career served as a Consultant to the WHO-Headquarters (Geneva) and the Regional Office for Europe (Copenhagen). He was also a Scientific Advisor to the NIH, Bethesda, Maryland (USA) until his death. He played an important role in either devising or directing several other epidemiological studies in the USA or on a global scale, and in formulating public policy on prevention, also in his seminal publications (the last was a monograph on mortality trends in 27 countries (1996)). He was an invited speaker at countless national and international scientific gatherings; a member of many scientific Societies and an honorary member of other similar bodies; served on a number of Editorial Boards of Scientific Journals (Chief Editor of one), and was Chairman of the Council on Epidemiology of the American Heart Association (1968 and 1969).

In 1980 Epstein received an honorary degree from the Rupterto Carola University, Heidelberg, Germany, and in 1991 became a Member of the Royal College of Physicians, London, UK.

This outstanding scientist was also a very special human being: highly cultured and knowledgeable far beyond the area of his expertise, he showed a genuine compassion for and interest in people, always remaining kind, humble and noble.

Fred's friends mourn his loss with his beloved wife Doris and their four children. He shall be remembered, always.

Hermann Esterbauer

Hermann Esterbauer was born in Ach, Austria on 30 July 1936 and died in Graz, Austria on 7 January 1997. Fully aware of his progressing malignant disease he nevertheless organized a scientific International Symposium only 6 months prior to his death (Styria, Austria; July, 1996). He bore his condition with dignity, stating to his friends: "I now live day by day".

After completing his undergraduate education, Esterbauer stayed on as a postdoctoral fellow and Assistant Professor in the Institute of Physical Chemistry of the Karl-Franzens-University (KFU) in Graz (1963–1968), moving subsequently as an Assistant Professor to the Institute of Biochemistry at KFU where he was habilitated in 1970. He was a postdoctoral fellow in the School of Public Health at the University of Pittsburgh in 1973 and in the Department of Biochemistry at the University of Michigan, Ann Arbor, in 1974. Upon his return to Graz he was promoted to Professor of Biochemistry at the KFU, a post he held from 1974 to 1990, i.e., until he was made a Full Professor (Ordinarius) of Biochemistry. In 1988 he took over the directorship of the Institute of Biochemistry at the KFU and held it until his death. Esterbauer was a Guest Professor in the Departments of General Pathology at the University of Turin (1984–1989) and of Siena (1989), and a Visiting (Honorary) Professor in the Department of Biochemistry, the Brunel University, West London, UK (1987–1993). He received an honorary degree in Medicine and Surgery from the University of Turin in 1992.

Esterbauer was best known as the scientist who first synthesized 4-hydroxynonenal (HNE) (and related aldehydes); throughout his career he worked on the elucidation of the biological function and activity of HNE in addition to other large projects, e.g., the development of a biotechnological process for enzymatic biomass conversion. However, investigators in the field of atherosclerosis will remember him for his important contributions to the area of lipid peroxidaton and the chemistry of oxygen radicals. Towards the end of his life he became particularly fascinated with the relation between the oxidative stress, LDL and atherosclerosis. Many of his over 350 publications address this relation.

For his novel contributions to science Esterbauer earned an international acclaim. He was a member of a number of national and international scientific societies and of editorial boards of scientific journals. He was considered to be an outstanding but also a very generous scientist who shared his material (e.g., free samples of various 4-hydroxyalkenals) and his original thoughts with investigators around the world. He was an unpretentious person, and a congenial host and entertainer. He enjoyed good food, and good wine, and loved nature-hikes. His many colleagues and friends at home and abroad mourn his loss.

Gotthard Schettler

Gotthard Schettler was born in Falkenstein, Germany on 13 April 1917 and died unexpectedly in Heidelberg, Germany on 20 April 1996, after a brief hospital stay.

Schettler studied medicine (1936—1942) at the Universities of Jena, Leipzig, Vienna and finally in Tubingen, obtaining his MD-degree in 1942. He continued there his postdoctoral education (Pathology: 1942—1945; Internal Medicine: 1945—1950). Following his habilitation (1950; Thesis: "Nutrition and Cholesterol Metabolism: Experimental, Chemico-Analytical and Morphological Investigations"), he moved with his admired teacher, Prof H.F. Bock to the University of Marburg (Assistant Professor: 1950—1955; Associate Professor: 1955—1956). He became Director of Medicine in the Hospital of Stuttgart-Bad Cannstatt (1956—1961) and later of the 2nd Department of Medicine at the Free University of Berlin (1961—1963). Finally he held the post of Professor and Head of Medicine at the Ruperto Carola-University and Director of the Ludolf-Krehl Clinic in Heidelberg (1963—1986). Upon his official retirement he continued here his investigative and scholarly work until his death.

Schettler was one of the most outstanding medical scientists in post-WWII Germany and later of the world who pioneered the investigations in lipid metabolism and cholesterol. The broad scientific basis he acquired during his postgraduate education provided him with a life-long insight into his basic investigations, clinical research-trials and epidemiology. He began his studies by standardization of cholesterol measurements, and on the effect of nutrition on blood cholesterol levels in animal models, at a time when little was known on the relation of lifestyle, lipid metabolism and atherosclerosis (see above subject of his habilitation). Already in the late 40s he showed that the intake of vegetable oils lead to lowering of blood cholesterol whereas animal fat intake increased its level. Later he concentrated his work on lipoproteins pioneering their separation by starch gel electrophoresis. In the last decade of his life he concerned himself with epidemiological studies, and with the molecular and genetic basis of atherosclerosis. All of his research was ultimately directed towards the benefit of patients.

Schettler was also an outstanding educator and teacher whose "disciples" are today prominent scientists in their own rights. His textbook for medical students was translated into several languages. He was a prolific writer whose scientific and educational publications numbered almost 1,000, not counting the many books he wrote, and chapters he contributed. He was a member of Editorial Boards of several scientific journals. Of the many scientific gatherings organized and hosted by Schettler notable are the two International Symposia on Atherosclerosis, Berlin (1973 and 1982) and the Congresses of the German Association of Postgraduate Medical Education held by him annually in Berlin for almost three decades (1962—1990).

In recognition for his outstanding scientific and scholastic contributions Schettler was elected to many prestigious offices. In this limited space it would be impossible to cite them all as he served as Chairman, Director or President of 12 national or international scientific bodies. Most notable amongst these were: Chairman of the Scientific Council on Arteriosclerosis (1977—1985) and Scientific Board (1985—1988) of the International Society and Federation of Cardiology, WHO, Geneva; President of the Academy of Humanities and Sciences, Heidelberg (1986—1990) and the (Founding) President of the International Atherosclerosis Society (IAS) (1979—1985) (As Past-President he remained active in the IAS until the end of his life.)

Schettler was made a member of three Academies of Sciences (Swedish; New York; "Leopoldina" in Halle), an Honorary Member of six scientific Societies and was the recipient of 15 Medals, Prizes and Awards from scientific bodies, Universities and States around the globe. The last, (Gold) Ernst-von Bergmann-Medaille of the German Society for Internal Medicine, was awarded to him just days prior to his death. He also received honorary degrees from eight Universities at home and abroad (Munich; Edinburgh, UK; Padova, Italy; Montpellier, France; Berlin; Budapest, Hungary; Wuhan, China; and Kingston, Canada).

It is questionable whether Schettler would have achieved so much in his life without his personal human attributes. His gifts and versatile personality were characterized by his abilities as well as sensitivity, his open-mindedness for communication and friendship and his thinking ahead of times — combined with vigor, determination and honesty. His unique spirit of flexibility and never ceasing creativity kept him forever youthful. A man of broad education, Schettler was in command of several languages and knowledgeable in art and music. He displayed a unique quality of wit. His generosity towards young and struggling colleagues has been legendary.

Gotthard Schettler has been missed painfully by his wife Gina and their three children with respective families. Those of us who had the pleasure and privilege of sharing a segment of his path are now so much poorer by his loss. We shall never forget Gotthard.

Acknowledgements

The author wishes to thank Ms Kristine Milne BA, for her patient, competent and meticulous preparation of the manuscript and for photographic work; Ms Barbara Gordin and Ms Andrea Larsen (both of the Baylor College of Medicine, Houston, Texas) for their kind assistance in providing some photographs of archival items necessary for the completion of the history. A warm appreciation is conveyed to Mrs Bruna Avogaro, Mrs Doris Epstein and Mrs Gina Schettler who generously furnished the data or the photographs of their departed husbands for inclusion in this writing. I wish to express my pleasure of having had the opportunity of working closely with Dr Louis Smith (since 1985) and (since 1990) with Ms Barbara Gordin (whom we shall miss sorely after her leaving the Office in October, 1997).

In closing, my deep gratitude is directed to Dr Antonio Gotto Jr, our current

President, not only for the 20-year-long congenial work together, but also for his wisdom and efforts in leading the IAS to its rightful place of today.

References

1. Editorial. Council on Arteriosclerosis, American Heart Association, NEWSLETTER-SC-83-A, 1983 (January):10—11.
2. Haust MD. Notes on International Atherosclerosis (IAS). Council on Arteriosclerosis, American Heart Association, NEWSLETTER-SC-83-A, 1983 (July): 8—11.
3. Haust MD. A brief "History" and aims of the International Atherosclerosis Society (IAS). Atherosclerosis 1988;73:273—275.
4. Gotto AM Jr. Presentation of the 1994 Distinguished Service Award of the IAS and the establishment and naming of M. Daria Haust-Fellowship. In: Woodford FP, Davignon J, Sniderman A (eds) Atherosclerosis X. Amsterdam: Elsevier Science B.V. (International Congress Series 1066), 1995;7.

EDUCATIONAL LECTURES

Naked cDNA encoding secreted proteins for intra-arterial and intramuscular gene transfer

Takayuki Asahara, Yukio Tsurumi, Satoshi Takeshita and Jeffrey M. Isner
Departments of Medicine (Cardiology) and Biomedical Research, St. Elizabeth's Medical Center, Tufts University School of Medicine, Boston, Massachusetts, USA

Abstract. Experience with intra-arterial and intramuscular gene transfer of VEGF illustrates in pro-totypical fashion how features of the gene, protein and target tissue may all contribute to phenotypic modulation of the host, despite the low-transfection efficiency typical of naked plasmid DNA. These features include the fact that VEGF is naturally secreted, binds to cell-surface heparin sulfates, is generated by hypoxic-endothelial cells, reduces apoptosis, and binds to high-affinity receptors that are upregulated by hypoxia. Thus the success of gene therapy is not solely a function of vectors or transfection efficiency.

Despite major advances in both surgical and percutaneous revascularization techniques, therapeutic options for patients with lower extremity vascular obstructive disease are limited [1]. Conventional drug therapy is of no proven benefit for these patients. When vascular obstruction is lengthy and widespread, percutaneous revascularization may not be feasible. Surgical therapy is complicated by a variable morbidity and mortality and is dependent on long-term graft patency.

Recent investigations have established the feasibility of using recombinant formulations of angiogenic growth factors to expedite and/or augment collateral artery development in animal models of myocardial and hindlimb ischemia [2—9]. This strategy has been termed "therapeutic angiogenesis" and constitutes a potential alternative approach for patients with vascular insufficiency of the heart, lower extremities and other vascular districts as well.

Among the various growth factors which have been shown to promote angiogenesis, vascular endothelial growth factor (VEGF) [10] (also known as vascular permeability factor [11] and vasculotropin (VAS) [12]) is an endothelial-cell-specific mitogen. Because endothelial cells represent the critical cell type responsible for new vessel formation [13], and because smooth muscle cells (one of the critical cell types responsible for the development of certain vascular lesions [14—16]) would not be directly activated, endothelial-cell specificity has been regarded as an important advantage of VEGF for therapeutic angiogenesis.

Four homodimeric species of VEGF have been identified, each monomer having 121, 165, 189 or 206 amino acids, respectively [17]. The secretion pattern of

Address for correspondence: Jeffrey M. Isner MD, St. Elizabeth's Medical Center, 736 Cambridge St, Boston, MA 02135, USA. Tel.: +1-617-789-2392. Fax: +1-617-789-5029. E-mail: VeJeff@aol.com

the four isoforms differs markedly. $VEGF_{121}$ is a weakly acidic polypeptide that does not bind to heparin, and is freely soluble in the conditioned medium of transfected cells. The heparin-binding capabilities of the remaining three isoforms are progressively augmented as the result of a step-wise enrichment in basic residues. Thus $VEGF_{165}$, the predominant form secreted by a variety of normal and transformed cells [18], is a basic heparin-binding glycoprotein with an isoelectric point of 8.5; while secreted, a significant portion remains bound to the cell surface or extracellular matrix. The $VEGF_{189}$ isoform includes 24 additional amino acids and has been shown not to be freely secreted, but instead remains nearly completely bound to the cell surface and/or extracellular matrix [19]. $VEGF_{206}$ is a rare isoform so far identified only in a human fetal liver cDNA library.

No recombinant VEGF protein formulation of any of the three principal isoforms is currently approved or available for human clinical application. Arterial gene transfer constitutes an alternative strategy for accomplishing therapeutic angiogenesis in patients with limb ischemia. In the case of VEGF this is a particularly appealing strategy because the VEGF gene encodes a signal sequence which permits the protein to be naturally secreted from intact cells [17]. Previous studies from our laboratory [20,21] indicated that arterial gene transfer of cDNA encoding for a secreted protein potentially yield meaningful biological outcomes in spite of a low-transfection efficiency. Site-specific transfection of rabbit-ear arteries with the plasmid pXGH5 encoding the gene for human growth hormone, for example, was found to generate physiologic levels of human growth hormone, despite immunohistochemical evidence of gene expression among < 1% of cells in the transfected arterial segment [20]. While the three principal VEGF isoforms differ markedly with regard to heparin avidity, all include the secretory signal sequence. Therefore, we performed preclinical animal studies to establish the feasibility of site-specific gene transfer of $phVEGF_{121}$, $phVEGF_{165}$ and $phVEGF_{189}$ applied to the hydrogel-polymer coating of an angioplasty balloon [22], and delivered percutaneously to the iliac artery of rabbits in which the femoral artery had been excised to cause unilateral hindlimb ischemia [23].

Arterial gene transfer was achieved using "naked DNA", i.e., DNA not associated with viral or other adjunctive vectors such as liposomes [24]. The feasibility of using naked DNA for arterial gene transfer was initially documented in studies employing reporter genes [22,25]; using the hydrogel-polymer-coated balloon catheter, all rabbit arteries transfected with the luciferase gene (33/33, 100%) expressed luciferase activity. Moreover, luciferase activity was detectable for a minimum of 2 weeks posttransfection [22]. The use of DNA alone clearly simplifies the transfection protocol, obviating, for example, concerns regarding the potential toxicity of viral vectors [26].

Among control animals in which hydrogel-coated balloons were used to deliver pGSVLacZ, gene expression was limited < 0.5% of total arterial cells [22]. Presuming a similarly low-transfection efficiency in animals transfected with phVEGF$_{165}$, the demonstration that naked DNA encoding for VEGF could achieve phenotypic modulation of the host circulation confirms previous work suggesting that gene products which are secreted may have profound biologic effects, even when the number of successfully transfected cells remains low. Whether adjunctive use of liposomes or adenoviral vectors might further optimize the functional and/or anatomic results reported to date requires additional study.

Evidence of transgene expression in our animal model of arterial gene transfer has been documented for both VEGF mRNA and protein. Analysis by RT-PCR established that the time course of gene expression in this animal model is < 30 days. This duration of gene expression was nevertheless sufficient to permit augmented collateral vessel development and is consistent with the time course of collateral development reported previously in this animal model, following administration of the recombinant protein [7]. Cessation of gene expression by 30 days may be considered to represent a safety feature of the strategy proposed in this report, in that the recipient is not exposed indefinitely to increased levels of the gene product. The basis for extinction of gene expression in the present case, along with similar observations made by others using nonviral vectors [27], remains enigmatic. To date, no evidence of an immunological basis has been recognized in animal experiments performed using naked DNA [28,29].

Analysis of gene expression at the protein level, using an ELISA assay to evaluate blood samples obtained from the rabbit-ear artery, documented systemic circulation of the gene product. Thus while gene transfer was site-specific (no evidence of VEGF mRNA was detected at remote sites), expression of the protein was not. Light microscopic evidence of angiogenesis nevertheless appeared limited to the ischemic hindlimb. The basis for such a site-specific effect may be related to VEGF receptor expression: high-affinity VEGF receptors, particularly KDR [30−32], are expressed at relatively low levels in quiescent endothelial cells of most adult tissues [33−35], but are upregulated as much as 13-fold when endothelial cells are exposed to media conditioned by hypoxic myocytes [36].

Augmented vascularity in our animal investigations was documented in vivo by serial angiographic analyses, and ex vivo by analysis of the capillary/myocyte ratio in sections of skeletal muscle obtained from the ischemic limb at the time of necropsy examination. Previous studies from our laboratory [37] documented extensive proliferative activity among endothelial cells comprising the neovasculature of the ischemic hindlimb following administration of recombinant VEGF protein, consistent with the interpretation that angiogenesis contributes to augmented collateral development in the rabbit ischemic hindlimb model following phVEGF$_{165}$ gene transfer.

In vivo studies of blood pressure and blood flow performed pre- and postgene transfer documented that angiogenesis led to improvement in these physiologic indices [24]. The ratio of blood pressure measured in the ischemic vs. the normal limb improved to a statistically significant degree among animals transfected with plasmid DNA encoding for all three isoforms compared to LacZ. Likewise, blood flow measured in the ischemic limb with an intra-arterial Doppler guide-wire at rest as well as following vasodilator provocation improved in all three VEGF-transfected groups vs. the LacZ group. The magnitude of improvement observed in both these hemodynamic and flow indices following arterial gene transfer compares favorably with results obtained previously in this animal model following administration of recombinant $VEGF_{165}$ protein [7,38].

The teleologic basis for the 121, 165 and 189 isoforms which result from alternative splicing of the VEGF transcript has remained enigmatic. Although $VEGF_{121}$ lacks heparin-binding ability, all three isoforms bind to the flk-1 receptor which transduces the mitogenic signal [39] including $VEGF_{121}$, which binds exclusively to flk-1 [40]. Plate et al. speculated that the three principal isoforms might mediate distinct endothelial cell functions [35]. We considered that angiogenesis induced by VEGF may be differentially dependent upon the extent to which each particular isoform employed is freely secreted and soluble. The magnitude of freely secreted $VEGF_{121}$ isoform which reaches the ischemic focus from the site of synthesis, for example, might be superior to that achieved with the $VEGF_{165}$ isoform; alternatively, avid binding of the $VEGF_{189}$ isoform to the basement membrane and/or extracellular matrix [41] might result in more protracted bioavailability, and thereby yield an outcome superior to $VEGF_{165}$.

Because it has proved difficult to express affinity-purified recombinant $VEGF_{189}$ protein from mammalian and bacterial systems, we investigated the possibility of hierarchial efficacy among these three isoforms by performing arterial gene transfer of $phVEGF_{121}$, $phVEGF_{165}$, and $phVEGF_{189}$ in the rabbit ischemic hindlimb model. Remarkably, no differences with regard to anatomic or physiologic evidence of angiogenesis could be demonstrated — although all three isoforms yielded statistically significant improvement in every parameter measured compared to the LacZ controls. Moreover, separate experiments performed using 100, 200 and 400 μg of each plasmid failed to disclose a differential dose-response curve among the three isoforms with respect to angiographic score, calf blood pressure ratio, resting/maximum flow or capillary/myocyte ratio (Y. Tsurumi, unpublished data).

These findings represent what is to our knowledge, the first demonstration of biological equivalency among the three principal VEGF isoforms for in vivo angiogenesis, and may be interpreted to support the observation made previously by Houck et al. [19] regarding the proteolytically clipped VEGF species which result from the action of plasmin on the 165 and 189 isoforms. The size of the resulting monomers, which in each case are mitogenic for endothelial cells and enhance vascular permeability in a Miles assay [42], is similar to the size of the intact 121 isoform. It is, therefore, possible that the proteolytic cascade of plasminogen activation (a key step during angiogenesis [43]) cleaves the longer forms of VEGF, releasing a soluble $VEGF_{121}$-like species that is the final common mediator of angiogenesis in vivo.

Clinical application of arterial gene transfer of phVEGF$_{165}$

We have used our animal studies to develop clinically applicable strategies for therapeutic angiogenesis employing phVEGF$_{165}$. Because recombinant VEGF protein is not yet available for human application, clinical trials of human gene therapy involving percutaneous arterial gene transfer of phVEGF$_{165}$ [44] for patients with critical limb ischemia were undertaken in December 1994.

Using a dose-escalating design, treatment was initiated with 100 µg of phVEGF$_{165}$. Three patients presenting with rest pain (but no gangrene) and treated with 1,000 µg were subsequently shown at 1-year follow-up to have improved blood flow to the ischemic limb and remain free of rest pain. We considered the possibility that VEGF could produce flow augmentation simply as a result of its ability to act as a potent stimulus for the release of nitric oxide [45]; this explanation, however, seemed unlikely in view of the demonstration that augmented flow was documented on serial studies performed well beyond the time (21−30 days) that the transferred gene is actively expressed [24]. With the increase in dose of phVEGF$_{165}$ to 2,000 µg, angiographic evidence of new blood vessel formation became apparent [46]. Moreover, patient 8 developed three spider angiomata in the foot and ankle distal to the site of gene transfer; immunohistochemical staining of the lesion which was resected documented extensive proliferative activity among the endothelial cells comprising the lesion. These lesions were first observed 1 week postgene transfer and regressed completely 8 weeks later. The lesions were limited to the distal portion of the ischemic extremity. The time-course and distribution of these lesions strongly suggests that these vascular malformations developed as a consequence of phVEGF$_{165}$ expression. These lesions are in fact reminiscent of supernumerary vessels described previously following injection of VEGF recombinant protein into quail embryos [47,48]. The development of these lesions constitutes strong (albeit indirect) evidence of gene expression in this patient. These lesions, although benign and in this case self-limited, may be considered evidence of unwanted angiogenesis, and thus warrant careful monitoring in future patients receiving angiogenic therapy.

These findings thus established proof of the principle for two concepts. The first is the potential for the administration of angiogenic growth factors to promote development of new collateral blood vessels in human patients. The second concept is the feasibility of arterial gene transfer of naked DNA.

In the patient with angiographic and histologic evidence of neovascularization, as in several of the patients treated with the 1,000 µg dose of plasmid DNA, lower-extremity edema developed for the first time postgene therapy and resolved by week 5 postgene transfer (1 week beyond the 21−30 days during which the transgene has been shown to be actively expressed [49]) suggesting that this finding was a consequence of phVEGF$_{165}$ gene transfer. VEGF increases vascular permeability when assessed by the Miles assay [42], accounting for its alternative designation, vascular permeability factor or VPF [11,18,50]. The association between neovascularity and edema in this patient is consistent with previously reported evidence [18,48] linking functions of VEGF as a vascular growth factor and permeability factor.

Because the technique employed for local gene delivery in this case involves balloon inflation and thus the potential for endothelial disruption of the arterial wall, the gene transfer site was serially examined by intravascular ultrasound (IVUS). In neither of the examinations performed postgene therapy was there evidence that hydrogel balloon arterial gene transfer provoked intimal thickening. It is indeed likely that phVEGF$_{165}$ gene transfer accelerates re-endothelialization, and thereby obviates luminal compromise of the transfected segment [51,52].

Intramuscular gene transfer of phVEGF$_{165}$

Despite these encouraging preliminary findings, evaluation of candidates for phVEGF$_{165}$ arterial gene therapy exposed certain potential limitations of arterial gene transfer, particularly for lower-extremity ischemia. By definition, arterial gene transfer requires access to a satisfactory arterial donor site in the lower extremity circulation. In patients with critical limb ischemia, several factors may conspire to compromise such access. Lower extremity vascular disease is often so extensive that conventional sites for arterial puncture cannot be accessed percutaneously. Arterial sites which are patent may be nevertheless diffusely diseased by atherosclerosis [53]. Even in the absence of a thickened neointima, extensive calcific deposits at the intimal/medial interface (so-called "Monckeberg's disease" [54]) may limit gene transfer to the smooth muscle cells of the arterial media and/or make the vessel so brittle that balloon inflation fractures the calcified vessel [55], leading to unpredictable abrupt vessel closure; this complication may be devastating if the involved artery is the major donor of pre-existing collaterals or the only patent vessel supplying the ischemic limb. Even if arterial access is possible in such patients, it is often limited to the uppermost portion of the limb, 60 cm or more from sites in the distal limb where ischemia and/or necrosis is most profound. Because recent studies have demonstrated evidence of paracrine mediated endothelial cell upregulation of VEGF receptors by conditioned media of hypoxic muscle [36], there may be a tactical advantage to positioning the putative sites of constitutive VEGF synthesis in closer proximity to the ischemic focus.

Intramuscular (IM) gene transfer, pioneered by Wolff and colleagues [56—58], represents a less invasive alternative to arterial transfection. Striated muscle has been shown to take up and express foreign genes transferred in the form of "naked" plasmid DNA, i.e., DNA not associated with viral or other adjunctive vectors. As indicated above, IM gene transfer of naked plasmid DNA would be potentially advantageous since it obviates immunologic concerns associated with adenoviral vectors [26]. Because naked plasmid DNA injected IM remains in a nonreplicative, unintegraded, circular form [56], this strategy also is unlikely to be complicated by insertional mutagenesis.

While IM gene transfer of naked DNA would thus appear to address the technical limitations of arterial gene transfer in particular, and certain safety issues relevant to cardiovascular gene therapy in general, the magnitude of gene expression resulting from IM transfection has been a subject of further concern. Wolff et al. documented reporter gene expression up to 19 months following IM transfection with naked DNA [58], but concluded that the use of this approach for Duchenne's myopathy did not achieve satisfactory levels of dystrophin [59]. Subsequent investigators have been more optimistic when naked DNA was administered IM for use as a vaccine [60−64]. In the case of phVEGF$_{165}$, we considered that the secreted features of the gene product might permit a level of gene expression sufficient to achieve therapeutic angiogenesis. Accordingly, we again used the rabbit model of hindlimb ischemia to test the hypothesis that IM injection of naked plasmid DNA encoding the 165-amino acid isoform of VEGF could augment collateral development and tissue perfusion in the setting of experimentally induced hindlimb ischemia. In fact, we documented successful transfer and expression of phVEGF$_{165}$ in skeletal muscles of the ischemic limb, with evidence of increased collateral vessel development, and consequent amelioration in hemodynamic and physiologic deficits induced by ischemia [65]. Previous studies have shown that such improvements in perfusion are associated with improved performance of skeletal muscle groups in the treated limb [66]. These findings thus demonstrated for the first time the feasibility of the intramuscular (IM) gene transfer with naked DNA encoding VEGF for therapeutic angiogenesis in particular, and for the first time indicated bioactivity of naked DNA following IM transfection for cardiovascular gene therapy in general. From a clinical standpoint, these findings suggest that IM transfection represents a suitable alternative to arterial gene transfer of phVEGF$_{165}$ in patients with proximal obstruction of the lower extremity vasculature which precludes catheter access.

Many of the previous successful applications of IM gene transfer were achieved in young (4−6 weeks) mice, in which transgene uptake appears to be highest [67]. Our findings suggest that IM transfer of naked DNA is neither age nor species specific. VEGF expression was sufficient to yield augmented collateral vessel development associated with improved pressure, flow and perfusion in adult rabbits with hindlimb ischemia. The increase in angiographically apparent vessels and capillary density has been previously shown to result from a VEGF-induced increase in endothelial cell proliferation [37]. Consequently, the magnitude of improvement in calf blood pressure, blood flow (measured by intravascular Doppler analysis) and tissue perfusion (measured by an increase in microsphere distribution to the ischemic thigh and calf muscles) were all statistically significant in comparison to controls.

Several factors likely contributed to the success of phVEGF$_{165}$ IM gene transfer. As was the case with intra-arterial gene transfer, the secreted nature of the gene product constitutes the most important factor. This is further facilitated in the case of skeletal muscle by the inherently well-vascularized nature of this tissue.

Second, plasmid DNA was delivered in a relatively large volume of fluid, directly into the target muscle; the injection was performed slowly to prevent fluid loss from the epimysium. This approach may have allowed for more uniform distribution of the transgene. Wolff et al. previously demonstrated that higher and less variable levels of gene expression could be achieved by injecting a larger rather than a smaller volume of plasmid [57]. Similarly, Davis et al. showed that preinjection of muscles with a relatively large volume of hypertonic sucrose facilitated more uniform distribution and less variable expression of reporter genes [68].

Third, the skeletal muscle which was the site of gene transfer was ischemic. Recent work by Takeshita et al. [69] has shown that the transfection efficiency of IM gene transfer is augmented more than 5-fold when the injected muscle is ischemic. This finding may be the result of the skeletal muscle regeneration, including stem cell (myoblast) proliferation. Vitadello et al. [70] have reported an 80-fold increase in chloramphenicol acetyltranferase (CAT) activity following transfection of regenerating vs. control muscle. Consistent with this concept, Danko et al. [71] found that bupivacaine, which produces myonecrosis followed by satellite cell (muscle stem cell) proliferation and myotube formation 1–3 days later, may be used to enhance the expression of naked DNA injected IM into striated muscles.

Interestingly, the histological features of muscle retrieved from the ischemic limbs of animals used for the current series of experiments were similar in many respects to findings reported previously for bupivavaine-treated muscle, featuring myonecrosis, mononuclear cell infiltration, muscle cell proliferation and myotube formation [72]. Evidence of myocyte regeneration was in fact demonstrable in the current experiments at the time of IM plasmid administration; this finding may be related to the nearly 7-fold higher transfection efficiency suggested by morphometric analysis β-galactosidase gene expression. Taken together, it is likely that ischemic myonecrosis (a predictable feature of hindlimb ischemia in this animal model [2]) led to spontaneous muscle regeneration and coincidently augmented uptake of the transgene.

The ischemic milieu of the transfected hindlimb muscle further contributes to the success of therapeutic angiogenesis, independent of transgene uptake, by modulating VEGF receptor expression. Recent work from our laboratory has demonstrated paracrine induction of the KDR receptor (13-fold increase in KDR receptor/cell) in endothelial cells exposed to media conditioned by hypoxic myoblasts [36]. This finding presumably acts not only to amplify the impact of any given concentration of VEGF, but potentially accounts as well for the site-specific nature of the angiogenic response in this animal model [73].

Expression of the human VEGF transgene was detected by RT-PCR for up to 14 days after gene transfer in the present study. It is assumed, although not yet documented, that expression at the protein level is limited to a similar time frame. This relatively brief duration of transgene expression is likely related to the CMV promoter employed in the phVEGF$_{165}$ plasmid construct. Previous work by Wolff et al. [56,58] and others [67,71] demonstrated that naked DNA constructs which include the Rous sarcoma virus (RSV) promoter appear to express for considerably longer periods of time, although the level of expression obtained may be lower than that obtained with CMV. Addition of selected introns and/or regulatory sequences in the 3' noncoding region of CMV constructs, however, may augment both the magnitude and temporal stability of transgene expression [74,75].

Use of a skeletal muscle-specific promoter represents another potential consideration for enhancing the efficiency of IM gene transfer. It is not clear, however, that this strategy would necessarily augment gene expression for the application described in the current series of experiments. Buttrick et al. [76], for example, have previously shown that cardiac-specific expression from the rat myosin heavy chain gene was 20-fold less active than expression from RSV regulatory sequences. Likewise, Vincent et al. [77] have documented similar levels of expression for a pRSV-CAT construct and an MCK-CAT construct (containing the promoter and enhancer of the rabbit creatinine kinase-M gene) in transfection of rat cardiac and skeletal muscles. More recently, Vincent and Walsh (unpublished data) have found that 198.3 chicken skeletal actin promoter (-198 to -1 and $+1-313$ fragment) was 1% as active as RSV-LTR or CMV promoters in direct IM injection of rat heart. Thus, constitutive viral regulatory sequences (vs. tissue-specific muscle promoter) may be optimal even for IM expression of exogenous genes due to their inherently higher activity. It is possible, however, that applying modifications cited above [74,75] to the CMV vector used here might yield more robust gene expression.

The duration of gene expression in the current series of experiments was nevertheless sufficient to permit augmented collateral vessel development. This is consistent with the time course of collateral development reported previously in this animal model following administration of the recombinant protein, in which maximal endothelial cell proliferation is observed within 5 days following VEGF therapy [37]. Provided that a satisfactory clinical benefit has been realized, early cessation of gene expression may represent a safety feature of the strategy proposed in this report, in that the recipient is not exposed indefinitely to increased levels of the transgene product.

Role of protein in determining the success of gene transfer

In summary, experience with intra-arterial and intramuscular gene transfer of VEGF to date illustrates in prototypical fashion how features of the gene, protein and target tissue may all contribute to phenotypic modulation of the host despite a low-transfection efficiency.

First, rhVEGF contains at its amino terminus the signal sequence which permits it to be actively secreted by intact cells.

Second, heparin-avidity of the intermediate and longer VEGF isoforms, $VEGF_{165}$ and $VEGF_{189}$, respectively, promotes binding to cell surface and matrix heparin sulfates that may create a biological reservoir of the secreted pro-

190

tein, enhancing the temporal opportunity for bioactivity.

Third, while ECs were previously viewed solely as the target for VEGF, it is now clear that ECs under stress, in particular hypoxia, can synthesize VEGF as well [78]. This autocrine feature of VEGF creates the opportunity for amplifying the effects of even a small amount of exogenous VEGF, as EC proliferation in the ischemic territory creates additional potential sites of VEGF synthesis and secretion.

Fourth, VEGF inhibits apoptosis (D.W. Losordo, unpublished data), apparently by upregulating EC expression of fibronectin and $\alpha v \beta 3$ and thus promoting the critical step of EC attachment to the extracellular matrix. Such reduction in EC apoptosis would be expected to complement the mitogenic effect of VEGF, resulting in a further net increase in EC viability.

Fifth, with regard to the target of gene therapy, it has been noted [24,46,79] that VEGF-induced angiogenesis is not indiscriminate or widespread, but is instead restricted to sites of ischemia. This appears to result from paracrine upregulation of the principal high-affinity VEGF receptor (Kdr) in response to factors released from hypoxic skeletal myocytes [36]. Receptor upregulation on ECs within the region of lower limb or myocardial ischemia thus enables these cells to act as magnets for any VEGF secreted into the ischemic milieu.

These considerations underscore the notion that the success of gene therapy is not solely a function of vectors or transfection efficiency. While it is clear that better vectors with which to augment transfection efficiency should remain a principal goal of gene therapy, features of the gene and target may independently increase or decrease the likelihood of a favorable outcome. Modifications in any of these respects, including the use alone or in combination of other angiogenic growth factors, will receive intensive scrutiny in the coming months to optimize angiogenesis as a useful treatment option for lower extremity and myocardial ischemia.

References

1. European Working Group on Critical Leg Ischemia. Second European consensus document on chronic critical leg ischemia. Circulation 1991;84:IV-1—IV-26.
2. Baffour R, Berman J, Garb JL, Rhee SW, Kaufman J, Friedmann P. Enhanced angiogenesis and growth of collaterals by in vivo administration of recombinant basic fibroblast growth factor in a rabbit model of acute lower limb ischemia: dose-response effect of basic fibroblast growth factor. J Vasc Surg 1992;16:181—191.
3. Banai S, Jaklitsch MT, Shou M et al. Angiogenic-induced enhancement of collateral blood flow to ischemic myocardium by vascular endothelial growth factor in dogs. Circulation 1994;89: 2183—2189.
4. Yanagisawa-Miwa A, Uchida Y, Nakamura F et al. Salvage of infarcted myocardium by angiogenic action of basic fibroblast growth factor. Science 1992;257:1401—1403.
5. Banai S, Jaklitsch MT, Casscells W et al. Effects of acidic fibroblast growth factor on normal and ischemic myocardium. Circ Res 1991;69:76—85.
6. Pu LQ, Sniderman AD, Brassard R et al. Enhanced revascularization of the ischemic limb by means of angiogenic therapy. Circulation 1993;88:208—215.

7. Takeshita S, Zheng LP, Brogi E et al. Therapeutic angiogenesis: a single intra-arterial bolus of vascular endothelial growth factor augments revascularization in a rabbit ischemic hindlimb model. J Clin Invest 1994;93:662—670.

8. Asahara T, Bauters C, Zheng LP et al. Synergistic effect of vascular endothelial growth factor and basic fibroblast growth factor on angiogenesis in vivo. Circulation 1995;92:II-365—H-371.

9. Pearlman JD, Hibberd MG, Chuang ML et al. Magnetic resonance mapping demonstrates benefits of VEGF-induced myocardial angiogenesis. Nature Med 1995;1:1085—1089.

10. Ferrara N, Henzel WJ. Pituitary follicular cells secrete a novel heparin-binding growth factor specific for vascular endothelial cells. Biochem Biophys Res Comm 1989;161:851—855.

11. Keck PI, Hauser SD, Krivi G et al. Vascular permeability factor, an endothelial cell mitogen related to PDGF. Science 1989;246:1309—1312.

12. Plouet J, Schilling J, Gospodarowicz D. Isolation and characterization of a newly identified endothelial cell mitogen produced by AtT-20 cells. EMBO J 1989;8:3801—3806.

13. Folkman J. Clinical applications of research on angiogenesis. N Engl J Med 1995;333: 1757—1763.

14. Ross R. The pathogenesis of atherosclerosis: a perspective for the 1990s. Nature 1993;362: 801—805.

15. Clowes AW, Reidy MA, Clowes MM. Kinetics of cellular proliferation after arterial injury. Smooth muscle growth in the absence of endothelium. Lab Invest 1983;49:327—333.

16. Pickering JG, Weir L, Jekanowski J, Kearney MA, Isner JM. Proliferative activity in peripheral and coronary atherosclerotic plaque among patients undergoing percutaneous revascularization. J Clin Invest 1993;91:1469—1480.

17. Tischer E, Mitchell R, Hartmann T et al. The human gene for vascular endothelial growth factor: multiple protein forms are encoded through alternative exon splicing. J Biol Chem 1991; 266:11947—11954.

18. Dvorak HF, Brown LF, Detmar M, Dvorak AM. Vascular permeability factor/vascular endothelial growth factor, microvascular hyperpermeability, and angiogenesis. Am J Pathol 1995;146: 1029—1039.

19. Houck KA, Leung DW, Rowland AM, Winer J, Ferrara N. Dual regulation of vascular endothelial growth factor bioavailability by genetic and proteolytic mechanisms. J Biol Chem 1992; 267:26031—26037.

20. Losordo DW, Pickering JG, Takeshita S et al. Use of the rabbit ear artery to serially assess foreign protein secretion after site specific arterial gene transfer in vivo: evidence that anatomic identification of successful gene transfer may underestimate the potential magnitude of transgene expression. Circulation 1994;89:785—792.

21. Takeshita S, Losordo DW, Kearney M, Isner JM. Time course of recombinant protein secretion following liposome-mediated gene transfer in a rabbit arterial organ culture model. Lab Invest 1994;71:387—391.

22. Riessen R, Rahimizadeh H, Blessing E, Takeshita S, Barry JJ, Isner JM. Arterial gene transfer using pure DNA applied directly to a hydrogen-coated angioplasty balloon. Hum Gene Ther 1993;4:749—758.

23. Pu LQ, Jackson S, Lachapelle KJ et al. A persistent hindlimb ischemia model in the rabbit. J Invest Surg 1994;7:49—60.

24. Takeshita S, Tsurumi Y, Couffinhal T et al. Gene transfer of naked DNA encoding for three isoforms of vascular endothelial growth factor stimulates collateral development in vivo. Lab Invest (In press).

25. Chapman GD, Lim CS, Gammon RS et al. Gene transfer into coronary arteries of intact animals with a percutaneous balloon catheter. Circ Res 1992;71:27—33.

26. Yang Y, Nunes FA, Berencsi K, Furth EE, Gonczol E, Wilson JM. Cellular immunity to viral antigens limits E1-deleted adenoviruses for gene therapy. Proc Natl Acad Sci USA 1994; 91:4407—4411.

27. Lemarchand P, Jones M, Yamada I, Crystal RG. In vivo gene transfer and expression in normal

uninjured blood vessels using replication-deficient recombinant adenovirus vectors. Circ Res 1993;72:1132–1138.

28. Nabel EG. Gordon D, Yang Z-Y et al. Gene transfer in vivo with DNA-liposome complexes: lack of autoimmunity and gonadal localization. Hum Gene Ther 1992;3:649–656.

29. Nabel G. Proposed amendment to Appendix D of the NIH guidelines regarding a human gene therapy protocol entitled immunotherapy of malignancy by in vivo gene transfer into tumors. Hum Gene Ther 1994;5:236–240.

30. Terman BI, Dougher-Vermazen M, Carrion ME et al. Identification of the KDR tyrosine kinase as a receptor for vascular endothelial cell growth factor. Biochem Biophys Res Commun 1992;187:1579–1586.

31. Millauer B, Wizigmann-Voos S, Schnurch H et al. High-affinity VEGF binding and developmental expression suggest Flk-1 as a major regulator of vasculogenesis and angiogenesis. Cell 1993;72:835–846.

32. Waltenberger J, Claesson-Welsh L, Siegbahn A, Shibuya M, Heldin C-H. Different signal transduction properties of KDR and Flt-1, two receptors for vascular endothelial growth factor. J Biol Chem 1994;269:26988–26995.

33. Detmar M, Brown LF, Claffey KP et al. Overexpression of vascular permeability factor/vascular endothelial growth factor and its receptors in psoriasis. J Exp Med 1994;180:1141–1146.

34. Brown LF, Yeo K-T, Berse B et al. Expression of vascular permeability factor (vascular endothelial growth factor) by epidermal keratinocytes during wound healing. J Exp Med 1992;176:1375–1379.

35. Plate KH, Breier G, Weich HA, Mennel HD, Risau W. Vascular endothelial growth factor and glioma angiogenesis: coordinate induction of VEGF receptors. Distribution of VEGF protein and possible in vivo regulatory mechanisms. Int J Cancer 1994;59:520–529.

36. Brogi E, Schatteman G, Wu T et al. Hypoxia-induced paracrine regulation of VEGF receptor expression. J Clin Invest 1996;97:469–476.

37. Takeshita S, Rossow ST, Kearney M et al. Time course of increased cellular proliferation in collateral arteries following administration of vascular endothelial growth factor in a rabbit model of lower limb vascular insufficiency. Am J Pathol 1995;147:1649–1660.

38. Bauters C, Asahara T, Zheng LP et al. Physiologic assessment of angiogenesis induced by vascular endothelial growth factor in a rabbit ischemic hindlimb model. Am J Physiol 1994;36:H1263–H1271.

39. Keyt BA, Nguyen HV, Berleau LT et al. Identification of vascular endothelial growth factor determinants for binding KDR and FLT-1 receptors. J Biol Chem 1996;271:5638–5646.

40. Gitay-Goren H, Cohen T, Tessler S et al. Selective binding of VEGF121 to one of the three vascular endothelial growth factor receptors of vascular endothelial cells. J Biol Chem 1996;271:5519–5523.

41. Park JE, Keller G-A, Ferrara N. The vascular endothelial growth factor (VEGF) isoforms: differential deposition into the subepithelial ECM and bioactivity of ECM-bound VEGF. Molec Cell Biol 1993;4:1317–1326.

42. Miles AA, Miles EM. Vascular reactions to histamine, histamine liberators or leukotoxins in the skin of the guinea pig. J Physiol 1952;118:228–257.

43. Pepper MS, Montesano R. Proteolytic balance and capillary morphogenesis. Cell Dif Dev 1990;32:319–328.

44. Isner JM, Walsh K, Symes J et al. Arterial gene transfer for therapeutic angiogenesis in patients with peripheral artery disease. Hum Gene Ther 1996;7:959–988.

45. van der Zee R, Zollman F, Passeri J, Lekutat C, Silver M, Isner JM. Vascular endothelial growth factor (VEGF)/vascular permeability factor (VPF) augments nitric oxide release from quiescent rabbit and human vascular endothelium. Circulation (In press).

46. Isner JM, Pieczek A, Schainfeld R et al. Early report: clinical evidence of angiogenesis following arterial gene transfer of phVEGF$_{165}$. Lancet 1996;348:370–374.

47. Drake CJ, Little CD. Exogenous vascular endothelial growth factor induces malformed and

hyperfused vessels during embryonic neovascularization. Proc Natl Acad Sci USA 1995;92: 7657—7661.

48. Ingo F, von Reutern M, Drexler HCA, Syed-Ali S, Risau W. Overexpression of vascular endothelial growth factor in the avian embryo induces hypervascularization and increased vascular permeability without alterations of embryonic pattern formation. Dev Biol 1995;171: 399—414.

49. Minutes Recombinant DNA Advisory Committee (RAC) of National Institutes of Health, 13 Sept 1994. RAC #9409—088 approved in final form 11/15/94.

50. Connolly DT, Hewelman DM, Nelson R et al. Tumor vascular permeability factor stimulates endothelial cell growth and angiogenesis. J Clin Invest 1989;84:1470—1478.

51. Asahara T, Bauters C, Pastore CJ et al. Local delivery of vascular endothelial growth factor accelerates re-endothelialization and attenuates intimal hyperplasia in balloon-injured rat carotid artery. Circulation 1995;91:2793—2801.

52. Asahara T, Chen D, Kearney M et al. Accelerated re-endothelialization and reduced neointimal thickening following catheter transfer of phVEGF$_{165}$. J Am Coll Cardiol 1996;27:1A(Abstract).

53. Feldman LJ, Steg PG, Zheng LP et al. Low-efficiency of percutaneous adenovirus-mediated arterial gene transfer in the atherosclerotic rabbit. J Clin Invest 1995;95:2662—2671.

54. Lachman AS, Spray TL, Kerwin DM, Shugoll GI, Roberts WC. Medial calcinosis of Monckeberg. Am J Med 1977;63:615—622.

55. Fitzgerald PJ, Ports TA, Yock PG. Contribution of localized calcium deposits to dissection after angioplasty. An observational study using intravascular ultrasound. Circulation 1992;86:64—70.

56. Wolff JA. Malone RW, Williams P et al. Direct gene transfer into mouse muscle in vivo. Science 1990;247:1465—1468.

57. Wolff JA, Williams P, Acsadi G, Jiao S, Jani A, Chong W. Conditions affecting direct gene transfer into rodent muscle in vivo. BioTechniques 1991;11:474—485.

58. Wolff JA, Ludtke JJ, Acsadi G, Williams P, Jani A. Long-term persistence of plasmid DNA and foreign gene expression in mouse muscle. Hum Mol Genet 1992;1:363—369.

59. Acsadi G, Jani A, Massie B et al. A differential efficiency of adenovirus-mediated in vivo gene transfer into skeletal muscle cells of different maturity. Hum Mol Genet 1994;3:579—584.

60. Ulmer JB, Donnelly JJ, Parker SE et al. Heterologous protection against influenza by injection of DNA encoding a viral protein. Science 1993;259:1745—1749.

61. Tang DJ, DeVit M, Johnston SA. Genetic immunization is a simple method for eliciting an immune response. Nature 1992;356:152—154.

62. Hsu C-H, China K-Y, Tao M-H et al. Immunoprophylaxis of allergen-8-induced immunoglobulin E synthesis and airway hyperresponsiveness in vivo by genetic immunization. Nature Med 1996;2:540—544.

63. McDonnell WM, Askari FK. DNA vaccines. N Engl J Med 1996;334:42—45.

64. Donnelly JJ, Friedman A, Maretinez D et al. Preclinical efficacy of a prototype DNA vaccine: enhanced protection against antigenic drift in influenza virus. Nature Med 1995;1:583—587.

65. Tsurumi Y, Takeshita S, Chen D et al. Direct intramuscular gene transfer of naked DNA encoding vascular endothelial growth factor augments collateral development and tissue perfusion. Circulation 1996;(In Press).

66. Walder CE, Errett CJ, Ogez J et al. Vascular endothelial growth factor (VEGF) improves blood flow and function in a chronic ischemic hind limb model. J Cardiovasc Pharmacol 1996;27: 91—98.

67. Wells DJ, Goldspink G. Age and sex influence expression of plasmid DNA directly injected into mouse skeletal muscle. FEBS Lett 1992;305:203—205.

68. Davis HL, Whalen RG, Demeneix BA. Direct gene transfer into skeletal muscle in vivo: factors affecting efficiency of transfer and stability of expression. Hum Gene Ther 1993;4:151—159.

69. Takeshita S, Isshiki T, Sato T. Increased expression of direct gene transfer into skeletal muscles observed after acute ischemic injury in rats. Lab Invest 1996;74:1061—1065.

70. Vitadello M, Schiaffino M, Picard A, Scarpa M, Schiaffino S. Gene transfer in regenerating

muscle. Hum Gene Ther 1994;5:11—18.

71. Danko I, Fritz JD, Jiao S, Hogan K, Latendresse JS, Wolff JA. Pharmacological enhancement of in vivo foreign gene expression in muscle. Gene Therapy 1994;1:114—121.

72. Hall-Craggs ECB. Early ultrastructural changes in skeletal muscle exposed to the local anaesthetic bupivacaine (marcaine). Br J Exp Pathol 1980;61:139—149.

73. Bauters C, Asahara T, Zheng LP et al. Site-specific therapeutic angiogenesis following systemic administration of vascular endothelial growth factor. J Vasc Surg 1995;21:314—325.

74. Coleman ME, DeMayo F, Yin KC et al. Myogenic vector expression of insulin-like growth factor I stimulates muscle cell differentiation adn myofiber hypertrophy in transgenic mice. J Biol Chem 1995;270:12109—12116.

75. Manthorpe M, Cornefert-Jensen F, Hartikka J et al. Gene therapy by intramuscular injection of plasmid DNA: studies on firefly luciferase gene expression in mice. Hum Gene Ther 1993;4:419—431.

76. Buttrick PM, Kass A, Kitsis RN, Kaplan ML, Leinwand LA. Behavior of genes directly injected into the rat heart in vivo. Circ Res 1992;70:193—198.

77. Vincent CK, Gualberto A, Patel CV, Walsh K. Different regulatory sequences control creatine-kinase-M gene expression in directly injected skeletal and cardiac muscle. Molec Cell Biol 1993;13:1264—1272.

78. Namikl A, Brogi E, Kearney M et al. Hypoxia induces vascular endothelial growth factor in cultured human endothelial cells. J Biol Chem 1995;270:31189—31195.

79. Takeshita S, Zheng LP, Asahara T et al. Therapeutic angiogenesis: a single intra-arterial bolus of vascular endothelial growth factor augments collateral vessel formation in a rabbit ischemic hindlimb. Circulation 1993;88:I—370(Abstract).

Atherosclerosis XI.
B. Jacotot, D. Mathé and J.-C. Fruchart, editors.

Fish oils, lipids and coronary artery disease

Paul J. Nestel
Cardiovascular Nutrition Laboratory, Baker Medical Research Institute, Melbourne, Australia

Abstract. The fish oil n-3 fatty acids modify key risk factors for coronary disease. This is partly related to effects on lipid metabolism and partly to effects on vascular function, which are influenced by plasma and tissue lipids.

The antiatherogenic outcomes of eating fish oil include reduced triglyceride-rich lipoproteins and raised HDL cholesterol which together constitute the high-risk phenotype in the metabolic syndrome and diabetes. Clearance of chylomicron remnants and thus of postprandial lipids is enhanced. ApoB production and LDL density are reduced.

The in vitro raised oxidizability of LDL may not represent in vivo events, since atherogenesis declines. Nevertheless, potentially raised oxidant status remains a concern, but it is correctable with vitamin E and none of the in vivo correlates of high-oxidized LDL are seen. For instance, vascular vasodilatation and arterial compliance are improved with fish oil, reflecting the favorable lipoprotein profile rather than any oxidant effect. Reduced thrombogenicity occurring through fish oil is in part related to lower triglyceride levels.

Some effects of fish oil are mediated through raised fatty acid oxidation, inhibition of fatty acid and cholesterol synthesis, reduced FFA outflow from fat stores and reduced assembly of VLDL in liver. The relative potency of EPA and DHA is unclear.

Thus fish oils, by modifying lipid metabolism, reduce coronary risk through multiple mechanisms. In this respect they resemble benefits of eating fish but may be the preferred source of n-3 fatty acids in people with coronary disease and those at high risk. Intervention trials are in progress to determine the benefit on clinical outcomes.

Introduction

The active molecules of fish oil fatty acids, the n-3 EPA and DHA (and possibly other minor fatty acids) are highly multipotent compounds. Their potential to counter atherosclerotic vascular diseases has been supported by an increasingly lengthy list of functions. Some relate to lipid metabolism, but many other effects that may reduce cardiovascular disease are mediated through nonlipid parameters.

The underlying support for fish oil in the management of cardiovascular risk is the apparent protection by eating fish. At least four large prospective studies have documented such benefit from relatively small amounts of fish eaten regularly. That this was not observed in two other population studies was ignored until a further negative experience with a very large US study, The Health Professionals Follow-up Study published in 1995 [1]. The most plausible explanation is that the average consumption of fish was already high in these individuals reducing the likelihood of showing a "dose-related" response. The current consensus is that fish eating is beneficial, at surprisingly modest intakes and probably depends to a major degree on its fatty acid profile. Two recent reports, one from Seattle [2] and the other from Honolulu [3] indicate that about two fish meals weekly

196

are protective, halving the risk of sudden cardiac death [2] and largely preventing the high risk from smoking [3].

We have reported that when similar amounts of n-3 fatty acids (4 g) are eaten as fish or as fish oil, the risk reduction may even be greater with fish [4]. A recent report of Tanzanian villagers showed that eating fish (3–5 g n-3 fatty acid daily) outperformed vegetarianism in risk factor reduction [5]. Recently, Mori et al. [6] have also found similar benefits from eating fish or fish oil, on platelet aggregability (3.65 g/d n-3 fatty acid).

However, it is not clear whether the apparent protection against CHD is directly related to antiatherogenic functions of these fatty acids or mediated through their modification of the risk factors through mechanisms not directly related to lipids.

The multipotent effects of n-3 fatty acids on arterial function and disease include:
1) reduction in cardiovascular risk factors;
2) inhibition of atherogenic processes within the artery; and
3) improved endothelial function.
These are summarized in Table 1.

Risk factor reduction includes lowering of arterial pressure especially in hypertensive subjects [7]. Although the effect is modest, more importantly, the overall reduction in cardiovascular risk enhances the usefulness of fish oil as adjunct therapy in hypertension.

Endothelial dysfunction is now a well-recognized cause of clinical symptomatology in CHD and its reversal improves prognosis. Endothelium-dependent dilatation of arteries is enhanced by fish oils which also inhibit the vasoconstrictive effects of sympathetic overactivity and norepinephrine. We have shown that the vascular resistance in the microcirculation of the forearm (which mimics that in the coronary circulation) when norepinephrine or angiotensin II are infused, is attenuated by taking fish oil [8]. The improvement might have partly been due to the better lipid profile, since dyslipidemia impairs endothelial function. Enhancement of acetylcholine-mediated dilatation of the coronary circulation has also been reported [9].

Another index of arterial function is compliance, a measure of the elasticity of large arteries including the thoracic aorta. Compliance has been reported to be improved by treating diabetics (in whom compliance is low as arteries stiffen) with fish oil [10].

Table 1. Fish oil and arterial disease.

Epidemiological evidence
Experimental atherosclerosis
Risk factor reduction
Modification of atherogenic processes
Protection of endothelial function
Protection of myocardial function

Table 2. Role of lipid modification.

Pluses:
Increased HDL cholesterol
Reduced TG-rich lipoproteins
Reduced postprandial lipemia
Reduced remnant concentration
Minuses:
Raised LDL cholesterol
Increased LDL oxidizability

A major question concerns the importance of lipid modification, which is a potent outcome of fish oil supplementation (Table 2). On balance, it is likely to represent a significant antiatherogenic factor. The benefits include increased HDL_2 cholesterol levels, reduced triglyceride-rich lipoproteins, reduced postprandial lipemia and reduced remnant concentrations. In contrast, low-density lipoprotein (LDL) cholesterol levels have often been noted to rise, and the potential of increased oxidizability of LDL is clearly adverse, but can be overcome by vitamin E. The characteristic lipid changes and the underlying mechanisms will now be reviewed.

Effect on triglyceride

Modification of dyslipidemia has been the most characteristic effect of fish oils. Triglyceride rich lipoproteins are almost invariably reduced by mechanisms which are now mostly understood. Postprandial lipemia is reduced and potentially atherogenic remnants are cleared. The reduction in triglyceride is one of the modifications in the risk profile. Raised triglycerides are now widely recognized as an independent risk for CHD although the coexistence of a low HDL or a high LDL augments the risk substantially. The atherogenicity of IDL (the remnant of VLDL catabolism) is being rediscovered [11].

The concentrations of endogenously-derived triglyceride-rich lipoproteins, VLDL and IDL, have been almost uniformly reported as lowered. Fish oils have been effective in normal subjects and in patients with common phenotypes of hyperlipidemia in which VLDL levels are raised. The minimal effective dose of n-3 FA appears to be slightly more than 1 g per day. At intakes of more than 2 g per day, the fall in VLDL averages 25% in normal subjects and is greater in hypertriglyceridemic subjects; it is approximately 50% in those with types 4 or 5 phenotype and approximately 40% for those with combined hyperlipoproteinemia [12]. Furthermore, this response is maintained. In more severe forms of hypertriglyceridemia (such as type 5 hyperlipoproteinemia) in which both VLDL and chylomicrons are present, excess n-3 FA can be highly effective. Whether this result reflects enhanced removal of chylomicrons is uncertain. Catabolized VLDL and chylomicrons compete for similar removal mechanisms, diminished chylomicron removal may therefore, occur whenever VLDL overproduction increases the need for VLDL removal as in type 5 hyperlipoproteinemia. Chylomicronemia after a fatty meal is diminished when fish oil is eaten over weeks [13] but not after a single meal. Remnants in type 3 hyperlipoproteinemia are partly cleared with fish-oil treatment [14].

Dietary fish oils also modify the hypertriglyceridemia that is inducible by carbohydrate which stimulates while fish oil inhibits VLDL production.

The nature of the predominant n-3 FA (EPA or DHA) does not seem important in determining plasma-triglyceride lowering in humans. Fish oils vary considerably in their content of EPA and DHA as well as of long-chain monoenes and DEPA. An urgent need is a dose-response trial comparing EPA and DHA. Reduced triglyceride formation is ascribed largely to reduced fatty acid availability in the liver (for review see [15]).

Key factors include:
1) increased oxidation of fatty acids by peroxisomal as well as mitochondrial routes;
2) reduced fatty acid synthesis (suppression of key enzymes);
3) diversion of fatty acids into phospholipid;
4) reduced plasma FFA flux;
5) downregulation of esterifying enzymes; and
6) increased apo B degradation.

Chylomicron assembly and secretion are reduced in isolated intestinal cells incubated with EPA. The mechanisms appear to include less apoB formation and diversion of EPA from triglyceride to phospholipid [15]. This partly explains the reduction in postprandial lipemia.

Effects on LDL

This represents the more controversial aspects of the n-3 fatty acid effects. Why does the LDL cholesterol concentration sometimes rise, when cholesterol synthesis is depressed, biliary cholesterol secretion may rise, and the absorption of cholesterol may even be reduced. There is as some evidence for downregulation of the LDL receptor in hepatic cells [15]. Abnormal LDL binding to the receptor in human monocytes and to skin fibroblasts has been reported. Changes in the LDL particle are minor, but tend to larger cholesterol-enriched LDL [16]. LDL size relates to exchange of lipid between LDL, VLDL and HDL and fish oil would reduce such exchange and favor larger LDL.

The n-3 enrichment renders LDL susceptible to oxidation, as has been demonstrated in several studies, with some exceptions.

The evidence comprises increased in vitro copper-oxidized and macrophage-modified changes in LDL that led to their increased uptake by macrophages [17]. These findings define a potential atherogenic property of dietary fish oil, although it must be emphasized that these are in vitro observations and that the sum of the metabolic outcomes of marine n-3 fatty acids appears to be anti-atherogenic in life. Nevertheless, there is a need for more antioxidant capacity, such as α-tocopherol, if large amounts of fish oil are to be taken. We have shown that the addition of vitamins E and C to n-3 fatty acid enriched macrophages inhibits the capacity to oxidize LDL [18]. In a recent study with pigs fed atherogenic diets, atherosclerosis was not increased in animals fed fish oil despite evidence of raised LDL oxidizability [19].

Effects on HDL

Most reports indicate a favorable effect of fish oil on HDL. Larger cholesterol-rich HDL, in the HDL_2 range, increase at the expense of HDL_3 [16]. This reflects reduced CETP activity [16].

Potential clinical uses of fish oils

These have been summarized in Table 3.

The indications relate to the proven triglyceride-lowering capacity of n-3 fatty acids and extend this to supplementing lipid-lowering drugs.

Secondly, small dose fish oil might form part of the secondary prevention strategy for coronary heart disease.

Thirdly, it would appear useful as adjunct therapy in treating people with the metabolic, or insulin resistance, syndrome.

With the rising incidence of obesity worldwide, managing its major consequence has become the major challenge in preventing CHD. Three of the charac-

Table 3. Clinical targets for fish oil.

Part of hypolipidemic therapy

Sole option for mild hypertriglyceridemia
With fibrate for severe hypertriglyceridemia
With statin for combine hyperlipoproteinemia
1—6 g n-3 fatty acid daily

Part of secondary prevention in coronary heart disease — adjunct therapy goals

Antiarrhythmogenicity
Antithrombogenicity
Normal endothelial function
Normal lipid profile
1 g n-3 fatty acid daily

Part of managing metabolic syndrome

Improves raised Tg low HDL
Mildly hypotensive
Antithrombogenic
Probably no adverse effect on insulin sensitivity
1 g n-3 fatty acid daily

teristics of this syndrome, the dyslipidemia, increased thrombogenicity and raised blood pressure are susceptible to improvement with fish oil. There is no longer serious concern that n-3 fatty acids will increase insulin resistance [20].

References

1. Ascherio A, Rimm EB, Stampfer MN et al. Dietary intake of marine n-3 fatty acids, fish intake, and the risk of coronary disease among men. N Engl J Med 1995;332:977—982.
2. Siscovick DS et al. Dietary intake and cell membrane levels of long-chain n-3 polyunsaturated fatty acids and the risk of primary cardiac arrest. JAMA 1995;274:1363—1367.
3. Rodriguez BL et al. Fish intake may limit the increase in risk of coronary heart disease morbidity and mortality among heavy smokers. Circulation 1996;94:952—956.
4. Cobiac L, Clifton PM, Abbey M, Belling GB, Nestel PJ. Lipid, lipoprotein and homeostatic effects of fish vs. oil n-3 fatty acids in mildly hyperlipidemic males. Am J Clin Nutr 1991; 53:1210—1216.
5. Pauletto P, Puato M, Caroli MG, Casiglia E, Munhambo AE et al. Blood pressure and atherogenic lipoprotein profiles of fish-diet and vegetarian villagers in Tanzania: the Lugalawa study. Lancet 1996;348:784—788.
6. Mori TA, Beilin LJ, Burke V, Morris J, Ritchie J. Interactions between dietary fat, fish and fish oils and their effects on platelet function in men at risk of cardiovascular disease. Arterioscl Thromb Vasc Biol 1997;17:279—286.
7. Morris MC, Sacks F, Rosner B. Does fish oil lower blood pressure? A meta-analysis of controlled trials. Circulation 1993;88:523—533.
8. Chin JPF, Gust AP, Nestel PJ, Dart AM. Marine oils dose-dependently inhibit vasoconstriction of forearm resistance vessels in humans. Hypertension 1993;21:22—28.
9. Fleischhauer FJ, Yan WD, Fischell TA. Fish oil improves endothelium-dependent coronary vasodilation in heart transplant recipients. J Am Coll Cardiol 1993;21:982—999.
10. McVeigh GE, Brennan GM, Cohn JN, Finkelstein SM, Hayes RJ et al. Fish oil improves arterial compliance in noninsulin-dependent diabetes mellitus. Arterioscl Thromb 1994;14:1425—1429.
11. Nestel PJ. New lipoprotein profiles and coronary heart disease. Circulation 1990;82:649—651.
12. Harris WS. Fish oils and plasma lipid and lipoprotein metabolism in humans. J Lipid Res 1989;30:785—807.
13. Weintraub MS, Zechner R, Brown A, Eisenberg S, Breslow JL. Dietary polyunsaturated fats of the ω-6 and ω-3 series reduce postprandial lipoprotein levels. J Clin Invest 1988;82:1884—1893.
14. Dallongeville J, Boulet L, Davignon J, Lussier-Cacan S. Fish oil supplementation reduces β very low density lipoprotein in type III dysbetalipoproteinemia. Arterioscl Thromb 1991;11: 864—871.
15. Nestel PJ. Effects of n-3 fatty acids on lipid metabolism. Ann Rev Nutr 1990;10:149—167.
16. Abbey M, Clifton P, Kestin M, Belling B, Nestel PJ. Effect of fish oil on lipoproteins, lecithin: cholesterol acyltransferase, and lipid transfer protein activity in humans. Arteriosclerosis 1990; 10:85—94.
17. Suzukawa M, Abbey M, Howe PRC, Nestel PJ. Effects of fish oil fatty acids on low-density lipoprotein size, oxidizability, and uptake by macrophages. J Lipid Res 1995;36:473—484.
18. Suzukawa M, Abbey M, Clifton P, Nestel PJ. Enhanced capacity of n-3 fatty acid-enriched macrophages to oxidize low-density lipoprotein mechanisms and effects of antioxidant vitamins. Atherosclerosis 1996;124:157—169.
19. Whitman SC, Fish JR, Rand ML, Rogers KA. n-3 fatty acid incorporation into LDL particles renders them more susceptible to oxidation in vitro but not necessarily more atherogenic in vivo. Arterioscl Thromb 1994;14:1170—1176.
20. Sirtori CR et al. n-3 fatty acids do not lead to an increased diabetic risk in patients with hyperlipidemia and abnormal glucose tolerance. Am J Clin Nutr 1997;65:1874—1881.

Atherosclerosis XI.
B. Jacotot, D. Mathé and J.-C. Fruchart, editors.

New insights into the mechanisms of atherosclerosis

Russell Ross
Department of Pathology, University School of Medicine, Seattle, Washington, USA

Keywords: endothelium, lipoprotein, macrophage, smooth muscle, T lymphocyte.

Introduction

The advanced lesions of atherosclerosis represent the culmination of a series of cellular and molecular events in which there is replication of both smooth muscle cells and macrophages, which had previously entered the artery wall [1,2]. The interactions among these cells (with the overlying endothelium and T lymphocytes also in the lesion) may lead to a massive fibroproliferative response. Smooth muscle cells lay down relatively large amounts of connective tissue and form a fibrous cap which covers the advanced lesion of atherosclerosis (or fibrous plaque), the deeper portions of which consist of macrophages, T lymphocytes, smooth muscle cells, connective tissue, necrotic debris and varying amounts of lipids and lipoproteins. Terminal events such as myocardial or cerebral infarction, are usually derived from secondary changes within the fibrous plaque that lead to the formation of an occlusive thrombus. These changes include fissuring, cracking or ulceration in the surface of the lesion, which can become subjected to altered rheologic forces.

The protective response

Examination of the earliest cellular events that occur during atherogenesis has demonstrated that the cells involved are classical components of a specialized type of chronic inflammatory response that precedes migration and proliferation of arterial smooth muscle cells. The first observable events include increased accumulation of lipid and lipoprotein particles beneath the endothelium, presumably due to increased transport and/or permeability of the lining endothelial cells. This is rapidly followed by attachment, adherence and spreading of peripheral blood monocytes and T lymphocytes at sites throughout the arterial tree, particularly at branches and bifurcations. These cells adhere due to the formation of adhesive cell-surface glycoproteins by the endothelium and the leukocytes, which interact in a ligand-receptor manner. Thus, one of the earliest changes induced by hypercholesterolemia and hypertension appears to be altered endothelial per-

---

Address for correspondence: Prof Russell Ross PhD, Department of Pathology, University of Washington School of Medicine, P.O. Box 357470, Seattle, WA 98195-7470, USA.

meability together with the adherence of leukocytes, representing the first phase of an inflammatory response.

The leukocytes migrate across the surface of the endothelium, probe between the junctions of the endothelial cells, and are chemotactically attracted into the subendothelial space where they begin to accumulate within the intima. In the presence of oxidized low-density lipoprotein (ox LDL), the monocytes become converted to activated macrophages (and via their scavenger receptors and ox LDL receptors) take up the modified lipoprotein particles and become foam cells. The formation of foam cells and their continued accumulation in the intima lead to the first ubiquitous lesion of atherosclerosis, the fatty streak. If the offending agent (such as hypercholesterolemia or other risk factors) continues, then the inflammatory response will also continue. What may begin as a protective, inflammatory response can become sufficiently deleterious to the cells of the artery wall.

This condition may lead to an expanded, intermediate (or fibrofatty) lesion that may contain multiple layers of smooth muscle, connective tissue, macrophages and T lymphocytes. Eventually, if the conditions that induce the response continue long enough, remodeling of the lesion may occur with the formation of a fibrous cap. The cap covers the numerous proliferated smooth muscle cells and macrophages, together with varying amounts of necrotic cell debris, intracellular and extracellular lipid and potentially massive amounts of new connective tissue. The advanced lesion, or fibrous plaque, can then intrude into the artery wall. Changes in the fibrous cap that covers the fibrous plaque may lead to fissuring or rupture, with formation of a thrombus that can cause sudden death, or organize itself and lead to further lesion progression and compromise the flow at the local site.

The response-to-injury hypothesis of atherosclerosis

The response-to-injury hypothesis of atherosclerosis states that the initial, inflammatory response followed by the formation of a fibroproliferative response begins as a protective mechanism, which with time and continuing insult may become excessive. In its excess, both the inflammation and the fibrous connective tissue proliferation become (in themselves) the disease process. This is the essence of the process of atherogenesis [2].

Gene expression by the cells

As one examines the lesions of atherosclerosis during the different stages of lesion formation, it becomes apparent that the intercellular networking, which occurs among macrophages, T lymphocytes, endothelium and smooth muscle, is critical to determine the direction the lesions will go. For example, gene expression in macrophages can lead to synthesis and secretion of many growth-stimulatory molecules (e.g., platelet-derived growth factor (PDGF), fibroblast growth factor (FGF), heparin-binding epidermnal growth factor-like growth factor (HB-EGF), monocyte-colony stimulating factor (M-CSF), granulocyte-monocyte colony stimulating factor (GM-CSF)) and growth-inhibitory molecules (e.g., transforming growth factor β (TGFβ), interleukin-1 (IL-1), tumor necrosis factor α (TNFα)). However, the cytokines formed by macrophages, including TGFβ, IL-1 and TNFα, can also induce secondary gene expression in smooth muscle cells for PDGF-AA and in some cases HB-EGF, thus inducing the cells to make growth-stimulatory molecules. Whether or not a lesion will progress, remain static or undergo regression may be in part a reflection of which of these genes is expressed in the different cell types.

Macrophage replication can occur through the action of CSFs formed by endothelium, smooth muscle, or the macrophages themselves. Studies have demonstrated that macrophage replication occurs during all phases of lesion progression in atherogenesis and that macrophage replication may be as prominent a feature of lesion progression as is smooth muscle replication.

The matrix surrounding the cells regulates their responses to mitogens

The connective tissue matrix surrounding the smooth muscle cells in the media of the artery profoundly impacts the cells' ability to respond to mitogenic stimuli. Recently, we have shown that smooth muscle cells bind to collagen in vitro via α2β1 integrins and apparently, in vivo via α1β1 integrins. When human type 1 collagen is in fibrillar form in vitro (as is the case when the fibrils surround the smooth muscle cells in the media of the artery) the smooth muscle cells are nonresponsive to mitogens, such as PDGF or to fetal calf serum [3]. This occurs because integrin-mediated signaling leads to upregulation of two cell cycle inhibitors, p27 and p21. As smooth muscle cells enter the G1/S interface, cyclin E binds to cyclin-dependent kinase 2 (cdk2). The cdk2 molecule is phosphorylated on a specific threonine moiety in cdk2. This cyclin E/cdk2 phosphorylated complex permits the cells to traverse into S. This activity happens when smooth muscle cells are cultured on collagen that does not polymerize to fibrils but remains in a monomeric state. Monomeric collagen forms when the collagen is solubilized in dilute acetic acid and air dried on the plate. Cells that attach to this monomeric substrate when cultured respond logarithmically to mitogens, such as PDGF. In sharp contrast, when the cells are cultured on the same type of collagen in fibrillar form, the cell cycle inhibitor p27 is markedly upregulated, binds to the cyclin E/cdk2 complex, and prevents phosphorylation of the cdk2 molecule. This complex then prevents cell cycle traverse and keeps the cells in G1/G0 and thus prevents smooth muscle proliferation. Observations and approaches such as these may help to explain why medial smooth muscle cells are nonresponsive to mitogens and neointimal smooth muscle cells (such as those residing in the lesions of atherosclerosis) are markedly responsive. Thus, the matrix plays a key role in determining whether these cells can undergo cell cycle traverse and proliferate. The same may be true for macrophages that find themselves surrounded by matrix and for endothelial cells. Further experiments need to be done to determine if this is the case.

Summary

Thus, the lesions of atherosclerosis represent a protective, inflammatory-fibroproliferative response against the different agents that can cause the disease. If the injury continues chronically over a long period of time, it may become excessive and in its excess becomes the disease itself. It has been shown that this excessive, inflammatory, fibroproliferative response can be reversed, given sufficient opportunity for the injurious factors to be modified. Approaches to modifying specific cellular interactions, growth-regulatory molecules, or intracellular signaling molecules may afford opportunities to modify these processes and lead to lesion prevention or regression.

Acknowledgements

This work is supported in part by the National Heart, Lung and Blood Institute, National Institutes of Health, grant HL18645, and by Bristol-Myers Squibb Company, an unrestricted grant for cardiovascular research.

References

1. Ross R. The pathogenesis of atherosclerosis — an update. N Engl J Med 1986;314:488—500.
2. Ross R. The pathogenesis of atherosclerosis: a perspective for the 1990s. Nature 1993;362: 801—809.
3. Koyama H, Raines EW, Bornfeldt KE, Roberts JM, Ross R. Fibrillar collagen inhibits arterial smooth muscle proliferation through regulation of CDK2 inhibitors. Cell 1996;87:1069—1078.

A preventive and therapeutic approach in atherosclerosis

William W. Parmley
University of California, San Francisco, California, USA

Death from heart disease (principally coronary artery disease) remains the number one cause of mortality in the USA, although the death rate from heart disease has been going down since around 1968. Coronary disease remains a similar problem in other Western and developed countries. The Framingham study coined the term "risk factor" to describe those factors which statistically appeared to contribute to the development of coronary artery disease in their long-term study. Results have shown that these risk factors are additive to one another, and that appropriate attention to all of them must be given in order to minimize the risk of developing atherosclerosis and coronary artery diseases [1]. Despite this knowledge regarding risk factors for coronary disease, it appears that the known risk factors can perhaps account for only half of the cases of coronary artery disease. Thus, genetic factors remain an important cause of disease and have yet to be fully elucidated. For the clinician caring for patients with heart disease, however, it is apparent that control of risk factors is the primary approach to protecting patients against the development of disease. Table 1 lists some of the standard risk factors for coronary artery disease. Those at the top have been felt to be of considerable importance. Those at the bottom represent risk factors over which we have no control. Those in the middle appear to be intermediate in terms of the magnitude of risk. Each of these risk factors will be touched on briefly, relative to the evaluation and management of patients with preclinical and clinical disease.

Lipoprotein abnormalities

Lipid abnormalities are major risk factors for the development of coronary artery disease [2]. These include an elevated low-density lipoprotein (LDL) cholesterol, a reduced high-density lipoprotein (HDL) cholesterol, the level of LPa and perhaps additional contributions of elevated triglycerides and other lipoprotein factors. Epidemiologic evidence clearly relates the level of these lipid risk factors to the development of coronary artery disease. There have been considerable attempts, therefore, to prevent disease or reverse existing disease by appropriately

Address for correspondence: William W. Parmley MD, Professor of Medicine, 1186 Moffitt Hospital, 505 Parnassus Avenue, San Francisco, CA 94143-0124, USA.

206

Table 1. Risk factors for coronary artery disease

Lipoprotein abnormalities
Smoking
Hypertension

Diabetes
Lack of exercise
Homocysteine
Hypercoagulability
Stress — type A
Coronary artery calcification

Positive family history
Age
Sex

altering the lipoprotein abnormalities. A number of quantitative coronary angiographic studies have shown that although one can produce dramatic reductions in elevated LDL cholesterol, it has been more difficult to cause considerable regression of actual lesions [3]. Despite this inability to change lesions very much, there appears to be a 50% or more reduction in clinical events such as acute myocardial infarction [4]. This suggests that lipid lowering has an independent effect on stabilizing plaque and thus reducing the number of myocardial infarctions. It is unclear whether this stabilization of plaque occurs by reversing endothelial dysfunction, removing lipid pools from the soft plaques which are at risk for rupture, or other undefined mechanisms of benefit. Nevertheless, the data is convincing that lowering lipids is one of the most powerful protectors against acute myocardial infarction and subsequent mortality. Several recent trials have pointed out the advantages of the statins in producing benefit. In the 4S trial in patients with known vascular disease [5], simvastatin was effective in reducing morbidity and mortality. The divergence of the placebo and simvastatin treated curves suggests that this effect is a continuing one. In the prevention trial from the west of Scotland with pravastatin [6], there was similar benefit on morbidity and mortality in patients with considerable risk factors but no overt evidence of disease. In the CARE trial, postmyocardial infarction pravastatin [7] also was effective in reducing subsequent events in patients with known disease following a recent cardiac event. These and other trials point out the considerable benefit which can accrue from reducing elevated lipids. There is some controversy as to how low lipids should be reduced, and what the benefit is at high and low lipid levels, but the overall benefit of lipid reduction appears to be clear-cut.

Smoking

Tobacco use kills over 400,000 Americans each year including about 174,000 from heart disease. In addition, environmental tobacco smoke kills about 50,000 nonsmokers per year [8]. Active and passive smoking together, therefore, are the most preventable cause of premature death in the USA. A variety of mechanisms contribute to the adverse effects of smoking which can be addictive because of the nicotine content. Smoking alters lipoproteins, may increase heart rate and blood pressure, enhances platelet activation and clotting, produces vasoconstriction by altered endothelial function, increases carbon monoxide and oxygen free radicals and has other chemicals which may contribute to atherosclerosis [8]. Like other risk factors, cigarette smoke damages endothelial cells and worsens endothelial function. In lipid-fed rabbits exposed to environmental tobacco smoke, we showed that its adverse effects on endothelial function were markedly blunted by the simultaneously administration of dietary L-arginine [9]. Since L-arginine is an amino acid precursor for the vasodilator nitric oxide, it may be that L-arginine in the future could have a preventive role or treatment role in the management of patients with risk factors.

The clinical challenge is to get patients to stop smoking [10]. There has been a substantial reduction in the smoking rate among physicians in the USA, with a similar but less impressive reduction in nurses. It is unclear, however, that this trend with physicians applies in many other countries. Limiting tobacco sales to minors would be an effective way of reducing the risk. In addition, mandating smoke-free work places, schools and public places would also be helpful. In the USA there are approximately 3,000 new smokers per day which generally come from teenagers. Approximately 2,000 Americans stop smoking each day and another 1,000 die from smoke-related diseases.

Hypertension

Hypertension is a major modifiable risk factor for the development of coronary disease. It is of interest, however, that control of blood pressure causes a 40% reduction in stroke with only about a 15% reduction in the rate of myocardial infarction [11]. The precise difference between these two circulations and their response to reduction in blood pressure is not clear. There has been recent controversy about the use of short-acting calcium entry blockers for treating patients with hypertension. Overall, I believe the data suggest that short-acting calcium entry blockers should not be used but that long-acting calcium entry blockers are safe and effective for the management of hypertension. A number of drugs are effective in managing blood pressure. Although the joint national commission recommended that β-blockers and diuretics should be first-line therapy in patients for hypertension [12], in the USA the ACE-inhibitors and calcium blockers are by far and away the most preferred monotherapy for treating hypertension.

Patients who have hypertension and evidence of left ventricular hypertrophy (LVH) on the electrocardiogram appear to be at even greater increased risk for the development of coronary artery disease [13]. It is unclear whether attempts at regression of LVH in these patients will be effective. The ACE-inhibitors and calcium blockers appear to be preferable in reducing left ventricular hypertrophy, although all drugs which lower blood pressure are effective. Controversy still exists about how low blood pressure should be reduced. The literature has some suggestions of a J shaped curve [14] with an increase in mortality as diastolic pressure is lowered below 85 down to 80 and 75 mmHg. Long-term, ongoing trials will help to answer this important question. Salt restriction appears to be an important management issue for controlling blood pressure although only about half the USA population is salt-sensitive.

Diabetes

Diabetes may increase the risk for coronary disease [15] in part because of the associated dyslipidemia, hypertension and elevated insulin levels with insulin resistance. The microangiopathy affecting the retina and kidney can be reduced by maintaining more normal levels of glucose [16]. It is unclear whether strict control of diabetes has a marked favorable effect on the development of coronary artery disease.

Exercise

There is controversy about the effects of physical inactivity as a contributing factor to coronary artery disease [17]. Physical activity is important in maintaining an appropriate body weight and blood pressure and in reducing high lipid levels. In general, it appears prudent to suggest a regular exercise pattern including walking. Such exercise can be helpful in lowering blood pressure, improving glucose tolerance, reducing lipids, reducing weight, training the cardiovascular system and perhaps decreasing plasma renin levels.

Obesity

There remains some controversy about the independent risk that obesity provides for the development of coronary artery disease [18]. Because it is frequently associated with other risk factors such as hypertension, glucose intolerance and elevated lipids, its independent adverse effects are less clear. There is evidence that central accumulation of abdominal fat has a higher risk for the development of coronary artery disease than peripheral accumulation [19]. In general, there are a number of health reasons for patients to avoid obesity and maintain a reasonable exercise program.

Homocysteine

Homocysteineria is a rare disease with high total levels of plasma homocysteine and a high incidence of coronary disease in adolescents [20]. A number of studies have suggested that high homocysteine levels may lead to the development of coronary disease [21], presumably because of their adverse effects on endothelial function. Homocysteine levels are not a routine measurement in all laboratories. Treatment with folic acid [22] perhaps in a regular multivitamin, is very effective in countering this increased risk.

Hypercoagulability

There is a relationship between the risk of developing coronary artery disease and fibrinogen concentrations [23]. The beneficial effects of aspirin and other platelet inhibitors suggest that excess platelet activation may contribute to acute coronary events [24]. Data with the new IIb-IIIa inhibitors in acute coronary syndromes again suggest benefit [25]. Other anticoagulants such as low molecular weight heparin, heparin or coumadin have shown benefit in patients with known coronary artery disease. Although there is an increased risk of bleeding with these agents which interfere with coagulation, it appears that they should be given serious consideration in the management of patients with coronary artery disease. Certainly, the routine use of 81–325 mg of aspirin per day may provide protection against acute myocardial infarction [24].

Stress

There is controversy about the role of emotional stress and personality type in relation to risk factors for coronary artery disease [26]. It does appear that acute emotional stress can precipitate coronary events. The risks of personality types, however, are less clear. It is also unclear whether stress management can have an important effect on this potential risk.

Coronary artery calcification

The use of ultrafast CT scanning to examine the presence and location of calcification in coronary arteries has provided interesting new information in patients [27]. Premature coronary calcification appears to signal an increased risk for developing coronary artery disease. Frequently, it occurs long before a positive treadmill test and thus provides an individualized marker of where a person is relative to the development of coronary disease. It is unclear whether this test should be considered routinely, but in selected patients it may provide important information about risk.

Family history, age and gender

It is clear that a positive family history [28], advanced age and male gender also increase the risk of developing coronary artery disease. Women tend to delay their development of coronary disease by about 10 years with some catch-up after menopause [29]. It is presumed that protection by female hormones, principally estrogen, delays the onset of coronary disease. This is the rationale for giving estrogen postmenopausally which does appear to reduce the risk of coronary events. However, estrogen can also increase the risk of endometrial cancer and may have an adverse effect on breast cancer in patients with a family history of breast cancer. Nevertheless, the protective benefits on the development of coronary disease and osteoporosis suggest that estrogen is an effective preventive therapeutic strategy [30].

It should be apparent from the preceding that all risk factors may work through promoting endothelial dysfunction and that reduction of risk factors can protect against endothelial dysfunction. This provides an attractive common final pathway for the interaction of risk factors in the development of coronary disease.

ACE-inhibitors and calcium blockers

There is interesting recent data that the ACE-inhibitors may be protective in patients with known coronary artery disease. In many of the ACE-inhibitor trials, including those postmyocardial infarction, there has been a reduction in infarction rate in the patients treated with ACE-inhibitors compared with placebo [31]. There is considerable evidence that angiotensin 2 may worsen endothelial dysfunction and set in motion a number of events which promote atherosclerosis [32]. Alternatively, reduction of angiotensin 2 levels, and an increase of bradykinin released nitric oxide appear to have the opposite beneficial effects. In the TREND trial, the administration of the ACE-inhibitor quinapril over a 6-month period was effective in reversing adverse coronary endothelial function in patients with established coronary artery disease [33]. Whether ACE-inhibitors would have a similar beneficial role in prevention of disease, for example, in patients with hypertension is less clear. Ongoing long-term studies will help to answer this question.

Interestingly, the calcium entry blockers have shown important antiatherogenic effects in animal models of atherosclerosis [34]. However, the clinical trials which have been carried out primarily with the short-acting calcium entry blockers have not shown benefit, and in some cases suggested harm [35]. It is unclear whether the long-acting calcium entry blockers might show some clinical benefit. It could be argued that the rise and fall of heart rate, blood pressure and neurohormones two or three times a day in patients with potential coronary disease may be adverse risk factors for the development of acute events. A long-acting calcium entry blocker with a relatively constant plasma level should be able to avoid this kind of adverse oscillation of cardiac factors.

Final thoughts

The reduction in death rate from coronary artery disease in the USA from the mid-1960s to the present is presumed to be mostly due to a reduction in risk factors in the population at large. There certainly has been some additional benefit from both medical and surgical therapy but this may be less than that achieved by generalized risk factor reduction. It appears that many physicians have paid less attention to patients with known coronary disease in terms of continued risk factor reduction. Hopefully, the new information about the beneficial effects of risk factor reduction on endothelial function will motivate physicians to be more aggressive in this area.

References

1. Stamler J. Epidemiology, established major risk factors, and the primary prevention of coronary heart disease. In: Parmley WW, Chatterjee K (eds) Cardiology. Philadelphia: J.B. Lippincott Co., 1994;chapter 2-1.
2. Mahley RW, Bersot TP. Lipid abnormalities: mechanisms, clinical classifications, and manager. In: Parmley WW, Chatterjee K (eds) Cardiology. Philadelphia: J.B. Lippincott Co., 1994;chapter 2-2.
3. Rossouw JE. Lipid lowering interventions in angiographic trials. Am J Cardiol 1995;76:86C—92C.
4. Holme I. Cholesterol reduction and its impact on coronary artery disease and total mortality. Am J Cardiol 1995;76:10C—17C.
5. Scandinavian Simvastatin Survival Study Group. Randomized trial of cholesterol lowering in 4444 patients with coronary heart disease. The 4S Trial. Lancet 1994;344:1383—1389.
6. Shepherd J, Cobbe SM, Ford I et al. Prevention of coronary heart disease with pravastatin in men with hypercholesterolemia. N Engl J Med 1995;333:1301—1307.
7. Sacks FM, Pfeffer MA, Moye LA et al. The effect of pravastatin on coronary events after myocardial infarction in patients with average cholesterol levels. N Engl J Med 1996;335:1001—1009.
8. Glantz SA. Tobacco: Biology and Politics. Waco: Health EDCO (Division of WRS Group Inc.), 1992.
9. Sun Y, Zhu BQ, Sievers RE, Glantz SA, Deedwania PC, Parmley WW. L-arginine preserves endothelial-dependent relaxation during environmental tobacco smoke in lipid fed rabbits. Circulation 1994;90(4):I—459.
10. Transdermal Nicotine Study Group. Transdermal nicotine for smoking cessation. JAMA 1991;266:3133—3138.
11. Kaplan NM. Cardiovascular risk reduction: the role of antihypertensive treatment. Am J Med 1991;90:19S.
12. Fifth Report of the Joint National Committee on Detection, Evaluation and Treatment of High Blood Pressure. National Institutes of Health. NIH Publication, 1993.
13. Levy D, Garrison RJ, Savage DD, Kannel WB, Castelli WP. Prognostic implications of echocardiographically determined left ventricular mass in the Framingham heart study. N Engl J Med 1990;322:1561—1566.
14. Safar M. Therapeutic trials and large arteries in hypertension (review). Am Heart J 1988;115:702.
15. Garcia MJ, McNamara PM, Gordon T, Kannel WB. Sixteen year follow-up study. Morbidity and mortality in diabetics in the Framingham population. Diabetes 1976;23:105.
16. Clark CM Jr. Risks and benefits of intensive management in non-insulin-dependent diabetes mellitus. Ann Int Med 1996;124:184—186.
17. Slattery ML, Jacobs DR Jr, Nichaman MZ. Leisure time physical activity and coronary heart disease death. The US Railroad Study. Circulation 1989;79:304.
18. Kannel WB, Gordon T. Physiological and medical concomitants of obesity: The Framingham Study. In: Bray GA (ed) Obesity in America. Washington, D.C.: US Department of Health, Edu-

212

cation and Welfare, 1979;125—163(NIH Publication No. 79—359).

19. Lapidus L, Bentsson C, Larsson B. Distribution of adipose tissue and body fat and risk of cardiovascular disease. A 12-year follow-up of participants in the population study of women in Gothenburg, Sweden. Br Med J Clin Res 1984;289:1257.

20. Mudd SH, Levy HL, Skovby F. Disorders of transulfuration. In: Scriver CR, Beaudet AL, Sly WS et al. (eds) The Metabolic Basis of Inherited Disease. New York: McGraw-Hill Book Co., 1989;693—734.

21. Veland PM, Refsum H, Brattstrom L. Plasma homocysteine and cardiovascular disease. In: Francis RJ (ed) Atherosclerotic Cardiovascular Disease, Hemostasis and Endothelial Function. New York: Marcel Dekker Inc., 1992;183—236.

22. Selhub J, Jaques PF, Wilson PWF, Rush D, Rosenberg IN. Vitamin status and intake as primary determinants of homocysteinemia in an elderly population. JAMA 1993;270:2693—2698.

23. Yarnell JWG, Baker IA, Sweetnam PM et al. Fibrinogen, viscosity, and white blood cell count are major risk factors for ischemic heart disease. The Caerphilly and Speedwell collaborative heart disease studies. Circulation 1991;83:836.

24. Antiplatelet Trialists' Collaboration. Collaborative overview of randomized trials of antiplatelet treatment. Part I: Prevention of vascular death, MI, and stroke by prolonged antiplatelet therapy in different categories of patients. Br Med J 1994;308:81—106.

25. Evolution of the clinical applications of glycoprotein IIb/IIIa inhibitors. J Inv Cardiol 1996; 8(Suppl B):1B—80B.

26. Jenkins CD. Psychosocial and behavioral factors. In: Kaplan NM, Stamler J (eds) Prevention of Coronary Heart Disease: Practical Management of the Risk Factors. Philadelphia: W.B. Saunders Co., 1983;99.

27. Fallavollita JA, Brody AS, Bunnell IL, Kumar K, Canty JM Jr. Fast computed tomography detection of coronary calcification in the diagnosis of coronary artery disease. Comparison with angiography in patients < 50 years old. Circulation 1994;89:285—290.

28. Sinaiko AR, Wells TG. Childhood hypertension. In: Laragh JH, Brenner BM (eds) Hypertension, vol 2. New York: Raven Press, 1990;1855—1868.

29. Matthews KA, Meilahn E, Kuller LH et al. Menopause and risk factors for coronary artery disease. N Engl J Med 1989;321:641.

30. Stampfer MJ, Willett EC, Colditz GA et al. Past use of oral contraceptives and cardiovascular disease: a meta-analysis in the context of the Nurses' Health Study. Am J Obst Gynecol 1990; 163:285.

31. Lonn EM, Yusuf S, Jha P et al. Emerging role of ACE-inhibitors in cardiac and vascular protection. Circulation 1994;90:2056—2069.

32. Gibbons GH, Dzau VJ. The emerging concept of vascular remodeling. N Engl J Med 1994;330:1431—1438.

33. Mancini GBJ, Henry GC, Macaya C et al. ACE-inhibition with quinapril improves endothelial vasomotor dysfunction in patients with coronary artery disease: the TREND study. Circulation 1996;94:258—265.

34. Parmley WW. Can calcium antagonists alter the course of atherosclerosis. J Myocardial Isochem 1991;3:11—26.

35. Yusuf S. Calcium antagonists in coronary artery disease and hypertension. Time for re-evaluation. Circulation 1995;92:1079—1082.

Primary prevention program in North Karelia: predicting mortality from changes in CHD risk factors

Matti J. Tikkanen[1] and Erkki Vartiainen[2]

[1] *Department of Medicine, University of Helsinki; and* [2] *Department of Epidemiology and Health Promotion, National Public Health Institute, Helsinki, Finland*

Abstract. This review summarizes the history and current situation of the community interventions carried out since 1972 in North Karelia, Finland. Continuous monitoring of risk factor levels and coronary heart disease (CHD) mortality trends in the population has made it possible to evaluate the relationship between changes in risk factors and those in CHD mortality. Recent analyses indicate that CHD mortality could be predicted relatively accurately on the basis of risk factor changes up to the early 1980s, after which the observed mortality declined more rapidly than predicted. The gap between predicted and observed mortality may reflect improved secondary preventive measures and introduction of effective new treaments.

Keywords: blood pressure, cholesterol, smoking.

Introduction

By about 1970, Finland was characterized by a record-high coronary heart disease (CHD) mortality in middle-aged men [1], and the province of North Karelia located in the eastern part of the country, had even higher mortality than the other areas. Recognition of this serious public health problem led to initiation in 1972 of the community-based North Karelia project, a primary prevention program aimed at preventing CHD by changing lifestyle and reducing risk factors. The scientific basis had been established in the Seven Countries [2] and Framingham [3] studies demonstrating that elevated blood pressure, high serum cholesterol and cigarette smoking were major CHD risk factors. Thereafter, similar programs were started in other areas, and the North Karelia pilot project was gradually converted into a nationwide preventive effort. Now, 25 years later it is possible to evaluate to what extent risk factor changes could predict changes in CHD mortality.

Lines of intervention in North Karelia

The first targets of the North Karelia Project were to reduce smoking, serum cholesterol levels and high blood pressure which were regarded as the three major

Address for correspondence: Matti J. Tikkanen MD, Department of Medicine, Helsinki University Central Hospital, FIN-00290 Helsinki, Finland. Tel.: +358-9-4712210. Fax: +358-9-4714013. E-mail: matti.j.tikkanen@helsinki.fi

214

causative risk factors for CHD, and to promote early diagnosis, treatment and rehabilitation of patients with cardiovascular disorders. Based on the evidence available it was assumed that achieving these targets would lead to the goal of decreasing morbidity and mortality of CHD.

Several lines of community-based intervention were started, all aimed at reducing CHD risk factor levels in the population, with emphasis on a healthy lifestyle:

1. Existing community services and special support services were reorganized in order to improve the efficacy of risk factor detection and reduction. For example, mass hypertension screening was added to obligatory X-ray screening for tuberculosis and cytological screening for cervical cancer in women. Physicians and nurses in health centers were instructed to give dietary and antismoking advice to their patients. Voluntary organizations were encouraged to promote healthier lifestyles by arranging "long life" parties in their villages.

2. A particular effort was made to inform and educate the public by programs on television and radio as well as articles and interviews in the newspapers. In the late 1980s the dairy industry started a counteroffensive claiming that intake of dairy fats was not related to elevated cholesterol and increased risk of CHD. This advertizing campaign backfired, the public at large became aware of the issue, and dietary habits started to change more rapidly resulting in a dramatic reduction in consumption of saturated fats.

3. Information systems were created, such as registers of patients with hypertension, myocardial infarction and stroke, and systems were developed for continuous monitoring of the community prevention program.

4. "Environmental" changes with particular emphasis on lifestyle were generated, e.g., by antismoking measures and promotion of healthier diet.

5. Importance was attached to training personnel participating in the project at all levels, physicians, nurses and nonprofessional volunteers.

The project was started in 1972 by surveying random population samples for CHD risk factors in North Karelia and also in the Kuopio area, which was chosen as reference area for the study [4]. The surveys were repeated every 5 years in independent random samples drawn from the population register, and other samples were later drawn in southwestern and southern Finland.

Observed changes in CHD risk factors

Serum cholesterol

Serum cholesterol levels decreased gradually during the 20-year period starting in 1972 (Fig. 1). In men, total serum cholesterol fell by 16% in North Karelia and by 12% in the Kuopio reference area. The corresponding reductions for women were 18 and 17% [4]. The decreasing trend has continued also after 1992.

The most probable reason for the decreasing serum cholesterol levels in the population has been the changing Finnish diet. In the late 1960s, 23% of energy intake was from saturated fats. During the 20-year period starting in 1972, the

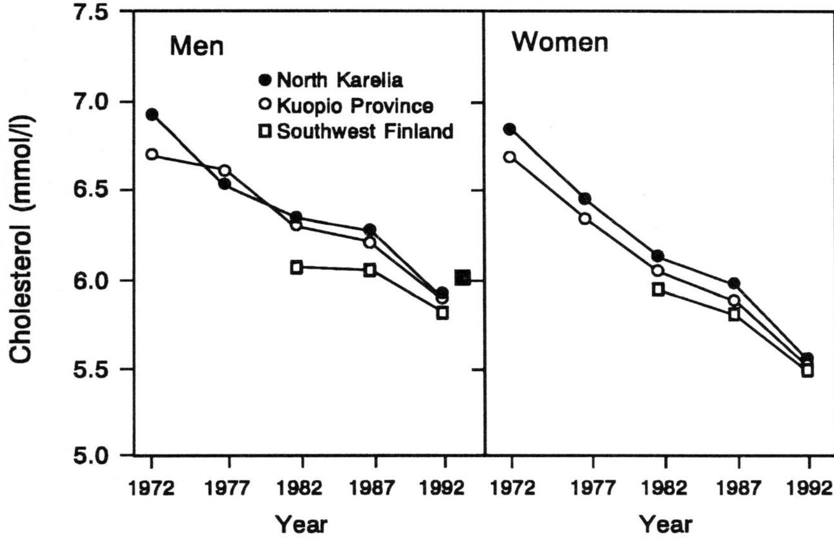

Fig. 1. Mean cholesterol in men and women in different regions in Finland between 1972 and 1992 (adapted from [4]).

consumption of full-fat milk and butter has gradually decreased, while that of low-fat milk and margarine has increased [5] resulting in a continuous increase in the ratio of polyunsaturated:saturated fats in the diet. This change was accelerated after a dairy industry-sponsored media campaign backfired (see above), and the consumption of vegetable oils, margarines and fat-free milk increased rapidly. Also total fat consumption decreased. In 1982, 38.5% of energy intake in men was derived from fat, but in 1992 only 34.4%, a reduction by 4.1%. The corresponding reduction in women was from 36.7 to 33.8% [5]. These dietary changes are thought to explain the changes in cholesterol levels relatively well.

Blood pressure

The mean diastolic blood pressure in men fell by 8.1% in North Karelia and by 10.2% in Kuopio, the corresponding decreases in women being 13.9 and 12.9% (Fig. 2) [4]. The cuff size used for blood pressure measurements was increased in the 1982 survey, probably causing slight overestimation of the reduction between 1977 and 1982.

It is not completely clear what caused the favorable trend in blood pressure between 1972 and 1992, which is still continuing. As the consumption of alcohol has increased, and the mean body mass index is on the rise [6], other factors must be involved. Likely explanations are the decreased salt consumption in the 1980s [5], and the switch from use of saturated fats to polyunsaturated ones, a dietary alteration claimed to have an antihypertensive effect [7], in addition to

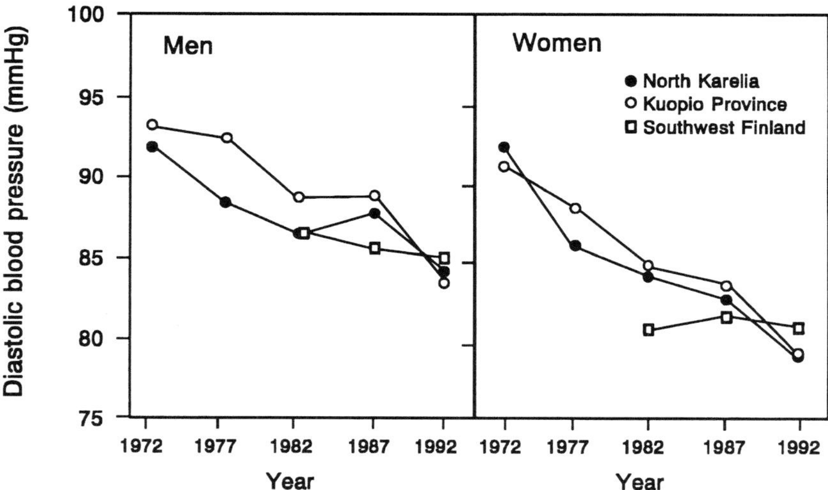

Fig. 2. Mean diastolic blood pressure in men and women in different regions in Finland between 1972 and 1992 (adapted from [4]).

cholesterol lowering. One contributing factor is the expansion of use of antihypertensive medications during the study period.

Cigarette smoking

During the period between 1972 and 1992, cigarette smoking in men decreased from 52 to 32% in North Karelia, and from 50 to 37% in the Kuopio reference area [4]. In women, however, smoking increased during the same time period from 10 and 11% in the North Karelia and Kuopio areas to 17 and 19%, respectively. The North Karelia investigators have reported that study participation rates fell during the 20-year period, which could have caused overestimation of the decline in smoking. In their survey they contacted 50% of the nonparticipants and found out that the smoking rate was 53% among nonparticipants compared to 38% in participants [4].

Changes in CHD mortality in relation to changes in major CHD risk factors

The North Karelia project was originally aimed at testing the feasibility and efficacy of a community-based program of risk factor reduction to prevent cardiovascular disease [8]. This pilot program was later actively converted into a nationwide program, with North Karelia and Kuopio remaining as "core" activities.

Risk factor changes were correlated with CHD mortality trends in a recent analysis, which used pooled data from the North Karelia and Kuopio areas [9]. Pooling of data was possible because of the similarity of risk factor changes after the 5 years, except for cigarette smoking in men which continued to fall more rapidly in North Karelia.

Trends in age-standardized mortality from CHD in men and women aged 35—65 years are shown in Fig. 3. The mortality in middle-aged men fell from 647 per 100,000 to 289 per 100,000 between 1969 and 1992. The corresponding decline in women was from 114 per 100,000 to 36 per 100,000 [9]. Using logistic regression models, the investigators calculated predicted mortality changes for each risk factor separately as well as for all three combined (Fig. 4). For men, the predicted reduction in mortality between 1972 and 1992 based on all risk factors was 44%, which was smaller than the observed 55% decline in mortality (Table 1). The predicted decrease in women was 49%, also smaller than the observed 68% reduction in CHD mortality. The increase in smoking among women resulted in a smaller predicted mortality reduction. Alterations in the three major causative risk factors of CHD seemed to explain two-thirds of the mortality decrease. Starting in the 1980s, mortality decreased at a faster rate than predicted on the basis of risk factor changes. Presumably, increased use of thrombolytic treatment for myocardial infarction, coronary revascularization procedures and prophylactic use of acetylsalicylic acid [9] as well as other secondary preventive measures such as use of β-blockers and cholesterol-lowering agents, may have contributed to this accelerated decline in CHD mortality. It is not clear to what extent the decline in mortality reflected reduced incidence of CHD and to what extent a possible decrease in case fatality. A long-term analysis of the myocardial infarction register in North Karelia has indicated a marked decrease in occurrence of the first event (incidence) between 1972 and 1981 [10]. During the subsequent decade, incidence fell relatively little while recurrent coronary attacks and mortality decreased more.

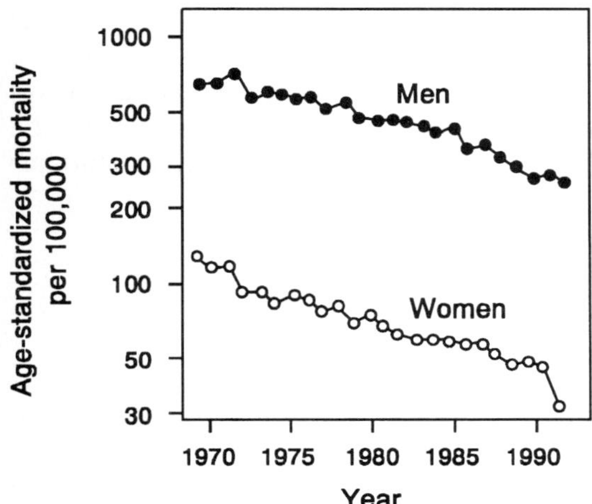

Fig. 3. Trends in age-standardized mortality from CHD in men and women aged 35—64 years in Finland, 1969—1992. (Adapted from [9].)

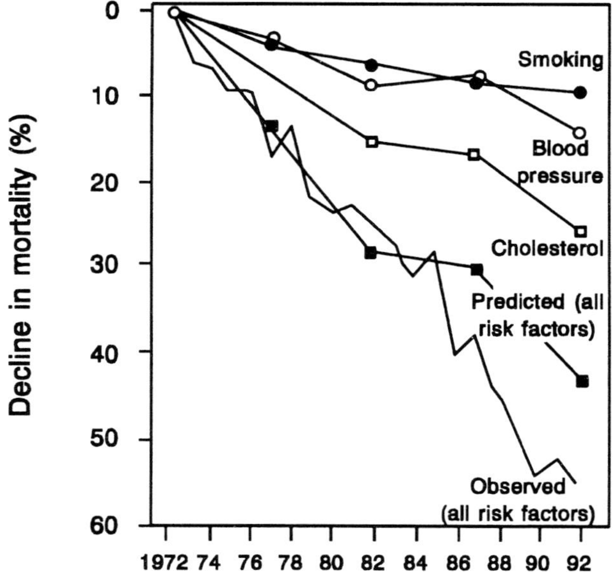

Fig. 4. Observed and predicted mortality from CHD in men aged 35—64 years in Finland between 1972 and 1992 (adapted from [9]).

Summary

The data obtained from North Karelia and other study areas are of importance for public health planning. They show that CHD mortality trends can to a relatively large extent be predicted on the basis of changes occurring in three major CHD risk factors — elevated blood pressure, high serum cholesterol and cigarette smoking. Accordingly, despite the existence of many other important risk factors, it is useful to maintain emphasis on the three major ones. Preventive strategies employed in North Karelia and later in other regions have probably reduced the incidence of first myocardial infarctions (primary prevention) as well as reinfarc-

Table 1. Percent observed and predicted decline in mortality from CHD (1972—1992) in men and women in Finland. Numbers represent percent decline from baseline values in 1972.

	Men		Women	
	Observed	Predicted	Observed	Predicted
1997	7	14	28	22
1982	25	28	41	32
1987	38	30	45	38
1992	55	44	68	49

Adapted from [9].

tions (secondary prevention). It is not clear to what extent reductions in mortality can be explained by diminished case fatality due to improved availability of new effective treatments. Further measures to intensify the process of risk factor reduction in the population will probably result in further reduction in CHD mortality. Reversal of unfavorable trends in risk factors, such as increases in body mass index and smoking in women, would probably result in further benefit.

References

1. Pisa Z, Uemura K. Trends of mortality from ischaemic heart disease and other cardiovascular diseases in 27 countries, 1968-1977. World Health Stat Q 1982;35:11—17.
2. Keys A. Coronary Heart Disease in Seven Countries. American Heart Association Monograph No. 29, New York, 1970.
3. Kannel WB, Gordon T. The Framingham Study: an epidemiological investigation of cardiovascular disease. 18 year follow-up. DHEW Publ. No. (NIH) 74-599, 1974.
4. Vartiainen E, Puska P, Jousilahti P, Korhonen HJ, Tuomilehto J, Nissinen A. Twenty-year trends in coronary risk factors in North Karelia and in other areas of Finland. Int J Epidemiol 1994; 23:495—504.
5. Pietinen P. Changing dietary habits in the population: the Finnish experience. In: Ziant G (ed) Lipids and Health. Amsterdam: Elsevier Science Publishers B.V., 1990;243—256.
6. Pietinen P, Vartiainen E, Männistö S. Trends in body mass index and obesity among adults in Finland from 1972 to 1992. Int J Obesity 1996;20:114—120.
7. Iacono JM, Puska P, Dougherty RM, Pietinen P, Vartiainen E, Leino U, Mutanen M, Moisio S. Effect of dietary fat on blood pressure in a rural Finnish population. Am J Clin Nutr 1983;38: 860—869.
8. Puska P, Nissinen A, Tuomilehto J, Salonen JT, Koskela K, McAlister A, Kottke TE, Maccoby N, Farquhar JW. The community-based strategy to prevent coronary heart disease: conclusions from the ten years of the North Karelia Project. Ann Rev Pub Health 1985;6:147—193.
9. Vartiainen E, Puska P, Pekkanen J, Tuomilehto J, Jousilahti P. Changes in risk factors explain changes in mortality from ischaemic heart disease in Finland. Br Med J 1994;309:23—27.
10. Jousilahti P, Vartiainen E, Tuomilehto J, Pekkanen J, Puska P. Effect of risk factors and changes in risk factors on coronary mortality in three cohorts of middle-aged people in eastern Finland. Am J Epidemiol 1995;141:50—60.

STATE-OF-THE-ART SYMPOSIA

The concept of the vulnerable plaque in coronary heart disease

M.J. Davies
St George's Hospital Medical School, London, UK

Keywords: atherosclerosis, myocardial infarction, thrombosis, unstable angina, vulnerable plaque.

Mechanisms of clinical expression of coronary heart disease

Unstable angina and regional myocardial infarction have now been established by autopsy atherectomy, angiographic and angioscopic studies [1–4] to be due to acute coronary thrombosis on a culprit plaque. In contrast, stable exertional angina is associated with chronic stenoses which are flow limiting on exercise.

The American Heart Association has produced a standard nomenclature for plaque types [5]. Stage V is the advanced or fibrolipid plaque which is an elevated hump when viewed enface on the intima of coronary arteries. Plaques range from yellow to white depending on the proportions of lipid and collagen present. The type Va plaque has a lipid core separated from the lumen of the artery by a cap of fibromuscular tissue. The lipid core is a space within the connective tissue of the plaque containing an acellular mass of lipid including crystalline cholesterol. The plaque cap consists of a regular network of type I collagen within which lacunae contain smooth muscle cells. These smooth muscle cells produce and maintain the cap collagen. Plaques are increasingly being seen as dynamic structures. The lipid core is formed to a large extent by the death of lipid containing macrophages at its margins. The core may be expanding due to this lipid accumulation and the release of metalloproteinases which lead to further destruction of the plaque connective tissue. Within the fibrous cap connective tissue matrix synthesis and degradation are balanced.

Plaques which are designated as type Va show considerable heterogeneity (Fig. 1). The core may occupy a small or a large proportion of the overall plaque volume. The cap may be thick or thin and is often variable in thickness. Another variable is the degree of stenosis that such plaques cause. Type Va plaques can cause high-grade stenosis but are more often angiographically invisible. The seminal work of Glagov [6] elucidated the mechanisms by which large plaques remain undetected. The vessel wall is a dynamic structure and when a plaque develops the external diameter of the artery increases (compensatory dilatation) to accommodate the plaque without compromising the lumen dimensions.

Address for correspondence: M.J. Davies, Professor of Cardiovascular Pathology, Department of Cardiovascular Pathology, St. George's Hospital Medical School, Cranmer Terrace, London SW17 ORE, UK. Tel.: +44-181-6729178. Fax: +44-181-7670268.

224

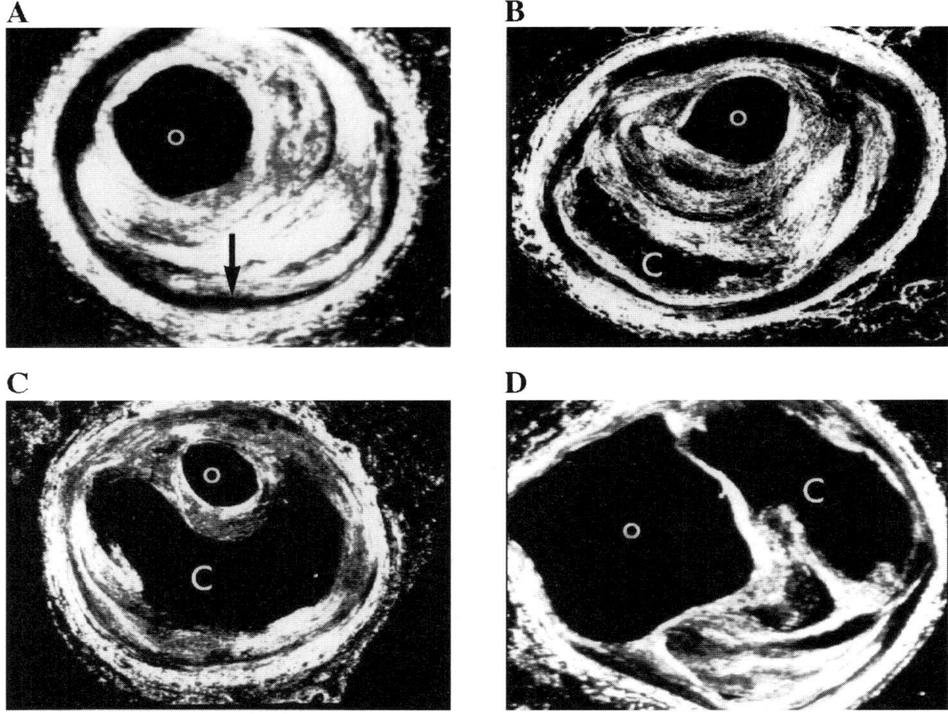

Fig. 1. Cross-sectional images of coronary plaques have been generated by staining with Sirius Red which binds only to collagen. Under polarised light images of plaques very similar to intravascular ultrasound can be produced. Plaque A is solid without a lipid core (AHA Type Vc). Plaque B is multilayered (Type Vb) but has a small core deep in the intima. Plaque C has a large lipid core but a thick cap and is causing very high-grade stenosis. Plaque D is most vulnerable to thrombosis and has a large core and a thin cap. In all the pictures O = arterial lumen, C = lipid core.

Mechanisms of thrombosis on atherosclerotic plaques

Two mechanisms (Fig. 2) cause thrombosis on plaques. In endothelial loss (erosion or denudation) the subendothelial connective tissue is exposed which leads to platelet adhesion. The thrombus is laid down on the surface of the plaque. Endothelial denudation is not an initiating event for plaque formation but over plaques of grade IV and above small foci of endothelial cell loss are common. The great majority of such thrombi are ultramicroscopic [7]. Larger areas of endothelial loss are associated with heavy infiltration of the subendothelial tissues with activated macrophages and a generalised inflammatory response with smooth muscle cells being activated to express class II MHC antigens [8]. These larger areas of endothelial loss may cause thrombi of sufficient size to compromise blood flow and produce acute ischemic symptoms.

The second form of thrombosis is due to plaque disruption (rupture) (Figs. 2

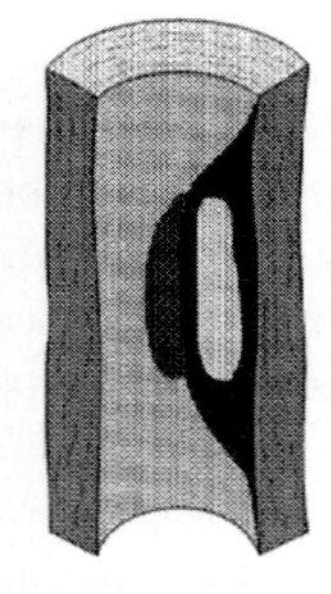
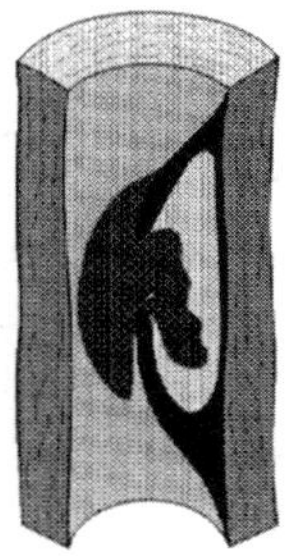

Fig. 2. The two mechanisms of thrombus initiation. In plaque disruption there is an element of thrombus within the lipid core itself.

and 3). In this process the fibrous cap of a plaque tears allowing blood from the lumen of the artery to enter the lipid core. The lipid core contains tissue factor and is intensely thrombogenic; thrombus forms within the plaque itself which is expanded from within. Thrombus may then extend into the lumen and will initi-

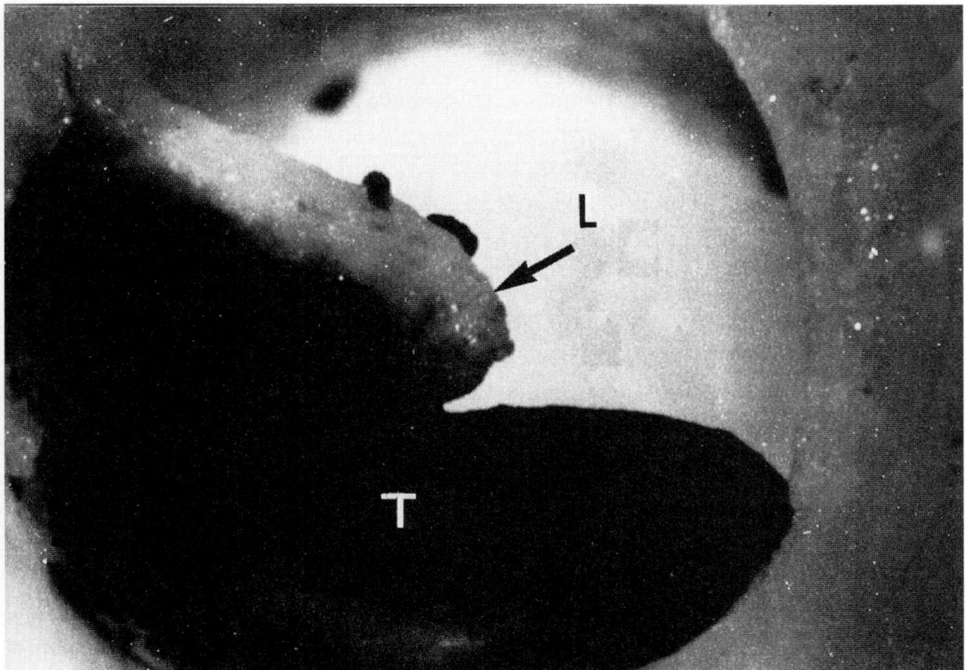

Fig. 3. Human coronary artery with a plaque disruption in which the torn cap projects into the lumen. Thrombus fills (T) the core and also projects into the lumen (L).

ally be mural with antegrade flow continuing, and then may become occlusive. The thrombosis which follows plaque disruption is therefore a staged process which can proceed at widely different rates in different individuals and can be stopped or reversed at any point. The surface of nonoccluding intraluminal thrombus typical of unstable angina is covered by activated platelets which give rise to microemboli into the myocardium causing small foci of myocardial necrosis [9,10].

Autopsy studies suggest that in a high proportion of episodes of plaque disruption the thrombotic process is arrested at an early stage and no clinical sequelae occur. The plaque will, however, have been expanded in size and thrombotic material will stimulate smooth muscle growth increasing the degree of chronic stenosis.

Characteristics of plaques at risk of thrombosis

Disrupted plaques when compared to intact plaques in the same individual [11,12] have lipid cores which occupy a high proportion of the overall plaque volume, a thin cap with a reduced number of smooth muscle cells and high concentrations of activated macrophages. Cap thinning is related to macrophage numbers. By implication, plaques which have these same characteristics but are at present stable (no thrombosis) are at a high risk of becoming unstable in the future. Such plaques have been called vulnerable and the risk of acute ischemic events for an individual is determined by their number. Individual patients vary widely in the number of such plaques they possess and the challenge is to stratify risk. The blood levels of C reactive protein may be a marker of those with a high number of inflammatory vulnerable plaques [13]. Any systemic or local factor which potentates inflammation such as infection with chlamydia would increase the risk of further events [14].

Dynamics of the plaque cap

The tensile strength of the plaque cap is dependent on the connective tissue matrix proteins including collagen, elastin and proteolycans. The question arises over the balance between synthesis and degradation of connective tissue matrix proteins in the cap. Smooth muscle cells synthesise these proteins under the influence of growth factors but synthesis may be inhibited by substances such as interferon Y released by lymphocytes in the plaque [15]. Degradation of collagen is mediated by a range of metalloproteinases. A major source of metalloproteinases is the macrophage. Under the influence of cytokines such as TNFα macrophages secrete inactive metalloproteinases which are then activated in the tissues by plasmin. A number of studies [16—18] now show that some of the metalloproteinases are present and active in disrupted plaques. The current view, therefore, is that plaque cap tears represent an autodestructive phenomenon largely mediated by the inflammatory activity of activated macrophages.

Mechanisms of production of chronic high-grade coronary stenosis

High-grade stenosis is the end result of several processes. Some type Va plaques grow to encroach sufficiently on the lumen to cause high-grade stenosis. In part this may be due to a failure of compensatory dilatation and the external diameter of the vessel has not increased. It is not known if this is due to unusually rapid plaque growth or whether individuals differ in their capacity to remodel their artery wall. Other stenoses appear to be due to concordance of more than one plaque forming at the same site. Another form of stenosis, however, arises from the healing of an episode of plaque disruption and thrombosis. In the healing phase after disruption lysis of thrombus in the lumen occurs but the thrombus in the plaque is often not lysed and induces smooth muscle proliferation followed by the formation of new collagen. This process solidifies the plaque and restores stability. The new connective tissue, however, may encroach onto the lumen increasing the degree of stenosis for some weeks after the acute event.

The concept that the disruption of vulnerable plaques with a lipid core can cause both acute ischemic syndromes and contribute to silent progression is in accord with the clinical observations that angiographic progression predicts acute events in the future [19,20].

Therapeutic implications of the concept of plaque vulnerability

If the vulnerable plaque could be treated in some way to improve its stability, disease progression would be slowed. The major affect would be a reduction in the number of acute ischemic events in the future. Another affect would be to reduce the number of clinically silent plaque disruptions leading to a reduction in the appearance of new angiographic stenoses. Four trials, 4S WOSCOPS. CARE [21—23] and the Lipid Study are consistent in showing a reduction in acute ischemic events following therapeutic lowering of plasma lipids. Angiographic trials of regression show far less marked affects on already established stenotic lesions. Such results can only mean that the risk of episodes of plaque disruption has been diminished; the most logical explanations include a qualitative change in vulnerable plaques or an inhibition of the evolution of new vulnerable lesions. The exact mechanisms by which lowering plasma lipids stabilises plaques is as yet unknown. There is some evidence from animal models that while not all the lipid in the core can be removed, smooth muscle proliferation can once more become dominant solidifying the plaque and restoring its mechanical efficiency [24—25]. It is, however, possible that lipid lowering simply reduces macrophage recruitment and activity limiting the inflammatory autodestructive mechanisms that initiate plaque disruption.

References

1. Levin DC, Fallon JT. Significance of the angiographic morphology of localized coronary steno-

228

sis: histopathologic correlations. Circulation 1982;66:316—320.

2. Ambrose JA, Winters SL, Arora RR. Angiographic evolution of coronary artery morphology in unstable angina. J Am Coll Cardiol 1986;7:472—478.

3. Davies MJ, Thomas AC. Plaque fissuring — the cause of acute myocardial infarction, sudden ischemic death and crescendo angina. Br Heart J 1985;53:363—373.

4. White CJ, Ramee SR, Collins TJ, Escobar AE, Karsan A, Shaw D, Jain SP, Bass TA, Heuser RR, Teirstein PS, Bonan R, Walter PD, Smalling RW. Coronary thrombi increase PTCA risk. Angioscopy as a clinical tool. Circulation 1996;93:253—258.

5. Stary HC, Chandler AB, Dinsmore RE, Fuster V. A definition of advanced types of atherosclerotic lesions and a histological classification of atherosclerosis. A report from the Committee on vascular lesions of the council on Atherosclerosis, American Heart Association. Circulation 1995;92:1355—1374.

6. Glagov S, Weisenberd E, Zarins CK, Stankunavicius R, Kolettis GJ. Compensatory enlargement of human atherosclerotic coronary arteries. N Engl J Med 1987;316:1371—1375.

7. Davies MJ, Woolf N, Rowles PM, Pepper J. Morphology of the endothelium over atherosclerotic plaques in human coronary arteries. Br Heart J 1988;60:459—464.

8. van der Wall AC, Becker AE, van der Loos CM, Das PK. Site of intimal rupture or erosion of thrombosed coronary atherosclerotic plaques is characterised by an inflammatory process irrespective of the dominant plaque histology. Circulation 1994;89:36—44.

9. Falk E. Unstable angina with fatal outcome: dynamic coronary thrombosis leading to infarction and/or sudden death. Circulation 1985;71:699—708.

10. Davies MJ, Thomas AC, Knapman PA, Hangartner R. Intramyocardial platelet aggregation in patients with unstable angina suffering sudden ischemic cardiac death. Circulation 1986;73:418—427.

11. Falk E. Morphological features of unstable atherothrombotic plaques underlying acute coronary syndromes. Am J Cardiol 1989;63:114E—120E.

12. Davies MJ. Stability and instability: Two faces of coronary atherosclerosis. The Paul Dudley White Lecturer 1995. Circulation 1996;94:2013—2020.

13. Ridker PM, Cushman M, Stampfer MJ, Tracy RP, Hennekens CH. Inflammation, aspirin, and the risk of cardiovascular disease in apparently healthy men. N Engl J Med 1997;336:973—979.

14. Gurfinkel G, Bozovich G, Daroca A, Beck E, Mautner B, for the ROXIS Study Group. Randomised trial of roxthromycin in non-Q wave coronary syndromes: ROXIS pilot study. Lancet 1997;350:404—407.

15. Libby P. Molecular bases of the acute coronary syndromes. Circulation 1995;91:2844—2850.

16. Henney AM, Wakeley PR, Davies MJ, Foster K, Hembry R, Murphy G, Humphries S. Localization of stromelysin gene expression in atherosclerotic plaques by in situ hybridization. Proc Natl Acad Sci USA 1991;88:8154—8158.

17. Galis ZS, Sukhova GK, Lark MW, Libby P. Increased expression of matrix metalloproteinases and matrix degrading activity in vulnerable regions of human atherosclerotic plaques. J Clin Invest 1994;94:2493—2503.

18. Brown DL, Hibbs MS, Kearney M, Loushin C, Isner JM. Identification of 92-kD gelatinase in human coronary atherosclerotic lesions: association of active enzyme synthesis with unstable angina. Circulation 1995;91:2125—2131.

19. Azen SP, Mack WJ, Cashin-Hemphill L, LaBree L, Shircore AM, Selzer RH, Blankenhorn DH, Hodis HN. Progression of coronary artery disease predicts clinical coronary events. Long-term follow-up from the cholesterol lowering atherosclerosis study. Circulation 1996;93:34—41.

20. Waters D, Higginson L, Gladstone P, Boccuzzi S, Cook T, Lesperance J. Smoking accelerates the progression of coronary atherosclerosis as assessed by serial quantitative coronary arteriography. Circulation 1993;88:I—344(Abstract).

21. Anonymous. Randomised trial of cholesterol lowering in 4444 patients with coronary heart disease: The Scandinavian Simvastatin Survival Study (4S). Lancet 1994;344:1383—1389.

22. Shepherd J, Cobb SM, Ford I. Prevention of coronary heart disease with pravastatin in men with

hypercholesterolemia. N Engl J Med 1955;333:1301—1307.

23. Sacks FM, Pfeffer MA, Moye LA, Rouleau JL, Rutherford JD, Cole TG, Brown L, Warnica JW, Arnold JM, Wun CC, Davis BR, Baunwald E. The effect of pravastatin on coronary events after myocardial infarction in patients with average cholesterol levels. Cholesterol and Recurrent Events Trial investigators. N Engl J Med 1996;335:1001—1009.

24. Small DM, Bond MG, Waugh D, Prack M, Sawyer JK. Physicochemical and histological changes in the arterial wall of nonhuman primates during progression and regression of atherosclerosis. J Clin Invest 1984;73:1590—1605.

25. Kaplan JR, Manuck SB, Adams MR, Williams JK, Register TC, Clarkson TB. Plaque changes and arterial enlargement in atherosclerotic monkeys after manipulation of diet and social environment. Arterioscl Thromb 1993;13:254—263.

The Long-Term Intervention with Pravastatin in Ischaemic Disease (LIPID) Study

Andrew M. Tonkin[1] and Paul P. Glaziou[2] on behalf of the LIPID Study Group
[1]*National Heart Foundation, Melbourne, Victoria; and* [2]*University of Queensland Medical School, Herston, Queensland, Australia*

Abstract. *Background.* Clinical research aims to produce appropriate widespread changes in patient management. The Long-Term Intervention with Pravastatin in Ischaemic Disease (LIPID) Study was designed to determine the long-term benefits and risks of lipid lowering in patients with coronary heart disease (CHD). Its pragmatic trial design allowed for open-label lipid-lowering therapy, individual management decisions at the clinician's discretion and the widespread dissemination of the results of other secondary prevention trials, which avoided possible ethical dilemmas.

Methods. A total of 9,014 patients in 87 centres in Australia and New Zealand were randomized between June 1990 and December 1992, stratified according to an entry diagnosis of acute myocardial infarction (two-thirds) or unstable angina pectoris (one-third) in the preceding 3 months to 3 years. The range of baseline cholesterol at randomisation (155–271 mg/dl (4–7 mmol/l)) was chosen because most patients with CHD in Australia and New Zealand have cholesterol levels similar to those of the general population.

Results. The LIPID study is the largest secondary prevention lipid-lowering trial to have completed recruitment, and its number of end points should clarify many important questions about lipid-lowering therapy. A meta-analysis of its data with that from the West of Scotland Coronary Prevention Study and the Cholesterol and Recurrent Events Study will provide additional information.

Conclusions. Application of results from clinical trials and meta-analysis extends beyond mere examination of trials' inclusion and exclusion criteria. Treatment should be individualised based on available evidence concerning potential modifiers of effect such as age, sex, other risk factors, magnitude of effect; the effect of baseline risk or predictors of risk (e.g., low-density lipoprotein cholesterol) on relative risk reduction; noncardiac effects of pravastatin treatment; and net benefits and cost-effectiveness of treatment in particular subgroups.

Keywords: cholesterol, coronary heart disease, lipid lowering, meta-analysis.

Introduction

The Long-Term Intervention with Pravastatin in Ischaemic Disease (LIPID) Study [1] was designed in the late 1980s, when there was still considerable scepticism in the medical community about the long-term benefits and safety of lipid lowering. The availability of more potent new agents, the 3-hydroxy-3-methylglutaryl coenzyme (HMG-CoA) reductase inhibitors, enabled the study of the effect of more aggressive cholesterol lowering. The LIPID study was designed to have

---

Address for correspondence: Dr A.M. Tonkin, Director of Medical Scientific Affairs, National Heart Foundation, King Street, Melbourne, Victoria 3084, Australia.

adequate power by including a very large number of patients of a heterogeneous nature and a long follow-up period, and its design anticipated and allowed for the analysis and publication of other trials during the follow-up period. However, health care is now being delivered during a period of major change, in a more sophisticated scientific and economic climate. Cardiovascular disease is still the major cause of death and morbidity in industrialised countries and is increasing rapidly in countries that previously had low rates. Funding and other considerations have dictated the need for optimisation and individualisation of treatment.

Materials and Methods

Trial design and initial rationale

The LIPID study is a randomized, double-blind, placebo-controlled trial of cholesterol lowering with pravastatin 40 mg per day. A total of 9,014 patients aged 31–75 years were randomised in 87 centres in Australia and New Zealand between June 1990 and December 1992. Patients were stratified at randomisation according to an entry diagnosis of acute myocardial infarction (two-thirds) or unstable angina pectoris (one-third) in the preceding 3 months to 3 years.

Full details of the design, management, and baseline characteristics of the patients in the LIPID study have been published [1]. The range of total cholesterol at baseline (155–271 mg/dl (4–7 mmol/l)) deserves comment. Although compelling epidemiologic data have related the incidence of coronary heart disease (CHD) to a raised cholesterol level [2], in Australia [3], New Zealand [4], and the USA [5] most patients with manifest CHD have "average" cholesterol levels similar to those of the general population.

The primary end point of the LIPID study is CHD mortality, and the study was designed to continue until 700 CHD deaths occur. Secondary end points include total mortality, total and nonhaemorrhagic stroke, combined incidence of fatal CHD and nonfatal myocardial infarction, revascularisation procedures, effects on lipid fractions and relationship of these effects to CHD mortality and other end points, and total days of hospitalisation.

Ongoing management

The LIPID study allowed the primary clinician to individualise treatment, including open use of lipid-lowering therapy when indicated. This aspect, and the widespread dissemination of the results of other studies to LIPID investigators and their institutional ethics committees, to clinicians, and to enrolled patients, has avoided ethical dilemmas. The study's data and safety monitoring committee recommended after an interim analysis that the study terminate because of a clear and significant decrease in total mortality in patients treated with pravastatin. Final patient visits were on 30 September 1997.

Discussion

Other studies have shown the benefit of cholesterol lowering for secondary prevention in patients with elevated baseline cholesterol levels [6] and normal or low cholesterol levels [7], but the LIPID study and others [8,9] can contribute additional information on the following issues. Treatment should be individualised based on recently suggested approaches [10].

Are there potential modifiers of effect?
Patient age, sex, baseline total cholesterol, baseline low-density lipoprotein (LDL) cholesterol, baseline triglyceride level, qualifying event and time since this event, hypertension, diabetes, smoking, ancillary treatments, or magnitude of effect of the intervention could potentially modify the effects of treatment. Risk increases with age, and the absolute benefits of intervention are greater in the elderly. However, comorbidity might negate the net benefit of a "targeted" therapy. At the same age, women have a lower risk of CHD than men; however, diabetes partially removes this difference, and in postmenopausal women, triglyceride levels are an important predictor of risk.

The Scandinavian Simvastatin Survival Study (SSSS) [6] excluded patients with initial high-density lipoprotein (HDL) cholesterol (<1 mmol/l) or serum triglyceride level >2.5 mmol/l. Total serum cholesterol was elevated; although there was no difference in relative risk reduction in SSSS in diabetics and nondiabetics, these selection criteria tend to exclude patients with typical diabetic phenotype. The Cholesterol and Recurrent Events (CARE) Study [7] criteria were broader, and relative risk reduction by pravastatin was similar for diabetics and nondiabetics. The LIPID study includes 1,346 patients aged >75 years, 1,511 women, and 774 diabetics and will further address these issues.

The "intensity" of intervention may be crucial and is currently under discussion. Whether to treat to an absolute level of LDL cholesterol or only to a certain fixed percentage reduction may depend on how much the other properties of the HMG-CoA reductase inhibitors (e.g., haemostatic) are relevant to benefit.

Does the relative risk reduction vary with baseline risk or predictors of baseline risk?
A meta-analysis of "older" randomised, controlled studies of cholesterol lowering has shown that risk reduction depended on the event rate in the trials' control limb [11]. The SSSS cohort had elevated baseline total cholesterol levels. Subgroup analysis did not show any differences in relative risk reduction in different quartiles of baseline total, HDL, or LDL cholesterol [12]. In the CARE study, however, treatment did not reduce risk in patients with initial LDL cholesterol levels <125 mg/dl, but its power to examine this issue was low. The LIPID study and the Prospective Pravastatin Pooling (PPP) Project [8] will provide further data on whether relative risk reduction is attenuated at a lower LDL cholesterol level and lower risk.

234

What effects does statin treatment have on the incidence of stroke? Does it affect mood or increase the risk of cancer?
Older meta-analyses, particularly of primary intervention trials, suggested that cholesterol-lowering therapy may have resulted in and increased the rate of non-CHD deaths (mostly cancer and violent causes). However, further analysis of these studies showed no increase in non-CHD deaths with increased cholesterol reduction [13]. A relationship was found between non-CHD mortality and the particular intervention used [13]. Only fibrates (clofibrate and gemfibrozil) and hormone therapy (particularly in men) increased the incidence of non-CHD deaths. Only haemorrhagic stroke may have increased due to cholesterol reduction. The recently published large-scale intervention trials [6,7,14] showed no increase in violent deaths, but other publications may again fuel these controversies.

The possible link between cholesterol-lowering agents and cancer has again been raised because these agents are associated with carcinoma in rodents [15]. However, very high doses were often used, rats have a high spontaneous rate of cancer, and these mechanisms, particularly peroxisome proliferation, probably do not apply to humans. In the CARE study [7], there was an increase in breast cancer in patients randomised to pravastatin, but this may have been due to an imbalance in risk factors for breast cancer among pravastatin- and placebo-treated patients. No such excess of breast cancer was found in a preliminary analysis of the large cohort of women in the LIPID study after an average follow-up period of 4 years. Cholesterol levels $\leqslant 4.14$ mmol/l have been associated with an increased rate of cancer [16]. The LIPID study will provide more information on this vexing issue, for which longer term follow-up is required.

Recent studies [17,18] have reopened discussion on whether lipid-lowering treatment affects mood, but Law [19] has cautioned against these data. One study showed no difference in mood scores between psychologically healthy patients with increased coronary risk treated with simvastatin or placebo [20]. A LIPID substudy of 1,000 patients has shown no significant change in mood scores with pravastatin [21].

Whether and by how much cholesterol reduction prevents stroke is becoming increasingly important. Stroke is a leading cause of death and morbidity in developed countries. Recent unpublished data from the Asia-Pacific region suggest a significant relationship between serum cholesterol level and risk of nonhaemorrhagic stroke (A. Rodgers and S. MacMahon, personal communication). This is consistent with previous studies in which the incidence of stroke was decreased by a diet high in polyunsaturated fat [22] and nicotinic acid [23]. Recent ultrasound data have demonstrated that treatment with pravastatin reduces carotid atherosclerosis [24].

What are the net benefits and cost-effectiveness in particular subgroups?
Higher risk patients with no major modifiers of effect are likely to have the greatest net benefit, therefore, they should be treated. Net benefit usually increases as

Table 1. Number needed to treat (5 years) to prevent CHD death.

End points	SSSS [6]	CARE [7]	WOSCOPS [14]
	Secondary	Secondary	Primary
Average LDL (mg/dl)	186	139	192
CHD deaths (control/treated) (%)	8.5/5.0	5.7/4.6	1.9/1.3
Relative risk reduction (%)	41	19	32
Absolute risk reduction (%)	3.5	1.1	0.6
Number needed to treat	29	90	167

CARE = Cholesterol and Recurrent Events Study; CHD = coronary heart disease; LDL = low-density lipoprotein; SSSS = Scandinavian Simvastatin Survival Study; WOSCOPS = West of Scotland Coronary Prevention Study.

risk increases, provided the magnitude of harmful effects is constant and not dependent on risk. Table 1 shows relative and absolute risk reduction and number needed to treat in three studies [6,7,14].

Above what level of risk and cholesterol is lipid-lowering therapy indicated? The absolute benefits should clearly outweigh any potential adverse effects, and the net benefit should be reasonable value for the money. The adverse effects of statin therapy appear to be minimal and therefore, their cost-effectiveness is likely to be an issue, with different thresholds used for different risk groups. However, the risk-benefit equation is complex, and lipid-lowering therapy can achieve a number of cost offsets, particularly in high-risk groups (e.g., fewer CHD events, less hospitalisation and revascularisation). Moreover, primary prevention with pravastatin may be more cost-effective than medication for mild hypertension [14].

The ideal of individualised multivariate risk prediction in evaluating individual clinical worth and cost-effectiveness is being developed and incorporated into guidelines for lipid-lowering therapy by including other risk factors for CHD [25]. The LIPID study and its collaborative analysis in the PPP project will provide needed data. In addition, the LIPID study has incorporated a prospective cost-effectiveness substudy.

Acknowledgements

The LIPID study is being conducted under the auspices of the National Heart Foundation and is supported by a grant from Bristol-Myers Squibb Pty., Ltd. It is independent of these groups; neither group has voting members on the study's management committee.

References

1. The LIPID Study Group. Design features and baseline characteristics of the LIPID (long-term intervention with pravastatin in ischaemic disease) study: a randomised trial in patients with

previous myocardial infarction and/or unstable angina pectoris. Am J Cardiol 1995;76: 474–479.

2. Law MR, Wald NJ, Thompson SG. By how much and how quickly does reduction in serum cholesterol concentration lower risk of ischaemic heart disease? Br Med J 1994;308:367–372.
3. Bennett S, Magnus P. Trends in cardiovascular risk factors in Australia. Results from the National Heart Foundation's Risk Factor Prevalence Study 1980–1989. Med J Aust 1994;161: 519–527.
4. Jackson R, Beaglehole R, Lay Yee R et al. Trends in cardiovascular risk factors in Auckland 1982–1987. NZ Med J 1990;103:363–365.
5. Rubins HB, Robins SJ, Collins D et al. Distribution of lipids in 8,500 men with coronary artery disease. Am J Cardiol 1995;75:1196–1201.
6. Scandinavian Simvastatin Survival Study Group. Randomised trial of cholesterol lowering in 4444 patients with coronary heart disease: the Scandinavian Simvastatin Survival Study (4S). Lancet 1994;344:1383–1389.
7. Sacks FM, Pfeffer MA, Moye LA et al. The effect of pravastatin on coronary events after myocardial infarction in patients with average cholesterol levels. N Engl J Med 1996;335: 1001–1009.
8. PPP Project Investigators. Design, rationale, and baseline characteristics of the Prospective Pravastatin Pooling (PPP) Project – a combined analysis of three large scale randomised trials: Long-Term Intervention with Pravastatin in Ischaemic Disease (LIPID), Cholesterol and Recurrent Events (CARE), and West of Scotland Coronary Prevention Study (WOSCOPS). Am J Cardiol 1995;76:899–905.
9. Cholesterol Treatment Trialists' (CTT) Collaboration. Protocol for a prospective collaborative overview of all current and planned randomized trials of cholesterol treatment regimens. Am J Cardiol 1995;75:1130–1134.
10. Glazsiou PP, Irving LM. An evidence-based approach to individualising treatment. Br Med J 1995;311:1356–1359.
11. Davey Smith G, Song F, Sheldon TA. Cholesterol lowering and mortality: the importance of initial level of risk. Br Med J 1993;306:1367–1373.
12. Scandinavian Simvastatin Survival Study Group. Baseline serum cholesterol and treatment effect in the Scandinavian Simvastatin Survival Study (4S). Lancet 1995;345:1274–1275.
13. Gould AL, Rossouw JE, Santanello NC et al. Cholesterol reduction yields clinical benefit: a new look at old data. Circulation 1995;91:2274–2282.
14. Shepherd J, Cobbe SM, Ford I et al. Prevention of coronary heart disease with pravastatin in men with hypercholesterolemia. N Engl J Med 1995;333:1301–1307.
15. Newman TB, Hulley SB. Carcinogenicity of lipid-lowering drugs. JAMA 1996;275:55–60.
16. Kritchevsky SB, Kritchevsky D. Serum cholesterol and cancer risk: an epidemiologic perspective. Ann Rev Nutr 1992;12:391–416.
17. Zureik M, Courbon D, Ducimetière P. Serum cholesterol concentration and death from suicide in men: Paris Prospective Study I. Br Med J 1996;313:649–651.
18. Ploeckinger B, Dantendorfer K, Ulm M et al. Rapid decrease of serum cholesterol concentration and postpartum depression. Br Med J 1996;313:664–679.
19. Law M. Having too much evidence (depression, suicide, and low serum cholesterol). Commentary. Br Med J 1996;313:651–652.
20. Wardle J, Armitage J, Collins R et al. Randomised placebo controlled trial of effect on mood of lowering cholesterol concentration. Br Med J 1996;313:75–79.
21. Stewart RA, Sharples KJ, Scott D et al. Long-term assessment of "psychological" status in a randomised trial of cholesterol reduction. Circulation 1996;94(Suppl I):I–540.
22. Dayton D, Pearce ML, Hashimoto S et al. A controlled clinical trial of a diet high in unsaturated fat in preventing complications of atherosclerosis. Circulation 1969;40(Suppl II-II-I-II):63.
23. The Coronary Drug Project Research Group. Clofibrate and niacin in coronary heart disease. JAMA 1975;231:360–381.

24. Crouse JR III, Byington RP, Bond MG et al. Pravastatin, lipids, and atherosclerosis in the carotid arteries (PLAC II). Am J Cardiol 1995;75:455—459.
25. Johnson B, Johannesson M, Kjekshus J et al. Cost-effectiveness of cholesterol lowering. Eur Heart J 1996;17:1001—1007.

New insights in diabetes and coronary artery disease

Richard W. Nesto

Beth Israel Deaconess Medical Center, Harvard Medical School, Boston, Massachusetts, USA

Keywords: coronary artery disease, diabetes.

In addition to the increased clinical incidence of CHD, the extent of the disease in the coronary arteries is greater among diabetic patients [1]. Autopsy studies have reported that diabetic patients, compared to nondiabetics, have a higher incidence of two- and three-vessel disease (83 vs. 17% in one report) and a lower incidence of one-vessel disease [2].

Retrospective analyses of patients undergoing elective percutaneous transluminal coronary angioplasty (PTCA) support these data. One study, for example, retrospectively analyzed data on 1,133 diabetic and 9,300 nondiabetic patients undergoing PTCA [3]. The diabetic patients had more multivessel disease. Furthermore, the likelihood of remaining free of infarction or additional revascularization at 5 years was much lower in diabetic (36 vs. 53%).

These findings are supported by two large-scale thrombolytic trials that have provided coronary angiographic data obtained during an acute myocardial infarction [4,5]. The Thrombolysis and Angioplasty in Myocardial Infarction (TAMI) trial included 148 diabetics and 923 nondiabetic patients in whom cardiac catheterization was performed at 90 min and 7–10 days after thrombolytic therapy [4]. Compared to the nondiabetics, the diabetic patients had a greater incidence of multivessel disease (66 vs. 46%, p = 0.0001) and a greater number of diseased vessels.

Silent myocardial ischemia

In addition to the increased frequency of symptomatic CHD, another important aspect of diabetes is a blunted appreciation of ischemic pain, often resulting in silent ischemia or even silent infarction [6]. The scope of this problem can be illustrated by the following observations in which diabetic patients are compared to nondiabetics:
1. An increased frequency of unrecognized myocardial infarction (39 vs. 22%) [7].

Address for correspondence: R.W. Nesto MD, 110 Francis Street, Suite 4B, Boston, MA 02215, USA. Tel.: +1-617-632-9202. Fax: +1-617-632-7533. E-mail: RNESTO@BIDMC.HARVARD.EDU

240

2. An increased frequency of silent ST segment depression and coronary perfusion abnormalities during exercise testing and thallium scintigraphy (69 vs. 35%) [8,9].
3. Prolongation of the anginal perceptual threshold during exercise testing, i.e., the time from onset of ischemic changes on the electrocardiogram to the onset of angina [10].

Silent ischemia in diabetes is thought to be caused by autonomic denervation of the heart due to an alteration in the normal link between the afferent and efferent limbs of the autonomic system [11–13]. In support of this hypothesis is the observation that the norepinephrine analogue metaiodobenzylguanidine (MIBG) is taken up to a lesser extent and in an abnormal fashion in diabetic patients with silent ischemia [14].

Parasympathetic fibers are affected before sympathetic fibers. Thus, there may initially be a relative increase in sympathetic tone, possibly leading to an increase in blood pressure and exaggerated or inappropriate vasoconstriction [15].

Autonomic dysfunction can promote the development of ischemia and infarction by several mechanisms, in addition to elimination of the early warning symptoms of ischemia:

1. Increased heart rate at rest, thereby increasing myocardial oxygen demand.
2. Increased coronary vascular tone, thereby reducing myocardial blood flow.
3. Reduced coronary perfusion pressure during hypotension.

Atherogenesis and thrombogenesis in diabetes

Numerous factors, including hyperlipidemia, hypertension and platelet and coagulation abnormalities contribute to the process of accelerated atherosclerosis in diabetes.

Dyslipidemia

There are a number of differences in the lipid profile between diabetics and nondiabetics which may contribute to the increase in atherosclerosis [16,17]. These differences constitute the rationale for considering hypolipidemic therapy in selected diabetic patients, particularly those with evidence of CHD. The 4S trial conclusively showed that LDL lowering with simvastatin produced a survival benefit in diabetics similar to that observed in nondiabetics.

In the Framingham Study, the serum concentrations of very low-density lipoprotein (VLDL) and triglycerides were higher and high-density lipoprotein (HDL) were lower in diabetic patients compared to nondiabetics [17,18]. In this report and in MRFIT [19], there were no differences between the two groups in the serum concentrations of total cholesterol or low-density lipoprotein (LDL) levels. However, for a lipoprotein level, diabetic patients have more significant CHD than do nondiabetic persons. This may be due to qualitative differences in the lipoprotein fractions or to the presence of other proatherosclerotic metabolic changes in diabetics. Two such changes are increases in the serum concentrations of small dense LDL [17] and perhaps in lipoprotein(a) [16,20].

In addition, the oxidation of lipoproteins, in particular LDL, seems to be enhanced in diabetics, especially in the setting of poor glucose control, hypertriglyceridemia, and microvascular disease. Oxidation of LDL results in a moiety that is cytotoxic to vascular endothelial and smooth muscle cells, probably contributing to atherogenesis. Diabetic patients have increased levels of oxidized lipoprotein fractions that is in part due to hypertriglyceridemia. In addition, LDL incubated with glucose exhibits greater oxidative properties than LDL alone, a change can be suppressed by antioxidants such as α-tocopherol and probucol [21].

It has been proposed that glycation (i.e., the nonenzymatic attachment of glucose to an amino group) of apoB is increased in diabetic individuals and may contribute to the development of atherosclerosis [22,23]. According to this theory, glycation causes impaired recognition of LDL by its receptor on hepatocytes, thereby increasing its half-life. The glycated LDL is then taken up preferentially by macrophages via a separate receptor and is degraded. Cholesterol ester accumulates within the macrophages which are converted into foam cells. In contrast to these effects on LDL, glycation of HDL increases its clearance, thereby decreasing its half-life. Immunohistochemical analysis of coronary arteries obtained from patients with type 2 diabetes showed high levels of reactivity of advanced glycosylation end products (AGE) within atherosclerotic plaques stained with anti-AGE antibodies [24]. This observation is consistent with a link between hyperglycemia, hyperlipidemia and atherosclerosis in diabetes.

The lipid abnormalities in diabetes may promote lipid uptake by the vascular wall. In one report, for example, in vitro arterial smooth muscle cells and macrophages took up cholesterol and converted it into cholesterol ester more readily from VLDL obtained from diabetic subjects than from nondiabetics [25]. The increased atherogenicity of VLDL and LDL remnants of diabetic patients may be due to increased apolipoprotein E (apoE) in the lipoprotein fractions of diabetic patients which is then recognized by cell surface receptors, allowing uptake of the lipoprotein into the cell.

Platelet abnormalities

Diabetes has a number of effects on platelet function that may predispose to coronary thrombosis.
1. More primary aggregation in response to ADP (adenosine diphosphate); this effect is independent of insulin administration [26].
2. Increased sensitivity to secondary aggregation in response to platelet agonists including ADP, collagen, arachidonic acid, platelet activating factor (PAF) and thrombin [27].
3. Increased release of the contents of α-granules, including thromboglobulin and platelet factor 4 [28].

242

4. Increased synthesis of thromboxane A2 with increased serum levels most often being found in those with poor glycemic control or vascular complications [27,29].
5. Enhanced binding of fibrinogen to the glycoprotein IIb/IIIa complex, located on the platelet surface, an effect which may be due in part to an increase in the number of glycoprotein IIb/IIIa receptors on the platelet surface.

Coagulation and fibrinolysis abnormalities

In addition to the abnormalities in platelet function, diabetes also predisposes individuals to abnormalities in the various pathways involved in coagulation, hemostasis and fibrinolysis [20].

As an example, diabetes is associated with an increase in serum fibrinogen levels [29,30], and an impairment of fibrinolytic activity [30,31]. Circulating tissue-type plasminogen activator (tPA0) levels are normal or increased in plasma of diabetic persons, but its activity is decreased because of enhanced binding to its inhibitor, suggesting that glycemic control directly influences fibrinolysis. The relative protein C deficiency seen in the diabetic state also may impair fibrinolysis by decreasing tPA release [29].

The exact mechanisms by which these alterations in fibrinolysis occur in the diabetic state are unclear. Administration of precursors of insulin cause synthesis of PAI-1 by hepatic cells in culture, suggesting that insulin resistance with subsequent hyperinsulinemia may in part explain the impaired fibrinolysis observed in clinical studies [32]. This observation also provides some insight into the many epidemiologic studies that link insulin resistance, hyperinsulinemia, hypertension and coronary disease [33,34]. One study, for example, reported that among 1,263 elderly nondiabetic patients, hyperinsulinemic microalbuminuria strongly predicted cardiac events and mortality during a 3.5-year follow-up, even when corrected for other risk factors [35]. The risk was 6 times as great as that in patients with normal insulin levels.

Treatment of coronary heart disease in diabetes mellitus

The treatment of CHD in patients with diabetes mellitus is often similar to that in nondiabetics. There are, however, a number of issues that must be considered in the management of acute myocardial infarction and in the performance of coronary revascularization by percutaneous transluminal coronary angioplasty or coronary artery bypass graft.

Acute myocardial infarction

Thrombolytic therapy

Thrombolytic therapy has dramatically changed the course of acute myocardial infarction. Subgroup analysis of some of the large thrombolytic trials has yielded interesting data about the outcomes of diabetic patients with acute myocardial infarction.

Firstly, diabetic patients appear to derive the same or more benefit from thrombolysis as nondiabetics. This was demonstrated in the International Study of Infarct Survival-II (ISIS-II) trial which found that diabetic patients receiving streptokinase had a 31% improvement in survival compared with the placebo group [36]. This was greater than the 23% improvement seen in nondiabetics.

Secondly, although diabetic patients respond to thrombolytic therapy, they have more severe pre-existing disease and have a worse outcome. This relationship can be illustrated by the results of three large trials: TAMI; GUSTO-1, and GIS-SI-2:

The TAMI trial involved 1,078 patients with acute myocardial infarction and 148 with diabetes, who underwent coronary angiography within 90 min of the administration of a thrombolytic agent [37]. The diabetics were older and were more likely to have hypertension and multivessel disease (66 vs. 46%). Diabetic and nondiabetic patients had similar infarct-related artery patency rates (71 vs. 70%). However, the latter response did not translate into equivalent outcomes. The in-hospital mortality was higher among diabetics (11 vs. 6%, p = 0.02), especially in diabetic women.

The GUSTO-1 trial (almost 2,500 patients, 13% of whom were diabetic) found that the diabetic patients were more likely to be elderly and to have hypertension and congestive heart failure [38]. They also had a higher number of prior infarctions and more CABG procedures. There were no significant differences between diabetics and nondiabetics in the infarct-related arterial patency rates (TIMI flow grade III) at 90 min (40.3 vs. 37.6%), reocclusion rates (9.2 vs. 5.3%), or in the left ventricular ejection fraction at 90 min or at 5—7 days. Despite these similarities, the diabetic patients had a significantly higher 30-day mortality rate (11.3 vs. 5.9%, p < 0.001). After adjustment for clinical and angiographic variables, diabetes remained an independent determinant of 30-day mortality.

The TIMI-II trial also found an increase in mortality in diabetic patients [39]. In this study, a history of diabetes doubled the relative risk for mortality within the first 42 days after an acute myocardial infarction.

Severity of complications

During an acute myocardial infarction, patients with diabetes present in acute pulmonary edema more commonly than do nondiabetic patients (11 vs. 4% in TAMI, p = 0.001), often despite similar infarct sizes and left ventricular ejection fractions [37,40—42]. This observation suggests that the left ventricle in diabetes tolerates infarction poorly, regardless of infarct size and the left ventricular ejection fraction.

Factors accounting for the higher incidence of congestive heart failure at the time of myocardial infarction in diabetics may include one or more of the follow-

244

ing:
1. A greater extent of coronary disease (i.e., more multivessel disease) which affects myocardial performance by limiting blood flow to noninfarcted myocardium [37,43].
2. Intrinsic myocardial dysfunction.
3. Neurohormonal factors.
4. An increased incidence of prior infarction [38].
Diabetic patients also may have a higher risk of other complications. These include arrhythmias, cardiogenic shock and recurrent infarction [41,44,45].

The decrease in insulin availability can impair energy-independent transport of glucose across the cell membrane. The most important glucose transporter in cardiac myocytes is GLUT4, the insulin responsive glucose transporter. In the presence of insulin, GLUT4 is translocated from the intracellular pool, where it is inactive, to the plasma membrane where it results in an increased glucose uptake by the myocardial cells in response to an increased workload [46]. The ischemic myocardium and metabolism during acute myocardial ischemia are necessary for maintenance of myocardial function [47,48]. Diminished insulin activity limits glucose availability, resulting in a shift toward fatty acid metabolism reducing the compensatory capacity of noninfarcted myocardium [49]. Positron emission tomography using the glucose analogue F18-flurodeoxyglucose demonstrates that myocardial glucose uptake can be substantially improved or normalized in both type 1 and type 2 diabetes if adequate insulin is present [50,51].

Long-term prognosis

As noted above, 30- and 42-day mortalities were increased in diabetic patients in GUSTO-I and GISSI-2, respectively [38,40]. The increase in mortality among diabetic patients, largely the result of reinfarction and congestive heart failure, extends well into the postdischarge period. In the Norwegian timolol trial, for example, diabetic patients in the placebo group had twice the mortality of nondiabetic patients during a mean follow-up of 18 months [52]. Similarly, in GISSI-2, the mortality at 180 days remained higher for diabetics compared to nondiabetics [40]. The risk was greatest in insulin-dependent diabetic women whose 14% mortality was 3 times that of nondiabetic women and more than 4.5 times that of nondiabetic men.

During long-term, postinfarction follow-up, congestive heart failure develops more commonly in diabetic patients. One study performed in the prethrombolytic era, involved 500 patients with an acute myocardial infarction, 85 of whom were diabetic [41]. There was a higher incidence of congestive heart failure in diabetic compared to nondiabetic patients at 3 and 6 month follow-up despite preserved left ventricular systolic function at the time of acute MI suggesting poor remodelling of the right ventricle.

Au — does this mean diastolic dysfunction?

Patients with diabetes surviving an acute myocardial infarction also have a higher incidence of recurrent nonfatal and fatal infarction compared to nondiabetics [53]. Consistent with this hypothesis are the findings in a study in which technetium pyrophosphate scintigraphy was performed in diabetic and nondiabetic patients in the acute phase and 3 months after infarction [54]. A persistently positive scan was present in 62% of diabetics compared to only 12% of nondiabetics [54]. In addition, angioscopy has documented that diabetic patients have a significant increase in plaque ulceration and thrombosis.

Factors accounting for the poorer prognosis after an infarction and higher reinfarction rate in diabetic patients include the severity and extent of coronary artery disease, the higher frequency of left ventricular dysfunction and congestive heart failure and the thrombotic-thrombolytic equilibrium at the time of plaque rupture [55]. The clotting and fibrinolytic profile of patients with diabetes (high concentrations of fibrinogen and plasminogen activator inhibitor type I) leave the patient at high risk for future cardiovascular events.

References

1. Robertson WW, Strong J. Atherosclerosis in persons with hypertension and diabetes mellitus. Lab Invest 1968;18:538.
2. Waller B, Palumbo P, Robert W. Status of the coronary arteries at necropsy in diabetes mellitus with onset after age 30 years. Am J Med 1980;69:498.
3. Stein B, Weintraub W, King S. Influence of diabetes mellitus on early and late outcome after percutaneous transluminal coronary angioplasty. Circulation 1995;91:979.
4. Granger C, Califf R, Young S et al. Outcome of patients with diabetes mellitus and acute myocardial infarction treated with thrombolytic agents. J Am Coll Cardiol 1993;21:920.
5. Mueller HS, Braunwald E and the TIMI Investigators. Predictors of early morbidity and mortality after thrombolytic therapy of acute myocardial infarction. Analysis of patient subgroups in the Thrombolysis in Myocardial Infarction (TIMI) trial, phase II. Circulation 1992;85:1254.
6. Niakan E, Harati Y, Rolak L et al. Silent myocardial infarction and diabetic cardiovascular autonomic neuropathy. Arch Int Med 1986;146:2229.
7. Margolis JR, Kannel W, Feinlab M et al. Clinical features of unrecognized myocardial infarction — silent and symptomatic. Am J Cardiol 1973;32:1.
8. Nesto R, Phillips R, Kett K et al. Angina and exertional myocardial ischemia in diabetic and nondiabetic patients: assessment by exercise thallium scintigraphy. Ann Int Med 1988;108:170.
9. Nesto R, Watson F, Kowalchuk G et al. Silent myocardial ischemia and infarction in diabetics with peripheral vascular disease: assessment with dipyridamole thallium-201 scintigraphy. Am Heart J 1990;120:1073.
10. Ranjadayalan K, Umachandran V, Ambeptiyla G et al. Prolonged angina perceptual threshold in diabetes: effects on exercise capacity and myocardial ischemia. J Am Coll Cardiol 1990; 16:1120.
11. Watkins P, Mackay J. Cardiac denervation in diabetic neuropathy. Ann Int Med 1980;92:304.
12. Faerman I, Faccio E, Milei J et al. Autonomic neuropathy and painless myocardial ischemia in diabetic patients: histologic evidence of their relationship. Diabetes 1977;26:1147.
13. Lloyd-Mostyn R, Watkins P. Defective innervation of heart in diabetic autonomic neuropathy. Br Med J 1975;25:15.

14. Langer A, Freeman M, Josse R et al. Metaiodobenzylguanidine imaging in diabetes mellitus: assessment of cardiac sympathetic denervation and its relation to autonomic dysfunction and silent myocardial ischemia. J Am Coll Cardiol 1995;25:610.
15. Kahn J, Zola B, Juni J et al. Decreased exercise heart rate and blood pressure response in diabetic patients with cardiac autonomic neuropathy. Diabet Care 1986;9:389.
16. Garg A, Grundy SM. Management of dyslipidemia in NIDDM. Diabet Care 1990;13:153.
17. Siegel RD, Cupples A, Schaefer EJ, Wilson PW. Lipoproteins, apolipoproteins, and low-density lipoprotein size among diabetics in the Framingham offspring study. Metabolism 1996;45:1267.
18. Kannel W, McGee D. Lipids, diabetes and coronary heart disease: insights from the Framingham Study. Am Heart J 1985;110:1100.
19. Stamler J, Vaccaro O, Neaton J et al. Diabetes, other risk factors and 12-year cardiovascular mortality for men screened in the Multiple Risk Factor Intervention Trial. Diabet Care 1993;16:434.
20. Haffner SM. Lipoprotein(a) and diabetes. An update. Diabet Care 1993;16:835.
21. Chisolm GM, Irwin KC, Penn MS. Lipoprotein oxidation and lipoprotein-induced cell injury in diabetes. Diabetes 1992;41:61.
22. Lyons T. Lipoprotein glycation and its metabolic consequences. Diabetes 1992;41:67.
23. Bucala R, Makita A, Vega G et al. Modification of low-density lipoprotein by advanced glycation end products contributes to the dyslipidemia of diabetes and renal insufficiency. Proc Natl Acad Sci USA 1994;91:9441.
24. Nakamura Y, Horil Y, Nishino T et al. Immunohistochemical localization of advanced glycosylation end products in coronary atheroma and cardiac tissue in diabetes mellitus. Am J Pathol 1993;143:1649.
25. Bierman E. Atherosclerosis in diabetes. Arterioscl Thromb 1992;12:647.
26. Winocour P. Platelet abnormalities in diabetes mellitus. Diabetes 1992;41:26.
27. Davi G, Catalano I, Averna M et al. Thromboxane biosynthesis and platelet function in type II diabetes mellitus. N Engl J Med 1990;322:1769.
28. Rosove M, Harrison F, Harwig M. Plasma B-thromboglobulin, platelet factor 4, fibrinopeptide A, and other hemostatic functions during improved short-term glycemic control in diabetes mellitus. Diabet Care 1984;7:174.
29. Osterman H, van de Loo J. Factors of the hemostatic system in diabetic patients. Hemostasis 1986;16:386.
30. Badawi H, El-Sawy M, Mikhail M et al. Platelets, coagulation, and fibrinolysis in diabetic and nondiabetic patients with quiescent coronary heart disease. Angiology 1970;21:511.
31. Small M, Lowe G, MacCuish A et al. Thrombin and plasmin activity in diabetes mellitus and their association with glycemic control. Q J Med 1987;248:1025.
32. Nordt T, Schneider D, Sobel B. Augmentation of the synthesis of plasminogen activator inhibitor type I by precursors of insulin. Circulation 1994;89:321.
33. Reaven GM. Role of insulin resistance in human disease (syndrome X): an expanded definition. Ann Rev Med 1993;44:121.
34. Depres JP. The insulin resistance-dyslipidemia syndrome: the most prevalent cause of coronary artery disease. Can Med Assoc J 1993;148:1339.
35. Kuusisto J, Mykkanen L, Pyorala K et al. Hyperinsulinemic microalbuminuria: a new risk indicator for coronary heart disease. Circulation 1995;90:831.
36. ISIS-2 Collaborative Group. Randomized trial of intravenous streptokinase, oral aspirin, both, or neither a month 17, 187 cases of suspected acute myocardial infarction: ISIS-2. Lancet 1988;2:349.
37. Granger C, Califf R, Young S et al. Outcome of patients with diabetes mellitus and acute myocardial infarction treated with thrombolytic agents. J Am Coll Cardiol 1993;21:920.
38. Woodfield SL, Lundergan CG, Reiner JS et al. for the GUSTO-I Angiographic Investigators. Angiographic findings and outcome in diabetic patients treated with thrombolytic therapy for acute myocardial infarction: the GUSTO-I experience. J Am Coll Cardiol 1996;28:1661.

39. Mueller HS, Braunwald E, TIMI Investigators. Predictors of early morbidity and mortality after thrombolytic therapy of acute myocardial infarction. Analysis of patient subgroups in the Thrombolysis in Myocardial Infarction (TIMI) trial, phase II. Circulation 1992;85:1254.

40. Zuanetti G, Latini R, Maggioni AP et al. Influence of diabetes on mortality in acute myocardial infarction: data from the GISSI-2 study. J Am Coll Cardiol 1993;22:1788.

41. Stone PH, Mueller J, Hartwell T et al. The effect of diabetes mellitus on prognosis and serial left ventricular function after acute myocardial infarction: contribution of both coronary disease and left ventricular dysfunction to the adverse prognosis. The MILIS Study Group. J Am Coll Cardiol 1989;14:49.

42. Jaffe AS, Spadaro JJ, Schechtman K et al. Increased congestive heart failure after myocardial infarction of modest extent in patients diabetic mellitus. Am Heart J 1984;108:31.

43. Stein B, Weintraub W, King S. Influence of diabetes mellitus on early and late outcome after percutaneous transluminal coronary angioplasty. Circulation 1995;91:979.

44. Savage MP, Krolewski A, Kemien G et al. Acute myocardial infarction in diabetes mellitus and significance of congestive heart failure as a prognostic factors. Am J Cardiol 1988;62:665.

45. Yudkin JS, Oswald GA. Determinants of hospital admission and case fatality in diabetic patients with myocardial infarction. Diabet Care 1988;11:351.

46. Rensing BJ, Hermans WR, Vos J et al. Luminal narrowing after percutaneous transluminal coronary angioplasty. A study of clinical, procedural, and lesional factors related to long-term angiographic outcome, Coronary Artery Restenosis Prevention on Repeated Thromboxane Antagonism (CARPORT) Study Group. Circulation 1993;88:975.

47. Weintraub W, Wenger N, Kosinski A et al. Percutaneous transluminal coronary angioplasty in women compared with men. J Am Coll Cardiol 1994;24:81.

48. Carrozza J, Kuntz R, Fishman R et al. Restenosis after arterial injury caused by coronary stenting in patients with diabetes mellitus. Ann Intern Med 1993;118:344.

49. Salomon N, Page U, Okies J et al. Diabetes mellitus and coronary artery bypass. J Thorac Cardiovasc Surg 1983;85:264.

50. Higgins T, Estafanous F, Loop F et al. Stratification of morbidity and mortality outcome of preoperative risk factors in coronary artery bypass patients. JAMA 1992;267:2344.

51. Morris J, Smith R, Jones R et al. Influence of diabetes and mammary artery grafting on survival after coronary bypass. Circulation 1991;84(Suppl 3):275.

52. Gunderson T, Kjekshus J. Timolol treatment after myocardial infarction in diabetic patients. Diabet Care 1983;6:285.

53. Gilpin E, Ricon F, Dittrich H et al. Factors associated with recurrent myocardial infarction within one year after acute myocardial infarction. Am Heart J 1991;121:457.

54. Nicod P, Lewis S, Corbett J et al. Increased incidence and clinical correlation of persistently abnormal technetium pyrophosphate scintigrams following acute myocardial infarction in patients with diabetes mellitus. Am Heart J 1982;103:822.

55. Fuster V, Badimon L, Badimon JJ et al. The pathogenesis of coronary artery disease and the acute coronary syndromes. N Engl J Med 1992;326:242.

Molecular mechanisms of action in fenofibrate

Bart Staels, Johan Auwerx and Jean-Charles Fruchart
Department of Atherosclerosis — U325 Inserm, Institut Pasteur, Lille, France

Abstract. Treatment with fenofibrate, a widely used lipid-modifying agent, results in a substantial decrease in plasma triglycerides, reduced low-density lipoprotein cholesterol (LDL-C) and increased high-density lipoprotein cholesterol (HDL-C) concentrations. Fenofibrate induces marked changes in the physicochemical characteristics of lipoprotein particles, which include a reduction in atherogenic dense LDL, resulting in increased resistance of LDL to oxidation. These alterations in lipoproteins are linked to changes in their apolipoprotein (apo) content, such as decreased apo C-III in triglyceride-rich lipoproteins and increased apo A-I and apo A-II in HDL. These effects of fenofibrate are due to alterations in the transcription of genes controlling lipoprotein metabolism. Fenofibrate activates specific transcription factors belonging to the nuclear receptor superfamily, termed peroxisome proliferator-activated receptors (PPARs). PPARs bind as heterodimers with the retinoid X receptor (RXR) to specific response elements, thus altering the transcription rate of target genes. Among the different PPARs, the PPARα form mediates fenofibrate action on HDL-C levels via the transcriptional induction of the major HDL apolipoproteins, apo A-I and apo A-II. The hypotriglyceridemic action of fenofibrate also involves PPARs, and is in part due to increased lipoprotein-lipase-mediated (LPL) lipolysis (due to a transcriptional repression of hepatic apo C-III synthesis), followed by enhanced cellular uptake, conversion to acyl-CoA derivatives and catabolism by the β-oxidation pathways of fatty acids. Furthermore, a reduction in fatty acid and triglyceride synthesis and a decrease in very low density lipoprotein (VLDL) production have been documented. In conclusion, both enhanced catabolism and reduced synthesis of triglycerides underlie the hypotriglyceridemic effect of fenofibrate, whereas their effect on HDL metabolism is associated with changes in HDL apolipoprotein expression. These effects are mediated by PPARs, key messengers responsible for the translation of fenofibrate activity into changes in gene expression.

Keywords: gene expression, hypolipidemic drugs, lipoprotein metabolism, nuclear receptors.

Fenofibrate is effective in lowering plasma concentrations of atherogenic lipoproteins, and in increasing lipoproteins which confer protection against coronary artery disease [1]. This effect has recently be attributed to the activation of specific nuclear receptors that belong to the steroid hormone receptor superfamily [2]. The first member of this family of transcription factors, PPARα, has been discovered due to its role in mediating the peroxisome proliferation response in rodent liver. These receptors have, therefore, been called "peroxisome proliferator-activated receptors" or PPARs. PPARs have a modular structure consisting of six domains termed A-F. The N terminal A/B domain includes

---

Address for correspondence: J.-C. Fruchart, Dépt. d'Athérosclérose — U325 INSERM, Institut Pastuer, 1 rue du Pr Calmette, BP 245, 59019 Lille Cedex, France.

a ligand-independent transactivation function. The DNA binding or C domain contains two zinc finger complexes and targets the receptor to specific DNA sequences. In addition, the C domain participates in heterodimerization with the retinoid X receptor (RXR). The E domain contains a transactivation function, whose activity depends on ligand binding and dimerization. Recent data suggest that the hypolipidemic activity of fenofibrate is primarily mediated by the PPARα form.

PPARα is predominantly expressed in tissues metabolizing a high amount of fatty acids, such as liver and muscle. Unequivocal evidence for a direct implication of PPARα in lipid metabolism has been demonstrated in mice, in which targeted disruption of this gene renders them resistant to the pleiotropic effects of peroxisome proliferators [3]. Once activated, PPARα heterodimerizes with RXR and binds to specific DNA recognition sequences termed peroxisome proliferator response elements (PPREs). PPREs consist of a direct repeat of the classic nuclear receptor hexameric DNA recognition motif (PuGGTCA; Pu: any purine) spaced by one nucleotide (DR-1). Once bound to a PPRE, the receptor complex can activate or repress the expression of a target gene. Transactivation or repression can occur through direct interaction with components of the transcription preinitiation complex, or via specific proteins, adaptors or coactivators, which bridge the receptor to the transcription machinery [2].

The role of PPARα in mediating fenofibrate action on lipid metabolism in rodents

In rodents, fenofibrate induces the expression of genes (such as acyl-CoA oxidase and medium-chain acyl-CoA dehydrogenase) implicated in the peroxisomal and mitochondrial β-oxidation pathways of fatty acids, and in the ω-hydroxylation of a variety of substrates such as fatty acids and prostaglandins, and as such enhances the rate of fatty acid β-oxidation. Furthermore, fenofibrate enhances the rate of ketogenesis (an effect which may be PPAR-mediated via the induction of the expression of HMG-CoA synthase, a mitochondrial enzyme with a key role in ketogenesis). In addition, certain cytosolic proteins are activated following treatment with fenofibrate. These include palmitoyl-CoA hydrolase, malic enzyme and a number of fatty acid binding proteins. In several of the above mentioned genes functional PPRE sequences have been identified and the role of PPARα in mediating the effects of fenofibrate on their expression has been clearly established (Table 1). By contrast, very little data are available on the regulation of their human counterparts, and it awaits further study to determine whether fenofibrate also regulates the expression of any of these genes in humans. However, in contrast to rodents, there is no evidence that fenofibrate would induce peroxisome proliferation in humans and primates. These data are corroborated by the lack of induction of Acyl-CoA oxidase gene expression by fibrates in human hepatocytes [4].

Table 1. Genes regulated by fenofibrate.

Gene	Species	Induction/ Reduction	PPRE	Function: localization
Acyl-CoA oxidase	Rodent	Induction	Yes	β-oxidation; peroxisomes
	Human	No effect	?	β-oxidation; peroxisomes
Hydratase dehydrogenase	Rodent	Induction	Yes	β-oxidation; peroxisomes
3-ketoacyl-CoA thiolase	Rodent	Induction	?	β-oxidation; peroxisomes
CYP4A6	Rodent	Induction	Yes	ω-oxidation; microsomes
Medium-chain acyl-CoA dehydrogenase	Rodent	Induction	Yes	β-oxidation; mitochondria
HMG-CoA synthase	Rodent	Induction	Yes	Ketogenesis; mitochondria
Liver fatty acid binding protein	Rodent	Induction	Yes	Liver fatty acid binding; cytosol
aP2	Rodent	Induction	Yes	Adipocyte fatty acid binding; cytosol
Acyl-CoA-binding protein	Rodent	Induction	?	Acyl-CoA binding protein; cytosol
Phosphoenolpyruvate carboxykinase	Rodent	Induction	Yes	Gluco- and glyco-neogenesis; cytosol
Malic enzyme	Rodent	Reduction	Yes	Fatty acid synthesis; cytosol
Acetyl-CoA carboxylase	Rodent	Induction	?	Fatty acid synthesis; cytosol
Fatty acid synthase	Rodent	Induction	?	Fatty acid synthesis; cytosol
Lipoprotein lipase	Rodent	Induction	Yes	Lipoprotein and energy metabolism
	Human	Induction	Yes	Lipoprotein and energy metabolism
Apo A-I	Rodent	Reduction	No	Lipoprotein metabolism
	Human	Induction	Yes	Lipoprotein metabolism
Apo A-II	Rodent	Reduction	?	Lipoprotein metabolism
	Human	Induction	Yes	Lipoprotein metabolism
Apo C-III	Rodent	Reduction	?	Lipoprotein metabolism
	Human	Reduction	Yes	Lipoprotein metabolism
Lecithin:cholesterol acyltransferase	Rodent	Reduction	?	Lipoprotein metabolism
Heptic lipase	Rodent	Reduction	?	Lipoprotein metabolism
Acyl-CoA synthetase	Rodent	Induction	Yes	Fatty acid metabolism; mitochondria, peroxisomes
Fatty acid transport protein	Rodent	Induction	?	Fatty acid transporter; membrane

The role of PPARα in mediating fenofibrate action on the metabolism of triglyceride-rich lipoproteins

In humans the role of PPARα in mediating triglyceride-lowering activity of fenofibrate can be attributed to [5]:
1. The hypotriglyceridemic action of fenofibrate involves combined effects on LPL and apo C-III expression resulting in increased lipolysis (Fig. 1). In

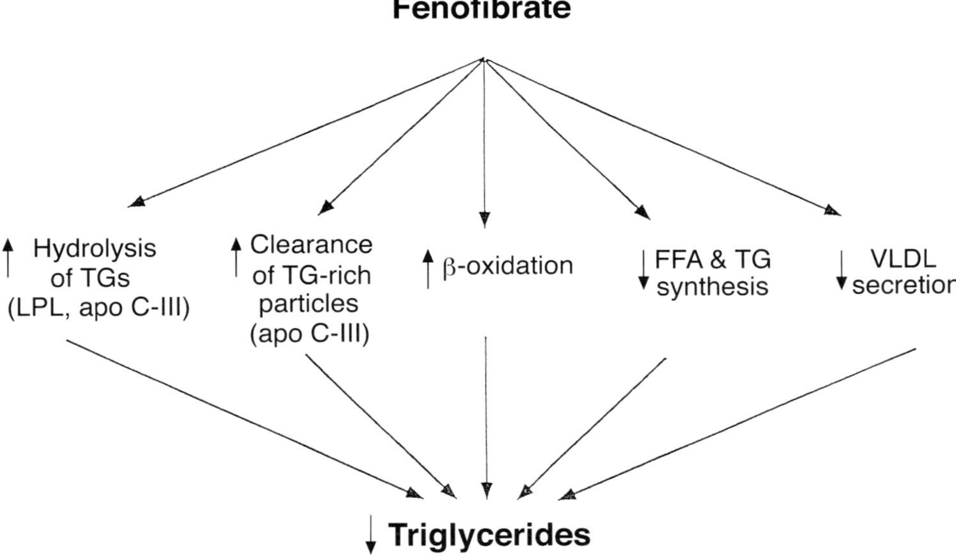

Fig. 1.

man, fenofibrate increases postheparin plasma LPL activity [1]. This is most likely due to the induction of LPL expression at the transcriptional level, an effect mediated by PPAR which binds to a PPRE present in the human LPL gene promoter [2]. In contrast to LPL, transcription of the apo C-III gene is inhibited by fenofibrate, resulting in a decreased production of apo C-III in the liver [4]. The repression of apo C-III gene expression by fenofibrate may be mediated by a PPRE located in the apo C-III gene promoter, which has previously been shown to mediate transregulation by other members of the nuclear receptor superfamily, such as the strong liver-specific transcription factor HNF-4. Consistent with the repression of apo C-III expression, turnover studies in humans indicate that fenofibrate reduce apo C-III synthesis. The fenofibrate-induced reduction in apo C-III levels enhances the LPL-mediated lipolysis of lipoprotein triglycerides and results in both an increased catabolism of VLDL particles and an increased apo E-dependent clearance of VLDL-remnants. Consequently, this dual action of fibrates on LPL and apo C-III gene expression may cause a reduction in plasma triglyceride concentrations and have thereby a beneficial effect on postprandial hypertriglyceridemia [5].

2. Recent animal studies suggest that fibrates exert their hypolipidemic action not only by enhancing the catabolism of triglyceride-rich lipoproteins but also by increasing the hepatic uptake and degradation of FFA [2]. The cellular uptake of long-chain fatty acids may be facilitated by fatty acid transporters, such as the fatty acid transporter protein (FATP) and the fatty acid transporter

(FAT). Preliminary studies indicate that the expression of these fatty acid transporters in the liver of rodents is enhanced by fenofibrate treatment [6]. While membrane transporters facilitate the passage of FFA across the plasma membrane, the induction of the acyl CoA synthetase (ACS) gene by fenofibrate [7] results in an enhanced esterification of the FFA to acyl-CoA derivatives thereby preventing their efflux from the cell. Through the action of this enzyme FFA able also activated for utilisation in both catabolic (β-oxidation) and/or anabolic pathways (conversion into more complex cellular lipids). ACS gene expression and activity is induced by fenofibrate in a variety of tissues and cells via PPAR interacting with a PPRE located in the C-ACS promoter [7]. Moreover, fenofibrate not only increases β-oxidation, but also decreases triglyceride synthesis, as well as apo B and VLDL production. As a consequence, a reduced secretion of VLDL particles together with an enhanced catabolism of triglyceride-rich particles most likely accounts for the hypolipidemic effect of fibrates. Further studies are required, however, to determine whether all these mechanisms are operative in man also.

The role of PPARα in mediating the effect of fenofibrate on HDL metabolism

A large number of clinical studies in humans have demonstrated that fenofibrate exerts a beneficial, inductive action on plasma concentrations of HDL, which is a protective factor against atherosclerosis development [1]. Fenofibrate increases plasma levels of apo A-I and apo A-II and stimulates their production in human hepatocytes [8,9]. In vitro studies have demonstrated that the induction of human apo A-I gene expression after fibrates may be mediated by the interaction of PPAR with a functional PPRE, localised in the A site of the human apo A-I promoter [10]. The lack of induction of apo A-I expression by fibrates in rodents is due to minor sequence differences between the human and rodent A-sites, which prevents the rodent A-site from being activated by PPARα. These in vitro observations have been corroborated in vivo by studies using transgenic animals overexpressing the human apo A-I gene under control of its homologous promoter containing the PPRE containing A-site [9]. In mice, treatment with fenofibrate results in the transcriptional induction of human apo A-I gene expression, whereas the endogenous mouse apo A-I gene is repressed [9]. Furthermore, fibrate treatment increases plasma concentrations of HDL containing human apo A-I in these mice. These opposite effects on apo A-I gene expression in rodents and humans are due to differences in regulatory elements in their respective genes.

Contrary to rodents and similar to man, rabbits are much less sensitive to peroxisome proliferators. Furthermore, they are resistant to the hypolipidemic activity of fenofibrate since administration of fenofibrate at a high dose for 3 weeks did not influence serum lipid or high-density lipoprotein (HDL) concentrations in normal rabbits. By contrast, in rabbits overexpressing the human apo A-I gene under control of its homologous promoter (including its PPAR-response elements), administration of fenofibrate increases serum HDL and human apo A-I concentrations due to an increased expression of the human apo A-I gene in liver (manuscript submitted for publication). However, in these transgenic rabbits, liver weight or activity of ACO (the rate-limiting enzyme of peroxisomal β-oxidation whose activity is significantly induced in rodents by peroxisome proliferators (*cf.* supra)) remains unchanged after fenofibrate. Thus, expression of the human apo A-I transgene in the rabbit liver suffices to confer fibrate-responsiveness to HDL. These data provide, therefore, in vivo evidence that the beneficial effects of fibrates on plasma lipoprotein metabolism can mechanistically be dissociated from any possible deleterious activity on peroxisome proliferation.

In addition to apo A-I, human apo A-II plasma concentrations increase after fenofibrate treatment. This is a consequence of the induction of hepatic apo A-II synthesis by fenofibrate, and is mediated through PPAR/RXR heterodimers which bind to an imperfect DR-1 in the apo A-II J site [8]. Fenofibrate increases apo A-II mRNA levels and protein secretion in human hepatocytes [8].

Mechanism of fenofibrate action on lipoprotein modification

Fenofibrate is effective in lowering plasma triglycerides and LDL cholesterol. It is now well-established that fenofibrate, by activating LPL, promotes the fractional clearance rate of triglyceride-rich lipoproteins (*cf.* supra). Activation of ultravascular lipolysis causes surface components of chylomicrons and VLDL to be released to HDL, leading to an increase in the plasma concentration of these lipoproteins.

Conversely, the downregulation of liver apo C-III gene expression by fenofibrate contributes to the hypotriglyceridemic action of this drug. The lowered secretion of apo C-III, along with unchanged apo E secretion by the liver leads to a decreased apo C-III/apo E ratio of triglyceride-rich particles which then can be more efficiently cleared from the plasma [5]. Furthermore, the decrease in apo C-III production observed after fibrate treatment results in a decrease in the plasma concentration of the LpC-III: B particles which are of the most atherogenic lipoprotein particles [11].

The decrease in apo C-III and the increase in LPL gene expression results also in modification of LDL structure and metabolism. In hypertriglyceridemic subjects, large VLDL particles lead to the formation of small dense LDL which are metabolized more slowly than large buoyant LDL and are more resistant to catabolism by the normal LDL receptor pathway [1]. These small dense LDL are more readily oxidised and are more likely to be taken up by macrophages, generating foam cells and atherosclerosis. Fenofibrate treatment leads to modification of LDL composition with changes in the conformation of apo B, fully restoring the capacity of LDL to interact with the LDL receptor. This is postulated to result from the fenofibrate-induced decrease in the size of VLDL particles made by the liver favouring the formation of more buoyant LDL particles, which are more readily catabolized via the LDL receptor pathway. Thus, through its qualitative effects on LDL subfractions, fenofibrate is more efficient than one would assume from its quantitative effects on plasma LDL concentrations. In a recent investigation of the relation between fenofibrate and LDL heterogeneity in hypercholesterolemia, it has been shown that fenofibrate decreases LDL cholesterol by 36% and small dense atherogenic LDL by 43% [12].

The fenofibrate-induced reduction in small dense LDL has also been shown in patients suffering from combined hyperlipidemia and in hypertriglyceridemic patients with non-insulin-dependent diabetes mellitus (NIDDM) [1].

The elevation of plasma HDL concentrations could be attributed partially to the lipolysis of triglyceride-rich lipoproteins and the redistribution of lipid components from these particles to HDL. However, experiments done recently in transgenic apo A-I rabbits which show no hypotriglyceridemic response after fenofibrate treatment suggests that an increased production of HDL is a major mechanism of fenofibrate action on HDL metabolism (manuscript submitted for publication). In most of the clinical studies, fenofibrate favours the appearance of a HDL profile consisting of an increase of LpA-I:A-II particles associated with a decrease of LpA-I particles. It has been shown that LpA-I levels are inversely correlated with the production rate of apo A-II which appears, therefore, to be a determinant factor in the distribution of apo A-I among LpA-I and LpA-I: A-II. The fenofibrate-induced apo A-II production through a PPARα-dependent mechanism offers a mechanism explaining the altered HDL distribution after fenofibrate treatment. In view of the evidence coming from transgenic animal studies linking elevated human apo A-I and apo A-II expression to a protective effect against atherosclerosis, these data suggest that the fenofibrate-induced increase of HDL cholesterol should result in a decreased risk of coronary artery disease.

Fenofibrate action and atherosclerosis risk factors modification

Numerous scientific investigations have shown that LDL cholesterol reduction between 28 and 38% can reduce heart disease events by 30%, particularly in people with high blood cholesterol concentrations. Micronised fenofibrate reduces LDL cholesterol by 28—34% in patients with hypercholesterolemia. Unfortunately, LDL cholesterol measurement does not provide any information concerning the LDL distribution pattern between large (pattern A) and small (pattern B) particles. Since patients with pattern B have a 3 times higher risk for developing heart disease compared to patients with pattern A, it is useful to know what type of lipid-lowering medication is best suited for a pattern B individual. Micronised fenofibrate decreases small dense atherogenic LDL by 43% and promotes LDL catabolism via the receptor mediated pathway.

Recent critical appraisal of epidemiological data, and a better understanding of risk factor modulation and interaction suggest that triglycerides are an important independent risk factor [1]. This view has recently been strengthened by a meta-analysis of population-based prospective studies showing that triglycerides are a

256

risk factor for coronary artery disease in both men and women [1]. Micronised
fenofibrate has a pronounced decreasing effect on plasma triglycerides
(40—50%). Recent results of the prospective cardiovascular Münster (PROCAM)
study have helped to define a subset of individuals at high risk which are likely
to respond optimally to fenofibrate. These patients with a high LDL/HDL cholesterol ratio (more than 5) and high plasma triglycerides (more than 2.3 nmol/
l) had the highest risk of developing coronary artery disease. It was suggested several years ago that postprandial lipoprotein remnants are potentially atherogenic
[1]. Several case-control studies have indicated that postprandial lipemia is a significant risk factor for coronary artery disease. Postprandial lipoprotein clearance is markedly improved with micronised fenofibrate administration. Among
triglyceride-rich lipoprotein remnants, apo B and apo C-III-containing particles
(LpB:C-III) are a strong predisposing factor for the development of atherosclerotic vascular disease [11]. Furthermore, genetic studies have identified several apo
C-III gene polymorphisms which may be associated with increased apo C-III
levels and hypertriglyceridemia [11]. Marked atherosclerosis was documented in
animals heterozygote for LDL receptor deficiency and overexpressing apo C-III,
while animals with a targeted disruption of the apo C-III gene were protected
from postprandial lipemia. Treatment of patients with micronised fenofibrate
results in a 40—50% reduction of LpB:C-III due to a decrease in synthesis rate
of apo C-III [5].

Increased plasma levels of HDL are correlated with lowered risk for coronary
artery disease. It has been recently demonstrated that cholesterol-loaded foam
cells (due to excessive LDL uptake) secrete a number of factors that fragilize the
lipid-rich plaque. In order to decrease the formation of these foam cells, one
needs to be able to increase HDL which can enter the arterial wall, pull out
foam cell cholesterol and allow it to be returned for excretion to the liver.

Transgenic animal studies indicate that overexpression of apo A-I and apo A-II
(the two most important proteins of human HDL) confers resistance to atherosclerosis. Micronised fenofibrate increases HDL cholesterol by 16—38%.

In hypertriglyceridemic patients with low HDL cholesterol, improvement of
LPL mediated lipolysis and increase of apo A-I and apo A-II synthesis may all
contribute to the rise in HDL levels upon treatment with fenofibrate. The lowering of the pool of triglyceride-rich lipoproteins decreases the availability of triglycerides for cholesterol ester transfer protein (CETP) mediated exchange with
the cholesteryl ester of HDL. The resulting reduction in net CE transfer from
HDL to triglyceride-rich lipoproteins ultimately leads to an increase in cholesteryl ester and a decrease in triglyceride content of HDL. Although no direct correlation has been observed between the magnitude of changes in plasma triglycerides and HDL cholesterol, the extent of HDL rise upon treatment with
micronised fenofibrate appears to depend on the distinct primary metabolic
defect, and on the levels of plasma triglycerides attained after treatment.

Acknowledgements

Research in the laboratory of the authors is supported by INSERM, CNRS, Institut Pasteur de Lille, la région Nord-Pas de Calais, la Fondation de la Recherche Médicale. Bart Staels and Johan Auwerx are members of the CNRS.

References

1. Davignon J. Fibrates: a review of important issues and recent findings. Can J Cardiol 1994;10: 61B–71B.
2. Schoonjans K, Staels B, Auwerx J. Role of the peroxisome proliferator-activator receptor (PPAR) in mediating the effects of fibrates and fatty acids on gene expression. J Lipid Res 1996;37:907–925.
3. Lee SST, Pineau T, Drago J, Lee EJ, Owens JW, Kroetz DL, Fernandez-Salguero PM, Westphal H, Gonzalez FJ. Targeted disruption of the α isoform of the peroxisome proliferator-activated receptor gene in mice results in abolishement of the pleiotropic effects of peroxisome proliferators. Molec Cell Biol 1995;15:3012–3022.
4. Staels B, Vu Dac N, Kosykh V, Saladin R, Fruchart JC, Dallongeville J, Auwerx J. Fibrates down-regulate apolipoprotein C-III expression independent of induction of peroxisomal Acyl Coenzyme A Oxidase. J Clin Invest 1995;95:705–712.
5. Auwerx J, Schoonjans K, Fruchart JC, Staels B. Transcriptional control of triglyceride metabolism: fibrates change the expression of the LPL and apo C-III genes by activating the nuclear receptor PPAR. Atherosclerosis 1996;124:529–537.
6. Martin G, Schoonjans K, Lefebvre AM, Staels B, Auwerx J. Coordinate regulation of the expression of the Fatty Acid Transporter Protein (FATP) and Acyl CoA Synthetase (ACS) genes by PPARα and PPARγ activators. J Biol Chem 1997;(In press).
7. Schoonjans K, Watanabe M, Suzuki H, Mahfoudi A, Krey G, Wahli W, Grimaldi P, Staels B, Yamamoto T, Auwerx J. Induction of the Acyl-Coenzyme A synthetase gene by fibrates and fatty acids is mediated by a peroxisome proliferator response element in the C promoter. J Biol Chem 1995;270:19269–19276.
8. Vu Dac N, Schoonjans K, Kosykh V, Dallongeville J, Fruchart JC, Staels B, Auwerx J. Fibrates increase human apolipoprotein A-II expression through activation of the peroxisome proliferator-activated receptor. J Clin Invest 1995;96:741–750.
9. Berthou L, Duverger N, Emmanuel F, Langouët S, Auwerx J, Guillouzo A, Fruchart JC, Rubin E, Denèfle P, Staels B, Branellec D. Opposite regulation of human vs mouse apolipoprotein A-I by fibrates in human apo A-I transgenic mice. J Clin Invest 1996;97:2408–2416.
10. Vu Dac N, Schoonjans K, Laine B, Fruchart JC, Auwerx J, Staels B. Negative regulation of the human apolipoprotein A-I promoter by fibrates can be attenuated by the interaction of the peroxisome proliferator-activated receptor with its response element. J Biol Chem 1994;269: 31012–31018.
11. Luc G, Fiévet C, Arveiler D, Evans A, Bard JM, Cambien F, Fruchart JC, Ducimetière P. Apolipoproteins C-III and E in apo B and non apo B containing lipoproteins in two populations at contrasting risk for myocardial infarction: the ECTIM Study. J Lipid Res 1996;37:508–517.
12. Caslake MJ, Packard CJ, Gaw A et al. Fenofibrate and LDL metabolic heterogeneity in hypercholesterolemia. Arterioscl Thromb 1993;13:702–711.

Atherosclerosis XI.
B. Jacotot, D. Mathé and J.-C. Fruchart, editors.

Insulin resistance, compensatory hyperinsulinemia and dyslipidemia in syndrome X

Gerald M. Reaven

Stanford University School of Medicine, Stanford and Shaman Pharmaceuticals Inc., South San Francisco, California, USA

Keywords: liver, triglycerides, very low density lipoproteins.

Introduction

Reports published approximately 30 years ago demonstrated a significant relationship between plasma insulin and triglyceride (TG) concentrations [1], and subsequent data defined a direct relationship between resistance to insulin-mediated glucose disposal, compensatory hyperinsulinemia, hepatic very low density lipoprotein (VLDL)-TG secretion rate, and plasma TG concentration in nondiabetic subjects with both elevated and normal plasma TG concentrations [2,3]. It was postulated that the more insulin resistant these normoglycemic individuals were, and the higher their plasma insulin concentrations, the greater would be the increase in hepatic VLDL-TG synthesis and secretion and plasma TG concentration. The goal of this review is to critically evaluate available experimental data concerning this formulation.

Relationship between insulin resistance, compensatory hyperinsulinemia, increased hepatic VLDL-TG secretion and hypertriglyceridemia.

The schema outlined in Fig. 1 is adapted from the results of two studies. Figure 1A depicts the relationship between the four variables in question in a population of 34 nondiabetic individuals whose baseline plasma TG concentration ranged from 69 to 546 mg/dl, whereas Fig. 1B is based upon the study of 16 individuals with plasma TG concentration < 175 mg/dl. Although there appears to be reasonable consensus as to the existence of these relationships, controversy exists as to the causal roles played by insulin resistance and compensatory hyperinsulinemia in the genesis of the increased hepatic VLDL-TG secretion.

Hyperinsulinemia as an inhibitor of VLDL-TG secretion

It was proposed in a recent review [4] that hypertriglyceridemia (HTG) occurs in

Address for correspondence: G.M. Reaven MD, 213 East Grand Avenue, South San Francisco, CA 94080-4812, USA. Tel.: +1-415-952-7070. Fax: +1-415-873-8377. E-mail: greaven@shaman.com

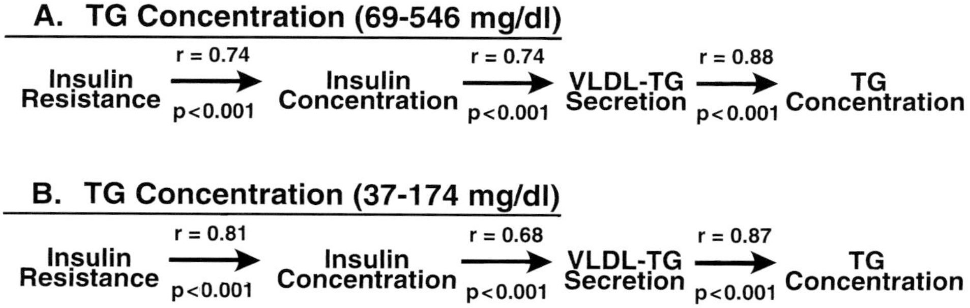

260

A. TG Concentration (69-546 mg/dl)

Insulin Resistance $\xrightarrow[p<0.001]{r = 0.74}$ Insulin Concentration $\xrightarrow[p<0.001]{r = 0.74}$ VLDL-TG Secretion $\xrightarrow[p<0.001]{r = 0.88}$ TG Concentration

B. TG Concentration (37-174 mg/dl)

Insulin Resistance $\xrightarrow[p<0.001]{r = 0.81}$ Insulin Concentration $\xrightarrow[p<0.001]{r = 0.68}$ VLDL-TG Secretion $\xrightarrow[p<0.001]{r = 0.87}$ TG Concentration

Fig. 1. Summary of correlation coefficients between resistance to insulin-mediated glucose disposal, plasma insulin response to oral glucose, very low density lipoprotein (VLDL)-triglyceride (TG) secretion, and plasma TG concentration over a range of fasting plasma TG concentrations from 69 to 546 mg/dl (**A**) or 37–174 mg/dl (**B**). Adapted from data published in A) American Journal of Medicine (1974;52:551) and B) Metabolism (1981;30:165) with permission of the authors and the journal.

insulin-resistant, nondiabetic individuals because the normal ability of insulin to inhibit hepatic VLDL-TG secretion is deficient. In the absence of this postulated inhibition of hepatic VLDL-TG secretion by insulin, it is suggested that there is an increase in the ability of FFA to promote hepatic VLDL-TG synthesis and secretion. Evidence that HTG in nondiabetic, insulin-resistant individuals results from hepatic resistance to insulin inhibition of VLDL-TG secretion is derived primarily from acute experiments. For example, results of several studies have recently been reviewed [5] demonstrating that insulin acutely inhibits VLDL-TG secretion from cultured rat and human hepatocytes and HepG2 cells. The acute infusion of insulin has also been shown to suppress hepatic VLDL-TG secretion in human [6,7], associated with a substantial decrease in plasma FFA concentration. An obvious explanation for the ability of an acute insulin infusion to decrease VLDL-TG secretion is the profound decrease in adipose tissue lipolysis that occurs secondary to the hyperinsulinemia. Indeed, elevation of plasma FFA levels significantly attenuated the decrease in VLDL-TG secretion associated with the acute infusion of insulin. On the other hand, since VLDL-TG secretion was still lower under these conditions, it was concluded that the decrease in VLDL-TG secretion was not entirely explained by the antilipolytic effect of insulin.

Hyperinsulinemia as an enhancer of VLDL-TG secretion

As noted above, results of in vitro studies are usually cited to support the view that insulin acts to suppress hepatic VLDL-TG secretion. On the other hand reports published many years ago indicated that the addition of insulin to perifused [8] and perfused [9] rat liver actually stimulated TG secretion. More recently, evidence has been presented showing that the addition of insulin plus oleate to HepG2 cells led to an increase in VLDL secretion above baseline [10].

If we now focus on experiments which have evaluated the chronic effects of hyperinsulinemia on hepatic VLDL-TG secretion, a different picture emerges. In particular, these results provide support for a unifying hypothesis describing the interaction between muscle insulin resistance, compensatory hyperinsulinemia, ambient FFA concentrations, and VLDL metabolism. Experimental support for this formula can be seen in Fig. 2. This figure is the summary of a series of experiments comparing the ability of increases in perfusate FFA concentration to stimulate VLDL-TG secretion by perfused rat livers as a function of differences in the chronic metabolic state of the liver donor [11]. It can be seen that increases in perfusate FFA concentration are essentially incapable of increasing VLDL-TG secretion by livers of streptozotocin-injected, insulin-deficient animals (insulin = 6 ± 1 µU/ml). Since severely insulin-deficient rats are known to be insulin resistant [12], putative inhibitory effect of insulin on hepatic VLDL-TG secretion should be lacking. Then why are grossly elevated perfusate FFA concentrations incapable of stimulating hepatic VLDL-TG secretion? The obvious answer is that variations in the chronic insulin concentration play a crucial role in the ability of the liver to use FFA for TG synthesis.

At the other end of the spectrum, we have the sucrose-fed, hyperinsulinemic rat (insulin = 48 ± 4 µU/ml). It can be seen that livers from these rats secrete more VLDL-TG in response to increases in the perfusate FFA concentration (the hepatic TG secretion curve has been shifted to the left) than do livers from control

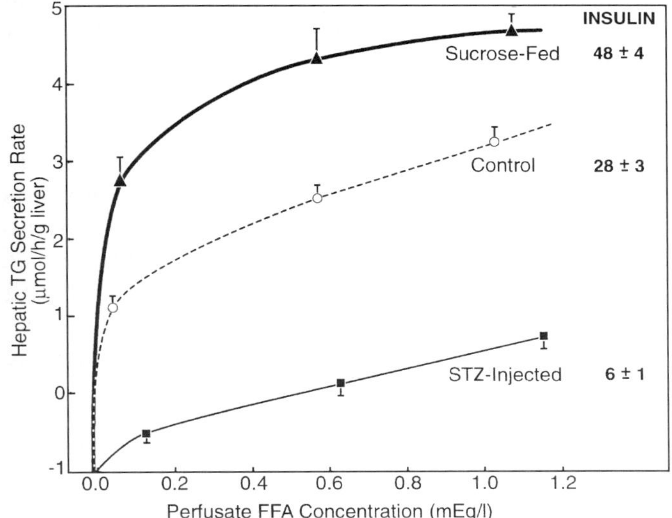

Fig. 2. Hepatic TG secretion by perfused rat livers as a function of perfusate FFA concentrations. The plasma insulin concentrations of the donor animal at the time that the liver perfusions begin are listed on the far right. The studies were performed 7–10 days after the induction of insulin deficiency with streptozotocin (STZ) or being placed on a sucrose-enriched diet. Adapted from data published in Hormone and Metabolic Research (1984;16:230) with permission of the authors and the journal.

262

rats (insulin = 28 ± 3 μU/ml). Since these rats are known to have higher than normal insulin levels [13], it might be predicted that they would secrete less VLDL-TG than normal at any given perfusate level if the view that insulin "normally" suppresses hepatic VLDL-TG secretion is correct.

I believe there is another way to think about the relationship between insulin resistance, circulating insulin and FFA concentrations, and VLDL metabolism that is more consistent with available data. Stated simply, and in reference to Fig. 2, it is argued that the circulating levels of insulin the liver is chronically exposed to determine the shape of the FFA-hepatic VLDL-TG dose response curve. The degree to which differences in FFA flux to the liver increase VLDL-TG secretion is a function of this metabolic set. Thus, the liver from animals that have been exposed to chronic hypoinsulinemia cannot increase VLDL-TG secretion in response to a massive influx of FFA. In contrast, livers from sucrose-fed rats, animals that have been exposed to chronic hyperinsulinemia, secrete more VLDL than do normal animals at a given FFA concentration.

Evidence for the above formulation can be seen in the results shown in Fig. 3. The top panel compares the plasma TG concentrations from 8am—4pm in insulin-resistant individuals with endogenous HTG to insulin sensitive, normal volunteers [14]. The results in the middle and lower panels show that day-long plasma insulin and FFA concentrations are higher (p < 0.001) in those with HTG. Multivariate analysis indicated that the increases in both insulin and FFA concentrations were independent predictors of the plasma TG concentration. Although the plasma FFA levels were certainly higher in those with HTG, the increases in plasma TG concentrations were disproportionately elevated — a finding consistent with the view that the livers of insulin-resistant, hyperinsulinemic individuals are more effective in converting FFA to TG.

Further evidence for that compensatory hyperinsulinemia does not inhibit hepatic VLDL-TG secretion can be derived from the effects of dietary manipulations. It has been known for more than 30 years that high-carbohydrate diets increase plasma TG concentrations [15]. Such diets have also been shown to increase plasma insulin levels and increase insulin sensitivity [16]. If HTG is due to the inability of insulin to inhibit VLDL-TG secretion from insulin resistant individuals, high-carbohydrate diets (by increasing both insulin levels and sensitivity) should lead to a decrease, not an increase, in hepatic VLDL-TG secretion. The fact that just the opposite is seen provides further evidence that chronic hyperinsulinemia, in insulin-resistant individuals, leads to hypertriglyceridemia by enhancing hepatic FFA esterification, and stimulating VLDL-TG secretion as outlined in Fig. 2.

Conclusion

There is extremely compelling evidence that both insulin resistance and compensatory hyperinsulinemia are associated with increases in hepatic VLDL-TG secretion and elevated plasma TG concentration in nondiabetic individuals.

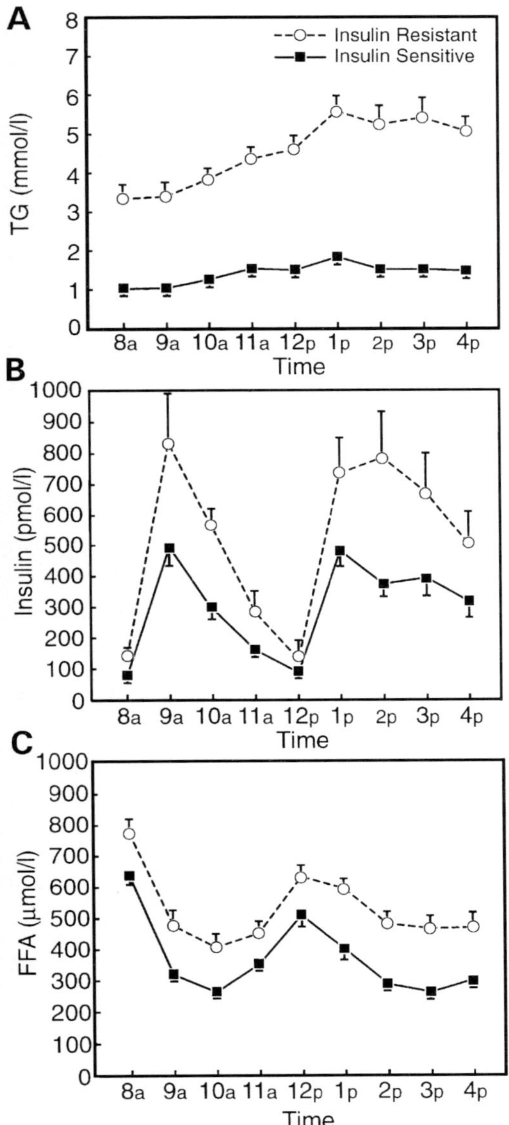

Fig. 3. Plasma TG (**A**), insulin (**B**), and FFA (**C**) concentrations from 8 am to 4 pm in nondiabetic volunteers, divided into insulin-resistant, hypertriglyceridemic (o–o) or insulin-sensitive, normotriglyceridemic groups. Breakfast was given at 8 am and lunch at 12 pm. Adapted from data published in Endocrinology and Metabolism (1994;1:15) with permission of the authors and the journal.

Indeed, it is likely that these changes in VLDL metabolism are the most common manifestation of insulin resistance and compensatory hyperinsulinemia, as well as the events most responsible for the increased risk of CHD in these individuals

264

[17]. In contrast, controversy continues as to the causal link between insulin resistance, compensatory hyperinsulinemia, and hepatic VLDL-TG secretion. Evidence has been presented suggesting that circulating insulin and FFA concentrations act in concert to enhance hepatic VLDL-TG secretion. In this formulation, ambient insulin concentrations modulate the FFA-hepatic VLDL-TG secretion dose response curve; the higher the insulin level the liver is chronically exposed to, the greater the hepatic VLDL-TG secretion rate at any given level of FFA. At the other extreme is the insulin-deficient subject, in whom even extreme elevations of FFA are incapable of increasing hepatic VLDL-TG secretion rates. Although this view is in conflict with the results of acute studies carried out in vitro and in vivo, I think it is the most likely explanation of chronic studies performed in both man and animals.

References

1. Reaven GM, Lerner RL, Stern MP, Farquhar JW. Role of insulin in endogenous hypertriglyceridemia. J Clin Invest 1967;46:1756—1767.
2. Olefsky JM, Farquhar JW, Reaven GM. Reappraisal of the role of insulin in hypertriglyceridemia. Am J Med 1974;57:551—560.
3. Tobey TA, Greenfield M, Kraemer F, Reaven GM. Relationship between insulin resistance, insulin secretion, very low density lipoprotein kinetics and plasma triglyceride levels in normotriglyceridemic man. Metabolism 1981;30:165—171.
4. Lewis GF. Fatty acid regulation of very low density lipoprotein production. Curr Opin Lipidol 1997; 8:146—153.
5. Sparks JD, Sparks CE. Insulin regulation of triacylglycerol-rich lipoprotein synthesis and secretion. Biochim Biophys Acta 1994;1215:9—32.
6. Lewis GF, Uffelman KD, Szeto LW, Steiner G. Effects of acute hyperinsulinemia on VLDL triglyceride and VLDL apoB production in normal weight and obese individuals. Diabetes 1993;42:833—842.
7. Lewis GF, Uffelman KD, Szeto LW, Weller B, Steiner G. Interaction between free fatty acids and insulin in the acute control of very low density lipoprotein production in humans. J Clin Invest 1995;95:158—166.
8. Tulloch BR, Dyal K, Fraser TR. Increased lipid synthesis by liver slice in a superfusion system following raised glucose or insulin concentration. Diabetologia 1972;8:267—273.
9. Topping DL, Mayes PA. The immediate effects of insulin and fructose on the metabolism of the perfused liver. Biochem J 1972;126:295—311.
10. Dashti N, Wolfbauer G. Secretion of lipids, apolipoproteins, and lipoproteins by human hepatoma cell line, HepG2: effects of oleic acid and insulin. J Lipid Res 1987;28:423—436.
11. Reaven GM, Mondon CE. Effect of in vivo plasma insulin levels on the relationship between perfusate free fatty acid concentration and triglyceride secretion by perfused rat livers. Horm Metab Res 1984;16:230—232.
12. Karnieli E, Hissin PJ, Simpson IA, Salans LB, Cushman SW. A possible mechanism of insulin resistance in the rat adipose cell in streptozotocin-induced diabetes mellitus. Depletion of intracellular glucose transport systems. J Clin Invest 1981;68:811—814.
13. Reaven GM, Risser TR, Chen Y-DI, Reaven EP. Characterization of a model of dietary-induced hypertriglyceridemia in young, nonobese rats. J Lipid Res 1979;20:371—378.
14. Jeng C-Y, Fuh MM-T, Sheu WH-H, Chen Y-DI, Reaven GM. Hormone and substrate modulation of plasma triglyceride concentration in primary hypertriglyceridemia. Endocrinol Metab 1994;1:15—21.

15. Farquhar JW, Frank A, Gross RC, Reaven GM. Glucose, insulin and triglyceride responses to high and low carbohydrate diets in man. J Clin Invest 1966;45:1648—1656.
16. Koltermann OG, Reaven GM, Olefsky JM. Relationship between in vivo insulin resistance and decreased insulin receptors in obese man. J Clin Endocrinol Metab 1979;48:487—494.
17. Reaven GM. Hypertriglyceridemia: the central feature of Syndrome X. Cardiovasc Risk Factors 1996;6:29—35.

The Diabetes Atherosclerosis Intervention Study (DAIS)

The DAIS Project Group (prepared by G. Steiner)
DAIS Project Office, WHO Collaborating Centre for the Study of Atherosclerosis in Diabetes, University of Toronto; and Toronto Hospital (General Division), Toronto, Canada

Keywords: clinical trial, coronary artery disease, men, population, women.

The Diabetes Atherosclerosis Intervention Study (DAIS)

DAIS is a multinational study testing the hypothesis that the long-term correction of dyslipoproteinemia with micronized fenofibrate will reduce the angiographic progression or increase the regression of pre-existing coronary atherosclerosis in type II diabetes. The study is being carried out in 11 clinical centres (six Canadian, three Finnish, one Swedish and one French) and is conducted in collaboration with the World Health Organization [1].

This paper presents a brief, preliminary description of the baseline characteristics of the DAIS population. These are compared to the characteristics of those with diabetes in the 4S study, a study of secondary intervention with simvastatin in a population of hypercholesterolemic individuals, some of whom had diabetes. The baseline characteristics are also separately examined for those DAIS participants from Europe and those from Canada.

The rationale for DAIS

There are many reasons for conducting this study. Atherosclerotic cardiovascular disease is the most common complication of diabetes [2]. It accounts for the death of nearly 75% of those with diabetes in North America, a figure that contrasts with about 30% for those without diabetes. The risk of coronary artery disease in diabetes is 2—4 times greater in those with diabetes than it is in those without. This is regardless of the basal incidence and prevalence of CAD in the population examined. In those without diabetes it is well-established that the risk of CAD increases with hypercholesterolemia, with a high LDL [3,4] and with a low HDL [5]. There is also increasing evidence that hypertriglyceridemia increases the risk of CAD [6]. Clinical trials conducted have demonstrated, both angiographically and by clinical events (including total mortality) that cor-

---

Address for correspondence: Dr George Steiner, Room NUW9-112, The Toronto Hospital (General Division), 200 Elizabeth Street, Toronto, Ontario, Canada, M5G 2C4. Tel.: +1-416-340-4538. Fax: +1-416-340-3473.

recting hypercholesterolemia will reduce CAD [7—9]. Recently a clinical trial has come to the same conclusion with respect to hypertriglyceridemia [10]. However, the study populations for most of these have excluded those with diabetes. In three trials some of the population had diabetes. Their data was subjected to post-hoc subgroup analysis. One, the Helsinki Heart Study, had too few people with diabetes to show any statistical significance [11]. The other two, the 4S [12] and the CARE [9] studies, showed a benefit to reducing cholesterol levels with an HMG CoA reductase inhibitor. However, in the former, individuals with triglycerides over 2.5 mmol/l were excluded. As the major form of dyslipoproteinemia in diabetes is hypertriglyceridemia, this resulted in the 4S study examining a very select group of people with diabetes. There are not enough details yet published about the CARE population to know about the subgroup with diabetes. Furthermore, it appears that neither study used diabetes as one of the strata in randomizing the participants. Thus, the hypothesis has not yet been tested by a study specifically designed to examine those with diabetes.

Summary of DAIS protocol

The DAIS protocol has been published and is only summarized below [1]. Men and women with type II diabetes and ranging from 40 to 65 years of age are recruited. Some have had either a PTCA or coronary bypass (called the intervened group) others have not. Some will have had a myocardial infarct, while others will not. All have mild dyslipoproteinemia (LDL-cholesterol 3.5—4.5 mmol/l and triglyceride $\leqslant 5.2$ mmol/l; or triglyceride 1.7—5.2 mmol/l and LDL-cholesterol $\leqslant 4.5$ mmol/l; and total-/HDL-cholesterol $\geqslant 4$). Diabetes control should be that in usual clinical practice (i.e., HbA1c $\leqslant 170\%$ of upper normal limit). This is not a test of glycemic control and individuals are allowed to continue under the care of their usual physician as long as the control does not deteriorate beyond this. All undergo standardized coronary angiography and must have at least one minimally detectable lesion. Those who meet the study criteria are randomized to either placebo or active micronized fenofibrate (200 mg per day) with randomization being stratified by gender, previous coronary intervention (PTCA or CABG) and clinical centre. Prior to commencing recruitment we calculated the sample requirements to be 260 individuals to give a 90% power of detecting a difference in average segment diameter as small as 0.15 mm with an α of 2.5% (one-sided) and allowing for a 20% drop out. We also wished to have at least 100 from each gender. It will be indicated than we exceeded these numbers.

The DAIS population

There were 731 people who entered the baseline period during which they followed the study diet and were given placebo, in a single-blind manner. During that period they also had a series of examinations and biochemical tests to determine their eligibility. Out of 731 individuals 313 were found, mainly because of some biochemical parameter, to be ineligible for randomization. They were, however, comparable in terms of a number of lifestyle parameters to the 418 who were randomized to active fenofibrate or placebo.

In order to increase the randomization of the target number of women, a total of 418 individuals were randomized. This was 60% more than the sample size estimated to be required for the study. The population was made up of 305 men and 113 women. In Canada, 168 were randomized. The balance, 250 individuals, were in Europe (Finland, Sweden and France). In 218 cases there was no history of a prior myocardial infarct, coronary intervention coronary bypass (CABG), angioplasty (PTCA), or angina. The remaining 200 had had one or more of these as evidence of previous clinical coronary disease. There were 132 cases who had had a prior PTCA or CABG and 286 who had not. Gender, previous coronary intervention (PTCA or CABG) and clinical centre were used for randomization into groups treated with active or placebo drug. The numbers recruited per centre ranged from eight to 76. The participants' diabetes was treated with diet alone, or diet plus oral hypoglycemic agents or insulin or a combination of both. More Europeans than Canadians were treated with the combination of an oral agent plus insulin. Despite this, the Europeans' hemoglobin A1c was barely higher (p = 0.022) than that of the Canadians. There were no gender differences. All fell within the inclusion limits. The mean level for plasma cholesterol was 5.57 mmol/l, for plasma triglyceride was 2.42 mmol/l, for HDL cholesterol was 1.03 mmol/l and for calculated (according to the approach of Friedewald et al.) LDL was 3.43 mmol/l [13]. These values were similar in the four different diabetes treatment groups. The mean body mass index was 28.8 and did not differ between the genders. However, as expected, men had a higher waist/hip ratio than did women. The lipid values above were not correlated with either of these anthropometric parameters. Fifteen percent of the participants smoked at the time of recruitment. This number was similar for men and women, and for Europeans and Canadians. Both systolic and diastolic blood pressures were similar in the subgroups categorized by gender or prior PTCA or CABG. The mean blood pressures in Europe were minimally higher than those in Canada. Except for a greater proportion of individuals in the age range 61—65 years among those who had had prior coronary intervention, the age distributions were similar in the study population subgroups. Approximately one-half of the population took some aspirin at the time of entry to DAIS. This was similar in women and men, and in Canadians and Europeans. However, the figure was closer to 95% among those who had had a PTCA or CABG and 30% among those who had not.

The average age of the DAIS population (56.8 ± 5.9 years (mean ± SD)) was similar to that of those with diabetes in the 4S population (59.9 ± 6.6 years) [12]. As noted above, 218 of the DAIS population had no clinical evidence of coronary artery disease. This was in contrast to the 4S study in which one of the entry criteria required all to have a history of angina or a myocardial infarction [8]. Both studies had similar numbers of smokers, ex-smokers and people who had never smoked. The average blood pressure of those randomized in DAIS was 140.0/69.9, whereas that in 4S was 147.1/85.1. However, in both a similar proportion of participants had a history of hypertension. As a result of its eligibility criteria [8] (total cholesterol 5.5 to 8.0 mmol/l and serum triglyceride $\leqslant 2.5$ mmol/l), the average levels of cholesterol and LDL cholesterol were higher, and the average levels of triglyceride were lower in the 4S study than they were in DAIS.

Interpretation

The characteristics of the DAIS population should not be interpreted as applying to all individuals with type II diabetes, or to those with type II diabetes in either region or of either gender. They represent the population who met the eligibility criteria and were randomized into the Diabetes Atherosclerosis Intervention Study. The data indicate that the population is quite homogeneous. The similarity of those in Canada to those in Europe suggests that when the study is completed its information will be applicable to people with type II diabetes in both regions. DAIS will differ from both the CARE [9] and the 4S [8,12] studies in a number of respects. It is aimed at testing the "lipid hypothesis" specifically in diabetes, rather than being a posthoc subgroup analysis. DAIS will do so using angiography, 4S and CARE used clinical endpoints. It is examining a population with dyslipoproteinemias representative of those observed in most people with diabetes, whereas the other two studies focussed greater attention on hypercholesterolemic people. Two different classes of drugs are being studied. DAIS is using a fibrate, whereas both CARE and the 4S studies used HMG CoA reductase inhibitors. DAIS plans to report on women with diabetes.

References

1. Steiner G. The Diabetes Atherosclerosis Intervention Study (DAIS): a study conducted in cooperation with the World Health Organization. Diabetologia 1996;39:1655−1661.
2. Steiner G. Atherosclerosis, the major complication of diabetes. In: Vranic M, Hollenberg CH, Steiner G (eds) Comparison of Type I and Type II Diabetes. Plenum Press: New York, 1985; 277−297.
3. Castelli WP. The epidemiology of blood lipids. In: Steiner G, Shafrir E (eds) Primary Hyperlipoproteinemias. New York: McGraw Hill, 1991;119−128.
4. Stamler J, Vaccaro O, Neaton JD, Wentworth D. Diabetes, other risk factors, and 12-yr cardiovascular mortality for men screened in the multiple risk factor Intervention Trial. Diabet Care 1993;16:434−444.
5. Assmann G, Schulte H. Relation of high-density lipoprotein cholesterol and triglyceride to the incidence of atherosclerotic coronary artery disease (the PROCAM experience) Am J Cardiol 1992;70:733−737.
6. Hokanson JE, Austin MA. Plasma triglyceride level is a risk factor for cardiovascular disease independent of high-density lipoprotein cholesterol level: a meta-analysis of population-based prospective studies. J Cardiovasc Risk 1996;3:213−219.
7. Shepherd J, Cobbe SM, Ford I et al. Prevention of coronary heart disease with pravastatin in

men with hypercholesterolemia. West of Scotland Coronary Prevention Study Group. N Engl J Med 1995;333:1301—1307.

8. The Scandinavian Simvastatin Survival Study Group. Randomized trial of cholesterol lowering in 4444 patients with coronary heart disease: the Scandinavian Simvastatin Survival Study (4S). Lancet 1994;344:1383—1389.

9. Sacks FM, Pfeffer MA, Moye LA et al. The effect of pravastatin on coronary events after myocardial infarction in patients with average cholesterol levels. N Engl J Med 1996;335:1001—1009.

10. Ericsson C-G, Hamsten A, Nilsson J, Grip L, Svane B, de Faire U. Angiographic assessment of effects of bezafibrate on progression of coronary artery disease in young male postinfarction patients. Lancet 1996;347:849—853.

11. Koskinen P, Manttari M, Manninen V, Huttunen JK, Heinonen OP, Frick MH, Tenkanen L. Coronary heart disease incidence in NIDDM patients in the Helsinki Heart Study. Joint effects of serum triglyceride and LDL cholesterol and HDL cholesterol concentrations on coronary heart disease risk in the Helsinki Heart Study. Implications for treatment. Diabet Care 1992;85:37—45.

12. Pyorälä K, Pedersen TR, Kjekhus J, Faergeman O, Olsson AG, Thorgeirsson G. Cholesterol lowering with simvastatin improves prognosis of diabetic patients with coronary heart disease. Diabet Care 1997;20:614—620.

13. Friedewald WT, Levy RI, Fredrickson DS. Estimation of the concentration of low-density lipoprotein cholesterol in plasma without use of the preparative ultracentrifuge. Clin Chem 1972;18:499—502.

Results of the Lipoprotein and Coronary Atherosclerosis Study (LCAS)

Christie M. Ballantyne[1], J. Alan Herd[1], Jeffrey R. Schein[2], Peter H. Jones[1], John A. Farmer[1] and Antonio M. Gotto Jr[3]

[1]*Department of Medicine, Baylor College of Medicine, Houston, Texas;* [2]*Novartis Pharmaceuticals Corporation, East Hanover, New Jersey; and* [3]*Department of Medicine, Cornell University Medical College, New York, New York, USA*

Abstract. *Background.* Despite abundant evidence in patients with severely elevated low-density lipoprotein cholesterol (LDL-C), the benefit of reducing mildly to moderately elevated LDL-C in coronary artery disease (CAD) patients has not been well studied.

Methods. In the Lipoprotein and Coronary Atherosclerosis Study, 429 CAD patients with LDL-C of 115–190 mg/dl were randomized to fluvastatin 20 mg bid or placebo; patients with prerandomization LDL-C $\geq$ 160 mg/dl were also assigned cholestyramine. The primary endpoint was change in minimum lumen diameter from baseline to 2.5-year coronary angiography.

Results. At 2.5 years, LDL-C was reduced by 24% in all fluvastatin patients and by 22.5% in fluvastatin monotherapy patients to levels of 111 and 106 mg/dl, respectively. For the primary endpoint, fluvastatin patients had significantly less CAD progression, 0.028 vs. 0.100 mm with placebo (p = 0.005), with similar results in the respective monotherapy subgroups (0.024 vs. 0.094 mm, p = 0.02). Consistent angiographic benefit was seen across the range of baseline LDL-C concentrations in the study.

Conclusions. CAD patients with mildly to moderately elevated LDL-C received similar angiographic benefits to those reported in CAD patients with severely elevated LDL-C. The benefits obtained with fluvastatin were similar to those obtained with other statins.

Keywords: angiography, cholesterol, fluvastatin, lipid lowering, statins.

Introduction

Lipid-lowering therapy has been shown to reduce coronary artery disease (CAD) progression and events in patients with CAD and severely elevated low-density lipoprotein cholesterol (LDL-C) in a large number of clinical trials. However, the benefit of reducing LDL-C in CAD patients with only mild to moderate elevations has not been well studied, even though most CAD patients have LDL-C in this category [1]. The only previously published angiographic study in this population reported no significant difference between treatment groups for the primary endpoint [2].

New data on this large group of patients are provided by the Lipoprotein and

Address for correspondence: Christie M. Ballantyne MD, Baylor College of Medicine, 6565 Fannin, M.S. A-601, Houston, TX 77030, USA. Tel.: +1-713-798-5034. Fax: +1-713-798-7885. E-mail: cmb@bcm.tmc.edu

Coronary Atherosclerosis Study (LCAS) [3], which addresses two major questions:

1. Does treatment with fluvastatin produce benefits in patients with either mildly or moderately elevated LDL-C?
2. Does fluvastatin treatment lead to similar angiographic changes such as slowing progression, reducing new lesion formation, and inducing regression compared with angiographic trials with other 3-hydroxy-3-methylglutaryl coenzyme A (HMG-CoA) reductase inhibitors (statins)?

Material, Methods and Patients

LCAS was a double-blind, placebo-controlled trial designed to determine whether lipid-regulating therapy with fluvastatin reduces progression, and/or induces regression of coronary atherosclerotic lesions, and/or reduces new coronary lesion formation in patients with CAD and mildly to moderately elevated LDL-C [3]. Eligibility criteria included at least one coronary artery lesion causing 30—75% diameter stenosis by caliper measurement and LDL-C of 115—190 mg/dl on diet. Randomization was to fluvastatin 20 mg bid or placebo; patients with prerandomization LDL-C $\geqslant$ 160 mg/dl also received open-label adjunctive cholestyramine up to 12 g/day, begun 12 weeks after randomization. Subgroups were defined by prerandomization LDL-C $<$ 160 mg/dl (mildly elevated; three-quarters of patients) or $\geqslant$ 160 mg/dl (moderately elevated; one-quarter of patients). The primary endpoint was within-patient per-lesion change in minimum lumen diameter (MLD) assessed by quantitative coronary angiography at baseline and after 2.5 years of treatment.

Results

Lipids

In the 429 patients (19% women) randomized in the study, mean baseline LDL-C was 146 mg/dl. From baseline to 12 weeks before the initiation of cholestyramine, total cholesterol decreased by 18.1%, LDL-C decreased by 26.5%, HDL-C increased by 5.5% and triglyceride decreased by 10.1% with fluvastatin. From baseline to 2.5 years, LDL-C decreased by 24% in all fluvastatin patients, by 22.5% in fluvastatin monotherapy patients, and by 28% in fluvastatin-plus-cholestyramine patients, to final concentrations of 111, 106 and 124 mg/dl, respectively.

Minimum lumen diameter and percent diameter stenosis

Analysis of the primary endpoint indicated significantly less CAD progression in all fluvastatin patients, 0.028 vs. 0.100 mm in all placebo patients (p = 0.005). Comparable results were also seen with fluvastatin monotherapy: 0.024 vs.

0.094 mm with placebo monotherapy (p = 0.02). A similar but nonsignificant trend was observed among the adjunctive cholestyramine subgroups, in which MLD was reduced by 0.041 mm with fluvastatin plus cholestyramine vs. 0.117 mm with placebo plus cholestyramine (p = 0.1).

By design, mean baseline LDL-C was lower in the monotherapy subgroups (136 mg/dl) and higher in the adjunctive cholestyramine subgroups (173 mg/dl). Yet comparison of the treatment effect of fluvastatin (defined as the difference between change in MLD with fluvastatin and change in MLD with placebo) indicated consistent angiographic benefit across the range of baseline LDL-C concentrations in the study (Fig. 1). Among all patients with evaluable angiography (n = 340), the monotherapy subgroups (n = 261) and the adjunctive cholestyramine subgroups (n = 79), fluvastatin patients had 0.07−0.08 mm less progression than placebo patients. Similar angiographic benefit with fluvastatin was also seen in a posthoc subgroup defined by LDL-C < 130 mg/dl (n = 84), that is, below the recommended initiation level for drug therapy in the treatment guidelines of the US National Cholesterol Education Program (NCEP) [4].

Fluvastatin treatment also reduced progression as measured by change in percent diameter stenosis. Among all patients, percent diameter stenosis increased 0.6% in all fluvastatin patients vs. 2.8% in all placebo patients (p = 0.01), and among the monotherapy subgroups, percent diameter stenosis increased 0.5% with fluvastatin monotherapy vs. 2.5% with placebo monotherapy (p = 0.04).

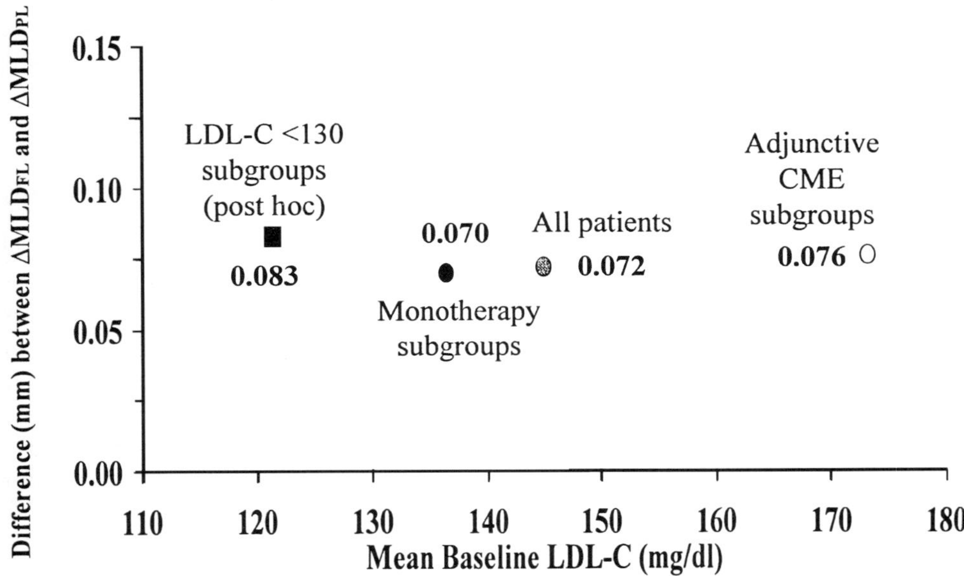

Fig. 1. Across the range of baseline low-density lipoprotein (LDL-C) concentrations included in LCAS, the difference between minimum lumen diameter (MLD) change with fluvastatin and with placebo was consistent. Reprinted with permission [3].

Progression, regression and new lesions

Definite progression was defined as at least one lesion with MLD decrease $\geqslant 0.4$ mm, including new total occlusions, and no lesion with MLD increase $\geqslant 0.4$ mm. Definite regression was defined as at least one lesion with MLD increase $\geqslant 0.4$ mm, no lesion with MLD decrease $\geqslant 0.4$ mm and no new total occlusion.

Comparison of the distribution of all patients among the three categories of definite progression, definite regression and mixed change or no response indicated significant benefit with fluvastatin (p = 0.02). Of all fluvastatin patients, 28.7% had definite progression, 14.6% had definite regression and 56.7% had mixed response or no change, vs. 39.1, 8.3 and 52.7%, respectively, of all placebo patients. Similarly, among the predefined subgroups, fewer fluvastatin patients had progression and more had regression compared with placebo, but these differences were not statistically significant.

New lesions were defined as lesions with an increase in lesion size of $\geqslant 0.4$ mm and reference lumen diameter minus MLD < 0.8 mm at baseline and $\geqslant 0.8$ mm at follow-up. The number of patients with new lesions was significantly reduced by 41% with fluvastatin therapy (22 fluvastatin vs. 37 placebo patients; p = 0.03). The number of patients with new total occlusions was reduced by 36% with fluvastatin therapy (7 fluvastatin vs. 11 placebo patients), but the difference was not statistically significant.

Clinical events

LCAS was not specifically designed to detect statistical differences in clinical events; however, consistent trends toward clinical benefit with fluvastatin were observed. Cardiac morbid events — defined as definite or probable myocardial infarction, percutaneous transluminal coronary angioplasty (PTCA), coronary artery bypass grafting (CABG), and unstable angina pectoris requiring hospitalization — or any fatal event occurred in 24.1% fewer fluvastatin patients: 31 (14.5%) of all fluvastatin vs. 41 (19.1%) of all placebo patients (p = 0.2). Similarly, the reduction in events was 32.8% with fluvastatin monotherapy, with events occurring in 20 (12.7%) fluvastatin monotherapy patients vs. 31 (18.9%) placebo patients (p = 0.1). Three fluvastatin patients and five placebo patients died.

Fluvastatin also reduced the need for revascularization procedures, although the difference was not statistically significant. Among all patients, 25.9% fewer fluvastatin patients required any revascularization procedure (myocardial revascularization (PTCA, CABG, coronary stent, atherectomy, or transcatheter revascularization)), carotid endarterectomy, peripheral angioplasty or peripheral bypass graft): 25 (11.7%) fluvastatin patients vs. 34 (15.8%) placebo patients. Among monotherapy patients, 35.8% fewer fluvastatin patients had revascularization procedures, 16 (10.2%) vs. 26 (15.9%) placebo monotherapy patients.

In a posthoc analysis, a proportional-hazards model was used to evaluate baseline patient characteristics as potential confounding factors affecting time to first cardiac morbidity or any fatal event. After adjustment for the disproportional distribution of high baseline plasma glucose and low baseline HDL-C levels between treatment groups, fluvastatin was found to have a significant treatment effect on event-free survival in monotherapy patients [5].

Discussion

LCAS demonstrated that CAD patients with mild to moderate elevations of LDL-C received similar angiographic benefits, including decreased progression, increased regression and reduced new lesion formation, as did CAD patients with more severe elevations of LDL-C. In addition, the benefits obtained with fluvastatin were similar to those obtained with other statins. In recent angiographic trials using statin therapy, treatment benefit (defined as the difference in MLD change between drug and placebo patients) was similar regardless of baseline LDL-C, except in HARP (Fig. 2). In the majority of these trials, including the randomized treatment groups and the subgroups in LCAS, the difference in

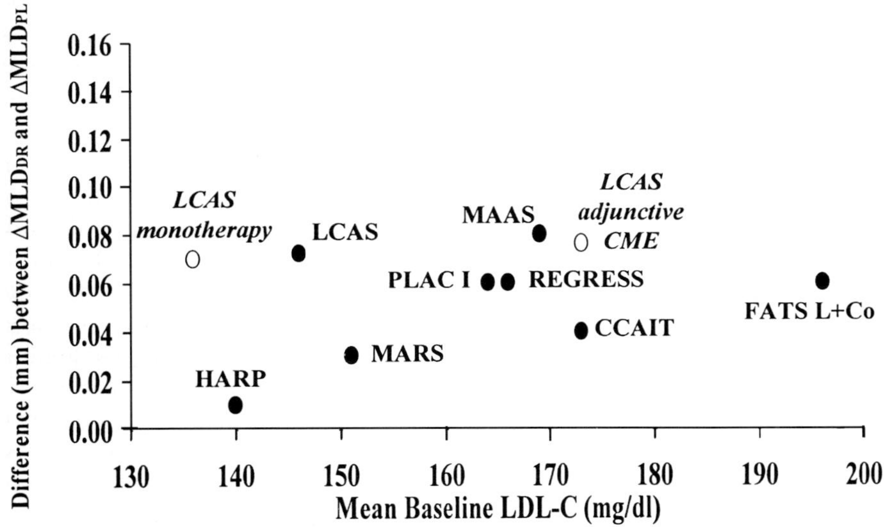

Fig. 2. In recent angiographic trials of statin therapy, the difference between change in minimum lumen diameter (MLD) with statin therapy and change in MLD with placebo was comparable regardless of baseline LDL-C, except in the Harvard Atherosclerosis Reversibility Project (HARP) [2]. The Canadian Coronary Atherosclerosis Intervention Trial (CCAIT) [6], the Familial Atherosclerosis Treatment Study (FATS) [7] and the Monitored Atherosclerosis Regression Study (MARS) [8] used lovastatin; the Multicentre Anti-Atheroma Study (MAAS) [9] used simvastatin; HARP, the Pravastatin Limitation of Atherosclerosis in the Coronary Arteries (PLAC I) [10] and Regression Growth Evaluation Statin Study (REGRESS) [11] used pravastatin; and the Lipoprotein and Coronary Atherosclerosis Study (LCAS) [3] used fluvastatin. Follow-up angiography was performed at 2 years in CCAIT, MARS and REGRESS; 2.5 years in HARP and LCAS; 3 years in PLAC I; and 4 years in MAAS. Adapted and reprinted with permission [3].

MLD change between drug and placebo was 0.06—0.08 mm. Reductions in new lesions and new total occlusions in LCAS were also similar to those in the other trials.

Plaque rupture may be the biological process that explains the relation between CAD progression rate as assessed by angiography and myocardial infarction event rate. Although the vast majority of myocardial infarctions are caused by plaque rupture, the majority of plaques that rupture do not cause clinical events but do cause lesion progression. Therefore, clinical event trials are a relatively insensitive method of assessing the influence of therapy on plaque rupture, whereas coronary angiography assesses changes in plaque size regardless of whether they cause symptoms. The biology of plaque rupture may also clarify the apparent discrepancy between the modest average change in MLD or percent diameter stenosis and the more impressive event reductions seen in clinical event and angiographic trials. Plaque rupture is a relatively infrequent event that causes a large decrease in MLD. The vast majority of lesions did not change appreciably in LCAS, and for this reason, the average change in MLD may not be the best reflection of plaque rupture. Instead, plaque rupture may be better measured by reductions both in marked progression of individual lesions (defined in LCAS as reduction in MLD of $\geqslant 0.4$ mm) and in percentage of patients with new lesion formation, which are similar to the percent reduction in events reported in clinical event trials. Reductions in new lesions and per-lesion progression may better reflect plaque stabilization that results in reduced plaque rupture.

Although LCAS was not designed specifically to measure changes in clinical event rates, the trends toward benefit seen in LCAS are consistent with the 24% reduction in risk for CAD death or nonfatal myocardial infarction noted in CARE, which enrolled CAD patients with similar LDL-C levels (115—174 mg/dl) [12]. Together, the results of LCAS and CARE demonstrate that statin therapy in patients with mild to moderate LDL-C elevations slows CAD progression and reduces clinical events as has previously been determined in patients with more severely elevated LDL-C.

The results of LCAS extend the angiographic and clinical benefit documented in patients with severely elevated LDL-C to patients whose LDL-C is mildly to moderately elevated. The treatment benefit with fluvastatin on CAD progression measured by change in MLD was consistent with results of angiographic trials using other statins, suggesting that these drugs act as a class, producing similar beneficial effects.

Acknowledgements

Funding for the Lipoprotein and Coronary Atherosclerosis Study was provided by Novartis Pharmaceuticals Corporation Grant No. B351 and NIH GCRC Grant No. 5M01RR00350. The authors acknowledge Kerrie Jara for editorial assistance.

References

1. Kannel WB. Range of serum cholesterol values in the population developing coronary artery disease. Am J Cardiol 1995;76:69C−77C.
2. Sacks FM, Pasternak RC, Gibson CM, Rosner B, Stone PH, for the Harvard Atherosclerosis Reversibility Project (HARP) Group. Effect on coronary atherosclerosis of decrease in plasma cholesterol concentrations in normocholesterolaemic patients. Lancet 1994;344:1182−1186.
3. Herd JA, Ballantyne CM, Farmer JA, Ferguson JJ III, Jones PH, West MS, Gould KL, Gotto AM Jr, for the LCAS Investigators. Effects of fluvastatin on coronary atherosclerosis in patients with mild to moderate cholesterol elevations (Lipoprotein and Coronary Atherosclerosis Study (LCAS)). Am J Cardiol 1997;80:278−286.
4. National Cholesterol Education Program. Second report of the Expert Panel on Detection, Evaluation and Treatment of High Blood Cholesterol in Adults (Adult Treatment Panel II). Circulation 1994;89:1329−1445.
5. Herd JA, West MS, Ballantyne CM, Farmer JA, Ferlic LL, Jones PH, Gotto AM Jr. Beneficial effects of fluvastatin on clinical cardiac and all fatal events in patients with mild cholesterol elevations (Abstract). J Invest Med 1997;45:222A.
6. Waters D, Higginson L, Gladstone P, Kimball B, Le May M, Boccuzzi SJ, Lespérance M, the CCAIT Study Group. Effects of monotherapy with an HMG-CoA reductase inhibitor on the progression of coronary atherosclerosis as assessed by serial quantitative arteriography: the Canadian Coronary Atherosclerosis Intervention Trial. Circulation 1994;89:959−968.
7. Brown G, Albers JJ, Fisher LD, Schaefer SM, Lin J-T, Kaplan C, Zhao X-Q, Bisson BD, Fitzpatrick VF, Dodge HT. Regression of coronary artery disease as a result of intensive lipid-lowering therapy in men with high levels of apolipoprotein B. N Engl J Med 1990;323:1289−1298.
8. Blankenhorn DH, Azen SP, Kramsch DM, Mack WJ, Cashin-Hemphill L, Hodis HN, DeBoer LWV, Mahrer PR, Masteller MJ, Vailas LI, Alaupovic P, Hirsch LJ, and the MARS Research Group. Coronary angiographic changes with lovastatin therapy: the Monitored Atherosclerosis Regression Study (MARS). Ann Int Med 1993;119:969−976.
9. MAAS Investigators. Effect of simvastatin on coronary atheroma: the Multicentre Antiatheroma Study (MAAS). Lancet 1994;344:633−638.
10. Pitt B, Mancini GBJ, Ellis SG, Rosman HS, Park J-S, McGovern ME, for the PLAC I Investigators. Pravastatin Limitation of Atherosclerosis in the Coronary Arteries (PLAC I): reduction in atherosclerosis progression and clinical events. J Am Coll Cardiol 1995;26:1133−1139.
11. Jukema JW, Bruschke AVG, van Boven AJ, Reiber JHC, Bal ET, Zwinderman AH, Jansen H, Boerma GJM, van Rappard FM, Lie KI, on behalf of the REGRESS Study Group. Effects of lipid lowering by pravastatin on progression and regression of coronary artery disease in symptomatic men with normal to moderately elevated serum cholesterol levels: the Regression Growth Evaluation Statin Study (REGRESS). Circulation 1995;91:2528−2540.
12. Sacks FM, Pfeffer MA, Moye LA, Rouleau JL, Rutherford JD, Cole TG, Brown L, Warnica JW, Arnold JMO, Wun C-C, Davis BR, Braunwald E, for the Cholesterol and Recurrent Events Trial Investigators. The effect of pravastatin on coronary events after myocardial infarction in patients with average cholesterol levels. N Engl J Med 1996;335:1001−1009.

Statins and coronary artery disease; it's the clinical endpoints that count

Graham Jackson
Department of Cardiology, Guy's Hospital, London, UK

It is perhaps not fully appreciated that 80% of individuals who develop coronary artery disease (CAD) have a total plasma cholesterol level that is within a similar range to those who do not develop CAD [1]. In other words, most people who develop CAD do not have very high cholesterol levels.

Taking each patient with CAD as an individual, a reasonable approach might be to say that the level of cholesterol at which CAD develops is too high for that individual. This would then lead to an approach to lowering cholesterol from its initial level by a percentage change rather than by an absolute number.

To advocate this we would need evidence that the lowering of cholesterol (LDL cholesterol in particular) was of similar benefit whatever the baseline as long as a similar percentage fall in LDL cholesterol was achieved. That evidence should be within the major clinical and angiographic trials (Table 1).

CARE trial

The cholesterol and recurrent events (CARE) trial [2] was a double-blind trial of pravastatin 40 mg daily or placebo, designed to determine if lipid-lowering therapy with an HMGCoA reductase inhibitor (statin) would reduce the risk of recurrent myocardial infarction (MI) or CAD death in patients with a previous MI and a total cholesterol level of less than 6.2 mmol/l. The LDL cholesterol had to be 3.0–4.5 mmol/l and the triglycerides less than 4.0 mmol/l.

A total of 4,159 patients were randomised, 3,583 (86%) men and 576 (14%) women. At 5 years, pravastatin had reduced total cholesterol by 20%, LDL cholesterol by 28%, raised HDL cholesterol by 5% and lowered triglycerides by 14%. The baseline mean total cholesterol was 5.4 mmol/l, LDL 3.6, HDL 1.0 and triglycerides 1.8 — by any standards, levels that are not at all impressive and most probably often dismissed as "OK" — which is what makes the trial so important because it deals with "typical" patients.

The clinical endpoints were impressive, confirming the view that what is all right for some is not for others. Pravastatin significantly reduced the risk of CAD death or nonfatal recurrence MI by 24%, total MI (fatal or nonfatal) by 25%, the need for angioplasty or coronary artery bypass surgery by 27% and for the first time in any of the lipid lowering CAD trials, stroke was reduced by a significant 31% (p = 0.03). Importantly there was also a significant benefit for

282

Table 1. Double-blind, placebo-controlled trials of the effect of HMGCoA reductase inhibitors on coronary events.

Study	Length (years)	Type	Subjects	Total cholesterol	Outcomes ($p < 0.05$)
4S [3]	4.9—6.3	Secondary prevention, dose titration with simvastatin 20—40 mg od	3617 men, 827 women aged 35—70 years	Entry 5.5—8.0 mmol/l, reduction 25%	Overall mortality reduced 30%, CHD deaths reduced 42%, coronary events reduced 34%
WOSCOPS [5]	4.9 (mean)	Primary prevention, pravastatin 40 mg od	6595 men aged 45—64 years	Entry > 6.5 mmol/l, reduction 20%	Cardiovascular deaths reduced 32%, coronary events reduced 31%
CARE [2]	4.0—6.2	Secondary prevention, pravastatin 40 mg od	3583 men, 576 women aged 21—75 years	Entry < 6.2 mmol/l, reduction 20%	Coronary events reduced 24%, revascularisation procedures reduced 26%

women as well as men.

Of particular interest was the comparison between baseline LDL cholesterol, clinical benefit and different degrees of LDL lowering (Fig. 1). The change in CAD risk was maximal when a 10—20% reduction in LDL had been achieved, but no benefit was seen when the baseline LDL was 3.2 mmol/l or less (Table 2).

4S Trial

The Scandinavian simvastatin survival study (4S) [3] enrolled 4,444 patients with

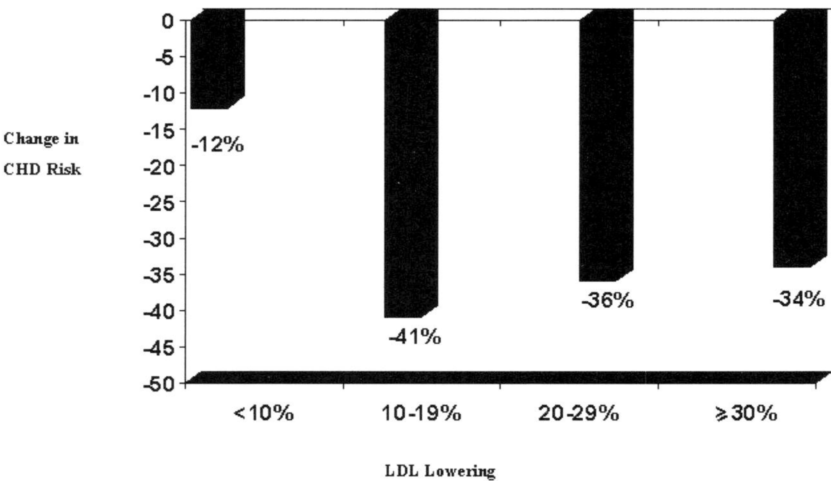

Fig. 1. Comparison between %LDL lowering and change in CHD risk in the CARE trial. No advantage is seen beyond 20%.

Table 2. Reduction in coronary events as a function of baseline plasma LDL cholesterol in the two large secondary prevention trials.

	Baseline LDL-cholesterol (mmol/l)	Reduction in coronary events
4S [3]	3.5—4.4	35%
	4.4—4.8	33%
	4.8—5.3	32%
	> 5.3	36%
CARE [2]	< 3.2	Nil
	3.2—3.8	24%
	3.8—4.5	37%

angina or previous MI and a mean total cholesterol level of 6.7 mmol/l (range 5.5—8.0). Compared with placebo over a follow-up period of 5.4 years, simvastatin reduced total cholesterol and LDL cholesterol by 25 and 35%, respectively. HDL rose by 8% and triglycerides fell by 10%. Simvastatin reduced all-cause mortality by 30% and there were marked and significant reductions in cardiovascular events, need for angioplasty and coronary artery bypass graft (CABG) as in the CARE trial (Table 1).

In the follow-up report [4] the authors looked at the relationship between the baseline cholesterol and treatment outcome. Simvastatin significantly reduced the risk of major CAD events by the same degree no matter what the baseline. In short, the percentage change in levels was an important determinant of outcome as the benefits were similar whether the cholesterol was 5.5 or 7.5 mmol/l at the start of therapy (Table 2).

WOSCOPS

The West of Scotland Coronary Prevention Study (WOSCOPS) [5] was a primary prevention trial of 6,595 high-risk Scottish men. After a period of diet, if the LDL cholesterol was greater than 4.0 but less than 6.0 mmol/l they were randomised to pravastatin (40 mg) or placebo. The mean total cholesterol at entry was 7.03 mmol/l and the LDL 4.96.

Over the average follow-up of 4.9 years, pravastatin reduced total cholesterol by 20%, LDL by 26% and raised HDL by 5%. Nonfatal MI or death from CAD was significantly reduced by 31% and death from all causes by 22%. The benefit was independent of baseline levels of total cholesterol or LDL cholesterol and appears maximal at an LDL reduction of 20% (Table 1).

Angiographic trials

We now accept that there is convincing evidence that treating hyperlipidemia slows the progression of CAD, and to a lesser extent results in some regression of CAD [6]. This angiographic evidence is associated with a reduction in clinical events, cardiovascular and overall mortality.

There have been several excellent and thoughtful reviews of the literature [6—8]. Progression of CAD can be reduced in most patients with regression occurring in 20—40%. However, in spite of "adequate therapy" progression continues in up to 40% of those treated. Most of the regression occurs in the first 2 years or so and is probably related to the modifiable lipid content of the plaque. Clinical benefits continue, almost certainly due to stabilisation of the plaque and any delay may in part be due to the time it takes for lipid lowering to be effective as a plaque stabiliser. At the clinical level it would be helpful to know if any particular groups are more or less likely to benefit and what our targets for LDL lowering are.

The Harvard project

The Harvard atherosclerosis reversibility project (HARP) [9] was designed to test whether lowering cholesterol from average (cholesterol 4.65—6.47 mmol/l) levels to low levels would slow the progression of CAD and induce regression. These baseline levels were similar to those in the Cholesterol and Recurrent Events (CARE) trial [2]. The HARP trial found coronary stenoses were not affected by therapy. At that time HARP had the lowest average LDL baseline of all regression trials (3.54 mmol/l) with most other studies reporting increased regression with LDL levels above 4.4 mmol/l. It remains important, however, not to exclude plaque stabilisation in the absence of angiographic change in HARP so that clinical benefit could still follow. A discrepancy between angiographic endpoints and clinical endpoints can be partly explained this way. However, we need to remember our priority is to reduce clinical events which is what ultimately makes the CARE trial so relevant and important.

Meta-analysis

An interesting review of the angiographic trials by Rossouw [8] noted that the average LDL reduction in the treatment groups was 26% and this related to a reduction in angiographic progression of 49%, increased odds for no change of 33% and increased odds of regression of 219% with cardiovascular clinical events reduced by 47%. He hypothesised that a minimum reduction of LDL is needed to slow the progression of CAD and that most trials achieved it. He suggested a decrease in LDL levels of 0.8 mmol/l or 20% is sufficient to modify the course of CAD.

This would fit well with the clinical event findings in CARE where the baseline LDL was 3.0—4.5 mmol/l and thus typical of most patients with CAD. In the HARP study which was small (79 patients) there was an interesting nonsignificant reduction of 33% in clinical cardiovascular events in treated patients.

LCAS

In November 1996 at the American Heart Association, the Lipoprotein and Coronary Atherosclerosis Study (LCAS) was presented [10]. This is a placebo controlled angiographic study of the effect of fluvastatin in 429 men and women with an LDL cholesterol between 3.0 and 4.95 mmol/l — a similar group to the CARE population. Fluvastatin (40 mg daily) significantly reduced LDL cholesterol by 22.5% and raised HDL cholesterol by 8.7%. The treated group experienced a significant reduction in progression of CAD, increased regression of CAD and fewer new lesions developed.

Though the study was not designed to detect differences in clinical endpoints after 130 weeks of treatment there was a nonsignificant reduction in cardiac events of 32.8% and the need for myocardial revascularisation of 33.6% (Fig. 2). LCAS is a much bigger trial than HARP and demonstrates favourable angiographic benefits in mild to moderate hypercholesterolemic patients. The benefits were seen at LDL cholesterol levels of over 4 mmol/l and below 3.4 mmol/l.

The LCAS trial and the CARE trial fit neatly together and are representative of the majority of patients with CAD. The divergence between biochemical and angiographic endpoints and clinical endpoints can be in part explained by knowing the point at which biochemical benefit is maximal and the effect of plaque stabilisation rather than the visible degree of angiographic stenosis change.

Evidence of clinical benefit

The evidence for the clinical benefits of statin therapy is overwhelming. However, the CARE trial did identify a baseline level of LDL (3.2 mmol/l) below which

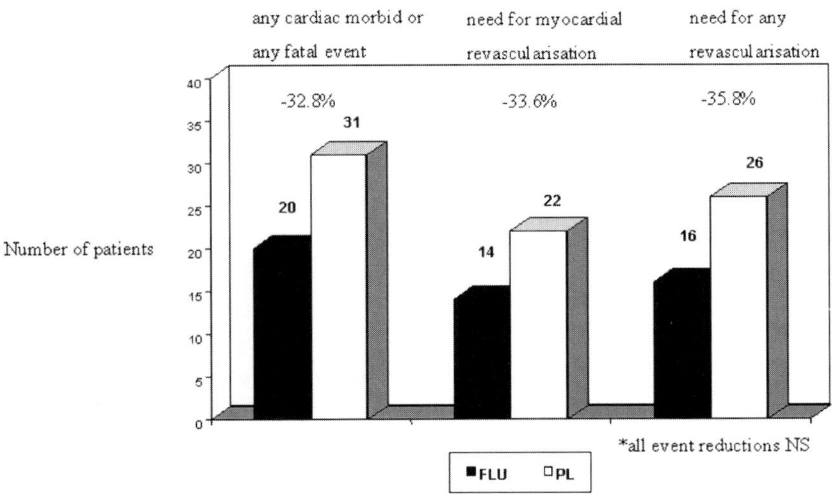

Fig. 2. LCAS trial. Clinical event reductions* in monotherapy groups.

286

there was no clear benefit from therapy. These patients may well be at risk by having a low HDL (<1.0 mmol/l) and elevated triglycerides (>2.0 mmol/l) and thereby possibly benefit from alternative therapy (e.g., fibrates).

It should also be added that CABG patients have been reported to benefit from lipid-lowering therapy with reduced progression of atherosclerosis in vein grafts when a target LDL of 1.6–2.2 mmol/l (aggressive therapy) was set compared with a "moderate" 3.4–3.6 mmol/l [11]. Using lovastatin primarily, the percentage changes for the former "aggressive" lipid-lowering group were an LDL reduction of 37–40% compared with 13–15% for the "moderate" treatment group. We do not have data for between 15 and 37% so cannot assess the effectiveness of a 20% reduction.

If we focus on the majority of patients as represented in CARE, 4S and WOSCOPS, we should be aiming to reduce LDL cholesterol by 20% and have a target LDL cholesterol of 3.2 mmol/l as the baseline for initiating (not stopping or reducing) therapy. We cannot extend this observation to those whose baseline total cholesterol is over 8.0 mmol/l or at present CABG patients, though I suspect with the latter a 20% reduction in LDL will in the majority mean a level below 3.0 mmol/l.

The statins have beneficial actions other than lowering LDL cholesterol [12] and there are differences between them in terms of potency, drug interactions and blood brain barrier penetration (with possible side effect implications). However, what is consistent between them is that they are generally safe and effective biochemically and clinically, and after all the clinical endpoints are what matters. The newest statin, atorvastatin reduces LDL cholesterol by 25–60% and triglycerides by up to 30% [13]. However, as can be seen from the above, this will not be relevant to the average patient who makes up 80% of those eligible for therapy.

It is vitally important to remember that the clinical not the biochemical benefit is our endpoint and we must not be seduced by bigger and better biochemical results if they have no clinical meaning. A sledgehammer is rarely needed to crack a nut. While atorvastatin will be of undoubted value in the more severe cases there will be no mandate to change from the tried and tested statins (fluvastatin, lovastatin, pravastatin and simvastatin) as they have been shown to, and will continue to benefit the majority. The only mandate for change would be evidence on the scale of CARE, 4S and WOSCOPS that atorvastatin was superior due to its potency and that will mean head-to-head trials.

Major trial needed

One of the remaining problems of treating hyperlipidaemia is the lack of evidence for treating those with low HDL cholesterol, elevated triglycerides and increased small dense LDL. The major weakness of the statins is the small impact on elevating HDL cholesterol which, in contrast, is a strength of the fibrates. There must be a compelling argument for a major trial comparing a statin with a statin/fibrate combination concentrating on clinical event benefits.

Table 3. Major interactions with HMG-CoA reductase inhibitors.

	Fluvastatin	Simvastatin	Pravastatin	Lovastatin	Atorvastatin	Cerivastatin
Warfarin	No	Yes	No	Yes	Yes	No
Digoxin	No	Yes	No	No	Yes	No
Nicotinic acid	No	No	No	Yes	Yes	No
Erythromycinll No		Yes	Yes	Yes	Yes	No

Based on Jokubaitis (1994).

Fluvastatin or cerivastatin with their reduced incidence of drug interactions and muscular aches would be the logical statin choices (Table 3).

We also need to know targets for benefit. Two recent excellent reviews gave no endpoint guidelines [14,15]. It looks as if most of the benefit in the baseline LDL range of 3.0—4.9 mmol/l occurs when the baseline LDL is lowered by 20%. It is helpful that this figure is applicable clinically and angiographically. Treating and preventing atheroma is a more complex entity than just lowering LDL cholesterol and more specific and targeted therapy will be advocated in the future, but it will remain vital that this complex subject is kept as simple as possible at the clinical level. While we need to know more about the effects of raising HDL cholesterol and reducing triglycerides, for the time being most patients with CAD and a baseline LDL of 3.2 mmol/l or greater should routinely be placed on a statin.

Conclusion

The cholesterol at which CAD develops in any individual is too high for that individual, the angiographic and clinical benefits of treatment demand action. It remains, however, the clinical benefit that matters and optimal treatment to achieve that should be our primary objective.

References

1. Kannel WB, Castelli WP, Gordon T. Cholesterol in the prediction of atherosclerosis disease. New perspectives based on the Framingham Study. Ann Int Med 1979;90:85—91.
2. Sachs FM, Pfeffer MA, Moye LA et al. The effect of pravastatin on coronary events after myocardial infarction in patients with average cholesterol levels. N Engl J Med 1996;335: 1001—1009.
3. Scandinavian Simvastatin Survival Study Group. Randomised trial of cholesterol lowering in 4444 patients with coronary heart disease: the Scandinavian Simvastatin Survival Study (4S). Lancet 1994;344:1383—1389.
4. Pedersen TR, Kjekshus J, Berg K et al. Baseline serum cholesterol and treatment effect in the Scandinavian Simvastatin Survival Study (4S) Lancet 1995;345:1274—1275.
5. Shepherd J, Cobbe SM, Ford I et al. Prevention of coronary heart disease with pravastatin in men with hypercholesterolemia. N Engl J Med 1995;333:1301—1307.

6. Superko HR, Krauss RM. Coronary artery disease regression: convincing evidence for the benefit of aggressive lipoprotein management. Circulation 1994;90:1056—1069.
7. Sacks FM, Gibson M, Rosner B et al. The influence of pretreatment low-density lipoprotein cholesterol concentrations on the effect of hypocholesterolemic therapy on coronary atherosclerosis in angiographic trials. Am J Cardiol 1995;76:78C—85C.
8. Rossouw JE. Lipid lowering interventions in angiographic trials. Am J Cardiol 1995;76:86C—92C.
9. Sacks FM, Pasternak RC, Gibson CM et al. Effect on coronary atherosclerosis of decrease in plasma cholesterol concentrations in normo-cholesterolaemic patients. Lancet 1994;344:1182—1186.
10. Herd JA, Ballantyne CM, Farmer JA et al. The effect of fluvastin on coronary atherosclerosis; the lipoprotein and coronary atherosclerosis study (LCAS). Am Heart Assoc 1996.
11. The Post Coronary Artery Bypass Trial Investigators. The effect of aggressive lowering of low-density lipoprotein cholesterol levels and low-dose anticoagulation on obstructive changes in saphenous vein coronary artery bypass grafts. N Engl J Med 1997;336;153—162.
12. Vaughan CJ, Murphy MB, Buckley BM. Statins do more than just lower cholesterol. Lancet 1996;348:1079—1082.
13. Nawrocki JW, Weiss SR, Davidson MH et al. Reduction of LDL cholesterol by 25% to 60% in patients with primary hypercholesterolemia by atorvastatin, a new HMGCoA reductase inhibitor. Arterioscl Thromb Vasc Biol 1995;15:678—682.
14. Oliver MF, Pyorala K, Shepherd J. Management of hyperlipidemia: why, when and how to treat. Eur Heart J 1997;18:371—375.
15. Anon. Management of hyperlipidemia. OTB 1996;34:89—93.

Optimal reduction in cardiovascular risk: who should we treat with HMG-CoA reductase inhibitors?

J.J.P. Kastelein
Department of Medical Genetics, University of British Columbia, Vancouver, British Columbia, Canada

When all the excitement and controversy ebbed away after the doubts that were raised about preventing coronary heart disease with lipid-lowering drugs by the British Medical Journal in 1992, we soon came to realize that with the advent of the HMG-CoA reductase inhibitors a new era in the treatment of atherosclerotic vascular disease had begun. Initially, all effects of these intriguing new compounds were predicted to arise from the rather simple concept of lowering plasma LDL cholesterol by upregulating LDL receptor expression at the liver cell surface [1]. Now, 10 years of study and millions of patient years later, we are beginning to doubt whether the spectacular efficacy of these drugs is indeed the sole consequence of decreasing LDL cholesterol in the circulation. Notably, a recent study demonstrated that the early use of pravastatin decreased the incidence of major rejection episodes and reduced the development of coronary vasculopathy in the 1st year after heart transplantation [2].

These effects are thought to stem from immune modulation rather than from changes in plasma lipoproteins, as was suggested by in vitro and in vivo models of natural killer-cell cytotoxicity and enhancement factor [3,4].

Since HMG Co-A reductase inhibitors not only reduce the cellular content of cholesterol but also influence a number of mevalonate-dependent processes and farnesylation of cellular proteins such as the ras oncoprotein, the cholesterol biosynthetic pathway could even be envisaged as a target for chemoprevention of cancer [5]. It is, therefore, not inconceivable that these drugs, which also act at the level of immunemodulation, cell growth, cell proliferation, monocyte chemotaxis and cytokine release, derive their benefit in the protection against the clinical sequelae of atherosclerosis partly from these processes [6—9].

In the modulation of risk factors for atherosclerotic vascular disease, proof of principle that HMG-CoA reductase inhibitors are efficacious can be provided at different levels.

Firstly, these cholesterol synthesis inhibitors produce substantial decreases in plasma total, LDL- and VLDL-cholesterol levels, and do so over a prolonged period of time. In addition, they produce a mild decrease in triglyceride levels

---

Address for correspondence: J.J.P. Kastelein MD, PhD, Department of Medical Genetics, University of British Columbia, Vancouver, British Columbia, Canada.

and a modest increase in HDL-cholesterol levels. Fortunately, the latter prospect might improve with the recent registration of atorvastatin, the latest branch on the statin tree which can reduce triglyceride levels up to 50% [10].

Secondly, evidence is rapidly accumulating to the effect that statins can significantly influence the hemostatic balance into the right direction [11]. They have also been shown to decrease platelet deposition and inhibit tissue-factor expression on human macrophages [12]. Overall, these effects might partly explain the rapid reduction in clinical events seen in prevention trials with lipid-lowering therapy and provide additional support for their use in patients with established coronary and cerebral atherosclerosis [13].

Thirdly, HMG-CoA reductase inhibitors are now thought to have the ability to re-establish endothelial function. In this hypothesis, reduction of plasma LDL-cholesterol leads to the restoration of nitric-oxide (NO) production by endothelial cells which in turn improves vasodilation and local blood flow. This has now been demonstrated conclusively in both brachial and coronary arteries [14,15]. With regard to the latter, these compounds have even recently been shown to improve silent myocardial ischemia as assessed by Holter-monitoring [16]. These findings advocate the use of these drugs in patients suffering from angina. Therefore, we should address the next question, which is whether statins can indeed decrease the incidence or severity of angina.

Apart from all these more or less "functional" changes brought about by this new class of drugs, different levels of morphological changes have also become evident.

Firstly, lipid lowering with statin therapy leads to a decrease in intimal-medial thickness of extracoronary arteries over the course of only a few years [17]. Whether this "regression" of thickened arterial wall is paralleled by similar changes in the coronary vasculature and can accurately predict clinical outcome remains to be investigated.

Secondly, at a next and undoubtedly more clinically relevant level, cholesterol synthesis inhibitors have been shown to retard the progression of coronary atherosclerosis in a number of so-called "regression" trials [18]. Slowing down the progression of coronary atherosclerosis was associated in these trials with a 30% decrease in cardiac endpoints, although the absolute difference in millimeters (often around 0.04 mm) was hardly impressive [19]. So, although these drugs induce modest anatomical changes over the course of a few years, they are much better at preventing the clinical consequences of coronary atherosclerotic vascular disease.

This really brings the next important consequence of the use of these compounds into focus, which is plaque stabilization and prevention of myocardial infarction and death [20,21]. Plaque stability is governed by both plaque morphology and lipid composition, properties which are now thought to be influenced by statin therapy [22]. With this knowledge, these medications have now become pivotal in our thinking with regards to both primary and secondary prevention of coronary artery disease.

Table 1. Priorities for lipid lowering.

Familial lipoprotein disorders.
Patients with any sign of atherosclerotic vascular disease.
Patients with diabetes or hypertension.
Persons at high risk for clinical events, e.g., asymptomatic hypercholesterolemia, postmenopausal dyslipidemic women, etc.

The notion that patients with diabetes mellitus seem to derive an even greater benefit from a statin than their nondiabetic counterparts, and the fact that these drugs also reduce stroke incidence in essentially nonhypertensive patients, also offers great hope for the prevention of cardiovascular endpoints in both diabetic and hypertensive subjects [23,24] (Table 1).

It is, therefore, not so much the question of whom to treat, but much more when to begin and when to end. We know we should treat patients with genetic lipoprotein disorders, any patient with a clinical manifestation of atherosclerotic vascular disease, patients with hypertension or diabetes and generally patients with a high overall risk for clinical events. The latter, however, is much more a question of gain of life years, long-term safety, cost-effectiveness issues and how much we are prepared to pay for prevention rather than for intervention in a later stage of the disease [25].

The next question, therefore, becomes what more is there left to strive for, have we not reached the optimum yet? The answer to that question is a very simple no. An impressive reduction of 40% in myocardial infarctions also entails that 60% of these potentially lethal occurrences were not prevented.

Fortunately, there is evidence that decreases in LDL-cholesterol of 50% or more are associated with more regression of disease and a better outcome [26]. It remains, however, to be demonstrated that LDL reductions of 60%, which now can be achieved by the newer statins, will also result in greater reductions in cardiovascular endpoints. Since statins such as atorvastatin also lower triglycerides and raise HDL-cholesterol to a significant extent, the next trials should encompass designs as far-reaching as lipid lowering vs. revascularization, an idea whose time for testing has come as Forrester and Shah so eloquently put it [27].

References

1. Summary of the second report of the National Cholesterol Education Program (NCEP) expert panel on detection, evaluation, and treatment of high blood cholesterol in adults (Adult Treatment Panel II). JAMA 1993;269:3015–3023.
2. Kobashigawa JA, Katznelson S, Laks H et al. Effect of pravastatin on outcomes after cardiac transplantation. N Engl J Med 1995;333(10):621–627.
3. McPherson R, Tsoukas C, Baines MG et al. Effects of lovastatin on natural killer cell function and other immunological parameters in man. J Clin Immunol 1993;13:439.
4. Kakkis JL, Ke B, Dawson S et al. Pravastatin increases survival and inhibits natural killer cell

enhancement factor in liver transplanted rats. J Surg Res 1997;69:393–398.

5. Casey PJ, Solski JA, Der CJ, Buss JE. p21ras is modified by a farnesyl isoprenoid. Proc Natl Acad Sci USA 1989;86:8323–8327.

6. Cutts JL, Scallen TJ, Watson J, Bankhurts AD. Role of mevalonic acid in the regulation of natural killer cell cytoxicity. J Cell Physiol 1990;139:550.

7. Vincent TS, Wulfert E, Merler E. Inhibition of growth factor signalling pathways by lovastatin. Biochem Biophys Res Commun 1991;180:1284–1289.

8. Kreuzer J, Bader J, Jahn L, Hautmann M, Kubler W, Von Hodenberg E. Chemotaxis of the monocyte cell line U937: dependence on cholesterol and early mevalonate pathway products. Atherosclerosis 1991;90:203–209.

9. Terkeltaub R, Solan J, Barry M Jr, Santoro D, Bokoch GM. Role of the mevalonate pathway of isoprenoid synthesis in IL-8 generation by activated monocytic cells. J Leuk Biol 1994;55:749–755.

10. Bakker-Arkema R, Davidson M, Goldstein R et al. Efficacy and safety of a new HMG-CoA reductase inhibitor, atorvastatin, in patients with hypertriglyceridemia. JAMA 1996;275:128–133.

11. Jerling JC, Vorster HH, Oosthuizen W, Vermaak WJH. Effect of simvastatin, a 3-hydroxy-3-methylglutaryl coenzyme A reductase inhibitor, on the haemostatic balance of familial hypercholesterolaemic subjects. Fibrinolysis 1997;11:91–97.

12. Colli S, Eligini S, Lalli M, Camera M, Paoletti R, Tremoli E. Vastatins inhibit tissue factor in cultured human macrophages. Arterioscl Thromb Vasc Biol 1997;17(2):265–272.

13. Pearson TA, Marx HJ. The rapid reduction in cardiac events with lipid-lowering therapy: mechanisms and implications. Am J Cardiol 1993;72:1072–1073.

14. Stroes ESG, Koomans HA, De Bruin TWA, Rabelink TJ. Vascular function in the forearm of hypercholesterolaemic patients off and on lipid-lowering medication. Lancet 1995;346:467–471.

15. Treasure CB, Klein JL, Weintraub WS et al. Beneficial effects of cholesterol-lowering therapy on the coronary endothelium in patients with coronary artery disease. N Engl J Med 1995;332(8):481–487.

16. Andrews TC, Raby K, Barry J et al. Effect of cholesterol reduction on myocardial ischemia in patients with coronary disease. Circulation 1997;95:324–328.

17. Fuberg CD, Adams HP Jr, Applegate WB et al. Effect of lovastatin on early carotid atherosclerosis and cardiovascular events. Circulation 1994;90(4):1679–1687.

18. de Vos J, Ruigrok PN, de Feyter PJ. Retardation of angiographic progression of coronary atherosclerosis results in improved clinical outcome. In: Fuster V (ed) Syndromes of Atherosclerosis: Correlations of Clinical Imaging. Armonk, NY: Futura Publishing Company, 1996.

19. Jukema JW, Bruschke AV, van Boven AJ et al. Effects of lipid lowering by pravastatin on progression and regression of coronary artery disease in symptomatic men with normal to moderately elevated serum cholesterol levels. The Regression Growth Evaluation Statin Study (REGRESS). Circulation 1995;91:2528.

20. Scandinavian Simvastatin Survival Study Group. Randomised trial of cholesterol lowering in 4444 patients with coronary heart disease: the Scandinavian Simvastatin Survival Study (4S). Lancet 1994;344:1383.

21. Shepherd J, Cobbe SM, Ford I et al. Prevention of coronary heart disease with pravastatin in men with hypercholesterolemia. N Engl J Med 1995;333:1301.

22. Felton CV, Crook D, Davies JM, Oliver MF. Relation of plaque lipid composition and morphology to the stability of human aortic plaques. Arterioscl Thromb Vasc Biol 1997;17(7):1337–1345.

23. Pyörälä K, Pedersen TR, Kjekshus J et al. Cholesterol lowering with simvastatin improves prognosis of diabetic patients with coronary heart disease. Diabetes Care 1997;20(4):614–620.

24. Blauw GJ, Lagaay AM, Smelt AHM, Westendorp RGJ. Strokes, statins and cholesterol: a meta-analysis of randomized, placebo-controlled, double-blind trials with HMG-CoA reductase in-

hibitors. Stroke 1997;28(5):946—950.

25. Kellett J. Likely gains in life expectancy of patients with coronary artery disease treated with HMG-CoA reductase inhibitors, as predicted by a decision analysis model. Eur J Surg 1997; 163:539—546.

26. Thompson GR. What targets should lipid-modulating therapy achieve to optimise the prevention of coronary heart disease? Atherosclerosis 1997;131:1—5.

27. Forrester JS, Shah PK. Lipid lowering vs revascularization. An idea whose time (for testing) has come. Circulation 1997;96:1360—1362.

WORKSHOPS

Extracellular matrix of the vessel and cell matrix interactions during atherogenesis

Collagens and atherosclerosis: cell-collagen interaction

Michael J. Barnes[1], C. Graham Knight[1] and Richard W. Farndale[2]
[1]Strangeways Laboratory; and [2]University Department of Biochemistry, Cambridge, UK

Abstract. Atherosclerotic disease of arteries is associated with thrombosis arising as a consequence of rupture of the atherosclerotic plaque. Thrombus formation can be attributed to the activation of blood platelets by collagens exposed as a result of plaque rupture. Our recent studies have allowed us to define a two-step mechanism of collagen-platelet interaction, involving firstly the recognition of specific sequences in collagen by the platelet collagen receptor, integrin $\alpha2\beta1$ which leads to capture of the platelet at the collagen fibre surface. Subsequent recognition of Gly-Pro-Hyp sequences in collagen by a second platelet collagen receptor, glycoprotein VI, leads to a series of specific signalling events, including activation of Fc receptor γ chain, p72syk, phospholipase Cγ2 and of p125fak, culminating in platelet activation and aggregation. The Gly-Pro-Hyp collagen sequence may provide a basis for a novel antithrombotic agent.

Keywords: collagen peptides, integrins, platelets, platelet GP VI, platelet signalling, thrombosis.

There are 19 collagens known to date, several of which occur in the vasculature. By far the most abundant of these in the blood vessel wall are the fibrous collagens, I and III.

Collagens in general fulfil a structural or mechanical role, imparting tensile strength and defining the architecture of a tissue. This structural role is particularly important as regards the stability of the atherosclerotic plaque. Plaque rupture commonly precedes heart attack or stroke. Rupture, it is considered, may occur in plaques of relatively low collagen content or as a consequence of disruption of the collagenous framework through the action of metalloproteinases [1,2].

Atherosclerosis involves the migration of smooth muscle cells (SMCs) from the media to the site of lesion development in the intima where they proliferate and produce new extracellular matrix including collagens. The latter, simply through their space-filling property, contribute to the occlusion of the lumen resulting from intimal thickening. In a similar way, they contribute to restenosis commonly occurring after angioplasty or occlusion in vein grafts, since in both cases there is movement of SMCs from media to intima where their proliferation and deposition of new matrix leads to intimal thickening.

Apart from their mechanical role, collagens provide a support or scaffold for cells and define or modulate cell function through their specific recognition of cells by interaction with collagen receptors on the cell surface. Of particular importance here in the context of this article, collagens I and III react with blood

Address for correspondence: Dr M.J. Barnes, Strangeways Laboratory, Worts Causeway, Cambridge CB1 4RN, UK. Tel.: +44-1223-234231. Fax: +44-1223-411609.

300

platelets causing their aggregation. Collagens may also play a crucial role in the regulation of SMC behaviour in the vessel wall.

Platelet activation by collagens is important in haemostasis but may also be a cause of thrombosis, the pathological expression of the haemostatic process. In particular, rupture of the atherosclerotic plaque leads to acute thrombosis resulting in unstable angina, myocardial infarction, or stroke. In our view, and that of others [3], this is a consequence of platelet activation by collagen exposed as a result of plaque rupture. Likewise, thrombosis associated with angioplasty or thrombolytic treatment of an occlusive clot may also involve platelet activation by collagens exposed at a damaged vessel surface. Restenosis after angioplasty is considered to involve platelet activation, arguably again by vessel wall collagens.

SMCs in the media are normally in a quiescent, contractile state. The advent of atherosclerotic disease involves the appearance in the intima of a set of cells expressing the undifferentiated, synthetic phenotype, which have migrated from the media. These cells proliferate and produce new matrix, leading to intimal thickening. A similar process underlies restenosis after angioplasty and intimal thickening in vein grafts. There is evidence that collagen IV in the basal lamina around the SMC may maintain the differentiated contractile phenotype through contact with the cell via the collagen receptor, the integrin $\alpha 1\beta 1$. Expression of the synthetic phenotype may involve the disruption of the basal lamina by metalloproteinases. These cells, released from the constraints of the basal lamina, may come to express a different collagen receptor, the integrin $\alpha 2\beta 1$, which allows migration of the cells into the intima along the surface of fibres of collagens I and III [4—8].

This article will focus in particular on the interaction of vessel wall collagens I and III with platelets and we will describe recent advances in our understanding of the mechanism of collagen-platelet interaction that could provide a basis for a specific inhibitor of the interaction that might serve as a novel antithrombotic agent.

Collagen interaction with platelets involves firstly their adhesion to the collagen fibre surface. Platelets then spread on the surface and undergo a process of activation, leading to the secretion of platelet products, the synthesis and release of thromboxane A_2 and a conformational change in the receptor integrin $\alpha IIb/\beta 3$ (glycoprotein (GP) IIb/IIIa) which allows binding of fibrinogen, essential for platelet-platelet interaction (platelet aggregation). We have been concerned in the past to define platelet-reactive amino acid sequences in collagen. Fragmentation studies pointed to the existence of different domains in collagen recognizing separate receptors for adhesion and aggregation and raised the possibility of a two-step process of interaction involving a primary adhesive receptor with subsequent activatory signalling through a second receptor which culminates in platelet aggregation [9,10].

Fragmentation studies were unable to pinpoint platelet-reactive loci in collagen precisely and we resorted to the use of synthetic peptides to define the nature of collagen's platelet-reactive sequences. At the outset, we synthesized very simple collagen-like peptides (CRPs, collagen-related peptides) comprising basically a repeat Gly-Pro-Hyp sequence. Since this sequence is common in all collagens and since we anticipated that highly specific sequences in collagen would be required for platelet reactivity, we assumed these peptides would be inactive. We prepared two peptides, GCP*(GPP*)$_{10}$GCP*G (single letter amino acid nomenclature; P* = Hyp) and a similar peptide with lysine (K) in place of cysteine (C). The introduction of C and K residues permitted the formation of a polymeric structure by cross-linking. These peptides spontaneously formed a highly stable collagen triple-helical conformation. Molecules associated to form microaggregates which were stabilized by cross-linking. To our surprise, these peptides proved highly platelet-reactive, even more potent than collagen fibres. Like collagen, platelet reactivity was dependent on both the tertiary (triple-helical) and quaternary (polymeric) structures. The monomeric (uncross-linked) peptide inhibited aggregation by both collagen fibres and cross-linked peptide indicating recognition by the peptide of a collagen receptor essential for platelet activation by collagen [11].

Several platelet surface proteins have been implicated as collagen receptors including integrin $\alpha2\beta1$, GP IV (CD36), GP VI and GP IIb/IIIa [12]. In particular, $\alpha2\beta1$ was commonly viewed as a crucial receptor [13]. However, several lines of evidence indicated that the reactivity of CRPs was not dependent on this receptor. Anti-$\alpha2\beta1$ monoclonal antibodies (mAbs) did not prevent platelet adhesion to CRPs nor aggregation induced by these peptides [11]. There was no binding of CRPs to the isolated A domain of $\alpha2\beta1$ known to be involved in the recognition of collagen by $\alpha2\beta1$ [14]. No binding of $\alpha2\beta1$ to CRPs immobilized on affinity columns was observed (authors' unpublished data). Furthermore, there was no adhesion of platelets to CRPs under flow conditions [15]. $\alpha2\beta1$ is known to be essential for platelet adhesion to collagen under flow so the implication was that CRPs do not react with $\alpha2\beta1$. Finally, platelet signalling in response to CRPs, which, as discussed below, closely resembles signalling induced by collagen, is unaffected by anti-$\alpha2\beta1$ mAbs [16,17].

The question, therefore, arises as to the identity of the signalling receptor recognized by CRPs. In collaborative studies with B. Kehrel (Münster) and M. Okuma (Kyoto), we sought to identify the receptor by investigating the interaction of CRPs with platelets having defined receptor deficiencies. These studies indicated that neither CD36, GP IIb/IIIa, nor von Willebrand factor (vWf) (which serves as an indirect receptor by bridging between collagen and the platelet receptor GP Ib) were the primary binding site for CRP interaction with platelets. However, GP VI-deficient platelets were totally unreactive towards CRP. There was no aggregation, no secretion, as measured by the surface expression of CD 62 and CD 63, and no activation of GP IIb/IIIa, as measured by the surface binding of fibrinogen. Likewise collagen failed to aggregate or cause secretion in GP VI-deficient platelets, although interestingly, fibrinogen binding was not totally absent [18]. In confirmation of the recognition of CRP by GP VI, we have found that adhesion to CRP, largely divalent cation-independent, is totally blocked by an anti-GP VI antiserum [19] even though the antibody concerned is an activatory antibody and stimulates activation-dependent adhesion to collagen fibres (Table 1). Likewise adhesion is blocked by the Fab fragment derived from the activatory antibody (data not shown). In contrast, adhesion to monomeric collagen immobilized on plastic is totally prevented by anti-$\alpha2\beta1$ mAbs but is enhanced by the anti-GP VI antiserum, presumably due to the deposition of platelet aggregates formed as a consequence of activation by the antiserum.

Confirmation of the importance of GP VI as a signalling receptor essential for platelet activation has come from recent signalling studies undertaken in collaboration with S.P. Watson and colleagues in Oxford. These studies have revealed that CRP signals in the same specific manner as collagen. A sequence of signalling events has been delineated involving firstly an association of GP VI, following ligand binding, with the Fc receptor (FcR) γ chain, which following its activation by tyrosine phosphorylation associates with the intracellular kinase p72syk which in turn, after activation, induces the activation of phospholipase Cγ2 [16,17,20] and, further downstream still, the activation of p125fak [21]. Signalling by CRP is $\alpha2\beta1$-independent [16,17]. Activation of p72syk and PLCγ2 by collagen is partially reduced by anti-$\alpha2\beta1$ mAbs but this may reflect simply impaired or reduced binding of collagen to platelets because of the blocking of $\alpha2\beta1$ [17]. Fak activation by both collagen and CRP is unaffected by anti-$\alpha2\beta1$ mAbs (Fig. 1). Collagen provides the first example of a nonimmune physiological stimulus acting through an immune receptor signalling mechanism (involving activation of FcR γ chain), and GP VI represents the first nonimmune receptor to be reported associating with FcR γ chain. Consistent with platelet activation by CRP via GP VI, M. Okuma and colleagues in Kyoto have found a total absence of protein tyrosine phosphorylation in GP VI-deficient platelets stimulated with CRP [22].

We are presently investigating whether the recognition of GPP* in collagen by GP VI is basically a recognition of the collagen triple helix per se or whether GPP* represents a specific recognition sequence. CRP may provide a basis for

Table 1. Platelet adhesion to CRP: affect of anti-GP VI.

		% Adhesion	
		2 mM Mg^{2+}	2 mM EDTA
CRP	Control	19	17
	+ 6F1	22	17
	+ anti-GP VI	4	3
Collagen	Control	16	4
	+ 6F1	3	ND
	+ anti-GP VI	61	ND
BSA		3	ND

Note: Adhesion was measured in 96-well plates for 1 h at 37°C. 6F1 (2 µg/ml) is an anti-integrin $\alpha2\beta1$ mAb. Anti-GP VI was an anti-GP VI antiserum (10%).

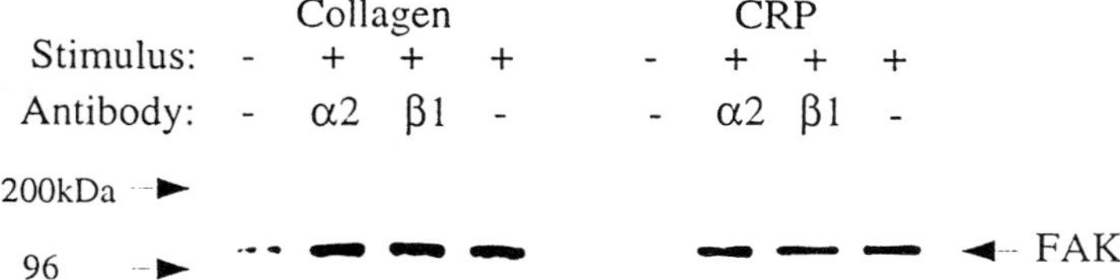

Fig. 1. Activation of p125fak stimulated by either collagen or CRP is α2β1-independent. Platelets were incubated with either type I collagen fibres (25 µg/ml) or cross-linked CRP (5 µg/ml) for 5 min, then lysed. p125fak was immunoprecipitated, separated by SDS-PAGE and immunodetected using antiphosphotyrosine. Platelets used to prepare lanes marked α2 or β1 were preincubated with antibodies directed against these integrin subunits (authors' unpublished data with M. Achison).

the construction of a highly specific inhibitor of collagen-platelet interaction.

Whilst GP VI can be seen as an essential activatory receptor for collagen, there is no doubt of the importance also of α2β1 [13] which we regard as basically an adhesive receptor essential for attachment of platelets under flow. At present, details of signalling through α2β1 and its difference to signalling via GP VI are unclear [23].

On the basis of the inhibitory activity of short, linear, collagen-based peptides, an α2β1 recognition sequence in collagen I has been attributed to the DGEA sequence representing residues 435—438 of the α1(I) chain, occurring in the collagen fragment α1(I)CB3 [24]. However, we have been unable to obtain inhibition with DGEA-containing peptides. The equivalent fragment in collagen III is α1(III)CB4. We have synthesized this fragment as a series of seven overlapping triple-helical peptides and have located an α2β1-recognition sequence involving residues 522—528 of the α1(III) chain comprising the sequence GGPP*GPR (in bovine collagen III) [25]. An antibody raised against human collagen III and blocking collagen III-induced platelet aggregation recognizes precisely this same locus in the human collagen [26]. This region of the collagen III molecule would seem to be crucial for its platelet reactivity since there may be close by a binding site for vWf and one for LAPP (leech antiplatelet protein) [27], which specifically blocks collagen-induced platelet aggregation (unpublished data of M. Verkleij and J.J. Sixma in collaboration with C.G. Knight and M.J. Barnes).

In summary, considerable advance has been made recently in our understanding of collagen-platelet interaction which has allowed us to propose a two-step mechanism, as presented in Fig. 2, in which adhesion is mediated firstly via vWf bridging between collagen and platelet GP Ib and by the recognition of specific α2β1-binding sites in collagen which allows the complete arrest of platelets on the fibre surface under flow. This is followed by a second activatory step involving recognition of GPP* sequences in collagen by GP VI, leading to specific signalling culminating in platelet activation and aggregation [15]. It is a matter of some interest as to whether other instances of cell-collagen interaction may involve sequential recognition of two or more receptors.

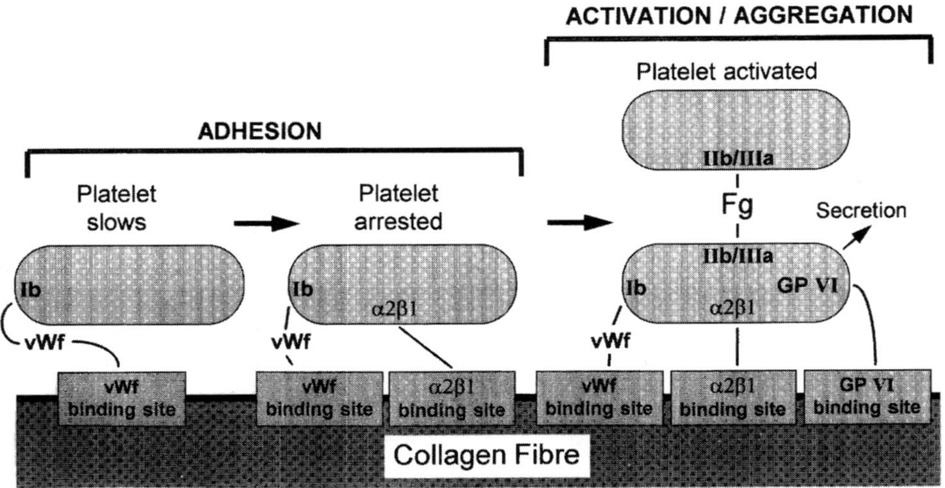

Fig. 2. Two-step mechanism of collagen-platelet interaction. Interaction involves firstly platelet adhesion to collagen under flow, mediated by vWf and the platelet receptor α2β1, and then activation through platelet receptor GP VI culminating in platelet aggregation. Based on [15] and Verkleij et al., submitted to Blood.

Acknowledgements

The authors are grateful for financial support from the British Heart Foundation and the Medical Research Council of which M.J. Barnes is a member of the External Scientific Staff. Acknowledgements are also expressed to our colleagues M. Achison, L.F. Morton and A.R. Peachey and to our collaborators M.J. Humphries (Manchester), B. Kehrel (Münster), M. Okuma (Kyoto), J.J. Sixma (Utrecht) and S.P. Watson (Oxford). We are grateful to B. Coller for the gift of 6F1 and to M. Okuma and H. Takayama for gifts of anti-GP VI antiserum.

References

1. Fuster V, Fallon JT, Badimon JJ, Nemerson Y. The unstable atherosclerotic plaque: clinical significance and therapeutic intervention. Thromb Haemost 1997;78:247–255.
2. Newby AC. Molecular and cell biology of native coronary and vein-graft atherosclerosis: regulation of plaque stability and vessel-wall remodelling by growth factors and cell-extracellular matrix interactions. Cor Artery Dis 1997;8:213–224.
3. van Zanten GH, de Graaf S, Slootweg PJ, Heijnen HFG, Connolly TM, de Groot PG, Sixma JJ. Increased platelet deposition on atherosclerotic coronary arteries. J Clin Invest 1994;93: 615–632.
4. Skinner MP, Raines EW, Ross R. Dynamic expression of α1β1 and α2β1 integrin receptors by human vascular smooth muscle cells: α2β1 integrin is required for chemotaxis across type I collagen-coated membranes. Am J Pathol 1994;145:1070–1081.
5. Gotwals PJ, Chi-Rosso G, Lindner V, Yang J, Ling L, Fawell SE, Koteliansky VE. The α1β1 integrin is expressed during neointima formation in rat arteries and mediates collagen matrix

reorganization. J Clin Invest 1996;97:2469—2477.

6. Seki J, Koyama N, Kovach NL, Yednock T, Clowes AW, Harlan JM. Regulation of $\beta1$-integrin function in cultured human vascular smooth muscle cells. Circ Res 1996;78:596—605.

7. Pickering JG, Uniyal S, Ford CM, Chau T, Laurin MA, Chow LH, Ellis CG, Fish J, Chan BMC. Fibroblast growth factor-2 potentiates vascular smooth muscle cell migration to platelet-derived growth factor: upregulation of $\alpha2\beta1$ integrin and disassembly of actin filaments. Circ Res 1997;80:627—637.

8. Thyberg J, Blomgren K, Roy J, Tran PK, Hedin U. Phenotypic modulation of smooth muscle cells after arterial injury is associated with changes in the distribution of laminin and fibronectin. J Histochem Cytochem 1997;45:837—846.

9. Morton LF, Peachey AR, Barnes MJ. Platelet-reactive sites in collagens type I and type III: evidence for separate adhesion and aggregatory sites. Biochem J 1989;258:157—163.

10. Zijenah LS, Barnes MJ. Platelet-reactive sites in human collagens I and III: evidence for cell-recognition sites in collagen unrelated to RGD and like sequences. Thrombos Res 1990; 59:553—566.

11. Morton LF, Hargreaves PG, Farndale RW, Young RD, Barnes MJ. Integrin $\alpha2\beta1$-independent activation of platelets by collagen: collagen tertiary (triple-helical) and quaternary (polymeric) structures are sufficient alone for activity. Biochem J 1995;306:337—344.

12. Kehrel B. Platelet receptors for collagens. Platelets 1995;6:11—16.

13. Santoro SA, Zutter MM. The $\alpha2\beta1$ integrin: a collagen receptor on platelets and other cells. Thromb Haemost 1995;74:813—821.

14. Tuckwell DS, Reid KBM, Barnes MJ, Humphries MJ. Integrin $\alpha2$ A-domain binds specifically to a range of collagens but is not a general receptor for the collagenous motif. Eur J Biochem 1996;241:732—739.

15. Verkleij MW, Morton LF, Barnes MJ, Gralnick HR, de Groot PG, Sixma JJ. Simple collagen-like peptides support platelet adhesion under static but not under flow conditions: interaction via $\alpha2\beta1$ with specific collagen sequences is a requirement to withstand shear forces. Thromb Haemost 1997;77(Suppl):11 (Abstract).

16. Gibbins J, Asselin J, Farndale R, Barnes M, Law C-L, Watson SP. Collagen stimulates tyrosine phosphorylation of the Fc receptor γ chain in platelets. J Biol Chem 1996;271:18095—18099.

17. Asselin J, Gibbins JM, Achison M, Lee YH, Morton LF, Farndale RW, Barnes MJ, Watson SP. A collagen-like peptide stimulates tyrosine phosphorylation of syk and phospholipase $C\gamma2$ in platelets independent of the integrin $\alpha2\beta1$. Blood 1997;89:1235—1242.

18. Kehrel B, Wierwille S, Clemetson KJ, Anders O, Steiner M, Knight CG, Farndale RW, Okuma M, Barnes MJ. Glycoprotein VI is a major collagen receptor for platelet activation: it recognizes the platelet-activating quaternary structure of collagen, whereas CD36, GPIIb/IIIa and VWf do not. Blood 1997;(In press).

19. Sugiyama T, Okuma M, Ushikubi F, Sensaki S, Kanaji K, Uchino H. A novel platelet aggregating factor found in a patient with defective collagen-induced platelet aggregation and autoimmune thrombocytopenia. Blood 1987;69:1712—1720.

20. Gibbins JM, Okuma M, Farndale R, Barnes M, Watson SP. Glycoprotein VI is the collagen receptor in platelets which underlies tyrosine phosphorylation of the Fc receptor γ-chain. FEBS Lett 1997;413:255—259.

21. Achison M, Knight CG, Barnes MJ, Farndale RW. Activation by collagen and a collagen-related peptide of the intracellular tyrosine kinase, p125fak, in human platelets which is independent of the integrin $\alpha2\beta1$. Thromb Haemost 1997;77(Suppl):156(Abstract).

22. Okuma M, Ichinohe T, Takayama H, Kehrel B, Knight CG, Farndale RW, Barnes MJ. Defective activation of GP VI-deficient platelets by triple-helical collagen-like peptides. Thromb Haemost 1997;77(Suppl):376 (Abstract).

23. Keely PJ, Parise LV. The $\alpha2\beta1$ integrin is a necessary coreceptor for collagen-induced activation of syk and the subsequent phosphorylation of phospholipase $C\gamma2$ in platelets. J Biol Chem 1996;271:26668—26676.

24. Staatz WD, Fok KF, Zutter MM, Adans SP, Rodriguez BA, Santoro SA. Identification of a tetra-peptide recognition sequence for the $\alpha 2\beta 1$ integrin in collagen. J Biol Chem 1991;266: 7363—7367.
25. Morton LF, Peachey AR, Knight CG, Farndale RW, Barnes MJ. The platelet reactivity of synthetic peptides based on collagen III fragment $\alpha 1$(III)CB4: evidence for an integrin $\alpha 2\beta 1$ recognition site involving residues 522—528 of the $\alpha 1$(III) collagen chain. J Biol Chem 1997; 272:11044—11048.
26. Glattauer V, Werkmeister JA, Kirkpatrick A, Ramshaw JAM. Identification of the epitope for a monoclonal antibody that blocks platelet aggregation induced by type III collagen. Biochem J 1997;323:45—49.
27. Connolly TM, Jacobs JW, Condra C. An inhibitor of collagen-stimulated platelet activation from the salivary glands of the Haementeria officinalis leech. J Biol Chem 1992;267: 6893—6898.

Proteoglycan — lipoprotein interactions

Magdolna Bihari-Varga
First Department of Pediatrics, Haynal I. University of Health Sciences, Budapest, Hungary

Abstract. Proteoglycans (PGs), biopolymers containing proteins and polysaccharide subunits (glycosaminoglycans (GAGs)) are enriched in the arterial wall and accumulate during the early phases of atherosclerosis. This accumulation predisposes the intima to lipid deposition, due to the specific ability of PGs to interact with serum lipoprotein (LPs). Altered length or molecular weight of the GAG chain or modification of core-protein structure, may exhibit different affinities for LPs. Complex formation with PGs induces further changes in the physical structure, mobility and susceptibility to oxidation of LP molecules, enhancing their deposition into the extracellular space. The complexes, taken up by endothelial and smooth muscle cells, influence the proliferation and differentiation of the cells. Interaction of modified LPs with monocytes, and their transformation into the foam cells, may also depend on interactions with PGs.

Keywords: arterial proteoglycans, atherogenesis, lipoproteins.

Proteoglycans (PGs) are biologically very active substances. They are involved in the activation and inhibition of a wide variety of enzymes, as well as in anticoagulative actions, and influence hemopoietic cell functions and immune reactions. Also, the migration, adhesion and proliferation of cells by various mechanisms, are essential in lipid clearance, in binding of fibrillar proteins, water and electrolytes (stable assembly of extracellular matrix).

Synthesis of specific families of PGs by arterial smooth muscle cells (SMC) or endothelial cells (EC) is under the control of a specific set of cytokines and growth factors. The regulation involves both the core-protein synthesis and the glycosaminoglycan (GAG) synthetic machinery.

Vascular PGs can be classified according to the GAG component of the molecule, e.g., chondroitin sulfate (CSA) could be identified in versican/aggrecan; dermatan sulfate (DS) was found in decorin and biglycan; perlecan and sindecans consist of heparan sulfate (HS), whereas lumican is built up of keratan sulfate (KS) chains.

The PG macromolecules differ in size, localization (matrix, cell surface, basement membrane, cell), number of GAG chains, degree of sulfation, link- and core-protein structure, gene organization and transcriptional control. Changes induced in the concentration, composition, structure or metabolism of PGs influence their biological activity and might initiate various pathological pro-

Address for correspondence: M. Bihari-Varga, First Department of Pediatrics, Haynal I. University, Heim Pál Hospital, H-1089 Budapest, Üllõi út 86, Hungary.

308

cesses or diseases.

In atherosclerosis the total amount of GAG/PG increases in the plasma and in certain areas of the arterial wall. Concerning the relative content of PGs, atherosclerotic arteries contain higher CS and DS amounts, whereas HSPGs are decreased [1]. Changes in the pattern or structure of GAG within PGs accumulated in the intimal lesions result in SMC proliferation, increase in the permeability and decrease in antithrombogenic activity.

Focal metabolic and biochemical alterations in PG may contribute to the development of atherosclerotic plaques since these molecules are capable of specifically binding and holding LDL that insudates into the arterial wall after endothelial dysfunction.

The formation of in vitro GAG/PG-LDL complexes was studied exhaustively in the last 40 years through a variety of techniques [2–4]. These complexes are supposed to be formed by electrostatic forces between negatively charged groups of GAG chains and charged components of lipoproteins [5], but might also be stabilized by interactions between the hydrophobic portions of the reacting molecules [6,7]. Altered GAG chain structure induced by TGF-β 1 and PDGF may exhibit different affinities for serum lipoprotein (LP). For example, CSAPGs isolated from proliferating SMC bind with greater affinity to LDL than those isolated from quiescent SMC. Length and molecular weight of CS chains have been positively correlated with their ability to complex to LDL.

Evidence for the existence in vivo of PG-LDL complexes has been obtained by biochemical and histochemical studies, clearly supporting the idea that PGs may play a role in atherogenesis by physically trapping LDL. CSAPG-LP complexes have been isolated from atherosclerotic lesions [8] and specific regions within the apolipoprotein moiety of the LPs interact with CS chains isolated from vascular tissue. CSA has been colocalized with apoB in the extracellular matrix of atherosclerotic arteries and colocalization of apoE-containing LPs with biglycan had been demonstrated as well.

Extensive research provided proof that genetic, humoral or tissue modifications of LDL increase their reactivity with PGs. Such modifications might be caused by the absorption of GAG circulating in soluble form in human plasma, especially when the concentration or activity of natural inhibitors is changed [9], or when Lp (a) level is elevated [10]. Biological modification might occur via freeradical induced peroxidation initiated by EC [11].

On the other hand, interaction with PG is able to modify LDL structure. LDL alterations involve a loss of lipid-protein organization, alterations in the thermotropic properties of the LP core and increased susceptibility to proteolysis or oxidation [12–14].

Modified LP preparations, as well as their PG complexes, taken up by EC and SMC, via the small PG receptor, the LDL receptor and/or the scavenger receptor, influence the proliferation and differentiation of cells and proved to be cytotoxic to EC in culture [15]. Furthermore, they are increasingly taken up by macrophages and contribute to foam-cell formation [16,17].

Conclusion

This short review concentrated on the role that PGs play in vascular wall pathology. We now know that a number of factors contribute to alterations of the PG content and composition of the arteries. Such alterations may, in turn, generate conditions in which PGs can form complexes with LPs. Among the several forms of LDL the small dense TG-rich particles, oxidised LDL and Lp (a) are supposed to be the most atherogenic, partially because of their stronger affinity to PGs.

Acknowledgements

This study was supported by a Hungarian Scientific Research Programme Grant No. OTKA 016111.

References

1. Cherchi GM, Coinu R, Demuro P, Formato M. Structural and functional modifications of human aorta proteoglycans in atherosclerosis. Matrix 1990;10:362—372.
2. Bihari-Varga M, Gergely J, Gerő S. Further investigations on complex formation in vitro between aortic mucopolysaccharides and beta-lipoproteins. J Atheroscl Res 1964;4:106—110.
3. Hollander W. Unified concept of the role of acidic mucopolysaccharides and connective tissue proteins in the accumulation of lipids, lipoproteins and calcium in the atherosclerotic plaque. Exp Mol Pathol 1976;25:106—120.
4. Camejo G. The interaction of lipids and lipoproteins with the extracellular matrix of arterial tissue. Adv Lipid Res 1982;19:1—53.
5. Bihari-Varga M, Végh M. Quantitative studies on the complexes formed between aortic mucopolysaccharides and serum lipoproteins. Biochim Biophys Acta 1967;144:202—210.
6. Camejo G, Ponce E, Lopez F, Starosta R, Hurt E, Romano M. Partial structure of the active moiety of lipoprotein complexing proteoglycan from human aorta. Atherosclerosis 1983;48: 241—254.
7. Wegrowski J, Moczar M, Robert L, Dachet C. Comparative study of the precipitation of low density lipoprotein by aortic proteodermatan sulphate and heparin. Int J Biol Macromol 1990; 12:213—217.
8. Srinivasasn SR, Yost C, Bhandaru RR, Radhakrishnamurthy B, Berenson GS. Lipoprotein-glycosaminoglycan interactions in aortae of rabbits fed atherogenic diets containing different fats. Atherosclerosis 1982;43:289—301.
9. Kempen HJM, Buytenhek M, Gruber E, Bihari-Varga M. Factor, present in plasma, inhibiting the interaction of low density lipoprotein with arterial proteoglycan. Atherosclerosis 1989; 78:137—144.
10. Bihari-Varga M, Gruber E, Rothender M, Zechner R, Kostner GM. Interaction of Lp (a) and low density lipoprotein with glycosaminoglycans from human aorta. Arteriosclerosis 1988;8: 851—857.
11. Steinbrecher VP, Zhang H, Lougheed M. Role of oxidatively modified low density lipoprotein in atherosclerosis. Free Radic Biol Med 1990;9:155—168.
12. Bihari-Varga M, Sztatisz J, Gál S. Changes in the physical behavior of low density lipoprotein in the presence of glycosaminoglycans and high density lipoproteins. Atherosclerosis 1981;39: 19—23.
13. Bihari-Varga M, Camejo G, Horn MC, Szabó D, Lopez F, Gruber E. Structure of low density lipoprotein in complexes formed with arterial matrix components. Int J Biol Macromol 1983:

5:58—62.
14. Cherchi GM, Formato M, Demuro P, Masserini M, Varani J, DeLuca G. Modifications of low density lipoprotein induced by the interaction with human plasma glycosaminoglycan-protein complexes. Biochim Biophys Acta 1994;1212:345—352.
15. Bihari-Varga M. Lp (a) and the arterial wall. In: Woodford FP, Davignon J, Sniderman A (eds) Atherosclerosis X. Amsterdam: Elsevier Science B.V., 1995;898—902.
16. Suzu S, Inaba T. Proteoglycan form of macrophage colony-stimulating factor binds low density lipoprotein. J Clin Invest 1994;94:1637—1641.
17. Srinivasan SR, Xu JH, Vijayagopal P, Radhakrishnamurthy B, Berenson GS. Low density lipoprotein binding affinity of arterial chondroitin sulfate proteoglycan variants modulates cholesterol ester accumulation in macrophages. Biochim Biophys Acta 1995;1272:61—67.

The elastin-laminin receptor in atherogenesis

Marie Paule Jacob
UFR de Médecine, Paris, France

Introduction

The formation of atherosclerotic plaque is described as a process where deposition of lipids, entry of circulatory and inflammatory cells, proliferation and migration of smooth muscle cells are the major events. However, the modification and alteration of the extracellular matrix are also important. In the young normal aorta, the endothelial cells are layered on well-organized basement membrane and subendothelial space; and smooth muscle cells are interspersed between well-defined elastic lamella. Early in the atherosclerotic process, the alteration and fragmentation of the internal elastic lamina and innermost elastic lamella are observed.

Elastin itself participates in the lipid deposition during the fatty steak formation [1,2]. This deposition is potentiated by calcium. The binding of lipids and calcium to elastin increase its susceptibility to elastolytic enzymes. As the elastin degradation occurs, elastin peptides are produced. These elastin peptides can act on adjacent cells or on blood cells as elastin peptides are detectable in blood [3,4].

The elastin receptor and transduction mechanism

A high-affinity receptor for elastin peptides has been detected on blood cells and cells of the arterial wall: monocytes, polymorphonuclear neutrophils, fibroblasts, smooth muscle cells and endothelial cells [5—7]. The elastin receptor is composed of three proteic components: two transmembrane subunits of 61 and 55 kDa and one extracellular subunit of 67 kDa. This latter subunit brings the binding site for elastin peptides as well as a galactoside binding site. The binding of lactose or other galactosides like N-acetylgalactosamine glycosaminoglycans (chondroitin sulfate or dermatan sulfate) to the 67 kDa elastin subunit induces a lower affinity of this subunit for elastin peptides, as well as for the two transmembrane subunits [8—10]. In presence of galactosides, the 67 kDa subunit is thus eluted from the cell surface. The receptor is coupled to a phospholipase C through a pertussis toxin-sensitive G protein. The binding of elastin peptides to

Address for correspondence: M.P. Jacob, Inserm U 460, UFR de Médecine X. Bichat, 16 rue H. Huchard, 75870 Paris Cedex 18, France.

its receptor triggers several intracellular events: increase of free calcium and inositol phosphate concentrations [5], modifications of ion fluxes (increase of calcium and sodium influxes, decrease of calcium efflux and potassium influx) [11] and production of NO (in endothelial cells).

Biological properties of elastin peptides

The presence of the elastin receptor on several cell types confers to elastin peptides several biological functions: chemotactic activity in monocytes [12], fibroblasts [13] and smooth muscle cells [14], stimulation of elastin fiber adhesion to vascular smooth muscle cells [15] and fibroblasts [16], release of lytic enzymes (elastase and β-glucuronidase) and oxygen-free radicals from leukocytes [17].

The elastin receptor acts also as a chaperon protein during the elastin synthesis process and direct tropoelastin to a site on the cell surface for assembly into the extracellular matrix. At that site, after the binding of galactosides to the 67 kDa subunit, the receptor-bound tropoelastin is released (possibly using the lectin nature of the elastin receptor) and incorporated into the extracellular matrix [8–10].

The two more recently described effects of elastin peptides were their effects on the vascular tone and on lymphocytes.

Effect of elastin peptides on vascular tone

Added to rat aortic rings, elastin peptides induce a dose- and endothelium-dependent relaxant action which is higher on aortic rings precontracted with noradrenaline 10^{-6} M than on rings tested at their resting tone [18,19]. As L-Name 10^{-5} M and indomethacin 10^{-5} M completely inhibit the effect of elastin peptides, it can be concluded that elastin peptides induce vasodilation through the synthesis of prostanoids and the production of NO. Thus, elastin peptides released during the degradation of elastin may contribute to the control of vascular tone in physiological and pathological conditions.

Detection of the elastin receptor on lymphocytes

Resting lymphocytes isolated from tonsils do not express the elastin receptor [20–22]. When they are nonspecifically stimulated by phytohemagglutin P, they expressed the receptor: $\approx 30\%$ of cells express it after 4 days in culture, $\approx 70\%$, after 5 days in culture; these percentages are slightly increased when 2 µg/ml of elastin peptides are added in the culture medium [20]. It appears that the helper (CD4+) and memory (CD45RO+) T cells exhibit the strongest increase of expression of elastin receptor in the presence of 2 µg/ml elastin peptides [21].

In the presence of 0.2–10 µg/ml elastin peptides, lymphocytes show increased proliferation and increased production of an elastase-type serine protease. At higher concentrations (1–5 mg/ml), elastin peptides induce death of lymphocytes. At the higher concentration tested (5 mg/ml), it could be shown, using the TUNEL method, that this death is predominantly due to apoptosis.

As lymphocytes are present in atherosclerotic plaques, it was interesting to visualize if these lymphocytes possess the elastin receptor. Using double immunolabelling, it can be shown that 50—60% of lymphocytes express the 67 kDa subunit of the elastin receptor. Adjacent smooth muscle cells also express the receptor.

Sequences of elastin recognized by the elastin receptor

Several oligopeptides mimic the effect of elastin peptides [23—31] (Table 1). Several of them have been tested using the chemotaxis assay. Although desmosine, a specific cross-link of elastin, is not required for elastin chemotaxis, it is itself,

Table 1. Sequences of elastin and analogues recognized by the elastin receptor.

A	V G V A P G	Fibroblastes [24], monocytes [24], endothelial cells [25], neutrophils [26]
B	L G T I P G [Laminin]	Fibroblasts [27]
C	P G A I P G	Fibroblasts [28]
	V G A M P G V G M A P G V G S L P G V G L S P G A G A I P G P G A V P G	Fibroblasts, neutrophils [29] (67 kDa, monoclonal antibody BA-4)
D	G L V P G F G V G G V A P G V G A P G	Monocytes [30]
E	G F G V G.A G V P A G V P.G F G V G G F G V G	Endothelial cells [25], fibroblasts [31]
F		Polymorphonuclear neutrophils [26]: increases of $[Ca^{2+}]_i$ and $O_2{}^-$ production:
	V G V A P G	+++
	P G V G V A	+++
	V G V G V A	+
	G V G V A	—
	V G V A	—
	V G V	—

Note: see the description of this table in the text.

a chemoattactant [23]. The other amino acid sequences of elastin involved in the interaction with different cell types are hydrophobic. The most extensively tested sequence is the hexapeptide VGVAPG, a sequence which is repeated several times in human and bovine elastins (Table 1 (A)) [24—26]. In addition to interacting with elastin, the 67 kDa elastin receptor also binds laminin. Several experimental data suggest that the elastin receptor and the 67 kDa laminin receptor are the same protein [27]. The hexapeptide sequence LGTIPG of the human laminin B1 chain has hydrophobic properties similar to VGVAPG, binds to the elastin receptor and induces a chemotactic response in fibroblasts (Table 1 (B)) [27].

Through their ability to induce lactose-sensitive chemotaxis in fibroblast and to bind the monoclonal antibody BA4 to VGVAPG, several related sequences were selected from an "epitope library" [28,29]. Some of the selected sequences are not present in the elastin molecule, especially those containing methionine residues, but all present structural similarities (Table 1 (C)). It should be noted that while amino acid substitutions can be made within the binding sequence, to date successful substitutions have involved only the small nonpolar or uncharged amino acids. The ability of the receptor to recognize several related sequences is a common feature of chaperon proteins.

Isolating chemotactic sequences from an elastolytic digest of elastin and synthesizing tetra- and pentapeptides homologous to the isolated peptides and VGVAPG, Tamburro et al. tried to identify a structure-activity relationship for the elastin-derived chemoattractant peptides (Table 1 (D)) [30]. All the active chemoattractant peptides are characterized by rather extended and flexible conformations without evidence of any folded structures.

Long et al. used longer peptides to test their chemotactic activity (Table 1 (E)) [25,31]. One interesting observation in their study is that a polynonapeptide is less active in the chemotaxis assay than the monomeric units probably because the polynonapeptide has less conformational freedom.

Testing properties of elastin peptides other than the chemotactic activity, Fülöp et al. studied tri-, tetra-, penta- and hexapeptides similar to, or shorter than VGVAPG (Table 1 (F)) [26]. The two hexapeptides VGVAPG and PGVGVA have similar effects on receptor-linked effects of elastin peptides, i.e., increase in free-calcium concentration and stimulation of superoxide anion production. The substitution of the proline residue with valine seems to reduce the biological effect of the hexapeptide PGVGVA. Shorter peptides have no activity.

In conclusion, the binding of elastin-related peptides to the receptor is not sequence-specific. Amino acid substitutions are tolerated as long as the hydrophobic nature of the peptide is maintained.

The elastin receptor in atherosclerosis

As elastin peptides are chemotactic for monocytes and smooth muscle cells, they can participate in the attraction of the circulatory cells in the fatty streaks and the migration of smooth muscle cells from the media to the intima [22]. The release of free radicals, superoxide anion and nitric oxide, during the activation of the elastin receptor might also be a crucial factor in atherogenesis. Finally, in more advanced atheromatous plaque, the presence of elastin peptides near the different cell types (monocytes/macrophages, lymphocytes, smooth muscle cells) activates the elastin receptor and induces further production and secretion of proteases like elastases. The activity of these proteases on the surrounding extracellular matrix may generate further extracellular matrix degradation products. These contribute to the chronicity and the progression of the lesion.

References

1. Jacob MP, Hornebeck W, Robert L. Studies on the interaction of cholesterol with soluble and insoluble elastins. Int J Biol Macromol 1983;5:275—278.
2. Kramsch DM, Franzblau C, Hollander W. The protein and lipid composition of arterial elastin and its relationship to lipid accumulation in the atherosclerotic plaque. J Clin Invest 1971;50: 1666—1677.
3. Fülöp T Jr, Wei SM, Robert L, Jacob MP. Determination of elastin peptides in normal and arteriosclerotic human sera by ELISA. Clin Physiol 1990;8:273—282.
4. Wei SM, Erdei J, Fülöp T, Robert L, Jacob MP. Elastin peptide concentration in human serum: variation with antibodies and elastin peptides used for the enzyme-linked immunosorbent assay. J Immunol Meth 1993;164:175—187.
5. Varga Z, Jacob MP, Robert L, Fülöp T Jr. Identification and signal transduction mechanism of elastin peptide receptor in human leukocytes. FEBS Lett 1989;258:5—8.
6. Wrenn DS, Hinek A, Mecham RP. Kinetics of receptor-mediated binding of tropoelastin to ligament fibroblasts. J Biol Chem 1988;263:2280—2284.
7. Perdomo JJ, Gounon P, Schaeverbeke M, Schaeverbeke J, Groult V, Jacob MP, Robert L. Interactions between cells and elastin fibers: an ultrastructural and immunocytochemical study. J Cell Physiol 1994;158:451—458.
8. Hinek A, Wrenn DS, Mecham RP, Barondes SH. The elastin receptor: a galactoside-binding protein. Science 1988;239:1539—1541.
9. Mecham RP. Receptors for laminin on mammalian cells. FASEB J 1991;5:2538—2546.
10. Hinek A, Mecham RP, Keeley F, Rabinovitch M. Impaired elastin fiber assembly related to reduced 67-kD elastin-binding protein in fetal lamb ductus arteriosus and in cultured aortic smooth muscle cells treated with chondroitin sulfate. J Clin Invest 1991;88:2083—2094.
11. Jacob MP, Fülöp T Jr, Foris G, Robert L. Effect of elastin peptides on ion fluxes in mononuclear cells, fibroblasts, and smooth muscle cells. Proc Natl Acad Sci USA 1987;84:995—999.
12. Senior RM, Griffin GL, Mecham RP. Chemotactic activity of elastin-derived peptides. J Clin Invest 1980;66:859—862.
13. Senior RM, Griffin GL, Mecham RP. Chemotactic responses of fibroblasts to tropoelastin and elastin-derived peptides. J Clin Invest 1982;70:614—618.
14. Ooyama T, Fukuda K, Oda H, Nakamura H, Hilita Y. Substratum-bound elastin peptide inhibits aortic smooth muscle cell migration in vitro. Arteriosclerosis 1987;7:593—598.
15. Hornebeck W, Tixier JM, Robert L. Inducible adhesion of mesenchymal cells to elastic fibers: elastonectin. Proc Natl Acad Sci USA 1986;83:5517—5520.
16. Groult V, Hornebeck W, Ferrari P, Tixier JM, Robert L, Jacob MP. Mechanisms of interaction between human skin fibroblasts and elastin: differences between elastin fibres and derived peptides. Cell Biochem Funct 1991;9:171—182.
17. Fülöp T Jr, Jacob MP, Varga Z, Foris G, Leovey A, Robert L. Effect of elastin peptides on human monocytes: Ca^{2+} mobilization, stimulation of respiratory burst and enzyme secretion. Biochem Biophys Res Commun 1986;141:92—98.

18. Faury G, Ristori MT, Verdetti J, Jacob MP, Robert L. Rôle du récepteur de l'élastine-laminine dans la vasorégulation. CR Acad Sci Paris 1994;317:807—811.
19. Faury G, Ristori MT, Verdetti J, Jacob MP, Robert L. Effect of elastin peptides on vascular tone. J Vasc Res 1995;32:112—119.
20. Péterszegi G, Robert AM, Robert L. Presence of the elastin-laminin receptor on human activated lymphocytes. CR Acad Sci Paris 1996;319:799—803.
21. Péterszegi G, Texier S, Robert AM, Robert L. Human helper and memory lymphocytes exhibit an inducible elastin-laminin receptor. Int Arch Allergy Immunol (In press).
22. Robert L. Aging of the vascular wall and atherogenesis: role of the elastin-laminin receptor. Atherosclerosis 1996;123:169—179.
23. Kunimoto M, Jay M. Elastin fragment-induced monocyte chemotaxis. The role of desmosines. Inflammation 1985;9:183—188.
24. Senior RM, Griffin GL, Mecham RP, Wrenn DS, Prasad KU, Urry DW. Val-Gly-Val-Ala-Pro-Gly, a repeating peptide in elastin, is chemotactic for fibroblasts and monocytes. J Cell Biol 1984;99:870—874.
25. Long MM, King VJ, Prasad KU, Freeman BA, Urry DW. Elastin repeat peptides as chemoattractants for bovine aortic endothelial cells. J Cell Physiol 1989;140:512—518.
26. Hauck M, Seres I, Kiss I, Saulnier J, Mohacsi A, Wallach J, Fülöp T Jr. Effects of synthesized elastin peptides on human leukocytes. Biochem Mol Biol Int 1995;37:45—55.
27. Mecham RP, Hinek A, Griffin GL, Senior RM, Liotta LA. The elastin receptor shows structural and functional similarities to the 67-kDa tumor cell laminin receptor. J Biol Chem 1989;264:16652—16657.
28. Grosso LE, Scott M. PGAIPG, a repeated hexapeptide of bovine tropoelastin, is a ligand for the 67-kDa bovine elastin receptor. Matrix 1993;13:157—164.
29. Grosso LE, Scott M. Peptide sequences selected by BA4, a tropoelastin-specific monoclonal antibody, are ligands for the 67-kilodalton bovine elastin receptor. Biochem 1993;32:13369—13374.
30. Bisaccia F, Castiglione Morelli MA, De Biasi M, Traniello S, Spisani S, Tamburro AM. Migration of monocytes in the presence of elastolytic fragments of elastin and in synthetic derivates. Structure-activity relationships. Int J Pept Protein Res 1994;44:332—341.
31. Long MM, King VJ, Prasad KU, Urry DW. Chemotaxis of fibroblasts toward nonapeptide of elastin. Biochim Biophys Acta 1988;968:300—311.

Elastase and elastase inhibitors and pulmonary and coronary artery disease

Marlene Rabinovitch

Division of Cardiovascular Research, The Hospital for Sick Children; and Departments of Pediatrics, Pathology and Medicine, University of Toronto, Toronto, Canada

Abstract. *Background.* Increased elastolytic activity is associated with development and progression of pulmonary hypertension in experimental animals. Elastase inhibitors prevent the development of pulmonary vascular disease in experimental models. Endogenous vascular elastase appears to be an enzyme 20 kD in molecular weight, is expressed by smooth muscle cells (SMC) and is a serine proteinase related structurally to the adipocyte enzyme, adipsin.

Methods. We used cell-culture systems to determine the mechanisms whereby elastase is released and induces vascular disease in pulmonary as well as coronary arteries.

Results. Elastase is induced by serum factors including apolipoprotein A1 (apo A1). The signalling mechanisms involve induction of the MAP-kinase pathway with increased expression of the transcription factor AML1. Increased activity of elastase results in the release of mitogens from the extracellular matrix such as basic fibroblast growth factor (FGF-2). Elastases in concert with matrix metalloproteinases can proteolyze collagen leading to the upregulation of the glycoprotein, tenascin, which is necessary to amplify the proliferative response to growth factors. The mechanism involves β_3-integrin-mediated signalling of the matrix glycoprotein tenascin. Elastin peptides upregulate fibronectin production, which is necessary for smooth muscle cell migration. Elastin peptides synergize with the cytokine interleukin 1β in inducing fibronectin in coronary artery SMC.

Conclusions. Since our other studies have shown that elastase inhibitors prevent the development of coronary artery disease experimentally induced after cardiac transplant, these enzymes might be implicated in other conditions with rapid development of neointimal formation such as restenosis.

Keywords: basic fibroblast growth factor, coronary artery disease, elastase inhibitors, pulmonary hypertension, tenascin.

Increased elastase activity and pulmonary hypertension

Our evidence that elastase might be involved in the pathophysiology of pulmonary vascular disease came from the ultrastructural study of lung-biopsy tissue from patients with congenital heart defect [1]. That is, there was fragmentation of the internal elastic lamina as a feature which preceded the development of pulmonary vascular disease. This was reinforced when the same process appeared to be evident (structurally) in the pathogenesis of experimentally induced pulmonary hypertension in rats injected with the toxin, monocrotaline [2]. Subsequent studies in experimental rats showed that early increase in activity of a ser-

Address for correspondence: Marlene Rabinovitch MD, Division of Cardiovascular Research, The Hospital for Sick Children, 555 University Avenue, Toronto, Ontario M5G 1X8, Canada. Tel.: +1-416-813-5918. Fax: +1-416-813-7480.

ine elastase was present prior to development of hypoxia or monocrotaline-induced pulmonary hypertension in rats. It was interesting that sustained activity of this enzyme was observed with the progressive form of pulmonary hypertension induced by monocrotaline [3]. A cause and effect relationship was further established in studies in which we used elastase inhibitors [4,5] and largely prevented the development and the progression of pulmonary hypertension. An endogenous vascular elastase was isolated with some structural relationship to the serine proteinase, adipsin [6]; it is 20 kD in molecular weight localized to smooth muscle cells, and therefore, is similar to the elastase enzyme reported in aortic smooth muscle cells and in atherosclerotic tissues [7].

Mechanism of induction of elastase activity

We had proposed that in response to a perturbing stimulus such as hypoxia, a toxin, or the high flow and pressure of the congenital defect, the endothelial cells would be the first causality. Structural and functional alterations in endothelium would lead to loss of barrier properties (Fig. 1). This could induce an increased leak of a plasma factor into the subendothelium which is not normally present in that location in high concentration. We subsequently showed that serum did induce increased elastase activity in vascular smooth muscle cells. The elastase was a serine proteinase. This serum inducing factor which included apolipoprotein A1 adhered to elastin and to the cell surface and appeared to induce binding of the elastin to the elastin-binding protein and also to integrins. A signal transduction mechanism was initiated whereby tyrosine kinase activity was expressed. There was phosphorylation of focal adhesion kinase (FAK) and members of the MAP-kinase family (ERK or extracellular regulated kinase-1) (Fig. 2) [8]. The phosphorylation of ERK results in the increased expression of the transcription factor AML1. AML 1 is the transcription factor for neutrophil elastase and is a

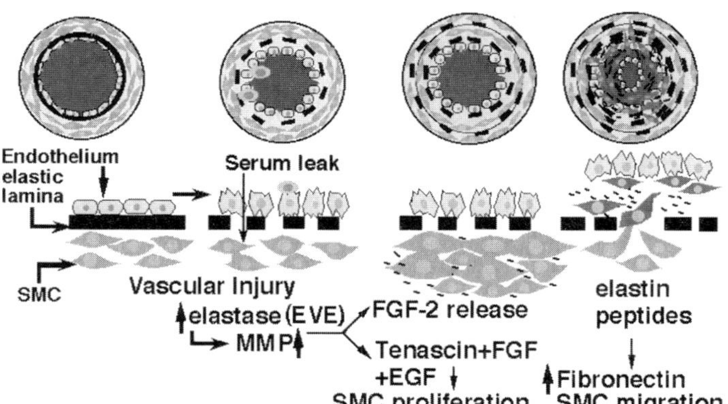

Fig. 1. A proposed schema linking vascular injury, elastase and matrix metalloproteinase activity with growth factors and tenascin in vascular pathobiology.

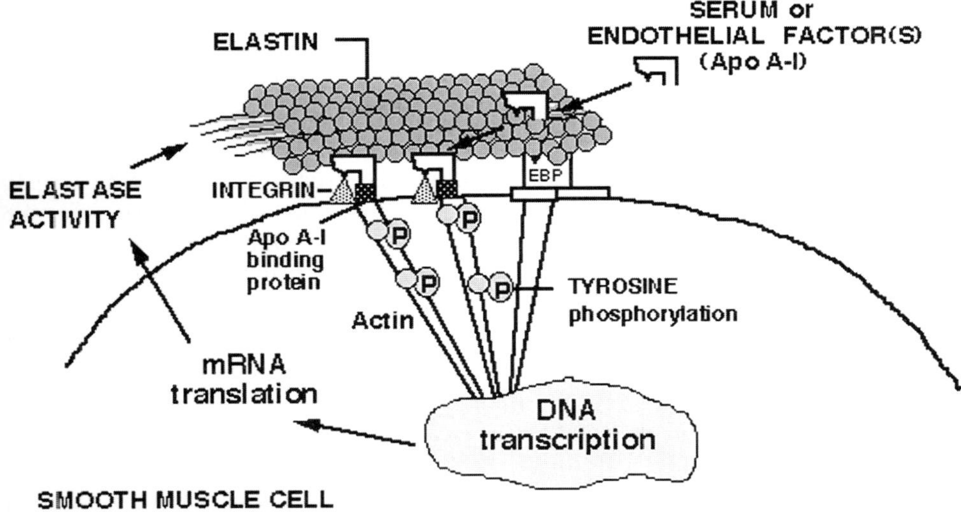

Fig. 2. A proposed schema indicating how serum factor(s) or endothelial factor, i.e., apo A1, tethers elastin to the smooth muscle cell surface, permitting engagement of the elastin-binding protein (EBP) and cooperative interaction with integrin-receptors resulting in tyrosine kinase activity. The subsequent promotion of DNA transcription and mRNA translation culminate in the induction of vascular elastase. (Reproduced with permission from Thompson K et al., J Cell Physiol, 1997;(In press).)

candidate transcription factor for vascular elastase [9]. We have documented by immunohistochemistry that AML1 is present in smooth muscle cells and expression is prominent in the nucleus with serum stimulation. On gel mobility shift assay AML1 is evident in nuclear extracts following serum-treated elastin-induced elastase activity and forms a binding complex with radiolabelled oligonucleotides containing the AML1 consensus sequence. Moreover, AML1 antisense nucleotides effectively repress serum-treated elastin-induction of elastase activity (unpublished).

Elastase activity linked to smooth muscle cell proliferation

Studies were further carried out to establish whether (as has been shown for other serine proteinases) expression of endogenous vascular elastase (EVE activity) would lead to the release of mitogenic smooth muscle cell growth factors [10]. We showed that both human leukocyte elastase and EVE induced by serum-treated elastin were effective in liberating FGF-2 from the extracellular matrices of smooth muscle cells. In our assays, we measured release of radiolabelled and endogenous FGF-2 into the conditioned medium by densitometry of autoradiographs and Western immunoblots, respectively. The FGF-2 released was mitogenically active as judged by the proliferation of "reader" smooth muscle cells with conditioned media enriched but not depleted of the liberated FGF-2.

Unpublished studies have also suggested that induction of EVE can also liberate TGF-β.

Amplification of the proliferative response with tenascin-C

Since FGF-2 can induce production of the matrix glycoprotein tenascin (TN)-C and since TN-C has been implicated in the pathology of atherosclerosis, we sought to determine whether it was also upregulated in pulmonary vascular disease and its role vis-à-vis cell proliferation. We examined lung-biopsy sections obtained for routine diagnostic purposes from children with congenital heart defects [11] and identified, by immunohistochemistry, the progressive increase in TN-C expression with severity of vascular lesion. When there was only medial hypertrophy, TN-C was observed primarily in the adventitial-medial border or diffusely throughout the media. However, with neointimal formation, TN-C was expressed in the neointima as judged by immunoperoxidase staining, where it colocalized with proliferating cells (positive for proliferating cell nuclear antigen) and epidermal growth factor (EGF). It was interesting that fibronectin accumulated largely in the periendothelial region of the hypertrophied artery and was also seen in the neointima with advanced disease. This supported an FN gradient as of potential importance in stimulating SMC migration and inflammatory cell transendothelial migration. There were, however, only a few macrophages in the neointima of advanced lesions.

Further studies were carried out to establish the relationship of TN-C expression in the evolution of pulmonary vascular disease in experimentally induced pulmonary hypertension in monocrotaline-injected rats [12]. It was interesting that, with the advent of medial hypertrophy (day 14 after injection) TN-C expression was evident in the outer adventitial-medial border colocalizing with proliferating smooth muscle cells. With progressive disease, at 21 days after injection of the toxin monocrotaline, TN-C was observed throughout the media and in the evolving neointima, associated with proliferating SMC. Endothelial cell apoptosis was noted as early as 7 days after monocrotaline injection and preceded expression of TN-C in the vessel wall. Northern blot analysis showed that there was also increased mRNA for TN-C in the lung and in the PA as early as 14 days after injection of monocrotaline. In situ hybridization localized TN-C in the lung to the arterial SMC. To assess the functional significance of TN-C in cell proliferation, rat PA SMC were cultured on collagen gels supplemented with TN-C. There was no change in PA SMC number on either substrate, but upon addition of FGF-2, TN-C increased cell proliferation and, in fact, supplementation with TN-C appeared to be a prerequisite for EGF-dependent PA SMC proliferation.

Mechanism of tenascin-C-induced SMC proliferation

We further investigated the mechanism whereby TN promotes SMC proliferation

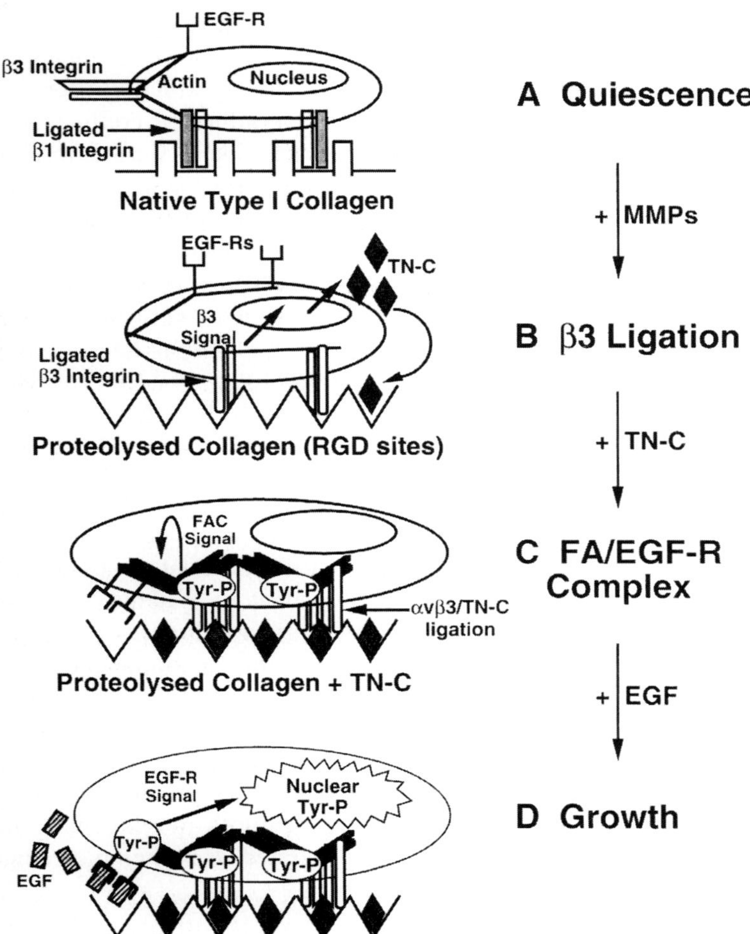

Fig. 3. Hypothetical model for the regulation and function of tenascin-C (TN-C) in vascular smooth muscle cells. **A:** Vascular smooth muscle cells attach and spread on native type I collagen using β1 integrins. Under serum-free conditions, the cells withdraw from the cell cycle and become quiescent. **B:** Degradation of native type I collagen by matrix metalloproteinases (MMPs) leads to the exposure of cryptic RGD sites that preferentially bind β3 subunit containing integrins. In turn, occupancy and activation of β3 integrins signals the production of TN-C. **C:** Incorporation of multivalent TN-C protein into the underlying substrate leads to further aggregation and activation of β3-containing integrins (αvβ3), and the accumulation of tyrosine phosphorylated (Tyr-P) signalling molecules and actin into a focal adhesion (FA) complex. Note that even in the absence of the EGF ligand, the TN-C-dependent reorganization of the cytoskeleton leads to clustering of actin-associated epidermal growth factor receptors (EGF-Rs). **D:** Addition of EGF ligand to clustered EGF-Rs results in rapid and substantial tyrosine phosphorylation of the EGF-R, and activation of downstream pathways culminating in the generation of nuclear signals leading to cell proliferation. (Reproduced with permission from Jones PL, J Cell Biol 1997;(In press).)

[13] (Fig. 3). We showed that on type I collagen SMC are relatively quiescent, but with degradation of collagen, cryptic RGD sites are exposed which ligate $\beta3$ integrins. These appear to signal the upregulation of TN-C which clusters $\beta3$ integrins leading to formation of actin cytoskeleton focal adhesion contacts and tyrosine phosphorylation of a 125 kD protein which is likely focal adhesion kinase. Upon ligation with EGF there is brisk phosphorylation of the EGF receptor and transmission of a nuclear phosphorylation signal which is reflected in cell growth. We then showed that expression of MMP-2 by gelatin zymography and Western immunoblot correlated with expression of TN-C and that inhibition of MMPs with GM-6001 could suppress TN-C expression selectively. We also showed that MMPs were suppressed and TN-C was downregulated with PA SMC cultured on floating compared to attached collagen gels and that this was associated with PA SMC apoptosis. Thus, TN-C appeared to be a SMC survival factor.

Elastase in systemic vascular disease

We had carried out further studies to investigate whether the elastase associated with pulmonary vascular disease might also be prevalent in systemic vascular disorders and, if so, how it might be related to the structural changes observed. We used an organ culture model [14] to determine whether or not there was a correlation between increased activity of the serine elastase and the development of neointimal formation in the aorta. We were able to correlate the expression of elastase activity with the increase in the number of intimal smooth muscle cells in this model. Moreover, inhibition of elastase activity with $\alpha1$ proteinase inhibitor markedly repressed the proliferation of neointimal smooth muscle cells. The elastase activity on the substrate gel appeared to be related to higher molecular weight species than EVE.

Elastase and postcardiac transplant coronary artery disease

We have also investigated the possibility that either EVE or serine elastases from invading inflammatory cells might be important in the pathophysiology of accelerated coronary artery disease that occurs after cardiac transplant. Using a heterotopic cardiac transplant model in the piglet, we measured an increased number of breaks in the internal elastic lamina in association with the progressive development of neointimal formation in the coronary arteries and correlated this with increased activity of a serine elastase of approximately 23 kD (Fig. 4). This serine elastase was inhibited by a specific inhibitor, elafin, which is a naturally occurring serine proteinase inhibitor [15]. In further studies, [16] we went on to show that elafin was highly effective when given intravenously in suppressing the development of coronary arteries with neointimal lesions in rabbits after heterotopic heart transplants (Fig. 5). Also, elafin suppressed the myocardial necrosis and dysfunction that occurred in association with acute rejection. The

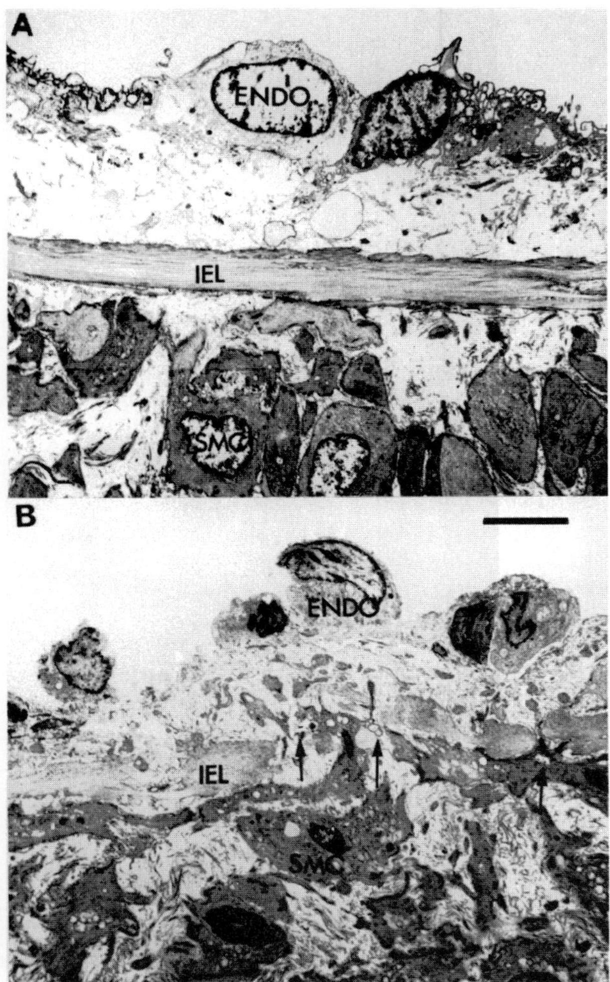

Fig. 4. Representative electron photomicrographs of host (**A**) and donor (**B**) coronary artery. No breaks are seen in the IEL of host coronary artery, whereas the IEL of the donor coronary artery is tortuous and few breaks (arrows) can be seen. ENDO, endothelial cell, SMC, smooth muscle cell. Magnification × 3760; scale bar = 5μ. (Reproduced with permission from Oho S et al, Am J Pathol 1994,145:202–210.)

latter feature was also attributed to its elastase inhibitory activities.

In vitro studies have gone on to address the mechanism whereby elafin might be preventing neointimal formation in coronary arteries (Fig. 6). It is anticipated that the mechanism which is associated with the development of smooth muscle cell proliferation, i.e., the release of growth factors by elastase, is also operational in the coronary arteries. This is evidenced by the fact that there is an increase in expression of the proliferating cell nuclear antigen in the coronary arteries of

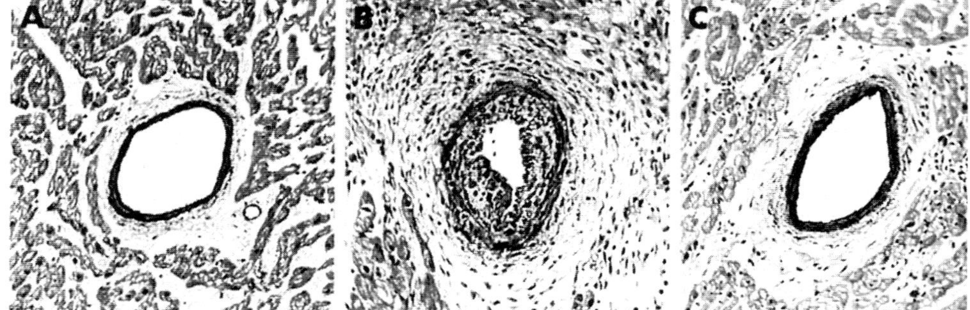

Fig. 5. Effect of recombinant human elafin treatment on cellular proliferation in coronary arteries as assessed by positive staining for PCNA in host and donor hearts from control and elafin-treated animals. There was a >3-fold increase in the number of proliferating cells in both medium (>100 ≤ 500 μm diameter) and small (≤100 μm diameter) size vessels of the donor control group relative to the host (p < 0.0001 and p < 0.0005, respectively, not indicated on Figure). The number of proliferating cells was significantly reduced in large (>500 μm diameter) (p < 0.0001) medium (p < 0.0001) and small arteries (p < 0.02) of donor hearts in elafin-treated animals and large (p < 0.0001) and medium vessels (p < 0.005) of elafin-treated host hearts. (Reproduced with permission from Cowan B et al., J Clin Invest 1996, 97:2452–2468.)

control animals but a relative decrease in those treated with the serine proteinase elafin. In addition, elastase appears to act in concert with cytokines via elastin peptides [17] to upregulate production of the matrix glycoprotein, fibronectin. Indeed, we have shown when interleukin 1β (IL-β) induction of fibronectin in coronary artery smooth muscle cells can be abrogated by elafin, it can be overridden by the addition of the elastin peptides. Indeed, elastin peptides appear to synergize with this cytokine in mediating the increase in fibronectin. Previous

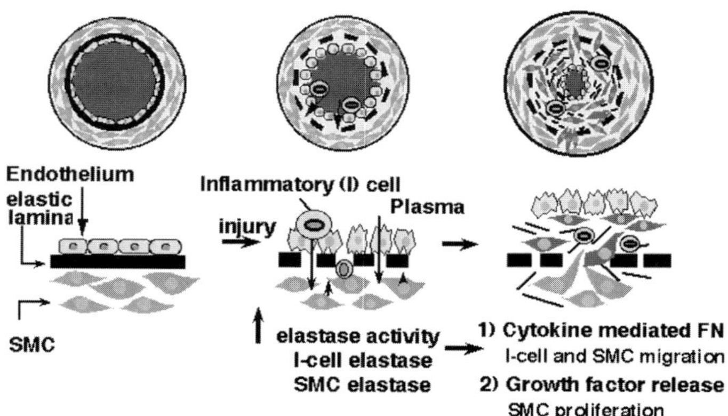

Fig. 6. Proposed schema showing how endogenous vascular and leukocyte elastase activity can lead to the development of postcardiac transplant coronary artery disease through both liberation of growth factors and mediation of elastin peptide modulation of cytokine-induced fibronectin production.

studies have shown that fibronectin is critical for smooth muscle cell migration and also for transendothelial T cell migration in the coronary arteries [18,19]. Further studies are now addressing how elastin peptides function in concert with cytokines in upregulating fibronectin. Initial studies indicate that while the induction of fibronectin by cytokines appears to involve an increase in mRNA levels, the elastin peptide-mediated induction of fibronectin is likely occurring at a posttranscriptional level. We have linked posttranscriptional regulation of fibronectin to increased efficiency of translation of the fibronectin mRNA in ductus arteriosus smooth muscle cells and more specifically, to the increased expression of a light chain 3 microtubular associated protein (LC-3)1A and B which binds a conserved AU rich element in the fibronectin 3' untranslated region (UTR) of the messenger RNA [20]

Potential therapeutic targets

These studies suggest novel therapeutic targets to prevent the development of vascular diseases of the serum factors that stimulate the process that needs to be identified and selectively targeted in the vessel wall. This will involve knowing more about the mechanism whereby apo A1 induces the upregulation of elastase. The signal transduction pathways need selectively to be targeted, as does the upregulation of the transcription factor AML1. The elastase gene needs to be cloned so that its regulation can be studied in order for it to be inhibited. In addition, the effects of this enzymatic activity, specific growth factors, fibronectin and tenascin can all be targets of therapeutic interventions.

References

1. Rabinovitch M, Bothwell T, Hayakawa BN, Williams WG, Trusler GA, Rowe RD, Olley PM, Cutz E. Pulmonary artery endothelial abnormalities in patients with congenital heart defects and pulmonary hypertension: a correlation of light with scanning electron microscopy and transmission electron microscopy. Lab Invest 1986;55:632—653.
2. Todorovich-Hunter L, Johnson DJ, Ranger P, Keeley FW, Rabinovitch M. Altered elastin and collagen synthesis associated with progressive pulmonary hypertension induced by monocrotaline: a biochemical and ultrastructural study. Lab Invest 1988;58:184—195.
3. Todorovich-Hunter L, Dodo H, Ye C, McCready L, Keeley FW, Rabinovitch M. Increased pulmonary artery elastolytic activity in adult rats with monocrotaline-induced progressive hypertensive pulmonary vascular disease compared with infant rats with nonprogressive disease. Am Rev Respir Dis 1992;146:213—223.
4. Maruyama K, Ye C, Woo M, Venkatacharya H, Lines LD, Silver MM, Rabinovitch M. Chronic hypoxic pulmonary hypertension in rats and increased elastolytic activity. Am J Physiol 1991;261:H1716—H1726.
5. Ye C, Rabinovitch M. Inhibition of elastolysis by SC-37698 reduces development and progression of monocrotaline pulmonary hypertension. Am J Physiol 1991;261:H1255—H1267.
6. Zhu L, Hinek A, Wigle D, Kobayashi J, Zuker M, Dodo H, Rabinovitch M. The vascular elastase which governs the development and progression of pulmonary hypertension is related to adipsin. Molec Biol Cell 1993;4:410a.
7. Hornebeck W, Brechemier D, Soleilhac JM, Bourdillon MC, Robert L. Studies on rat aorta

smooth muscle cells' elastase activity. In: Reddi AH (ed) Extracellular Matrix: Structure and Function. New York: Alan R Liss, 1985;269–282.

8. Thompson KE, Jones PL, Rabinovitch M. Induction of vascular elastase requires extracellular signal regulated kinase 1 and nuclear expression of transcription factor AML1. J Biol Chem 1997 (Submitted).

9. Nuchprayoon I, Meyers S, Scott LM, Suzoe J, Hiebert S, Friedman AD. PEBP2/CBF, the murine homolog of the human myeloid AML1 and PEBP2β/CBFβ proto-oncoproteins, regulates the murine myeloperoxidase and neutrophil elastase genes in immature myeloid cells. Molec Cell Biol 1994;14:5558–5568.

10. Thompson K, Kobayashi J, Childs T, Wigle D, Rabinovitch M. Endothelial and serum factors which include apolipoprotein A1 tether elastin to smooth muscle cells inducing serine elastase activity via tyrosine kinase-mediated transcription and translation. J Cell Physiol 1997;174:(In press).

11. Jones PL, Cowan KN, Rabinovitch M. Induction of tenascin and fibronectin are features associated with increased smooth muscle cell proliferation during the development of progressive pulmonary hypertension in children. Am J Pathol 1997;150:1349–1360.

12. Jones PL, Rabinovitch M. Tenascin-C is induced with progressive pulmonary vascular disease in rats and is functionally related to increased smooth muscle cell proliferation. Circ Res 1996; 79:1131–1142.

13. Jones PL, Crack J, Rabinovitch M. Regulation of tenascin-C, a vascular smooth muscle cell survival factor that interacts with the $\alpha_v\beta_3$ integrin to promote epidermal growth factor receptor phosphorylation and growth. J Cell Biol 1997;139:(In press).

14. Oho S, Daley SJ, Koo EWY, Childs T, Gotlieb AI, Rabinovitch M. Increased elastin-degrading activity and neointimal formation in porcine aortic organ culture. Reduction of both features with a serine proteinase inhibitor. Arterioscl Thromb Vasc Biol 1995;15:2200–2205.

15. Sallenave J-M, Silva A. Characterization and gene sequence of the precursor of elafin, an elastase-specific inhibitor in bronchial secretions. Am J Respir Cell Mol Biol 1993;8:439–453.

16. Cowan B, Baron O, Crack J, Coulber C, Wilson GJ, Rabinovitch M. Elafin, a serine elastase inhibitor, attenuates postcardiac transplant coronary arteriopathy and reduces myocardial necrosis in rabbits following heterotopic cardiac transplantation. J Clin Invest 1996;97: 2452–2468.

17. Hinek A, Molossi S, Rabinovitch M. Functional interplay between interleukin-1 receptor and elastin binding protein controls fibronectin synthesis in coronary artery smooth muscle cells. Exp Cell Res 1996;225:122–131.

18. Molossi S, Elices M, Arrhenius T, Diaz R, Coulber C, Rabinovitch M. Blockade of very late antigen-4 integrin binding to fibronectin with connecting segment-1 peptide reduces accelerated coronary arteriopathy in rabbit cardiac allografts. J Clin Invest 1995;95:2601–2610.

19. Boudreau N, Turley E, Rabinovitch M. Fibronectin, hyaluronan and a hyaluronan binding protein contribute to increased ductus arteriosus smooth muscle cell migration. Devel Biol 1991; 143:235–247.

20. Zhou B, Hammarback J, Rabinovitch M. Post-transcriptional mechanism upregulating fibronectin synthesis in ductus arteriosus smooth muscle is related to the UUAUUUAU sequence in the 3′ untranslated region of fibronectin mRNA and its binding protein. Circulation 1996; 94(Suppl):I–645.

Physicochemical interaction between plasma lipoproteins and the endothelial cell membrane and vascular matrix proteoglycans

G. Siegel[1], M. Malmsten[2], D. Klüßendorf[1], W. Leonhardt[3], A. Schmidt[4] and E. Buddecke[4]

[1]*Institute of Physiology, Berlin;* [2]*Institute of Surface Chemistry, Stockholm, Sweden;* [3]*Institute and Policlinic of Clinical Metabolic Research, Dresden; and* [4]*Institute of Arteriosclerosis Research, Münster, Germany*

Abstract. Proteoheparan sulfate can be adsorbed to a methylated silica surface in a monomolecular layer via its transmembrane hydrophobic protein core domain. Due to electrostatic repulsion, its anionic polysugar side chains are stretched out into the blood substitute solution representing the scavenger receptor for specific lipoprotein binding through basic amino acid-rich residues within their apolipoproteins. The binding process was studied by ellipsometric techniques showing that oxLDL has a deleterious effect on HS-PG binding and conformation. On the other hand, HDL bound to HS-PG protects against LDL docking and completely suppresses calcification of the proteoglycan lipoprotein complex.

Keywords: calcification, ellipsometry, heparan sulfate proteoglycan, lipoprotein binding, methylated silica surface, scavenger receptor.

Introduction

The polyanionic and hydrophilic glycosaminoglycan (GAG) chains dominate the physical properties of proteoglycans (PGs) such as endothelial cell membrane syndecan and vascular matrix perlecan. They have a strong influence not only on tissue hydration and elasticity, but also on counteraction attraction by their negative fixed charges. Thus, pericellular compartments with concentrated PGs and ions can influence spatiotemporally controlled reaction rates and concentration-dependent interactive physical processes. Under physiological ion concentrations and pH, the specific binding of GAGs to proteins such as proteases and antiproteases, growth factors and other cytokines, matrix proteins and glycoconjugates, cell adhesion molecules, lipoproteins and lipases allows PGs to intervene in cell and tissue development in numerous ways. Under pathophysiological conditions, chondroitin sulfate (CS)/heparan sulfate (HS) proteoglycans may initiate increased LDL/oxLDL binding and form an extracellular preatheromatous lipid deposition in the intima and inner media. Stretches of basic amino acid-rich residues within apoB and apoE constituting the predominant protein moiety of

Address for correspondence: Prof Dr med Günter Siegel, Institute of Physiology, Biophysical Research Group, The Free University of Berlin, Arnimallee 22, D-14195 Berlin, Germany.

LDL display a high electrostatic binding affinity to PGs. Thus, we measured first the individual adsorption rates of HS-PG, LDL, oxLDL, and HDL from Ca^{2+}-free Krebs solutions with normal pH at methylated silica surfaces by ellipsometric techniques.

Materials and Methods

Preparations and solutions [1—4], ellipsometry [5], surface force [6], and $^{23}Na^+$ nuclear magnetic resonance [7] measurements were described in detail in previous publications.

Results

HS-PG deposition at a methylated silica surface is initiated by its transmembrane hydrophobic core domain. The GAG side chains are stretched out into the blood substitute solution because of its negative fixed charges giving rise to electrostatic repulsion [8]. A lipoprotein particle may interact with the GAG chains on occasion of its positive amino acid residues. Thus, the situation reflects physiological conditions.

Figure 1 demonstrates HS-PG adsorption from pure water to a methylated silica surface over time [9]. The adsorbed amount (Γ) is depicted on the ordinate. Since Ca^{2+} ions screen the negative GAG chains, this ion species tremendously promotes proteoheparan sulfate adsorption, even with a physiological Ca^{2+} concentration of only 1.25 mmol/l. In principle, the adsorption of HS-PG from Ca^{2+}-free Krebs solution was the same. Again, addition of Ca^{2+} ions enhanced the deposition of these macromolecules [3]. On the other hand, LDL and oxLDL adsorption at methylated silica exhibited a quite different time course (Fig. 2).

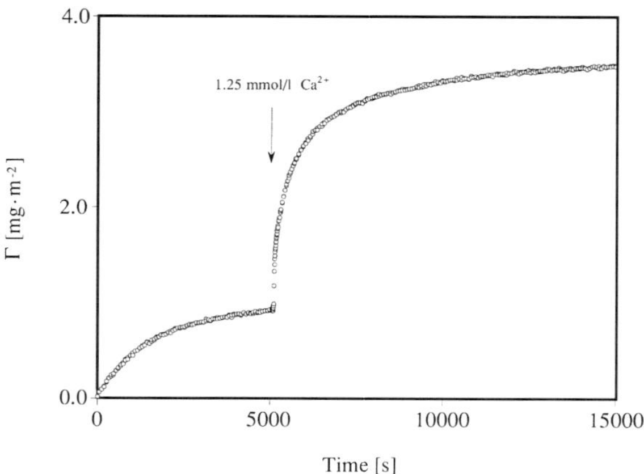

Fig. 1. Amount of proteoheparan sulfate adsorbed at hydrophobic silica from a 0.1 mg/ml aqueous solution as a function of time. The arrow indicates addition of 1.25 mmol/l $CaCl_2$. The pH was 5.6 [9].

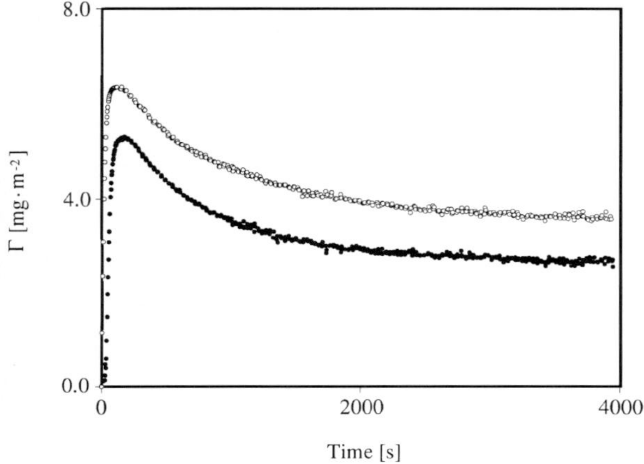

Fig. 2. Amount of LDL (○) and oxLDL (●) adsorbed at hydrophobic silica from 1.25 mmol/l physiological blood substitute solutions as a function of time. The pH was 7.3 [10].

After a fast initial adsorption, a desorption period of approximately 1 h followed [10]. After that time, the adsorption was constant. Now, we were interested to learn whether Ca^{2+} ions would influence LDL adsorption from a Ca^{2+}-free Krebs solution as could be demonstrated for HS-PG. Ca^{2+} ions in a physiological concentration of 2.5 mmol/l did not change or slightly increased the LDL adsorption, whereas 10 mmol/l Ca^{2+} accelerated the adsorption dramatically, probably by creating aggregates and thus increasing particle size.

In a second step, the physiological scenario was simulated. Lipoprotein binding to HS-PG preadsorbed from a Ca^{2+}-free Krebs solution at methylated silica resulted in no additional adsorbed amount for LDL during the first 25 min; thereafter, with LDL aggregation, the adsorbance increased to 14 mg/m^2 within 95 min (Fig. 3). In contrast, oxLDL steadily reduced the adsorbed amount of the HS-PG/oxLDL complex to 0.65 mg/m^2 within 2 h [10]. Furthermore, it was striking that after oxLDL addition, the scatter in the measurement rose significantly which may reflect a broad scope in HS-PG/oxLDL particle size. Thus, oxLDL seems to bind strongly to proteoheparan sulfate and to alter its polyanionic GAG binding sites, possibly by the intervention of oxygen free radicals. Summarizing the results of Fig. 3, one can easily conclude that LDL and oxLDL binding to preadsorbed HS-PG exhibits a large divergence. While LDL strongly increases the adsorbance, oxLDL diminishes the amount of the adsorbed HS-PG/oxLDL complex by reducing its hydrophobic interaction with the silica surface. This aggressive effect of oxLDL was again demonstrated in another experiment. HS-PG adsorbance from Ca^{2+}-free Krebs solution was strongly pronounced by the addition of Ca^{2+} ions, thus screening the electrostatic interplay which counteracts adsorption. The intervention of oxLDL initiated an immediate desorption that proceeded progressively over several hours.

In a further experimental design, we wanted to find out how these effects are

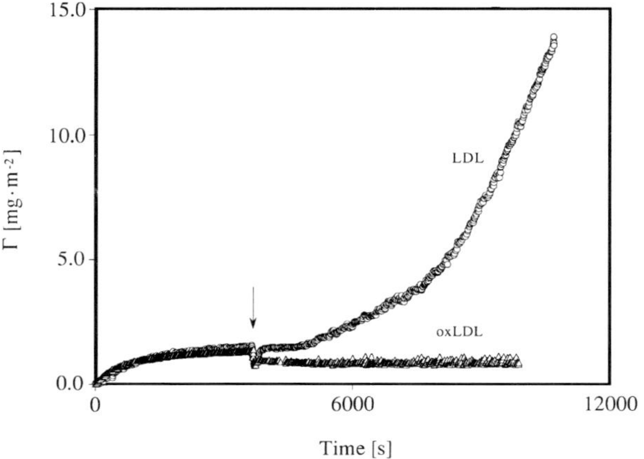

Fig. 3. Amount of proteoheparan sulfate adsorbed at hydrophobic silica from a 0.1 mg/ml physiological blood substitute solution as a function of time. The arrow indicates addition of 1.25 mmol/l LDL (O) or oxLDL (Δ). The pH was 7.3 [10].

modified by calcium ions, and if calcification of the proteoglycan/lipoprotein complexes takes place. HDL binding to HS-PG was only slightly increased by stepwise additions of Ca^{2+} ions. Furthermore, HDL seemed to strongly bind to HS-PG by reducing its hydrophobicity. In contrast, Ca^{2+} ions dramatically changed the HS-PG/LDL interaction. After preadsorbance of HS-PG, LDL did not significantly alter the adsorbed amount. However, the addition of 2.5 mmol/l Ca^{2+} increased this quantity by a factor of five [10]. Therefore, Ca^{2+} ions interfered decisively with the proteoheparan sulfate/LDL interplay.

In this context, the known protective role of HDL was examined. After HS-PG adsorption from a Ca^{2+}-free Krebs solution, HDL induced a desorption already described which was not affected by the addition of LDL in physiological concentrations. Most surprisingly, Ca^{2+} ions had no effect at all, not even in a concentration of 10 mmol/l. Moreover, the repeated addition of LDL (double-serum concentration) likewise did not change the adsorption [10].

Discussion

In earlier experiments, we could show that HS-PG in physiological salt solution is adsorbed to a hydrophobic silica surface in such a way, that its in situ conformation corresponds directly to the in vivo conformation of the hybrid HS/CS-proteoglycan syndecan in the vascular endothelial cell membrane, and of the uniform HS-proteoglycan perlecan in the basement membrane and vascular connective tissue matrix [6]. Its interaction with Ca^{2+} ions and other mono- and divalent-cations is sustained by an electrostatic screening and an electrosteric interplay of the GAG side chains [4]. In the present work, it has been highlighted that various lipoproteins can specifically bind to these PGs, probably via stretches of basic amino acid-rich residues within their apolipoproteins [10]. However, the docking domain on the polysugar side chains is still unknown. Thus, the transmembrane and vascular matrix PGs represent the scavenger receptor for the lipid docking to endothelial cell and basement membranes as well as to vascular connective tissue matrices, at least one scavenger receptor with specific heterophilic interaction. Furthermore, the proteoglycan-lipoprotein complex can massively calcify depending on lipoprotein species, ionic microenvironment of the complex, physicochemical conditions (e.g., pH, pCO_2, pO_2) in the extrachenary space, and previous history of the proteoglycanic interplay and conformational state. It is illustrated, for example, that the specific HDL-binding to HS-PG allows a molecular interpretation of the protective and beneficial effects of HDL in blood with high concentrations of LDL and calcium. Thus, we conclude that HDL binds with high affinity to HS-PG and excludes LDL from its electrostatic attraction to the polyanionic PGs. Furthermore, the calcification of the HS-PG/LDL complex seems to be prohibited [10]. Therefore, this experiment underscores the direct antiathero/arteriosclerotic effect of high-density lipoproteins.

References

1. Leonhardt W, Pietzsch J, Nitzsche S. Very-fast ultracentrifugation of human plasma lipoproteins: influence of the centrifugal field on lipoprotein composition. Clin Chim Acta 1994;224:21—32.
2. Schmidt A, Buddecke E. Cell-associated proteoheparan sulfate from bovine arterial smooth muscle cells. Exp Cell Res 1988;178:242—253.
3. Siegel G, Malmsten M, Klüßendorf D, Walter A, Schnalke F, Kauschmann A. Blood-flow sensing by anionic biopolymers. J Auton Nerv Syst 1996;57:207—213.
4. Siegel G, Walter A, Kauschmann A, Malmsten M, Buddecke E. Anionic biopolymers as blood flow sensors. Biosensors & Bioelectronics 1996;11:281—294.
5. Malmsten M, Siegel G. Electrostatic and ion-binding effects on the adsorption of proteoglycans. J Colloid Interface Sci 1995;170:120—127.
6. Malmsten M, Claesson P, Siegel G. Forces between proteoheparan sulfate layers adsorbed at hydrophobic surfaces. Langmuir 1994;10:1274—1280.
7. Siegel G, Walter A, Rückborn K, Buddecke E, Schmidt A, Gustavsson H, Lindman B. NMR studies of cation induced conformational changes in anionic biopolymers at the endothelium-blood interface. Polymer J 1991;23:697—708.
8. Siegel G, Malmsten M, Klüßendorf D, Walter A, Schmidt A. Chemistry, recognition and function of a natural shear stress biosensor. ACS Polym Mat Sci Eng 1997;76:573—575.
9. Malmsten M, Siegel G, Buddecke E, Schmidt A. Cation-promoted adsorption of proteoheparan sulphate. Coll Surf B: Biointerfaces 1993;1:43—50.
10. Siegel G, Malmsten M. Physicochemical interaction between plasma lipoproteins and vascular proteoglycans. Nature 1997 (Submitted).

Restenosis and remodelling

Remodeling rather than neointima formation explains restenosis: insights from experimental studies in pigs

Henning Rud Andersen
Department of Cardiology, Århus, Denmark

Background

Renarrowing after otherwise successful coronary angioplasty remains a major problem, occurring in 30—50% of cases within 3—6 months. An injury-induced exuberant healing response mediated by smooth muscle cell proliferation and matrix synthesis has traditionally been considered to play the key role in late restenosis, but recent data indicate that remodeling could be even more important [1,2]. Many drugs have proved effective in preventing or reducing the proliferative healing response after arterial injury in experimental rat and rabbit models, but until recently only stenting has proven effective in reducing postinterventional restenosis in humans. However, new studies indicate that radiation or treatment with antioxidants may also be effective [3,4]. The failure of antiproliferative treatment in humans could indicate that results obtained in smaller experimental animals are not readily translated to the clinical setting, or the reason could be that cell proliferation is not critical for development of restenosis in humans. Contrary to results obtained in the rat and rabbit models, those obtained in the pig coronary model appear to reflect the human experiences much better and the pig is now widely used to study the restenosis process after coronary interventional procedures. Also in the porcine models, research efforts have focused on smooth muscle cell proliferation, and the two models most commonly used to induce a proliferative healing response have been the coronary balloon overdilatation and oversized stenting [5,6]. Although the healing response may look impressive microscopically, only very modest angiographic stenosis develops after these procedures. Thus, the most important component in the restenotic process (luminal narrowing) is lacking in currently used porcine models of postinterventional coronary artery restenosis.

The purpose of the present study was to describe the development of luminal narrowing and the vascular response after deep vessel wall injury in a new coronary (re)stenosis model in the pig [7]. The focus was to study the influence of both remodeling and neointima formation on luminal narrowing.

Address for correspondence: H.R. Andersen MD, DMSc, Department of Cardiology, Skejby University Hospital, 8200 Århus, Denmark. Tel.: +45-89495566. Fax.: +45-89496002.

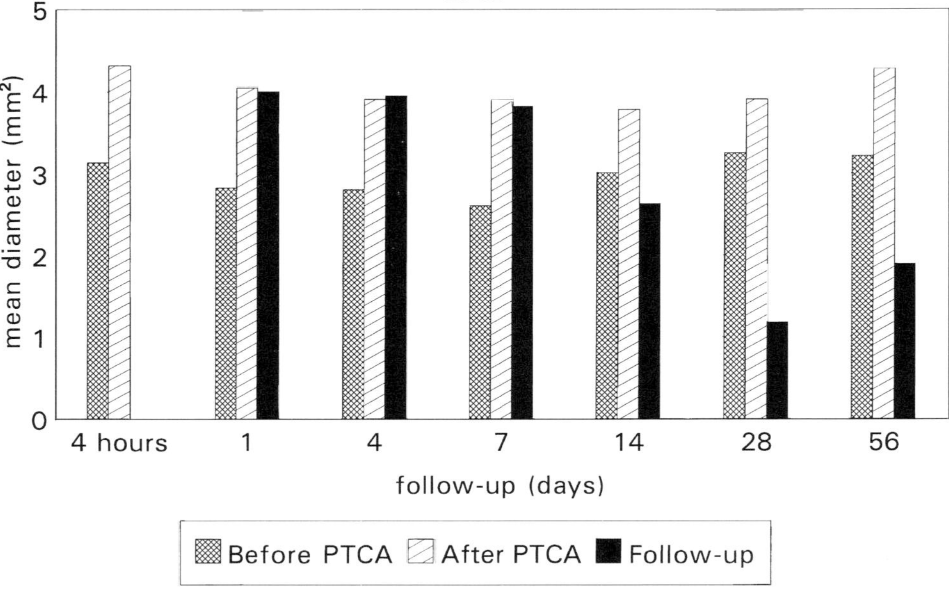

Fig. 1. Coronary angiography before and immediately after coronary angioplasty (PTCA) and at late follow-up (n = 5 in each group). The figure demonstrates that the lumen becomes narrowed after 14 days follow-up. LAD: left anterior descending coronary artery.

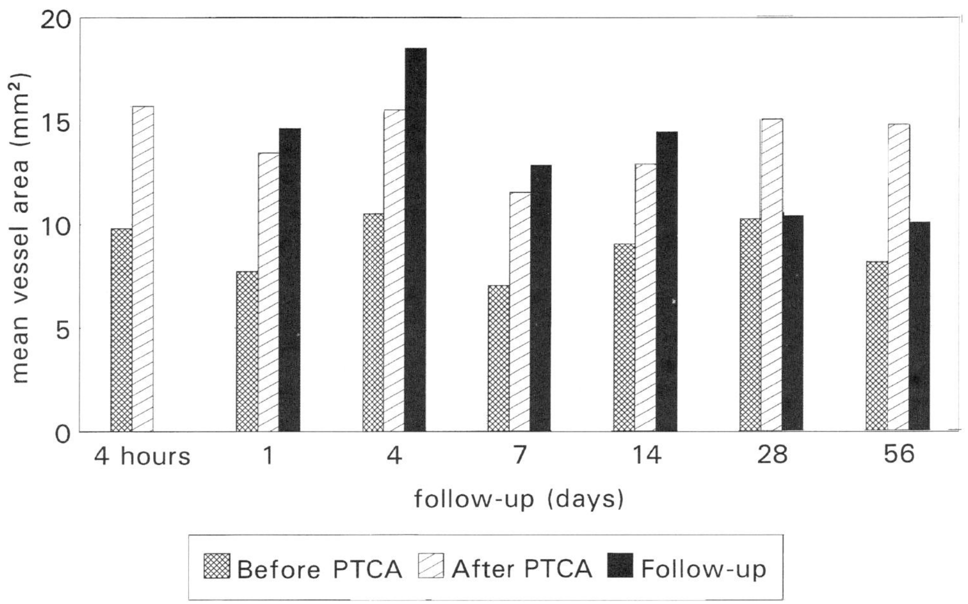

Fig. 2. Intracoronary ultrasound before and immediately after coronary angioplasty (PTCA) and at late follow-up (n = 5 in each group). The figure demonstrates that the vessel becomes smaller (constricted) after 28 days follow-up. LAD: left anterior descending coronary artery.

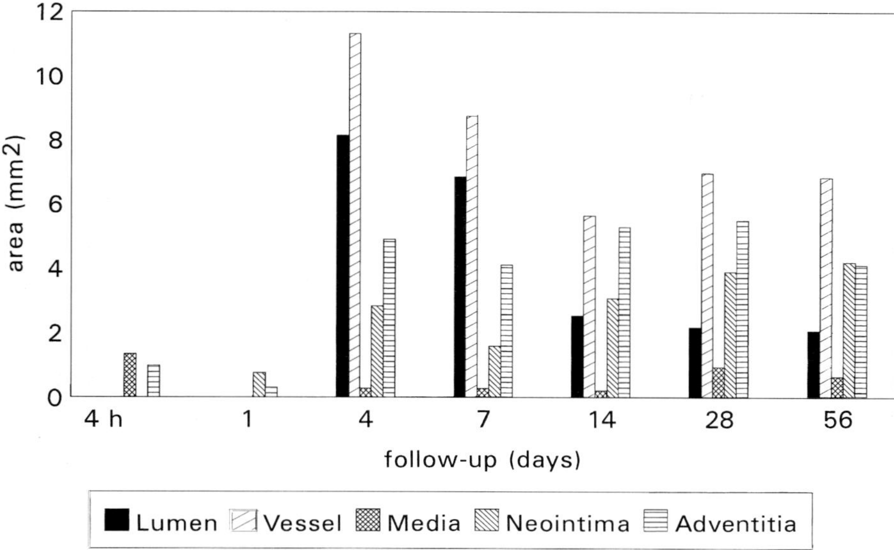

Fig. 3. Lumen area, vessel area and areas of the different vessel wall components measured by histology at follow-up (n = 5 in each group). In the two first follow-up groups (4 h and 1 day) it was not possible to measure the lumen area and the vessel area because the artery was collapsed. Therefore, only tissue areas for the vessel wall components are reported for these two groups. The figure demonstrates that the lumen and the vessel become smaller after 14 days follow-up. At 4 days follow-up the neointima is composed of 100% thrombus without cell proliferation. At 7 days follow-up the neointima is a mixture of thrombus and cell proliferation and at a later follow-up it is composed of 100% cells and extracellular matrix. The largest new formation of tissue in the vessel wall is neoadventitia formation.

Methods

Pigs weighing 75 kg were used. Before angioplasty (PTCA), coronary angiography and intracoronary ultrasound were performed. Immediately after PTCA the pigs were reinvestigated by coronary angiography, intracoronary ultrasound and intracoronary angioscopy. At the later follow-up, after 4 and 24 h, 4, 7, 14, 28 and 56 days (n = 5 in each group), the pigs were examined by coronary angiography and intracoronary ultrasound. Furthermore, intracoronary angioscopy was used at follow-up from 4 h to 14 days but not at later stages because at 14 days the luminal surface had healed again. Finally, the heart was excised and examined by pathology to correlate the follow-up measurements with the pathology.

Results

Angiography showed that the coronary arteries remained dilated for 7 days. Luminal narrowing was seen after 14 days and stenosis formation increased further at 28 and 56 days (Fig. 1). Intracoronary ultrasound revealed that stenosis was caused by vessel constriction (strangulation), i.e., the external perimeter of the stenotic vessel at late follow-up became smaller than it was immediately after PTCA (Fig. 2). The degree of vessel constriction correlated very strongly with the size of the lumen late after intervention; i.e., the bigger the postinterventional vessel size (no or only modest constriction), the better the lumen size. Pathology and coronary angioscopy revealed that thrombus formation (maximum at day 4) was small and thrombus organization explained only a small fraction of late neointima formation (Fig. 3). Pathology further demonstrated that neoadventitial formation was massive already at day 4 and preceded neointima formation which first appeared at day 7 and was maximal at days 28 and 56 (Fig. 3). Thus, addition of new mass (thrombus or neointima) inside the vessel could only explain a small fraction of the late lumen loss seen by angiography whereas constrictive vascular remodeling (strangulation) was the most important mechanism causing angiographic luminal narrowing.

Conclusion

In this pig model, late luminal narrowing was predominantly caused by constrictive remodeling (vessel strangulation) and not by addition of new mass (thrombus organization or neointimal proliferation). Thus, remodeling rather than neointima formation is most critical for restenosis in this pig model. These findings indicate that the pig-restenosis model reflects the pathophysiology of restenosis observed clinically.

References

1. Mintz GS, Popma JJ, Pichard AD et al. Atrerial remodeling after coronary angioplasty: a serial intravascular ultrasound study. Circulation 1996;94:35—43.
2. Kimura T, Kaburagi S, Tamura T et al. Remodeling of human coronary arteries undergoing coronary angioplasty or artherectomy. Circulation 1997;96:475—483.
3. Teirstein PS, Massullo V, Jani S et al. Catheter-based radiotherapy to inhibit restenosis after coronary stenting. N Engl J Med 1997;336:1697—1703.
4. Tardif JC, Côté G, Lespérance et al. Probucol and multivitamins in the prevention of restenosis after coronary angioplasty. N Engl J Med 1997;336:365—372.
5. Carter AJ, Laird JR, Farb A, Kufs W, Wortham DC, Virmani R. Morphologic characteristics of lesion formation and time course of smooth muscle cell proliferation in a porcine proliferative restenosis model. J Am Coll Cardiol 1994;24:1398—1405.
6. Schwartz RS, Murphy JG, Edwards WD, Camrud AR, Vlietstra RE, Holmes DR. Restenosis after balloon angioplasty. A practical proliferative model in porcine coronary arteries. Circulation 1990;82:2190—2200.
7. Andersen HR, Mæng M, Thorwest M, Falk E. Remodeling rather than neointima formation explains luminal narrowing after deep vessel wall injury. Insight from a new porcine (re)stenosis model. Circulation 1996;93:1716—1724.

Atherosclerosis XI.
B. Jacotot, D. Mathé and J.-C. Fruchart, editors.

Platelets and arterial remodeling

L. Badimon[1] and J.J. Badimon[2]

[1]*Cardiovascular Research Center, CSIC-HSCSP-UAB, Barcelona, Spain; and* [2]*Cardiovascular Institute, Mount Sinai Medical Center, New York, New York, USA*

Abstract. Remodeling and restenosis are reparative processes activated in response to injury induced by angioplasty. Luminal narrowing postangioplasty has been related to the accretion of a new mass of cells, proteins and glycans (thrombus and neointimal masses) and to remodeling, produced by early recoil, local vasoconstriction and late contraction not associated to compensatory enlargement. The contribution of SMC activation and matrix synthesis, traditionally considered essential in restenosis, has been questioned in favor of remodeling. In the porcine model of coronary angioplasty we observed that they are not excluding phenomena. However, fibrocellular hyperplasia and thrombosis are the predominant mechanisms responsible for late luminal narrowing after angioplasty. Acute platelet deposition is associated with thrombin generation and ultimately thrombus. Thrombin, procoagulant and mitogenic, is generated in large amounts at the time of arterial injury and persists for some time. Prolonged specific thrombin inhibition seems to reduce neointima formation on diverse animal models. Thrombi contain attractants and mitogens for smooth muscle cells and function as a matrix for the migration and proliferation of smooth muscle cells.

Keywords: restenosis, thrombin, thrombus.

Introduction

Despite procedural and technical advances in percutaneous transluminal coronary angioplasty (PTCA), the major drawback of the procedure, restenosis within 6 months, remains largely unchanged. Restenosis is a complex reparative process that involves several redundant and overlapping mechanisms. The sequence of events leading to restenosis after balloon angioplasty includes recoil which tends to occur within the first 24 h; remodeling; mural thrombus formation with subsequent organization by connective tissue which occurs within the first 2 to 3 weeks; and smooth muscle cell activation, migration, proliferation and increased synthesis of extracellular matrix. They are not exclusive events but tend to overlap to varying degrees. The underlying dilated vessel is an important determinant of the vessel response to injury. Numerous growth factors originating from the thrombus, the vessel wall and circulating cells contribute to the complex series of events involved in restenosis [1]. The angiographic presence of an intraluminal thrombus has been associated most consistently with an increased risk of early

---

Address for correspondence: Prof Lina Badimon, Cardiovascular Research Center, CSIC-HSCSP-UAB, Jordi Girona, 18-26, 08034 Barcelona, Spain. Tel.: +34-3-4006146. Fax: +34-3-2045904. E-mail: lbmucv@cid.csic.es

340

adverse outcome after PTCA. Intracoronary angioscopy, providing direct images of the endoluminal surface of the culprit lesions, has shown that, indeed, yellow color (disrupted plaque) and thrombus at the culprit lesion site before PTCA can identify patients at high risk of early adverse outcome (a major complication or a recurrent ischemic event) post-PTCA [2,3]. Thus, platelets and thrombosis play a central role in human vessel dilatation, and may regulate the diverse phases in which the pathogenesis of restenosis has been subdivided.

Stent (matched to vessel size) implantation demonstrated that the greater initial luminal gain obtained by the vessel scaffolding contributed to a significantly lower restenosis rate in the stented group compared with the balloon angioplasty group [4]. Implantation of oversized stents (resetting the vessel size into undiseased conditions) has also shown to produce enforced mechanical remodeling of the coronary vessel with subsequent reduction in subacute occlusion and improved accommodation of reactive intimal hyperplasia and a restenosis rate of 16% [5]. Although periprocedural complications and the oversized stent clinical effects should still be tested from a pathophysiological standpoint these results indicate that the enforced mechanical scaffolding, and hence controlled remodeling, results in the prevention of acute occlusion and chronic recoil of the vessels (lower local blood shear stress with lower platelet deposition than in nonscaffolded arteries). Both factors that reduce acute thrombosis seem to result in improved restenosis at follow-up [5].

Natural history of restenosis: platelet involvement

Recoil
An immediate increase of the vascular lumen is observed after percutaneous coronary interventions. However, spontaneous coronary artery vasoconstriction after PTCA occurs routinely at, and distal to, the site of balloon dilatation despite pretreatment with aspirin [6]. Recoil that develops within minutes to hours of the intervention may be the predominant contributor to restenosis in vessels where the dilated plaque is composed mainly of fibrotic or sclerotic tissue. Decreases in luminal diameter angiographically detected 24 h after successful PTCA are present in lesions that are more likely to develop restenosis at follow-up [7]. However, recoil may play a lesser role than thrombosis in restenosis of lipid-rich plaques where the high content of tissue factor and increased thrombogenicity make them more prone to develop luminal and intraluminal thrombi.

Mural thrombus formation
Balloon angioplasty causes significant vascular injury, as evidenced by the significant fracture and compression of the atherosclerotic plaque. Exposure of subendothelial and medial constituents to flowing blood leads to activation of the hemostatic system resulting in platelet deposition and extensive fibrin deposition [8,9]. Platelets through receptor-ligand interaction, coat the newly injured vessel wall with platelet-rich thrombus. Occupation of platelet receptors ultimately

results in discharge of α-granules (ADP, serotonin, thromboxane A_2, growth factors and prostaglandins) which promote further platelet activation and aggregation. These events begin instantaneously after injury [8]. Thrombi contain attractants and mitogens for smooth muscle cells and function as a matrix for the migration and proliferation of smooth muscle cells. Thrombin which is generated via the intrinsic and extrinsic coagulation systems accumulate in the thrombi. After arterial injury, exposed tissue factor (TF) in the atherosclerotic plaque interacts with factor VII with subsequent activation of factor X resulting in the conversion of prothrombin to thrombin. Thrombin is the most potent activator of platelets, furthermore it converts fibrinogen to fibrin, activates several coagulation factors and stabilizes the thrombus by cross-linking fibrin. Thrombin has also been shown to stimulate growth factor release and SMC proliferation. Thrombin shares with other growth factors, especially PDGF, the ability to activate numerous transmembrane signaling pathways.

Activated monocytes, which are recruited to the dilated area, are sources of TF and may play a role in the modulation of thrombus formation. By analyzing samples obtained at atherectomy it has recently been reported that there is an increased macrophage content in coronary plaques [10]. Atherosclerotic lesions display diverse morphology and composition, varying from highly lipid-rich to fibrotic. The exposed substrate after balloon angioplasty is therefore dependent on plaque composition, and the atheromatous (lipid-rich and TF-rich) core is the most thrombogenic component of human atherosclerotic plaques [11,12]. Therefore, angioplasty of plaques with a high content of lipid material will be associated with a significant acute thrombotic response as compared with the other plaque types and geometrical changes to the vessel wall after the procedure will also modulate thrombus formation [13]. Normal coronary arteries respond to increased shear stress by vasodilating; but this compensatory endothelium-dependent vasodilatation does not occur in atherosclerotic segments. Platelet-dependent vasoconstriction occurs in the absence of endothelium, suggesting a direct effect of platelet-secreted vasoconstrictors on the underlying muscle cells [14]. Angioplasty disrupts the antithrombotic properties of intact endothelium. Production of nitric oxide, and other antithrombotic and growth inhibitors such as heparin sulfate are no longer produced sufficiently to counteract the effects of platelets, thrombin and fibrin at the site of injury [8].

Smooth muscle cells activation and extracellular matrix synthesis
SMC hypertrophy and hyperplasia play a key role in the understanding of morphological changes and cellular rearrangements, or remodeling, after angioplastia. SMC migration and proliferation significantly contribute to restenosis through autocrine and paracrine mediators. Arterial narrowing results from increased synthesis of extracellular matrix by activated SMC. Immediately after injury, SMC leave their quiescent state and enter the cell cycle, associated with the induction of early response genes. Cell division and growth is tightly controlled by a series of positive and negative regulators which act at sequential

342

points throughout the cell cycle.

Numerous vasoconstrictors (including thromboxane, serotonin and prostaglandins) and mitogenic factors are released by activated platelets. The most important growth factors released by platelets are PDGF, EGF and TGF-β [15]. Stretching of the arterial wall by itself induces SMC activation and growth by stimulating the release of growth factors, specifically FGF from damaged EC and SMC. Additionally the existence of an active thrombotic stimulus will increase the local concentration of growth factors such as thrombin and PDGF.

There is controversy on the origin of the proliferative population of smooth muscle cells in restenotic plaques [16]. Human atherosclerotic intima is extremely rich in smooth muscle cells, as is the underlying media. Following angioplasty the smooth muscle cells observed in the neointima may originate either from remnant intima, media or a combination of both [17]. The duration of migration and whether cellular replication is required before migration are not known. In vitro data suggest that PDGF is a potent smooth muscle cell mitogen and chemoattractant; however, increasingly abundant data from in vivo studies indicate that PDGF may be more important for cell migration than proliferation. PDGF-BB also stimulates SMC to release plasmin, protein involved (in addition to fibrinolysis) in the digestion of extracellular matrix creating space for the migration of smooth muscle cells from the media to the intima. SMC arriving into the intima may undergo replication for different time following balloon angioplasty. Cellular proliferation in the intima is identifiable in human histological sections as soon as 5 days after angioplasty and appears to stabilize by the 3rd to 4th month after balloon angioplasty [18]. As SMC lose their capacity to proliferate, they begin to deposit large quantities of extracellular matrix including proleoglycans, collagen and elastin. TGF-β is a powerful regulator of extracellular matrix production [19]. TGF-β activates genes responsible for proteoglycan, collagen and elastin production, and decreases the synthesis of proteolytic enzymes.

Proliferation winds down and the new endothelium begins to produce larger quantities of the inhibitory proteoglycan, heparin sulfate, and nitric oxide. It is not known when neoendothelialization occurs but it seems that it occurs during the final phase. It is not known at what moment the new endothelium is functionally normal, but it passivates the angioplasty exposed vessel surface ending the constant interaction of platelets and platelet-derived products with the vessel wall.

Acknowledgements

This work has been made possible with funding from FIS 95-0917, CDTI/BMS 96-0035 and Cardiovascular Research Foundation, Catalana Occidente.

References

1. Ip J, Fuster V, Israel D et al. The role of platelets, thrombin and hyperplasia in restenosis after

coronary angioplasty. J Am Coll Cardiol 1991;17:77B—88.

2. Waxman S, Sassower MA, Mittleman MA et al. Angioscopic predictors of early adverse outcome after coronary angioplasty in patients with unstable angina and non-Q-wave myocardial infarction. Circulation 1996;93:2106—2113.

3. White CJ, Ramee SR, Collins TJ et al. Coronary thrombi increase PTCA risk. Circulation 1996;93:253—258.

4. Fischman DL, Leon MB, Baim DS et al. A randomized comparison of coronary stent placement and balloon angioplasty in the treatment of coronary artery disease. N Engl J Med 1994;331:496—501.

5. Ozaki Y, Keane D, Ruygrok P et al. Six-month clinical and angiographic outcome of the new, less shortening wallstent in native coronary arteries. Circulation 1996;93:2114—2120.

6. Fischell TA, Derby G, Tse TM et al. Coronary artery vasoconstriction routinely occurs after percutaneous transluminal coronary angioplasty. Circulation 1988;78:1323—1334.

7. Rodriguez A, Santaera O, Larribeau M et al. Early decrease in minimal lumen diameter after succesful PTCA predicts late restenosis. Am J Cardiol 1993;71:1391—1395.

8. Steele P, Chesebro JH, Stanson AW et al. Balloon angioplasty-natural history of the pathophysiological response to injury in a pig model. Circ Res 1985;57:105—112.

9. Badimon L, Alfon J, Royo T et al. Cell biology of restenosis post-angioplasty. Z Kardiologie 1995;84(Supp 4):145—149.

10. Moreno P, Falk E, Palacios I et al. Macrophage infiltration in acute coronary syndromes. Circulation 1994;90:988—996.

11. Fernandez-Ortiz A, Badimon JJ, Falk E et al. Characterization of the relative thrombogenicity of atherosclerotic plaque components. J Am Coll Cardiol 1994;23:1562—1569.

12. Toschi V, Fallon J, Gallo R et al. Tissue factor predicts the thrombogenicity of human atherosclerotic plaques. Circulation 1995;92:I—112.

13. Badimon L, Badimon JJ. Mechanism of arterial thrombosis in non-parallel streamlines: platelet-thrombi grow on the apex of stenotic severely injured vessel wall. J Clin Invest 1989;84:1134—1144.

14. Lam JYT, Chesebro JH, Steele PM et al. Is vasospasm related to platelet deposition? Relationship in a porcine preparation of arterial injury in vivo. Circulation 1987;75:243—248.

15. Schwartz SM, Reidy MA, O'Brian ERM. Assessment of factors important in atherosclerotic occlusion and restenosis. Thromb Hemost 1995;74:541—551.

16. Clowes AW, Schwartz SM. Significance of quiescent smooth muscle cell migration in the injured rat carotid artery. Circ Res 1985;56:139—145.

17. Schwartz SM, deBlois D, O'Brien ERM. The intima-Soil for atherosclerosis and restenosis. Circ Res 1995;77:445—465.

18. Gravanis MB, Roubin GS. Histopathologic phenomena at the site of percutaneous transluminal coronary angioplasty. Hum Pathol 1989;20:477—485.

19. Roberts AB, Sporn MB. Physiological actions and clinical applications of TGF-β. Am J Physiol 1993;264:G179—G186.

Arterial smooth muscle cell phenotypic modulation after angioplasty

Huguette Louis, Pascale Dufourcq, Julie Lavie, Danielle Daret, Jacques Bonnet and Jean-Marie Daniel Lamazière
INSERM, Unité 441 Athérosclérose, Pessac, France

Abstract. *Background.* Vascular smooth muscle cells (SMC) play an important role during the atherosclerosis process as well as restenosis after angioplasty. In order to better understand the role of SMC reactivity at the onset of intimal hypertrophy after angioplasty, we measured phenotypic variation of the tunica media before and after the intimal thickening.

Methods. We measured the SMC reactivity in a kinetic model of rabbit angioplasty between 2 and 30 days after ballooning.

Results. We focused our study on the reactivity of medial SMC. We measured antigenic distribution of markers of differentiation. Adhesion molecule VCAM-1 and its counterreceptor VLA4 were expressed in some cells of the internal part of the media; at the same time most cells re-expressed nonmuscle myosin-B (nm-MHC-B), and smooth muscle myosin heavy chain (sm-MHC).

Conclusion. The control of SMC differentiation is a key event for both the prevention and regulation of inflammation processes of arterial intima. New therapeutic targets can be proposed such as cytokine regulation (TGF-β) or control of SMC transcriptional factors.

Introduction

Atherosclerosis and restenosis after angioplasty implicated remodelling of the arterial wall. Most modifications of the arterial wall involved SMC reactivity. Medial smooth muscle cells (SMC) modified their phenotype and invaded the intimal space. Proliferation and migration of SMC in the vessel intima are well characterised for restenosis following angioplasty. Most SMC phenotypic modulations describe intimal cells; there is very little information concerning cell reactivity of the media before the initiation of the inflammatory process. Therefore the attempts to reveal specific characteristics of medial SMC are quite essential. Adhesion and signalling molecules found on the cell surface, such as the β1 integrins [1,2] and vascular cell adhesion molecule-1 [3,4] influence many disease processes, including atherogenesis [5,6] and have also been implicated in modulation of SMC function.

In order to better understand the key events which lead to intimal hyperplasia the present study examined, in a rabbit model of balloon injury, VCAM-1 and

---

Address for correspondence: Jean-Marie Daniel Lamaziere, INSERM U. 441, Avenue du Haut-Lévêque, 33600 Pessac, France. Tel.: +33-05-57-89-19-79. Fax: +33-05-56-36-89-79.
E-mail: Jean-Marie.D-Lamaziere@bordeaux.inserm.fr

346

the α-4 subunit of VLA-4 integrin expression by SMC, and SMC phenotypic modulation during neointimal formation. We showed that VCAM-1 and α-4 are coexpressed by SMC at the beginning of neointimal formation when SMC are activated and that this expression precedes the intimal thickening.

Materials and Methods

Experimental model

Briefly, under general anesthesia, a balloon angioplasty catheter (3F) was introduced through the femoral artery and advanced into the abdominal aorta. The endothelium of the descending thoracic aorta was denuded by passages of balloon catheter. The rabbits were killed between 2 and 45 days postinjury; the aortas were removed, conserved immediately in liquid nitrogen, freeze-dried with a tissue dryer (ETD4 Edwards), and embedded in paraffin.

Monoclonal antibody

Monoclonal antibody (MAb) 1A4, which recognizes α-smooth muscle actine; MAb HP2/1, which recognizes α4 subunit of VLA4; and MAb h SM-V against human smooth muscle myosin heavy chain, that cross-reacts with rabbit, was kindly provided by Dr M. Glukhova [7]. MAb 2P1A2, specific for activated rabbit smooth muscle cells of the plaque and not correlated with proliferation, was described previously [8,9]. MAb Rb 1/9, which recognizes rabbit VCAM-1, was a generous gift of Dr Cybulsky.

Immunohistochemistry

Immunohistochemistry was performed using the classical method and revealed by streptavidin biotinylated peroxidase complex.

Probes

The following primer sequence was used for polymerase chain reaction amplification: 5′AAGCCAAGAGCTTGGAAGC and 3′TCCTCCTCAGAACCATCTGC for smooth muscle myosin heavy chain (sm-MHC); 5′CTTCTCCCATGAAGATTCTGTCA; and 3′TCTCTGGACGCTTGGGAGGACCA for nonmuscle myosin-B (nm-MHC-B). Sequencing of the cDNA probes used in the present experiments indicates that the sm-MHC probe encodes a 3′ region of the sm-MHC gene and that it is 98% homologous to rabbit sm-MHC, and also that the probe nm-MHC-B encodes for a 5′ region of nm-MHC-B gene. The specificity of these probes for rabbit sm-MHC and nm-MHC-B were confirmed by northern blot analysis (data not shown).

In situ hybridization

In situ hybridisation using digoxigenin U-labelled riboprobes was performed as previously described. Hybridisation was performed overnight at 50°C in a humid chamber. After hybridisation sections were incubated twice with 50% formamide, 2XSSC at 55°C, treated with RNase A (20 µg/ml) for 30 min, and washed twice in 2XSSC, followed by 1XSSC washes. To detect the specific hybrids, the slides were incubated for 90 min at 37°C with an antidigoxigenin antibody conjugated to alkaline phosphatase. Staining was allowed to develop overnight in the dark with nitroblue tetrazolium salt and 5-bromo-4-chloro-3-indol phosphate. Slides were dehydrated, mounted in DPX and observed under a light microscope. The antigenic expression of SMC markers were quantified by color video image analysis using an IBM personal computer [10].

Results

SMC activation

VCAM-1 and VLA4 expression
Expression of VCAM-1 and VLA-4 using indirect immunohistochemistry is shown in Fig. 1A and B. Two days after balloon injury VCAM-1 and VLA-4 were expressed by SMC in the internal part of the media. We could show a great heterogeneity of the vascular response, only 30% of the cells were stained by both antibodies. This expression increased to 50% at 4 days. At 7 days after balloon injury, when an intimal thickening is present, VCAM-1 and VLA-4 expression decreased in the media, however, intimal SMC expressed VCAM-1 and VLA-4. This expression decreased up to the 10th day. Meanwhile most medial SMC expressed an antigen, 2P1A2, specific for activated SMC [8,9]

Myosin expression
Using immunohistochemistry for sm-MHC, we studied the phenotypic modulation of SMC in the media and intima layer. Until the 4th day, when no intima thickening was detected, SMC of the media expressed a high level of sm-MHC (40%) similar to a normal aorta (data not shown). Between 7 and 10 days postangioplasty sm-MHC decreased in the media (5%) and was absent in the neointima (Fig. 1C). After 15 days SMMHC increased in the media (39%) and the intima (29%), and returned to normal values after the 20th day. Since immunochemistry is not sensitive enough to demonstrate variation of protein synthesis, we analysed these variations of sm-MHC and we studied mRNA expression of sm-MHC and nm-NHC-B by in situ hybridisation (Fig. 1A—D).

In situ hybridisation for nm-MHC-B in uninjured arteries showed expression of this gene predominantly in the adventitial layer. A markedly elevated nm-MHC-B mRNA expression was detected 2 days after injury (Fig. 1A). Control hybridisations were negative. Seven days after balloon angioplasty, nm-MHC-B

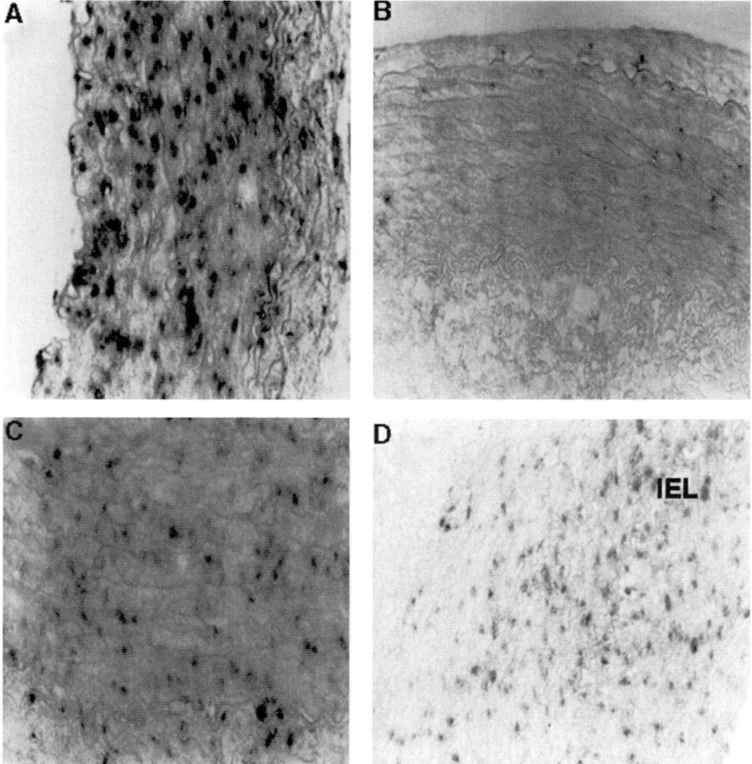

Fig. 1. **A:** In situ hybridisation of nm-MHC-B 2 days after injury. **B:** In situ hybridisation of nm-MHC-B 10 days after injury. **C:** In situ hybridisation of sm-MHC 2 days after injury. **D:** In situ hybridisation of sm-MHC 20 days after injury. IEL = internal elastic lamina.

mRNA expression was found primarily in the developing neointima and the medial expression decreased. Ten days after injury we could not detect any expression of nmMHC in both intimal and tunica media (Fig. 1B).

During this time course, as observed for protein, sm-MHC gene expression varied greatly. Sm-MHC mRNA decreased as soon as the 4th day (Fig. 1C) and was quasi undetectable until the 7th. At 10 days expression was found in the media. After 15 days mRNA expression of sm-MHC increased both in the media and in the intima layers and returned to normal values for the media at 20 days (Fig. 1D).

Discussion

Inflammation processes have been demonstrated to play major roles in intimal extension during intimal hypertrophy and hyperplasia. Pathological intima is invaded by circulating macrophages as well as by activated T lymphocytes. Moreover the possibility of SMC participating in the inflammatory process has been demonstrated. Some of them can express the class II antigen HLA-DR which is normally present at the surface of immunological cells, and SMC are able to synthesise adhesion molecules such as ICAM-1 and VCAM-1 implicated in the cellular recruitment during the inflammatory process.

We have shown in this paper the expression of VCAM-1 and its counterreceptor, VLA4, by SMC of the tunica media 2 days after angioplasty. We demonstrated that at the same time medial SMC dedifferentiate by the synthesis of nonmuscle myosin-B heavy chain. This form is normally synthesised during embryogenesis [11]. During the 1st week after ballooning, the dedifferentiation pattern is largely expressed throughout the media, meanwhile, the expression of adhesion molecules is restricted to some cells inside the internal part of the media. Activated SMC express antigens which are implicated into the inflammatory process, although this represents only a part of the dedifferentiated SMC.

With regards sm-MHC, we found, by in situ hybridisation, a large decrease in mRNA expression from the 4th to the 10th day postangioplasty. Moreover we detected a strong expression of this mRNA inside the intima after the 15th day postangioplasty, just before the intima stopped progressing. We can conclude that in order to prevent or stabilise intimal remodelling, new strategies of treatment should involve the control of SMC differentiation.

References

1. Clyman R, Turner DC, Kramer RH. An $\alpha 1/\beta 1$-like integrin receptor on rat aortic smooth muscle cells mediates adhesion to laminin and collagen types I and IV. Arterioscl Thromb 1990; 10:402−409.
2. Koyama N, Seki J, Vergel S, Mattsson E, Yednock T, Kovach NL, Harlan JM, Clowes AW. Regulation and function of an activation-dependent epitope of $\beta 1$ integrins in vascular cells after balloon injury in baboon arteries and *in vitro*. Am J Pathol 1996;148:749−761.
3. O'Brien KD, Allen MD, McDonald TO, Chait A, Harlan JM, Fishbein D, McCarty J, Ferguson M, Hudkins K, Benjamin CD, Lobb R, Alpers CE. Vascular cell adhesion molecule-1 is expressed in human coronary atherosclerotic plaques. J Clin Invest 1993;92:945−951.
4. Couffinhal T, Duplàa C, Moreau C, Daniel Lamazière JM, Bonnet J. Regulation of vascular cell adhesion molecule-1 in human vascular smooth muscle cells. Circ Res 1994;74:225−234.
5. Cybulsky M, Gimbrone J. Endothelial expression of a mononuclear leukocyte adhesion molecule during atherogenesis. Science 1991;251:788−791.
6. Duplàa C, Couffinhal T, Dufourcq P, Llanas B, Moreau C, Bonnet J. The integrin VLA-4 is expressed on human smooth muscle cell: involvement of $\alpha 4$ and VCAM-1 during smooth muscle cell differentiation. Circ Res 1997;80:159−169.
7. Glukhova MA, Frid MG, Koteliansky VE. Phenotypic changes of human aortic smooth muscle cells during development and in the adult vessel. Am J Physiol 1991;261:72−77.
8. Daniel Lamazière JM, Desmouliere A, Pascal M, Larrue J. Detection of atherosclerosic plaque with two monoclonal antibodies. Atherosclerosis 1988;74:115−126.
9. Desmoulière A, Daniel Lamazière JM, Larrue J. Phenotypic expression of surface antigens of rabbit aortic smooth muscle cells in culture. Atherosclerosis 1990;85:25−35.
10. Daniel Lamazière JM, Lavallée J, Zunino C, Larrue J. Semiquantitative study of the distribution

of two cellular antigens by computer-directed color analysis. Lab Invest 1993;68:248–252.
11. Sartore S, Chiavegato A, Rafaella F, Faggin E, Pauletto P. Myosin gene expression and cell phenotypes in vascular smooth muscle during development, in experimental model, and in vascular disease. Arterioscl Thromb 1997;17:1210–1215.

Atherosclerosis XI.
B. Jacotot, D. Mathé and J.-C. Fruchart, editors.

Role of specific smooth muscle cell populations in atherosclerosis and restenosis

P. Pauletto[1], E. Faggin[1], M. Puato[1], M. Zoleo[1], A. Chiavegato[2] and S. Sartore[2]
Departments of [1]Clinical and Experimental Medicine and [2]Biomedical Sciences, University of Padova, Italy

Abstract. Myointimal proliferation very often underlies the restenosis process which complicates almost all revascularisation procedures. A key role in this process is played by vascular smooth muscle cells (SMC). The use of myosin isoforms as markers of SMC differentiation allows the characterisation of different developmental stages. Based on smooth muscle (SM) and nonmuscle (NM) myosin heavy chain (MyHC) expression, SMC of rabbit aorta display three maturational stages: adult, postnatal, and fetal. These cell types can be identified in vivo and in vitro using monoclonal antibodies and molecular probes specific to the different MyHC isoforms. In rabbit carotid arteries, fetal-type SMC represent the bulk of the restenosis lesion 3 weeks after balloon injury despite the fact that these cells are absent in the normal adult vessel. In restenotic human carotid arteries, fetal SMC are also markedly expressed. The follow-up of patients who underwent carotid endarterectomy has shown that the number and the phenotypic characteristics of SMC found in the primary atheroma are predictive of the extent of intima-media thickness developed after surgery. Balloon injury experiments in animal models have revealed that an extensive transition from fibroblast to myofibroblast, and probably to SMC occurs also in the adventitia. This phenotypic transition might also play a potentially relevant role in humans.

Keywords: carotid arteries, differentiation, isomyosins, vascular disease.

Background

Recent results obtained using the nonmuscle (NM) myosin isoform as a marker of aortic smooth muscle cells (SMC) differentiation during development indicate that in the rabbit the mature cell phenotype is achieved through a three-step maturational process. In fact, at least two myosin isoform transitions take place: from fetal to postnatal, and from postnatal to adult. The second transition is, however, incomplete and depending upon the aortic level, a variable number of postnatal-type SMC persist in the vascular tissue of the adult animal. While the large conduit vessels display such developmental-specific phenotypical transitions, the peripheral resistance arterial vessels do not. They, in fact, possess a "fetal-type" pattern of myosin isoform expression, i.e., coexpression of NM and SM isomyosins (for review, see [1]).

Changes in the SMC composition of the rabbit and human aortic SM tissue are

Address for correspondence: P. Pauletto MD, Associate Professor, Dipartimento di Medicina Clinica e Sperimentale, Università di Padova, Via Giustiniani 2, 35126 Padova, Italy. Tel.: +39-49-8212272. Fax: +39-49-8754179. E-mail: pauletto@ux1.unipd.it

paralleled by modifications in the pattern of isomyosin expression. For example, the expression of the 200 kDa NM-MyHC is down-regulated with development, whereas the SM-type 200 kDa isoform (SM2) appears around birth and then increases markedly thereafter [1].

The size of the partially differentiated medial SMC population changes if chemical, hormonal, or mechanical insults are applied to the arterial wall [1]. For example, endogenous or exogenous hypercholesterolemia markedly increases the number of the postnatal SMC in the adult rabbit aortic media. This phenotypic change is accompanied by a marked accumulation of fetal-type SMC in the atherosclerotic plaque. Thus, both the increase of NM-MyHC expression and the down-regulation of SM2 are peculiar events of developing aortic SM tissue.

It is interesting to note that in the endothelial-injured carotid artery the medial SMC develop a fetal-type myosin isoform pattern (possibly due to a dedifferentiation process) before proliferation and migration in the neointima, but concomitantly with a burst of bromodeoxyuridine incorporation in the adventitia. After the first wave of proliferation in the media has occurred and the second one in the neointima has subsided, the majority of accumulated SMC in the neointima show the postnatal-type pattern of myosin isoform expression (partial recovery of a differentiated cell phenotype). Two months after surgery, part of the neointimal SMC acquire a fully differentiated phenotype. Polyunsaturated n-3 fatty acids (PUFA) administration to rabbits with endothelial-injured carotid arteries causes a slowing down of neointima formation, but in hypercholesterolemic rabbits which undergo endothelial lesion, administration of PUFA has no effect on plaque development. This preventive effect of PUFA occurs in absence of substantial modifications of the differentiation pattern of media/intimal SMC, indicating that the mechanism affecting neointima formation might be related to the antithrombotic effect of PUFA or by alteration of levels of reactive oxygen species, cytokines, and growth factors. It is also interesting that:
1. In the rabbit, atherosclerotic lesions occur only in those arterial sites which contain postnatal-type SMC.
2. In rabbit microvasculature (where vascular rarefaction seems to be the predominant response to hypertension), the fetal-type SMC do not increase with the increase of blood pressure levels.
3. The resistance of the rat to atherosclerosis can be correlated to lack of expansion of the "immature"-type SMC population of the media [1].

Taken together, these data stress the importance of the "immature"-type SMC in the cellular growth-response which follows a number of stimuli and indicate that in rabbit vascular SM tissue the pattern of SMC growth and the differentiation profile can be strictly related.

Vascular smooth muscle cell differentiation and the restenosis process

In most cases, restenosis after revascularization is due to myointimal proliferation [2] which is almost unrelated to the classical risk factors [3]. This peculiar aspect has been often neglected, so that many unsuccessful efforts have been made to prevent restenosis using the same approaches which were proven to be valid for primary (atherosclerotic) lesions. In addition, it is not clear whether, after removing the atherosclerotic lesion, medial SMC maintain the same characteristics displayed before plaque formation. Moreover, given the well-known low proliferation index displayed by human SMC [4], it is of fundamental importance to ascertain the existence of a cell conversion process in the adventitial layer which might add new SMC to the medial (and intimal?) layer(s). In fact, a phenotypic change occurs in the adventitial fibroblasts after endothelial injury in rabbit carotid arteries. In concordance with data of Shi et al. [5], we have found that adventitial fibroblasts become in part myofibroblasts soon after injury, and express NM-MyHC, vimentin and SM α-actin. According to the nomenclature proposed by Sappino et al. [6], these cells would correspond to the VA myofibroblast subtype. Interestingly, the E-11 antibody specific for the 22 kDa calponin-like, SM-specific SM22 polypeptide [7] is reactive with adventitial myofibroblasts. Since SM22 is expressed at early stages of development, when other SMC markers such as SM-MyHC are absent, the immunoreactivity found with this antibody in the adventitial layer of injured carotid arteries can represent a sort of recapitulation of the earliest stages of SMC lineage.

On this ground, a number of questions can be raised:

1. Are medial SMC homogeneous structurally and functionally?
2. Does a unique SMC population, with stable and heritable structural and functional properties, exist in the medial layer which might account for proliferation/migration from this compartment to the intima?
3. Are these committed medial SMC involved in the primary and/or the secondary lesion formation?
4. Are the same factors at work in the atherosclerosis lesion formation and in the development of myointimal proliferation after revascularization?
5. Can an experimental model be set up to study the phenotypical changes both in the atherosclerotic lesion/restenosis and in the underlying media?
6. Could specific markers for myofibroblast identification be prepared in order to confirm a possible incorporation of such cells into the human medial layer?
7. Can be evaluated to what extent such a process influences the size of medial/intimal layer in the atherosclerotic lesion formation and restenosis?

It must be emphasized that the "myosin" approach might give some advantages in this respect. For example, some authors [8] using a molecular probe for the NM myosin isoform B (MyHC-B) have identified SMC containing mRNA coding for this myosin isoform in biopsies obtained by directional atherectomy. In coronary arteries, while only 7% of SMC from primary lesions contained MyHC-B, about 80% of the cells were found to express this myosin isoform in restenosis specimens [9]. The presence of MyHC-B mRNA in SMC from primary coronary lesions represents a major determinant for restenosis after coronary atherectomy. Almost all patients who underwent atherectomy and whose sample hybridized with the probe for MyHC-B were prone to develop restenosis within 6 months of the procedure [9]. This is attributable to the peculiar propensity of SMC expressing this myosin isoform to migrate/proliferate [10]. A platelet myosin heavy chain (MyHC-A$_{pla1}$), B-like isoform, has also been found in the intimal thickening developed in the larger arteries of humans and the expression of this marker has been interpreted as an example of a recapitulation of an "immature" SMC phenotype in the intimal SMC [1]. The use of molecular probes [11] and monoclonal antibodies [7] to SM22 also seem to be promising to study the above-mentioned problems.

Other factors potentially involved in restenosis

For a better understanding of the restenosis process, some other relevant issues should be considered, namely the role of human cytomegalovirus infection (HCMV) and of the apoptotic process.

A latent HCMV infection has recently been associated with myointimal proliferation and restenosis of coronary arteries after percutaneous angioplasty [12]. Sequences from the HCMV immediate-early (IE) genes were found in the restenosis tissue [12]. In addition, the HCMV protein IE84, an inhibitor of the growth suppressor protein p53, was highly expressed by SMC growing from the lesion [12]. This data raised the hypothesis of the occurrence of an uncontrolled SMC proliferation induced by HCMV. Since data for a role of HCMV in restenosis of carotid arteries are lacking, and the presence of HCMV DNA was only partially tested in the previous reports on coronary arteries, we studied the restenosis tissue of internal carotid artery for the presence of HCMV genome [13]. Notwithstanding the high sensitivity of our PCR method, HCMV DNA could not be amplified in the different samples tested. Even if the number of restenosis specimens collected was limited, the lack of HCMV detection both in media and intima could be due to intrinsic resistance of this arterial segment to HCMV. In turn, this event might be related to the specific differentiation pattern displayed by SMC. Further studies are needed to clarify the relationship between HCMV and restenosis in different arterial segments.

As far as apoptosis is concerned, immunohistochemical studies on specimens retrieved from patients undergoing directional atherectomy for primary atherosclerotic or restenosis lesions have been recently carried out [14]. These studies showed that specimens from patients with restenosis contained foci of apoptosis more frequently than those from patients with primary atherosclerotic lesions. Among peripheral arterial specimens from patients with restenosis 93% contained foci of apoptosis. Conversely, apoptosis was observed in only 43% of peripheral specimens from patients with primary lesions. Moreover, in coronary arterial specimens apoptosis was observed in 86% of specimens from patients with restenosis vs. 29% of specimens from patients with primary lesions. Hence, apoptosis may modulate the cellularity of lesions that produce vascular narrowing, and particularly restenosis. In addition, other studies [15] have shown that the cytoplasmic changes of apoptosis as detected by transmission electron micro-

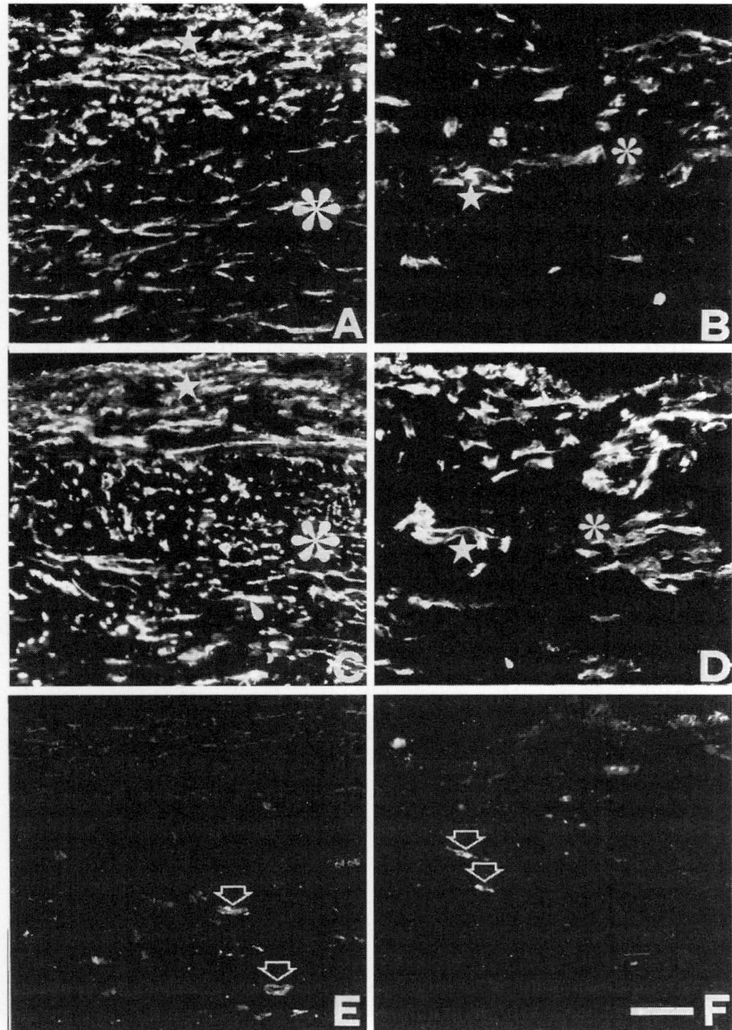

Fig. 1. Micrographs showing the immunofluorescence staining patterns of a lipidic atherosclerotic lesion (**A,C,E**) and restenotic tissue (**B,D,F**) from the same patient with SM-E7 anti-SM myosin (**A,B**), NM-F6 anti-NM myosin (**C,D**), and HAM-56 antimacrophage (**E,F**) antibodies. Note that in the atherosclerotic tissue the majority of cells are fetal-type SMC (i.e., coexpressing SM and MyHC-A_{pla1} myosin; in panels **A,C**), whereas in the restenotic tissue this SMC type represents the minority of cells (* in panels **B,D**). Noninflammatory-type MyHC-A_{pla1} containing cells are largely expressed in both tissues (* in panels **A—D**). Macrophages (in panels **E,F**) and T-lymphocytes (not shown) are barely detectable. Bar = 50 μm.

scopy are more frequent than the nuclei labeled by in situ endlabeling technique (ISEL). This suggests that SMC may undergo apoptosis without DNA fragmenta-

356

tion, and thus, the extent of apoptotic cell death in vascular lesion as evaluated by standard techniques might be underestimated.

Conclusions

On the whole, it appears that different factors are of potential importance in the process of myointimal proliferation which underlies restenosis. A more appropriate way to establish the clinical relevance of each of them is to undertake a study on medium-sized arteries using a reliable, noninvasive approach. In this view, the carotid segment is the optimal candidate for the following reasons: a number of patients undergo carotid endarterectomy for severe atherosclerosis, a large amount of tissue is removed at endarterectomy and is available for study, the morphology of the different layers of the carotid artery wall is reliably evaluated by ultrasound. In our university, more than 200 patients are being examined by ultrasound follow-up in order to define the degree of neointima developed after surgery. Our preliminary data on carotid endarterectomy specimens, obtained from fibrous or lipid-laden plaque and restenosis specimens suggest that myointimal proliferation leading to restenosis is accompanied by marked changes in the size of two specific cell populations: MyHC-A$_{pla1}$/SM myosin containing cells (fetal type SMC of our nomenclature) and noninflammatory-type MyHC-A$_{pla1}$ expressing cells (Fig. 1). Some cellular features of the primary lesion retrieved at endarterectomy appear to be relevant for predicting the degree of intima-media thickness (IMT) detected at 6-month ultrasound follow-up. In particular, a higher amount of fetal-type SMC and MyHC-A$_{pla1}$ containing cells, along with a lower content of macrophages and T lymphocytes was found in the lesion of patients displaying IMT $\geqslant$ 1.3 mm vs. those with normal intima (IMT $<$ 1.0 mm). Moreover, the degree of IMT at follow-up was inversely related with the SMC number in the media underlying the lesion. This approach might be useful for identifying patients at risk for developing relevant neointima after carotid artery surgery.

Acknowledgements

These studies are supported by a grant from the Regione Veneto, Venezia, Contract no. 708/02/96.

References

1. Sartore S et al. Myosin gene expression and cell phenotypes in vascular smooth muscle during development, in experimental models, and in vascular disease. Arterioscl Thromb Vasc Biol 1997;17:1210–1215.
2. Pauletto P, Sartore S, Pessina AC. Smooth-muscle-cell proliferation and differentiation in neointima formation and vascular restenosis. Clin Sci 1994;87:467–479.
3. Rensing BJ et al. Luminal narrowing after percutaneous transluminal coronary angioplasty. A study of clinical, procedural, and lesional factors related to long-term angiographic outcome. Circulation 1993;88:975–985.

4. Gordon D, Schwartz SM. Cell proliferation in human atherosclerosis. Trends Cardiovasc Med 1991;1:24—28.
5. Shi Y et al. Adventitial remodeling after coronary arterial injury. Circulation 1996;93:340—348.
6. Sappino AP, Schurch W, Gabbiani G. Differentiation repertoire of fibroblastic cells: expression of cytoskeletal proteins as marker of phenotypic modulations. Lab Invest 1990;63:144—161.
7. Duband JL et al. Calponin and SM22 as differentiation markers of smooth muscle: spatio-temporal distribution during avian embryonic development. Differentiation 1993;55:1—11.
8. Leclerc G et al. Evidence implicating nonmuscle myosin in restenosis. Use of in situ hybridization to analyze human vascular lesions obtained by directional atherectomy. Circulation 1992;85:543—553.
9. Simons M et al. Relation between activated SMC in coronary artery lesions and restenosis after atherectomy. N Engl J Med 1993;328:608—613.
10. Simons M, Rosemberg RD. Antisense nonmuscle myosin heavy chain and c-myb oligonucleotides suppress smooth muscle cell proliferation in vitro. Circ Res 1992;70:835—843.
11. Li L et al. SM22α, a marker of adult smooth muscle, is expressed in multiple myogenic lineages during embryogenesis. Circ Res 1996;78:188—195.
12. Speir E et al. Potential role of human cytomegalovirus and p53 interaction in coronary restenosis. Science 1994;265:391—394.
13. Pauletto P et al. Human cytomegalovirus and restenosis of the internal carotid artery. Stroke 1996;27:1669—1671.
14. Isner JM et al. Apoptosis in human atherosclerosis and restenosis. Circulation 1995;91:2703—2711.
15. Leszczynski D et al. Apoptosis of vascular smooth muscle cells: protein kinase C and oncoprotein Bcl-2 are involved in regulation of apoptosis in nontransformed rat vascular smooth muscle cells. Am J Pathol 1994;145:1265—1270.

Proliferation and death in monoclonal atherosclerotic lesions

Stephen M. Schwartz[1], Charles E. Murry[1], David Han[1], Ick-Mo Chung[1], Michael Rosenfeld[1], Leo Hofstra[2] and Martin Bennett[3]

[1]*Department of Pathology, University of Washington, Seattle, Washington, USA;* [2]*Department of Cardiology, University Hospital Maastricht, Maastricht, The Netherlands; and* [3]*Department of Medicine, University of Cambridge, Cambridge, UK*

Abstract. Until recently most attention to smooth muscle in atherosclerosis has focused on plaque smooth muscle replication. Recent findings, however, suggest that smooth muscle replication is mainly important as an etiologic process in the earliest stages of lesion formation, accounting for lesion clonality. At late stages proliferation may be a protective event, maintaining integrity of the fibrous cap. In contrast, loss of the cap may reflect apoptosis. In this brief article we review what is known about proliferation and death in the atherosclerotic lesion.

Keywords: apoptosis, necrosis, plaque rupture, programmed death.

Since Virchow's lectures in the 1850s, the conventional wisdom has been that the atherosclerotic lesion is defined by a proliferative response to toxic products that accumulate in the vessel wall, as a reaction to insudation of lipid. This now conventional view of replication of smooth muscle as a central event in atherosclerosis is problematic for three reasons. Firstly, numerous studies of smooth muscle proliferation in human atherosclerotic lesions have failed to show evidence of extensive replication [1–6]. Secondly, there is a major conceptual problem with the Virchow hypothesis. A proliferative response to injury should be polyclonal. We have, however, known for 20 years that atherosclerotic lesions are "clonal" [7]. That is, we know that the lesions in females heterozygotic for an X-linked marker, G6PD, usually express only one or the other allele. Thirdly, proliferation of plaque SMC may be beneficial rather than harmful. Recent concepts of the end stages of atherosclerosis suggest that loss of plaque integrity, rather than increase in plaque mass is the critical feature in atherosclerotic progression. Thus, cell proliferation may be beneficial by creating the matrix that prevents plaque rupture while programmed cell death may be the critical process leading to death of the individual with atherosclerotic vessels.

Clonality is the most direct evidence we have that plaques arise by proliferation. It is important, however, to realize that evidence of clonality does not necessarily mean neoplasia. Even though there is evidence that plaque smooth muscle have microsatellite instability [8,9], the marker used to detect clonality, including

Address for correspondence: S.M. Schwartz, Department of Pathology, Box 357335, University of Washington, Seattle, WA 98195-7335, USA.

somatic mutations, may not have etiologic significance. Using an X-linked CAG polymorphism in the human androgen receptor, we now know that large patches of single allotype exist even in normal arterial wall [10]. This implies that clonal expansion (defined as focal replication without mixing with neighboring clones) must, at least to some extent, be a normal feature of the human arterial wall and that plaques may arise in pre-existing intimal masses. Knowing when clonal expansion occurs then, may be useful as an "archaeological tool" to tell us about a very early event in the formation of these critical lesions. Autopsy studies suggest that intimal mass, present near birth, are the progenitors of the plaque smooth muscle.

If pre-existing intimal masses are the progenitor of the plaques, does proliferation become less interesting? Ironically, it is the death of proliferative plaque cells that now seems important in plaque progression. The identification of smooth muscle cells as the mesenchymal cells responsible for forming atherosclerotic lesions was accomplished when plaques were examined by electron microscopy by Haust et al. [11], Geer [12] and Parker and colleagues [13] in the 1960s. These workers, followed by Ross, Wissler, the Campbells and others made the reasonable assumption that the accumulation of smooth muscle was a response to injury in a smooth muscle rich tissue, just as gliosis is characteristic of responses to injury in the brain [14–16]. The studies of these investigators, however, occurred about the same time as the discovery of clonality and it was difficult to reconcile a response to injury hypothesis with the fact of monoclonality [17]. We now know that Benditt was correct about clonality of the lesions. Our recent data, however, using a definitive microdissection method to determine clonal expansion of X-linked methylated genomic DNA polymorphisms, shows that Benditt was correct and that the atherosclerotic plaque smooth muscle cell is a clone [10,18].

The only mechanistic study attempting to explain clonality was done by Thomas. He used cell-kinetic studies of pigs responding to a high-fat diet. These studies showed extensive perimitotic death of plaque smooth muscle and Thomas suggested that monoclonality might arise by selection of a subset of cells, or by some mechanism involving death of the plaque cells with overgrowth of the few remaining cells in any manner similar to dilute plate cloning in vitro [16,19,20]. Consistent with Thomas' view, we found that human plaque smooth muscle cells have an extraordinarily high level of apoptosis in vitro [21] implying that one of the unique properties of the plaque clone may be a programmed proclivity to die. This propensity is linked to the replication of these cultured cells [22].

The relevance of apoptosis of cultured plaque cells to clonal expansion in vivo is hard to explain since it reflects behavior of cells in a late, largely nonreplicative plaque. Perhaps the cells that comprise the plaque are postmitotic and those cells we obtain in vitro represent a subset that has not been selected because it has not been made to replicate. In support of this line of reasoning, numerous studies of cultured plaque smooth muscle cells have shown that these cells have a shortened replicative life span. We were able to lengthen the replicative life span by transforming the plaque cells with the antiapoptotic oncogene, bcl2 [21,23—26] suggesting that the short replicative life span reflects a need for more generations to overcome high rates of apoptosis [21,27—29]. As a clone, the plaque must be the result of repeated episodes of replication, but our and others' data have shown that plaque smooth muscle cells are not especially proliferative [1,3,6,30—36]. Indeed most of the data suggests that death, as indicated by classical morphological markers or more modern indicators of nuclear fragmentation, especially use of TUNEL, suggest that plaque smooth muscle cell are marked by high levels of death rather than replication [21,30,37—46].

The in vitro studies suggest that cell death may be a normal property of the intimal smooth muscle cell and may contribute to clonal selection in the intimal mass. Our own, now 20-year-old data in the developing intima of the rat showed high rates of spontaneous cell death [47]. Alternatively apoptosis of plaque smooth muscle may represent a response to the injury and inflammation induced by lipid accumulation. Similarly the high frequency of apoptotic cells seen during intimal thickening in the rat carotid injury model [30,38] indicate that death is "programmed" in that cells die in the absence of potentially cytotoxic leukocytes but does not rule out other paracrine phenomena. While our data do show an intrinsic p53-dependent death mechanism in plaque smooth muscle, the difficulty in studying mechanisms in poorly defined death pathways controlled by p53, led us to explore the role of the Fas/FasL pathway in these cells. The Fas receptor is part of the TNFα R1 receptor superfamily. In general, these death receptors signal death in response to cytokines. Apoptosis mediated by cytokines is likely to be an important issue in the inflammatory milieu of the atherosclerotic plaque [38,48]. In addition to interferons, IL-1β, and TNFα, the plaque contains growth factors and vasoactive agents also able to promote or inhibit apoptosis, including platelet-derived growth factor (PDGF), ET-1, angiotensin II, nitric oxide (NO) and TGF-β [21,49—51]. Geng and colleagues have suggested that plaque rupture could occur via the confluence of activated lymphocytes, and the release of cytokines able to kill smooth muscle cells at the shoulder of the plaque [48] and apoptosis via Fas/FasL have been implicated in transplant rejection arteritis [52].

We have been able to show that smooth muscle cells have all the components of the Fas/FasL pathway and that they die when Fas is activated. This death, as in some other cell types, is dependent on the absence of serum and the presence of inhibitors of protein synthesis. The relevance of these results to possible death mechanisms in vivo, however, was supported by four findings. First, Dr. Han used TUNEL to show that apoptosis was a frequent event in atherosclerotic plaque and rat neointima [38]. Second, Dr Conrad Lyles showed that macrophages [53], can locally release FasL. We have also observed FasL in the macrophage comprising a fatty lesion in monkeys, and, at least in the atherosclerotic coronary artery, we find FasL in the overlying endothelium. These observations raise the intriguing possibility that interactions between FasL and intimal smooth muscle cells can determine the death of intimal cells, perhaps explaining the

362

spontaneous death seen as intima forms spontaneously in the aging rat [47]. Third, we used western and northern blots as well as immunocytochemistry to establish that smooth muscle cells in vivo in the arterial media and at certain sites in the intima as well as all smooth muscle cells in vitro have Fas, FADD, FLICE, ICE, and YAMA. We were able to stimulate cell death by either FasL or anti-Fas IgM. Fourth, to our surprise, we found that endothelial cells also express FasL and, when cocultured with smooth muscle cells, the endothelial cell FasL could kill the smooth muscle cells in a manner that could be blocked by recombinant FasFc. Moreover, when we looked at atherosclerotic plaques by immunocytochemistry, we found areas of endothelium expressing FasL and in collaboration with Dr Lyles we found that activated macrophage can kill smooth muscle cells even in the absence of cycloheximide and the presence of serum. A large part of this effect is attributable to soluble FasL released by the activated macrophage. We also showed by χ^2 analysis that there was a very high degree of correlation between regions of the plaque showing cell death and regions showing presence of FasL. In summary, as originally proposed by Thomas [54], this could mean that clonal expansion to form the cap is due to apoptotic escape and that plaque rupture is due to activation of a Fas-mediated death pathway [55].

Finally, in thinking about the roles of death and replication in atherosclerotic progression it is important to realize that vascular narrowing, along with plaque rupture is the hallmark of advanced lesions. Narrowing, contrary to conventional wisdom, cannot be attributed to plaque growth. Instead, in both mice and men, as the plaque grows, the lumen enlarges by a poorly defined process of accommodation. We have recently shown that accommodation fails at certain sites in the vasculature of the apoE KO mouse and that this failure is correlated with loss of medial cells. This medial atrophy, presumably due to apoptosis, may be a significant factor in vascular narrowing [56].

References

1. Rekhter MD, Gordon D. Does platelet-derived growth factor-A chain stimulate proliferation of arterial mesenchymal cells in human atherosclerotic plaques? Circ Res 1994;75:410—417.
2. Conroy SC et al. Characterization of human aortic smooth muscle cells expressing HPV16 E6 and E7 open reading frames. Am J Pathol 1995;147:753—762.
3. Gordon D et al. Cell proliferation in human coronary arteries. Proc Natl Acad Sci USA 1990; 87:4600—4604.
4. Spagnoli LG et al. Autoradiographic studies of the smooth muscle cells in human arteries. Arterial Wall 1981;7:107—112.
5. O'Brien ER et al. Proliferation in primary and restenotic coronary atherectomy tissue: implications for antiproliferative therapy. Circ Res 1993;73:223—231.
6. Katsuda S et al. Human atherosclerosis IV. Immunocytochemical analysis of cell activation and proliferation in lesions of young adults. Am J Pathol 1993;142:1787—1793.
7. Benditt EP, Benditt JM. Evidence for a monoclonal origin of human atherosclerotic plaques. Proc Natl Acad Sci USA 1973;70:1753—1756.
8. Spandidos DA et al. Microsatellite instability in human atherosclerotic plaques. Biochem Biophys Res Commun 1996;220:137—140.

9. Hatzistamou J et al. Loss of heterozygosity and microsatellite instability in human atherosclerotic plaques. Biochem Biophys Res Commun 1996;225:186—190.
10. Chung IM et al. Monoclonality in atherosclerosis may arise by expansion of a preexisting clone of smooth muscle cells. Circulation 1996;94:1—238.
11. Haust MD et al. The role of smooth muscle cells in the fibrogenesis of arteriosclerosis. Am J Pathol 1960;37:377—389.
12. Geer JC. Fine structures of human aortic intimal thickening fatty streaks. Lab Invest 1965; 14:1764—1783.
13. Parker F, Odland GF. A corrective histochemical, biochemical and electron microscopic study of experimental atherosclerosis in the rabbit aorta with special references to the myo-intimal cell. Am J Pathol 1966;48:197—239.
14. Campbell GR et al. Arterial smooth muscle. A multifunctional mesenchymal cell. Arch Pathol Lab Med 1988;112:977—986.
15. Fischer-Dzoga K et al. The proliferative effect of platelets and hyperlipidemic serum on stationary primary cultures. Atherosclerosis 1983;47:35—45.
16. Ross R. The pathogenesis of atherosclerosis: a perspective for the 1990's. Nature 1993;362: 801—813.
17. Ross R. Atherosclerosis: a defense mechanism gone awry. Am J Pathol 1993;143:987—1002.
18. Murry CE et al. Monoclonality of smooth muscle cells in human atherosclerosis. Am J Pathol 1997;(In press).
19. Janakidevi K et al. Mosaicism in female hybrid hares heterozygous for glucose-6-phosphate-dehydrogenase. VI. Production of monotypism in the aortas of four of 10 mosaic hares fed cholesterol oxidation products. Exp Mol Pathol 1984;41:354—362.
20. Zavala C et al. Evidence for selection in cultured diploid fibroblast strains. Exp Cell Res 1978; 117:137—144.
21. Bennett MR et al. Apoptosis of human vascular smooth muscle cells derived from normal vessels and coronary atherosclerotic plaques. J Clin Invest 1995;95:2266—2274.
22. Bennett MR et al. Increased sensitivity of human vascular smooth muscle cells from atherosclerotic plaques to p53 mediated apoptosis. Circ Res 1997;(Submitted).
23. Moss NS, Benditt EP. Human atherosclerotic plaque cells and leiomyoma cells: comparison of in vitro growth characteristics. Am J Pathol 1975;78:175—190.
24. Dartsch PC et al. Growth characteristics and cytoskeletal organization of cultured smooth muscle cells from human primary stenosing and restenosing lesions. Arteriosclerosis 1990;10: 62—75.
25. Bierman EL. The effect of donor age on the in vitro life span of cultured human arterial smooth muscle cells. In Vitro 1978;14:951—955.
26. Dartsch PC et al. Human vascular smooth muscle cells in culture: growth characteristics and protein pattern by use of serum-free media supplements. Eur J Cell Biol 1990;51:285—294.
27. Bennett MR et al. Apoptosis of rat vascular smooth muscle cells is regulated by p53-dependent and -independent pathways. Circ Res 1995;77:266—273.
28. Bennett MR et al. Cell cycle activation and p53 induce apoptosis of smooth muscle cells in human atherosclerosis. Circ Res 1997;(In press).
29. Bennett MR et al. Increased sensitivity of human vascular smooth muscle cells from atherosclerotic plaques to P53-induced apoptosis. Circ Res 1997;(Submitted).
30. Isner JM et al. Apoptosis in human atherosclerosis and restenosis. Circulation 1995;91: 2703—2711.
31. Leclerc G et al. Assessment of cell kinetics in human restenotic lesions by in vitro bromodeoxyuridine labeling of excised atherectomy specimens. Clin Res 1993;41:343A (Abstract).
32. Pickering JG et al. Proliferative activity in peripheral and coronary atherosclerotic plaque among patients undergoing percutaneous revascularization. J Clin Invest 1993;91:1469—1480.
33. O'Brien ER et al. Angiogenesis in human coronary atherosclerotic plaques. Am J Pathol 1994; 145:883—894.

34. Rekhter M et al. Cell proliferation in human arteriovenous fistulas used for hemodialysis. Arterioscl Thromb 1993;13:609—617.
35. Rekhter MD, Gordon D. Cell proliferation and collagen synthesis are two independent events in human atherosclerotic plaques. J Vasc Res 1994;31:280—286.
36. Rekhter MD, Gordon D. Active proliferation of different cell types, including lymphocytes, in human atherosclerotic plaques. Am J Pathol 1995;147:668—677.
37. Bjorkerud S, Bjorkerud B. Apoptosis is abundant in human atherosclerotic lesions, especially in inflammatory cells (macrophages and T cells), and may contribute to the accumulation of gruel and plaque instability. Am J Pathol 1996;149:367—380.
38. Han DK et al. Evidence for apoptosis in human atherogenesis and in a rat vascular injury model. Am J Pathol 1995;147:267—277.
39. Arbustini E et al. Coronary atherosclerotic plaques with and without thrombus in ischemic heart syndromes: A morphologic, immunohistochemical, and biochemical study. Am J Cardiol 1991;68:36B—50B.
40. Geng YJ, Libby P. Evidence for apoptosis in advanced human atheroma. Colocalization with interleukin-1 beta-converting enzyme. Am J Pathol 1995;147:251—266.
41. Han DKM et al. Evidence for presence and function of Fas and Fas-ligand in the vessel wall: Mediation of smooth muscle cell apoptosis in human coronary atherosclerosis. J Biol Chem 1997;(Submitted).
42. Hofstra L et al. Monocyte induced apoptosis of vascular smooth muscle cells is mediated by Fas ligand: implications for the atherosclerotic plaque. Manuscript in preparation, 1997.
43. Kockx M, De Meyer G. Apoptosis in human atherosclerosis and restenosis (Letter to the Editor). Circulation 1995;91:394—395.
44. Kockx MM et al. Distribution of cell replication and apoptosis in atherosclerotic plaques of cholesterol-fed rabbits. Atherosclerosis 1996;120:115—124.
45. Lendon CL et al. Atherosclerotic plaque caps are locally weakened when macrophages density is increased. Atherosclerosis 1991;87:87—90.
46. Crisby M et al. Cell death in human atherosclerotic plaques involves both oncosis and apoptosis. Atherosclerosis 1997;130:17—27.
47. Schwartz SM, Benditt EP. Postnatal development of the aortic subendothelium in rats. Lab Invest 1972;26:778—786.
48. Geng Y-J et al. Apoptosis of vascular smooth muscle cells induced by in vitro stimulation with interferon-gamma, tumor necrosis factor-α, and interleukin-1β. Arterioscl Thromb Vasc Biol 1996;16:19—27.
49. Pollman MJ et al. Vasoactive substances regulate vascular smooth muscle cell apoptosis — Countervailing influences of nitric oxide and angiotensin II. Circ Res 1996;79:748—756.
50. O'Brien ER et al. βig-H3, a transforming growth factor-β-inducible gene, is overexpressed in atherosclerotic and restenotic human vascular lesions. Arterioscl Thromb Vasc Biol 1996;16:576—584.
51. Gibbons G et al. Vascular smooth muscle cell hypertrophy vs. hyperplasia. Autocrine TGF-beta-1 expression determines growth response to angiotensin II. J Clin Invest 1992;90:456—461.
52. Dong C et al. Human transplant coronary artery disease: pathological evidence for Fas-mediated apoptotic cytotoxicity in allograft arteriopathy. Lab Invest 1996;74:921—931.
53. Kiener PA et al. Characterization of the function and cellular distribution of Fas ligand in human monocytes and macrophages. Manuscript in preparation, 1997.
54. Thomas WA et al. Cell population kinetics in atherogenesis. Cell births and losses in intimal cell mass-derived lesions in the abdominal aorta of swine. Ann NY Acad Sci 1985;454:305—315.
55. Gerrity RG. The role of the monocyte in atherogenesis. I. Transition of blood-borne monocytes into foam cells in fatty lesions. Am J Pathol 1981;103:181—190.
56. Seo H-S et al. Peripheral vascular stenosis in Apo E-deficient mice: Potential roles of medial atrophy and adventitial inflammation. Arterioscl Thromb Vasc Biol 1997;(Submitted).

Development and progression of the atherosclerotic lesion

Evolution, progression and reversal of human atherosclerotic lesions

B. Greg Brown[1], Xue-Qiao Zhao[1], Drew Poulin[1] and John J. Albers[2]

[1]*Department of Medicine, Cardiology Division and the* [2]*Division of Metabolism, Endocrinology, and Nutrition, University of Washington School of Medicine, Seattle, Washington, USA*

Abstract. The dominant pathologic processes in the early stages of coronary lesion formation are an inflammatory macrophage infiltration and intimal lipid accumulation. Lipid-lowering therapy, as assessed by angiography, appears to benefit the arterial disease process. For example, in intensively treated FATS patients, the frequency of definite ($\geqslant 10\%$S) progression, per lesion at risk, was reduced by 75%, while regression frequency was doubled in mild and moderate lesion subgroups and quadrupled in the severe lesion subgroup. Clinical events were reduced by 73% in FATS; this was entirely due to a reduction in the likelihood that a mildly or moderately diseased arterial segment would undergo abrupt and substantial progression to a severe lesion at the time of the clinical event. It has been shown that the process of plaque fissuring is predicted by the size of the core lipid pool and the abundance of lipid-laden macrophages in the fibrous cap of the atheroma. Experimentally, lipid-lowering therapy virtually abolishes foam cells and more slowly depletes core cholesteryl ester deposits. Thus data presented here supports the idea that lipid-lowering therapy selectively depletes (regresses) that relatively small subgroup of lesions containing a large lipid core and abundant intimal macrophages. By doing so, the lipid-rich lesions, most vulnerable to fissuring, are stabilized and the clinical event risk is accordingly decreased.

Keywords: lipid-lowering therapy, plaque disruption, plaque regression, quantitative angiography.

Introduction

The first goal of therapy for ischemic heart disease (IHD) is to improve the symptoms of arterial obstruction, in which the blood supply is inadequate for the peak myocardial oxygen demands. Current medical management relieves symptoms by favorably altering the O_2 supply-demand imbalance. Symptom relief may also be achieved through more direct structural and/or physiological changes favorably affecting the diminished vascular flow reserve. Among these, regression has been debated as a possible mechanism for symptom relief. This report will review evidence for the promotion of regression by lipid-lowering.

A second goal of therapy in IHD is to prevent the anticipated progression to a clinical event such as sudden death, myocardial infarction or worsening angina requiring bypass surgery or angioplasty. We now appreciate that most clinical events are precipitated by an episode of plaque disruption. Data are presented in

Address for correspondence: B. Greg Brown MD, PhD, Division of Cardiology, P.O. Box 356422, University of Washington, 1959 NE Pacific Street, Seattle, WA 98195, USA. Fax: +1-206-543-3057.

this report which indicate a linkage between lipid-lowering and stabilization of plaque structure.

Histopathologic evolution of coronary lesions

The American Heart Association Committee on Vascular Lesions [1] has summarized the evolution of human coronary lesions. Briefly, there are six histological lesion classifications, with three variants of end-stage severe obstructive disease:

Type I: occurring in the first decade, contains increased monocytemacrophages in minimally thickened intima.

Type II: also first decade, many macrophages and a few smooth muscle cells are transformed to foam cells. Intima is minimally thickened without lumen encroachment.

Type III: as in type I and II, but with scattered, isolated pools of extracellular lipid.

Type IV: as in type I—III, but with confluent core of extracellular lipid and necrotic cell debris. Wall thickness is minimally increased by fibrous cap thickening (SMC, matrix, collagen) and by lipid core volume, and lumen encroachment is minimal. Types III and IV are typically seen in or after the third decade.

Type V: a progressive form of type IV in which smooth muscle collagen and core lipid accumulation thicken the plaque cap and there is progressive encroachment. The lumenal remodeling reserve [2] is exhausted. These lesions may also grow by fibrotic organization of thrombus.

Type VI: lesions of type IV and V, but with superimposed thrombosis, plaque disruption and intraplaque hemorrhage.

Type VII: an end stage plaque type in which calcification predominates.

Type VIII: an end stage version in which fibrosis predominates. There is some evidence that the latter two types evolve from the earlier advanced lesions as a phenomenon of plaque aging and remodeling.

Thus the evolution of the coronary plaque is dominated in its early stages (I—IV) by lipid accumulation [3] and a monocytic inflammatory response [4] with foam cell formation and followed by necrosis leading to extracellular lipid accumulation. Subsequent developments are a consequence of structural disruption, thrombosis [5] and remodeling of this basic fibrolipid plaque. The extent to which this progressive obstructive process can be retarded or reversed has been the subject of intense experimental and clinical investigation over the past three decades, as briefly summarized in this report.

Regression and progression of coronary lumen obstruction

The recanalization of a previously obstructed coronary artery, and the improvement of ordinary lesions are occasionally observed in a later arteriogram. Thus the critical question is not "does regression happen in patients?" (it does), but, "can it be promoted with sufficiently great magnitude and frequency to favorably alter the clinical course of the disease?" The emerging evidence regarding this question is extremely encouraging.

Experimental observations

That atherosclerosis can regress with lipid-lowering has been convincingly shown in studies in cholesterol-fed primates [6—10]. Such "atherogenic" diets increase coronary artery collagen (3 ×), elastin (4 ×), and cholesterol (7 × , mostly esterified). Cholesterol gradually accumulates in foam cells, and deep in the intimal lipid pool as ester droplets and monohydrate crystals. When the animals are changed to a vegetarian "regression" diet, serum cholesterol returns to normal (140 mg/dl), and the arterial lipid and connective tissue changes partially regress over 20—40 months. Collagen content does not decrease much from its peak value (− 20%), but elastin (− 50%) and cholesterol (− 60%, mostly esterified) do; and the plaques shrink [7,9].

Evidence of regression in patients

Regression in patients has been defined indirectly in terms of arteriographic lumen improvement and may occur in several ways. Plaque lipid may be depleted [5] as, to a lesser extent, may its connective tissues [8,10]. Lysis of fully occlusive thrombi or of mural thrombi is commonly seen. Remodeling of the underlying vascular architecture or relaxation of excess vasomotor tone may improve lumen size independently of changes in plaque size [2]. The importance of endothelial dysfunction as a basis for abnormal vasomotor and thrombogenic states, and the relationship(s) of therapy to functional recovery are becoming clarified in many of these processes [11].

Beginning in 1984, a series of randomized clinical arteriographic trials has documented the magnitude of, frequency of, and conditions under which regression can occur in patients. These have been summarized in detail [12]. Of interest, in only about half of these trials was there an entry requirement for even modest hyperlipidemia. Despite the heterogeneity among these studies in clinical presentation, lipid entry requirements, treatment regimens and methods for arteriographic analysis, their results are surprisingly consistent. The control group in each study had minimal (< 10%) LDLc reduction in virtually all cases and no change in HDLc. The LDLc reductions were substantial in all treated groups; HDLc also rose when niacin was used. Each study demonstrated an arterial treatment benefit. As a generalization from all these studies, less than one-twelfth of the control group patients were judged to have any improvement in arterial obstruction ("regression") during the study period. By contrast, more than one-quarter of treated patients were improved (a 3- to 4-fold increase). Furthermore, averaged estimates of coronary disease severity, per patient, worsened (pro-

370

gressed) by about 3% stenosis among the controls, while improving (regressing) by 1−2% stenosis among the treated patients. In nearly every study the frequency of clinical cardiovascular events was decreased substantially with therapy, although due to their small sizes, the reductions achieved statistical significance in only half of these trials.

Regression among lesions

As seen in Fig. 1, the likelihood that a given lesion will regress was surprisingly low. In FATS, only 5% of control group and 12% of treated group lesions were

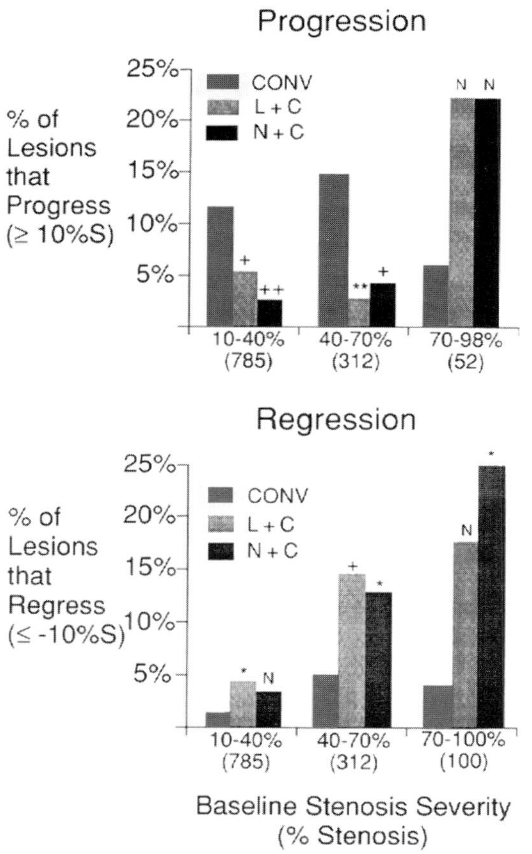

Fig. 1. Frequency of definite lesion progression and regression in FATS [12], expressed as the percentage of lesions that change in severity (regress) by a measured 10% stenosis, or more. Lesions (n = 1,197) from 120 patients are subgrouped by baseline severity into mild (10−40%S), moderate (40−70%S) and severe (70−100%S). χ^2 statistical comparisons vs. control group (CONV) frequency: *p < 0.05; +p < 0.02; N = not significant. L: lovastatin 20−40 mg bid; N: niacin 1−1.5 g qid; C: colestipol 10 g tid with meals.

seen to improve by the criterion amount of $\leqslant -10\%S$, which we consider "definite" regression with our method. Thus very few lesions undergo natural, or spontaneous regression. This number can be increased significantly by lipid-lowering therapy; nevertheless a large majority of lesions are unaltered by therapies which can be characterized as "intensive" and which result in marked alterations in the lipid and lipoprotein profile. Paradoxically, these regimens are commonly associated with substantial reductions in clinical event rate. We will return to this apparent paradox below.

Retarding progression of CAD

Data supporting the idea that lipid-lowering therapy can effectively retard progression of atherosclerotic arterial obstruction are detailed in [12] and Fig. 1. Again, despite the diversity of these trials, the evidence for reduced disease progression with therapy is surprisingly consistent. Over one-half of the control group, but only one-quarter of treated patients, were judged to have worsening arterial obstruction during the study periods.

Preventing plaque disruption and clinical events

Prevention of clinical events

Large clinical and small angiographic trials have confirmed that lipid-altering therapy will substantially reduce the frequency of cardiovascular events [13–17]. The amount of risk reduction seems out of keeping with the average $1–2\%S$ regression in lesion severity and with the fact that only about 12% of all intensively treated lesions actually regress. To understand this, we must understand the series of events in the plaque that turn a stable quiescent lesion into an unstable ischemia-provoking culprit lesion.

Determinants of plaque disruption

Two evolving insights have altered our understanding of the precipitation of clinical coronary events. First, mild and moderate coronary lesions ($<70\%$ stenosis) may abruptly progress to severe obstruction, with resulting unstable angina, myocardial infarction, or death. In fact, a majority of clinical events occur under these circumstances [18,19]. A second insight is that, for the great majority of ischemic coronary events, a "culprit" lesion can be identified with one or more of the following morphologic features at histologic examination: 1) a fissured, torn, or vented fibrous cap [20–22], 2) mural thrombus adherent at the site of the fissure [23], 3) bleeding into a large core lipid region [22], and 4) severe arterial obstruction secondary to the aggregate mass of expanded plaque and thrombus. Thus the histologic findings of a large lipid pool, and of an abundance of lipid-laden foam cells in a thinned fibrous cap and in the shoulder region of the atheroma each predispose to plaque fissuring and to subsequent plaque disruption, hemorrhage, and coronary events [23]. Based on experimental studies showing the principal mechanism of plaque regression to be lipid depletion, we propose that this small subpopulation of such fatty lesions accounts for most of the 12% frequency of lesion regression with therapy.

Prevention of plaque disruption

Reduction of plasma LDL might be expected to reduce the likelihood of fissuring because of the experimentally demonstrated favorable effects of LDL-reduction on the above predictors [9]. A consequence of such protection against fissuring would be a decline in the frequency of abrupt progression to clinical events among patients in whom LDL has been therapeutically reduced. Indeed, this has been the case. Analysis of the 13 coronary events among the 146 FATS [24] patients reveals that all were associated with a culprit coronary lesion in the distribution of worsening ischemia which had progressed substantially in severity from the baseline stenosis measurement to that at the time of the event. Furthermore, the progression of mild and moderately narrowed lesions to clinical events was virtually abolished by intensive lipid-lowering therapy, as shown in Fig. 2. Eight of nine clinical events among the conventionally treated patients arose

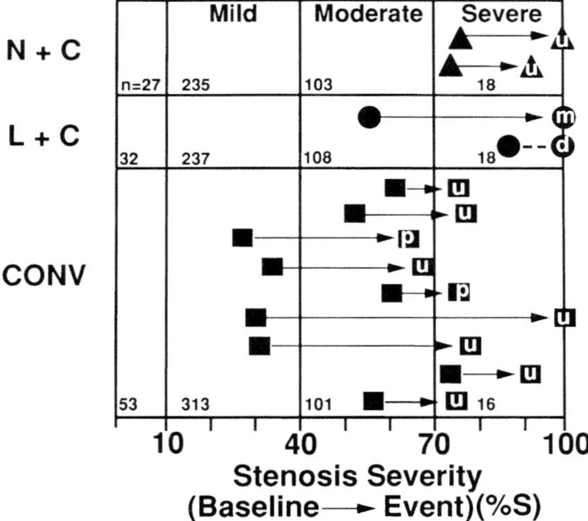

Fig. 2. Lesion changes associated with the 13 coronary events as measured from 1,316 lesions in FATS patients. Among lesions exposed to intensive lipid-lowering therapy, only one of 638 mild or moderate lesions, at baseline, among 74 such patients progressed to a clinical event while eight of 414 such lesions among 46 conventionally treated patients did so (p < 0.005). N = niacin, C = colestipol, L = lovastatin, CONV = conventional therapy, U = unstable angina event, M = myocardial infarction, D = death, P = progressive angina, %S = percent diameter stenosis. The number in each panel represents the number of lesions at risk, at baseline, in each subgroup.

from lesions less than 65% stenosis at baseline; the eight associated episodes of plaque disruption occurred among a pool of 414 mild or moderate lesions. Only one of 683 such lesions progressed to an event in the two intensively treated groups of patients (p < 0.005, per patient or per lesion). Thus, reduction in clinical events is strongly linked with stabilization of mild and moderate coronary lesions.

Acknowledgements

This manuscript is a substantially modified and abbreviated version of a previous publication [12]. Supported in part by NIH Grants R01 HL 19451, P01 HL 30086, and R01 HL 42419 from the National Heart, Lung and Blood Institute and in part by a grant from the John L. Locke, Jr. Charitable Trust, Seattle, WA.
We are grateful for the efforts of Brad Sousa in preparing this manuscript.

References

1. Stary HC, Chandler AB, Dinsmore RE, Fuster V, Glagov S, Insull W, Rosenfeld ME, Schwartz CJ, Wagner WD, Wissler RW. A definition of advanced types of atherosclerotic lesions and a histological classification of atherosclerosis. Circulation 1995;92:1512–1531.
2. Glagov S, Weisenberg E, Zarins CK, Stankunavicias R, Kolettis GJ. Compensatory enlargement of human atherosclerotic coronary arteries. N Engl J Med 1987;316:1371–1375.
3. Guyton JR, Klemp KF. Development of the atherosclerotic core region. Arterioscl Thromb 1994;14:1305–1314.
4. Henry AM, Wakeley PR, Davis MJ, Foster K, Hembry R, Murphy G, Humphries S. Localization of stromelysin gene expression in atherosclerotic plaque by in-sita hybridization. Proc Natl Acad Sci USA 1991;88:8154–8158.
5. Bini A, Fenoglio JJ, Mesa-Tejada R, Kudryk B, Kaplan KL. Identification and distribution of fibrinogen, fibrin, and fibrin(ogen) degradation products in atherosclerosis. Use of monoclonal antibodies. Arteriosclerosis 1989;9:109–121.
6. Wissler RW, Vesselinovitch D. Can atherosclerotic plaques regress? Anatomic and biochemical evidence from non-human animal models. Am J Cardiol 1990;65:33–40.
7. Armstrong ML, Megan MB. Lipid depletion in atheromatous coronary arteries in rhesus monkeys after regression diets. Circ Res 1972;30:675–680.
8. Clarkson TB, Bond MG, Bullock BC, Marzetta CA. A study of atherosclerosis regression in *Macaca mulatta*. IV. Changes in coronary arteries from animals with atherosclerosis induced for 19 months and then regressed for 24 or 48 months at plasma cholesterol concentrations of 300 or 200 mg/dl. Exp Mol Pathol 1981;34:345–368.
9. Small DM, Bond MG, Waugh D, Prack M, Sawyer JK. Physiochemical and histological changes in the arterial wall of non-human primates during progression and regression of atherosclerosis. J Clin Invest 73;1950–2605.
10. Armstrong MC, Megan MG. Arterial fibrous protein in cynomolygous monkeys after atherogenic and regression diets. Circ Res 1975;36:256–261.
11. Harrison DG, Armstrong ML, Freeman PC, Heistad DD. Restoration of endothelium-dependent relaxation by dictory treatment of atherosclerosis. J Clin Invest 1987;80:808–811.
12. Brown BG, Zhao X-Q, Sacco DE, Albers JJ. Lipid lowering and plaque regression. New insights into prevention of plaque disruption and clinical events in coronary disease. Circulation 1993; 87:1781–1791.
13. The Lipid Research Clinics Program. The Lipid Research Clinics Coronary Primary Prevention

Trial Results: I. Reduction in incidence of coronary heart disease. JAMA 1984;251:351—364.

14. Manninen V, Elo MO, Frick MH et al. Lipid alterations and decline in the incidence of coronary heart disease in the Helsinki Heart Study. JAMA 1988;260:641—651.

15. The 4S Investigators. Randomized trial of cholesterol-lowering in 4,444 patients with coronary heart disease: The Scandanavian Simvastatin Survival Study (4S). Lancet 1994;1383—1389.

16. Shepherd J, Cobbe SM, Ford I, Isles CG, Lorimer AR, McFarlane PW, McKillop JM, Packard CJ. Prevention of coronary heart disease with pravastatin in men with hypercholesterolemia. N Engl J Med 1995;333:1301—1307.

17. Sachs FM, Pfeffer MA, Moye LA, Rouleau JL, Rutherford JD, Braunwald E et al. The effect of pravastatin on coronary events after myocardial infarction in patients with average cholesterol levels. N Engl J Med 1996;335:1001—1009.

18. Ambrose JA, Tannenbaum MA, Alexopoulos D et al. Angiographic progression of coronary artery disease and the development of myocardial infarction. J Am Coll Cardiol 1988;12:56—62.

19. Brown BG, Gallery CA, Badger RS, Kennedy JW, Mathey D, Bolson EL, Dodge HT. Incomplete lysis of thrombus in the moderate underlying atherosclerotic lesion during intracoronary infusion of streptokinase for acute myocardial infarction: Quantitative angiographic observations. Circulation 1986;73:653—661.

20. Constantinides P. Plaque fissures in human coronary thrombosis. J Athero Res 1966;61:1—17.

21. Lendon CL, Davies MJ, Born GVR, Richardson PD. Atherosclerotic plaque caps are locally weakened when macrophage density is increased. Atherosclerosis 1991;87:87—90.

22. Richardson PD, Davies MJ, Born GVR. Influence of plaque configuration and stress distribution on fissuring of coronary atherosclerotic plaques. Lancet 1989;iii:941—944.

23. Davies MJ, Richardson PD, Woolf N, Katz DR, Mann J. Risk of thrombosis in human atherosclerosis plaques: role of extracellular lipid, macrophage, and smooth muscle cell content. Br Heart J 1993;69:377—381.

24. Brown BG, Albers JJ, Fisher LD et al. Regression of coronary artery disease as a result of intensive lipid-lowering therapy in men with high levels of apolipoprotein B. N Engl J Med 1990; 323:1289—1298.

Pathobiology of directional atherectomy specimens from de novo and restenotic coronary lesions

Javier Escaned[1] and Patrick W. Serruys[2]

[1] Hospital Universitario San Carlos, Madrid, Spain; and [2] Thoraxcenter, Erasmus University, Rotterdam, The Netherlands

Abstract. Biopsy of the atheromatous plaque in the course of percutaneous coronary revascularisation with directional atherectomy constitutes a unique opportunity of obtaining human, biologically viable, coronary atheroma from ongoing coronary syndromes. We have performed a number of studies comparing atheromatous plaques in both de novo and restenotic coronary atheroma. Valuable information on plaque histology, smooth muscle cell biology and characteristics of the extracellular matrix produced by SMC was obtained, and combined with clinical and angiographic data obtained at baseline and follow-up. Our findings highlight the potential use of atherectomy-retrieved tissue for research purposes in the field of atherosclerosis.

Introduction

The advent of percutaneous transluminal revascularisation techniques introduced a radical change in the treatment of coronary artery disease. First applied in patients by Gruentzig in 1977, dilation of coronary stenosis with balloon catheters proved feasible and successful in treating angina pectoris nonsurgically. However, it soon became evident that the long-term effect of this treatment was hampered by the reappearance of luminal narrowing in the treated segment, a phenomenon named restenosis [1]. Widespread use of balloon angioplasty confirmed that restenosis constitutes the main limitation of the method, appearing in 30—40% of patients in the 6-month period after angioplasty [2]. In the search for ways of avoiding this problem, new methods of percutaneous revascularisation were developed, including ablative, laser and scaffolding techniques. While these techniques contributed to further application and widespread use of percutaneous revascularisation, restenosis was not abolished (Fig. 1). Multiple trials on drug therapy aimed to reduce the restenosis rate have shown negative results. Given the tremendous relevance for further application of nonsurgical coronary revascularisation and reduction of health care costs, prevention of coronary restenosis currently constitutes a research priority for hundreds of investigators around the world.

Address for correspondence: Dr Javier Escaned, Hospital Universitario San Carlos, Hemodinámica Cardíaca, Prof. Martin Lagos s/n, 28040 Madrid, Spain.

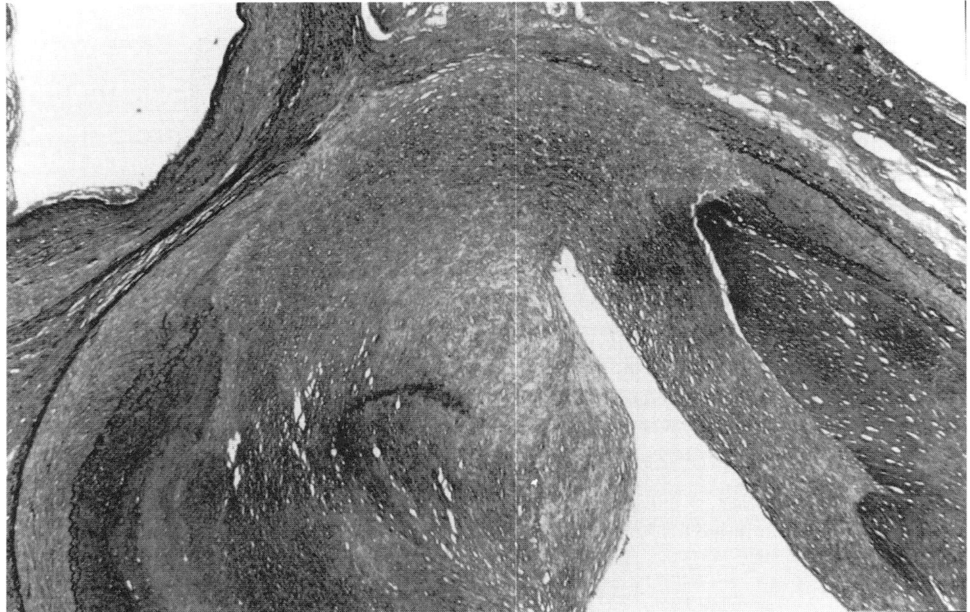

Fig. 1. Restenosis documented in a postmortem study 8 months after the performance of directional coronary atherectomy in the circumflex coronary artery. The original site of excision with the device can be identified by the lack of internal and external elastic lamina and media, resulting from the previous deep cut. From this site extensive proliferation of neointimal hyperplasia has developed into the lumen.

Directional atherectomy as an investigational tool

Since its introduction as a therapeutic device, directional coronary atherectomy attracted investigators of vascular biology as a potential tool for obtaining information on the constitution of atheromatous plaque treated with the device [3,4]. The main advantage of this source of knowledge is that the samples of atheroma provide information on an ongoing coronary syndrome, whereas the study of necropsy material is biased by restriction to the extreme of the clinical (and presumably pathological) spectrum of the syndrome. The topics of research have ranged from the biology of the cellular elements involved in atherosclerosis, particularly vascular smooth muscle cells and macrophages, to the expression of tissue factors [5—7].

Several groups [4,8], including ours [9,10], have reported on the feasibility of culturing smooth muscle cells present in atherectomy specimens using a miniaturized culture system. The use of this model has facilitated observations on the biological characteristics of smooth muscle cells from primary and restenotic lesions, and also on the factors influencing this phenomenon. When using such models, significant differences in the migratory velocity of smooth muscle cells from primary (de novo) and restenotic plaque were found by Bauriedel et al., restenotic cells having migratory velocities more than 2-fold greater than cells from primary lesion [11]. We also found that restenotic smooth muscle cells have increased proliferation rates, a phenomenon which is independent but as important as the migratory potential during the development of restenosis [10]. Growth curves obtained during smooth muscle cell culture were similar for de novo atheroma and medial substrate. On the contrary, growth curves for cells from established restenotic lesions revealed faster proliferation rates. Whether this is a result from persistent phenotypic modification, or is due to selection during the early stages of the restenotic process of specialized cell clones with increased proliferative potential remains to be determined.

Furthermore, we found that the combined proliferative and migratory ability of smooth muscle cells, assessed by the capacity to colonize the culture environment, was also significantly enhanced by the presence of thrombus organization in the retrieved tissue [9]. Histologically, thrombus organization was also associated with extensive neointimal fibrous proliferation. These findings, which suggest the presence of activated smooth muscle cells in the organizing thrombus, are particularly relevant to two clinical settings. Firstly, to the organization of mural thrombus resulting from spontaneous plaque rupture in complex atheroma (class VI in Stary classification), which may trigger the development of neointimal fibrous hyperplasia and result in acceleration of plaque growth. Secondly, to the organization of mural thrombi resulting from percutaneous coronary revascularisation, which are more frequent than suspected from angiography [12], and which may also promote neointimal hyperplasia formation. In this respect, a direct relationship between the presence of thrombus after revascularisation and the subsequent development of restenosis has been demonstrated using coronary angioscopy [13]. The development of neointimal proliferation (triggered by thrombus organisation) may explain the similarities in the histological substrate reported by Flugelman et al. between atherectomy samples in culprit lesions of unstable angina and restenosis [14].

Another novel concept derived from studies of atherectomy samples is that primary coronary stenotic lesions do not consist exclusively of atherosclerotic plaque. Neointimal hyperplasia, which was though to be characteristic of restenotic lesions, can be found in a significant proportion of de novo lesions. Interestingly, this finding occurs predominantly in young patients and is more frequent in the left anterior descending coronary artery. Several groups have reported on these findings [15,16], which fits with pathological observations by Corrado et al. in young individuals with sudden death due to coronary artery disease [17]. The cause of this intimal proliferative tissue remains controversial, although the possibility of having a different etiology compared to typical atherosclerosis (i.e., viral or bacterial infection triggering a response to injury phenomenon) cannot be ruled out.

One of the most relevant features of the phenotype of smooth muscle cells found in atherosclerotic plaques is its enhanced production of extracellular matrix, which in the long term constitute the largest part of plaque volume. Using a cell culture model, the production of collagen and glycosaminoglicans by smooth muscle cells obtained from de novo and restenotic plaques were compared. Cells from restenotic plaques produced a significantly larger amount of both matrix components than smooth muscle cells from de novo atheroma [18]. Furthermore, significant differences in the biological activities between the produced matrices can be observed. Based on previous observations by Sixma et al. suggesting a heterogeneous reactivity of extracellular matrix in atherosclerotic plaques towards blood platelets, we performed a cooperative work with the same authors in which we compared the reactivity of matrices synthesized by medial, restenotic and de novo plaque smooth muscle cells in a cell-culture model. The procoagulant activity of these matrices was also estimated from the rate of activated factor X generated after adding human coagulation factors VII and X. The results of the experiments showed a gradual and significant increase in the reactivity of matrices synthesized by medial, de novo atheroma, and restenotic SMC. In the latter the increase in area of matrix covered by platelets was typically due to an increase in platelet spreading. No increase in tissue factor activity was observed for matrices from atherosclerotic and restenotic SMC. An increased reactivity towards platelets by restenotic matrices may be important in order to explain the high trend to develop a second restenosis. Platelet spreading facilitates better platelet vessel wall interaction; contact platelets and small thrombi with little platelet spreading are swept away more easily by the arterial blood flow. Furthermore, the amount of growth factors delivered by platelets to the arterial wall is critically dependent on the surface covered by platelets, and not by the absolute number of platelets forming aggregates. These observations may be related to the higher restenosis rate observed in secondary (restenotic) lesions treated with a second angioplasty, and deserve further attention [19].

A distinct advantage of atherectomy retrieved tissue as research material in the field of restenosis is that the information obtained can easily be combined with patient follow up. Several groups have tried to identify predictors of restenosis in the excised tissue of the treated patients. Simons et al. reported that the expression of the β-isoform of nonmuscle myosin heavy chain in the retrieved specimens is associated with higher restenosis rate [20]. On the contrary, several groups (including ours) have demonstrated a negative or even inverse relationship between the presence of factors which might have enhanced neointimal proliferation (thrombus, activated SMC, etc.) [21–23]. A partial explanation of this biological paradox of restenosis is that successful extraction of intimal tissue with high biological activity (i.e., organizing thrombus) might have prevented the development of extensive neointimal hyperplasia (a reminder of Heisemberg's word of caution on the fact that the actual practice of observation itself introduces modification that invariably affect the interpretation of that observation).

It is foreseeable that atherectomy will continue being part of the repertoire of interventional techniques. We believe that a close, interdisciplinary work between cardiologists, pathologists and basic scientists should be undertaken to obtain the full benefit not only of the therapeutic value of atherectomy techniques, but also from this new access to coronary atheroma in the living man.

Acknowledgements

The following individuals are acknowledged for their active contribution to the work presented: Pim J. de Feyter, B.H. Strauss, D.C. MacLeod, A.G. Violaris, R.J. van Suylen, F.T. Bosman (Thoraxcenter, Rotterdam), J.J. Sixma, H. van Zanten and Y.E.G. Helmond (University Hospital Utrecht).

References

1. Ip JH, Fuster V, Badimon L, Badimon J, Taubman MB, Chesebro JH. Syndromes of accelerated atherosclerosis: role of vascular injury and smooth muscle cell proliferation. J Am Coll Cardiol 1990;15:1667—1687.
2. Serruys PW, Luijten HE, Beatt KJ et al. Incidence of restenosis after successful coronary angioplasty: a time related phenomenon. A quantitative angiographic study in 342 consecutive patients at 1, 2, 3, and 4 months. Circulation 1988;77:361—371.
3. Safian RD, Gelbfish JS, Erny RE, Schnitt SJ, Schmidt DA, Baim DS. Coronary atherectomy. Clinical, angiographic and histological findings and observations regarding potential mechanisms. Circulation 1990;82:69—79.
4. Dartsch PC, Voisard R, Bauriedel G, Hofling B, Betz E. Growth characteristics and cytoskeletal organization of cultured smooth muscle cells from human primary stenosing and restenosing lesions. Arteriosclerosis 1990;10:62—75.
5. Waller BF, Johnson DE, Schnitt SJ, Pinkerton CA, Simpson JB, Baim DS. Histological analysis of directional coronary atherectomy samples. A review of findings and their clinical relevance. Am J Cardiol 1993;72:80E—87E.
6. Hofling B, Heimerl J, Gonschior P, Bauriedel G. Analysis of atherectomy specimens. Am J Cardiol 1993;72:96E—107E.
7. MacLeod DC, de Jong M, Umans VAWM, Escaned J, van Suylen RJ, Serruys PW, de Feyter P. Directional coronary atherectomy: combining basic research and intervention. Am Heart J 1993;125:1748—1759.
8. Pickering GJ, Weir L, Rosenfield K, Stetz J, Jekanowski J, Isner JM. Smooth muscle cell outgrowth from human atherosclerotic plaque: implications from the assessment of lesion biology. J Am Coll Cardiol 1992;20:1430—1439.
9. Escaned J, de Jong M, Violaris AG, MacLeod DC, van Suylen RJ, Umans VA, Verdouw PD, de Feyter PJ, Serruys PW. Clinical and histological determinants of smooth muscle cell outgrowth in cultured atherectomy specimens: importance of thrombus organisation. Cor Artery Dis 1993;4:883—890.
10. MacLeod DC, Strauss BH, de Jong M, Escaned J, Umans VA, van Suylen RJ, Verkerk A, de Feyter PJ, Serruys PW. Proliferation and extracellular matrix synthesis of smooth muscle cells cultured from human coronary atherosclerotic and restenotic lesions. J Am Coll Cardiol 1993;23:59—65.
11. Bauriedel G, Windstetter U, DeMaio SJ, Kandolf R, Hofling B. Migratory activity of human smooth muscle cells cultivated from coronary and peripheral primary and restenotic lesions removed by percutaneous atherectomy. Circulation 1992;85:554—564.
12. den Heijer P, Foley DP, Escaned J, Hillege HL, van Dijk RB, Serruys PW, Lie KI. Angioscopic versus angiographic detection of intimal dissection and intracoronary thrombus. J Am Coll Cardiol 1994;24:649—654.
13. Bauters C, Labanche JM, McFaden EP, Hamn M, Bertrand ME. Relation of coronary angio-

scopy findings at coronary angioplasty to angiographic restenosis. Circulation 1995; 92:2473—2479.

14. Flugelman MY, Virmani R, Correa R, Yu ZX, Farb A, Leon MB, Elami A, Fu YM, Cascells W, Epstein SE. Smooth muscle cell abundance and fibroblast growth factors in coronary lesions of patients with nonfatal unstable angina. Circulation 1993;88:2493—2500.

15. Escaned J, van Suylen RJ, MacLeod DC, Umans VAWM, de Jong M, Bosman FT, de Feyter PJ, Serruys PW. Histological characteristics of tissue excised during directional coronary atherectomy in stable and unstable angina pectoris. Am J Cardiol 1993;71:1442—1447.

16. Miller MJ, Kuntz RE, Friedrich SP, Leidig GA, Fishman RF, Schnitt SJ, Baim DS, Safian RD. Frequency and consequences of intimal hyperplasia in specimens retrieved by directional coronary atherectomy of native primary coronary stenoses and subsequent restenosis. Am J Cardiol 1993;71:652—658.

17. Corrado D, Thiene G, Pennelli N. Sudden death as the first manifestation of coronary artery disease in young people (< 35 years). Eur Heart J 1988;8:139—144.

18. Violaris A, de Jong M, MacLeod MC et al. Extracellular matrix production by primary and restenotic smooth muscle cells. Am Heart J 1996;131:613—615.

19. Escaned J, van Zanten H, de Jong M, Helmond Y, Slootweg P, Serruys PW, Sixma JJ. Extracellular matrix and restenosis: abnormal reactivity towards blood platelets. Rev Esp Cardiol 1993; 46(Suppl I):5.

20. Simons M, Leclerc G, Safian MD, Isner JM, Weir L, Baim DS. Relation between activated smooth-muscle cells in coronary-artery lesions and restenosis after atherectomy. N Engl J Med 1993;328:608—613.

21. Depre C, Wijns W, Haine E, Renkin J, Hanet C, Havaux X. Risk of restenosis after directional coronary atherectomy: predictive value of structural analysis and cell labelling of atheromatous fragments. Circulation 1992;86(Suppl I):I—225.

22. Isner JM, Kearney M, Berdan LG, Keeler G, Califf RM, Topol EJ for the CAVEAT investigators. Core pathology lab findings in 425 patients undergoing directional atherectomy for a primary coronary artery stenosis and relationship to subsequent outcome: the CAVEAT STUDY 1993. J Am Coll Cardiol 1993;21:380A.

23. Escaned J, Violaris AG, de Jong M, Umans VA, de Feyter PJ, Serruys PW. A biological paradox of restenosis after directional coronary atherectomy: enhanced smooth muscle cell outgrowth and high cellularity of retrieved specimens is associated with less luminal loss. Circulation 1993;88(Suppl 4):551.

Atherosclerosis XI.
B. Jacotot, D. Mathé and J.-C. Fruchart, editors.

Role of thrombosis and hematoma in atherosclerosis progression

Hanne Berg Ravn, Steen Dalby Kristensen and Erling Falk
Department of Cardiology and Institute of Experimental Clinical Research, Aarhus University Hospital (SKS), Aarhus, Denmark

Abstract. Atherogenesis initially occurs beneath an intact but activated and probably dysfunctioning endothelium. Due to increased endothelial permeability, many blood-derived components, including hemostatic factors, are present in early as well as advanced atherosclerotic lesions. Therefore, the presence of fibrin(ogen) in plaques does not necessarily indicate previous thrombosis or hemorrhage. Fibrinogen, and other plasma macromolecules, may enter plaques through an intact but "leaky" endothelium.

In mature plaques endothelial denudation with platelet adhesion may contribute to lesion growth (platelet monolayer releasing growth factors), but thrombosis and hematoma play no role in the initiation and progression of early atherosclerosis. Aggregated platelets, fibrin(ogen), erythrocytes, and plasma proteins are, however, frequently found on or within mature plaques, and both thrombosis and hemorrhage may thus contribute significantly to the development of the mature plaque responsible for clinical disease.

All major plaque hemorrhages are associated with disruption of the plaque surface, whereas rupture of new and fragile adventitia-derived capillaries at the plaque base (neovascularization) is a frequent cause of small deeply located bleedings, unrelated to plaque disruption and thrombosis.

Plaque disruption is responsible for two-thirds to three-quarters of all major coronary thrombi. Beneath the rest of the thrombi plaque erosion is found, which refers to an endothelial denudation without exposure of the lipid-rich core.

Keywords: acute myocardial infarction, atherosclerosis, coronary thrombosis, plaque rupture, platelets, unstable angina pectoris.

Disruption of a plaque surface, often with hemorrhage into the plaque and/or with thrombosis superimposed, plays a fundamental role in the progression of atherosclerosis and is probably the most important mechanism for the development of arterial occlusion in acute coronary syndromes [1—4]. Atherosclerosis is in general a benign disease which starts early on in life, and it takes several decades to form the mature plaques responsible for the ischemic episodes that occur in patients with coronary artery disease.

The risk of thrombotic events in patients with atherosclerosis depends primarily on plaque type rather than plaque size. Lipid-rich and soft plaques are more dangerous than collagen-rich and hard plaques, because they are vulnerable to

Address for correspondence: Erling Falk, Department of Cardiology and Institute of Experimental Clinical Research, Aarhus University Hospital (SKS), DK-8200 Aarhus N, Denmark. Tel./Fax: +45-89496009.

rupture and are highly thrombogenic after disruption.

In this paper, a possible role of thrombosis and hematoma in atherosclerosis progression is considered, and the bleeding- and thrombus-mediated complications responsible for the development of acute coronary syndromes are discussed.

Atherogenesis

The initiation and growth of the atherosclerotic plaque are the result of a dynamic interaction between the vessel wall and the flowing blood, involving several pathological processes [5—7]. In lesion-prone areas, probably related to local hemodynamic factors, increased endothelial permeability leads to increased influx of macromolecules into the intima [7]. Most lipids deposited in atherosclerotic lesions are derived from plasma low-density lipoproteins (LDL), being transcytosed across the endothelium [6]. All major cell types within the intima can oxidize LDL, but the endothelial cell is probably the main place during early atherogenesis [8]. Mildly oxidized LDL may be an important factor for monocyte recruitment in early lesions, whereas tissue necrosis, peptide fragments of fibrin, elastin, collagen degradation products, fibronectin, and thrombin may be the predominant monocyte chemoattractants in more advanced stages. Finally, monocytes/macrophages themselves may release substances that enhance monocyte adhesiveness and chemotaxis thus amplifying their own recruitment [5,6]. Some of the modified LDL is trapped in the intima and endocytosed by the monocyte-derived macrophages, giving rise to the "hallmark cell" in atherogenesis: the lipid filled foam cell.

Simultaneously or subsequently, the damaged endothelium attracts platelets [6]. Platelets in combination with activated endothelium and macrophages release growth factors, which stimulate intimal smooth muscle cells (SMC) to proliferate, migrate and synthesize new matrix giving rise to an elevated intimal lesion: the mature atherosclerotic plaque.

Because of the increased endothelial permeability associated with atherogenesis, many blood-derived components, including albumin and fibrin(ogen) are found in early as well as in advanced lesions [9—11]. Using immunohistochemical technique, fibrin(ogen) is frequently found in areas rich in neovascularization (exudation from leaky capillaries) and in the shoulder region of the plaque with inflammatory cell infiltrates [10]. A similar staining pattern was also observed for albumin, indicating that increased endothelial permeability, rather than incorporation of thrombus material, is responsible for the occurrence of fibrin(ogen) in plaques [11].

Degeneration of the plaque takes place with lipid accumulation, preferentially LDL, and necrosis, which may be related to the cytotoxic effect of oxidized lipid. The lipid-rich core is avascular and usually also acellular, consisting mainly of debris with abundant cholesterol crystals. Foam-cells are often bordering the cavity, particularly at the luminal side, where they often are disintegrated with the cell constituents emptied into the lipid-rich core, indicating that cell death (apoptosis) occurs during plaque growth [12,13].

Calcification of the plaque has in the past been regarded as a mere passive process of absorption and precipitation of calcium phosphate crystals, but recent studies suggest that this may be a regulated process, involving expression of bone-regulating and -differentiating proteins within the plaque [14,15].

Mature plaques: two main components

In patients with ischemic heart disease, the coronary arteries are often diffusely involved with confluent "plaquing". There is no simple relation between the size of a plaque (or stenosis severity) and its vulnerability to rupture [16]. Moreover, the composition, vulnerability, and thrombogenicity of individual plaques vary greatly without any obvious relation to risk factors for clinical disease, except perhaps serum cholesterol. Recently, Burke et al. evaluated the association between various risk factors for ischemic heart disease and plaque morphology in the coronary arteries at autopsy, and found that abnormal serum cholesterol concentrations — particularly elevated ratios of total cholesterol to high-density lipoprotein cholesterol — was found in patients who died of plaque rupture. Hypertension, smoking status, age, glycosylated hemoglobin value, and race were not associated with the presence of vulnerable or ruptured plaques, but smoking seemed to predispose patients to acute coronary thrombosis regardless of the underlying plaque morphology [17].

As the name "atherosclerosis" implies, mature plaques consist typically of two main components: soft, lipid-rich atheromatous "gruel" and hard, collagen-rich sclerotic tissue (Fig. 1). The sclerotic component usually is by far the most voluminous but it is relatively innocuous because collagen secreted by SMC stabilizes a plaque against disruption. In contrast, the atheromatous component is by far the most dangerous because it destabilizes a plaque, making it vulnerable and susceptible to rupture and thrombosis [7]. The destabilizing atheromatous component or core lacks supporting collagen, is rich in extracellular lipids (predominantly cholesterol and its esters), is avascular and hypocellular, and is usually soft like gruel.

Disruption of vulnerable plaques occurs frequently. It is followed by a variable amount of luminal thrombosis and/or hemorrhage into the soft gruel, causing rapid growth of the lesion. Autopsy data indicate that 9% of apparently healthy persons have disrupted plaques (without superimposed thrombosis) in their coronary arteries [18]. The numbers increase to 22% in persons with diabetes or hypertension [18]. One or more disrupted plaques, with or without superimposed thrombosis, are usually present in coronary arteries of patients dying of ischemic heart disease [1,19].

The risk of plaque disruption depends on both intrinsic properties of individual plaques (their vulnerability) and extrinsic forces acting on plaques (rupture triggers). The former predispose plaques to rupture, while the latter may precipitate disruption if vulnerable plaques are present.

384

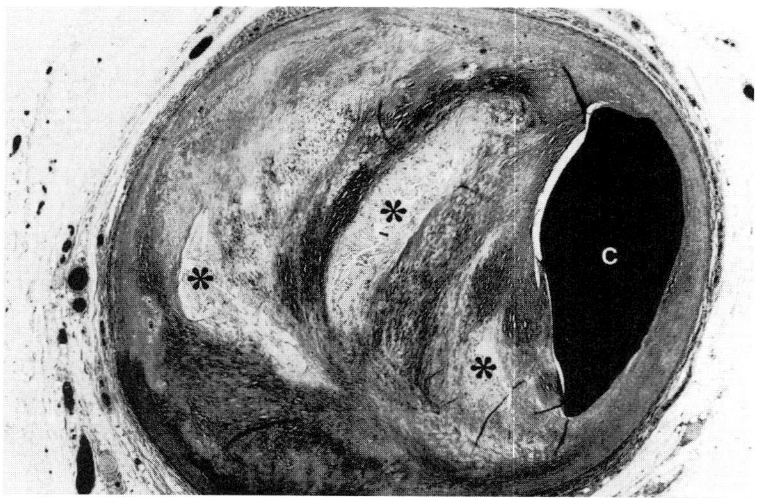

Fig. 1. Mature atherosclerotic plaque containing soft, lipid-rich atheromatous "gruel" (asterisks) and hard, collagen-rich sclerotic tissue. c = contrast medium injected postmortem.

Plaque vulnerability

The size and consistency of the atheromatous core are important factors for the stability of a plaque. The majority of plaques undergoing thrombosis have a lipid core occupying more than 40% of the cross-sectional area of the plaque [20]. Ruptured caps contain less collagen, more extracellular lipid, reduced number of smooth muscle cells, and increased density of macrophages. This leads to a reduced tensile strength and increased extensibility compared to intact caps [7].

Rupture of the fibrous cap occurs most frequently at the "shoulder region" where the cap joins the normal intima, being where the cap usually is thinnest [20]. In this area infiltration with monocyte-derived macrophages is often seen. These cells are capable of degrading extracellular matrix by phagocytosis or by secretion of proteolytic enzymes, such as metalloproteinases and plasminogen activators, whereby the cap is weakened and more prone to rupture. It is noteworthy that culprit lesions from patients with unstable coronary syndromes contain significantly more macrophages than do plaques from stable patients [21].

Coronary plaques are constantly stressed by a variety of mechanical and hemodynamic forces that may precipitate or "trigger" disruption of vulnerable plaques. Physical exertion and emotional stress could, for example, trigger plaque disruption via surges in sympathetic activity with an increase in blood pressure, pulse pressure, blood flow (shear forces), heart rate, and coronary tone [22].

Plaque progression

Proliferation of SMC, matrix synthesis, and lipid accumulation may gradually narrow the arterial lumen and ultimately lead to myocardial ischemia and anginal pain, but plaque progression is neither linear nor time-related. Serial angiography has revealed that new high-grade lesions often appear in segments of coronary arteries, which were normal at previous examinations [23]. This unpredictable and episodic progression can be explained by the occurrence of plaque rupture with subsequent hemorrhage into the plaque and/or mural thrombosis leading to stepwise plaque growth. Plaque disruption is common and in the majority of cases clinically silent [5]. However, if a major luminal thrombus evolves with subsequent flow impairment, this may turn a relatively benign disease into a life-threatening acute coronary syndrome [5].

Recent reports have suggested that inflammation may play an important role in the pathogenesis of atherothrombosis. High plasma fibrinogen levels as well as increased levels of other inflammatory mediators such as C reactive protein, amyloid A protein and interleukin 6 have also been associated with a higher risk of acute coronary events [24]. Data from the Physicians Health Study indicate that baseline plasma concentration of C-reactive protein can predict the risk of myocardial infarction and stroke not only in patients with ischemic heart disease, but also in apparently healthy men [25].

The reason for the increased levels of inflammatory mediators remains unknown. It cannot be attributed to the severity of atherosclerosis, as there is no correlation in patients with chronic stable angina; to minor degrees of myocardial necrosis, as troponin-T is not elevated; to prolonged ischemia, as C-reactive protein remains low in patients with variant angina; or to haemostatic activation, as thrombin does not stimulate increased synthesis of C-reactive protein [24]. This has led to an intense search for an infectious agent (cytomegalovirus, chlamydia, helicobacter, etc.), that could stimulate the synthesis of acute phase reactants, such as fibrinogen and C-reactive protein.

The most convincing evidence so far is the association between *Chlamydia pneumoniae*, an obligatory intracellular pathogen, and coronary artery disease. Significantly elevated antibody titres have been observed in patients with myocardial infarction compared to healthy controls. Moreover, elevated *C. pneumoniae* antibodies were strong predictors of cardiac events in a follow-up study in heart patients, independent of other risk factors [26]. *C. pneumoniae* has been identified in macrophages, interstitially in the lipid rich core in plaques and in smooth muscle cells, but not in normal tissue adjacent to the lesion [27]. Eradication therapy with antichlamydial macrolides has shown to reduce the risk of cardiovascular events not only in postmyocardial infarct patients, who were seropositive [26], but also in patients with unstable angina and non-Q-wave myocardial infarction irrespective of the patient's antibody titre [28]. Despite the accumulating evidence for an association between *C. pneumoniae* and coronary artery disease it remains unclear whether the organism is causal in itself. More than 50% of the population is seropositive at the age of 50, suggesting that reinfection is common.

Plaque hemorrhage

Thrombosis does, as already described, most frequently take place in atherosclerotic arteries, and the mechanisms through which it occurs has been intensively investigated. Serial sectioning of thrombosed atherosclerotic arteries has been of major value during this exploration, but before this method was introduced the insight into this process was rather limited. In the small number of cases where thrombi developed over ulcerated plaques with the whole cap torn off and blood clotting on top off the disrupted plaque surface, it was not difficult to understand the reaction. But in most cases the thrombus was found in association with a seemingly intact fibrous cap, and most frequently a hemorrhage was seen in the underlying lipid-rich gruel as described by Paterson in 1938 [29].

Three mechanisms have been proposed to explain thrombus formation over an intact, but often hemorrhagic plaque. Thrombosis could be caused by stasis and/or blood hypercoagulability, but when these theories were tested experimentally, extreme systemic hypercoagulability resulted in multiple small thrombi in the capillaries and venules of various viscera, and not in a single thrombus in a single artery over a single plaque [30]. Furthermore, these two theories did not explain the intraplaque hemorrhage. The third mechanism, the luminal capillary hemorrhage theory, suggested that thrombi were caused by rupture of the thin-walled, lumen-derived capillaries due to the high pressure from within the lumen. However, the fact that most plaques are capillarized from the adventitial vaso vasorum and not from the lumen lends little support to this hypothesis.

The importance of adventitial vaso vasorum has been studied by Barger et al., who suggested that neovascularization, in the region of the atherosclerotic plaque, plays an important role in the pathogenesis of atherosclerosis and thrombosis [31,32]. A dense capillary network of neovascular appearance is often found at the base of atherosclerotic plaques. According to their theory, rupture of these fragile vessels results in intraplaque hemorrhages, which during certain circumstances may lead to a "blow-in" lesion from the plaque to the lumen and extrusion of core material into the lumen causing thrombosis [31,32]. Microscopic examination of thrombosed arteries using serial sectioning technique indicates, however, that such a mechanism rarely if ever occurs.

Cap disruption nearly always occurs in avascular areas (i.e., no capillaries either at the break site or proximal or distal to it). Furthermore, cap disruption without any hemorrhage has been described indicating that the breaks can be sealed off before any blood enters the plaque. And finally, intraplaque hemorrhage originating from adventitia-derived capillaries is seen in the deep plaque regions and often found in combination with a major lumen-derived hemorrhage, but without any physical connection between the former and the latter [30,7]. Although capillarization of plaques from the lumen may occur during organisation of a mural thrombus, hemorrhages from these capillaries have not been associated with cap disruption and thrombosis [30].

Plaque thrombosis

About two-thirds to three-quarters of all thrombi responsible for acute coronary syndromes are precipitated by plaque disruption whereby the highly thrombogenic gruel is exposed to the flowing blood (Fig. 2). Superficial plaque inflammation with intimal erosion but no frank disruption (i.e., no deep injury) are found beneath the remaining fatal thrombi, usually in combination with a severe atherosclerotic stenosis [7].

Most disrupted plaques are resealed by a small mural thrombus (Fig. 3), and only sometimes does a major luminal thrombus evolve. Therefore, the thrombotic response to plaque disruption/erosion is a key event in the pathophysiology of acute ischemic syndromes. Several factors such as the thrombogenic substrate, local flow disturbances and, last but not least, the systemic thrombotic propensity are important.

The atheromatous "gruel" is not only the most vulnerable plaque component, it also appears to be the most thrombogenic component [33,34]. Recent data indicate that macrophage-derived tissue factor probably is responsible for the high thrombogenicity of the gruel [34,35]. Plaque content of tissue factor is increased in patients with unstable angina compared to patients with stable angina [36]. The content of tissue factor correlates with areas of macrophages and smooth muscle cells, suggesting a cell-mediated thrombogenicity in patients with acute coronary syndromes [35].

A severe stenosis and surface irregularities may activate platelets. A platelet-rich thrombus may indeed form and grow within a severe stenosis, where the

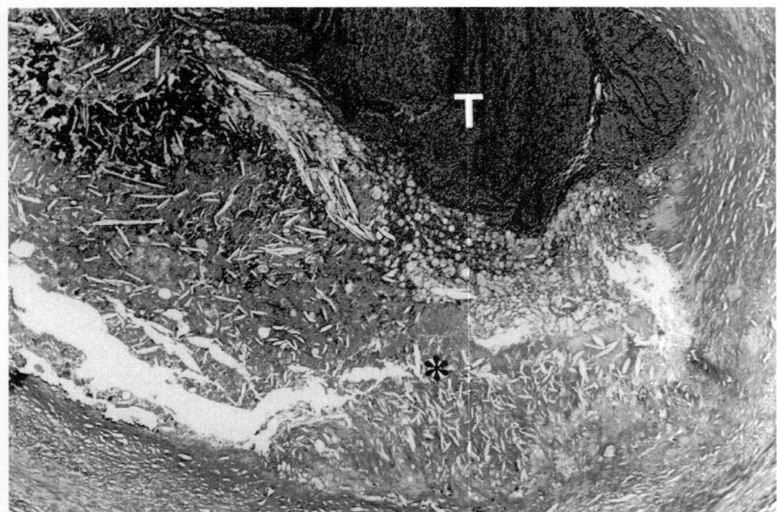

Fig. 2. Atherosclerotic plaque containing a lipid-rich atheromatous core (asterisk) that is covered by a thin, foam-cell infiltrated and disrupted fibrous cap (between arrows). An occlusive thrombus (T) is seen on top of the exposed highly thrombogenic "gruel".

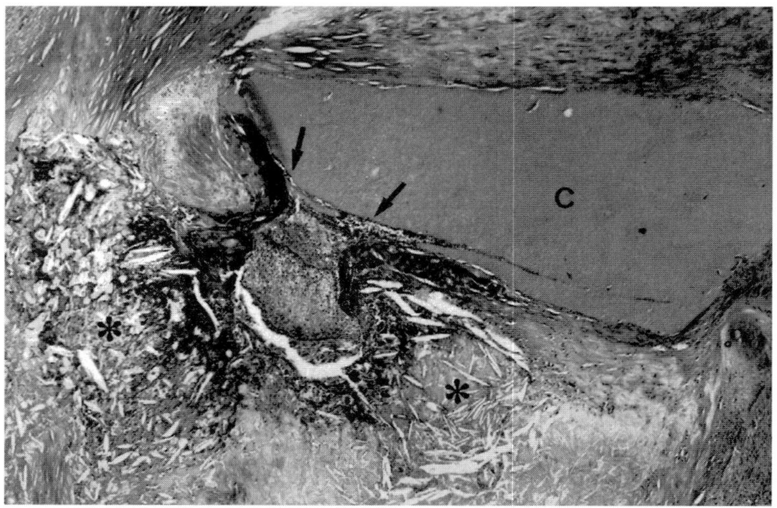

Fig. 3. Disrupted plaque surface (missing cap between arrows) associated with hemorrhage into the soft atheromatous core (asterisks) and mural thrombosis causing rapid nonocclusive growth of the plaque. c = contrast medium injected postmortem.

blood velocity and shear forces are highest, probably because of shear-induced platelet activation [7]. Irregularities of the exposed surface increase platelet deposition and thrombus formation [33].

The actual thrombotic-thrombolytic equilibrium at the time of plaque disruption does also influence the outcome. The concept of impaired fibrinolysis as a risk factor for cardiovascular disease has been supported by prospective studies in which endogenous fibrinolytic capacity assessed at baseline was found to predict future risk of cardiovascular morbidity and mortality. Plasma levels of tissue-type plasminogen activator antigen (t-PA:ag) and plasminogen activator inhibitor (PAI-1) are strongly correlated, but epidemiological studies indicate that the most useful marker for risk prediction seems to be t-PA:ag both in patients with coronary disease and in apparently healthy men, where an increase in baseline t-PA:ag was associated with an increased risk of future coronary thrombosis [37].

Several coagulation and platelet related parameters have also proven to be of predictive value in determining arterial thrombotic risk. Plasma levels of factor VII activity, von Willebrand factor antigen, prothrombin fragment$_{1+2}$, and thrombin-antithrombin complexes have all been proposed as additional markers of thrombotic risk [37]. There is substantial evidence that an increase in platelet reactivity occurs in the acute phase of a myocardial infarction and in unstable angina pectoris [38]. In prospective studies of platelet markers, a high platelet count [39] and an increased mean platelet volume [40], as well as increased platelet aggregability [41] have been associated with increased vascular risk. The importance of platelets is clearly documented by the protective effect of aspirin in patients with stable and unstable angina pectoris and in patients with acute myocardial infarction [42].

Conclusion

Progression of atherosclerosis from a relatively benign disease into a life-threatening condition occurs usually as a result of plaque disruption with superimposed thrombosis. The risk of plaque disruption depends more on plaque composition and vulnerability than on the number and size of plaques. There are three major determinants of plaque vulnerability, namely: 1) lipid-rich core size, 2) cap thickness, and 3) cap inflammation and repair. Plaque vulnerability (intrinsic disease) is a prerequisite for rupture, whereas rupture triggers (extrinsic forces) are external stimuli (mechanical, hemodynamic factors, etc.) that may precipitate or "trigger" rupture of the vulnerable plaque. The thrombogenicity of the atherosclerotic plaque is determined by the nature and extent of the plaque components exposed to blood flow together with local flow disturbances and the systemic thrombotic-thrombolytic equilibrium at the time of rupture.

Plaque disruption is a common event which often occurs during the development of atherosclerotic lesions and it is in the majority of cases clinically silent. It is likely to be the most important mechanism underlying sudden and rapid plaque progression. Erythrocytes, platelets, fibrin and other plasma proteins are often found on or within atherosclerotic plaques, indicating that thrombosis and hemorrhage, after plaque disruption, may contribute significantly to the evolution of mature plaques.

References

1. Falk E. Plaque rupture with pre-existing stenosis precipitating coronary thrombosis. Characteristics of coronary atherosclerotic plaques underlying fatal occlusive thrombi. Br Heart J 1983;50:127–134.
2. De Feyter PJ, Ozaki Y, Baptista J, Escaned J, Di Mario C, de Jaegere PT, Serruys PW, Roelandt JRTC. Ischemia-related lesion characteristics in patients with stable or unstable angina. Circulation 1995;92:1408–1413.
3. Davies MJ, Thomas AC, Knapman PA, Hamgartner JR. Intramyocardial platelet aggregation in patients with unstable angina pectoris suffering sudden cardiac death. Circulation 1986;73: 418–427.
4. Tabata H, Mizuno K, Arakawa K, Satumura K, Shibuya T, Kurita A, Nakamura H. Angioscopic identification of coronary thrombus in patients with postinfarction angina. J Am Coll Cardiol 1995;25:1282–1285.
5. Ross R. The pathogenesis of atherosclerosis: a perspective for the 1990s. Nature 1993;362: 801–809.
6. Fuster V. Lewis A. Conner Memorial Lecture. Mechanisms leading to myocardial infarction: insights from studies of vascular biology. Circulation 1994;90:2126–2146.
7. Falk E, Shah PK, Fuster V. Coronary plaque disruption. Circulation 1995;92:657–671.
8. Steinberg D, Workshop Participants. Antioxidants in the prevention of human atherosclerosis. Circulation 1992;85:2338.

390

9. Valenzuela R, Shainoff JR, DiBello PM, Urbanic DA, Anderson JM, Matsueda GR, Kudryk BJ. Immunoelectrophoretic and immunohistochemical characterizations of fibrinogen derivatives in atherosclerotic aortic intimas and vascular prothesis pseudointimas. Am J Pathol 1992; 141:861—880.

10. Zhang Y, Cliff WJ, Schoefl GI, Higgins G. Immunohistochemical study of intimal microvessels in coronary atherosclerosis. Am J Pathol 1993;143:164—172.

11. Zhang Y, Cliff WJ, Schoefl GI, Higgins G. Plasma protein insudation as an index of early coronary atherogenesis. Am J Pathol 1993;143:496—503.

12. Björkerud S, Björkerud B. Apoptosis is abundant in human atherosclerotic lesions, especially in inflammatory cells (macrophages and T cells), and may contribute to the accumulation of gruel and plaque instability. Am J Pathol 1996;149:367—380.

13. Geng YJ, Libby P. Evidence for apoptosis in advanced human atheroma. Am J Pathol 1995;147:251—266.

14. Demer LL, Watson KE, Boström K. Mechanism of calcification in atherosclerosis. Trends Cardiovasc Med 1994;4:45—49.

15. Wexler L, Brundage B, Crouse J, Detrano R, Fuster V, Maddahi J et al. Coronary artery calcification: Pathophysiology, epidemiology, imaging methods, and clinical implications. Circulation 1996;94:1175—1192.

16. Mann JM, Davies MJ. Vulnerable plaque. Relation of characteristics to degree of stenosis in human coronary arteries. Circulation 1996;94:928—931.

17. Burke AP, Farb A, Malcom GT, Liang YH, Smialek J, Virmani R. Coronary risk factors and plaque morphology in men with coronary disease who die suddenly. N Engl J Med 1997;336:1276—1282.

18. Davies MJ, Bland JM, Hangartner JRW, Angelini A, Thomas AC. Factors influencing the presence or absence of acute coronary artery thrombi in sudden ischaemic death. Eur Heart J 1989;10:203—208.

19. Davies MJ, Thomas AC. Thrombosis and acute coronary artery lesions in sudden cardiac death. N Engl J Med 1984;310:1137—1140.

20. Davies MJ, Richardson PD, Woolf N, Katz DR, Mann J. Risk of thrombosis in human atherosclerotic plaques: role of extracellular lipid, macrophage, and smooth muscle cell content. Br Heart J 1993;69:377—381.

21. Moreno PR, Falk E, Palacios IF, Newell JB, Fuster V, Fallon JT. Macrophage infiltration in acute coronary syndromes: implications for plaque rupture. Circulation 1994;90:775—778.

22. Muller JE, Abela GS, Nesto RW, Tofler GH. Triggers, acute risk factors and vulnerable plaques: the lexicon of a new frontier. J Am Coll Cardiol 1994;23:809—813.

23. Bruschke AVG, Kramer JR, Bal ET, Haque IU, Detrano RC, Goormastic M. The dynamics of progression of coronary atherosclerosis in 168 medically treated patients who underwent coronary arteriography three times. Am Heart J 1989;117:296—305.

24. Maseri A, Biasucci LM, Liuzzo G. Inflammation in ischaemic heart disease. Br Med J 1996; 312:1049—1050.

25. Ridker PM, Cushman M, Stampfer MJ, Tracy RP, Hennekens CH. Inflammation, aspirin, and the risk of cardiovascular disease in apparrently healthy men. N Engl J Med 1997;336:973—979.

26. Gupta S, Leatham EW, Carrington D, Mendall MA, Kaski JC, Camm AJ. Elevated *Chlamydia pneumoniae* antibodies, cardiovascular events, and azithromycin in male survivors of myocardial infarction. Circulation 1997;96:404—407.

27. Kuo C-C, Shor A, Campell LA, Fukushi H, Patton DL, Grayston JT. Demonstration of *Chlamydia pneumoniae* in atherosclerotic lesions of coronary arteries. J Infect Dis 1993;1667:841—849.

28. Gurfinkel E, Bozovich G, Daroca A, Beck E, Mautner B. ROXIS Study Group. Randomised trial of roxithromycin in non-Q-wave coronary syndromes: ROXIS pilot study. Lancet 1997; 350:404—407.

29. Paterson JC. Capillary rupture with intimal hemorrhage as a causative factor in coronary

thrombosis. Arch Pathol 1938;25:474—479.

30. Constantinides P. Cause of thrombosis in human atherosclerotic arteries. Am J Cardiol 1990;66:37G—40G.
31. Barger AC, Beeuwkes R III, Lainey LL, Silverman KJ. Hypothesis: vasa vasorum and neovascularization of human coronary arteries. N Engl J Med 1984;310:175—177.
32. Barger AC, Beeuwkes R III. Rupture of coronary vasa vasorum as a trigger of acute myocardial infarction. Am J Cardiol 1990;66:41G—43G.
33. Fernandez-Ortiz A, Badimon JJ, Falk E, Fuster V, Meyer B, Mailhac A, Weng D, Shah PK, Badimon L. Characterization of the relative thrombogenecity of atherosclerotic plaque components: implications for consequences of plaque rupture. J Am Coll Cardiol 1994;23:1562—1569.
34. Toschi V, Gallo R, Lettino M, Fallon JF, Gertz SD, Fernandez-Ortiz A, Cheseboro JH, Badimon L, Nemerson Y, Fuster V, Badimon JJ. Tissue factor modulates the thrombogenecity of human atherosclerotic plaques. Circulation 1997;95:594—597.
35. Moreno PR, Bernardi VH, López-Cuéllar J, Murcia AM, Palacios IF, Gold HK, Mehran R, Sharma SK, Nemerson Y, Fuster V, Fallon JT. Macrophages, smooth muscle cells, and tissue factor in unstable angina. Circulation 1996;94:3090—3097.
36. Ardissino D, Merlini PA, Ariëns R, Coppola R, Bramucci E, Manucci PM. Tissue-factor antigen and activity in human coronary atherosclerotic plaques. Lancet 1997;349:769—771.
37. Ridker PM. Fibrinolytic and inflammatory markers for arterial occlusion: the evolving epidemiology of thrombosis and hemostasis. Thromb Haemost 1997;78:53—59.
38. Kristensen SD. The platelet-vessel wall interaction in experimental atherosclerosis and ischaemic heart disease — with special reference to thrombopoiesis. Dan Med Bull 1992;39:110—127.
39. Thaulow E, Erikssen J, Sandvik L, Stormorken H, Cohen PF. Blood platelet count and function are related to total and cardiovascular death in apparently healthy men. Circulation 1991;84: 613—617.
40. Martin JF, Bath PM, Burr ML. Influence of platelet size on outcome after myocardial infarction. Lancet 1991;338:1409—1411.
41. Trip MD, Manger Cats V, van Capelle FJL, Vreeken J. Platelet hyperreactivity and prognosis in survivors of myocardial infarction. N Engl J Med 1990;322:1549—1554.
42. Collaborative overview of randomised trials of antiplatelet therapy-I: Prevention of death, myocardial infarction, and stroke by prolonged antiplatelet therapy in various categories of patients. Antiplatelet Trialists' Collaboration. BMJ 1994;308:81—106.

Natural history of atherosclerosis: the sequence of changes in lesion composition

Herbert C. Stary
Louisiana State University Medical Center, New Orleans, USA

Abstract. This article describes the cell- and intercellular-matrix components and the structures of successive atherosclerotic lesion types from the first (only microscopically visible) macrophage foam cell accumulations in susceptible locations of arteries to lesion forms that produce vascular occlusion. The likely effect of drastic therapeutic reduction of high plasma atherogenic lipoproteins on the components of the range of human lesion types is inferred from studies of regression of comparable lesions in rhesus monkeys after treatment.

Keywords: arterial locations susceptible to atherosclerosis, atherosclerosis progression, atherosclerosis regression.

Introduction

In the course of the development of atherosclerosis, lesions of greatly differing compositions are encountered in arteries. At every period of a human life, certain compositions (lesion types) are characteristic although by late middle age, most types of lesions may be present in a person. Lesions begin as minimal accumulations of lipid in the intima in susceptible locations of the arterial system. Lipid accumulations do not at first disorganize or deform the artery (lesion types I—III). However, by the third decade of life, accumulations may be large enough to disorganize the cell and matrix structure of the arterial wall and change the contours of the affected arterial segments (type IV lesion). After this stage has been reached, mechanisms and components additional to and less predictable than lipid influx and accumulation may accelerate wall thickening and lumen reduction (lesion types V—VIII). Lesion types IV—VIII are collectively regarded as advanced lesions because they include structural disorganization and thickening of a segment of artery. Although considered advanced by histological criteria, some type IV lesions may not narrow the arterial lumen or be visible by angiography and many histologically advanced lesions remain clinically silent for a lifetime.

Address for correspondence: H.C. Stary MD, Professor of Pathology, L.S.U. Medical Center, 1901 Perdido Street, New Orleans, LA 70112, USA. Tel.: +1-504-568-6048. Fax: +1-504-568-6037.

394

Fluid mechanical forces, adaptive intimal thickening and arterial locations that are susceptible to lesion formation

An artery adjusts to the normal segmental asymmetries in fluid mechanical forces along its course and around its circumference by adjusting the thickness of its wall (and so its lumen) in individual segments or regions. The aim is to maintain flow equally at all points along its course. Arteries, therefore, normally have both thin and thick segments. Increases occur through the activation of native intimal smooth muscle cells (adaptive intimal thickening), intimal cells clearly being quicker to respond than medial cells. Such increases in thickness are self-limited and cannot be considered as obstructions at any age. Focal adaptive increases begin to develop in fetal life and although variable in degree, are found in everyone at birth [1]. Focal and eccentric adaptive thickening occurs at and near bifurcations of arteries and at the mouths of even the smallest branch vessels. Adaptive thickening is also found in some parts not obviously related to a branch vessel where it is more diffuse.

From the first minimal beginning of lipid accumulation in early life, more is found in locations with adaptive intimal thickening. These are the same locations in which the first and largest advanced lesions are found if advanced lesions are found in later life. The explanation for the preferred development of lesions in specific locations are the mechanical forces in these regions. These forces give rise to adaptive thickening and they also independently enhance influx of lipoproteins.

Some authors view adaptive thickening as atherosclerosis. Others have speculated that adaptive thickening, while not a lesion itself, is a prerequisite for the retention and accumulation of lipid and thus for lesion formation. Neither assumption is likely because when atherogenic lipoproteins are very high, atheroma develops also in locations without adaptive thickening.

Since the characteristics of mechanical forces and their degree vary for different arteries and different segments and regions of arteries, the degree to which influx of lipid (and in hyperlipidemia — accumulation) occurs also varies. Simplified, we can distinguish three degrees of susceptibility to lipid accumulation and lesion formation:
1. Locations that generally are not susceptible.
2. Moderately susceptible locations (lesion types I and II develop but progression to advanced lesions, if it occurs at all, is relatively slow and late).
3. Highly susceptible locations (lesion types I and II develop and, if risk factors are high enough, advanced lesions appear first in these locations).

Composition of lesions at successive stages of development

Figure 1 indicates a main characteristic for each lesion type and it shows how they succeed one another. This view of the chronological order of lesion compositions is based on data from 1,400 people autopsied in New Orleans in the 1980s

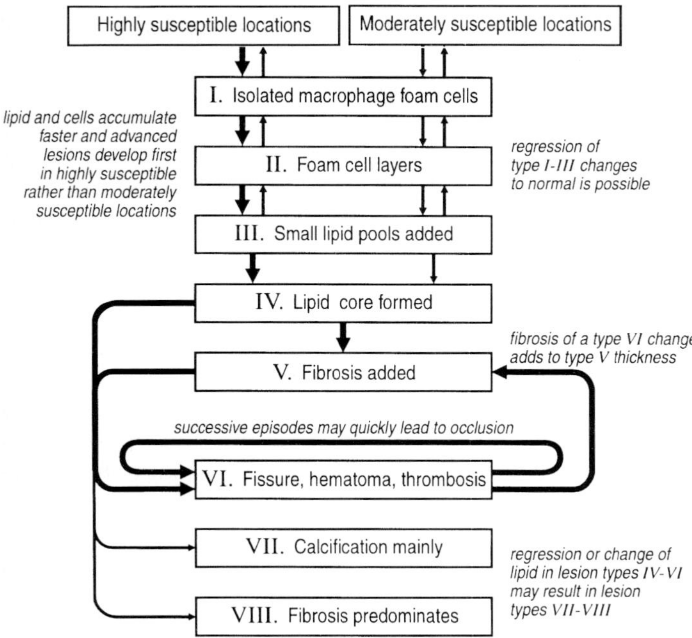

Fig. 1. Flow diagram indicating pathways in the progression and regression of human atherosclerotic lesions. The chronological order of lesion compositions is designated with the numerals I—VIII. The diagram lists a main histological characteristic for each sequential step (lesion type). Text and references contain fuller descriptions of the compositions of lesions.

following unexpected death mainly from accidents and violence [2—5].

The first chemically and microscopically detectable changes consist of the accumulation of lipoprotein and isolated macrophages and macrophages containing lipid droplets (macrophage foam cells) in susceptible locations of the intima. We call these changes the type I lesion. In the first 8 months of life, 45% of infants have type I changes in their coronary arteries [1,2].

After a temporary decline following infancy, macrophage foam cells, now more numerous and stratified in layers, reappear in the same spots in children at puberty (type II lesions). The intimal smooth muscle cells of the involved locations also contain lipid droplets. Of children aged 12—14 years, 65% have mostly type II lesions (a few still have only type I) in coronary arteries [2] and all have fatty streaks (histologically mainly type II lesions) in the aorta.

In many (and probably most) children, the type I and type II changes do not develop further or they regress. When I applied the term lesion to type I and type II changes it was not to advocate that the changes should be treated in all children. The use of the term lesion is justified, however, since the sequence of changes indicates that when clinical disease appears in later life, it developed from the initially minimal changes.

The manner of progression of type II to atheroma had not been clear and the assumption that clinical disease can develop from type II lesions had been questioned. The morphology of the usual type II lesions, traditionally viewed as several layers of foam cells in a thin intima, seemed too unlike that of atheroma. The ostensibly insurmountable difference in morphologies is explained by the fact that type IV lesions (atheroma) develop preferentially from the subgroup of type II lesions in narrowly delimited intima locations that normally contain layers of smooth muscle cells (i.e., adaptive thickening), and by the histological delineation of the type III lesion.

The type III lesion has a composition intermediate between minimal lesions and advanced lesions. In addition to the lipid droplet-laden cells of type II lesions, type III contains microscopically visible extracellular lipid droplets and particles to the extent that small pools of this material (in large part the contents of dead foam cells) are present. By this definition, multiple separate pools of extracellular lipid that begin to displace some smooth muscle cells and intercellular matrix of the intima (generally within a colocalized adaptive thickening) constitute progression beyond minimal (type I and II) changes.

Small separate pools of extracellular lipid may increase in size with time and fuse to form a single but extensive accumulation of extracellular lipid (a lipid core). We designate a lesion with a lipid core (but still without a fibrous tissue increase, surface defect, hematoma or thrombus) as a type IV lesion. The smooth muscle cells that normally occupy the core of the intima (actually the core of adaptive thickening) are dispersed or dead and lost because of the pressure on them of the lipid particles and droplets that now congest the core region. While the accumulated lipid thickens the wall significantly, a simultaneous loss in structural coherence (and thus resilience) may somewhat enlarge the circumference of the artery, and the lumen may, at least at first, not be narrowed much. Much of the tissue above the lipid core is the remaining native intima. It contains macrophages, macrophage foam cells and lymphocytes. Many of the remaining intimal smooth muscle cells have lipid droplet inclusions.

Lesions of like-composition vary in size and extent in the intima. In the larger of the lesions of type IV (and subsequent types V−VII) all or some of the pathological changes may extend into the adjacent part or throughout the thickness of the adjacent media layer. The adjacent adventitia may contain foam cells. In these instances, lymphocytes and macrophages are sometimes more numerous in the adventitia than in the intima.

A fibrous tissue change or increase may be superimposed on intima with a lipid core. We call this morphology the type V lesion. This additional component may represent repair of arterial structure disrupted by the accumulated lipid or incorporation of hematoma and thrombus. Smooth muscle and connective tissue that represent native intima must not be mistaken for fibrous tissue that is a reaction to tissue destruction or thrombosis. Thus, the fibromuscular component of a type V lesion represents a mixture of native intima and atherosclerosis or thrombosis-generated layers. Only appropriate microscopic methods distinguish between native and newly formed parts. With the formation of thick fibrous tissue layers, the lumen of an artery is increasingly reduced.

From about the fourth decade of life on, lesions may contain disruptions of the surface, hematoma and thrombotic deposits. Lesions with these components are designated as type VI. Thrombi may not be large at first but new layers of thrombus are often superimposed on old layers and an occlusion of the lumen may build up over a period of days, weeks or years. Thrombotic deposits that are not immediately dissolved or not immediately fatal are colonized by intimal smooth muscle cells and converted to collagen. The resulting fibrotic layer, although smaller than the original hematoma and thrombus is a lasting addition to the narrowing of the lumen. A lesion with an extracellular lipid accumulation usually underlies an intimal surface defect and/or thrombosis.

From the fifth decade of life on, many advanced lesions may have a predominantly mineral character. The term type VII lesion may be applied to such lesions. In addition to the calcified parts, the fibromuscular increase that is characteristic of type V lesions may also be present. Variable amounts of calcium are found in every lesion with a lipid core. With refined microscopic methods, even the type IV lesions of the youngest adults reveal small degrees of calcification. Only lesions in which most, or all of the lipid and necrotic components have become calcified qualify for designation as type VII.

Some intimal lesions are composed mainly of irregularly structured reparative fibrous tissue. Accumulated lipid is minimal, and sometimes there seems to be no lipid at all. We designate such lesions as type VIII. The regularly and predictably structured fibromuscular tissue of native intima, particularly that of adaptive intimal thickening, must not be mistaken for type VIII lesions. Type VIII changes could be the result of the incorporation of thrombi, the extension of the fibrous component of an adjacent type V lesion, or the resorption (regression) of a lipid accumulation.

Composition of lesions at successive stages of regression

There are no histological descriptions of the changes in the composition of human lesions that undoubtedly occur when high serum cholesterol is reduced to low levels. We obtained data that explain what might happen in human lesions in experiments in which groups of rhesus monkeys with either minimal (types I—III) or advanced (types IV—V) lesions were killed at intervals from a few weeks to 3.5 years after high serum cholesterol was reduced to levels below 180 mg/dl [6,7]. Histological studies of the regressing monkey lesions revealed the lengths of time that are required to remove or reduce individual lesion components. Some components regressed quickly and completely, some slowly, and some remained or increased.

Briefly, most accumulated macrophage foam cells were removed within a period of 3—6 months after high serum cholesterol levels had declined to below 180 mg/dl. The reduction of extracellular lipid that was pooled in large amounts at the cores of lesions required much more time. Still, the bulk of this component even disappeared after 1—2 years. As accumulated macrophages, foam cells and extracellular lipid progressively decreased in lesions comparable to human types IV and V, the vacated but disrupted spaces changed to relatively acellular fibrous tissue. Normal composition and structure of arteries were not entirely re-established and calcium deposits and increased thickness remained to a variable extent. Nevertheless, we may assume that if comparable changes in lesion composition can be achieved in humans, the lesions would be less susceptible to surface disruptions, hematoma, and thrombosis than before. Figure 1 indicates the directions in which various human lesion types might change when risk factors are drastically reduced. Normal arterial composition may be restored when lesions of types I—III regress. The size of lesion types IV—VI may be reduced somewhat while their residuals take the compositions of type VII or type VIII lesions.

References

1. Stary HC. Macrophages, macrophage foam cells, and eccentric intimal thickening in the coronary arteries of young children. Atherosclerosis 1987;64:91—108.
2. Stary HC. Evolution and progression of atherosclerotic lesions in coronary arteries of children and young adults. Arteriosclerosis 1989;9(Suppl I):19—32.
3. Stary HC. The sequence of cell and matrix changes in atherosclerotic lesions of coronary arteries in the first forty years of life. Eur Heart J 1990;11(Suppl E):3—19.
4. Stary HC. Composition and classification of human atherosclerotic lesions. Virchows Arch A 1992;421:277—290.
5. Stary HC. The histological classification of atherosclerotic lesions in human coronary arteries. In: Fuster V, Ross R, Topol EJ (eds) Atherosclerosis and Coronary Artery Disease. Philadelphia: Lippincott-Raven Publishers, 1996;463—474.
6. Stary HC. Regression of atherosclerosis in primates. Virchows Arch A 1979;383:117—134.
7. Strong JP, Bhattacharyya AK, Eggen DA, Stary HC, Malcom GT, Newman WP, Restrepo C. Long-term induction and regression of diet-induced atherosclerotic lesions in rhesus monkeys. II. Morphometric evaluation of lesions by light microscopy in coronary and carotid arteries. Arterioscl Thromb 1994;14:2007—2016.

Epidemiology: new risk factors

Alcohol consumption and coronary heart disease: some recent epidemiological data

Pierre Ducimetière
INSERM Cardiovascular Epidemiology Unit, Paris, France

Abstract. The epidemiological evidence in favour of the concept of a protective effect of light to moderate alcohol consumption on coronary heart disease risk is reviewed. While no epidemiological data give actual proof that additional protection is gained from wine drinking rather than other alcoholic beverages, regular intake opposed to "binge drinking" appears beneficial. Modifications of lipid metabolism, especially HDL lipoproteins, represent a major biological mechanism for explaining the associations, although possible gene-environment interactions might interfere. From the public health point of view, no general public recommendations favouring light to moderate alcohol consumption should be given, taking into account their likely consequences on the frequency of heavy drinkers.

The concept of a protective effect of moderate alcohol consumption on coronary heart disease (CHD), morbidity and mortality results from an enormous bulk of epidemiological knowledge even though a formal proof of the causal nature of this relationship has not yet been given [1].

New data on these topics are currently being published and it is important to review periodically the state of evidence. Four main questions should be addressed: how much benefit? Which types of alcoholic beverages? Which consumption habits? Which biological mechanisms? Finally, the problem of public health recommendations in the field of alcohol drinking should also be emphasized.

How much benefit?

Recent meta-analyses of case-control and cohort data (e.g., [1–3]) confirmed the lower CHD-death risk of drinkers as compared to nondrinkers with a U-shape relationship skewed towards higher consumption levels. Maximum protection with a relative risk in the range 0.6–0.8 seems to be obtained for an intake of an order of magnitude of 20 g ethanol/day (approximately two drinks) and remains more or less stable until 60 g/day [3]. Data in British doctors [4] follow exactly the same pattern but failed to show any increase of all-cause mortality in heavy drinkers (more than nine drinks/day) in comparison with teetotallers.

This finding is at variance with most observational studies which clearly indi-

Address for correspondence: Pierre Ducimetière, INSERM U 258, Hôpital Broussais, 96 rue Didot, F-75014 Paris, France.

cate the lower life duration of those people. For instance, men who were drinking more than 50 g/day alcohol in the Paris Prospective Study II had twice the risk of dying during a 9-year follow-up than those drinking less than 20 g/day, including the few abstinent present in that French population, after adjustment for tobacco smoking and other factors [5].

Even though CHD protection seems to be established for an intake up to 60 g/day, the fact that all causes mortality is rising in the interval 20—60 g explains why only moderate consumption (two-three drinks/day) may be considered as beneficial.

Which types of alcoholic beverages?

The nature of the type of alcoholic beverage which is dominantly consumed in one country is highly variable as it results from cultural habits. It has long been accepted that the negative correlation at the country level between CHD mortality rate and the average alcohol per capita intake is particularly evident when alcohol derived from wine only is considered [6]. However, as it has been recently reviewed by Rimm et al. [7], the relationships at the individual level do not reproduce these ecological findings. Most studies which tried to estimate the specific effect attached to each class of alcoholic beverages (classically, wine, beer and spirits) from case-control or cohort data found hardly any clear-cut differences between them. In the multicenter CORALI study which correlated atherosclerosis scores obtained from coronarography in various patient populations in France, with individual alcohol intake before disease onset estimated by a questionnaire, a significant decrease in the stenosis score was observed with an increase in both wine and nonwine consumption, the decrease being of the same order of magnitude [8]. The meta-analysis of six cohort studies reported by Maclure [1] yielded a relative risk of CHD mortality of drinkers/abstainers; 0.74, 0.78 and 0.79 for wine, beer and liquors, respectively. Recently, in a large cohort study in Shanghai, the same figures for total mortality comparing men with one to four drinks/day vs. abstainers were, respectively, 0.82, 0.86 and 0.83, after adjustment for multiple risk factors [9]. In the ECTIM population based case-control study on myocardial infarction, the adjusted odds ratios associated with an increase of 10 g of wine- and nonwine-related alcohol/day were, 0.74 and 0.82, respectively ($p < 0.05$ for both) [10]. In this analysis, wine was mostly consumed by cases and controls from France recruitment centers whereas nonwine was consumed by those from Northern Ireland.

The Copenhagen City Heart Study is the only recently published cohort study who gave different results: deaths from cardiovascular and cerebrovascular disease were less frequent in wine drinkers/never, as frequent in beer drinkers/never, and more frequent in spirit drinkers/never [11]. Specific conditions attached to beverage preferences in some countries might explain such discrepancies from the classical thesis which considers ethanol intake as the major contribution to the CHD protective effect.

Which consumption habits?

Cultural differences apply to evidence, not only of the type of alcoholic beverages, but also of the consumption habits. The question of their possible differential effects was addressed in the British Regional Heart Study which reported that weekend drinkers were at slightly higher risk (RR = 1.2) than daily drinkers with a similar week-averaged intake of one to two drinks/day [12]. However, a large enough observational study for giving a precise answer to this question yielded its results only recently [13]. In this case-control study in Australia with more than 10,000 myocardial infarction cases, it was shown that risk was lowest in men who reported one to four drinks daily over 5 or 6 days a week and for women reporting one or two drinks under the same conditions. The fact that moderate consumption of alcohol entails a risk reduction when it is regular over 5—6 days a week (at least in Australia), might contribute to the interpretation of the low coronary heart disease mortality seen in both men and women in France [14].

Which biological mechanisms?

Acute and chronic biological effects of alcohol drinking are innumerable. Chronic effects of alcohol have been reported on metabolic or physiological systems which might participate in the lowering of coronary disease risk both on the atherosclerosis and/or the thrombosis side of the disease. The increase in serum HDL cholesterol as a result of chronic alcohol ingestion represents the most often cited effect in that respect and following the 1987 LCR Follow-Up Study Report [15] a number of cohort studies appear consistent in estimating that 50% of alcohol consumption preventive effects might be "explained" by HDL cholesterol elevation [16,17]. This estimate, however, is purely statistical and no causality has been in fact demonstrated. Recent observations might have introduced some complications in this etiological relationship. HDL_3 rather than HDL_2 cholesterol [18] and $LpA_1:A_2$ rather than LpA_1 [19] concentrations increase with alcohol drinking, whereas the second rather than the first can be implicated in the "reverse cholesterol transport", the supposed mechanism of protection from atherosclerosis. However, all HDL fractions seem to increase with alcohol intake and the argument does not appear conclusive. The complex metabolic interplay of HDL particles and CETP activity can point out the latter as a possible link in the chain of causality [20]. More recently, an interaction of alcohol intake with HDL cholesterol, CETP level and risk of myocardial infarction according to a polymorphism of CETP gene has been described in the ECTIM Study [21]. More precisely, the effect of alcohol intake on HDL cholesterol level and MI risk was present only in male homozygotes for the TaqIB polymorphism of the CETP gene (16% of the population). The confirmation of such a gene-environment interaction would be an important step in understanding the biological mechanisms of the alcohol protection.

Other possible mechanisms include the effect of alcohol on thrombotic factors and fibrinolysis parameters, with emphasis also being put on the free radical and antioxidant biology. However, there seems to be no epidemiological data presently available in order to document these associations as far as coronary heart disease risk is concerned.

The public health recommendations

Keeping closely to a light to moderate regular alcohol consumption (up to three drinks/day), it might be tempting to recommend such a habit at the population level. In fact, much evidence favours the hypothesis that the resulting increase in the average consumption of the population would be accompanied by a larger proportion of heavy drinkers with serious health consequences. Coming from observations of S. Ledermann in the '50s, this concept has been recently reassessed in an ecological analysis in England [22]. The conclusions of the authors are unambiguous and should be clearly stated while economic interests try to promote alcohol drinking from health arguments. "...Our data suggest that policies that increase consumption of the general population may lead to an increase in the amount of problem drinking and related problems and are therefore not in the interest of public health" (Colhoun et al. [22]). The fact that, on the opposite, the decrease of the average per capita alcohol consumption in France during the last 20 years was associated with a dramatic decrease in premature mortality due to alcoholism and heavy drinking is on-line with these conclusions, especially when we observe that cardiovascular mortality also decreased regularly during that period in the country.

References

1. Maclure M. Demonstration of deductive meta-analysis: ethanol intake and risk of myocardial infarction. Epidemiol Rev 1993;15:328—351.
2. Poikolainen K. Alcohol and mortality: a review. J Clin Epidemiol 1995;48:455—465.
3. Mäkelä P et al. Estimated numbers of deaths from coronary heart disease "caused" and "prevented" by alcohol: an example from Finland. J Stud Alcohol 1997;58:455—463.
4. Doll R et al. Mortality in relation to consumption of alcohol: 13 years' observations on male British doctors. Br Med J 1994;309:911—918.
5. Zureik M, Ducimetière P. High alcohol-related premature mortality in France: concordant estimates from a prospective cohort study and national mortality statistics. Alcohol Clin Exp Res 1996;20:428—433.
6. Leger AS et al. Factors associated with cardiac mortality in developped countries with particular reference to the consumption of wine. Lancet 1979;i:1017—1020.
7. Rimm EB et al. Review of moderate alcohol consumption and reduced risk of coronary heart disease: is the effect due to beer, wine, or spirits? Br Med J 1996;312:731—736.
8. Ducimetière P et al. Arteriographically documented coronary artery disease and alcohol consumption in French men. The CORALI Study. Eur Heart J 1993;14:727—733.
9. Yuan JM et al. Follow up study of moderate alcohol intake and mortality among middle aged men in Shanghai, China. Br Med J 1997;314:18—23.
10. Marques-Vidal P et al. Alcohol consumption and myocardial infarction: a case-control study in

France and Northern Ireland. Am J Epidemiol 1996;143:1089—1093.

11. Gronbaek M et al. Mortality associated with moderate intakes of wine, beer, or spirits. Br Med J 1995;310:1165—1169.

12. Shaper AG et al. Alcohol and ischemic heart disease in middle aged British men. Br Med J 1987;294:733—737.

13. McElduff P, Dobson AJ. How much alcohol and how often? Population based case-control study of alcohol consumption and risk of major coronary event. Br Med J 1997;314:1159—1164.

14. Ducimetière P, Richard JL. Dietary lipids and coronary heart disease: is there a French paradox? Nutr Metab Cardiovasc Dis 1992;2:195—201.

15. Criqui MH et al. Lipoproteins as mediators for the effects of alcohol consumption and cigarette smoking in cardiovascular mortality: results from the Lipid Research Clinics Follow-up-Study. Am J Epidemiol 1987;126:629—637.

16. Langer RD, Criqui MH, Reed DM. Lipoproteins and blood pressure as biological pathways for effect of moderate alcohol consumption on coronary heart disease. Circulation 1992;85:910—915.

17. Suh I et al. Alcohol use and mortality from coronary heart disease: the role of high-density lipoprotein cholesterol. Ann Int Med 1992;116:881—887.

18. Gaziano JM et al. Moderate alcohol intake, increased levels of high-density lipoprotein and its subfractions, and decreased risk of myocardial infarction. N Engl J Med 1993;329:1829—1834.

19. Puchois P et al. Effect of alcohol intake on human apolipoprotein A-I-containing lipoprotein subfractions. Arch Int Med 1990;150:1638—1641.

20. Savolainen MJ et al. Increased high-density lipoprotein cholesterol concentration in alcoholics is related to low cholesteryl ester transfer protein activity. Eur J Clin Invest 1990;20:593—599.

21. Fumeron F et al. Alcohol intake modulates the effect of a polymorphism of the cholesteryl ester tranfer protein gene on plasma high density lipoprotein and the risk of myocardial infarction. J Clin Invest 1995;96:1664—1671.

22. Colhoun H et al. Ecological analysis of collectivity of alcohol consumption in England: importance of average drinker. Br Med J 1997;314:1164—1168.

New risk factors in the Atherosclerosis Risk in Communities Study

Aaron R. Folsom, for the Atherosclerosis Risk in Communities Study (ARIC) Investigators
Division of Epidemiology, School of Public Health, University of Minnesota, Minneapolis, Minnesota, USA

Abstract. *Background.* Although a number of cardiovascular (CVD) risk factors have been firmly established, several putative risk factors require further investigation of their role in CVD.

Methods. The Atherosclerosis Risk in Communities (ARIC) Study has examined several potential "new" risk factors in relation to carotid intima-media thickness (a subclinical marker of atherosclerosis) and to incident coronary heart disease (CHD) in a population-based sample.

Results. ARIC data have implicated fibrinogen, lipoprotein(a), and cellular adhesion molecules as markers of, or risk factors for, CVD. Fibrinolytic factors and platelet activation were associated with carotid atherosclerosis, but we do not yet have data for their associations with incident CHD. Notably, we do not find strong evidence that homocysteine or prior infection with *Chlamydia pneumoniae* or CMV are risk factors for incident CHD, though they were weakly associated with prevalent carotid atherosclerosis. The role of serum insulin as a CHD risk factor remains uncertain, given an association for women but not men in ARIC, and inconsistency in the literature.

Conclusions. The ARIC Study provides prospective evidence related to several potential new risk factors for CHD.

Keywords: cardiovascular disease, coronary disease, prospective study.

Introduction

Epidemiologic research over the past 40 years has clearly established that atherosclerotic cardiovascular disease (CVD) risk is greatly determined by several life-style and constitutional characteristics. Well-established risk factors include age, male sex, dyslipidemia, high blood pressure, cigarette smoking, diabetes, obesity, physical inactivity, and family history. Dietary imbalance plays a crucial role in determining several of these risk factors. Extensive clinical trial evidence shows that reduction of major risk factors, particularly hypercholesterolemia and high blood pressure, can reduce risk of CVD [1].

Established risk factors account for a majority, but not the totality, of CVD occurrence. Other characteristics of populations or individuals likely contribute to levels of CVD risk. Identification of new risk factors can help elucidate the pathogenesis of CVD, pinpoint subgroups at particular risk, and suggest possible strategies for primary or secondary prevention.

Address for correspondence: Dr Aaron R. Folsom, Division of Epidemiology, School of Public Health, University of Minnesota, Suite 300, 1300 South Second Street, Minneapolis, MN 55454-1015, USA.

One aim of the Atherosclerosis Risk in Communities Study (ARIC), begun in the mid-1980s, was to evaluate prospectively the role of several putative new CVD risk factors suggested in clinical and case-control studies. This manuscript reviews some of the major findings to date on new risk factors in ARIC, namely hemostatic factors, serum insulin, lipoprotein(a) (Lp(a)), homocysteine, infectious agents, and circulating adhesion molecules.

Methods

The ARIC study cohort consists of 15,782 adults aged 45–74 years at baseline level in 1987–89 [2]. ARIC selected probability samples from four US communities: Forsyth County, North Carolina; Jackson, Mississippi (blacks only); suburbs of Minneapolis, Minnesota; and Washington County, Maryland. Response rates to a baseline examination were 46% in Jackson and approximately 66% in the other three communities. ARIC conducted subsequent examinations in 1990–92, 1993–95, and 1996–98.

The baseline examination included standardized assessments of established and new CVD risk factors and of prevalent disease. We measured average carotid intima-media thickness as a marker of subclinical atherosclerosis using a standardized B-mode ultrasonographic technique [3,4]. Blood specimens were also stored for subsequent nested case-control studies. Among participants free of coronary heart disease (CHD) at baseline, ARIC ascertained CHD incidence (myocardial infarction or CHD death) during follow-up [5].

Results

ARIC has documented that the established risk factors, hypercholesterolemia, high blood pressure, cigarette smoking, diabetes, obesity, and physical inactivity, were all associated with greater carotid intima-media thickness at baseline [6,7]. These risk factors were also associated with greater progression of intima-media thickening longitudinally [8] and with CHD incidence [9]. Moreover, increased carotid intima-media thickness, itself, was associated with greater risk of incident CHD [9]. For example, adjusted for age, field center and race, the relative risk of CHD for carotid intima-media thickness ≥ 1.0 vs. < 0.6 mm was 18.9 (95% confidence interval (CI) = 7–48) in women and 4.2 (95% CI = 2–9) in men.

Findings for several new risk factors are discussed separately.

Hemostatic factors

The role of hemostatic factors in the causation of CVD is a matter of considerable debate. In the whole ARIC cohort, prevalent CVD and carotid intima-media thickness at baseline level were positively and strongly associated with plasma fibrinogen, but were essentially unassociated with levels of factor VIIc, factor VIIIc, von Willebrand factor, protein C antigen, and antithrombin III [10]. Carotid intima-media thickness was also strongly and positively associated with levels of β-thromboglobulin [11], plasminogen activator inhibitor-1 (PAI-1) antigen, tissue plasminogen activator (t-PA) antigen, and D-dimer [12].

Incident CHD in ARIC was also positively and strongly associated with baseline fibrinogen (multivariately adjusted relative risk per standard deviation increment = 1.48, 95% CI = 1.2−1.8). Incident CHD was also associated positively with von Willebrand factor and factor VIIIc, though these latter associations were not independent of other risk factors [13]. As with carotid intima-media thickness, CHD incidence was not associated with factor VIIc, protein C, or antithrombin III. The platelet and fibrinolysis markers are only now being studied in relation to incident CHD in ARIC.

Thus, ARIC data strongly support fibrinogen as a risk factor for CVD, and suggest that platelet and fibrinolysis markers may be also.

Insulin

Whether serum insulin, or insulin resistance, is a risk factor for CVD is controversial. Fasting serum insulin was modestly positively associated with carotid intima-media thickness at baseline level among ARIC participants free of diabetes [7]. Prospectively, serum insulin was associated positively with CHD incidence in women but not men [14]. Adjusted for age, race field center, smoking status, ethanol drinking status, education level, physical activity and hormone replacement, the relative risks across quintiles of fasting insulin were 1.00, 0.76, 2.08, 2.08, and 2.82 (p for linear trend = 0.02) for women, respectively.

Thus, ARIC data do not strongly support fasting insulin being an important risk factor for CVD.

Lipoprotein (a)

Considerable evidence suggests that Lp(a) is associated with increased risk of CVD. At baseline in ARIC, a one standard deviation difference in Lp(a) protein was associated with an odds ratio of 1.49 (95% CI = 1.2−1.9) for elevated carotid intima-media thickness, adjusted for age, LDL and HDL cholesterol, fibrinogen, hypertension, and cigarette smoking [15]. Prospectively, the relative risk of CHD was 1.20 (95% CI = 1.06−1.36) per one standard deviation increment of Lp(a) in whites. However, in blacks, this relative risk was 0.97 (0.82−1.15) [16].

Thus in ARIC, Lp(a) appears to be a stronger CHD risk factor in whites than in blacks.

Homocysteine

Plasma homocysteine has rapidly been implicated as a CVD risk factor in the 1990s. However, the number of prospective, population-based studies to show this are few. In ARIC at baseline, plasma homocysteine was associated positively with carotid atherosclerosis, as reflected by an elevated intima-media thickness [17]. However, the association between plasma homocysteine and carotid atherosclerosis was not statistically significant after adjustment for established risk factors. Moreover, preliminary evidence (A. Folsom et al., unpublished) suggests that there is no significant association prospectively between homocysteine and CHD incidence in ARIC, after adjustment for other risk factors.

ARIC data are most consistent with plasma homocysteine being elevated by atherosclerotic disease but not being an important risk factor for incident CHD.

Infectious agents

Several lines of evidence have suggested that certain infectious agents may contribute to CVD, particularly *Chlamydia pneumoniae* and the herpes viruses. In ARIC, *C. pneumoniae* seropositivity was associated positively with carotid atherosclerosis, independent of major risk factors [18], but it was not associated with incident CHD after adjustment for other risk factors [19]. Carotid atherosclerosis was not associated with antibody titers to herpes simplex virus type 1 or type 2, but was weakly associated with cytomegalovirus (CMV) seropositivity. The CMV odds ratio was 1.36 (95% CI = 0.8–2.3), adjusted for smoking, LDL cholesterol, education level, diabetes, hypertension, alcohol, and age [20]. Prospective data on CHD incidence in relation to the herpes viruses are not yet available in ARIC.

Thus, ARIC suggests possible weak associations of these infectious agents with subclinical atherosclerosis.

Adhesion molecules

Recruitment of circulating leukocytes at sites of atherosclerosis is mediated through adhesion molecules. ARIC therefore measured vascular cell adhesion molecule-1 (VCAM-1), endothelial-leukocyte adhesion molecule-1 (E-selectin) and intercellular adhesion molecule-1 (ICAM-1) in a sample of incident CHD cases, thickened carotid atherosclerosis cases, and controls [21]. VCAM-1 was not associated with either CVD endpoint. Adjusted for age, race, gender, body mass index, hypertension, diabetes, total and HDL cholesterol, smoking, triglycerides, fibrinogen von Willebrand factor, and white blood cell count, the odds ratio for the upper quartile vs. the lower quartile of ICAM-1 were 2.64 (95% CI = 1.4–5.0) for carotid atherosclerosis and 5.53 (95% CI = 2.5–12.2) for incident CHD. The respective odds ratios for E-selectin were 2.03 (95% CI = 1.1–3.6) and 1.60 (95% CI = 0.78–3.3).

Thus, circulating cellular adhesion molecules predict atherosclerotic disease in ARIC, though the causal role of these molecules needs to be established.

Discussion

The ARIC study is one of the most comprehensive epidemiologic prospective studies to date, affording the opportunity to associate new risk factors with both carotid atherosclerosis and incident CHD. Our findings implicate fibrinogen, Lp(a), and cellular adhesion molecules as markers of, or risk factors for, CVD. Fibrinolytic factors and platelet activation were associated with carotid atherosclerosis, but we do not yet have data for their associations with incident CHD. Notably, we do not find strong evidence that homocysteine or prior infection with *C. pneumoniae* or CMV are risk factors for CHD, though they were weakly associated with prevalent carotid atherosclerosis. The role of insulin as a CHD risk factor remains uncertain, given differences for women vs. men in ARIC, and in the literature.

Our data, and that of others, do not suggest that any of these risk markers, other than perhaps fibrinogen, deserve to be designated yet as major, established risk factors. Unfortunately, a number of these new physiologic risk markers may be elevated as a consequence of subclinical disease and therefore may not be true causes of CVD. Even ARIC prospective data on people without recognized CVD may suffer from this ambiguity about cause and effect. Other supportive data, including more prospective studies and clinical trials, where feasible, are needed to properly rate the importance of these putative new causes of CVD.

Acknowledgements

The ARIC Study is supported by contracts N01-HC-55015, N01-HC-55016, N01-HC-55018, N01-HC-55019, N01-HC-55020, N01-HC-55021, N01-HC-55022 from the US National Heart, Lung, and Blood Institute.

References

1. Yusuf S, Lessem J, Jha P, Lonn E. Primary and secondary prevention of myocardial infarction and strokes: an update of randomly allocated, controlled trials. J Hypertens 1993;11(Suppl 4):S61—S73.
2. ARIC Investigators. The Atherosclerosis Risk in Communities (ARIC) Study: Design and objectives. Am J Epidemiol 1989;129:687—702.
3. Bond MG, Barnes RW, Riley WA, Wilmoth SK, Chambless LE, Howard G, Owens B. High resolution B-mode ultrasound scanning methods in the Atherosclerosis Risk in Communities Study (ARIC). J Neuroimag 1991;1:68—73.
4. Riley WA, Barnes RW, Bond MG, Evans G, Chambless Le, Heiss G. High resolution B-mode ultrasound reading methods in the Atherosclerosis Risk in Communities Study (ARIC). J Neuroimag 1991;1:168—172.
5. White AD, Folsom AR, Chambless LE, Sharrett AR, Yang K, Conwill D, Higgins M, Williams OD, Tyroler HA, and the ARIC Investigators. Community surveillance of coronary heart disease in the Atherosclerosis Risk in Communities (ARIC) Study: Methods and initial two years' experience. J Clin Epidemiol 1996;49:223—233.
6. Heiss G, Sharrett AR, Barnes R, Chambless LE, Szklo M, Alzola C. Carotid atherosclerosis

412

measured by B-mode ultrasound in populations: associations with cardiovascular risk factors in the ARIC study. Am J Epidemiol 1991;134:250—256.

7. Folsom AR, Eckfeldt JH, Weitzman S, Ma J, Chambless LE, Barnes RW, Cram KB, Hutchinson RG, and the Atherosclerosis Risk in Communities (ARIC) Study Investigators. Relation of carotid artery wall thickness to diabetes mellitus, fasting glucose and insulin, body size, and physical activity. Stroke 1994;25:66—73.

8. Evans GW, Chambless LE, Szklo M, Folsom AR, Hutchinson RG, Heiss G. Risk factors for carotid atherosclerosis progression: The ARIC Study (Abstract). Circulation 1996;93:9.

9. Chambless LE, Heiss G, Folsom AR, Rosamond W, Szklo M, Sharrett AR, Clegg LX. Association of coronary heart disease incidence with carotid arterial wall thickness and major risk factors: The Atherosclerosis Risk in Communities (ARIC) Study 1987-1993. Am J Epidemiol (In press).

10. Folsom AR, Wu KK, Shahar E, Davis CE. Association of hemostatic variables with prevalent cardiovascular disease and asymptomatic carotid artery atherosclerosis. Arterioscl Thromb 1993;13:1829—1836.

11. Ghaddar HM, Cortes J, Salomaa V, Kark JD, Davis CE, Folsom AR, Heiss G, Stinson V, Wu KK, for the Atherosclerosis Risk in Communities Study Investigators. Correlation of specific platelet activation markers with carotid arterial wall thickness. Thromb Haemost 1995;74: 943—948.

12. Salomaa V, Stinson V, Kark JD, Folsom AR, Davis CE, Wu KK. The association of fibrinolytic parameters with early atherosclerosis: The Atherosclerosis Risk in Communities (ARIC) Study. Circulation 1995;91:284—290.

13. Folsom AR, Wu KK, Rosamond WD, Sharrett AR, Chambless LE. A prospective study of hemostatic factors and incidence of coronary heart disease: The Atherosclerosis Risk in Communities (ARIC) Study. Circulation (In press).

14. Folsom AR, Szklo M, Stevens J, Liao F, Smith R, Eckfeldt JH. A prospective study of coronary heart disease in relation to fasting insulin, glucose, and diabetes: The Atherosclerosis Risk in Communities (ARIC) Study. Diabet Care 1997;20:935—942.

15. Schreiner PJ, Morrisett JD, Sharrett AR, Patsch W, Tyroler HA, Wu K, Heiss G. Lipoprotein(a) as a risk factor for preclinical atherosclerosis. Arterioscler Thromb 1993;13:826—833.

16. Schreiner P, Chambless LE, Heiss G, Patsch W, Morrisett J, Sharrett AR, Watson R. Lipoprotein[a] as a risk factor for incident coronary heart disease: Early Results of the ARIC Study (Abstract). Abstracts from the 3rd International Conference on Preventive Cardiology, June 27—July 1, 1993, Oslo, Norway.

17. Malinow MR, Nieto FJ, Szklo M, Chambless LE, Bond G. Carotid artery intimal-medial wall thickening and plasma homocyst(e)ine in asymptomatic adults: The Atherosclerosis Risk in Communities Study. Circulation 1993;87:1107—1113.

18. Melnick SL, Shahar E, Folsom AR, Grayston JT, Sorlie PD, Wang SP, Szklo M, for the Atherosclerosis Risk in Communities (ARIC) Study Investigators. Past infection by *Chlamydia pneumoniae* strain TWAR and asymptomatic carotid atherosclerosis. Am J Med 1993;95:499—504.

19. Nieto FJ, Folsom AR, Sorlie P, Shahar E, Chambless LE, Szklo M. *Chlamydia pneumoniae* Infection and Incident Coronary Heart Disease: The Atherosclerosis Risk in Communities (ARIC) Study. Abstract presented at the 30th Annual Meeting of the Society for Epidemiologic Research, Edmonton, Alberta, Canada, June 12—14, 1997.

20. Sorlie PD, Adam E, Melnick SL, Folsom A, Skelton T, Chambless LE, Barnes R, Melnick JL, for the Atherosclerosis Risk in Communities (ARIC) Study Investigators. Cytomegalovirus/herpes virus and carotid atherosclerosis: The ARIC Study. J Med Virol 1994;42:33—37.

21. Boerwinkle E, Sharrett AR, Ballantyne CM, Davis CE, Gotto A Jr, Smith L. Circulating adhesion molecules predict atherosclerosis and incident CHD in the ARIC Study (Abstract). Circulation 1996;93:2.

413

von Willebrand factor, endothelial cell markers and arterial thrombosis

Andrew Blann

Haemostasis, Thrombosis and Vascular Biology Unit, University Department of Medicine, The City Hospital, Birmingham, UK

Abstract. Endothelial integrity is crucial to several physiological systems, such as renal function and may be assessed by the use of plasma markers which include von Willebrand factor, soluble thrombomodulin and soluble E-selectin. This communication summarises the evidence that these molecules may have clinical relevance in predicting which individuals are at risk of the development or progression of atherosclerosis. However, despite the importance of the endothelium, it is likely that other markers such as fibrinogen may have equal potency as markers of mortality in patients with existing vascular disease.

von Willebrand factor, endothelial cells and arterial thrombosis

Virchow was among the first to consider the pathogenesis of atherosclerosis. His triad hypothesised that the vascular lesions (atheroma) were the product of three distinct components: blood flow (which we now recognise as rheology and viscosity), the constituents of the blood (now known to include leucocyte, platelet and soluble coagulation factors such as fibrinogen), and the lining of the blood vessel wall. The importance of this latter aspect of the triad is currently demonstrated by an appreciation of the importance of the endothelium in areas such as haemostasis and the regulation of vascular tone, [1] and the view that damage to the endothelium is a primary event in the pathogenesis of atherosclerosis [2].

Consequently, good markers of endothelial cell integrity are likely to be useful as research tools for vascular biologists and for clinicians seeking to predict which of the large number of patients with atherosclerosis and its risk factors are at the greatest risk of disease progression to stroke, for example. Of the numerous candidates available, only a few have the required specificity, sensitivity and ease of measurement to justify assessment as endothelial markers. Much is known about the physiology of tissue plasminogen activator (tPA) in cardiovascular disease, but the presence of its inhibitor (PAI) and the possibility that antigenic activity (i.e., as defined by ELISA) may not equate to functional activity, implies difficulty in interpreting data [3]. For example, the immunological ELISA assay may measure not only free tPA but also (biologically inactive) tPA com-

---

Address for correspondence: Andrew Blann, Haemostasis, Thrombosis and Vascular Biology Unit, University Department of Medicine, The City Hospital, Dudley Road, Birmingham B18 7QH, UK. Tel./Fax: +44-121-507-5076.

414

plexed to PAI-1, whereas the bioassay is likely to measure only free tPA.

von Willebrand factor (vWf) has been studied for over 20 years, and considerable literature suggests that it is (although imperfect) the nearest we have to a gold standard for endothelial function. The levels of this molecule are raised in a wide series of inflammatory, autoimmune and atherosclerotic diseases, broadly reflecting disease activity. They can be reversed by treatment of the (generally injurious) stimulating factor (such as hypercholesterolaemia, and smoking). High levels can also predict cardiovascular endpoints (including death) in patients with frank atherosclerosis, its risk factors, and in health. vWf is also of interest as it may participate directly in thrombus and atheroma formation, having binding sites for platelet-membrane components and also for constituents of the subendothelium [4]. Membrane bound thrombomodulin (CD141) has anticoagulant properties by sequestering thrombin and promoting the activities of protein C and protein S. It follows that loss of membrane activity, and the appearance of inactive soluble forms in the plasma and urine carries with it a risk of inappropriate coagulation and possibly of thrombosis. Therefore, increased levels of this plasma form, soluble thrombomodulin, (sTM) (also reflecting endothelial cell damage) are frequently found in the same conditions as is raised vWf, and can also be related to disease activity (e.g., in diabetes) [5]. The relationship between sTM and the risk factors for atherosclerosis are incomplete as levels are lower in smokers, for example. Of the few follow-up studies of this molecule, raised levels indicate a poor prognosis in coronary artery disease (CAD), and also in subjects on long-term oral anticoagulant therapy [6,7]. Soluble E-selectin (CD62E) is also shed from the endothelium (but at times of cytokine-directed activation), and raised levels are found in, for example, sepsis, rheumatoid arthritis, and certain cancers [3]. The relationship between risk factors and this molecule is even less well understood, with some contradictions in respect of the influence of lipids; few follow-up studies have been performed. However, levels have been reported to predict patients with restenosis following peripheral angioplasty [8].

Most of the above have come from studies where only one, or at best, two markers have been examined in parallel. Comparative studies in this laboratory have shown that the three markers vary, in apparently healthy individuals, in response to smoking, according to sex, and also when analysed for ABO blood group [9]. In a case-control study of 116 patients with CAD, vWf and sTM were significantly (p < 0.001) raised, but soluble E-selectin was only weakly raised (p = 0.011) [10]. A follow-up of some of these subjects revealed that raised sTM, but not soluble E-selectin, predicted adverse outcome [6]. Similarly, in a cross-sectional study of 200 patients with peripheral artery disease (PAD), levels of soluble E-selectin were not raised relative to controls. However, raised sTM, but not raised vWf, was able to differentiate patients with more extensive disease (i.e., of only one locus, compared to disease at two or more loci) [11].

The prediction of disease progression

But which of these two promising endothelial cell markers is a better marker of disease advancement? This question is currently being addressed in a long-term follow-up of the 116 patients with CAD and 200 patients with PAD outlined above [6,10,11], and in 200 apparently healthy controls, excluding diabetics and subjects with a florid acute phase response (ESR > 20 mm/h). Preliminary studies of the follow-up (mean 44 months) of 81 of these subjects [10,11] (patients with CAD, PAD and some asymptomatic subjects) in which all three markers have been measured has classified 33 into a group with a cardiovascular endpoint (fatal and nonfatal MI and stroke, arterial surgery, and the appearance of disease as defined by the Rose protocol [12]). This group had higher von Willebrand factor (mean/SD 150 ± 38 IU/dl vs. 119 ± 38, t test p < 0.0001), higher sTM (60 ± 25 ng/ml vs. 47 ± 17, p = 0.011) but equivalent soluble E-selectin (56 ± 27 ng/ml vs. 54 ± 17, p = 0.68) relative to those free of an endpoint. Patients with endpoints were also more likely to have existing vascular disease on outset (82 vs. 56%, χ^2 = 5.735, p = 0.017), with higher triglycerides (median 2.2 mmol, range 1.0−5.5 vs. 1.6, 0.5−3.8, Mann-Whitney p = 0.0146), higher fibrinogen (3.9 ± 0.6 g/l vs. 3.2 ± 1.0, p = 0.0095) and lower HDL (1.08 ± 0.23 mmol/l vs. 1.30 ± 0.40, p = 0.0023). There were no differences in total and LDL-cholesterol, triglycerides, systolic or diastolic blood pressures, age or sex. However, in multivariate analysis to define outcome, only the difference in vWf, sTM, fibrinogen and HDL remained. Entering the two significant endothelial cell markers against outcome, only vWf remained significant (p = 0.01, sTM = 0.131), but entering those three factors with a univariate p < 0.01, only HDL predicted disease progression (p = 0.029, vWf p = 0.129, fibrinogen p = 0.196). These preliminary data indicate that vWf may be a better predictor of adverse events than sTM, and that measurement of soluble E-selectin has little to offer in long-term follow-up studies in either CAD or PAD. However, it seems also that lower levels of HDL are an even better predictor. The study is continuing and completed results will be published in the future.

Conclusions

The most flimsy conclusion of the proceeding paragraph is that although endothelial cell damage is undoubtedly present in atherosclerosis, and is a poor prognostic factor, levels of other markers may be more sensitive in predicting adverse outcome. This view supports the assertions by Ridker [13], who has indicated that several nonspecific markers, headed by tPA and fibrinogen may be better predictors of disease progression than endothelial markers, and also of Fowkes et al., who also arrived at a similar conclusion regarding cross-linked FDPs in patients with peripheral arterial disease [14]. However, it is likely that changes in no single risk factor will reduce the incidence of atherosclerosis, and that a multiple approach will be beneficial. This is likely to include the management of risk factors (correction of which will reduce vWf, as in smoking and a lipid-rich diet) as well as existing (e.g., aspirin) and new pharmacological approaches such as reducing the biological ability of vWf to promote thrombosis with novel heparins, monoclonal antibodies and inhibitory peptides [15–18].

References

1. Vogel RA. Coronary risk factors, endothelial function, and atherosclerosis: a review. Clin Cardiol 1997;20:426–32.
2. Ross R. The pathogenesis of atherosclerosis: a perspective for the 1990s. Nature 1993;362: 801–809.
3. Blann AD, Taberner DA. A reliable marker of endothelial cell dysfunction: does it exist? Br J Haematol 1995;90:244–248.
4. Lip GYH, Blann AD. von Willebrand factor: a marker of endothelial cell dysfunction in vascular disorders? Cardiovasc Res 1997;34:255–265.
5. Boffa MC. Considering cellular thrombomodulin distribution and its modulating factors can facilitate the use of plasma thrombomodulin as a reliable endothelial marker? Haemostasis 1996;26(Suppl 4):233–243.
6. Blann AD, Amiral J, McCollum CN. Prognostic value of increased soluble thrombomodulin and increased soluble E-selectin in ischaemic heart disease. Eur J Haematol 1997;58:115–120.
7. Jansson JH, Boman K, Brannstrom M, Nilsson TK. Increased levels of plasma thrombomodulin are associated with vascular and all-cause mortality in patients on long-term anticoagulant treatment. Eur Heart J 1996;17:1503–1505.
8. Belch JJF, Shaw JW, Kirk G, McLaren M, Robb R, Maple C, Morse P. The white blood cell adhesion molecule E-selectin predicts restenosis in patients with intermittent claudication undergoing percutaneous transluminal angioplasty. Circulation 1997;95:2027–2031.
9. Blann AD, Daly RJ, Amiral J. The influence of age, gender and ABO blood group on soluble endothelial cell markers and adhesion molecules. Br J Haematol 1996;92:498–500.
10. Blann AD, Amiral J, McCollum CN. Circulating endothelial cell/leucocyte adhesion molecules in ischaemic heart disease. Br J Haematol 1996;95:263–265.
11. Blann AD, Seigneur M, Steiner M, Boisseau MR, McCollum CN. Circulating endothelial cell markers in peripheral vascular disease: relationship to the location and extent of atherosclerotic disease. Eur J Clin Invest 1997;27:(In press).
12. Rose GA. The diagnosis of ischaemic heart pain and intermittent claudication in field surveys. Bull WHO 1962;27:645–658.
13. Ridker PM. Fibinolytic and inflammatory markers for arterial occlusion: the evolving epidemiology of thrombosis and haemostasis. Thromb Haemostas 1997;78:53–59.
14. Fowkes FGR, Lowe GDO, Housley E, Rattray A, Rumley A, Elton RA, MacGregor IR, Dawes J. Cross-linked fibrin degradation products, progression of peripheral arterial disease and risk of coronary heart disease. Lancet 1993;342:84–86.
15. Sobel M, Bird KE, Tyler-Cross R, Margues D, Toma N, Conrad HE, Harris RB. Heparins designed to specifically inhibit platelet interactions with von Willebrand factor. Circulation 1996;93:992–999.
16. Golino P, Ragni M, Cirillo P, Pascucci I, Ezekowitz MD, Pawashe A, Scognamiglio A, Pace L, Guarino A, Chiariello M. Aurintricarboxylic acid reduces platelet deposition in sterilised and endothelially injured rabbit carotid arteries more effectively than other antiplatelet interventions. Thromb Haemostas 1995;74:974–979.
17. Zahger D, Fishein MC, Garfinkel LI, Shah PK, Forrester JS, Regnstrom J, Yano J, Vercek B. VCL, an antagonist of the platelet GPIb receptor, markedly inhibits platelet adhesion and inti-

mal thickening after balloon injury in the rat. Circulation 1995;92:1269—1273.
18. Hoylaerts MF, Yamamoto H, Vermylen J. Platelet adhesion to nondamaged aorta endothelium of cholesterol-fed rabbits is mediated by von Willebrand factor. Thromb Haemostas 1997; 78(Suppl):PS1409 (Abstract).

Atherosclerosis XI.
B. Jacotot, D. Mathé and J.-C. Fruchart, editors.

Homocysteine as a risk factor for cardiovascular disease

Ian M. Graham[1-3] and Raymond Meleady[4]

[1] Department of Epidemiology and Preventive Medicine, Royal College of Surgeons in Ireland; [2] Department of Cardiology, Trinity College, Dublin; [3] Department of Cardiology, Adelaide & Meath Hospitals, Dublin; and [4] Department of Cardiology, Adelaide Hospital, Dublin, Ireland

Introduction

Thirty-five years ago, Carson in Northern Ireland [1] and Gerritsen in Wisconsin [2,3] described the finding of large amounts of homocystine in the urine of mentally retarded children. Two years later, Mudd identified the commonest enzyme defect causing this condition, deficiency of cystathionine B synthase [4]. Homocystinuric subjects suffer from skeletal abnormalities which are similar to those of the Marfan syndrome, and are prone to aggressive and life-threatening atherothrombotic events. These occur prematurely, often within the first two decades of life [5]. The observations that several other, distinct enzyme defects are similarly characterized by very high plasma homocysteine levels with homocystinuria and with premature vascular disease led McCully [6,7] to propose the homocysteine theory of atherosclerosis, in which the common link between the distinct metabolic defects and vascular disease is a raised plasma homocysteine level.

The relationship between relatively uncommon metabolic errors and vascular disease is of clinical interest but not of major public health significance. The question arises as to whether milder elevations in plasma homocysteine, which might be relatively frequent, are also related to vascular disease. It is now clear that this is so. The present paper examines homocysteine metabolism (Fig. 1), mechanisms whereby homocysteine may damage the vascular tree, and looks at the relationships between moderate hyperhomocysteinaemia and vascular disease.

Homocysteine metabolism

Homocysteine is a sulphur amino acid which exists as a pure disulphide, homocystine (homocysteine-homocysteine), or as a mixed disulphide, homocysteine-cysteine. These species are 70% protein bound. The collective term "total homocysteine" (tHcy) is used in this article to refer to the combined free and protein bound forms of all the above species.

Homocysteine is formed by the demethylation of methionine. Whereas methionine is an essential amino acid which acts as a methyl donor for the production

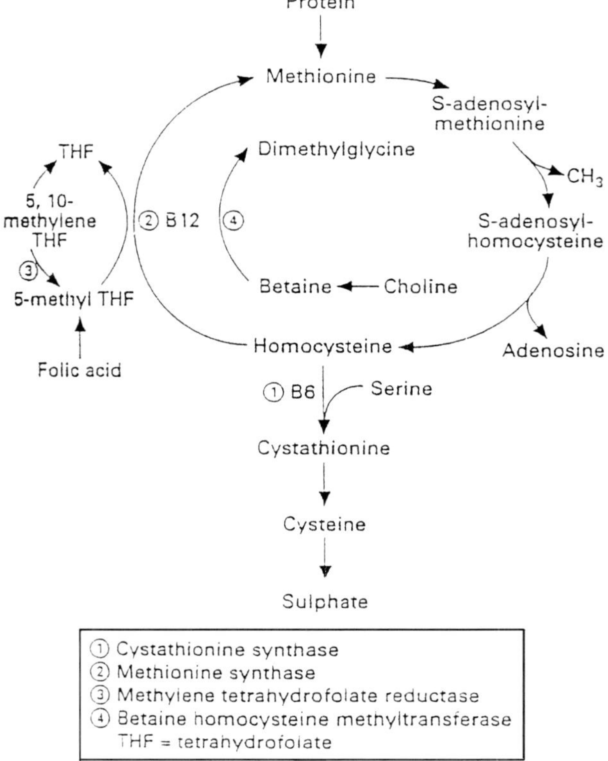

Fig. 1. Transsulphuration and remethylation of homocysteine.

of creatine and other substances, homocysteine has no known metabolic function.

Homocysteine may be irreversibly degraded using cystathionine B synthase, which requires vitamin B6 as a cofactor. Alternatively, methionine is conserved by the remethylation of homocysteine to methionine utilizing methylenetetrahydrofolate reductase (which requires folate as a cosubstrate) and methionine synthase, which requires vitamin B12 as a cofactor. It follows that a raised plasma homocysteine may result from either defects in the enzymes modulating its metabolism, or in deficiencies of the nutrients required for effective enzyme function. Diseases such as renal failure and certain medications, notably anticonvulsants and nitrous oxide, also raise plasma tHcy levels.

The classical enzyme defect causing severe hyperhomocysteinaemia with homocystinuria is homozygous cystathionine B synthase deficiency. Homozygous deficiency of methylenetetrahydrofolate reductase and defects in cobalamin metabolism are rarer causes of homocystinuria. A much more common mutation is the thermolabile variant of methylenetetrahydrofolate reductase which is present in perhaps 5—7% of normal subjects [8]. This enzyme variant is associated with raised plasma homocysteine levels in subjects with marginal or low folate status, but there is still dispute as to whether it constitutes a risk factor for vascular disease [9].

Plasma homocysteine is a sensitive marker of folate and B12 status, with levels rising at around about the median concentration of these substances in plasma, long before overt deficiency is present. If homocysteine is a risk factor for vascular disease, this may force reconsideration of desirable intakes.

Homocysteine and cardiovascular risk

There is no doubt that subjects with severe hyperhomocysteinaemia, such as that which occurs in homocystinuria, are at greatly increased risk of atherothrombotic events. It is now clear that milder elevations of plasma homocysteine also increase risk appreciably. The association between a raised plasma homocysteine and vascular risk has been shown in many case-control studies [9] and confirmed by prospective studies which indicate that the elevated plasma homocysteine precedes the development of disease. A 5 μmol/l increase in plasma homocysteine concentration has been estimated to increase the risk of coronary heart disease by as much as an increase in serum cholesterol concentration of 0.5 mmol/l [10].

The European Union Concerted Action Project, "Homocysteinaemia and Vascular Disease", indicated that, in 750 patients with vascular disease and 800 control subjects, a plasma homocysteine level above 12 μmol/l (the top fifth of the control distribution) doubled the risk of myocardial infarction, cerebral or peripheral vascular disease in both men and women [11]. The suggestion of a dose-response effect noted in the European Concerted Action Project has been convincingly confirmed by several prospective studies including the British Regional Heart Study in stroke subjects, and the Tromso Study.

In the European study, a plasma homocysteine level above 12 μmol/l conferred a risk similar to that associated with a cholesterol level of 6.5 mmol/l, or to that of cigarette smoking. Furthermore, strong interaction effects were noted in that a raised plasma homocysteine increased risk multiplicatively when combined with smoking or hypertension. This may have public health implications and it may be relevant to measure plasma homocysteine levels in subjects with other risk factors while similarly meticulous risk factor advice may be important in hyperhomocysteinaemic subjects.

Mechanisms whereby homocysteine may be atherogenic and prothrombotic have been reviewed in some detail [12]. These proposed mechanisms include altered platelet function, endothelial cell damage, enhancement of the binding of lipoprotein(a) to fibrin and effects on coagulation factors. More recently a reduction in the protective effect of endothelium derived relaxing factor has been proposed [13].

422

Preventive and therapeutic implications

The association between a raised plasma homocysteine and cardiovascular risk is only of public health or clinical relevance if the raised plasma homocysteine level can be treated, and if risk is reduced as a result. It is now clear that dietary supplementation with folic acid reduces plasma homocysteine concentrations by 25—30% in most subjects, with a stronger effect in those with higher homocysteine levels. Vitamin B12 has much less effect, except in those deficient in this vitamin. Vitamin B6 appears to be more effective in lowering the raised plasma homocysteine unmasked by a methionine loading test but the clinical implications of this observation are uncertain. The optimal dose of folic acid remains unknown despite considerable numbers of dose finding studies. It will probably emerge to be about 400—600 μg daily. Several large randomised control trials of folic acid supplementation are currently planned or starting to ascertain whether risk reduction will result from a lowering of homocysteine levels. In public health terms, a greater yield can probably be obtained by food fortification [10] based on the evidence that folic acid supplementation reduces the risk of neural tube defects, and on the proposed beneficial effects on cardiovascular risk, folate supplementation is becoming mandatory in some countries, notably the USA. Others are adopting a more conservative approach until randomised control trial evidence of reduction in vascular risk is available.

References

1. Carson NAJ, Neill DW. Metabolic abnormalities detected in a survey of mentally backward individuals in Northern Ireland. Arch Dis Child 1962;37:505—513.
2. Gerritsen T, Vaughan JG, Waisman HA. The identification of homocysteine in the urine. Biochem Biophys Res Commun 1962;9:493.
3. Gerritsen T, Waisman HA. Homocystinuria, an error in the metabolism of methionine. Pediatrics 1964;33:413—420.
4. Mudd SH, Finkelstein JD, Irreverre F, Laster L. Homocystinuria: an enzymatic defect. Science 1964;143:1443—1445.
5. Mudd SH, Levy HL, Skovby F. Disorders of transsulfuration. In: Scriver CR, Beaudet AL, Sly WS, Valle D (eds) The Metabolic Basis for Inherited Diseases. New York: McGraw-Hill, 1989; 693—734.
6. McCully KS. Vascular pathology of homocysteinemia: implications for the pathogenesis of arteriosclerosis. Am J Pathol 1969;56:111—128.
7. McCully KS, Wilson RB. Homocysteine theory of arteriosclerosis. Atherosclerosis 1975;22: 215—227.
8. Graham I, Meleady R. Heart attacks and homocysteine. Br Med J 1996;313:1419—1420.
9. Gallagher PM, Meleady R, Shields DC, Tan KS, McMaster D, Rozen R, Evans A, Graham IM, Whitehead AS. Homocysteine and risk of premature coronary heart disease. Evidence for a common gene mutation. Circulation 1996;94:2154—2158.
10. Boushey CJ, Beresford SAA, Omenn GS, Motulsky AG. A quantitative assessment of plasma homocysteine as a risk factor for vascular disease: probable benefits of increasing folic acid intake. JAMA 1995;274:1049—1057.
11. Graham IM, Daly LE, Refsum HM, Robinson K, Brattstrom LE, Ueland PM, Palma-Reis RJ,

Boers GHJ, Sheahan RG, Israelsson B, Uiterwaal CS, Meleady R, McMaster D, Verhoef P, Witteman J, Rubba P, Bellet H, Wautrecht JC, de Valk HW, Sales Luis AC, Parrot-Roulaud FM, Tan KS, Higgins I, Garcon D, Medrano MJ, Candito M, Evans AE, Andria G. Plasma homocysteine as a risk factor for vascular disease. The European Concerted Action Project. JAMA 1997;277:1775—1781.
12. Ueland PM, Refsum H, Brattstrom L. Plasma homocysteine and cardiovascular disease. In: Francis RB Jr (ed) Atherosclerotic Cardiovascular Disease, Hemostasis and Endothelial Function. New York: Marcel Dekker Inc; 1992;183—236.
13. Stamler JS, Osborne JA, Jaraki O, Rabbani LE, Mullins M, Singel D et al. Adverse vascular effects of homocysteine are modulated by endothelium-derived relaxing factor and related oxides of nitrogen. J Clin Invest 1993;91:303—318.

Atherosclerosis XI.
B. Jacotot, D. Mathé and J.-C. Fruchart, editors.

Advances in cardiovascular risk prediction: new biochemical and genetic markers

Jose M. Ordovas[1], L. Adrienne Cupples[2], Peter W.F. Wilson[3], Carlos Lahoz[1], Daniel Levy[3], James D. Otvos[4], Judith R. McNamara[1], Eric Gagne[5], Michael Hayden[5] and Ernst J. Schaefer[1]

[1]*Lipid Metabolism Laboratory, JM-USDA-HNRCA at Tufts University;* [2]*Department of Epidemiology and Biostatistics, Boston University School of Public Health, Boston, Massachussetts;* [3]*Framingham Heart Study, Framingham, Massachusetts;* [4]*Department of Biochemistry, North Carolina State University, Raleigh, North Carolina, USA; and* [5]*Department of Human Genetics, University of British Columbia, Vancouver, Canada*

Abstract. In clinical practice it is well-accepted that total plasma cholesterol is not the best indicator of a patient's risk of coronary heart disease (CHD). Furthermore, study of the established risk factors of high levels of low-density lipoprotein cholesterol (LDL-C) and low levels of high-density lipoprotein cholesterol (HDL-C) reveals a considerable overlap between CHD cases and controls. In this report, we present some preliminary results showing that lipoprotein remnants determined using a novel immunochemical technique can potentially improve CHD risk assessment. Moreover, we have shown that nuclear magnetic resonance spectroscopy could be used to examine the complexity of lipoprotein subclasses and to determine their precise value as CHD risk predictors. This technique allows for high sample throughput and automation; however, this instrumentation is not readily available to small laboratories. Regarding the use of genetic markers as CHD risk predictors, it is becoming evident that the apoE gene locus is a major determinant of CHD risk in the population. Moreover, common mutations at the LPL gene locus exert a significant effect on triglyceride and HDL-C levels.

Introduction

Determination of plasma cholesterol levels and their distribution among low-density (LDL) and high-density lipoproteins (HDL) have been used to identify subjects at risk for coronary heart disease (CHD); however, it is well-known that those measures have a significant overlap between CHD cases and controls [1]. Moreover, normal ranges for lipid and lipoprotein-related variables are based on fasting levels, and they might not reflect the postprandial lipid metabolism, the most common state in affluent societies. These postprandial lipid and lipoprotein levels could be highly informative in terms of CHD risk assessment [2]. However, the complexity and cost of measuring lipoprotein levels during the postprandial state have impaired the use of this information in the clinical routine. Therefore, there has been a continuous search for new markers that could increase our precision in the individual prediction of CHD risk.

Besides the search for new biochemical risk markers, we have seen dramatic improvements in molecular biology techniques, to the point that these techniques are now within the capacity of the clinical laboratory. Once adequate genetic markers are defined, we hope to be able to achieve a better prediction of CHD risk long before biochemical and clinical manifestations are present in the individual.

In addition to their possible use as CHD risk predictors, genetic markers can be used to identify responsiveness to dietary and pharmacological therapies [3—6]. In the future, this approach may allow the efficacy of hypocholesterolemic therapies to be maximized through designing an optimal approach for each subject.

In this work, we present some examples of biochemical and genetic markers currently being applied to the Framingham Heart Study. The purpose of this work is to determine whether any of these variables has an independent contribution to risk prediction, above and beyond that available from the traditional lipid-related CHD risk factors.

Biochemical factors

Lipoprotein remnants

Epidemiological studies have demonstrated a significant direct association between elevated plasma-triglyceride levels and CHD risk [7,8]. However, the statistical significance of these findings usually disappears in multivariate analysis after addition of HDL-C levels to the prediction model.

Following their intestinal synthesis, chylomicrons experience a fast lipolysis due to the action of lipoprotein lipase (LPL). During this process, triglyceride-rich lipoproteins (TRL) lose most triglycerides as well as C apolipoproteins. In addition, they become relatively enriched in cholesterol esters and acquire apolipoprotein E. These processes are mediated in part by the cholesteryl ester transport protein (CETP). These particles are known as chylomicron remnants and contain as major proteins apoB-48 and apoE. The final catabolism of these particles depends on their removal by the liver via receptors that recognize the apoE on these particles. There is growing evidence to suggest that these chylomicron remnants are atherogenic particles.

Another class of TRL is represented by the very low density lipoproteins (VLDL) synthesized in the liver. The processing of these particles is similar to that previously described for chylomicrons; however, unlike the particles of intestinal origin, VLDL particles have apoB-100 instead of apoB-48. Moreover, VLDL remnants have alternative catabolic pathways. They may be directly catabolized by the liver, or they may experience additional processing in the blood to generate intermediate-density lipoproteins (IDL) and finally LDL. All these intermediate particles, as well as their final product (LDL), are considered as atherogenic lipoproteins.

The isolation and measurement of remnant lipoproteins are carried out using techniques that are complex and beyond the capacity of the clinical laboratories. This difficulty is primarily due to the fact that both remnant and nascent lipoproteins share a large number of physical and chemical characteristics, including density and size as well as lipid and protein composition. Thus, there has always been a technical problem to differentiate nascent TRLs, probably nonatherogenic, from the remnants, possibly atherogenic. It is well-known that there is a dramatic interindividual variability in the levels and half-lives of these particles in plasma. This variability is often not well-reflected by the plasma lipid measurements carried out during the fasting state.

Recently, Nakajima et al. [9,10] have developed an immunological method that selectively isolates a subpopulation of particles with similar characteristics to those expected in lipoprotein remnants. The particles isolated using this approach are known in the literature as remnant-like particles (RLP). This method is based in the capture of particles containing apoA-I (mainly HDL) using a monoclonal antibody against human apoA-I, and most of the particles containing apoB (LDL and nascent chylomicrons and VLDL) using a monoclonal antibody against apoB. This antibody does not recognize apoB on those TRLs that are partially hydrolyzed and enriched on apoE. Incubation of plasma or serum with these agarose-immobilized antibodies results in a supernatant containing only remnant lipoproteins. Cholesterol and triglyceride concentrations can then be measured using conventional enzymatic methods. The reagents needed for this assay can be obtained from Otsuka America Pharmaceutical (Rockville, MD).

In order to determine normal levels of RLP in the general population, as well as gender and age effects, we are currently applying this assay to the Framingham Heart Study. Our final objective is to determine the clinical utility of this assay in CHD prediction. Our preliminary data in a population sample consisting of 1,607 men and 1,531 women indicate the following:

1. Men have RLP-C and RLP-TG levels that are significantly higher than those measured in women (23.9 and 26.1%, respectively).
2. RLP-C and RLP-TG levels change with age following profiles similar to those observed in this population for total plasma triglycerides. In brief, for men there is an increase with age until 50 years of age, followed by a decline. For women, the maximum levels are reached about 5 years later, and the decrease thereafter is less pronounced than in men.
3. When RLP-C and RLP-TG levels were compared among subjects with clinical evidence of CHD and those without any clinical manifestation, we observed that these variables are significantly elevated in cases over controls and the differences remain statistically significant after adjusting for other CHD risk factors.

Measurement of lipoprotein subclass profiles by nuclear magnetic resonance spectroscopy

In recent years, there has been a growing interest in the value of the different subfractions within the major lipoprotein families (VLDL, LDL and HDL) as mar-

428

kers of CHD risk. Most of the research has concentrated around the different LDL subpopulations. These particles have been classified into two major groups: small dense LDL and large buoyant LDL. The first group has been identified as the more atherogenic fraction [11−13]. So far, the methodology used to determine these subfractions has relied on their electrophoretic separation using gels that are relatively difficult to prepare and to standardize. It is not apparent in the foreseeable future that this technique will become routine in the clinical laboratory. We describe below some preliminary results using an alternative technique that allows the simultaneous separation and measurement of up to 15 different lipoprotein subfractions (6 VLDL, 4 LDL and 5 HDL) using nuclear magnetic resonance (NMR) [14,15].

One of the major advantages of NMR is that no previous treatment of the sample is required, thus decreasing the possibility of introducing artifacts from the physical or chemical treatments used by the most common separation methods (ultracentrifugation, electrophoresis, precipitation, etc.). This methodology is also highly efficient in terms of sample (only 0.5 ml is required), time (1 min per sample), and personnel (this technique can be highly automated). Moreover, this technique allows the quantitative measurement of plasma lipids and their distribution among the different subclasses.

Our preliminary results from applying this technique to the Framingham study demonstrate a high correlation between the concentrations of LDL-C and HDL-C determined by the classical methods and by NMR. Specifically, the correlation between LDL-C calculated using Friedewald equation and those obtained by NMR in 3,455 subjects is 0.850, whereas the correlation between HDL-C obtained after precipitation and that measured by NMR was 0.917, both being highly significant ($p < 0.0001$). We are currently exploring the usefulness of the different lipoprotein subfractions as independent CHD risk factors.

The instrumentation required to carry out these measurements is not usually available to the small laboratory; however, due to minimum needs for sample manipulation and the short assay time, it will be possible to carry out these assays in central laboratories able to process several thousands of samples per day in a totally automated manner.

Genetic factors

Apolipoprotein E gene

Apolipoprotein (apo) E has been the subject of increased interest since its discovery in the 70s. This has been the result of the association between its different isoforms with plasma lipid levels [16−18] as well as with CHD risk [19]. More recently genetic variability at this locus has also been associated with the risk of neurological disorders [20,21].

The apoE gene is located on the long arm of chromosome 19 close to the genes for the apolipoproteins CI, CIV and CII. This locus is highly polymorphic, with three common alleles and multiple rare mutations. The frequencies of the common alleles are on average, 0.07 for the E2, 0.83 for the E3 and 0.10 for the E4 alleles. However, these frequencies vary significantly among different ethnic groups.

This common heterogeneity is due to amino acid changes at residues 112 and 158. In the E2 allele, these amino acids are Cys/Cys; in the E3, Cys/Arg; and in the E4, Arg/Arg. Resulting from these changes, the protein has different affinity for the hepatic receptors (E2), or the lipoprotein particles (E4).

Population studies indicate that subjects with the apoE2 allele have lower LDL cholesterol levels than subjects with apoE3/3, while those with the apoE4 allele have higher levels. Moreover, the apoE2/2 phenotype has been associated with the expression of type III hyperlipidemia. With regard to CHD risk, we have shown that the E4 allele is associated with increased CHD risk [19], and these results are in agreement with a recent meta-analysis [22]. Moreover, we are currently analyzing 20-year follow-up data on the CVD risk associated with the presence of the apoE2 and apoE4 allele. Our data suggest that in men both the apoE2 and the apoE4 alleles are associated with increased risk. In the case of the apoE2, this is in part due to its association with higher triglycerides and delayed postprandial response, whereas for the E4 allele, the higher risk is partially mediated by increased LDL-C levels. In women, only the apoE4 allele was associated with increased risk. It is important to indicate that in women the apoE2 allele is not associated with the elevated triglyceride levels observed in men.

Our data suggest that the genetic variation at the apoE locus is one of the most important genetic determinants of CHD risk, and they account for a population attributable risk that is 7—14 times higher than that observed for the LDL receptor gene locus, the major gene for familial hypercholesterolemia.

Lipoprotein lipase

The importance of the enzyme lipoprotein lipase (LPL) in the development of dyslipidemia and atherosclerosis is clearly accepted. Common mutations in the LPL gene have been shown to be associated with lipid levels, usually triglycerides. Moreover, a large number of mutations have been associated with total elimination of the LPL activity; however, these mutations are present in a frequency less than 1% in the general population, and their overall impact is very limited. Other mutations such as the Asp9Asn and the Asn291Ser are more common with an allele frequency ranging from 3 to 5%. We have found these mutations to be associated with elevated triglycerides and reduced HDL-C levels. Moreover, these effects appear to be more marked in men than in women. These results are in agreement with those reported in European populations [23—25]. On the other hand, the Ser447Ter mutation has an allele frequency around 20% and it has been associated with a more protective lipoprotein profile, namely higher HDL-C and lower triglyceride levels [26]. In our population, a trend was

430

observed with both the Asp9Asn and Asn291Ser being associated with increased risk, whereas the Ser447Ter was associated with reduced CHD risk.

Acknowledgements

This work was supported by grants HL54776 and HL35243 and contract HV-83-03 from the National Institutes of Health and contract 53-K06-5-10 from the US Department of Agriculture Research Service.

References

1. Genest J Jr, McNamara JR, Ordovas JM, Jenner JL, Silberman SR, Anderson KM et al. Lipoprotein cholesterol, apolipoprotein A-I and B and lipoprotein (a) abnormalities in men with premature coronary artery disease. J Am Coll Cardiol 1992;19:792—802.
2. Zilversmit DB. Atherogenic nature of triglycerides, postprandial lipidemia, and triglyceride-rich remnant lipoproteins. Clin Chem 1995;41:153—158.
3. Mata P, Ordovas JM, Lopez-Miranda J, Lichtenstein AH, Clevidence B, Judd JT et al. ApoA-IV phenotype affects diet-induced plasma LDL cholesterol lowering. Arterioscl Thromb 1994;14:884—891.
4. Lopez-Miranda J, Ordovas JM, Espino A, Marin C, Salas J, Lopez-Segura F et al. Influence of mutation in human apolipoprotein A-1 gene promoter on plasma LDL cholesterol response to dietary fat. Lancet 1994;343:1246—1249.
5. Lopez-Miranda J, Ordovas JM, Mata P, Lichtenstein AH, Clevidence B, Judd JT et al. Effect of apolipoprotein E phenotype on diet-induced lowering of plasma low density lipoprotein cholesterol. J Lipid Res 1994;35:1965—1975.
6. Ordovas JM, Lopez-Miranda J, Perez-Jimenez F, Rodriguez CR, Park J, Cole T et al. Effect of apolipoprotein E and A-IV phenotypes on the low-density lipoprotein response to HMG-CoA reductase inhibitor therapy. Atherosclerosis 1995;113:157—166.
7. Austin MA. Plasma triglyceride and coronary heart disease. Arteriosclerosis 1991;11:2—14.
8. Assmann G, Schulte H, Von Eckardstein A. Hypertriglyceridemia and elevated lipoprotein(a) are risk factors for major coronary events in middle-aged men. Am J Cardiol 1996;77:1179—1184.
9. Nakajima K, Saito T, Tamura A, Suzuki M, Nakano T, Adachi M et al. Cholesterol in remnant-like lipoproteins in human serum using monoclonal anti apo B-100 and anti apo A-I immunoaffinity mixed gels. Clin Chim Acta 1993;223:53—71.
10. Nakajima K, Okazaki M, Tanaka A, Pullinger CR, Wang T, Nakano T et al. Separation and determination of remnant-like particles in human serum using monoclonal antibodies to apo B-100 and apo A-I. J Clin Ligand Assay 1996;19:177—183.
11. Campos H, Genest JJ Jr, Blijlevens E, McNamara JR, Jenner JL, Ordovas JM et al. Low-density lipoprotein particle size and coronary artery disease. Arterioscler Thromb 1992;12:187—195.
12. Austin MA, Hokanson JE. Epidemiology of triglycerides, small dense low-density lipoprotein, and lipoprotein(a) as risk factors for coronary heart disease. Med Clin North Am 1994;78:99—115.
13. Austin MA. Genetic and environmental influences on LDL subclass phenotypes. Clin Genet 1994;46:64—70.
14. Otvos JD, Jeyarajah EJ, Bennett DW, Krauss RM. Development of a proton nuclear magnetic resonance spectroscopic method for determining plasma lipoprotein concentrations and subspecies distributions from a single, rapid measurement. Clin Chem 1992;38:1632—1638.
15. Otvos J, Jeyarajah E, Bennett D. A spectroscopic approach to lipoprotein subclass analysis. J Clin Ligand Assay 1996;19:184—189.

16. Davignon J, Gregg RE, Sing CF. Apolipoprotein E polymorphism and atherosclerosis. Arteriosclerosis 1988;8:1—21.
17. Ehnholm C, Lukka M, Kuusi Y, Nikkila E, Utermann G. Apolipoprotein E polymorphism in the Finnish population: gene frequencies and relation to lipoprotein concentrations. J Lipid Res 1986;27:227—235.
18. Schaefer EJ, Lamon-Fava S, Johnson S, Ordovas JM, Schaefer MM, Castelli WP et al. Effects of gender and menopausal status on the association of apolipoprotein E phenotype with plasma lipoprotein levels. Results from the Framingham offspring study. Arterioscl Thromb 1994;14: 1105—1113.
19. Wilson PWF, Myers RH, Larson MG, Ordovas JM, Wolf PA, Schaefer EJ. Apolipoprotein E alleles, dyslipidemia, and coronary heart disease: the Framingham offspring study. JAMA 1994;272:1666—1671.
20. Myers RH, Schaefer EJ, Wilson PWF, D'Agostino RB, Bachman DL, Ordovas JM et al. Apolipoprotein E allele4 is associated with dementia in the Framingham study. In: Iqbal K, Mortimer JA, Winblsnd B, Wisniewski HM (eds) Research Advances in Alzheimer's Disease and Related Disorders. New York: John Wiley & Sons Ltd., 1995;64—69.
21. Myers RH, Schaefer EJ, Wilson PWF, D'Agostino R, Ordovas JM, Espino A et al. Apolipoprotein E4 association with dementia in a population-based study: the Framingham study. Neurology 1996;46:673—677.
22. Wilson PWF, Schaefer EJ, Larson M, Ordovas JM. Apolipoprotein E polymorphism and coronary heart disease: a meta-analysis. Arterioscl Thromb Vasc Biol 1996;16:1250—1255.
23. Mailly F, Fisher RM, Nicaud V, Luong LA, Evans AE, Marques-Vidal P et al. Association between the LPL-D9N mutation in the lipoprotein lipase gene and plasma lipid traits in myocardial infarction survivors from the ECTIM study. Atherosclerosis 1996;122:21—28.
24. De Bruin TWA, Mailly F, Van Barlingen HHJJ, Fisher R, Cabezas MC, Talmud P et al. Lipoprotein lipase gene mutations D9N and N291S in four pedigrees with familial combined hyperlipidaemia. Eur J Clin Invest 1996;26:631—639.
25. Jukema JW, Van Boven AJ, Groenemeijer B, Zwinderman AH, Reiber JHC, Bruschke AVG et al. The Asp_9 Asn mutation in the lipoprotein lipase gene is associated with increased progression of coronary atherosclerosis. Circulation 1996;94:1913—1918.
26. Kuivenhoven JA, Groenemeyer BE, Boer JMA, Reymer PWA, Berghuis R, Bruin T et al. Ser_{447}-stop mutation in lipoprotein lipase is associated with elevated HDL cholesterol levels in normolipidemic males. Arterioscl Thromb Vasc Biol 1997;17:595—599.

Molecular genetics of atherosclerosis

Structure and function of alleles in the 3′ end region of human apoB gene

B.S. Chen[1], Z.M. Guo[1], He Ping[1], Ye Ping[1], C. Buresi[2] and G. Roizes[2]

[1]*Institute of Basic Medical Science, CAMS, PUMC, Beijing, China; and* [2]*CNRS-INSERM, Montpellier, France*

Abstract. The main aim of this paper was to study the structure of alleles in the 3′ end of the apoB gene in Han, Mongolian and Tibetan populations in China as well as the role of alleles in the regulation of gene expression. From 303 Chinese individuals, 16 alleles with different sizes have been characterized. The distribution of alleles had two modes: one on allele34 (HVE34) and one on allele HVE48, with all the alleles varying from HVE22 to HVE52. In 258 alleles after digestion with Ssp1 and 4–12% acrylamide gel electrophoresis, the fragments of 266bp, 91bp, 61bp and 39bp were detected in almost all of the alleles. Some rare bands (196bp, 150bp, 55bp and 42bp) were observed in several samples as well. The assays in cultured cells suggested that alleles HVE30 and HVE36 were down-regulating gene expressions compared with control plasmids. In contrast, the plasmids containing HVE42 and HVE44 strongly stimulated the expression of pGL2-control and pGL2-promoter vectors in mammalian cells. These results open the possibility that the minisatellite in the 3′ end of apoB gene could control the expression of the gene itself.

Keywords: allele, apolipoprotein B gene, distribution, function, minisatellite, structure.

Variable number of tandem repeats (VNTR) loci, as highly polymorphic genetic markers, are powerful tools for constructing high-resolution genetic maps [1,2], as well as forensic and paternity identification [3,4]. The apoB minisatellite is located close to the 3′ end of the apoB gene and it consists of a series of tandemly repeated short A+T-rich DNA sequences exhibited by a large number of various sized alleles. C. Buresi et al. [5] have analyzed the internal structure of the apoB gene and confirmed the existence of four domains in the 3′ region of the apoB gene. The distributions of the allele frequencies are very different among White, Black and Asian populations [6–8]. Some laboratories [9,10] studied apoB matrix attachment regions (MACS) effects on the expression of transiently and stably transfected reporter genes in rat and human hepatoma cells [11]. In this paper, we reported the results of the distribution and the frequencies of alleles in the 3′ end of apoB gene as well as the structure and function of the various sized alleles.

Address for correspondence: Chen Bao-Sheng, Institute of Basic Medical Sciences, Chinese Academy of Medical Sciences, 5 Dong Dan San Tiao, 100005 Beijing, China. Tel.: +86-10-65296413. Fax: +86-10-65240529.

Materials and Methods

Blood samples of Hans, Mongolians and Tibetans were collected from Beijing City, Intermongolia and Qing Hai Provinces, respectively. DNA were obtained from leukocytes by phenol-chloroform extraction and ethanol precipitation. PCR were carried out in a 50 μl volume containing 50 ng of genomic DNA as a template. The Ssp1-digested products were loaded on a gradient acrylamids gel and run for 3 h. For the study of gene expression, the alleles of HVE22, HVE24, HVE26, HVE28, HVE30, HVE32, HVE34, HVE36, HVE38, HVE40, HVE42, HVE44, HVE46, HVE48 and HVE50 were cloned into the pGL2-control and pGL2-promoter plasmids. The constructs were tested in cultured HepG2 and HeLa cells using transient assays.

Results and Discussion

The alleles distribution and frequencies of the apoB gene 3′ minisatellite in Han, Mongolian and Tibetan Nationalities of China were analyzed. Sixteen alleles with different repeat numbers have been characterized. The distribution of alleles had two modes: one on allele 34 (hypervariable element, HVE34) and one on allele HVE48, with all of the alleles varying from HVE22 to HVE52. Allele HVE34 was the most common (58.4%), followed by allele HVE36 and HVE32 (13.8 and 10.5%, respectively). The structural analysis of alleles in the 3′ end region of the apoB gene was carried out by Ssp1 digestion. In the present study, 258 PCR products including 122, 64 and 72 alleles from Han, Mongolian and Tibetan nationalities, respectively, were digested with Ssp1 and running 4–12% acrylamide gel electrophoresis. We detected the fragments of 266bp, 91bp, 61bp and 39bp in almost all of the samples, otherwise some rare fragments, e.g., 296bp, 155bp and 150bp, were also detected in less samples. From this result, it

```
5' CCCCCTGTGGAGCGTTTAAAATATAGGTCCTGAAGTAATTGTGTTTTT

ATAATTAAATATTTT      ATAATTAAATATTTT      ATAATTAAAATATTT
       X                    X                    Y
ATAATTAAATATTTT      ATAATTAAAATATTT      ATAATTACATATTTT
       X                    Y                   Xii
ATAATTAAAATGTTT      ATAATTACATATTTT      ATAATTAAAATGTTT
      Yii                  Xii                  Yii
ATAATTACATATTTT      ATAATTACATATTTT      ATAAAGTATTT
      Xii                  Xii                 Yiii
ATAATTACATATTTT      ATAATTAAAGTATTT      ATAATTACATATTTT
      Xii                   Yi                  Xii
ATAATTAAAATATTT      ATAATTACATATTTT      ATAATTCAATATTTT
       Yi                  Xii                  Xi

ATAAAGTTAAAAAGACGAGGAAAATTTTTTAGGGGGTGCGAGGTTTTTTAGGG  3'
```

Sequence: X XY----(Xii Yii)2 Xii Xii Yiii (Xii Yi)2 Xii Xi---

Fig. 1. Nucleotide sequence of apoB gene VNTR allele 18.

HVE18	X XY (XY)--------- (XiiYii)2 Xii Xii Yiii (Xii Yi)2 Xii Xi
HVE20	XY X (XY)2 (X Yii)2 ------------ Xii Xii Yiii (Xii Yi) 2 Xii Xi
HVE30	XY X (XY)5 (X Yii) (Xii Yii)3 Xii Xii Yiii (Xii Yi) 2 Xii Xi
HVE32	XY X (XY)5 (X Yii)2 (Xii Yii)3 Xii Xii Yiii (Xii Yi) 2 Xii Xi
HVE34	XY X (XY)5 (X Yii)2 (Xii Yii)4 Xii Xii Yiii (Xii Yi) 2 Xii Xi
HVE36	XY X (XY)6 (X Yii) (Xii Yii)5 Xii Xii Yiii (Xii Yi) 2 Xii Xi
HVE38	XY X (XY)8 (X Yii) (Xii Yii)4 Xii Xii Yiii (Xii Yi) 2 Xii Xi
HVE40	XY X (XY)7 (X Yii) (Xii Yii)5 Xii Xii Yiii (Xii Yi) 2 Xii Xi
HVE42	XY X (XY)9 (X Yii) (Xii Yii)5 Xii Xii Yiii (Xii Yi) 2 Xii Xi
HVE44	XY X (XY)9 (X Yii) (Xii Yii)6 Xii Xii Yiii (Xii Yi) 2 Xii Xi
HVE48	XY X (XY)15 (XYii) (Xii Yii)2 Xii Xii Yiii (Xii Yi) 2 Xii Xi

Fig. 2. Sequence of apoB gene 3′ VNTR alleles.

suggested clearly that the nonvarying internal structure of the allele was detected in this group of Chinese populations as found in the other populations (Figs. 1 and 2).

The function of alleles in 3′ end minisatellite of human apoB gene was studied in cultured cells with transient expressive assay. The pGL2 with luciferase reporter vectors are designed to support rapid and convenient analysis of promoter and enhancer sequences using luciferase as the genetic reporter. Two vectors are available, containing different combinations of SV40 promoter and enhancer elements. We inserted alleles (HVE22 to HVE50) into the pGL2-control vectors and pGL2-promoter vectors at the 3′ end, respectively, after HepG2 and HeLa cells were transfected. The tested results indicated that if the inserted fragments were cloned into the pGL2-control vectors, the small alleles (including HVE22,

Table 1. The role of apoB gene 3′ minisatellite in regulation of HepG2 cells in expression.

Ratio of expression activity in pGL2-control plasmids (RLU)[a]

Without HVE	1.00	Without HVE	1.00
With HVE22	0.59	With HVE42	1.63
With HVE24	0.52	With HVE44	2.02
With HVE26	0.50	With HVE46	1.91
With HVE28	0.61	With HVE48	1.86
With HVE30	0.58	With HVE50	1.80

[a]RLU expresses the relative light unit (RLU) of the luciferase activity in the system of epG2 and HeLa cells. The ratio of the expression activity is the ratio of the expression activity between the plasmids with insertions (HVE) and the plasmids without insertions (HVE). The expression activity of the plasmids without insertions is defined as 1.00. If the value of RLU is bigger than 1.00, it means that the role of the insertion elevated the expression activity of HepG2 or HeLa cells. If the value of RLU is less than 1.00, it means that the role of the insertions decreased the expression activity of HepG2 or HeLa cells in vitro.

Table 2. The role of apoB gene 3′ minisatellite in regulation of HepG2 cells expression.

Ratio of expression activity in pGL2-promoter plasmids (RLU)[a]

Without HVE	1.00	Without HVE	1.00
With HVE 22	0.53	With HVE 42	1.02
With HVE 24	0.61	With HVE 44	1.52
With HVE 26	0.73	With HVE 46	1.89
With HVE 28	0.49	With HVE 48	1.77
With HVE 30	0.42	With HVE 50	1.82

[a]For table note see Table 1.

HVE24, HVE26, HVE28, HVE30, HVE32, HVE34 and HVE36) decreased the expression of the luciferase reporter activity. In comparison, the large alleles (including HVE44, HVE46, HVE48 and HVE50) obviously elevated the expressive activity of the luciferase reporter.

The same results were obtained using pGL2-promoter vectors containing alleles of the same size. In the system of HeLa cells, the expressive activity of pGL2-control and pGL2-promoter vectors containing the described alleles was similar to that of HepG2 cells.. From the results, we found that the alleles in the 3′ end minisatellite of human apoB gene could control the expression of the gene itself. One result of "the ECTIM" indicated that the allele HVE48 increased the mass of the patient body with hypercholesterolemia. Our results demonstrated further that the bigger alleles of apoB 3′ end minisatellite could enhance the expression of apoB gene itself in the patients with the high level of cholesterol in the blood. Otherwise the small alleles could have the negative role in the expression of the apoB gene. A more direct demonstration has been given by gene constructs containing several copies of the consensus A+T-rich sequence found in most of the MAR studied so far. This A+T-rich sequence was shown to strongly stimulate the expression of an integrated gene construct containing the SV-40 promoter and the luciferase reporter gene. However, some results indicated that A+T-rich MAR sequences do not have an insulating effect (Tables 1 and 2).

Acknowledgements

This work was supported by the grants from CNRS ERS115, France and from Natural Sciences Foundation of China (39270164), and from National Pan Deng Ji Hua of Beijing, China.

References

1. Weissenbach et al. A second-generation linkage map of the human genome. Nature 1992; 359:794–801.
2. Buetow KH et al. Integrated human gnome-wide maps constructed using the CHEF reference

panel. Nature Genet 1994;6:391—396.

3. Jeffreys AJ et al. Hypervariable "minisatellite" region in human DNA. Nature 1985;314:67—73.

4. Chakraborty R et al. The utility of DNA typing in forensic work. Science 1991;254:1735—1739.

5. Buresi C et al. Structural analysis of the minisatellite present at the 3' end of the human apolipo-protein B gene: new definition of the alleles and evolutionary implications. Human Mol 1996; 5:61—68.

6. Balazs IN et al. Human population genetic studies using hypervariable Loci. I. Analysis of Assamese, Australian, Cambodian, Caucasian, Chinese and Melanesian populations. Genetics 1992;131:191—198.

7. Deka R et al. Characteristic of polymorphism at a VNTR locus 3' to the apolipoprotein B gene in five human populations. Am J Hum Genet 1992;51:1325—1333.

8. Wall WJ et al. Variation of short tandem repeats within and between populations. Hum Mol Genet 1993;2:1023—1029.

9. Levy-Wilson B, Fortier C. The limits of the DNase 1-sensitive domain of the apolipoprotein B Gene coincide with the locations of chromosomal anchorage loops and define the 5' and 3' boundaries of the Gene. JBC 1989;264:21196—21204.

10. Attal J et al. The effect of matrix attached regions (MAR) 3' and specialized chromatin structure (SCS) on the expression of gene constructs in cultured cells and in transgene mice. Molec Biol Reports 1996;22(1):37—46.

11. Kalos M et al. Position-independence transgene expression mediated by boundary elements from the apolipoprotein B chromatin domain. Molec Cell Biol 1995;15:198—207.

A transracial analysis of common genetic variants that relate to coronary artery disease

Q. Zhang[1], Y. Liu[2], B.W. Liu[2], P. Fan[2], J. Cavanna[1] and D.J. Galton[1]

[1]*Department of Metabolism and Genetics, St Bartholomew's Hospital, London, UK; and* [2]*Apolipoprotein Research Unit, West China University of Medical Sciences, Chengdu, China*

Abstract. *Background.* The large ethnic differences in prevalence of coronary artery disease both between and within Chinese and European populations may relate to genetic and environmental differences. Therefore, to assess possible genetic factors we have studied the frequencies of disease-related variants of genes involved in lipid transport in Chinese, North and South European subjects. The loci studied include lipoprotein lipase (Asp9Asn, Asn291Ser, Ser447Ter and Thr361Thr); apolipoprotein AI (restriction sites at Msp-1, Xmn-1, and Pst-1); and apolipoprotein CIII (G3175C). All these variants have been shown in previous published literature to relate to either dyslipidaemia and/or premature coronary heart disease in Caucasians.

Results. Two disease-related genetic variants in Europeans (Asp9Asn and Asn291Ser) were not found in the Chinese subjects. The apo CIII G3175C variant was found more frequently in the upper tertile distributions for apolipoprotein CIII, apolipoprotein E and plasma triglyceride/HDL ratios ($p < 0.05$). The rare allele of the apo AI Msp-1 restriction site polymorphic variant was also found more frequently in the upper tertiles for apo CIII, apo E and plasma triglyceride/HDL ratios ($p < 0.04$).

Conclusion. Genetic differences between Chinese and Europeans may have an effect on the prevalence of coronary artery risk factors involved in lipid transport; therefore a further extended study is warranted.

Keywords: apolipoproteins, China, coronary artery disease, Europe, genetic variants, lipoprotein lipase, plasma lipids.

Introduction

The dyslipidaemic syndrome of raised plasma triglycerides and low HDL occurs commonly in European populations at frequencies of greater than 5% and is a well-established risk factor for premature coronary heart disease [1–3]. Several common genetic variants have been detected that associate with this dyslipidaemia and in some cases may constitute genetic determinants for the condition. For example a common G3175C transversion that is transcribed but not translated in exon 4 of the apolipoprotein CIII gene on chromosome 11p21 has been found in association [4,5] and pedigree studies [6] to link with dyslipidaemia; two apo-CIII promoter mutations at position C-482T and T-455C have also

---

Address for correspondence: Prof D. Galton, Department of Medicine, St. Bartholomew's Hospital, West Smithfield, London EC1A 7BE, UK. Tel.: +44-171-982-6018. Fax: +44-171-982-6064. E-mail: D.J.Galton@mds.qmw.ac.uk

been found to associate with hypertriglyceridaemia [7]. In addition, several common mutations in the gene encoding lipoprotein lipase on chromosome 8p have also been found to relate to dyslipidaemia [2,5]. For example, a C1595G transversion that converts serine 447 to a stop codon thereby prematurely truncating the enzyme protein by 2 amino acids has been shown to relate to low levels of plasma triglycerides and elevated levels of HDL in several studies [8,9]. Two other common mutations at lipoprotein lipase, namely Asp9Asn and Asp291Ser, have also been shown to associate with dyslipidaemia [10,11] and in vitro transfection studies show a decreased activity of both mutant enzymes.

There are large ethnic differences between Western Europe and China in the prevalence of coronary artery disease manifesting before the age of 60 years. For example, the UK standardized mortality rates in men aged 35—64 for coronary heart disease is approximately 350/100,000 compared to 30/100,000 in rural China and 60/100,000 in urban China for men aged 35—74 years in 1988 [12]. Part of this difference may be due to differences in the frequencies of environmental risk factors such as diabetes mellitus, hyperlipidaemia, hypertension and smoking habits. But all these cardiovascular risk factors occur commonly in China; diabetes mellitus (NIDDM) 2.5%, hyperlipidaemia 20% and hypertension 11.6% [13—15]. It is, therefore, of great interest to compare frequencies of the common genetic variants of the apo AI-CIII-AIV gene cluster and lipoprotein lipase genes that have been postulated to contribute to the atherogenic dyslipidaemia of raised plasma triglycerides/low HDL in Chinese and European populations to see if genetic factors may show such ethnic differences.

Subjects

Subjects (n = 881) under the age of 65 years were selected randomly from the staff members of Hong Guang Electron Tube Factory and four universities in the Chengdu area. Those with hepatic, renal and thyroid diseases were excluded from the study. The subjects were asked to fast 12—14 h before venous blood was taken. From this survey 69 subjects were identified with fasting plasma triglycerides > 204 mg/dl and selected for further study. None of them were taking medication known to affect levels of plasma lipids and they were considered to have a primary dyslipidaemia. Controls (n = 74) came from the same survey who had fasting plasma triglycerides < 177 mg/dl. The presence of other related diseases (diabetes mellitus, coronary artery disease, etc.) were established by a questionnaire. Full clinical details of the study groups are presented in Table 1.

Methods

Lipoprotein analysis

Total serum cholesterol and triglycerides were measured by the enzymatic method (kits, Zhong Sen Co., Beijing). HDL-C was determined after sodium phos-

Table 1. Clinical features (adjusted for age and BMI) of Chinese subjects with or without hyperlipideamia.

	Hyperlipideamia (n = 69)	Controls (n = 74)	p
Age (years)	54.69 ± 6.83	52.81 ± 8.03	NS[a]
Sex (male + female; No. & %)	64 + 5 (92.8 + 7.2%)	68 + 6 (91.9 + 8.1%)	NS[b]
Weight (kg)	70.32 ± 9.23	62.86 ± 8.67	<0.001[a]
BMI (kg/m^2)	25.42 ± 2.76	22.67 ± 2.76	<0.001[a]
Diabetes mellitus (No. & %)	5 (7.2%)	5 (6.8%)	NS[b]
Hypertension (>130 mmHg;No. & %)	15 (21.7%)	10 (13.5%)	NS[b]
Blood glucose (mg/dl)	101.64 ± 19.30	98.94 ± 30.42	NS
Triglycerides (mg/dl)	440.16 ± 363.16	125.55 ± 29.81	<0.0001
Cholesterol (mg/dl)	227.83 ± 223.80	184.70 ± 34.30	NS
HDL-C (mg/dl)	36.58 ± 9.52	50.58 ± 10.21	<0.0001
ApoAI (mg/dl)	108.05 ± 14.86	117.43 ± 19.85	0.004
ApoCIII (mg/dl)	18.95 ± 10.83	9.13 ± 2.44	<0.0001
ApoE (mgdl)	7.20 ± 5.19	3.97 ± 0.82	<0.0001
TG/HDL	13.54 ± 16.68	2.62 ± 0.91	<0.0001

BMI indicates body mass index. p values were analysed by Oneway ANOVA[a], χ^2 test[b] and analysis of covariance and triglycerides were $\log_{10}$ transformed before analysis.

photungstate/magnesium chloride precipitation of low-density lipoprotein by polyvinyl sulfate. Serum apolipoprotein AI, AII, B100, CII, CIII and E were quantified by the radial-immunodiffusion kits developed by the Apolipoprotein Research Laboratory in West China University of Medical Sciences, China [16].

DNA analysis

DNA was isolated from fresh or frozen EDTA whole blood cells using a Nucleon II Kit (Scotlabs Ltd., UK) and resuspended in TE buffer and stored at −20°C.

Digestion and electrophoresis

Five microliters of digestion mixture containing the manufacturer's recommended restriction buffer and 5 U restriction enzyme were added to the amplification product and incubated at 65°C for 3 h with Taq I for analysis of exon 2 of LPL gene; or incubated at 37°C overnight with HindIII (Gibco BRL) for analysis of the intron 8 RFLP and Mnl I for the Ser447-Ter mutation of exon 9 in the LPL gene; with Msp I for the exon 5 RFLP of hepatic lipase (HL) gene and apo-AI gene; and with Pst I and Xmn I for the apo AI, and with Sst I for apo CIII genes. Subsequently, the samples were electrophoresed in TBE buffer (89 mmol/Tris-borate, 2 mmol/L EDTA pH 8.3) in 2—3% agrose gels at 150 V for 1—1.5 h. DNA was visualized by staining the gels with ethidium bromide (0.5 µg/ml) and transillumination with UV light.

444

Statistical analysis

Genotype distributions between the study groups were analyzed by 2×2 and 3×2 contingency tables and by performing χ^2 analysis. Variations in the biochemical traits with respect to genotypes were analyzed by performing analysis of covariance. Similar comparisons of genotype distribution were undertaken using χ^2 analysis after biochemical traits were divided into tertiles. Analyses were performed using SPSS for Windows 6.1 statistical packages.

Results

The clinical and biochemical characteristics of the Chinese group are presented in Table 1. The hypertriglyceridaemic Chinese group had raised plasma levels of apolipoproteins -B, -CII, -CIII and -E due probably to the increased circulating levels of triglyceride rich lipoproteins compared to Chinese controls. They also had decreased levels of apolipoproteins -AI and -AII and HDL.

Allele frequencies

With regard to allele frequencies of common genetic variants that have been reported in European populations to relate to the hypertriglyceridaemic/low HDL syndrome, the Asn291Ser and Asp9Asn variants of lipoprotein lipase were not detected in the Chinese control group (n = 74). The Serine447Ter variant and the HindIII restriction length polymorphism in intron 8 of the lipase

Table 2. Observed distribution of allele frequencies for the LPL gene and apoAI-CIII gene mutations compared between Chinese and European controls.

Gene	Chinese (n = 74)		European (n = 54)		p
	Allele frequencies				
	Common allele	Rare allele	Common allele	Rare allele	
LPL					
Asp⁹-Asn	1.000 (140)	0.000 (0)	0.991 (107)	0.009 (1)	NS
Asn²⁹¹-Ser	1.000 (140)	0.000 (0)	0.963 (104)	0.037 (4)	<0.03
Ser⁴⁴⁷-Ter	0.893 (125)	0.107 (15)	0.880 (95)	0.120 (13)	NS
LPL-HindIII	0.771 (108)	0.229 (32)	0.704 (76)	0.296 (32)	NS
Thr³⁶¹-Thr (HaeIII)	0.886 (124)	0.114 (16)	0.870 (94)	0.130 (14)	NS
ApoAI					
AI-MspI	0.707 (99)	0.293 (41)	0.889 (96)	0.111 (12)	<0.0006
AI-XmnI	0.714 (100)	0.286 (40)	0.870 (94)	0.130 (14)	<0.004
AI-PstI	0.929 (130)	0.071 (10)	0.954 (103)	0.046 (5)	NS
ApoCIII					
CIII-SstI	0.721 (101)	0.279 (39)	0.880 (95)	0.120 (13)	<0.003

The number of observed alleles are presented in parentheses. Values for Caucasian controls are taken from our previous publication [9].

gene were found at similar frequencies to European groups (Table 2). The two disease-related restriction length polymorphisms of the apo-AI gene (detected with Msp 1 and Xmn 1) were also significantly different in frequencies between Chinese controls and Caucasian control groups; as were the apo-CIII G3175C variants (Table 2).

Disease associations

Apolipoproteins AI/CIII variants
The apolipoprotein AI/CIII variants (the apo AI-Msp1 and apo CIII poly-morphisms) that have shown disease relationships in European studies also appear in the Chinese group (Table 3). Thus the rare apo-CIII variant (G3175C) is found more frequently in the upper tertile for plasma apo CIII and TG/HDL ratios. The apo AI-MspI rare variant is also found more frequently in the upper tertile for plasma TG/HDL ratio. The similar results found with plasma apo-E tertiles probably reflect the increased amounts of apolipoprotein E carried on VLDL in lipaemic plasma. Within the European population the apo CIII variant (G3175C) related to the plasma triglyceride levels (after log transformation) with a p value = 0.05 (ANOVA); and the rare variant was found more frequently in the upper than lower tertiles of the HDL-triglyceride distribution ($p < 0.05$).

Lipoprotein lipase mutations

The frequencies of lipoprotein lipase mutants in Chinese hyperlipidaemic sub-

Table 3. Lipid and lipoprotein tertiles related to apoAI-CIII genotypes.

	Number of subjects represented by genotypes							
	ApoAI-MspI				ApoCIII-SstI			
	M1M2	M1M2	M2M2	p	S1S1	S1S2	S2S2	p
ApoCIII								
Lower tertile (<9.72 mg/dl)	26	17	4	NS	28	16	3	0.05
Higher tertile (>13.90 mg/dl)	25	14	11		25	13	12	
ApoE								
Lower tertile (<3.75 mg/dl)	20	24	6	0.03	20	24	6	0.03
Higher tertile (>5.15 mg/dl)	31	11	8		31	11	8	
TG/HDL								
Lower tertile (<3.06)	23	22	2	0.04	25	20	2	0.05
Higher tertile (>7.08)	25	15	10		25	15	10	

p values were analysed by χ^2 tests (2×2 contingency tables) and Fisher's exact test where appropriate.

Table 4. Observed distribution of allele frequencies for the LPL gene and apoAI-CIII gene mutations compared between Chinese patients and controls.

Gene	Controls (n = 70)		Patients (n = 68)	
	Allele frequencies			
	Common allele	Rare allele	Common allele	Rare allele
LPL				
Asp^9-Asn	1.000 (140)	0.000 (0)	1.000 (136)	0.000 (0)
Ala^{261}-Thr	1.000 (140)	0.000 (0)	0.993 (135)	0.007 (1)
Asn^{291}-Ser	1.000 (140)	0.000 (0)	1.000 (136)	0.000 (0)
Ser^{447}-Ter	0.893 (125)	0.107 (15)	0.926 (126)	0.074 (10)
LPL-HindIII	0.771 (108)	0.229 (32)	0.824 (112)	0.176 (24)
Thr^{361}-Thr (HaeIII)	0.886 (124)	0.114 (16)	0.904 (123)	0.096 (13)
ApoAI				
AI-MspI	0.707 (99)	0.293 (41)	0.647 (88)	0.353 (48)
AI-XmnI	0.714 (100)	0.286 (40)	0.721 (98)	0.279 (38)
AI-PstI	0.929 (130)	0.071 (10)	0.949 (129)	0.051 (7)
ApoCIII				
CIII-SstI	0.721 (101)	0.279 (39)	0.647 (88)	0.353 (48)

The observed alleles are presented in parentheses. Comparisons show no significant difference.

jects are presented in Table 4. The Ala261Thr variant was found more frequently in lipaemic subjects than Chinese controls but did not reach statistical significance, possibly because of small samples. None of the other common variants showed significant differences. The Serine447Ter variant showed a tendency to be found at lower frequencies in the lipaemic subjects. The Serine447Ter was found less frequently in the European subjects with proven coronary artery disease (n = 186) compared to controls (n = 110, p = 0.02).

Discussion

The question whether genetic variants at loci involved in lipid transport could in part account for differences in mortality rates from coronary heart disease between Chinese and European populations has been considered. In support of this hypothesis we have found that two common disease-related mutants of lipoprotein lipase in Caucasian groups do not occur in our Chinese samples. However, the Chinese group is small (n = 143) and a larger study is warranted to substantiate these results. If confirmed, the data may indicate that these mutations are of recent evolutionary origin, or that they have been exposed to positive selection pressures (possibly nutritional) in Caucasian populations. The Asn291Ser mutant [17] is found at increased frequencies in Caucasian male patients with premature atherosclerosis who have low levels of HDL. This variant results in a significant decrease in LPL catalytic activity and in vitro expression studies confirm that this variant is associated with a significant reduction in LPL activity [19]. The Asp9Asn variant [18] lowers lipoprotein lipase expression by about

25—30% and is found at higher frequencies in patients with hypertriglyceridaemia than in healthy controls. Healthy carriers of the mutation also have plasma triglyceride levels 25—30% higher than noncarriers; and survivors of myocardial infarction who were both obese and were carriers were found to have higher plasma triglyceride levels than noncarriers. The fact that these mutations were not observed in a Chinese sample may add weight to the hypothesis that they have an impact on the development of coronary heart disease.

No ethnic differences were found in other reported LPL variants (Ser447Ter, HindIII restriction length polymorphism) and no differences in allelic frequencies were found within the Chinese group (n = 143) between upper and lower tertiles for plasma triglyceride, or HDL. This, however, is a small sample and statistical significance may be lost as a result.

Acknowledgements

This work was supported by grants from the Royal Society (UK) to B.W. Liu; Overseas Research Fellowship to Q. Zhang; Joint Research Board of St. Bartholomew's Hospital to J. Cavanna; and the EU project PL 931211 to D.J. Galton (coordinator).

References

1. Carlson LA, Bottger LE, Ahfeldt PE. Risk factors for myocardial infarction in the Stockholm Prospective Study. Acta Med Scand 1979;206:351—360.
2. Austin MA. Plasma triglyceride as a risk factor for coronary heart disease. The epidemiologic evidence and beyond. Am J Epidemiol 1989;129:249—259.
3. Assmann GA, Gotto AM, Paoletti R. The hypertriglyceridaemias: risk and management. Am J Cardiol 1991;68:1A—42A.
4. Rees A, Stocks J, Shoulders CC, Galton DJ, Baralle FE. DNA polymorphism adjacent to the human apolipoprotein AI gene in relation to hypertriglyceridaemia. Lancet 1983;I:444—447.
5. Rees A, Stocks J, Shoulders CC, Baralle FE, Galton DJ. DNA polymorphism in the apo AI/CIII gene cluster: association with hypertriglyceridaemia. J Clin Invest 1985;76:1090—1095.
6. Wojciechowski AP, Farrall M, Cullen P, Wilson TE, Bayliss JD, Farren B, Griffen BA, Caslake MJ, Packard CJ, Shepherd J, Scott J. Familial combined hyperlipidaemia linked to the apolipoprotein AI-CIII-AIV gene cluster on chromosome 11_q23-_q24. Nature 1991;349:161—164.
7. Dammerman M, Sandkuijl LA, Halaas JL, Chung W, Breslow JL. An apolipoprotein CIII haplotype protective against hypertriglyceridemia specified by promoter and three untranslated region polymorphisms. Proc Natl Acad Sci USA 1995;90:4562—4566.
8. Stocks J, Thorn JA, Galton DJ. Lipoprotein lipase genotypes for a common premature termination codon detected by PCR medicated site-directed mutagenesis. J Lipid Res 1992;33:853—857.
9. Zhang Q, Cavanna J, Winkelmann BR, Shine B, Marz W, Galton DJ. Common genetic variants of lipoprotein lipase that relate to lipid transport in patients with premature coronary artery disease. Clin Genet 1995;48:293—298.
10. Mailly F, Fisher R, Nicaud V. Association between the LPL D9N mutation in the lipoprotein lipase gene and plasma lipid traits in myocardial infarction survivors from the ECTIM study. Atherosclerosis (In press).
11. Ma Y, Ooi TC, Liu M-S, Zhang H et al. Increased frequency of an Asn 291 Ser mutation in the

448

human LPL gene in patients with apo E2 deficiency and hyperlipidaemia including type III hyperlipoprotinaemia. Circulation 1993;88:175—179.

12. Tao S-q. Progress in epidemiology of cardiovascular disease. Chin J Cardiol 1993;21:340—342.
13. Pan XR. A preventive programme for diabetes mellitus in 1995. Chin J Diabet 1993;4:123—129.
14. Wang JL, Fang J, Wu TX. A cross-sectional study of hyperlipidemia of hypertensives (711 cases). Chin J Prevent Chronic Dis 1996;4:6—8.
15. Wu Xg, Duan XF, Giu DF, Hao JS, Tao SC, Fan DJ. Prevalence of hypertension and its trends in Chinese populations. Int J Cardiol 1995;52:39—44.
16. Liu BW. Immunoassays of human plasma apolipoproteins and clinical applications. In: Wang KQ (ed) Lipoproteins and Atherosclerosis. Chengdu: Beijing People's Health Press, 1995; 359—368.
17. Reymer P, Gagne E, Groenemeyer BE, Zhang H, Forsyth IJ, Jansen H, Seidel JC, Kromhout D, Lie KE, Kastelein JJP, Hayden MR. A lipoprotein lipase mutation (Asn 291 Ser) is associated with reduced HDL levels in patients with premature atherosclerosis. Nature Genet 1995;10: 28—34.
18. Mailly F, Olivecroma G, Tugrul Y, Reymer PWA, Bruin T, Seed M, Groenemeyer BF, Asplund-Carlson A, Vallance D, Winder AF, Miller GJ et al. A common variant in the gene for lipoprotein lipase (Asp 9 Asn): functional implications and prevalence in normal and hyperlipidaemic subjects. Arterioscl Thromb Vasc Biol 1995;15:465—472.
19. Hayden MR, Kastelein JJ, Funke H, Brunzell JD, Ma Y. Phenotypic variation in the human lipoprotein lipase gene. Biochem Soc Tranc 1993;21:506—509.

Lessons from molecular defects in secretion, transport and reverse transport of cholesterol

Hiroshi Mabuchi, Kouji Kajinami, Akihiro Inazu and Junji Koizumi
The Second Department of Internal Medicine, Kanazawa University School of Medicine, Kanazawa, Japan

Abstract. Genetic defects of cholesterol secretion, transport, reverse transport and recycling pathways produce dyslipidemias. Abetalipoproteinemia due to microsomal triglyceride transfer protein (MTP) deficiency produces severe hypolipidemia, and it is proposed that inhibition of MTP will provide a specific mechanism for lowering plasma cholesterol and triglyceride levels. The data of death in familial hypercholesterolemia (FH) showed a curve of incidence of coronary heart disease (CHD) in each cholesterol level, and this line separates benefit and no benefit areas by cholesterol-lowering therapy. Lecithin cholesterol acyltransferase (LCAT) deficiency produces a complete obstruction of the reverse cholesterol transport, but LCAT deficiency does not necessarily produce atherosclerosis, probably due to concomitant low level of LDL-cholesterol. An interruption of cholesterol recycling pathway by blocking cholesteryl ester transfer protein (CETP) activity will produce antiatherogenic lipoprotein profile observed in CETP deficiency. As a conclusion for the treatment of hypercholesterolemia, all the "physiological" pathways supplying cholesterol to low-density lipoprotein (LDL) should be blocked.

Keywords: abetalipoproteinemia, CETP deficiency, cholesterol-lowering therapy, familial hypercholesterolemia, LCAT deficiency.

Genetic defects of cholesterol secretion, transport, reverse transport and recycling pathways produce dyslipidemias, resulting in prominent clinical manifestations, such as atherosclerosis and xanthomas. Here we discuss how to manipulate serum cholesterol levels according to the lessons from these genetic diseases.

Defects in lipoprotein secretion: abetalipoproteinemia

Abetalipoproteinemia is a rare autosomal recessive disease characterized by a defect in the assembly or secretion of plasma lipoproteins containing apolipoprotein B. The molecular mechanism of this disease has been elucidated by Sherp et al. [1], their results indicated that microsomal triglyceride transfer protein (MTP) is required for the normal secretion of plasma lipoproteins containing apolipoprotein B, and that a defect in the MTP gene is the cause of abetalipoproteinemia.

The proband is a 29-year-old man, and his serum cholesterol, triglyceride,

---

Address for correspondence: Dr H. Mabuchi, The Second Department of Internal Medicine, Kanazawa University School of Medicine, Takara-machi 13-1, Kanazawa 920, Japan.

high-density lipoprotein (HDL) cholesterol and apolipoprotein B levels were 33, 0, 28 and 0 mg/dl, respectively. All fat-soluble vitamins were low in concentration. Clinically the proband showed cerebellar signs, such as dysmetria, ataxia and spastic gait. Ophthalmologic symptoms are retinitis pigmentosa, and decreased night and color vision. The patient had mild anemia with evidence of hemolysis. Most circulating red blood cells were acantocytes shown in the scanning electron micrograph. Malabsorption of fat began in infancy with steatorrhea and poor weight gain. Endoscopic examination showed pale yellowish intestine and the histopathology revealed normally formed intestinal villi with lipid-engorged enterozytes.

Sequence analysis of genomic DNA revealed a G-to-A mutation at the intron 9/exon 10 junction, and the proband's parents are heterozygous for the mutation. At present 15 mutants of the MTP gene have been reported. An intestinal biopsy was obtained from the proband, and total RNA was isolated and reversely transcribed into first-strand cDNA. The MTP cDNA showed a deletion of exon 10, skipping from exon 9 to 11. Thus, the defect of MTP produces destabilization of apolipoprotein B and the assembly and secretion of lipoprotein containing apolipoprotein B might be disturbed. As the defects in MTP can cause abetalipoproteinemia, it is proposed that inhibition of MTP will provide a specific mechanism for lowering plasma cholesterol and triglyceride levels. However, six heterozygotes in this family showed normal average cholesterol levels of 192 mg/dl.

Therefore, we suggest that MTP inhibitors will not be effective in reducing serum LDL-cholesterol levels even by 50% suppression of MTP activity.

LDL-receptor defect: familial hypercholesterolemia

LDL-receptor defects produce familial hypercholesterolemia (FH), which is characterized by severe hyper-LDL-cholesterolemia, tendon xanthomas and premature CHD. FH is a highly common disease in Japan as well as in the western countries, and we have collected 19 homozygotes and more than 1,500 heterozygotes in the Kanazawa district of Japan. More than 200 mutants of the LDL-receptor gene have been reported in the world and we have found nine mutants.

Nine of 19 homozygotes died, and their causes of death are shown in Table 1 [2]. One case died of leukemia, while all other eight patients died of CHD. Thus, 90% of the homozygotes die of CHD. The average age of death was 33 years, and the average serum cholesterol level was 704 mg/dl. 123 heterozygotes died during the past 20 years and the causes of death are shown in Table 2. Eighty-two heterozygotes (67%) died of CHD. Serum cholesterol levels were about 350 mg/dl, and the average age of death was 60 years in males, and 70 years in females.

As cholesterol-lowering therapy is principally aiming at the primary and the secondary prevention of cardiovascular disease, the highest benefit will be obtained in the FH homozygotes. Even in these patients, the percentage receiving

Table 1. Causes of death in homozygous FH patients.

Number	Case	Sex	Age (years)	Cause of death	Cholesterol (mg/dl)	Triglyceride (mg/dl)
1	KY	F	27	Sudden death	609	126
2	KM	F	42	Sudden death	610	180
3	SS	F	29	Sudden death	1004	784
4	YE	M	11	Heart failure	908	300
5	ST	M	18	Heart failure	781	189
6	MI	F	23	Sudden death	730	273
7	TT	M	57	Sudden death	558	388
8	MK	F	50	Leukemia	550	143
9	NY	F	38	Sudden death	590	93
Mean			33		704	275
SD			15		164	213

benefit from cholesterol-lowering therapy is 90%. In the FH heterozygotes whose mean serum cholesterol level is 350 mg/dl, the percentage of benefit is 67%. As the average serum cholesterol level in Japan is approximately 200 mg/dl, and the rate of death from CHD is about 6%, we suggest a curve from these data of incidence of CHD in each cholesterol level, and this line separates benefit and no benefit areas by cholesterol lowering therapy (Fig. 1).

Cholesterol reverse transport defect: LCAT deficiency

LCAT plays an important role in reverse cholesterol transport. LCAT deficiency blocks the reverse cholesterol transport at the gate of the pathway. We found a 37-year-old male patient with LCAT deficiency. His serum cholesterol, HDL-cholesterol and LCAT activity levels were 55 mg/dl, 2 mg/dl and 0%/40 min/3 µl, respectively. Clinically, slit-lamp examination showed minute dots in the cornea, proteinuria and mild anemia.

By gene analysis, the proband was identified as homozygotes of a G-to-A tran-

Table 2. Causes of death in heterozygous FH patients.

Cause of death	Number		Age (years)		Cholesterol (mg/dl)		Triglyceride (mg/dl)	
	Male	Female	Male	Female	Male	Female	Male	Female
CHD	51	31	59 ± 14	70 ± 8	350 ± 73	351 ± 64	145 ± 53	155 ± 79
Stroke	4	8	64 ± 5	71 ± 4	365 ± 143	345 ± 66	130 ± 72	151 ± 66
Cancer	10	5	61 ± 9	63 ± 13	345 ± 66	366 ± 88	192 ± 96	167 ± 35
Others	6	8	64 ± 18	72 ± 10	315 ± 89	361 ± 84	132 ± 53	148 ± 78
Total	71	52	60 ± 13	70 ± 8	348 ± 73	353 ± 76	151 ± 62	154 ± 72

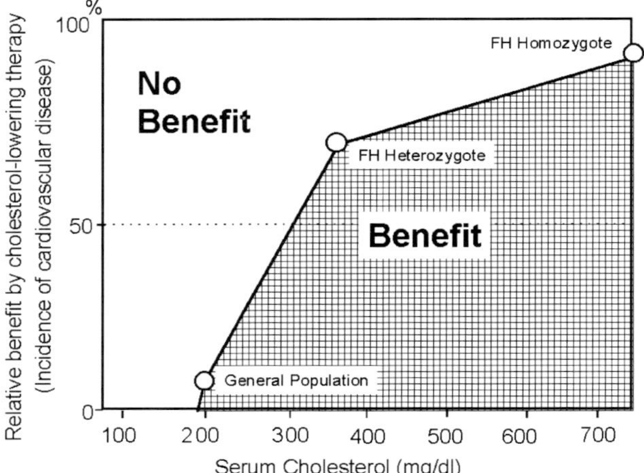

Fig. 1. Incidence of coronary heart disease in each cholesterol level in normal subjects, and heterozygous and homozygous patients with familial hypercholesterolemia. The curve separates benefit and no-benefit areas by cholesterol-lowering therapy.

sition at 1729 nucleotide in exon 2 of LCAT gene, causing the Gly-to-Ser substitution in amino acid codon 30 [3]. This mutation was found to cause complete LCAT deficiency. The proband's mother and sister were identified as heterozygous for the mutation. LCAT deficiency produces various clinical manifestations, such as corneal opacity, hemolytic anemia and renal failure. However, LCAT deficiency is not generally accompanied by premature atherosclerosis as much as in Tangier disease.

Thus, a complete obstruction of this pathway does not necessarily produce atherosclerosis, probably due to a concomitant low level of LDL-cholesterol.

Cholesterol recycling defect: CETP deficiency

In 1985 we reported the first case of CETP deficiency [4]. The proband is a 58-year-old Japanese man who was found to have hypercholesterolemia of 317 mg/dl and a HDL-cholesterol level of 247 mg/dl. Agarose gel electrophoresis of serum lipoprotein showed a pale β band of LDL and a dark α band of HDL. The serum lipoprotein pattern is similar to those found in rat serum, in which species CETP activity is deficient. Therefore, we studied CETP in this patient, and the CETP activity was found to be deficient in this patient.

By gene analysis, the proband was identified as the homozygotes of CETP gene defect [5]. At the 5′ splice donor of intron 14 (position +1) there was a G-to-A change altering the strictly conserved G-T intron splice donor to A-T (Int14 A), and the proband's wife was normal G at the site, his sister was also the homozygotes of A mutant. His children showed heterozygotes of the mutant. The proband was born to a consanguineous marriage, and three homozygotes and 10 heterozygotes were confirmed in this family [6].

Correlational analysis of lipoprotein and CETP levels using homozygotes, heterozygotes and unaffected revealed a strong inverse relation between CETP levels and the ratio of the HDL_2 levels to the sum of HDL_2 and HDL_3 levels, the correlation coefficient was -0.790. A positive correlation was found between CETP and LDL-cholesterol levels (r = 0.517). The lipoprotein profile of persons with CETP deficiency, that is high HDL and low LDL levels, is potentially antiatherogenic.

Thereafter, six mutants of CETP gene have been found in Japan and other Asian countries, and three mutants were identified in Caucasian people. D442G and Int 14-G-to-A are common mutants in Japan.

Thus, interruption of choleteryl recycling by blocking CETP will reduce LDL and increase HDL, which will be antiatherogenic.

There is much controversy as to whether CETP is proatherogenic or antiatherogenic. Therefore, we studied CHD in patients with double heterozygotes of FH and CETP deficiency, next, the incidence of CETP-deficiency in patients with old myocardial infarction, then control subjects, and finally, the effects of drugs on CETP activities.

We found several families with double heterozygotes of FH and CETP-deficiency [7]. Coronary stenosis determined by coronary angiography in double heterozygotes showed no differences from those of FH. From these findings we suggest that atherogenicity of hyper-LDL-cholesterolemia in FH is more powerful than antiatherogenicity of hyper-HDL-cholesterolemia in CETP deficiency.

Next we studied the frequency of CETP mutants in the general population and in the patients with old myocardial infarction. The incidence of CETP-deficiency in old myocardial infarction is 6.3%, while that in the general population is 10.9%. Although statistically insignificant, CETP-deficiency is thought not to be atherogenic, but rather antiatherogenic.

Finally we studied the effects of drugs on CETP activities and HDL-cholesterol levels. Probucol reduced HDL-cholesterol levels, while pravastatin did not. Probucol increased CETP levels by 23%, while pravastatin decreased CETP levels by 21%. Antiatherogenic effects of statins may be partially explained by their inhibiting CETP activity.

Sugano and Makino reported that after injecting rabbits with antisense oligonucleotide against rabbit CETP, plasma cholesterol levels and CETP activities decreased, whereas HDL-cholesterol levels increased [8]. A reduction in the hepatic CETP mRNA was also observed. They observed that atherosclerosis was greatly reduced in the rabbits treated by antisense oligonucleotide. We hear that a Japanese drug company developed a CETP inhibitor, which inhibited CETP activities by 50%, serum cholesterol and LDL-cholesterol levels decreased and HDL-cholesterol levels increased in animals.

Therefore, an interruption of the cholesterol recycling pathway by blocking CETP activity will produce antiatherogenic lipoprotein profile.

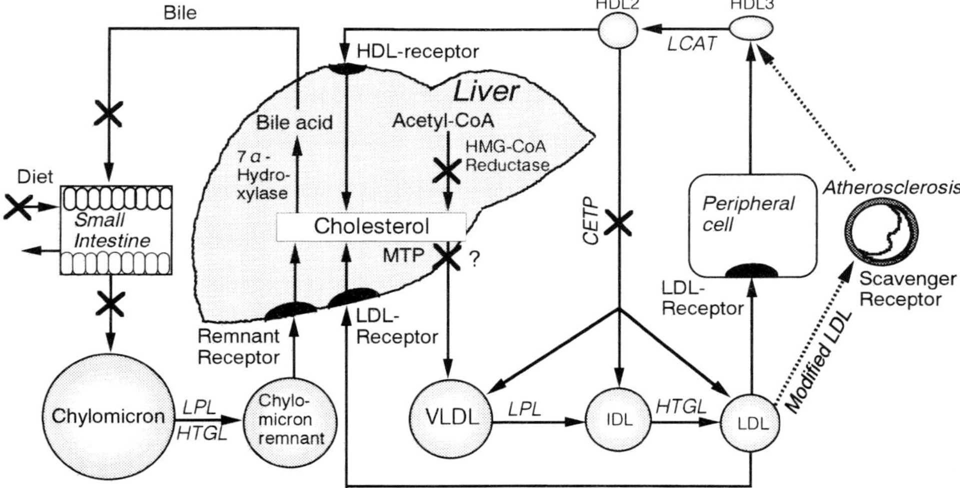

Fig. 2. For the treatment of hypercholesterolemia, all the "physiological" pathways supplying cholesterol to LDL should be blocked.

Conclusions: lessons from genetic dyslipidemias

As a result of the lessons learnt from genetic dyslipidemia, we have to block all pathways supplying cholesterol to LDL for the treatment of hypercholesterolemia. Thus, dietary restriction of cholesterol, blocking reabsorption of bile acid by resins, blocking cholesterol synthesis by HMG-CoA reductase inhibitors and blocking recycling cholesterol from HDL by inhibiting CETP activities is necessary (Fig. 2).

As a conclusion, for the treatment of hypercholesterolemia, all the "physiological" pathways supplying cholesterol to LDL should be blocked.

References

1. Sharp D, Blinderman L, Combs KA et al. Cloning and gene defects in microsomal triglyceride transfer protein associated with abetalipoproteinemia. Nature 1993;365:65—69.
2. Mabuchi H, Miyamoto S, Ueda K et al. Causes of death in patients with familial hypercholesterolemia. Atherosclerosis 1986;61:1—6.
3. Yang X-P, Inazu A, Honjo A et al. Catalytically inactive lecithin: cholesterol acyltransferase (LCAT) caused by a Gly 30 to Ser mutation in a family with LCAT deficiency. J Lipid Res 1997;38:585—591.
4. Koizumi J, Mabuchi H, Yoshimura A et al. Deficiency of serum cholesterol-ester transfer activity in patients with familial hyperalphalipoproteinemia. Atherosclerosis 1985;58:175—186.
5. Brown ML, Inazu A, Hesler CB et al. Molecular basis of lipid transfer protein deficiency in a family with increased high-density lipoproteins. Nature 1989;342:448—451.
6. Inazu A, Brown ML, Hesler CB et al. Increased high-density lipoprotein levels caused by a common cholesteryl-ester transfer protein gene mutation. N Engl J Med 1990;323:1234—1238.

7. Haraki T, Inazu A, Yagi K et al. Clinical characteristics of double heterozygotes with familial hypercholesterolemia and cholesteryl ester transfer protein deficiency. Atherosclerosis 1997; 132:229—236.
8. Sugano M, Makino N. Changes in plasma lipoprotein cholesterol levels by antisense oligodeoxy-nucleotides against cholesteryl ester transfer protein in cholesterol-fed rabbits. J Biol Chem 1996;271:19080—19083.

Genetic architecture of the quantitative lipoprotein(a) trait

Gerd Utermann and Hans Georg Kraft
Institute for Medical Biology and Human Genetics, University of Innsbruck, Innsbruck, Austria

Abstract. Lp(a) is a quantitative genetic trait in human plasma which is associated with athero-sclerotic disease and shows considerable interethnic variation. In Caucasians the major gene locus controlling Lp(a) concentration is the apolipoprotein(a) gene on chromosome 6q27. Sib-pair linkage and population genetic data suggest that apo(a) gene variation is also the major determinant of Lp(a) concentrations in other populations (e.g., African Blacks, Khoi-San) but that the relative and absolute contribution of intragenic variation in apo(a) to Lp(a) levels varies among groups. Three types of variation in apo(a) have been related to Lp(a) levels: 1) In all populations there exists a strong effect of kringle IV-2 repeat number on Lp(a) concentrations which is causal in nature. 2) In Caucasians and some Asian populations, though not in Africans, there exists an association of Lp(a) concentration with a pentanucleotide repeat polymorphism in the promoter. These associations are heterogeneous and reflect linkage disequilibria with unknown causal mutations. 3) A C→T substitution at +93 of apo(a) which introduces a new ATG start codon has a causal effect on Lp(a) levels but as a result of allele frequencies and linkage disequilibria this polymorphism has an impact on Lp(a) in Africans but not Caucasians. Finally there exist genetic effects on Lp(a) not linked to the apo(a) locus particularly in Africans.

Keywords: apolipoprotein(a), repeat polymorphism, sib-pair analysis.

Introduction

Lipoprotein(a) which is a covalent complex of low-density lipoprotein (LDL) and the distinguished apolipoprotein(a) is one of the most extreme quantitative traits in human plasma [1]. Concentrations in apparently healthy individuals cover a range from below 1 mg/dl to greater than 200 mg/dl. Large differences in the distributions and median concentrations exist also between human populations, where Africans have the highest average Lp(a) concentrations ([2] and references therein).

High concentrations of Lp(a) are associated with premature coronary heart disease and stroke in Asian and Caucasian populations (for review see [3]). This is believed to be due to both atherogenic and thrombogenic potential of Lp(a). Understanding the genetic control of Lp(a) concentrations may therefore be of considerable interest and may have practical therapeutic implications.

Address for correspondence: Prof Gerd Utermann, Institut für Medizinische Biologie und Humangenetik, Schöpfstrasse 41, 6020 Innsbruck, Austria. Tel.: +43-512-507-3450.

458

Apolipoprotein(a) polymorphism and Lp(a) concentrations

The apo(a) gene on chromosome 6q27 has been identified as a major gene controlling Lp(a) concentrations in Caucasians [4—7] but many aspects of the mechanism by which apo(a) determines Lp(a) concentrations are presently unclear. It is also not known whether differences in apo(a) allele frequencies, transacting factors and/or environmental agents are responsible for the large intraethnic differences, e.g., between Africans and Caucasians (Lp(a) concentrations are about 2- to 3-fold higher in Africans than in Caucasian populations).

The apo(a) gene has a unique structure among known human genes [8]. Primate apo(a) has evolved from plasminogen and contains a variable number (from 2 to > 40) of identical 5.6 kb repeats which contain exons coding for the so-called kringle IV type 2 domains in apo(a) [5,6,9]. Hence the apo(a) gene represents a transcribed VNTR the transcript of which is translated into protein resulting in the extraordinary size polymorphism of the apo(a) protein. More than 40 alleles coding for apo(a) isoforms of different sizes exist in the population [10,11]. In addition other polymorphisms have been detected in apo(a), both in coding and noncoding regions of the gene [12—18]. These include amongst others a pentanucleotide repeat polymorphism (PNRP) in the apo(a) promoter [13,14], and a C/T polymorphism at +93, where the presence of a T creates a new ATG start codon [15,17] (Fig. 1). The K-IV VNTR, the PNRP, and the +93 C/T polymorphism are associated with Lp(a) concentrations but as will be outlined here the mechanisms underlying these associations are fundamentally different.

K-VI VNTR and Lp(a) concentrations

An inverse association of apo(a) length with Lp(a) concentrations was first demonstrated by apo(a) isoform analysis [4]. This association exists in all populations studied so far and has been confirmed by analysis of the relation between the number of K-IV-2 repeats in the apo(a) gene (which determines the length of the protein) and Lp(a) plasma concentrations suggesting that it reflects a basic mechanism [6,10,11]. Although present in all populations the strength of the association varies across human populations and is weaker in Africans than in Caucasians or Asians [11]. Quantitative analysis of population data suggests that from 25 to 70% of the variance in Lp(a) concentrations is explained by the apo(a) size polymorphism (depending on the population and the type of analy-

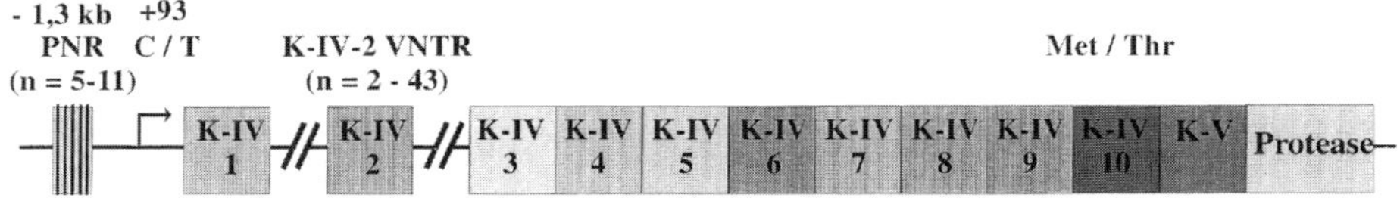

Fig. 1. Simplified scheme of the apo(a) gene with some polymorphisms (not drawn to scale).

sis). Against expectation differences in the frequencies of apo(a) size alleles between populations do not explain the differences in Lp(a) concentrations between them [10,11,19]. Hence this must be due to either apo(a) sequence variation, other genes, or environment. Notably the association of the K-IV repeat variation with Lp(a) concentrations reflects a causal relationship. Studies in baboon hepatocytes [20] and Hep G2 transfected with apo(a) cDNA [21] have demonstrated an effect of K-IV-2 repeat number on apo(a) processing and secretion by cells. Hence the effect of the K-IV VNTR is causal in nature and homogeneous across populations (Table 1).

Contribution of the apo (a) locus to Lp (a) level variance

The high degree of allelic variation at the apo(a) locus (95% heterozygosity for the K-IV VNTR) is ideal to determine the effect of the apo(a) locus on the variance of Lp(a) concentrations by sib-pair linkage analysis. Three independent studies have suggested that in Caucasians more than 90% of the variance is explained by variation at the apo(a) locus [5,7,22]. Together with the population data this implies that other variation in or around the apo(a) locus also contributes to Lp(a) variability. A recent reanalysis or our sib-pair data using a variance components model has, however, resulted in a considerably lower estimate of the effect of the apo(a) locus. According to this analysis about 70 to 75% of the variance in Lp(a) concentrations are explained by apo(a) genetic variation (M. Scholz, H.G. Kraft, A. Lingenhel, R. Delport, E.H. Vorster, H. Bickebōller and G. Utermann, unpublished). We further have extended our sib-pair/family analysis to African populations (South African Blacks and Khoi-San). This revealed significant differences in the genetic architecture of Lp(a) between Africans and Caucasians. First, the contribution of the genetic variation to Lp(a) variability was smaller in Africans ($\sim 65\%$). Second, the impact of the major gene (apo(a)) was also smaller and was not significant which probably reflects the weaker association of the K-IV- VNTR with Lp(a) concentrations in Africans. Consistent with the population data an estimate of the fraction of the Lp(a) variance explained by apo(a) resulted in an estimate of about 35%. The weaker effect of the apo(a) locus in Africans is also apparent from the intraclass correlation between siblings sharing two, one, or no apo(a) allele identical by descent (i.b.d.) (Fig. 2). In particular in sib-pairs with two alleles i.b.d. the correlation was

Table 1. Effects of apo(a) genetic variation on Lp(a) plasma concentrations.

Polymorphism	Type of effect	Effect across populations	Interpretation
K IV-2 VNTR	direct	homogeneous	causal effect
Promoter PNR	indirect	heterogeneous	reflects allelic associations
+93 C/T	direct	heterogeneous	causal, masked by allelic association in same populations

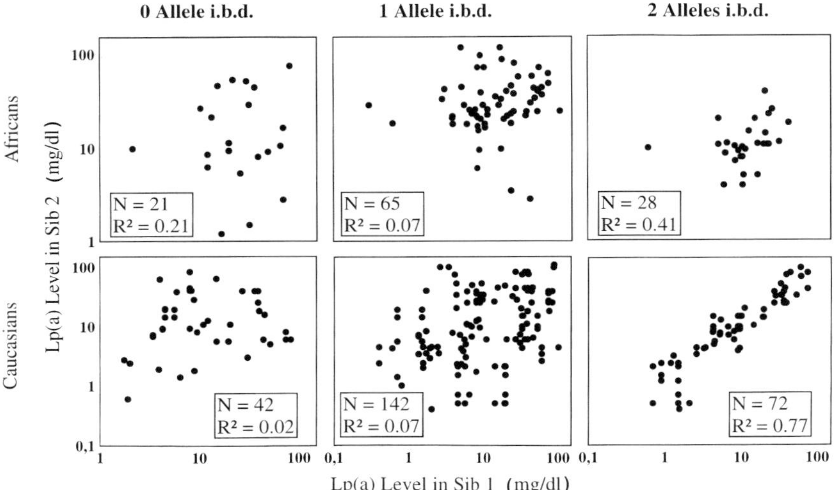

Fig. 2. Correlations of Lp(a) concentrations in sib-pairs i.b.d. for two, one, or no apo(a) alleles from African (upper pannels) and Caucasian (lower pannels) families.

much stronger in Caucasians than in Blacks (Fig. 2). Together our data suggest: 1) the existence of sequence variation in or around the apo(a) locus which affects Lp(a) levels; and 2) the existence of (a) transacting factor(s) influencing Lp(a) levels in Blacks. The latter conclusion is consistent with a recent sib-pair analysis of African Americans by Mooser et al. [2].

Pentanucleotide repeat polymorphism

A PNR in the apo(a) promoter has been identified by Wade et al. [17]. Family [13] and population [14] analyses which were considered and stratified for the K-IV VNTR effect both have demonstrated a significant association of the PNRP with Lp(a) concentrations. The population data further demonstrated that this effect is present in Caucasians but not in Blacks [14] suggesting that the PNR variation is not causal. This has been confirmed by direct analysis of apo(a) promoters from alleles containing different numbers of PNR repeats in luciferase reporter assays [13].

Recent studies of Asian populations have shown that the PNR is associated with Lp(a) levels but that the type of association is different (i.e., other alleles than in Caucasians are associated with high and low Lp(a), respectively (H.G. Kraft and G. Utermann, unpublished). Together we can state that the effect of the promoter PNR on Lp(a) is heterogeneous across populations and not causal. The associations therefore are likely caused by allelic associations with mutations which have yet to be identified.

C/T polymorphism

The +93 C/T polymorphism has been analyzed in different populations which were already characterized for K-IV VNTR and PNRP. This was essential for the evaluation and interpretation of the data. Surprisingly a significant effect was present in Africans but not in Caucasians (H.G. Kraft, M. Windegger, H.J. Menzel and G. Utermann, unpublished) This is explained by linkage disequilibrium. In Caucasians T alleles (which in vitro result in a 60% reduction in apo(a) translation [15] are in strong allelic association with 9 PNRs in the promoter and with intermediate size K-IV repeats. Such alleles are associated with very low Lp(a) in Caucasians anyhow. Therefore the effect is masked in Caucasians. The situation is different in Africans where the +93 T allele is present on alleles which are associated with rather high Lp(a). Here the T allele results in a lowering of about 50% (H.G. Kraft, M. Windegger, H.J. Menzel and G. Utermann, unpublished) which is consistent with the in vitro data [15].

Acknowledgements

This work was supported by grant P 11695 from the "Austrian Fonds zur Förderung der wissenschaftlichen Forschung" to G.U.

References

1. Utermann G. The mysteries of lipoprotein(a). Science 1989;246:904–910.
2. Mooser V et al. The apo(a) gene is the major determinant of variation in plasma Lp(a) plasma in African Americans. Am J Hum Genet 1997;61:402–417.
3. Utermann G. Lipoprotein (a). In: Scriver ChR, Beaudet AL, Sly WS, Valle D (eds) The Metabolic and Molecular Bases of Inherited Disease. New York: McGraw Hill Inc., 1995; 1887–1912.
4. Utermann G et al. Lp(a) glycoprotein phenotypes. Inheritance and relation to Lp(a)-lipoprotein concentrations in plasma. J Clin Invest 1987;80:458–465.
5. Kraft H et al. The apolipoprotein(a) gene: a transcribed hypervariable locus controlling plasma lipoprotein(a) concentration. Hum Genet 1992;90:220–230.
6. Lackner C et al. Molecular basis of apolipoprotein (a) isoform size heterogeneity as revealed by pulsed-field gel electrophoresis. J Clin Invest 1991;87:2153–2161.
7. Boerwinkle E et al. Apolipoprotein(a) gene accounts for greater than 90% of the variation in plasma lipoprotein(a) concentrations. J Clin Invest 1992;90:52–60.
8. McLean JW et al. cDNA sequence of human apolipoprotein (a) is homolgous to plasminogen. Nature 1987;300:132–137.
9. Lackner C, Cohen JC, Hobbs HH. Molecular definition of the extreme size polymorphism in apolipoprotein(a). Hum Mol Genet 1993;2:933–940.
10. Gaw A et al. Comparative analysis of the apo(a) gene, apo(a) glycoprotein, and plasma concentrations of Lp(a) in three ethnic groups. Evidence for no common "null" allele at the apo(a) locus. J Clin Invest 1994;93:2526–2534.
11. Kraft HG et al. Frequency distributions of apolipoprotein(a) kringle IV repeat alleles and their effects on Lp(a) levels in Caucasian, Asian, and African populations: the distribution of null alleles is non-random. Eur J Hum Genet 1996;4:74–87.
12. Cohen JC et al. Sequence polymorphisms in the apolipoprotein(a) gene. J Clin Invest 1993;

91:1630—1636.
13. Mooser V et al. Sequence polymorphisms in the apo(a) gene associated with specific levels of Lp(a) in plasma. Hum Mol Genet 1995;4:173—181.
14. Trommsdorff M et al. A pentanucleotide repeat polymorphism in the 5' control region of the apolipoprotein(a) gene is associated with lipoprotein(a) plasma concentrations in Caucasians. J Clin Invest 1995;96:150—157.
15. Zysow RR et al. C/T polymorphism in the 5t untranslated region of the apolipoprotein(a) gene introduces an upstream ATG and reduces in vitro translation. Arterioscl Thromb 1995;15:58—64.
16. Mancini FP et al. Sequence microheterogeneity in apolipoprotein(a) gene repeats and the relationship to plasma Lp(a) levels. Hum Mol Genet 1995;4:1535—1542.
17. Wade DP et al. 5' control regions of the apolipoprotein(a) gene and members of the related plasminogen gene family. Proc Natl Acad Sci USA 1993;90:1369—1373.
18. Van der Hoek YY et al. The apolipoprotein(a) kringle IV repeats which differ from the major repeat kringle are present in variably-sized isoforms. Hum Mol Genet 1993;2:361—366.
19. Sandholzer C et al. Effects of the apolipoprotein(a) size polymorphism on the lipoprotein(a) concentration in 7 ethnic groups. Hum Genet 1991;86:607—614.
20. White AL et al. Molecular basis for "null" lipoprotein(a) phenotypes and the influence of apolipoprotein(a) size on plasma lipoprotein(a) level in the baboon. J Biol Chem 1994;269:9060—9066.
21. Roingeard P et al. Immunocytochemical and electron microscopic study of hepatitis B virus antigen and complete particle production in hepatitis B virus DNA transfected HepG2 cells. Hepatology 1990;11:277—285.
22. DeMeester CA et al. Genetic variation in lipoprotein(a) levels in families enriched for coronary artery disease is determined almost entirely by the apolipoprotein(a) gene locus. Am J Hum Genet 1995;56:287—293.

Lipoprotein oxidation and atherosclerosis

Endothelial activation in atherogenesis — roles of oxidized LDL and lysophosphatidylcholine

Noriaki Kume and Toru Kita

Department of Geriatric Medicine, Kyoto University, Kyoto, Japan

Abstract. Endothelial activation, or dysfunction, elicited by oxidized low-density lipoprotein (Ox-LDL) and its lipid constituent, lysophosphatidylcholine (lyso-PC) have been implicated in the pathogenesis of atherosclerosis. In addition to transcriptional gene induction, lyso-PC can stimulate actin stress fiber formation and tyrosine phosphorylation of a cell surface adhesion molecule, PECAM-1. These might play a role in lyso-PC-induced signal transduction mechanisms. Furthermore, a novel endothelial receptor for Ox-LDL, designated lectin-like Ox-LDL receptor-1 (LOX-1) has been identified. LOX-1 expressed in arterial endothelium appears to be an Ox-LDL-specific receptor whose structure does not share any homology with other Ox-LDL receptors. Ox-LDL uptake by LOX-1 and subsequent endothelial activation may play an important role in atherogenesis.

Lyso-PC modulates various endothelial functions relevant to atherogenesis

Endothelial activation, or dysfunction, has been implicated in the pathogenesis of atherosclerosis [1–3]. Oxidatively modified low-density lipoprotein (Ox-LDL) appears to play a key role in atherogenesis. Lysophosphatidylcholine (lyso-PC), a polar phospholipid constituent of Ox-LDL, has been shown to modulate various endothelial functions relevant to atherogenesis [4,5]. Lyso-PC can impair nitric oxide release, stimulate production of hydrogen peroxide, inhibit cell migration and induce expression of vascular cell adhesion molecules-1 (VCAM-1), intercellular adhesion molecule-1 (ICAM-1) [4], heparin-binding epidermal growth factor-like factor (HB-EGF) [5], platelet-derived growth factor (PDGF) A- and B-chains [5], constitutive nitric oxide synthase and cyclooxygenase type 2. These functional changes elicited by lyso-PC are thought to be relevant to atherogenesis caused by hyperlipidemia.

Lyso-PC stimulates actin stress fiber formation in cultured vascular endothelial cells

Vascular endothelial cells, on the other hand, have been shown to form actin stress fibers in vivo, in response to a variety of pathophysiological stimuli.

Address for correspondence: Noriaki Kume MD, PhD, Department of Geriatric Medicine, Graduate School of Medicine, Kyoto University, 54 Kawahara-cho, Shogoin, Sakyo-ku, Kyoto 606, Japan. Tel.: +81-75-751-3465. Fax: +81-75-751-3574. E-mail: nkume@kuhp.kyoto-u.ac.jp

Increased formation of actin stress fibers has been detected in aortic endothelium covering atherosclerotic lesions in hypercholesterolemic animals in vivo. Therefore, we have examined the effect of lyso-PC on the organization of actin cytoskeleton in cultured vascular endothelial cells. Confluent monolayers of HUVEC were treated with lyso-PC, and actin cytoskeleton was visualized by staining with fluorescence-labeled phalloidin. Lyso-PC, as low as 10 μmol/l in serum-free culture media, stimulated formation of actin stress fibers aligned in parallel. In sham-treated HUVEC, in contrast, very few stress fibers were formed in cytoplasm and staining with phalloidin was localized to peripheral regions of cytoplasm and intercellular junctions.

To explore signal transduction pathways involved in lyso-PC-induced formation of actin stress fibers, roles of cyclic AMP and protein tyrosine phosphorylation were examined. Forskolin (a reagent that elevates intracellular cyclic AMP, as well as genistein, an inhibitor of tyrosine phosphorylation) efficiently blocked lyso-PC-induced actin stress fiber formation. Interestingly, lyso-PC-induced expression of PDGF-B chain also was suppressed by forskolin [6] and genistein.

We further explored the roles of rho, a ras-related small GTP-binding protein, on lyso-PC-induced actin stress fiber formation. Pretreatment of HUVEC with C3 exoenzyme, which inactivates rho by ADP-ribosylation [7] inhibited lyso-PC-induced actin stress fiber formation. In contrast, the expression of PDGF-B chain induced by lyso-PC was not significantly altered by pretreatment with C3 exoenzyme. These results suggest that actin stress fiber formation and expression of PDGF-B chain induced by lyso-PC may share (in part) the same signal transduction pathways; however, dependence upon rho appears to be different between actin stress fiber formation and PDGF-B chain gene expression.

Lyso-PC rapidly tyrosine phosphorylates PECAM-1

Since protein tyrosine events are involved in both lyso-PC-induced gene expression and actin stress fiber formation, we sought to identify proteins that can rapidly be tyrosine phosphorylated. We performed immunoblot analyses of whole cell lysates from lyso-PC-treated and untreated cultured bovine aortic endothelial cells (BAEC) using an antiphosphotyrosine monoclonal antibody. A protein with an approximate molecular mass of 130 kDd (designated p130) has been shown to be tyrosine phosphorylated by lyso-PC. The dose-response relationship showed that lyso-PC concentrations as low as 5 μmol/l can induce tyrosine phosphorylation of p130. Time course experiments revealed that tyrosine phosphorylation of p130 was detectable as early as 10 min after stimulation with lyso-PC, and remained for at least 1 h.

To identify p130, we carried out immunoprecipitation followed by immunoblotting with use of antibodies for proteins with a molecular mass of 130 kDa in combination with an antiphosphotyrosine monoclonal antibody. A band with a molecular mass of 130 kDa was detectable in lyso-PC-treated BAEC, but only if we first immunoprecipitated with an anti-PECAM-1 antibody and subsequently immunoblotted with an antiphosphotyrosine antibody. In addition, a similar 130 kDa band was shown in lyso-PC-treated BAEC, when we immunoprecipitated lyso-PC treated cell lysates with an antiphosphotyrosine antibody and subsequently carried out immunoblotting with an anti-PECAM-1 antibody. These results demonstrate that lyso-PC can rapidly tyrosine phosphorylates PECAM-1 in BAEC, although its role in lyso-PC-induced signal transduction remains to be elucidated.

LOX-1, a novel endothelial receptor for oxidized LDL

Previous studies have indicated that cultured vascular endothelial cells can internalize and degrade Ox-LDL presumably through specific receptors [8]; however, molecules involved in this process have not been fully clarified. By an expression-cloning strategy (a cDNA library from BAEC and diI-labeled Ox-LDL) we have identified a novel endothelial receptor for Ox-LDL [9]. The cloned receptor is a type II membrane glycoprotein with a approximate molecular mass of 50 kDa whose structure belongs to C-type lectin family. Human homologue of LOX-1 has also been cloned by screening human lung cDNA libraries by bovine LOX-1 cDNA as a probe. Amino acid sequences of human LOX-1 are 72% identical to bovine LOX-1. Interestingly, LOX-1 does not share any structural homology with other receptors for Ox-LDL including class A, B and C scavenger receptors. Binding and proteolytic degradation assays using radiolabelled Ox-LDL in CHO-K1 cells stably expressing both bovine and human LOX-1 revealed that LOX-1 can bind, internalize and degrade Ox-LDL but not significantly native LDL or acetylated LDL. RT-PCR and northern blot analysis showed that LOX-1 expression in vivo appears to be detectable arterial intima, including atherosclerotic lesions, as well as vascular-rich organs such as lung, liver and placenta. Furthermore, LOX-1 expression can be dynamically regulated by an inflammatory process. LOX-1, therefore, may play an important role in atherogenesis and inflammatory responses in the vascular wall, although further studies would be necessary to understand the pathophysiological significance in human diseases.

References

1. Gimbrone MA Jr, Cybulsky MI, Kume N, Collins T, Resnick N. Vascular Endothelium. An integrator of pathophysiological stimuli in atherogenesis. Ann NY Acad Sci 1995;748:122—132.
2. Ross R. The pathogenesis of atherosclerosis: a perspective for the 1990's. Nature 1993; 362:801—809.
3. Witztum JL, Steinberg D. Role of oxidized low-density lipoprotein in atherogenesis. J Clin Invest 1991;88:1785—1792.
4. Kume N, Cybulsky MI, Gimbrone MA Jr. Lysophosphatidylcholine, a component of atherogenic lipoproteins, induces mononuclear leukocyte adhesion molecules in cultured human and rabbit arterial endothelial cells. J Clin Invest 1992;90:1138—1144.
5. Kume N, Gimbrone MA Jr. Lysophosphatidylcholine transcriptionally induces growth factor

gene expression in cultured human endothelial cells. J Clin Invest 1994;93:907—911.

6. Ochi H, Kume N, Nishi E, Kita T. Elevated levels of cyclic AMP inhibit protein kinase C-independent mechanisms of endothelial platelet-derived growth factor-B chain and intercellular adhesion molecule-1 gene induction by lysophosphatidylcholine. Circ Res 1995;77:530—535.

7. Morii N, Narumiya S. Purification of native and recombinant *Clostridium botulinum* C3 ADP-ribosyltransferase and identification of rho proteins by ADP-ribosylation. Meth Enzymol 1995;256:196—206.

8. Kume N, Arai H, Kawai C, Kita T. Receptors for modified low-density lipoproteins in human endothelial cells: different recognition for acetylated low-density lipoprotein and oxidized low-density lipoprotein. Biochim Biophys Acta 1991;1091:63—67.

9. Sawamura T, Kume N, Aoyama T, Moriwaki H, Hoshikawa H, Aiba Y, Tanaka T, Miwa S, Katsura Y, Kita T, Masaki T. An endothelial receptor for oxidized low-density lipoprotein. Nature. 1997;386:73—77.

A role for macrophage scavenger receptors in atherosclerosis

Kenji Inoue, Hiroshi Suzuki, Takao Hamakubo and Tatsuhiko Kodama
*Department of Molecular Biology and Medicine, Research Center for Advanced Science and Technology,
University of Tokyo, Tokyo, Japan*

Abstract. Type I and II macrophage scavenger receptors are implicated in the pathologic deposition of cholesterol during atherogenesis through receptor-mediated uptake of modified low-density lipoproteins (mLDL). Type I and II receptors have an extraordinarily wide range of ligand-binding capability including the bacterial pathogens, and is also known to mediate cation-independent macrophage adhesion in vitro. Here we report that the targeted disruption of the type I and II receptor gene results in a reduction in the size of atherosclerotic lesions in an apolipoprotein E (apo E) deficient animal. Macrophages from type I and II receptor deficient mice exhibit a marked decrease in mLDL uptake in vitro, whereas mLDL clearance from plasma occurs at a normal rate, suggesting that there are alternative mechanisms for the uptake of mLDL from the circulation. In addition, these knockout mice show increased susceptibility to Listeria monocytogenes infection and herpes simplex virus type-1 (HSV-1) infection, indicating a role for scavenger receptors in host defense against various pathogens.

Introduction

After molecular cloning of type I and II macrophage scavenger receptors [1,2], several structurally and functionally related receptor proteins [3] were cloned (Fig. 1). After initial attempts to elucidate the role for scavenger receptors in atherosclerosis, we established the mice lacking type I and II receptors.

Results and Discussion

Binding and endocytosis of multiple ligands by type I and II receptor deficient macrophages

Type I and II receptor knockout mice [4] grow normally and are fertile. Peritoneal macrophages of homozygous mice have less than 20% activity of normal acetyl-LDL degradation. In contrast these macrophages still have a significant oxidized LDL degradation activity, 40—70% activity as compared with normal control. The uptake of advanced glycosilation product BSA by type I and II deficient macrophages was about one-third of normal control [5]. The specificity of oxidized LDL binding activity remaining in type I and II deficient macrophages is similar to the reported specificity of macrosialin/CD68 [6]. Acetyl- and oxidized LDL are rapidly cleared by the liver in mice deficient in type I and II

Address for correspondence: Kenji Inoue, Department of Molecular Biology and Medicine, Research Center for Advanced Science and Technology, University of Tokyo, 4-6-1 Komaba, Tokyo 153, Japan.

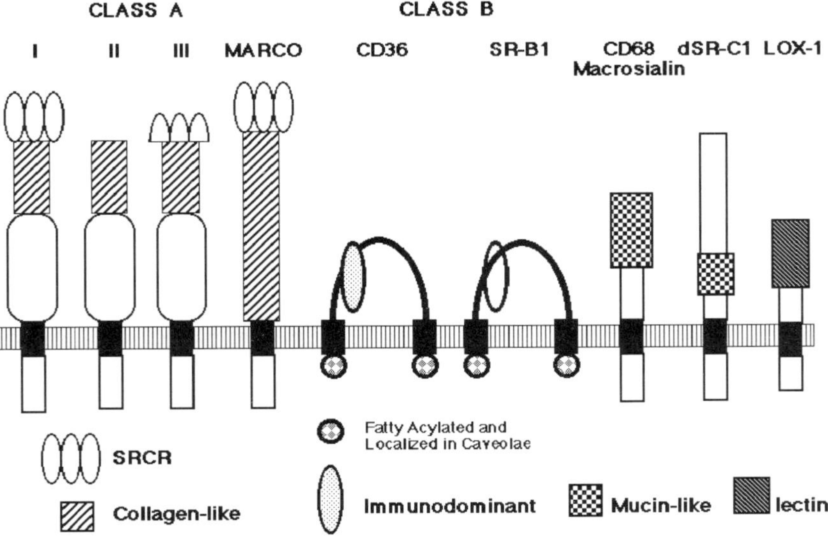

Fig. 1. Type I, II and III (P. Gogh and S. Gordon, personal communication) macrophage scavenger receptors are generated by an alternative splicing. MARCO has a longer collagenous domain but it lacks a coiled coil domain. A cluster of basic amino acids in a collagenous domain mediate the ligand binding. CD36 and SR-BI have two membrane spanning domains, and are concentrated in a plasma membrane microdomain, caveolae. In case of CD36, an immunodominant domain is essential for the ligand recognition. CD68/macrosialin has a mucin-like structure. dSR-CI has a Ser/Thr rich domain, which is a reminiscent of *Drosophila* mucins. LOX-1 is expressed in endothelial cells.

receptors and type I and II receptors do not play a major role in the clearance of acetyl-LDL from plasma (T.J.C. van Berkel, unpublished observation).

Phagocytosis of apoptotic cells

Uptake of steroid-treated apoptotic thymocytes by normal thymic macrophages is partially inhibited by monoclonal antitype I and II receptor antibody, 2F8 [8]. Type I and II deficient macrophages also show a 50% reduction in phagocytosis of apoptotic thymocytes in vitro [9]. In contrast, type I and II receptors do not mediate the uptake of oxidized red blood cell phagocytosis [10]. Other classes of receptors are also known to mediate phagocytosis of apoptotic cells and oxidized red blood cells.

Cell adhesion

The antimurine type I and II receptor monoclonal antibody, 2F8, inhibits divalent cation-independent adhesion of murine macrophage to plastic [7]. Peritoneal macrophages obtained after thioglycolate stimulation adhere tightly to a plastic tissue culture plate after overnight incubation and many protrusions and distortion in shape are apparent. Macrophages deficient in type I and II receptors are still round in shape and less adhesive after one overnight incubation (12—20 h). It takes more than 40 h for type I and II deficient macrophages to adhere to a plastic dish and change their shape [4]. The adhesion mediated by the type I and II receptors is prominent in an early phase of this process, less than 24 h after initiation of cultivation.

Host defense function

Macrophages play an important role in the host defense system in normal and pathological processes. Type I and II receptors can bind bacterial endotoxin, gram-positive bacteria and recognize lipoteichoic acid [11]. The binding of endotoxin to type I and II receptors did not mediate endotoxin signaling, and this pathway may serve as a route for the cleaning up of the excess endotoxin. Homozygout type I and II receptor deficient mice are more susceptible to injection of macrophage tropic pathogens, listeria monocytogenes and herpes simplex virus type 1. The clearance of L monocytogenes from plasma did not change in deficient mice, and the number of micro-organella in the host organ was increased. MARCO can also bind bacteria and is implicated in their clearance from plasma.

Atherosclerotic lesion in type I and II receptor knockout mice

Type I and II receptor proteins [12,13] as well as mRNA [14] are expressed in the macrophages in atherosclerotic lesions. We mated type I and II deficient mice to atherosclerosis model strains, LDL receptor deficient mice or apolipoprotein E (apoE) deficient mice [4]. In the case of apo E deficiency, plaque formation was observed without a high cholesterol diet. The plasma cholesterol level of the type I and II/apoE double knockout mice was slightly higher than the apoE single knockout mice. However, the average size of atherosclerotic lesion decreased by 60%. In the case of type I and II/LDL receptor knockout mice, a 1.25% high cholesterol diet was started at 10 weeks of age, and the lesion size was smaller than LDL receptor single knockout mice, but the difference (a decrease of 25%) was less prominent. MARCO and macrosialin were expressed by the macrophages in the atherosclerotic lesion in knockout mice (Sakaguchi et al., unpublished observation). Although the plasma cholesterol level and plasma clearance of acetyl- or oxidized LDL in type I and II deficient mice did not differ from that of wild-type controls, the lesion size diminished [4]. This result supports the hypothesis that modification in the vessel wall is essential for the lesion formation.

Type I and II receptors are known as major divalent cation independent macrophage adhesion molecule, and in atherosclerotic lesion, type I and II scavenger receptors may cause the accumulation of macrophage in lesion rich in modified LDL. Oxidized LDL is known to stimulate macrophage proliferation through the uptake mediated by type I and II receptors [15]. The signal is mainly mediated by the uptake of lysophosphatidyl choline.

The ligand specificity of oxidized LDL receptor remained in type I and II deficient macrophages is similar to that of CD68 [6]. CD36 is also expressed both in the monocytes and core of advanced lesion, suggesting that this receptor can also mediate the oxidized LDL uptake. Scavenger receptors mediate the phagocytosis and uptake of apoptotic cells [9]. During macrophage transmigration macrophages can uptake matrix proteins digested by macrophage metalloproteases. LDL attached to the matrix can be taken up at the same time. Many apoptotic cells are found in atherosclerotic lesions and macrophages uptake these cells by scavenger receptors [15]. This process also provides cholesterol to macrophages. Recent identification of SR-BI as an HDL receptor [16] suggest that SR-BI may rather involve reverse cholesterol transport. Further study will be necessary to clarify this point.

References

1. Kodama T, Freeman M, Rohrer L, Zabrecky J, Matsudaira P, Krieger M. Type I macrophage scavenger receptor contains alpha-helical and collagen-like coiled coils. Nature 1990;343: 531–535.
2. Rohrer L, Freeman M, Kodama T, Penman M, Krieger M. Coiled-coil fibrous domains mediate ligand binding by macrophage scavenger receptor type II. Nature 1990;343:570–572.
3. Kodama T, Doi T, Suzuki H, Takahashi K, Wada Y, Gordon S. Collagenous macrophage scavenger receptors. Curr Opin Lipid 1996;7:287–291.
4. Suzuki H, Kurihara Y, Takeya M, Kamada N, Kataoka M, Jishage K et al. A role for macrophage scavenger receptors in atherosclerosis and susceptibility to infection. Nature 1997;386: 292–296.
5. Araki N, Higashi T, Mori T, Shibayama R, Kawabe Y, Kodama T, Takahashi K. Macrophage scavenger receptor mediates the endocytic uptake and degradation of advanced glycation end products of the Maillard reaction. Eur J Biochem 1995;230:408–415.
6. Lougheed M, Lum CM, Ling W, Suzuki H, Kodama T, Steinbrecher U. High affinity saturable uptake of oxidized low density lipoprotein by macrophages from mice lacking the scavenger receptor class A type I/II. J Biol Chem 1997;272:12938–12944.
7. Ling W, Lougheed M, Suzuki H, Buchan A, Kodama T, Steinbrecher UP. Oxidized or acetylated low density lipoproteins are rapidly cleared by the liver in mice with disruption of the scavenger receptor class A type I/II gene. J Clin Invest 1997;100:244–252.
8. Fraser I, Hughes D, Gordon S. Divalent cation-independent macrophage adhesion inhibited by monoclonal antibody to murine scavenger receptor. Nature 1993;364:343–346.
9. Platt N, Suzuki H, Kurihara Y, Kodama T, Gordon S. Role for the class A macrophage scavenger receptor in the phagocytosis of apoptotic thymocytes in vitro. Proc Natl Acad Sci USA 1996; 93:12456–12460.
10. Terpstra V, Kondratenko N, Steinberg D. Macrophages lacking scavenger receptor A show a decrease in binding and uptake of acetylated low-density lipoprotein and of apoptotic thymocytes, but not of oxidatively damaged red blood cells. Proc Natl Acad Sci USA 1997; 94:8127–8131.
11. Krieger M, Herz J. Structure and functions of multiligand lipoprotein receptors: macrophage scavenger receptors and LDL receptor-related proteins. Annu Rev Biochem 1994;63:601–637.
12. Matsumoto A, Naito M, Itakura H, Ikemoto S, Asaoka H, Hayakawa I et al. Human macrophage scavenger receptors: primary structure, expression, and localization in atherosclerotic lesions. Proc Natl Acad Sci USA 1990;87:9133–9137.

13. Naito M, Suzuki H, Mori T, Matsumoto A, Kodama T, Takahashi K. Coexpression of type I and type II human macrophage scavenger receptors in macrophages of various organs and foam cells in atherosclerotic lesions. Am J Pathol 1992;141:591—599.
14. Ylä-Herttuala S. Expression of lipoprotein receptors and related molecules in atherosclerotic lesions. Curr Opin Lipid 1996;7:292—297.
15. Sakai M, Miyazaki A, Hakamata H, Kodama T, Suzuki H, Kobori S, Schichiri M, Horiuchi S. The scavenger receptor serves as a route for internalization of lysophosphatidylcholine in oxidized low density lipoprotein-induced macrophage proliferation. J Biol Chem 1996:271; 27346—27352.
16. Kozarsky KF, Donahee MH, Rigotti A, Iqbal SN, Edelman ER, Krieger M. Overexpression of the HDL receptor SR-BI alters plasma HDL and bile cholesterol levels. Nature 1997;387: 414—417.

Lipoprotein oxidation in human atherosclerosis

R. Stocker[1], J.M. Upston[1], X. Niu[1], A.C. Terentis[1], V. Zammit[1], L.J. Hazell[1], S. Fu[2] and R.T. Dean[2]

[1]*Biochemistry and* [2]*Cell Biology Groups, The Heart Research Institute, Camperdown, Australia*

Abstract. Intimal oxidation of low-density lipoprotein (LDL) may contribute to atherogenesis, although the nature of the in vivo oxidant(s) and the extent of oxidative modification of the lipid and protein moieties of lesion LDL remain largely unknown. Control human arteries and advanced carotid plaque samples were examined for the presence of vitamin E and "markers" for specific protein and lipid oxidation. Advanced lesions contain active myeloperoxidase and hypochlorite-modified proteins, as well as elevated levels of hydroxyvaline, DOPA, hydroxyleucine, ortho- and meta-tyrosine (i.e., markers of hydroxyl radical-induced damage). Early lesions present in control vessels also contain hypochlorite-modified proteins. In advanced lesions, a great proportion of the lipids are oxidised, yet the levels of vitamin E are normal. Preliminary results indicate that in such lesions oxidation products of cholesteryl linoleate show geometrical specificity, suggestive of their formation having taken place in the presence of vitamin E, by either enzymic or nonenzymic reactions. These results indicate that different types of protein damage may occur at different developmental stages of atherogenesis, and that oxidation of most plaque cholesteryl linoleate may not be the result of vitamin E deficiency.

Keywords: atherosclerosis, hydroxyl radical, hypochlorite, vitamin E.

Introduction

Oxidation of low-density lipoprotein (LDL) in the arterial intimal space is widely believed to participate in the process of atherogenesis [1,2], although the nature of the in vivo oxidant(s) and the extent of oxidative modification of the lipid and protein moieties of lesion LDL remain largely unknown. The presence of "markers" specific for particular oxidation pathways may be used to gain information on the nature of oxidants involved. For example, stereospecific lipid oxidation products of 15-lipoxygenase have been reported to be present in early stages of human atherogenesis [3]. This, the presence of 15-lipoxygenase mRNA and protein in lesions [4], together with the fact that 15-lipoxygenase can oxidise LDL in vitro [5], that transfer of the 15-lipoxygenase gene into rabbit iliac arteries results in the appearance of lipid-protein adducts characteristic of oxidised LDL [6], and that a specific inhibitor of 15-lipoxygenase inhibits atherosclerosis in rabbits [7], suggest that 15-lipoxygenase contributes to LDL oxidation early in atherogenesis. However, the above stereospecificity in lipid oxidation product is no longer observed in intermediate and advanced stages of atherogenesis [8], sug-

---

Address for correspondence: Dr Roland Stocker, Biochemistry Group, The Heart Research Institute, 145 Missenden Road, Camperdown NSW 2050, Australia.

476

gesting that additional oxidative pathways may also be important. Here we review evidence for the presence of such additional oxidative pathways, and discuss the extent of oxidative modification of lesion LDL in light of antioxidant intervention strategies.

Protein oxidation in human atherosclerosis

Heinecke et al. [9,10] recently reported elevated levels of dityrosine and 3-chlorotyrosine in early lesions obtained from postmortem aortic specimens that contained different stages of atherosclerosis, including advanced lesions. Both markers (Fig. 1) are thought to be specific for myeloperoxidase-derived tyrosyl radical and/or hypochlorite [9,10]. In further support of an involvement of myeloperoxidase as a relevant oxidant in atherogenesis, the protein and enzymic activity are present in human lesions [11]. Furthermore, hypochlorite-modified proteins are present in early, intermediate and advanced human lesions [12] with some of such modified protein being present in an apolipoprotein B-100-rich density fraction prepared from plaque [12]. In vitro hypochlorite-modified LDL can cause lipid accumulation when added to peritoneal mouse [13] and human macrophages (Hazell et al., unpublished). Importantly, this type of oxidative modification of LDL, which is largely directed to apolipoprotein B-100, has no requirement for lipid oxidation [13,14], and is unaffected by α-tocopherol (α-TOH) [15]. In contrast, tyrosyl radical-induced oxidation of LDL [16] is affected and, in fact can be mediated by α-TOH. Thus, LDL devoid of α-TOH is resistant to tyrosyl radical-induced oxidation and replenishment while the vitamin restores the "oxidisability" of the lipoprotein [17].

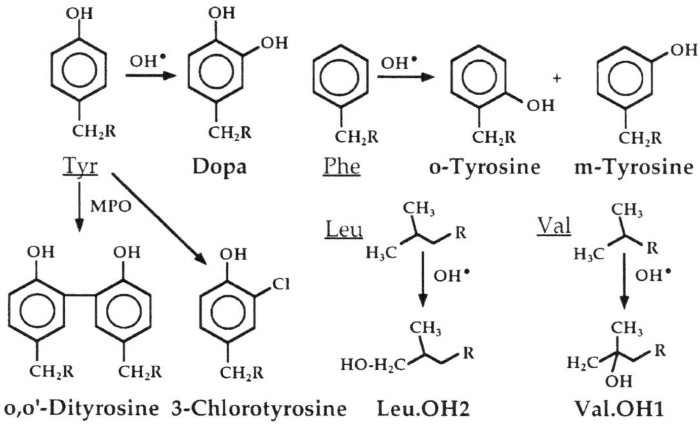

Fig. 1. Selected reaction pathways for the oxidation of protein-bound tyrosine, phenylalanine, valine and leucine by myeloperoxidase (MPO) and hydroxyl radical (OH•). Parent amino acid residues are underlined and the respective oxidation products given in bold. Leu.OH2, 4-hydroxyleucine; Val.OH1, 3-hydroxyvaline.

Advanced human carotid plaque also contains elevated levels of protein-bound DOPA, ortho- and meta-tyrosine, hydroxyleucine and hydroxyvaline when compared with control iliac arteries [18] (Fu et al., unpublished). Like other markers, these markers for hydroxyl radical-induced protein oxidation (Fig. 1) are conveniently expressed per respective parent amino acid, thereby allowing comparison with control and other diseased tissues. In apparent contrast to dityrosine and hypochlorite-modified proteins, the levels of ortho- and metatyrosine in postmortem aortic samples have been reported to be comparable in normal arteries vs. early and intermediate lesions [10] (Fig. 2). This has been interpreted by Heinecke et al. [10] as evidence for a preferential involvement of tyrosyl radical/hypochlorite during the early stages of atherogenesis. Together, these results suggest that different types of protein damage may occur at different developmental stages of atherogenesis.

Despite extensive literature documenting the presence of large quantities and different types of oxidised lipids in atherosclerotic lesions, the extent of oxidative modification of lipids in intimal LDL remains largely unknown. Such knowledge

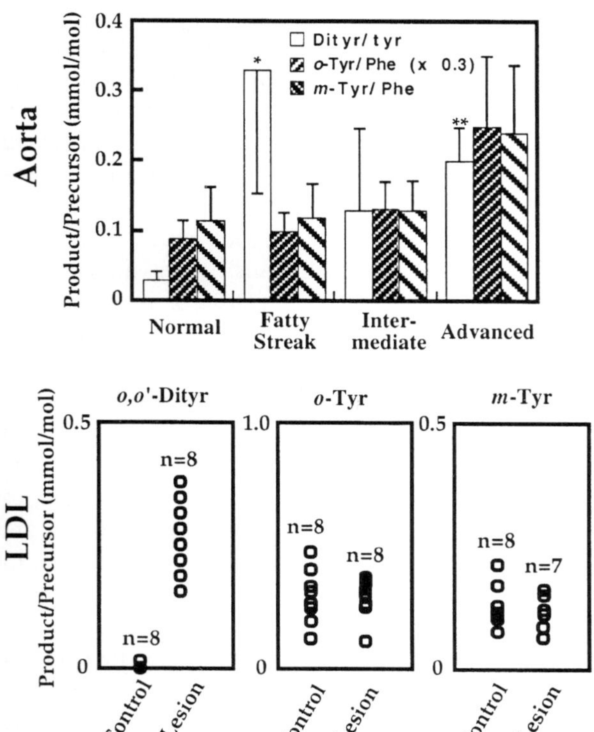

Fig. 2. Evidence for the preferential accumulation of o,o′-dityrosine in LDL of early atherosclerotic lesions. Adapted from [10].

is important, however, as different strategies may be chosen to attempt to prevent lipid (per)oxidation, depending on the degree of LDL oxidation. It is generally thought that formation of "high-uptake" LDL recognised by the scavenger receptor occurs only after depletion of LDL's α-TOH. This holds true for hydroxyl radicals [19] and probably other one-electron oxidants, but not necessarily for the nucleophilic (two-electron) oxidant hypochlorite [13]. Steinbrecher and Lougheed have demonstrated [20] that LDL isolated from postmortem human aorta with advanced lesions is not recognised by the scavenger receptor, although such lipoproteins contained oxidised protein and lipids and are taken up by mouse peritoneal macrophages more avidly than native LDL isolated from blood. These results suggest that in vivo oxidation of intimal LDL may not proceed beyond α-TOH depletion, and may be less than that achieved by the commonly used in vitro exposure of LDL to high concentrations and nonphysiological forms of copper.

Lipid peroxidation in human atherosclerosis

Determining the content of α-TOH in human necropsy samples of normal arterial wall and of atherosclerotic lesions, Carpenter et al. [21] reported that the ratio of α-TOH to cholesterol levels varies widely in normal arteries but is consistently low in lesions, especially those rich in macrophage foam cells. Studies from our laboratories [22] showed the presence of α-tocopheryl quinone (an oxidation product of α-TOH in advanced plaque) in support of oxidative activity in the lesion leading to oxidation of LDL's α-TOH. However, the ratio of unesterified to esterified cholesterol is increased substantially in human lesions when compared to plasma or LDL [21], and fatty acid moieties that contain bisallylic hydrogen(s) are more readily oxidised than cholesterol. Thus, expressing α-TOH per cholesteryl esters, particularly cholesteryl linoleate (Ch18:2 is the single most abundant, readily oxidisable lipid in human lipoproteins and atherosclerotic lesions) may be more relevant. It has been shown [22] that 10–15% of Ch18:2 is oxidised and contains either fatty acyl hydroxides, ketones, or hydroperoxides in homogenates prepared from advanced human plaque using conditions optimised for antioxidant recovery and minimal inadvertent oxidation. Despite this, however, the levels of α-TOH remain intact or even elevated when expressed per Ch18:2 and compared with LDL derived from plasma [22]. Similar results are obtained with apolipoprotein B-100-containing density fractions prepared from advanced carotid plaques (Zammit et al, unpublished), suggesting that there is no gross deficiency of α-TOH at the most advanced stage of atherogenesis.

A limitation of the assessment of human material is that it only provides a snapshot of information on what is a series of complicated and time-dependent processes. For example, the coexistence of both oxidised lipids and apparently normal levels of α-TOH in plaque may be the result of lipid peroxidation occurring at a time where the vitamin was deficient, with the lipid oxidation products remaining in the intima until α-TOH is replenished. However, α-TOH controls

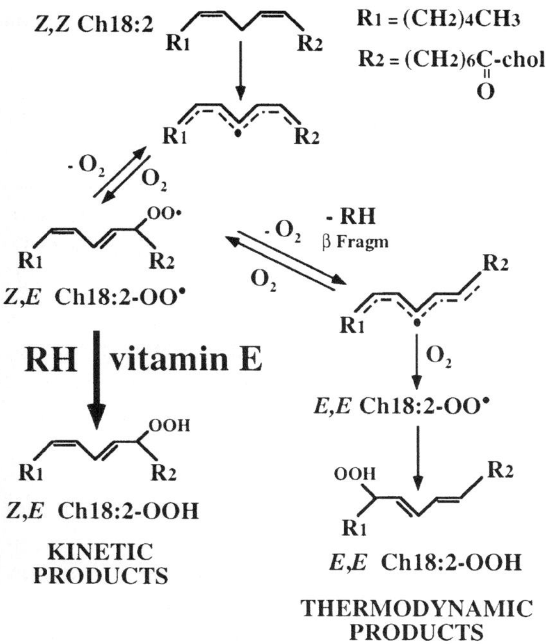

Fig. 3. Nonenzymic oxidation of cholesterol linoleate (Ch18:2). Cis,trans (Z,E) regioisomers predominate in the presence of strong H-donors (RH) such as vitamin E. In the absence of RH, $-fragmentation ($ Fragm) of the initially formed Ch18:2 peroxyl radical (Ch18:2-OO•) occurs to yield the thermodynamically more stable trans,trans (E,E) products of Ch18:2 hydroperoxides (Ch18:2-OOH). For simplicity reasons, distinction between formation of the 13- and 9-Ch18:2-OOH is not made. Chol: cholesterol moiety of cholesterol linoleate.

the pattern of the primary oxidation products of Ch18:2 formed in LDL exposed in vitro to nonenzymic, free radical-induced oxidation [23,24] (Fig. 3): during the α-TOH-containing period of oxidation, the kinetic products, i.e., the cis,trans (or Z,E) regioisomers of Ch18:2 hydroperoxides, predominate over the thermodynamically preferred trans,trans (or E,E) isomers. Once α-TOH is consumed, (E,E) Ch18:2 hydroperoxides accumulate at increased rates [24]. Therefore, we propose that determination of the Z,E to E,E ratio of Ch18:2 hydro(pero)xides in lesion materials may provide direct information on whether lipid oxidation occurs largely in the presence or absence of α-TOH. Indeed, preliminary results obtained with carotid plaque indicate that even in the most advanced stages of atherogenesis, a majority of the oxidised Ch18:2 show Z,E geometry (Table 1), suggesting that these oxidised lipids were formed predominantly in the presence of α-TOH. Also, carotid plaque appears to contain similar concentrations of 9- and 13-(Z,E) Ch18:2 hydroperoxide isomers, indicating that nonenzymic, free radical-induced reactions contribute significantly to this type of intimal lipid oxidation.

480

Table 1. Distribution of regioisomers of cholesteryl linoleate hydroperoxides in advanced human carotid plaques.

Sample	n	Z,E:E,E	Z,E:total[a]	13-(Z,E):9-(E,Z)
Plaque homogenate	8	1.8 ± 0.4	64.6 ± 5.3	1.1 ± 0.2

Plaques were obtained from patients undergoing carotid endarterectomy and frozen at $-80°C$ until analysis. Following thawing, plaques were homogenised [22], the homogenate extracted using acidified methanol and hexane, and the hexane phase analysed for regioisomers of Ch18:2 hydroxides (derived from the corresponding hydroperoxides after reduction of the samples with borohydride) by HPLC, as described previously [24]. [a]Z,E refers to the sum of 13Z,E plus 9E,Z, expressed as a percentage of the total, i.e., trans,trans plus cis,trans isomers of 13- and 9-Ch18:2 hydroxides.

Conclusions

There is growing evidence that intimal (lipo)proteins are exposed to different types of oxidants at different stages of atherogenesis. Presently available information suggests a role for myeloperoxidase in oxidative alterations to proteins occurring during the early stages of the disease, whereas at the more advanced stages, hydroxyl radicals/transition metals also appear to contribute to protein oxidation. There is also increasing evidence that 15-lipoxygenase and nonenzymic, free radical-induced processes contribute to intimal lipid (per)oxidation. The coexistence of Z,E oxidised lipids and α-TOH in intimal lipids may reflect lipid peroxidation proceeding in the presence of vitamin E. The latter can be explained mechanistically by tocopherol-mediated peroxidation, a process where α-TOH alone fails to prevent lipoprotein lipid peroxidation [25], if suitable reductants for α-tocopheroxyl radical are lacking [26], and intimal LDL experiences a low incidence of radical hits [25,27]. Recent studies indicate that tocopherol-mediated peroxidation can, to a greater or lesser extent, explain lipoprotein lipid peroxidation induced by different radical (though not nucleophilic) oxidants [17]. Therefore, rather than employing a single antioxidant, such as vitamin E, the restriction/prevention of intimal lipoprotein lipid and protein oxidation is likely to require a combination of different antioxidants, including inhibitors of tocopherol-mediated peroxidation, myeloperoxidase and 15-lipoxygenase.

Acknowledgements

This work was supported by the Australian National Heart Foundation Grant 94S4061.

References

1. Steinberg D, Parthasarathy S, Carew TE, Khoo JC, Witztum JL. Beyond cholesterol: modifications of low-density lipoprotein that increase its atherogenicity. N Engl J Med 1989;320:

915—924.

2. Berliner JA, Heinecke JW. The role of oxidized lipoproteins in atherogenesis. Free Radic Biol Med 1996;20:707—727.

3. Kühn H, Heydeck D, Hogou I, Gniwotta C. In vivo action of 15-lipoxygenase in early stages of human atherogenesis. J Clin Invest 1997;99:888—893.

4. Ylä-Herttuala S, Rosenfeld ME, Parthasarathy S, Sigal E, Sarkioja T, Witztum JL, Steinberg D. Gene expression in macrophage-rich human atherosclerotic lesions. 15-lipoxygenase and acetyl low-density lipoprotein receptor messenger RNA colocalize with oxidation specific lipid-protein adducts. J Clin Invest 1991;87:1146—1152.

5. Sparrow CP, Parthasarathy S, Steinberg D. Enzymatic modification of low-density lipoprotein by purified lipoxygenase plus phospholipase A2 mimics cell-mediated oxidative modification. J Lipid Res 1988;29:745—753.

6. Ylä-Herttuala S, Luoma J, Viita H, Hiltunen T, Sisto T, Nikkari T. Transfer of 15-lipoxygenase gene into rabbit iliac arteries results in the appearance of oxidation-specific lipid-protein adducts characteristic of oxidized low-density lipoprotein. J Clin Invest 1995;95:2692—2698.

7. Sendobry SM, Cornicelli JA, Welch K, Bocan T, Tait B, Trivedi BK, Colbry N, Dyer RD, Feinmark SJ, Daugherty A. Attenuation of diet-induced atherosclerosis in rabbits with a highly selective 15-lipoxygenase inhibitor lacking significant antioxidant properties. Br J Pharmacol 1997; 120:1199—1206.

8. Kuhn H, Belkner J, Zaiss S, Fahrenklemper T, Wohlfeil S. Involvement of 15-lipoxygenase in early stages of atherogenesis. J Exp Med 1994;179:1903—1911.

9. Hazen SL, Heinecke JW. 3-Chlorotyrosine, a specific marker of myeloperoxidase-catalyzed oxidation, is markedly elevated in low-density lipoprotein isolated from human atherosclerotic intima. J Clin Invest 1997;99:2075—2081.

10. Leeuwenburgh C, Rasmussen JE, Hsu FF, Mueller DM, Pennathur S, Heinecke JW. Mass spectrometric quantification of markers for protein oxidation by tyrosyl radical, copper, and hydroxyl radical in low-density lipoprotein isolated from human atherosclerotic plaques. J Biol Chem 1997;272:3520—3526.

11. Daugherty A, Dunn JL, Rateri DL, Heinecke JW. Myeloperoxidase, a catalyst for lipoprotein oxidation, is expressed in human atherosclerotic lesions. J Clin Invest 1994;94:437—444.

12. Hazell LJ, Arnold L, Flowers D, Waeg G, Malle E, Stocker R. Presence of hypochlorite-modified proteins in human atherosclerotic lesions. J Clin Invest 1996;97:1535—1544.

13. Hazell LJ, Stocker R. Oxidation of low-density lipoprotein with hypochlorite causes transformation of the lipoprotein into a high-uptake form for macrophages. Biochem J 1993;290:165—172.

14. Hazell LJ, van den Berg JJM, Stocker R. Oxidation of low-density lipoprotein by hypochlorite causes aggregation that is mediated by modification of lysine residues rather than lipid oxidation. Biochem J 1994;302:297—304.

15. Hazell LJ, Stocker R. α-Tocopherol does not inhibit hypochlorite-induced oxidation of apolipoprotein B-100 of low-density lipoprotein. FEBS Lett 1997;(In press).

16. Savenkova ML, Mueller DM, Heinecke JW. Tyrosyl radical generated by myeloperoxidase is a physiological catalyst for the initiation of lipid peroxidation in low-density lipoprotein. J Biol Chem 1994;269:20394—20400.

17. Witting PK, Upston JM, Stocker R. The molecular action of α-tocopherol in lipoprotein lipid peroxidation: pro- and antioxidant activity of vitamin E in complex heterogeneous lipid emulsions. In: Quinn P, Kagan V (eds) Subcellular Biochemistry: Fat-soluble Vitamins. London: Plenum Press, 1997;(In press).

18. Dean RT, Fu S, Stocker R, Davies MJ. Biochemistry and pathology of radical-mediated protein oxidation. Biochem J 1997;324:1—18.

19. Bedwell S, Dean RT, Jessup W. The action of defined oxygen-centered free radicals on human low-density lipoproteins. Biochem J 1989;262:707—712.

20. Steinbrecher UP, Lougheed M. Scavenger receptor-independent stimulation of cholesterol esterification in macrophages by low-density lipoprotein extracted from human aortic intima. Arter-

ioscl Thromb 1992;12:608—625.

21. Carpenter KL, Cheeseman KH, van der Veen C, Taylor SE, Walker MK, Mitchinson MJ. Depletion of alpha-tocopherol in human atherosclerotic lesions. Free Radic Res 1995;23:549—558.
22. Suarna C, Dean RT, May J, Stocker R. Human atherosclerotic plaque contains both oxidized lipids and relatively large amounts of α-tocopherol and ascorbate. Arterioscl Thromb Vasc Biol 1995;15:1616—1624.
23. Kenar JA, Havrilla CM, Porter NA, Guyton JR, Brown SA, Klemp KF, Selinger E. Identification and quantification of the regioisomeric cholesteryl linoleate hydroperoxides in oxidized human low-density lipoprotein and high-density lipoprotein. Chem Res Toxicol 1996;9: 737—744.
24. Upston JM, Neuzil J, Stocker R. Oxidation of LDL by recombinant human 15-lipoxygenase: evidence for α-tocopherol-dependent oxidation of esterified core and surface lipids. J Lipid Res 1996;37:2650—2661.
25. Bowry VW, Stocker R. Tocopherol-mediated peroxidation. The pro-oxidant effect of vitamin E on the radical-initiated oxidation of human low-density lipoprotein. J Am Chem Soc 1993; 115:6029—6044.
26. Bowry VW, Mohr D, Cleary J, Stocker R. Prevention of tocopherol-mediated peroxidation of ubiquinol-10-free human low-density lipoprotein. J Biol Chem 1995;270:5756—5763.
27. Neuzil J, Thomas SR, Stocker R. Requirement for promotion, or inhibition by α-tocopherol of radical-induced initiation of plasma lipoprotein lipid peroxidation. Free Radic Biol Med 1997;22:57—71.

Macrophages, LDL oxidation and atherosclerosis

Michael Aviram
Lipid Research Laboratory, Technion Faculty of Medicine, Rappaport Family Institute for Research in the Medical Sciences; and Rambam Medical Center, Haifa, Israel

Keywords: antioxidants, foam cells, HDL, lipid peroxidation, lipoproteins, paraoxonase, polyphenols.

LDL oxidation in the arterial wall is considered to be a key event during early atherogenesis, and all major cells in the arterial wall (endothelial cells, smooth muscle cells and macrophages) were shown to be able to oxidize LDL [1−3]. At an early stage of atherogenesis, macrophages play an important role in LDL oxidation. At this stage macrophage foam cell formation is characterized by the accumulation of ceroids which are oxidized cholesteryl-ester derivatives.

Cell-mediated oxidation of LDL depends on the oxidative state of both the lipoprotein and the cells. Therefore we analyzed the effect of pro-oxidants and antioxidants in the lipoprotein particle, as well as in the macrophages, on the oxidation of LDL (Fig. 1).

LDL-associated pro-oxidants and antioxidants

LDL, the major cholesterol carrier in human plasma, mainly contains polyunsaturated fatty acids in its cholesteryl ester (which are prone to oxidation) such as linoleic acid (C-18:2) and arachidonic acid (C-20:4). In hypercholesterolemic patients we have previously shown that the enhanced susceptibility of their LDL to oxidation is also related to increased levels of arachidonic acid in their lipoprotein cholesteryl ester moiety. Similarly, LDL from subjects supplemented with fish oil, which is rich in w-3 polyunsaturated fatty acids, showed a 2-fold increased susceptibility to oxidation. There was no significant alteration in the content of the LDL-associated antioxidant vitamins A, E and β-carotene. Thus, the pro-oxidative effect of fish oil ingestion must be taken into account whenever supplementing fish oil to the diet.

The monounsaturated fatty acid oleic acid (C-18:1), unlike the polyunsaturated fatty acids, was found to possess antioxidant properties. We tested the effect of olive oil supplementation (50 g/day) to the diet of 10 healthy male subjects, dur-

---

Address for correspondence: Prof Michael Aviram, Lipid Research Laboratory, Rambam Medical Center, Haifa 31096, Israel. Tel.: +972-4-8528986. Fax: +972-4-8542130.
E-mail: aviram@tx.technion.ac.il

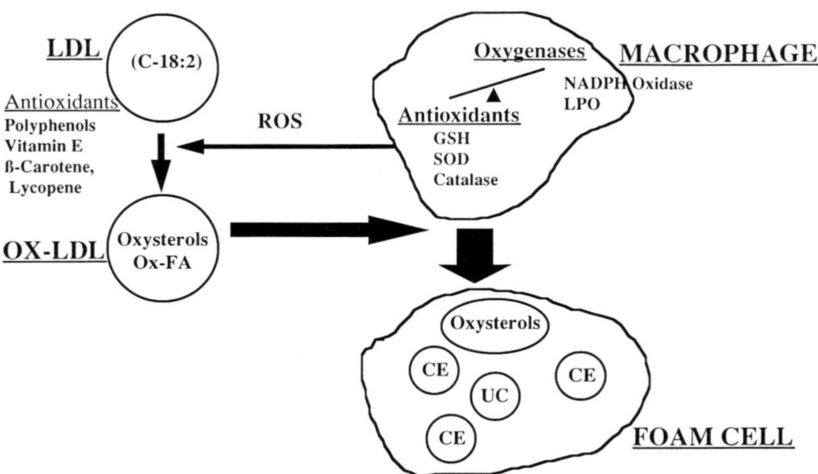

Fig. 1. The effect of the oxidative state of LDL and of macrophages on cell-mediated oxidation of LDL. C-18:2 = linoleic acid; Ox-FA = oxidized fatty acids; CE = cholesteryl ester; UC = unesterified cholesterol; GSH = glutathione; SOD = superoxide dismutase; and LPO = lipoxygenase.

ing a 2-week period, on the propensity of their LDL to oxidation. Olive oil supplementation to the diet modified the LDL lipid composition, and enriched the lipoprotein with oleic acid and with sitosterol. The olive-oil-induced modified lipoprotein was found to be resistant to in vitro peroxidation and showed reduced uptake by macrophages [4].

The LDL particle is protected from oxidation by several antioxidants which are associated to the lipoprotein (vitamin E, β-carotene, lycopene, ubiquinol and several lipophilic polyphenols), as well as by antioxidants in the LDL plasma environment (vitamin C, uric acid, albumin and several hydrophilic polyphenols). The carotenoids are lipid soluble antioxidants which are located in the core of the LDL.

We have previously shown [5—8] that both the all-trans and the 9-cis isomers of β-carotene can bind to plasma lipoproteins and affect LDL oxidation, with the all-trans isomer of β-carotene being more effective than the 9-cis isomer in inhibiting the susceptibility of the lipoproteins to lipid peroxidation and in reducing the cellular uptake of the oxidized LDL by macrophages. Furthermore, in healthy subjects we have demonstrated an inhibitory effect on the susceptibility of LDL to oxidative modification by both of these isomers of β-carotene. However, we found that not all subjects responded to β-carotene supplementation by inhibition of ex vivo LDL oxidation. Comparison of the antioxidant status in "responder" and "nonresponder" LDLs, revealed that the vitamin E content in the "responder LDLs" was significantly higher than that found in the "nonresponder LDLs". We thus analyzed the effect of carotenoids in combination with vitamin E, on the susceptibility of LDL to copper-ions-induced oxidation. A synergistic antioxidative effect against LDL oxidation was obtained when a combination of the carotenoids together with vitamin E was used, instead of using the individual antioxidants separately. Recently, we have also analyzed the antioxidative capabilities of lycopene against LDL oxidation. We have demonstrated a protective effect of tomato's lycopene against oxidative modification of LDL. This LDL protection by lycopene exceeded the protection exhibited by β-carotene, was selective only to LDLs with high vitamin E content and was shown when the carotenoids were present in combination with vitamin E, but not when the carotenoids were supplemented alone. Supplementation of vitamin E alone (25 μg/muse/day for 3 months) to the apolipoprotein E deficient (E$^\circ$) mice was found to be a potent antioxidant against LDL oxidation and also reduced the lesion size by 35% [9].

Polyphenolic flavonoids are most potent antioxidants. In olive oil, hydroxytyrosol was shown to contribute to the inhibitory effect on LDL oxidation (in addition to a major effect of the oleic acid). Other nutrient sources for polyphenols include licorice root ethanolic extract (rich with the isoflavan glabridin), red wine (rich with the flavonol quercetin and the flavanol catechin), ginger, and orange peels [4,10–13].

The Asian plant Licorice is a source of polyphenols antioxidants with the isoflavane glabridin being the major one.

In humans, licorice root ethanolic extract was shown to inhibit LDL oxidation in a dose-dependent manner. The mechanism responsible for the antioxidative effects of licorice and glabridin was shown to involve free radicals scavenging capacity. LDL isolated from the plasma of 10 normolipidemic subjects who were supplemented for a period of 2 weeks with 100 mg of licorice extract per day, was more resistant to copper-ions-induced oxidation, as well as to AAPH-induced oxidation, by 44 and 36%, respectively (in comparison to LDL isolated before licorice supplementation). In E$^\circ$ mice, dietary supplementation of licorice (200 μg/day/mouse), or of pure glabridin (20 μg/day/mouse), for 6 weeks resulted in 68 and 22% reduction in the susceptibility of their LDL to copper-ions-induced oxidation, respectively, and also resulted in a significant reduction in the atherosclerotic lesion area. These results show that glabridin, the polyphenol with lipophilic characteristics which is present in licorice ethanolic extract, is absorbed, binds to the LDL particle, and subsequently protects the LDL from oxidation in multiple modes of oxidative stress, as shown in humans and in the E$^\circ$ mice [12,13].

The effect of consuming red wine (11% alcohol) with meals, on the propensity of plasma and LDL to lipid peroxidation was studied in 17 healthy men. Red wine consumption reduced the propensity of the volunteers LDL to lipid peroxidation (in response to copper ions) as determined by a 46, 72 and 54% decrement in the content of the lipoprotein-associated aldehydes, lipid peroxides, and conjugated dienes, respectively, as well as by a substantial prolongation of the lag phase required for the initiation of LDL oxidation [10]. The antioxidant effect of dietary red wine on plasma lipid peroxidation was not secondary to changes

486

in plasma vitamin E or β-carotene content, but could be related to the elevation in polyphenol concentrations in plasma and LDL. Thus, some phenolic substances that exist in red wine are absorbed, bind to plasma LDL, and thus could be responsible for the antioxidant properties of red wine.

In E° mice that were supplemented with 50 μg of polyphenols/day/mouse for 6 weeks, plasma LDL isolated after red wine or quercetin, was less susceptible (30—80%) to oxidation induced by either copper ions, or by the free radical initiator 2,2′-azobis 2-amidinopropane hydrochloride (AAPH), or by J-774 A.1 macrophages in culture, in comparison to LDL isolated from a placebo E° mice group [11].

Cellular uptake of E° mice LDL that was derived after catechin, quercetin or red wine consumption was found to be reduced, by 31, 40 and 52%, respectively, in comparison to the cellular uptake of LDL derived from the placebo group. In agreement with these results, we found that the atherosclerotic lesions areas in E° mice that were treated with red wine, quercetin or catechin were significantly reduced, by 40, 38 and 32%, in comparison to the lesion areas in E° mice treated with placebo. We thus conclude that dietary consumption by E° mice, of red wine or of its polyphenolic flavonoids quercetin, and to a lesser extent catechin, leads to reduced susceptibility of their LDLs to oxidation and to attenuation in the development of atherosclerosis [11].

Macrophage-associated pro-oxidants and antioxidants

LDL oxidation is affected not only by the lipoprotein oxidative state (pro- vs. anti-LDL-associated oxidants). Macrophage-mediated oxidation of LDL is considerably affected also by the oxidative state in the cells. This oxidative state depends on the balance between cellular oxygenases and macrophage-associated antioxidants. Macrophage binding of LDL initiates the activation of cellular oxygenases.

LDL oxidation by arterial wall cells (a key event during early atherogenesis) was suggested to involve the activation of macrophage 15-lipoxygenase and of nicotinamide adenine dinucleotide phosphate (NADPH) oxidase. We sought to analyze the role of these oxygenases in macrophage-mediated oxidation of LDL under oxidative stress. Upon incubation of LDL with the J-774 A.1 macrophage-like cell line or with human monocyte-derived macrophages (HMDM) in the presence of 1 μM $CuSO_4$, the release of superoxide anions to the medium was demonstrated.

Under these conditions, the cytosolic protein components of the NADPH oxidase complex, P-47 and P-67, translocated to the plasma membrane, indicating LDL-mediated activation of the NADPH oxidase complex [14]. Under the above-mentioned experimental conditions, macrophage 15-lipoxygenase was also activated, as determined by the release of 15-hydroxy-5,8,11,13-eicosatetrenoic acid (15-HETE) and 13-hydroxyoctadecadienoic acid (13-HODE) to the medium. Inhibition of the macrophage NADPH oxidase with apocynin or dismutation of superoxide anions, the product of NADPH oxidase activation, with superoxide dismutase (SOD), significantly inhibited macrophage-mediated oxidation of LDL (by 61 to 89%, respectively) under these conditions. Phorbol myristate acetate (PMA), which causes NADPH oxidase activation in J-774 A.1 macrophages, had no significant effect on 15-lipoxygenase activity, but still resulted in cell-mediated oxidation of LDL. Finally, HMDM from two patients with chronic granulomatous disease (CGD) that were shown to lack active NADPH oxidase, but to possess almost normal 15-lipoxygenase activity, failed to oxidize LDL. We thus conclude that LDL-induced NADPH oxidase activation (under oxidative stress) is required for macrophage-mediated oxidation of LDL, whereas activation of 15-lipoxygenase may not be sufficient for LDL oxidation under these conditions [14]. On using J-774 A.1 macrophages, we have demonstrated that phospholipase A_2 as well as phospholipase D are involved in macrophage NADPH oxidase-mediated oxidation of LDL. Furthermore, the products of these phospholipases, arachidonic acid and phosphatidic acid (respectively) can induce NADPH oxidase activation, followed by cell-mediated oxidation of LDL. This LDL oxidation was shown to be dependent on extracellular calcium ions. We conclude that phospholipases A_2 and D can induce macrophage NADPH oxidase-dependent oxidation of LDL, and thus can contribute to the formation of atherogenic oxidized lipoprotein [15].

Macrophage-mediated oxidation of LDL can result also from an initial peroxidation of the cell lipids. When cultured macrophages were exposed to ferrous ions (50 μM $FeSO_4$) for 4 h at 37°C, cellular lipid peoxidation (measured by analyses of malondialdehyde (MDA), conjugated dienes (CD), and lipid peroxides (PD)), increased by 2- to 4-fold in comparison with nontreated cells. Incubation of LDL (0.2 mg of protein/ml) with these oxidized macrophages resulted in LDL lipids peroxidation, as evidenced by an 8-fold increase in LDL-associated MDA, in comparison with LDL that was incubated under similar conditions with nonoxidized macrophages. Furthermore, oxidation of LDL by macrophages that were oxidized by incubation with deoxycholic acid (DCA) or angiotensin II (ANG-II) can also induce oxidative modification of macrophages, via metal ion-independent mechanisms. Incubation of LDL (200 μg of protein/ml) for 24 h at 37°C with DCA, ANG-II or with $FeSO_4$-induced oxidized macrophages, resulted in a substantial oxidative modification of the lipoprotein. The oxidative modification of LDL by oxidized macrophages was found to be a progressive process. Incubation of LDL with oxidized macrophages for increasing periods of time (up to 24 h) resulted in a progressive increment of the electrophoretic mobility of LDL, the MDA formation in LDL, and the cellular uptake of LDL by the oxidized macrophages via the Ox-LDL receptor. The increased uptake of LDL by oxidized macrophages thus results from two routes including enhanced uptake via the LDL receptor due to increased LDL receptor activity in oxidized macrophages, and enhanced lipoprotein uptake via the Ox-LDL receptor [16—19].

As macrophage antioxidants may also contribute to the extent of cell-mediated oxidation of LDL, and since the glutathione is an important antioxidant system we analyzed the role of cellular reduced glutathione (GSH) content and of glutathione peroxidase (GPx) activity in this process [20]. Upon incubation of J-774 A.1 macrophages for 20 h at 37°C with 50 µM of buthionine sulfoximine (BSO) (an inhibitor of glutathione synthesis) cellular GSH content and GPx activity were reduced by 89 and 50%, respectively. This effect was associated with a 2-fold elevation in macrophage-mediated oxidation of LDL. The BSO-treated cells contained high levels of peroxides and released 39% more superoxide anions than nontreated cells in response to their stimulation with phorbol myristate acetate. In order to increase macrophage GSH content and GPx activity we have used L-2-oxothiazolidine-4-carboxylic acid (OTC) which delivers cysteine residues to the cells for GSH synthesis, and also selenium which activates GPx and increases cellular glutathione synthesis. GSH content and GPx activity in J-774 A.1 macrophages were increased by 80 and 50%, respectively, following cells incubation with 2 mM OTC for 20 h at 37°C, and this was paralleled by a 47% inhibition in LDL oxidation by these cells. An inverse correlation was found between the extent of macrophage-mediated oxidation of LDL and cellular GSH content (r = 0.97), or GPx activity (r = 0.95). Upon incubation of J-774 A.1 macrophages with selenomethionine (10 ng/ml) for 1 week, cellular GSH content and GPx activity were increased by about 2-fold as compared to control cells, and this effect was associated with a 30% reduction in cell-mediated oxidation of LDL. Dietary selenium supplementation (1 µg/day/mouse) to the atherosclerotic apolipoprotein E deficient mice for a 6 month period, increased GSH content and GPx activity in the mice peritoneal macrophages by 36 and 30%, respectively, and this effect was associated with a 46% reduction in cell-mediated oxidation of LDL. Finally, the atherosclerotic lesion area in the aortas derived from these mice after selenium supplementation was found to be reduced by 30% as compared to the lesion area found in nontreated mice. Our results demonstrate an inverse relationship between macrophage GSH content/GPx activity and cell-mediated oxidation of LDL. Intervention methods to enhance the macrophage GSH-GPx status may thus contribute to attenuation of the atherosclerotic process.

The relationship between the glutathione system and plasma lipid peroxidation in six renal transplanted patients (which are under oxidative stress, and thus at high risk for atherosclerosis), was also studied by using dietary selenium in order to activate the glutathione system. AAPH-induced plasma lipid peroxidation was increased by 60% in all six patients in comparison to normal subjects. Dietary selenium supplementation (0.2 mg/day for a period of 3 months) resulted in a 50% reduction in AAPH-induced plasma lipid peroxidation. The susceptibility of the patients plasma to lipid peroxidation returned toward baseline values 3 months after termination of the selenium treatment. Analyses of the patients red blood cell (RBC) glutathione system revealed low levels of reduced glutathione (GSH) and decreased activity of RBC glutathione peroxidase by 23 and 20%, respectively, in comparison to normal RBC. Selenium treatment resulted in a significant elevation in red blood cells GPx activity and in the GSH content by 64 and 11%, respectively [21].

Next we questioned whether macrophage enrichment with nutritional antioxidants such as β carotene, lycopene, vitamin E, or polyphenolic flavonoids can affect their ability to oxidize LDL. We investigated the effect of dietary supplementation of β-carotene on plasma lipid peroxidation (induced by AAPH) and on cell-mediated oxidation of LDL by human monocyte-derived macrophages (HMDM). Significant enrichment with β-carotene was noted in plasma (2-fold), in LDL (2.6-fold) and in HMDM (1.6-fold) 2 weeks after dietary supplementation with 180 mg/day of β carotene. In these subjects plasma lipids peroxidation decreased by 22% and LDL oxidation decreased by 40% in AAPH-induced oxidation system [7]. After β-carotene supplementation, LDL enrichment, but not enrichment of the cells with β-carotene, significantly reduced LDL oxidation. Thus, we suggest that β-carotene content of LDL, but not that of the macrophages, is responsible for the inhibition of LDL oxidation by the cells. Similarly, enrichment of mouse peritoneal macrophages with lycopene or with β-carotene did not effect cell-mediated oxidation of LDL. On the contrary, upon macrophage enrichment with vitamin E, cell-mediated oxidation of LDL was significantly inhibited. Following 18 h of macrophage incubation with 25 μM of vitamin E, macrophage-mediated oxidation of LDL was reduced by 59%. Similarly, the polyphenols glabridin, catechin or quercetin, accumulated in macrophages upon cell incubation with these purified polyphenols. Upon incubation of these antioxidant-enriched macrophages with native LDL under oxidative stress (1 μM $CuSO_4$), cells enrichment with these antioxidants resulted in up to 70, 45 and 90% inhibition in cell-mediated oxidation of LDL.

Possible mechanisms for the removal of Ox-LDL

The atherogenicity of Ox-LDL involves its stimulatory effect on macrophage cholesterol accumulation, as well as its atherogenic effects on blood and on arterial wall cells. Thus, removal of Ox-LDL from plasma or from the extracellular space, by cells of the arterial wall, may be beneficial as long as it does not cause massive cellular cholesterol accumulation and foam cell formation.

Other mechanisms which can contribute to the elimination of atherogenic Ox-LDL from entering the arterial wall cells are related to the balance among LDL-associated and cell-associated pro-oxidants and antioxidants. In addition, mechanisms for the elimination of Ox-LDL from the extracellular space may include hydrolysis of lipoprotein-associated peroxides (Fig. 2).

Plasma HDL was previously shown to inhibit LDL oxidation but the mechanism for this effect was not elucidated yet. It was suggested that human apolipoprotein A-I may possesses antioxidant properties which might affect LDL lipid peroxidation.

Plasma HDL from both normal mice and from the human apolipoprotein A-I transgenic mice, at similar concentrations, inhibits LDL lipid peroxidation, but

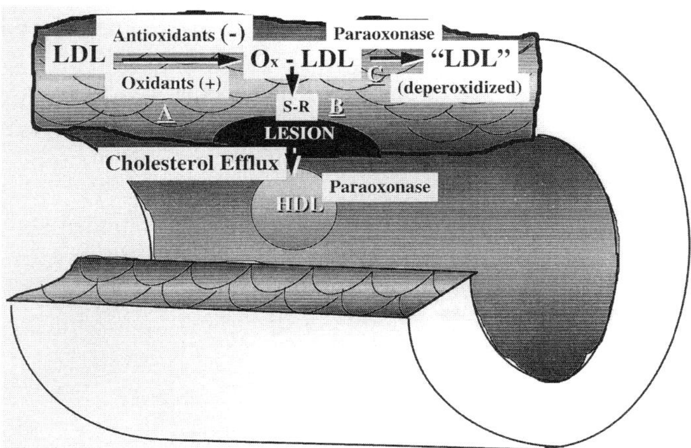

Fig. 2. Formation and elimination of atherogenic oxidized LDL. **A**: Role of oxidants and antioxidants (in the lipoprotein and in the cells). **B**: Role of Ox-LDL removal by cells of the arterial wall. **C**: Role of deperoxidation of Ox-LDL by paraoxonase.

the effect of the HDL from the human apolipoprotein A-I trangenic mice was 2-fold greater than that of HDL derived from control mice [22].

An additional possibility for the inhibitory effect of HDL on LDL oxidation is the presence of the enzyme paraoxonase (PON) in plasma HDL [23,24]. Serum PON activity was shown to be lower in atherosclerotic patients such as patients after myocardial infarction, patients with familial hypercholesterolemia or patients with diabetes mellitus. Although the physio/pathological role of serum PON is not known yet, evidence for a protective effect of PON against oxidative damage was shown.

As PON was suggested to be involved in atherogenesis via an inhibitory effect on lipoprotein oxidation, we have used the apolipoprotein E deficient mice (which develop accelerated atherosclerosis) to analyze the association among the atherosclerosis lesion size, serum lipid peroxidation and serum paraoxonase activity. Whereas both serum lipids peroxidation and the extent of the mice lesion area increased with age, serum PON activity significantly reduced. We next analyzed the effect of HDL-associated PON, as well as of purified PON, on HDL and on LDL oxidation, by using specific PON inhibitors, and could clearly demonstrate a significant inhibitory effect of PON on the oxidation of the lipoproteins in several oxidative systems. Furthermore, HDL-associated PON was found to directly act upon and hydrolyze lipoprotein-associated peroxides mainly in oxidized HDL, but to some extent also on oxidized LDL and hydrogen peroxides. These results suggest that paraoxonase have an important role in the removal of atherogenic oxidized lipoproteins and may thus be considered anti-atherogenic.

References

1. Aviram M. Oxidized low-density lipoprotein (Ox-LDL) interaction with macrophages in atherosclerosis and the antiatherogenicity of antioxidants. Eur J Clin Chem Clin Biochem 1996;34: 599—608.
2. Steinberg D, Parthasarathy S, Carew TE, Khoo JC, Witztum JL. Beyond cholesterol: modifications of low-density lipoprotein that increase its atherogenicity. N Engl J Med 1989;320: 915—924.
3. Berliner JA, Navab M, Fogelman AM, Frank JlS, Demer LL, Edwards PA et al. Atherosclerosis: basic mechanisms, oxidation, inflammation and genetics. Circulation 1995;91:2488—2498.
4. Aviram M, Kasem E. Dietary olive oil reduces the susceptibility of low-density lipoprotein to lipid peroxidation and inhibits lipoprotein uptake by macrophages. Ann Nutr Metabol 1993; 37:75—84.
5. Lavy A, Ben-Amotz A, Aviram M. Preferential inhibition of LDL oxidation by the all-transisomer of -carotene in comparison to the 9-cis-carotene. Eur J Clin Chem Clin Biochem 1993; 31:83—90.
6. Levy Y, Ben-Amotz A, Aviram M. Effect of dietary supplementation of B-carotene to humans on its binding to plasma LDL and on the lipoprotein susceptibility to undergo oxidative modification: comparison of the synthetic all transisomer with the natural algae B-carotene. J Nutr Envir Med 1995;5:13—22.
7. Levy Y, Kaplan M, Ben-Amotz A, Aviram M. The effect of dietary supplementation of β-carotene on human monocyte-macrophage-mediated oxidation of low-density lipoprotein. Isr J Med Sci 1996;32(6):473—478.
8. Fuhrman B, Ben-Yaish L, Attias J, Hayek T, Aviram M. Tomato's lycopene and β-carotene inhibit low-density lipoprotein oxidation and this effect depends on the lipoprotein vitamin E content. Nutr Metab Cardiovasc Dis 1997;7:433—443.
9. Maor I, Hayek T, Coleman R, Aviram M. Plasma LDL oxidation leads to its aggregation in the atherosclerotic apolipoprotein E deficient mice. Arterioscler Thromb Vasc Biol 1997;17: 2995—3001.
10. Fuhrman B, Lavy A, Aviram M. Consumption of red wine with meals reduces the susceptibility of human plasma and low-density lipoprotein to lipid peroxidation. Am J Clin Nutr 1995;61: 549—554.
11. Hayek T, Fuhrman B, Via J, Rosenblat M, Belinki P, Coleman R, Elis A, Aviram M. Reduced progression of atherosclerosis in the apolipoprotein E deficient mice following consumption of red wine, or its polyphenols quercetin, or catechin, is associated with reduced susceptibility of LDL to oxidation and to aggregation. Arterioscler Thromb Vasc Biol 1997;17:2744—2750.
12. Vaya J, Belinki P, Aviram M. Antioxidant constituents from licorice roots: isolation, structure elucidation and antioxidative capacity towards LDL oxidation. Free Radic Biol Med 1997;23: 302—313.
13. Fuhrman B, Buch S, Vaya J, Belinky PA, Coleman R, Hayek T, Aviram M. Licorice etanolic extract and its major polyphenol glabridin protect LDL against lipid peroxidation: in vitro and ex vivo studies in humans and in the atherosclerotic apolipoprotein E deficient mice. Am J Clin Nutr 1997;66:267—275.
14. Aviram M, Rosenblat M, Etzioni A, Levy R. Activation of NADPH oxidase but not of 15-lipoxygenase by low-density lipoprotein (LDL) in the presence of copper ions is required for LDL oxidation by macrophages. Metabolism 1996;45(9):1069—1079.
15. Aviram M, Rosenblat M. Phospholipase A_2 and phospholipase D are involved in macrophage NADPH oxidase-mediated oxidation of LDL. Isr J Med Sci 1996;32:749—756.
16. Fuhrman B, Oiknine J, Aviram M. Iron induces lipid peroxidation in cultured macrophages increases their ability to oxidatively modify LDL and affect their secretory properties. Atherosclerosis 1994;111:65—78.
17. Keidar S, Kaplan M, Hoffman A, Brook JG, Aviram M. Angiotensin II stimulates macrophage-

mediated lipid peroxidation of low-density lipoprotein. Atherosclerosis 1995;115:201—215.

18. Ljubuncic P, Fuhrman B, Oiknine J, Aviram M, Bomzon A. The effect of deoxycholic acid and ursodeoxycholic acid on lipid peroxidation in cultured macrophages. Gut 1996;39:475—478.

19. Fuhrman B, Oiknine J, Keidar S, Kaplan M, Aviram M. Increased uptake of low-density lipoprotein (LDL) by oxidized macrophages is the result of enhanced LDL receptor activity and of progressive LDL oxidation. Free Radic Biol Med 1997;23:34—46.

20. Rosenblat M, Aviram M. Macrophage glutathione content and glutathione peroxidase activity are inversely related to cell-mediated oxidation of LDL. Free Radic Biol Med (In press).

21. Hussein O, Rosenblat M, Refael G, Aviram M. Dietary selenium increases cellular glutahtione peroxidase activity and reduces the enhanced susceptibility to lipid peroxidation of plasma and low-density lipoprotein in kidney transplanted patients. Transplantation 1997;63:679—685.

22. Hayek T, Oiknine J, Dankner G, Brook JG, Aviram M. HDL apolipoprotein A-I attenuates oxidative modification of low-density lipoprotein: studies in transgenic mice. Eur J Clin Chem Clin Biochem 1995;33:721—725.

23. La Du BN. Structural and functional diversity of paraoxonases. Nature 1996;2(11):1186—1187.

24. Mackness MI, Mackness B, Durrington PN, Connelly PW, Hegele RA. Paraoxonase: biochemistry, genetics and relationship to plasma lipoproteins. Curr Opin Lipid 1996;7:69—76.

Elevated homocyst(e)ine increases the ability of human aortic cells to oxidize LDL

Marek Naruszewicz

Regional Center for Atherosclerosis Research, Pomeranian Academy of Medicine, Szczecin, Poland

Abstract. Current evidence indicates that hyperhomocysteinemia is an independent risk factor of premature cardiovascular disease but the mechanism involved remains unclear. Besides its direct toxic effect on endothelial cells homocyst(e)ine (HCY) can stimulate the oxidation of LDL in vitro in the presence of redox metals. The possibility that high levels of HCY also in vivo increase the ability of human aortic cells to oxidize LDL has now been studied.

Aortic biopsies were obtained from 35 CAD patients undergoing bypass surgery. Samples of 10 mg were incubated with LDL (100 µg protein/ml) for 18 h at 37°C, in DMEM supplemented with 1 µM $CuSO_4$. Aortic samples from hyperhomocyst(e)inemia patients (15.4 ± 3.5 µmol/l) oxidized markedly greater amounts of LDL than samples from patients with low plasma levels of HCY (8.2 ± 4.3 µmol/l), as shown by TBARS (15.2 ± 3.1 vs. 10.7 ± 2.3 mmol MDA/mg LDL protein). Interactions between HCY and lipoproteins contributing to the development of atherosclerosis are discussed.

Introduction

Elevated plasma levels of homocyst(e)ine (HCY) are considered a common risk factor of coronary artery disease, peripheral artery disease, stroke and venous thrombosis, and are deemed by some to be as potent as hypercholesterolemia and cigarette smoking [1—3]. In fact, a recent study has shown that HCY is a strong predictor of mortality in patients with angiographically confirmed coronary artery disease [4]. The mechanism for the acceleration of atherosclerosis by HCY appears to involve endothelial cell injury caused by hydrogen peroxide generated during the oxidation of the amino acid's sulfhydryl group [5]. It has also been shown that HCY inhibits intracellular glutathione peroxidase, the enzyme responsible for the reduction of hydrogen and lipid peroxides to their corresponding alcohols [4]. Taken together, the present evidence stands for a major role of free radical species in endothelial cell damage mediated by this sulphur-containing amino acid. It seems, therefore, highly probable that the same mechanism may be responsible for the oxidative modification of LDL in the extracellular space of the arterial wall. This issue has now been addressed by comparing the ability of normal and hyperhomocyst(e)inemic human aortic cells to oxidize LDL.

Address for correspondence: Marek Naruszewicz, Regional Center for Atherosclerosis Research, Pomeranian Academy of Medicine, al. Powstańców Wlkp 72, 70-111 Szczecin, Poland.

Subjects

35 patients (11 females and 24 males) with angiographically assessed CAD (stenosis $>90\%$ in one and $>40\%$ in another coronary artery) were divided into two groups according to fasting HCY concentration, taking 14.0 µmol/l as the cutoff point [5]. Clinical characteristics of the patients are presented in Table 1. Patients with diabetes, on calcium channel blockers or vitamin E were excluded.

Methods

Macroscopically normal (lesion-free) fragments of coronary arteries were obtained from patients undergoing bypass surgery. Fresh samples of 10 mg were incubated with LDL (100 µg protein/ml) for 18 h at 37°C, in DMEM supplemented with 1 µM $CuSO_4$ (Fig. 1). Lipid peroxidation in LDL was followed by thiobarbituric acid reactive substances (TBARS) released into the medium and the results were expressed as nmol malondialdehyde (MDA) equivalents per mg protein. Total homocysteine in plasma (being the sum of protein-bound and free HCY) was measured by high-performance liquid chromatography with fluorescence detection. Plasma cholesterol, triglyceride, LDL and high-density lipoprotein cholesterol levels were determined according to the Lipid Research Clinics Protocol.

Results

Table 2 shows that cells of the arterial wall from patients with hyperhomocyst(e)-inemia (HCY > 14.0 µmol/l) had a 40% greater ability to oxidize LDL than cells from individuals with homocyst(e)ine level normal. It should be mentioned that LDL obtained from subjects with low and high levels of HCY did not differ in their susceptibility to oxidation in the presence of copper (data not shown). How-

Table 1. Clinical characteristics of CAD patients with low and high homocysteine levels.

	Group	
	Control (n = 20)	Hyperhomocyst(e)inemia (n = 15)
Age (years)	51.8 ± 8.2	53.4 ± 4.5
Sex (M/F)	14/6	10/5
BMI	25.3 ± 2.8	26.1 ± 3.5
Cigarette smoking (n)	11	12
Hypertension (n)	5	4
Total cholesterol (mg/dl)	227 ± 23	224 ± 18
LDL (mg/dl)	167 ± 19	161 ± 13
HDL (mg/dl)	35.8 ± 2.4	34.2 ± 4.2
Homocyst(e)ine (mmol/l)	8.2 ± 4.3	15.4 ± 3.5

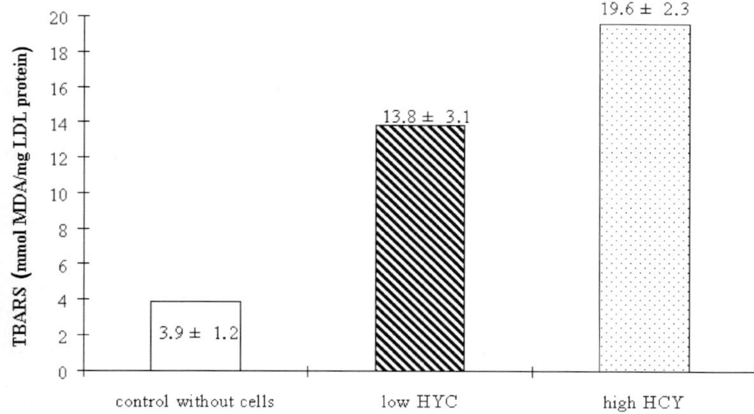

Fig. 1. Oxidation of LDL by monocyte-macrophages obtained from CAD patients with low and high levels of homocyst(e)ine. Ten milligrams of LDL protein were incubated with 2×10^6 cells in the presence of 1 mM Cu^{+2} for 18 h.

ever, fresh monocytes isolated from patients with hyper-HCY and stimulated with PMS showed a greater ability for oxidative modification of LDL.

Discussion

It is generally acknowledged that elevated plasma levels of homocysteine, independent of any genetic or dietetic background, are to a large extent responsible for premature or more severe atherosclerosis observed in a comparable risk factor setting. Reasons for this can certainly be traced to a variety of coagulation disorders caused by HCY that lead to the hypercoagulable state. Reduced levels of antithrombin III, factor VII and protein C have been reported [6]. An additional pathogenetic factor is the intensification by homocysteine of LDL modification inside the arterial wall. Subsequently, this can result in accelerated formation of foam cells which constitute the basis of fatty streaks.

We have previously demonstrated that homocysteine thiolactone is able to modify LDL by binding to free lysyl epsilon amino groups of apolipoprotein B and thereby increase the aggregation of these lipoprotein particles. LDL aggregates

Table 2. Oxidation of LDL by human aortic cells obtained from CAD patients with low and high levels of homocyst(e)ine.

Aortic cells — donor	TBARS (nmol MDA/mg LDL protein)	Electrophoretic mobility (cm)
Control	10.7 ± 2.3	1.4 ± 0.07
Hyperhomocyst(e)inemia	15.2 ± 3.1	1.8 ± 0.15
Without cells	3.1 ± 0.5	1.0 ± 0.09

496

are removed by phagocytizing macrophages, causing an accumulation of cholesterol esters in these cells [7].

The present study indicates that LDL oxidation is stimulated with higher levels of homocysteine in the arterial wall. This appears from our preliminary unpublished results to be a consequence of the reduced activity of antioxidative enzymes, such as superoxide dismutase. Our assumption is supported by a recent study of Young et al. [8] who have demonstrated that massive homocysteinemia induced in pigs results in an increased accumulation of lipid peroxide degradation products (i.e., MDA) in the organism, particularly in the heart. Further studies are necessary to elucidate the relationship between homocysteinemia and the decreased antioxidative barrier in the arterial wall, as well as the influence of this process on the pathogenesis of atherosclerosis.

References

1. Genest JJ, McNamara JR, Salem DN, Wilson PWF, Shaefer EJ, Malinow MR. Plasma homocyst(e)ine levels in men with premature coronary artery disease. J Am Coll Cardiol 1990;16: 1114–1119.
2. Fermo J, Vigano D'Angelo S, Paroni R, Mazzola G, Calori G, D'Angelo A. Prevalence of moderate hyperhomocyst(e)inemia in patients with early-onset venous and arterial occlusive disease. Ann Int Med 1995;123:747–753.
3. Ubbink JB, Vermaak WHJ, Bennett JM, Becker PJ, Van Staden DA, Bissbort S. The prevalence of homocysteinemia and hypercholesterolemia in angiographically defined coronary artery disease. Klin Wochenschr 1991;69:527–534.
4. Nygärd O, Nordrehaung JE, Refsum H, Ueland PM, Farstad M, Vollset SE. Plasma homocysteine levels and mortality in patients with coronary artery disease. N Engl J Med 1997;337: 230–236.
5. Starkebaum G, Harlan JM. Endothelial injury due to copper-catalyzed hydrogen peroxide generation from homocysteine. J Clin Invest 1986;77:1370–1376.
6. Rodgers GM, Conn MT. Homocysteine an atherogenic stimulus reduces protein C activation by arterial and venous endothelial cells. Blood 1990;75:895–901.
7. Naruszewicz M, Mirkiewicz E, Olszewslo AJ, Mc Cully KS. Thiolation of low-density lipoprotein by homocysteine thiolactone causes increased aggregation and altered interaction with cultured macrophages. Nutr Metab Cardiovasc Dis 1994;4:70–77.
8. Young PB, Kennedy S, Molloy AM, Scott JM, Weir DG, Kennedy DG. Lipid peroxidation induced in vivo by hyperhomocysteinemia in pigs. Atherosclerosis 1997;129:67–71.

Atherosclerosis XI.
B. Jacotot, D. Mathé and J.-C. Fruchart, editors.

Effect of α-tocopherol on scavenger receptor activity, mRNA expression and regulation in macrophages

Daniel Teupser, Joachim Thiery, Wolfgang Wilfert, Ulrike Haas and Dietrich Seidel

Institute of Clinical Chemistry, University of Munich, Munich, Germany

Abstract. *Background.* The aim of this study was to investigate the effect of α-tocopherol on scavenger receptor (SR) activity, SR class A (SR-A) mRNA expression and regulation in macrophages.

Methods. Scavenger receptor activity was determined by uptake of DiI-acLDL in rabbit peritoneal macrophages and human monocytes/macrophages incubated in the presence and absence of tocopherols. SR-A mRNA expression was determined by Northern blotting, the activity of the transcription factor activator protein-1 (AP-1) by electrophoretic mobility shift assay.

Results. We show for the first time, that in the presence of α-tocopherol scavenger receptor activity in macrophages is reduced in a dose-dependent manner. This was correlated with a reduced SR-A mRNA expression and AP-1 binding transcription factors in presence of α-tocopherol. Interestingly, γ-tocopherol which is an analog of α-tocopherol with a comparable antioxidative capacity showed only a weak suppression of SR activity, SR-A expression and AP-1 activity.

Conclusions. Our results point to the conclusion that the reduction of SR-A expression and activity in presence of α-tocopherol is not necessarily related to a general antioxidative effect but rather to a direct action on cell signaling.

Keywords: AP-1, DiI-acLDL, SR-A, vitamin E.

Introduction

Scavenger receptors (SRs) are cell membrane proteins which can bind chemically modified lipoproteins, such as acetylated (acLDL) and oxidized LDL [1]. It is hypothesized that LDL entering the arterial wall can be oxidized and recognized by SRs on the surface of macrophages. Oxidized LDL has also been shown to induce the immigration of monocytes into the arterial wall, and express SRs as they differentiate into macrophages. SRs then mediate the endocytosis of modified lipoproteins from the extracellular space, which can result in massive intracellular cholesterol accumulation and the transformation of macrophages into foam cells. On the other hand, SRs have also been linked with the initiation of immunity and host defense, because of their ability to bind a wide variety of pathogens. Though a number of different classes of scavenger receptors have been identified [1,2], the present paper will focus on class A scavenger receptors

Address for correspondence: Joachim Thiery MD, Institute of Clinical Chemistry, Klinikum Grosshadern, University of Munich, 81377 Munich, Germany.

(SR-A) in macrophages.

There is only limited information on the regulation of class A scavenger receptors. Recently, it has been shown that peroxides can induce protein kinase C (PKC) in smooth muscle cells [3]. PKC induces AP-1 binding transcription factors, which are thought to be involved in the upregulation of class A scavenger receptors in THP-1 monocytes/macrophages [4]. α-Tocopherol can inhibit PKC stimulation and the induction of AP-1 in rat smooth muscle cells [5,6]. Based on these observations, we hypothesized that α-tocopherol may also affect scavenger receptor activity (Fig. 1).

Methods

Isolation and cultivation of rabbit peritoneal macrophages

New Zealand White rabbits (n = 10) were killed by an overdose of pentobarbital 3 days after intraperitoneal injection of 40 ml mineral oil. Peritoneal macrophages were isolated by lavage with 800 ml 0.9% NaCl in tubes containing EDTA (final concentration 0.1 g/l). The cells were washed with HANKS salt solution (0.1 g EDTA/l), pooled in DMEM containing 10% FCS, penicillin/ streptomycin and diluted to a final concentration of 10^6 cells/ml. α-, β-, γ- or δ-tocopherol (a generous gift from Malton E, Münsing, Germany) were dissolved in ethanol at 0, 1, 5, 10, 50 and 100 mM and added to the cell suspension in a 1:1,000 dilution. The cells were plated on cell-culture dishes and incubated in the presence of the tocopherols for up to 20 h.

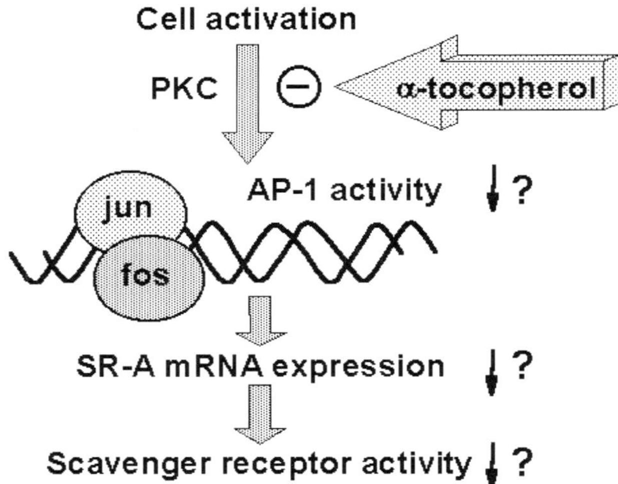

Fig. 1. Hypothesis of the effect of α-tocopherol on scavenger receptor activity.

Isolation and cultivation of human monocytes

Mononuclear cells were isolated from five healthy human donors by ficoll density gradient centrifugation using standardized tubes (Vacutainer CTP Cell Preparation Tubes, Becton Dickinson). The cells were washed with HANKS salt solution (0.1 g EDTA/l) and 10^7 cells were plated per 35 mm dish in DMEM (10% FCS). After 2 h of incubation (37°C, 5% CO_2), the nonadherent cells were removed. The adherent monocytes were incubated with DMEM (10% FCS, penicillin/streptomycin) containing 0 or 100 µM α-tocopherol. α-Tocopherol was dissolved in ethanol at 0 and 100 mM and added to the cells in a 1:1,000 dilution. The cells were incubated with and without α-tocopherol for 8 or 15 days.

Lipoproteins

LDL was prepared from human EDTA-plasma by ultracentrifugation. LDL was labeled with the fluorescent probe 1,1′-dioctadecyl-3,3,3′,3′-tetramethylindocarbocyanine perchlorate (DiI) (Molecular Probes, Eugene, OR, USA) as described by Innerarity et al. [7] and acetylated as described by Basu et al. [8]. Protein concentrations were determined by the method of Lowry et al. [9].

Quantitative analysis of scavenger receptor activity

After 20 h incubation of macrophages with or without tocopherols on 35 mm dishes, the cells were incubated with 10 µg DiI-acLDL/ml DMEM for 5 h. After incubation with DiI-acLDL the cells were washed and 2 ml of lysis reagent (SDS/NaOH) were added. This reagent allowed the determination of fluorescence intensity (FI) as well as cell protein in the same sample of lysed cells. FI was measured in the lysate on microtiter plates with excitation and emission wave length set at 520 and 580 nm, respectively. FI of the DiI-labeled lipoprotein diluted in the lysis reagent (1:2,000) was measured in order to determine the specific fluorescence intensity of the DiI-acLDL preparation used. The data were expressed as ng cell associated DiI-acLDL per mg of cell protein [10].

Northern blot

Total RNA was isolated with TRIzol (Gibco) from macrophages incubated with/ without tocopherols before or 1, 5 or 20 h after adherence of the cells on 10 cm culture dishes. RNA was separated by electrophoresis and blotted onto nitrocellulose membranes. A fragment of the collagenous domain of rabbit scavenger receptor corresponding to bp 833−1057 was PCR-amplified from rabbit cDNA [11]. It was radiolabeled with ^{32}P by random priming and hybridized to the membrane at 42°C in 50% formamide 5 × SSPE. The membranes were washed in 2 × SSC, 0.1% SDS at 42°C and exposed on storage phosphor screen. Subsequently the membranes were stripped of probe and rehybridized with a random

500

prime labeled fragment of rabbit GAPDH corresponding to bp 557–1258 or rabbit β-actin corresponding to bp 1284–1718. Storage phosphor screens were read with a phosphorimager and quantitatively analyzed using ImageQuaNT Software (Molecular Dynamics, Krefeld, Germany).

Electrophoretic mobility shift assay (EMSA)

Nuclear extracts were prepared as described by Schreiber et al. [12] from rabbit peritoneal macrophages before, 3, 5 or 20 h after adhesion of the cells to 10 cm culture dishes. AP-1 consensus oligonucleotides were labeled with ^{32}P according to the recommendations of the supplier (Promega, Madison, USA). 0.8 µg of nuclear protein was incubated on ice for 30 min with 50,000 cpm of the labeled AP-1 consensus oligo. Free AP-1 was separated by electrophoresis on a 5% acrylamide/bisacrylamide gel at 4°C. The gels were exposed on storage phosphor screens, read in a phosphorimager (Molecular Dynamics, Krefeld, Germany) and quantified using ImageQuaNT Software.

Results

We found a 4-fold increase in the activity of transcription factor AP-1 in freshly isolated rabbit peritoneal macrophages during the first 5 h of adhesion to culture dishes. This increase of AP-1 activity was significantly attenuated (50%) in the presence of α-tocopherol (data not shown). In addition, we observed a marked concentration-dependent reduction of AP-1 activity in adherent rabbit peritoneal macrophages in presence of α-tocopherol, in contrast to β-, γ- and δ-tocopherol, which had only little or no effect (Fig. 2). Chemically the four tocopherols differ only in the presence and position of two methyl groups and have a comparable antioxidative capacity. This suggests that the inhibitory effect of α-tocopherol on AP-1 activity is not necessarily related to its antioxidative effects.

In parallel with the data obtained for AP-1, we found an increase of SR-A mRNA expression after adhesion of the macrophages which was attenuated in the presence of α-tocopherol. The decrease of SR-A expression in presence of α-tocopherol was confirmed in additional experiments, as shown in Fig. 3. Interestingly, β-tocopherol showed an equally low SR-A expression, though it had a much weaker effect on AP-1 inhibition than α-tocopherol. In contrast, γ-tocopherol had little effect on both SR-A expression and AP-1 activity (Fig. 3).

The data obtained by Northern blotting were confirmed by a comparable pattern of scavenger receptor activity as measured by uptake of DiI-acLDL (Fig. 4). Scavenger receptor activity was significantly reduced in the presence of α- and β-tocopherol, but there was only a weak effect which was not significant in presence of γ-tocopherol. In a separate experiment, we studied if the reduction of scavenger receptor activity in rabbit peritoneal macrophages follows a concentration-dependent manner. We found a significant, concentration-dependent decrease of DiI-acLDL uptake of -13, -16, -18 and -24% after preincuba-

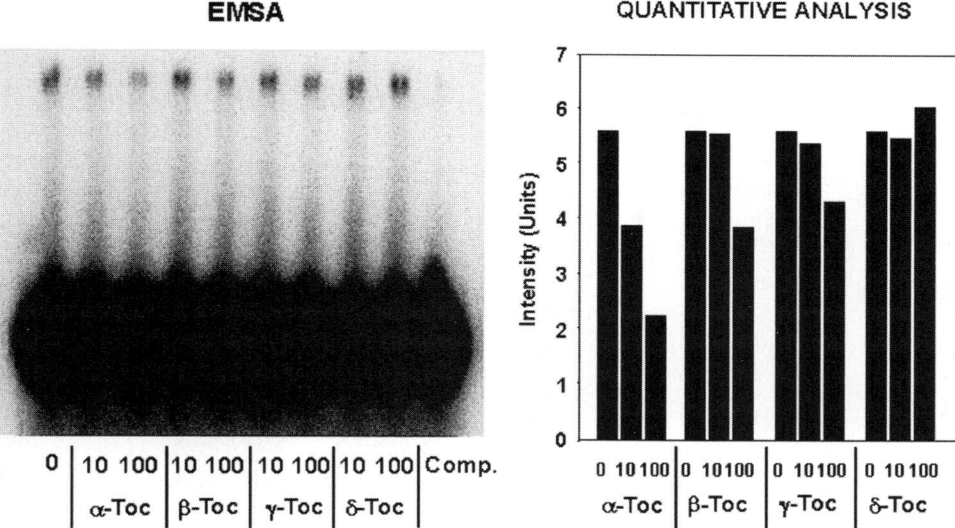

Fig. 2. Concentration-dependent effect of tocopherols (0, 10 and 100 μM) on AP-1 binding transcription factors. The specificity of binding (0 μM sample) was determined in the presence of an excess of unlabeled AP-1 (Comp.).

tion with α-tocopherol (1, 5, 10, 50 μM, respectively) for 20 h as compared to control.

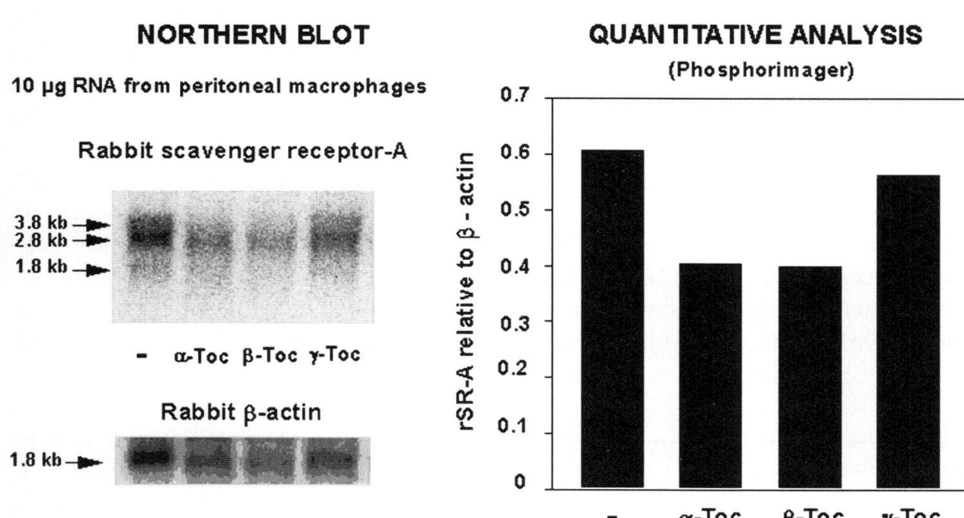

Fig. 3. Effect of different tocopherols (50 μM/20 h) on scavenger receptor-A expression in rabbit peritoneal macrophages. Rabbit SR-A was quantified by phosphorimager analysis and normalized to β-actin.

502

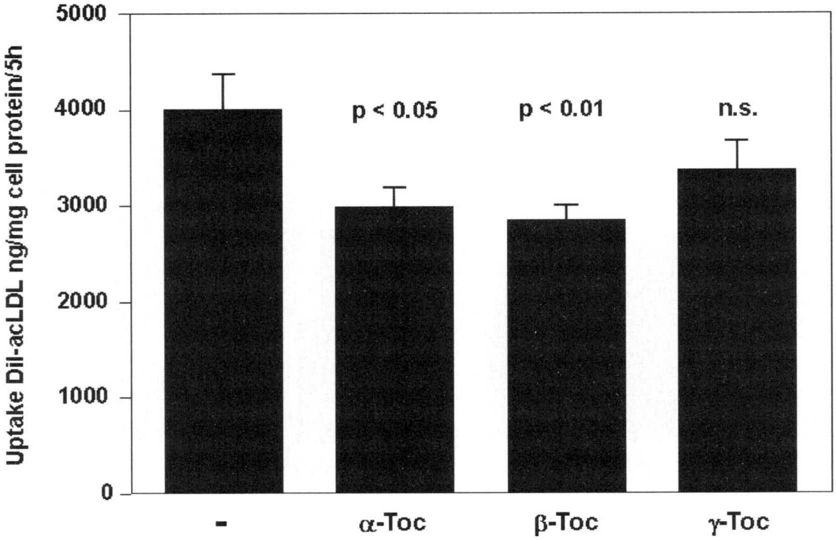

Fig. 4. Effect of different tocopherols (50 µM/20 h) on scavenger receptor-A activity in rabbit peritoneal macrophages as determined by uptake of DiI-acLDL (10 µg/ml/5 h), mean ± SD.

In an additional set of experiments, we studied if the effect of α-tocopherol on scavenger receptor activity in rabbit macrophages could also be seen in human monocytes/macrophages. As shown in Table 1, scavenger receptor activity was low in human-monocyte-derived macrophages after 8 days in culture and α-tocopherol had no significant effect. However, after 15 days in culture, there was a substantial increase in scavenger receptor activity which was significantly attenuated in the presence of 100 µM α-tocopherol (Table 1).

Discussion

The experiments presented here show for the first time that α-tocopherol suppresses scavenger receptor activity in rabbit macrophages and human monocytes/macrophages. The significant dose-response effect confirms the assumption that the inhibition of scavenger receptor is due to a specific action of α-tocopher-

Table 1.

Days in culture	8		15	
α-Tocopherol	0	100 µM	0	100 µM
Uptake DiI-acLDL ng/mg cell protein/5 h	316 ± 74	229 ± 131	1805 ± 1041[a]	680 ± 219[a]

Scavenger receptor activity in human monocyte derived macrophages cultivated for 8 and 15 days in presence (100 µM) and absence of α-tocopherol (mean ± SD). After 15 days of incubation, scavenger receptor activity was significantly lower ([a]p < 0.05) in cells incubated with α-tocopherol.

ol. In addition, these findings could be confirmed by a decreased scavenger receptor-A mRNA expression in macrophages incubated with α-tocopherol. One could speculate, that the reduction of SR-A expression is due to a delayed maturation of the macrophages in the presence of α-tocopherol. This is also in line with the reduced increase of the activity of transcription factor AP-1 in presence of α-tocopherol during adherence of freshly isolated rabbit macrophages to culture dishes. Indeed, transcription factor AP-1 has been shown to be involved in scavenger receptor activation [4]. Interestingly β-tocopherol had a comparable effect on scavenger receptor expression to α-tocopherol but only a weak effect on AP-1 activity. The findings of AP-1 activity in rabbit macrophages are well in line with the data obtained by Azzi et al., indicating that α-tocopherol may have a direct action on cellular signal transduction in rat smooth muscle cells by inhibition of PKC activity [5,6]. However, the surprisingly low SR-A expression in presence of β-tocopherol points to the hypothesis that in addition to AP-1, other transcription factors may be involved in the tocopherol-mediated reduction of scavenger receptor activity. On the other hand, the experiments with the different tocopherols, which have a comparable antioxidative capacity but show different effects on SR-A expression and SR-activity, point to the conclusion that the reduction of SR-A expression and activity in presence of α-tocopherol is not due to a general antioxidative effect but rather to a direct action on cell signaling.

Acknowledgements

This work was supported by a grant from the Deutsche Forschungsgemeinschaft (Th 374, 2-1) to Dr Thiery and by Malton E, Münsing, Germany.

References

1. Krieger M. The other side of scavenger receptors: pattern recognition for host defense. Curr Opin Lipid 1997;8:275—280.
2. Kodama T, Doi T, Suzuki H, Takahashi K, Wada Y, Gordon S. Collagenous macrophage scavenger receptors. Curr Opin Lipid 1996;7:287—291.
3. Mietus-Snyder M, Friera A, Glass CK, Pitas RE. Regulation of scavenger receptor expression in smooth muscle cells by protein kinase C. A Role of oxidative stress. Arterioscl Thromb Vasc Biol 1997;17:969—978.
4. Moulton KS, Semple K, Wu H, Glass CK. Cell-specific expression of the macrophage scavenger receptor gene is dependent on PU.1 and a composite AP-1/ets motif. Molec Cell Biol 1994; 14:4408—4418.
5. Tasinato A, Boscoboinik D, Bartoli GM, Maroni P, Azzi A. d-alpha-tocopherol inhibition of vascular smooth muscle cell proliferation occurs at physiological concentrations, correlates with protein kinase C inhibition, and is independent of its antioxidant properties. Proc Natl Acad Sci USA 1995;92:12190—12194.
6. Sträuble B, Boscoboinik D, Tasinato A, Azzi A. Modulation of activator protein-1 (AP-1) transcription factor and protein kinase C by hydrogen peroxide and D-alpha-tocopherol in vascular smooth muscle cells. Eur J Biochem 1994;226:393—402.
7. Innerarity TL, Pitas RE, Mahley RW. Lipoprotein-receptor interactions. Meth Enzymol 1986;129:542—565.

8. Basu SK, Goldstein JL, Anderson RGW, Brown MS. Degradation of cationized low density lipoprotein and regulation of cholesterol metabolism in homozygous familial hypercholesterolemia fibroblasts. Proc Natl Acad Sci USA 1976;73:3178−3182.

9. Lowry OH, Rosenbrough NJ, Farr AL, Randall RJ. Protein measurement with the Folin phenol reagent. J Biol Chem 1951;193:265−275.

10. Teupser D, Thiery J, Walli AK, Seidel D. Determination of LDL- and scavenger-receptor activity in adherent and nonadherent cultured cells with a new single-step fluorometric assay. Biochim Biophys Acta 1996;1303:193−198.

11. Bickel PE, Freeman MW. Rabbit aortic smooth muscle cells express inducible macrophage scavenger receptor messenger RNA that is absent from endothelial cells. J Clin Invest 1992;90: 1450−1457.

12. Schreiber E, Matthias P, Müller MM, Schaffner W. Rapid detection of octamer binding proteins with "miniextracts", prepared from a small number of cells. Nucl Acid Res 1989;17:6419.

Nutrition and CHD

Dietary composition and low-density lipoprotein (LDL) modifications

Rafael Carmena[1], Jose M. Ordovas[2], Juan F. Ascaso[1], German Camejo[3], Eva Hurt-Camejo[3] and Jose Martinez-Valls[1]

[1]Department of Medicine, University of Valencia, Spain; [2]Lipid Metabolism Laboratory, Tufts University, Boston, Massachusetts, USA; and [3]Wallenberg Laboratory, University of Gothenburg, Sweden

Several dietary factors influence plasma lipids and lipoproteins. Traditionally, the effects of diet on coronary heart disease (CHD) risk have been attributed to the effects of medium-chain fatty acids and dietary cholesterol on the plasma levels of low-density lipoproteins (LDL), which carry about three-quarters of the cholesterol in normal human plasma. In more recent years, the effect of individual fatty acids, antioxidant vitamins, and other nutrients on LDL plasma levels and composition have been investigated. In this review we shall focus on dietary components that have been shown to induce qualitative and quantitative modifications of the LDL particles. For reviews on the extensive literature published on this subject see [1—4].

Dietary cholesterol

The major effects of dietary cholesterol in man and nonhuman primates is to raise LDL-C levels. In humans, however, the effects of dietary cholesterol on plasma LDL-C levels are much less pronounced than in most primate species, and a marked variability in responsiveness does exist [5]. Recent publications have suggested that several plasma apolipoproteins (apo) play a role in the regulation of LDL-C response to dietary cholesterol and saturated fat [6,7]. A common genetic variant of apo A-IV (A-IV-2) has been associated with blunting of the response to dietary cholesterol, possibly by reducing intestinal fat absorption [6,7] although this mechanism was not substantiated in a recent report [8].

Dietary cholesterol not only elevates plasma LDL-C, but also relates independently to the risk of CHD and may render postprandial triglyceride-rich lipoproteins more atherogenic [9]. In a recent publication, Levy et al. [10] have shown that consumption of two eggs per day with meals for 3 weeks resulted in an 11% increase in plasma LDL-C and an enhanced susceptibility of these particles

Address for correspondence: Prof Rafael Carmena, Department of Medicine, Facultad de Medicina, Avd Blasco Ibanez 17, 46010 Valencia, Spain. Tel.: +34-6-386-2665. Fax: +34-6-386-4767. E-mail: Carmena@uv.es

to oxidation. Since the LDL content in polyunsaturated fatty acids (PUFA) was not changed, the enhanced propensity to oxidation could be related to the increment in LDL cholesterol content. Hence, a high-cholesterol diet becomes atherogenic by increasing the cholesterol content of LDL and by making these particles more susceptible to oxidation.

Saturated fatty acids and LDL levels

Using regression analysis of data collected from meticulously controlled feeding studies, Keys et al. [11] and Hegsted et al. [12] reported that saturated fatty acids (SFA) raised blood-cholesterol concentrations about twice as much as polyunsaturated fatty acids (PUFA) lowered them. These investigators also showed that the individual SFA had different effects on LDL levels. Lauric acid (C12:0), myristic acid (C14:0), and palmitic acid (C16:0) were shown to raise plasma total and LDL cholesterol, while stearic acid (C18:0) appeared to be neutral with regard to LDL-C levels.

Recently, the difference in the cholesterol-raising action of the different SFA has been further investigated. Using liquid formula diets rich in lauric, palmitic and oleic acids, Denke and Grundy [13] reported that the rise in LDL-C on the high lauric-acid diet was about two-thirds of that on the high palmitic-acid diet. These findings are compatible with those of Cox et al. [14] who compared the effects of coconut oil, butter and safflower oil on lipids and lipoproteins of moderately hypercholesterolemic subjects. Total and LDL cholesterol were higher on butter than coconut oil, the lowest being observed on the safflower diet, while apo B levels were higher on coconut oil and on butter than on safflower oil. Therefore, palmitic acid, the predominant fatty acid of butter, has a more marked total and LDL cholesterol-raising effect than lauric acid, which is found in high concentrations in coconut oil. Hence, a high saturated-fat diet modifies the LDL particles in two ways, by increasing their cholesterol content and by enlarging the size of the particle [15].

Medium chain (C8:0 and C10:0) fatty acids (MCT) diffuse rapidly into the portal circulation and after reaching the liver are β-oxidized into acetyl coenzyme A. In spite of being saturated, MCT have long been described as neutral dietary constituents that have no effect on plasma cholesterol concentrations but can raise triglycerides much like carbohydrates do [16]. In recent nutritional studies, however, MCT-oil feeding showed one-half the potency of palmitic acid at raising total and LDL-C concentrations [17].

One mechanism responsible for the increase in LDL-C during a diet rich in cholesterol and SFA seems to depend on downregulation of the hepatic LDL receptors. Extensive data obtained in both experimental animals and humans [18] demonstrate that the primary effect of cholesterol feeding is to expand the storage pool of cholesteryl esters in the hepatocyte and reduce the level of hepatic receptor activity. Addition of triacylglycerol containing long-chain SFA to the diet causes further suppression of receptor activity and a near doubling of the

LDL-C production rate. As mentioned before, there is much heterogeneity in the response of individuals to changes in dietary SFA and cholesterol [5]. Individuals considered as "nonresponders" to a high-fat, high-cholesterol diet would increase hepatic LDL receptor levels to the extent needed to maintain previous LDL levels, while "responders" would regulate LDL receptors incompletely or not at all. As stated above, apolipoproteins play a role in the LDL-C response to saturated fat. Individuals carrying the apo E4 allele seem to respond more to changes in the dietary content in SFA than E2 or E3 carriers [6,7].

Another mechanism that could be involved in the differences in LDL-C between individuals and in their response to dietary modifications is cholesteryl ester transfer protein (CETP) activity [19—21]. The data provided by these studies supports a causal contribution of increased CETP activity to the increased in LDL-C observed in response to saturated fat. It has been calculated that, in the case of response to saturated fat, CETP could be directly responsible for about one-third of the increase observed in LDL-C. In the case of response to transfatty acids (see below), the increased CETP activity seems to be responsible for the whole LDL-C increase [22].

Unsaturated fatty acids

In the previously mentioned experiments by Keys et al. [11] and Hegsted et al. [12] it was demonstrated that the polyunsaturated fatty acids linoleic acid (C18: 2 n-6) and α-linolenic acid (C18: 3 n-3), which are the essential fatty acids in our diet, lower serum cholesterol. The influence of monounsaturated fatty acids (MUFA) on total cholesterol levels was considered "neutral", similar to that of carbohydrates. In more recent years it has been demonstrated that oleic acid (C18:1 n-9 cis), the major MUFA in the diet, can significantly reduce LDL-C levels with no modification, or slight increase, in the HDL-C levels [23,24]. In addition, oleate-rich diets have been shown to generate LDL particles more resistant to in vitro oxidation [25—27].

Recent nutritional studies have confirmed that the effect of α-linolenic acid (C18: 3 n-3) is equivalent to n-6 oils vis-à-vis lipid and lipoprotein profiles [28], i.e., a reduction in total and LDL-C, without modifications in the triglyceride levels. The plant-derived C18:3 n-3 fatty acid (α-linolenic acid) is the metabolic precursor to the marine n-3 fatty acids and is found in high concentrations ($> 50\%$) in linseed oil. The marine n-3 fatty acids (C20:5 n-3 and C22:6 n-3), also referred to as fish oils, have been extensively studied in the last decade. They have a significant hypotriglyceridemic effect, as little as 3 g/day can reduce plasma triglycerides by 30%, through inhibition of VLDL and triglyceride synthesis in the liver [29]. On the other hand, contrary to what could be expected of PUFA, they can also raise LDL-C concentrations, especially in hypertriglyceridemic subjects, behaving in this respect like fibrates do. HDL-C is essentially unaffected by n-3 fatty acids [26].

Besides their effects on lipids and lipoproteins, fish oils alter eicosanoid metabolism in a favourable way, inhibiting the synthesis of thromboxane A in platelets, reducing platelet aggregation and increasing the bleeding time, and enhancing the production of the vasodilator prostacyclin [30]. In addition, fish oils also lessen postprandial lipemia. For these reasons, fish oil consumption, or a fish-rich diet, may play a critical role in the prevention of atherosclerosis [28]. Moreover, according to some studies [31], marine polyunsaturated n-3 fatty acids supplementation has no measurable effect on the susceptibility of LDL to lipid peroxidation, i.e., n-3 fatty acids do not seem to render the LDL particle more atherogenic. There is not, however, complete agreement on this point [26].

Transunsaturated FA

The double bonds of unsaturated fatty acids can occur in either of two configurations relative to the plane of the acyl chain, cis or trans. The majority of double bonds in fatty acids occurring in food are in the cis configuration. The transfatty acids in the diet come from the chemical hydrogenation of vegetable oils, that changes the physical characteristics of an oil from a liquid to a semisolid or solid state at room temperature [32]. Transfatty acids raise plasma LDL-C levels when exchanged for cis unsaturated fatty acids in the diet. The effect is similar to that of saturated fat and appears to be shared by transfatty acids from various sources and with different isomer compositions [33]. In addition, transfatty acids have unfavorable effects on other lipoproteins because they simultaneously decrease HDL-C and increase LDL-C levels. As stated above, the mechanism for these changes could be an increased CETP activity, that elevates LDL while reducing HDL-C levels [21]. Finally, the transconfiguration, being more stable than cis, should protect LDL particles from oxidation [34].

Carbohydrates

The effects of high-carbohydrate diets, which are necessarily low in fat, on LDL-C levels, composition, and physical properties have been the subject of numerous studies and debate during the past decades. It has been repeatedly shown that substantial decreases in fat and parallel increases in carbohydrate reduces LDL-C concentrations, associated with an increase in triglyceride and a reduction of HDL-C levels [35]. High-carbohydrate diets increase the liver production of triglycerides, without elevating that of cholesteryl esters or apo B [36]. The VLDL leaving the liver are larger and richer in triglycerides, with no elevation in the number of particles secreted nor in the apo B plasma levels.

It has been reported that consumption of a low-fat diet is associated with an increased concentration of the smaller, denser (pattern B) LDL particles, while during a high-fat diet most subjects exhibit LDL subclass A (large, buoyant LDL) [15]. On the other hand, individuals with the pattern B (small, dense LDL) had a greater lowering of LDL-C and plasma concentrations of apo B when consuming a low-fat (24%), high-carbohydrate (60%) diet than did pattern

A (large, buoyant LDL) individuals. The results suggest that the greater LDL-C response to low-fat diets in pattern B individuals can be explained by a reduced number of LDL particles. Hence, a low-fat, high-carbohydrate diet may preferentially benefit subjects with small, dense LDL, a high-risk lipoprotein profile [33].

Schaefer et al. [37] have studied free-living individuals while following an average US diet (35% total energy from fat), a low-fat (15%) high-carbohydrate (68%) diet with energy adjusted to keep body weight constant, and finally ad libitum low-fat diet in which the subjects were permitted to adjust their energy intake according to personal preference. The first diet was associated with a decrease in total, LDL-C and HDL-C, an increase in the total/HDL-C ratio and an increase in triglycerides. However, when participants were permitted to adjust their energy intake as desired, their LDL-C decreased still further, the total/HDL-C ratio improved and triglycerides fell in parallel with the reduction in body weight. The authors concluded that an ad libitum low-fat diet may promote weight loss and improve the lipid profile. A fat-restricted diet, when combined with weight loss, promotes lowering of LDL-C levels without adverse effects on the total/HDL-C ratio and triglyceride-rich particles.

The fact that low-fat, high-carbohydrate diets can lower HDL-C levels and increase fasting plasma triglyceride concentrations is a cause of concern for some, since theoretically it could increase the risk for CHD. Moreover, hypertriglyceridemia may be the primary event leading to the plurimetabolic syndrome and enhanced risk of atherosclerosis [38]. As stated above, this topic is still the subject of debate and controversy [39—41]

Soluble dietary fiber

It has long been established that soluble fibers (pectin, gums, oat bran) are able to lower LDL-C levels by 4—10% [42]. The mechanism of action is unclear but it seems related to their binding to bile acids and increased fecal excretion of cholesterol and bile acids.

Soy protein

In experimental animals, the ingestion of soy bean-rich diets leads to a reduction in plasma LDL-C levels. Evidence is accumulating indicating that the same occurs in humans [43]. A recent meta-analysis of dietary experiments concluded that soy-protein ingestion was associated with significant reductions in total- and LDL-cholesterol concentrations of −9.3 and −12.9%, respectively [44]. The precise mechanism to explain such changes has not been fully established. Moreover, the flavonoids present in soy may protect LDL particles from oxidation [45].

512

Other dietary components

Boiled coffee, as is traditionally done in Scandinavia, has been shown to raise total and LDL cholesterol, probably by its content in diterpenes like cafestol and kahweol [46]. The preparation method is critical, since diterpene levels in brewed coffee depend on it. Filtered or instant coffee do not contain diterpenes and have no effect on plasma cholesterol levels.

The effect of alcoholic beverages on lipid levels is (like carbohydrates) an elevation in triglycerides, particularly in individuals with an underlying defect in triglyceride metabolism. As component of the dietary energy intake, alcohol may contribute to obesity. Alcohol consumption is associated with increases in HDL-C but does not influence the concentrations of either LDL-C or apo B [47]. Due to its content in flavonoids, alcoholic beverages may protect LDL particles from oxidation [45].

Garlic powder, administered as pills at meal time to hyperlipidemic subjects, has been shown to prevent the LDL-C effect of fish-oil supplements, maintaining the triglyceride lowering effect [48]. In a recent meta-analysis, the ingestion of one half clove of garlic per day was shown to lower serum cholesterol by approximately 9% [49]. The mechanism involved in cholesterol reduction by garlic may be related to inhibition of hepatic cholesterol synthesis [50].

Overnutrition and obesity can raise plasma LDL-C levels, although significant interindividual variations do occur. In hypercholesterolemic individuals, weight loss causes a distinct reduction in LDL-C levels [51].

Antioxidants

The atherogenicity of LDL may be modulated by its serum levels, structure and affinity for components of the intima, all properties that can be altered by diet. In particular, diet can significantly affect the susceptibility of LDL to oxidation as the substrates of LDL oxidation (fatty acids and cholesterol moieties) are derived from dietary cholesterol and fatty acids. Other important determinants of LDL susceptibility to oxidation are a high PUFA and low antioxidants (vitamin E, β-carotene, etc.) content and the small, dense particles phenotype. Diets enriched in linoleate increase the content of linoleic fatty acid in LDL and may increase its sensitivity to oxidation. Vitamin E (α-tocopherol) enrichment of LDL reduces their susceptibility to oxidation. Several studies [52] have shown that vitamin E, but not β-carotene, has the capacity to protect LDL from oxidation.

We have studied [53] in healthy male volunteers the effect of two types of diet (rich in monousanturated or in polyunsaturated fatty acids) on LDL level, composition, size, oxidation and interaction with arterial proteoglycans. The fat and antioxidant content of the diets during the two experimental periods is presented in Table 1, and each dietary period lasted for 3 weeks. The dietary content of natural antioxidants during the sunflower-seed-oil (SFO) diet was triple that

Table 1. Fat and antioxidant content of the diets during the two experimental diets.

Parameter	Sunflower seed oil	Olive oil
SFA g/day (% daily energy)	18.4 ± 2.5 (6.8)	19.0 ± 3.3 (6.9)
MUFA g/day (% daily energy)	30.0 ± 4.4 (10.9)	59.0 ± 6.3 (21.6)
PUFA g/day (% daily energy)	36.6 ± 4.6 (13.3)	11.1 ± 1.4 (4.7)
Total fat g/day (% daily energy)	85.0 (31)	89.6 (30.5)
Total MUFA+PUFA g/day (% daily energy)	66.6 (24.2)	70.6 (25.6)
Vitamin E (mg/day)	27.0 ± 3.7	9.1 ± 1.4[a]
β-carotenes (μg/day)	6540.0 ± 705.0	4179.0 ± 795.4[a]
Vitamin C (mg/day)	261.9 ± 64.9	120.0 ± 60.6[a]

[a]$p < 0.001$.

found during the olive oil (OO) diet. No differences were found in BMI, waist/hip ratio, systolic and diastolic blood pressure at the end of the two dietary periods. Table 2 shows changes observed in plasma LDL levels and in LDL composition, oxidation, size and affinity for arterial proteoglycans after the two dietary periods. As expected, the content of linoleic fatty acid in LDL was significantly increased after the sunflower-seed-oil diet. When the two dietary periods were compared, LDL particles following the SFO diet became richer in cholesterol and triglyceride and were of the large, buoyant, less dense type, exhibiting more resistance to oxidation. Moreover, these LDL particles showed less affinity for arterial proteoglycans than those derived from OO diet with low-antioxidant content.

Table 2. Changes in LDL levels, composition, oxidation, size and affinity for arterial proteoglycans after the two dietary periods.

LDL parameters	Sunflower seed oil	Olive oil	p value
Serum LDL-C	3.36 ± 0.87	4.08 ± 1.13	<0.001
(C+TG) PR (mg/mg)	1.96 ± 0.35	1.81 ± 0.23	<0.01
Vit E (mol/particle)	10.9 ± 2.0	9.8 ± 1.3	<0.01
β-carot (mol/particle)	1.44 ± 0.83	1.20 ± 0.82	NS
Vit A (mol/particle)	0.029 ± 0.0014	0.023 ± 0.01	<0.001
Total antioxidants (mol/particle)	12.35 ± 2.57	11.10 ± 1.96	<0.003
PUFA/(S+MUFA)	1.06 ± 0.11	0.73 ± 0.06	<0.001
Total FA (mol/particle)	2166 ± 288	2036 ± 215	<0.05
TBARS (AUC)	581 ± 363	757 ± 384	<0.01
lnTBARS (AUC)	6.19 ± 0.59	6.51 ± 0.50	<0.01
Dienes	210 ± 65	561 ± 180	<0.01
lnDienes (AUC)	5.35 ± 0.55	6.33 ± 0.45	<0.01
Size LDL (relative mobility)	0.39 ± 0.06	0.41 ± 0.07	<0.01
Affinity for CSPG (Bt)	23.9 ± 7.4	29.3 ± 7.3	<0.05

C: total cholesterol; TG: triglycerides; PR: protein (apolipoprotein B); PUFA: polyunsaturated fatty acids; S: saturated fatty acids; MUFA: monounsaturated fatty acids; FA: fatty acids; Vit E: vitamin E, α-tocopherol; Vit A: vitamin A, retinol; β-carot: beta carotenes; and CSPG: chondroitin sulfate-rich versican proteoglycan.

The evidence presented indicates that in healthy male volunteers the consumption during 3 weeks of a diet rich in natural antioxidants and containing 31% of daily calories derived from fat (6.8% saturated, 13.3% PUFA and 10.9% MUFA) induces favourable changes in the lipid and lipoprotein profiles, lesser susceptibility of LDL to oxidation and lesser affinity for arterial wall proteoglycans. Taken together, these changes may diminish the atherogenic profile of LDL. Hence, the risk of increasing the sensitivity of LDL to oxidative modifications due to the high PUFA intake was counterbalanced by the changes induced in these particles and by the high content in the diet of natural antioxidants. Our results stress the complexity of the relation between LDL structure and oxidizability and suggest that further research is needed before we could safely incorporate conclusions about oxidation of lipoproteins into nutritional recommendations for the general population.

Concluding remarks

Dietary saturated fat and cholesterol raise LDL-C and contribute to excess cardiovascular risk. Excess cholesterol and saturated fat in the diet results in decreased LDL receptor activity. There is strong evidence that C18:0 (stearic acid) and C18:1 n-9cis (oleic acid) are neutral or can lower LDL-C relative to SFA or carbohydrates. Polyunsaturated fatty acids (C18:2 n-6 and C18:3 n-3) lower LDL-C, while eicosapentaenoic acid (C20:5 n-3) and docosahexanoic acid (C22:6 n-3) when given as fish oil lower triglycerides and can raise LDL-C. Transfatty acids have unfavorable effects on the lipid profile since they decrease HDL-C and increase LDL-C levels. A diet rich in PUFA renders LDL particles more susceptible to oxidation, while MUFA-rich diet are protective. We have shown that increasing the content in natural antioxidants of a PUFA-rich diet can counterbalance the susceptibility to oxidation. In addition, the LDL particles generated with such diets were larger and showed less affinity for arterial proteoglycans.

References

1. Grundy SM, Denke MA. Dietary influences on serum lipids and lipoproteins. J Lipid Res 1990; 31:1149−1172.
2. Denke MA. Review of human studies evaluating individual dietary responsiveness in patients with hypercholesterolemia. Am J Clin Nutr 1995;62:471S−477S.
3. Kris-Etherton PM, Yu S. Individual fatty acid effects on plasma lipids and lipoproteins: human studies. Am J Clin Nutr 1997;65(Suppl):1628S−1644S.
4. Mann JI. Dietary effects on plasma LDL and HDL. Curr Opin Lipid 1997;8:35−38.
5. Katan MB, Berns MAM, Glatz JFC, Knuiman JT, Nobels A, de Vries JHM. Congruence of individual responsiveness to dietary cholesterol and to saturated fat in humans. J Lipid Res 1988;29:883−892.
6. Ordovas JM, Lopez-Miranda J, Mata P, Perez-Jimenez F, Lichtenstein AH, Schaefer EJ. Gene-diet interaction in determining plasma lipid response to dietary intervention. Atherosclerosis 1995;118(Suppl):S11−S27.

7. Dreon D, Krauss RM. Diet-gene interactions in human lipoprotein metabolism. J Am Coll Nutr 1997;16:313—324.

8. Geissinger BW, Terry JG, Crouse JR, Stegner J, Weinberg RB. Effect of the apo A-IV-2 allele on intestinal cholesterol absorption and plasma lipoprotein response to a high-cholesterol/saturated fat diet. Circulation 1996;94(suppl):I—266(Abstract).

9. Grundy SM, Barret-Connor E, Rudel LL. Workshop on the impact of dietary cholesterol on plasma lipoprotein and atherogenesis. Atherosclerosis 1988;8:95—101.

10. Levy Y, Maor I, Presser D, Aviram M. Consumption of eggs with meals increases the susceptibility of human plasma and low-density lipoprotein to lipid peroxidation. Ann Nutr Metab 1996;40:243—251.

11. Keys A, Anderson JT, Grande F. Serum cholesterol response to changes in the diet. IV. Particular saturated fatty acids in the diet. Metabolism 1965;14:776—787.

12. Hegsted DM, McGandy RB, Myers ML, Stare FJ. Quantitative effects of dietary fat on serum cholesterol in men. Am J Clin Nutr 1965;17:81—295.

13. Denke MA, Grundy SM. Comparison of effects of lauric acid ans palmitic acid on plasma lipids and lipoproteins. Am J Clin Nutr 1992;56:895—898.

14. Cox C, Mann J, Sutherland W, Chisholm A, Skeaff M. Effects of coconut oil, butter, and sunflower oil on lipids and lipoproteins in persons with moderately elevated cholesterol levels. J Lipid Res 1995;36:1787—1795.

15. Krauss RM, Dreon DM. Low-density lipoprotein subclasses and response to a low-fat diet in healthy men. Am J Clin Nutr 1995;62:478S—487S.

16. Hill JO, Peters JC, Swift LL, Yang D, Sharp T, Abumrad N, Greene HL. Changes in blood lipids during 6 days of overfeeding with medium or long chain triglycerides. J Lipid Res 1990;31: 407—416.

17. Cater NB, Heller HJ, Denke MA. Comparison of the effects of medium-chain triacylglycerols, palm oil, and high oleic sunflower oil on plasma triacylglycerol fatty acids and lipid and lipoprotein concentrations in humans. Am J Clin Nutr 1997;65:41—45.

18. Spady DK, Woollett LA, Dietschy JM. Regulation of plasma LDL-Cholesterol levels by dietary cholesterol and fatty acids. Ann Rev Nutr 1993;13:355—381.

19. Tato F, Vega GL, Tall AR, Grundy SM. Relation between cholesteryl ester transfer protein activities and lipoprotein cholesterol in patients with hypercholesterolemia and combined hyperlipidemia. Arterioscl Thromb Vasc Biol 1995;15:112—120.

20. Groener JEM, van Ramshorst EM, Katan MB, Mensink RP, van Tol A. Diet-induced alteration in the activity of plasma lipid transfer protein in normolipidemic human subjects. Atherosclerosis 1991;87:221—226.

21. Schwab US, Maliranta HM, Sarkkinen ES, Savolainen MJ, Kesaniemi YA, Ussiitupa MIJ. Different effects on palmitic and stearic acid enriched diets on serum lipids and lipoproteins and cholesteryl ester transfer protein activity in healthy young women. Metabolism 1996;45: 143—149.

22. Fielding CJ. Response of low-density lipoprotein cholesterol levels to dietary change: contributions of different mechanisms. Curr Opin Lipid 1997;8:39—42.

23. Mattson FH, Grundy SM. Comparison of effects of dietary saturated, monounsaturated, and polyunsaturated fatty acids on plasma lipids and lipoproteins in man. J Lipid Res 1985;26: 194—202.

24. Carmena R, de Oya M, Ascaso JF, Mata P, Serrano S, Alvarez-Sala L, Martinez-Valls FJ, Rubio MJ. Monounsaturated fatty acids in the diet and plasma lipoproteins. In: Gotto AM Jr, Smith LC (eds) Drugs Affecting Lipid Metabolism X. Amsterdam: Elsevier, 1990;249—252.

25. Esterbauer H, Gebicki J, Puhl H, Juergens G. The role of lipid peroxidation and antioxidants in oxidative modification of LDL. Free Rad Biol Med 1992;13:341—390.

26. Parthasarathy S, Khoo J, Miller E, Barnett J, Witztum JL, Steinberg D. Low-density lipoprotein rich in oleic acid is protected against oxidative modification: implications for dietary prevention of atherosclerosis. Proc Natl Acad Sci USA 1990;87:3994—3998.

27. Bonanome A, Pagnan A, Biffanti S, Opportuno A, Sorgato F, Dorella M, Maiorino M, Ursini F. Effect of dietary monounsaturated and polyunsaturated fatty acids on the susceptibility of plasma low-density lipoprotein to oxidative modifications. Arterioscl Thromb 1992;12: 529–533.
28. Harris WS. n-3 fatty acids and serum lipoproteins: human studies. Am J Clin Nutr 1997; 65(Suppl):1645S–1654S.
29. Harris WS, Connor WE, Illingworth DR, Rothrock DW, Foster DM. Effect of fish oil on VLDL triglyceride kinetics in man. J Lipid Res 1990;31:1549–1558.
30. Connor WE. The beneficial effects of omega-3 fatty acids: cardiovascular disease and neuro-development. Curr Opin Lipid 1997;8:1–3.
31. Nenseter MS, Volden V, Tonstad S, Gudmundsen O, Ose L, Drevon CA. Modification of low-density lipoprotein in relation to intake of fatty acids and antioxidants. World Rev Nutr Diet 1994;75:144–148.
32. Lichtenstein AH, Ausman LM, Carrasco W, Jenner JL, Ordovas JM, Schaefer EJ. Hydrogenation impairs the hypolipidemic effect of corn oil in humans. Arterioscl Thromb 1993;13: 154–161.
33. Katan MB, Zock PL, Mensink RP. Transfatty acids and their effects on lipoproteins in humans. Ann Rev Nutr 1995;15:473–493.
34. Emken EA. Transfatty acids and coronary heart disease. Physicochemical properties, intake and metabolism. Am J Clin Nutr 1995;62(Suppl):659S–669S.
35. Ginsberg H, Oleksky JM, Kimmerling G, Crapo P, Reaven GM. Induction of hypertriglyceridemia by a low-fat diet. J Clin Endocrinol Metab 1976;42:729–735.
36. Cianflone K, Dahan S, Monge JC, Sniderman AD. Pathogenesis of carbohydrated-induced hypertriglyceridemia using HepG2 cells as a model system. Arterioscl Thromb 1992;12: 271–277.
37. Schaefer EJ, Lichtenstein AH, Lamon-Fava S, McNamara JR, Schaefer MM, Rasmussen H, Ordovas JM. Body weight and low-density lipoprotein cholesterol changes after consumption of a low-fat ad libitum diet. JAMA 1995;274:1450–1455.
38. Reaven GM. Do high-carbohydrate diets prevent the development or attenuate the manifestations (or both) of syndrome X? A viewpoint strongly against. Curr Opin Lipid 1997;8:23–27.
39. Purnell JQ, Brunzell JD. The central role of dietary fat, not carbohydrate, in the insulin resistance syndrome. Curr Opin Lipid 1997;8:17–22.
40. Connor WE, Connor SL. Clinical debate: The case for a low-fat diet. N Engl J Med 1997; 337:562–563.
41. Katan MB, Grundy SM, Willett WC. Clinical debate: beyond low-fat diets. N Engl J Med 1997; 337:563–566.
42. Truswell AS. Dietary fibre and blood lipids. Curr Opin Lipid 1995;6:14–19.
43. Potter SM. Soy protein and serum lipids. Curr Opin Lipid 1996;7:260–264.
44. Anderson JW, Johnstone BM, Cook-Newwell ME. Meta-analysis of the effects of soy protein intake on serum lipids. N Engl J Med 1995;333:276–282.
45. Howard BV, Kritchevsky D. Phytochemicals and cardiovascular disease: a statement for health-care professionals from the American Heart Association. Circulation 1997;95:2591–2593.
46. Urgert R, Katan MB. The cholesterol-raising factor from coffee beans. Ann Rev Nutr 1997;17: 305–324.
47. Crouse JR, Grundy SM. Effects of alcohol on plasma lipoproteins and cholesterol and triglyceride metabolism in man. J Lipid Res 1984;25:486–496.
48. Adler AJ, Holub BJ. Effect of garlic and fish-oil supplementation on serum lipid and lipoprotein concentrations in hypercholesterolemic men. Am J Clin Nutr 1997;65:445–450.
49. Warshaksky S, Kamer RS, Sivak SL. Effect of garlic on total serum cholesterol: a meta-analysis. Ann Intern Med 1993;119:599–605.
50. Sendl A, Schliack M, Loser R, Stanislaus F, Wagner H. Inhibition of cholesterol synthesis in vitro by extracts and isolated compounds prepared from garlic and wild garlic. Atherosclerosis

1992;94:79—85.
51. Davis TA, Anderson EC, Ginsberg AV, Goldberg AP. Weight loss improves lipoprotein lipid profiles in patients with hypercholesterolemia. J Lab Clin Med 1985;106:447—454.
52. Olson AG, Ming Yuan X. Antioxidants in the prevention of atherosclerosis. Curr Opin Lipid 1996;7:374—380.
53. Carmena R, Ascaso JF, Camejo G, Varela G, Hurt-Camejo E, Ordovas JM, Martinez-Valls J, Bergstom M, Wallin B. Effect of olive and sunflower oils on low-density lipoprotein level, composition, size, oxidation and interaction with arterial proteoglycans. Atherosclerosis 1996;125:243—255.

Nutrient composition and the metabolic syndrome

Scott M. Grundy
Departments of Clinical Nutrition and Internal Medicine; and Center for Human Nutrition, Dallas, Texas, USA

Keywords: carbohydrates, insulin resistance, monounsaturated fatty acids.

The diet has long been implicated in the development of coronary heart disease (CHD). Epidemiologic studies reveal that CHD rates vary greatly among different countries, particularly among those in which the nutrient composition of diet differs. The specific dietary factors underlying this connection have been intensely investigated. Most research has focused on the influence of particular nutrients on serum cholesterol levels; this is because an elevated serum cholesterol is a major risk factor for CHD, and serum cholesterol concentrations are influenced by the diet. Two constituents, saturated fatty acids and cholesterol, are well-established as serum cholesterol-raising nutrients. These two constituents primarily raise low-density lipoprotein (LDL), the major atherogenic lipoprotein. Higher intakes of saturated fatty acids and cholesterol (typical of high-risk populations) seemingly account for LDL-cholesterol levels that are about 15—20% above those of low-risk populations [1]; conversely, in the latter populations, lower LDL-cholesterol concentrations result largely from lower intakes of animal fats and eggs which are the major sources of saturated fatty acids and cholesterol. Over the short term (e.g., < 10 years), a 15% higher level of serum LDL-cholesterol translates into an approximate 15% higher risk for CHD [2]. Epidemiological data [3], on the other hand, suggest that a 15% higher LDL-cholesterol will raise CHD risk by about 45% when present over the long term (30—40 years). This latter estimate reveals just how dangerous the moderately raised levels of serum LDL cholesterol are that result from high intakes of saturated fatty acids and cholesterol. Thus, high intakes of saturated fatty acids and cholesterol should be reduced in high-risk populations. This can be achieved largely by decreasing the intakes of animal fats, and in some countries, tropical oils. This change will prompt a critical question: what is the most desirable replacement for saturated fatty acids in the diet? This question can be separated into two others:
1. Which nutrients produce the most desirable levels of serum LDL cholesterol?

Address for correspondence: Scott M. Grundy MD, PhD, Departments of Clinical Nutrition and Internal Medicine, University of Texas Southwestern Medical Center at Dallas, 5323 Harry Hines Boulevard, Dallas, TX 75235-9052, USA. Tel.:+1-214-648-2890. Fax: +1-214-648-4837.

520

2. Which nutrients lead to the lowest overall risk for CHD?
These two questions will be addressed under separate headings.

Differential effects of various nutrients on LDL cholesterol levels

Saturated fatty acids

Extensive evidence discloses that saturated fatty acids as a class raise LDL-cholesterol levels, relative to other nutrients. The predominant saturated fatty acid consumed by most high-risk populations is palmitic acid; and multiple studies, carried out in different laboratories, document that palmitic acid is a cholesterol-raising fatty acid [4]. Several recent investigations also shed light on how other saturated fatty acids affect serum LDL-cholesterol. Zock et al. [5], for example, reported that myristic acid is hypercholesterolemic, even more so than palmitic acid. In addition, both lauric acid [6] and medium-chain fatty acids [7], raise LDL-cholesterol levels, although less than palmitic acid does. Only one saturated acid, stearic acid, does not elevate the serum LDL-cholesterol [8].

Transfatty acids

When vegetable oils undergo hydrogenation, their unsaturated fatty acids are partially converted into transfatty acids. Recent investigation [9] documents that transfatty acids raise LDL-cholesterol levels in a similar manner to saturated fatty acids. Transfatty acids are found mainly in hard margarines, shortenings, and processed foods containing hydrogenated fats. Excessive consumption of transfatty acids in the American diet can be estimated to increase serum LDL-cholesterol by about 5 mg/dl [9]. Since saturated fatty acids and transfatty acids both raise serum LDL-cholesterol levels, together they can be called "cholesterol-raising" fatty acids.

Unsaturated fatty acids

The diet contains two major categories of unsaturated fatty acids: polyunsaturated and monounsaturated fatty acids. Polyunsaturates consist of omega-6 and omega-3 fatty acids. Omega-6 polyunsaturated fatty acids predominate in vegetable oils, such as corn oil and safflower oil; omega-3 polyunsaturates occur mainly in fish oil. The predominant monounsaturated fatty acid is oleic acid, which is present in both animal fats and vegetable oils. Oils especially rich in oleic acid include olive oil and canola oil. Both omega-6 polyunsaturated fatty acids and oleic acid lower LDL-cholesterol levels when substituted for saturated fatty acids in the diet. Early studies suggested that polyunsaturated fatty acids reduce serum cholesterol more than oleic acid does [4]. More recent investigations [10] in which lipoproteins were measured, observed less striking differences in LDL-cholesterol levels between the two kinds of unsaturated fatty acids; essentially both polyunsaturated and monounsaturated fatty acids reverse the actions of cholesterol-raising fatty acids when the latter are replaced. The unsaturated fatty acids do not possess unique LDL-lowering properties, as do certain cholesterol-lowering drugs.

Carbohydrate

A series of investigations have shown that substitution of carbohydrate for saturated fatty acids reduces LDL-cholesterol levels [4]. The degree of reduction in LDL-cholesterol concentrations approximates that observed with the unsaturated fatty acids.

Differential effects of various nutrients on other metabolic risk factors

Since omega-6 polyunsaturated fatty acids, monounsaturated fatty acids and carbohydrate have similar effects on LDL cholesterol when they replace cholesterol-raising fatty acids in the diet, the question arises as to which is the preferred replacement. To answer this question, the various metabolic effects of unsaturated fatty acids and carbohydrates must be taken into account. Among these three nutrients, polyunsaturated fatty acids are the most metabolically active. Low intakes of polyunsaturates (1—2% of calories) are required to maintain normal metabolism. On the other hand, because of the metabolic potential of polyunsaturates, concern has been expressed about possible adverse responses to high intakes. Moreover, few epidemiological data are available to certify the safety of high intakes (e.g., > 10% of total calories), when polyunsaturated fatty acids are consumed for many years. In laboratory animals, high intakes of polyunsaturates can suppress the immune system and can promote tumor development [4]. In humans, they may enhance the risk for cholesterol gallstones and promote oxidation of LDL. For these reasons, including a lack of epidemiological support for higher intakes, the current view is that dietary polyunsaturated fatty acids should be kept below 10% of total energy. Since present intakes in the US are about 7% of total calories, there is little leeway to increase polyunsaturates as replacements for saturated fatty acids.

Because of the ceiling on polyunsaturated fatty acids, consideration must be given to other nutrients, especially monounsaturated fatty acids and carbohydrates. Among various populations, percentage intakes of monounsaturates and carbohydrates vary widely. Since these two nutrients have similar effects on LDL-cholesterol levels, other considerations must define the desirable portions of monounsaturates and carbohydrate in the diet. One important consideration is whether other metabolic responses that affect CHD risk differ between these two nutrients. Of particular relevance is whether one or the other nutrient yields a more beneficial effect on the risk factors of the metabolic syndrome. To address this question, it will be necessary to review current concepts of the metabolic syndrome.

Metabolic syndrome

This disorder is characterized by a clustering of metabolic risk factors. These risk factors include:
1) the atherogenic lipoprotein phenotype, or lipid triad (raised triglycerides, abnormal LDL particles and low HDL-cholesterol levels);
2) raised blood pressure;
3) insulin resistance ($\pm$ glucose intolerance); and
4) a procoagulant state [11].
A cogent question is whether a single metabolic derangement can elicit this multiplicity of risk factors in a single individual. This question is clouded in uncertainty. It has been observed that many patients with the syndrome have a generalized metabolic disorder characterized by a dampened cellular response to insulin. A decrease in tissue responsiveness to insulin is called "insulin resistance". Since many patients with the metabolic syndrome manifest insulin resistance, it also has been called the "insulin-resistance syndrome". The term "metabolic syndrome" seems preferable, however, because it denotes a condition of metabolic origin, whereas insulin resistance is but one of the manifestations of the disorder. Insulin resistance thus can be viewed as one component of the metabolic syndrome.

There is currently great interest in the origins of the metabolic syndrome. One question under considerable research is whether genetic or acquired factors predominate in causing of this syndrome. Reaven [12] favors a predominant genetic basis; nonetheless, acquired factors clearly accentuate the syndrome. Further, interactions between genetic and acquired factors may be required to bring forth the various risk factors. So far a single cause has not been identified, and a multifactorial etiology is probably a stronger hypothesis. The major causative factors underlying the metabolic syndrome are obesity, physical inactivity, nutrient composition of the diet, ageing, and genetics. Patients who have truncal obesity are particularly susceptible to the metabolic syndrome; and since truncal obesity occurs more often in men than in women, the syndrome is more common in men.

There seems to be little doubt that the metabolic syndrome taken as a whole constitutes a major risk factor for CHD. What is less certain is that each component of the syndrome is an independent risk factor. Several epidemiological studies, which have focused on one or another component, support the "independence" of each as a risk factor. Still, because of the aggregation of risk factors in the metabolic syndrome, the likelihood of confounding between several factors in risk assessment is considerable. Even so, evidence of independence of each factor has been obtained through different monogenic disorders that affect one or another of the risk factors. Moreover, investigations in laboratory animals reinforce the concept that each component of the syndrome has some atherogenic potential.

Strong evidence indicates that the metabolic syndrome can be improved by changes in life habits. Both weight reduction and increased physical activity in obese patients reduce insulin resistance and mitigate all of the components of the metabolic syndrome. It must be further asked, however, whether the macronutrient composition of the diet also affects these metabolic risk factors. As noted before, the essential question with respect to macronutrient composition is: what is the desirable proportion of carbohydrates and monounsaturated fatty acids in the diet? In order to address this question, it will be necessary to compare the relative effects of these two nutrients on each component of the metabolic syndrome.

The atherogenic lipoprotein phenotype (the lipid triad)

A series of studies have been carried out to evaluate the influence of diet composition on serum levels of triglycerides and HDL and on characteristics of LDL particles. The results of these studies can be summarized briefly. Replacement of dietary saturated fat with carbohydrate causes a rise in serum-triglyceride levels [4]. This same response occurs when carbohydrates replace monounsaturates in the diet [13]. Although it was once speculated that carbohydrate-induced hypertriglyceridemia is a temporary response, more recent epidemiological surveys reveal that higher triglyceride levels persist over the long term [14]. The mechanism of this response is not fully understood. High-carbohydrate diets, which are synonymous with low-fat diets, may promote synthesis of excess triglycerides in the liver; these excess triglycerides may be incorporated into very low-density lipoproteins (VLDL). In addition, synthesis of lipoprotein lipase (LPL) may be reduced; if so, hydrolysis of VLDL triglycerides could be impaired.

One consequence of the rise in serum triglyceride levels is a fall in HDL-cholesterol concentrations. VLDL triglycerides replace cholesterol esters in HDL particles; this leads to depletion of HDL cholesterol and to formation of small HDL particles. Thus, low-fat, high-carbohydrate diets tend to lower HDL-cholesterol levels by raising serum triglyceride concentrations. In addition, low-fat diets appear to reduce the synthesis of apolipoprotein A-I (apo AI), the major apolipoprotein of HDL [15]. This change in apo AI synthesis probably contributes to the decrease in HDL-cholesterol levels. In contrast, diets high in monounsaturates maintain relatively high HDL-cholesterol levels. In addition, high intakes of carbohydrate at the expense of monounsaturates produce abnormalities in size and composition of LDL particles. LDL becomes partially depleted in cholesterol and more heterogenous in size. Smaller LDL particles predominate.

In aggregate, previous research denotes that high-carbohydrate diets (in contrast to diets high in monounsaturates) worsen the lipid triad. A crucial issue, therefore, is whether this apparently adverse change actually raises the risk for CHD. Although there is not certain proof that higher triglycerides, smaller LDL particles and lower HDL levels increase CHD risk when caused by high-carbohydrate diets, it must be a cause of some concern that accentuation of the lipid triad may occur through such a diet.

Hypertension

Hypertension is another component of the metabolic syndrome. There is little doubt the metabolic factors contribute to hypertension. Moreover, hypertension is commonly present in patients who have other components of the metabolic syndrome — dyslipidemia and insulin resistance [12]. Strong evidence points to hypertension being an independent risk factor for CHD. The general categories of causation of the metabolic syndrome also underlie the development of hypertension. Among these, the least investigated is the role of nutrient composition. Only a few studies [16] have examined the effects of nutrient variation on blood pressure, and definitive results have not been obtained. In particular, it is not known whether there are differential effects of dietary carbohydrates and monounsaturates on blood pressure in humans.

Insulin resistance

One feature of many patients with the metabolic syndrome is the presence of insulin resistance. This abnormality is expressed by an elevation of serum insulin concentrations, and in some patients by glucose intolerance. Epidemiological research [12] shows a positive association between insulin resistance and CHD risk. Insulin resistance commonly reflects a generalized biochemical disorder that may be responsible for several metabolic risk factors. In addition, hyperinsulinemia and/or glucose intolerance, which are the products of insulin resistance, may be independent risk factors. This is especially true when glucose intolerance deteriorates into frank hyperglycemia, because hyperglycemia per se has been identified as an independent risk factor. Hyperglycemia occurs when secretion of insulin falls below quantities required to overcome peripheral insulin resistance. One hypothesis holds that prolonged overstimulation of insulin secretion secondary to insulin resistance hastens the decline in insulin secretory capacity that typically occurs with aging. Finally, the metabolic abnormalities underlying insulin resistance may promote atherogenesis through mechanisms that are independent of the known risk factors.

Investigations in some animal models indicate that nutrient composition affects cellular responsiveness to insulin. In certain animal models, high-fat intakes, particularly those high in saturated fatty acids, worsen insulin resistance. The current question under consideration is whether insulin sensitivity in tissues increases or decreases when carbohydrates are exchanged for monounsaturates in the diet. Although some investigators [17] have reported that carbohydrates increase insulin resistance relative to monounsaturates, this difference has not been confirmed in all studies [16]. Therefore, further investigations are needed to define the functional consequences of differences in nutrient composition in humans.

A related issue is whether differences in nutrient composition affect 24 h levels of glucose and insulin differently. Studies in diabetic patients show that high-carbohydrate diets induce greater and more prolonged hyperglycemia than diets high in monounsaturates [16]. High-carbohydrate diets also induce higher insulin levels. Over the long term, these greater responses to high-carbohydrate diets could be detrimental.

Procoagulant state

Patients exhibiting the metabolic syndrome commonly have abnormalities in circulating coagulation factors. These include high serum levels of fibrinogen, factor VII, factor X, plasminogen activating inhibitor-1 (PAI-1) and possibly others. These abnormalities may increase risk for CHD in at least two ways: through enhanced atherogenesis and through thrombus extension at the time of acute coronary events. A procoagulant state has been noted to occur with obesity and the insulin resistance state. Limited research suggests that nutrient composition affects the coagulation system. A diet high in saturated fatty acids has been implicated in the development of a procoagulant state [18]. The possibility that nutrient composition influences the coagulation system in a way that alters CHD risk justifies further investigation. At present it is uncertain whether diet composition adds significantly to the procoagulant state occurring in obese patients, but this possibility cannot be discounted.

Nutrition composition and energy balance

There is a widely held view that nutrient composition is related to total energy balance. For example, some experimental animals develop obesity when they are allowed free access to diets with a high percentage of fat. This response appears to be influenced in part by genetic factors. Whether a high percentage of fat in the diet contributes to human obesity is a disputed and unresolved issue. Without doubt a low level of physical activity provides as substratum for development and maintenance of obesity; since physical inactivity independently increases insulin resistance, more energy-consuming exercise must be an integral part of any strategy to control the metabolic syndrome. Nonetheless, the fact remains that for any given level of physical activity, obese persons consume more food energy than they require. In most overweight persons, both fat and carbohydrate contribute to excess calories. The public health message to substitute low-fat foods for high-fat foods will not ensure weight reduction, particularly if carbohydrate replaces fat in this exchange. Consequently, a priority for curtailment of excess calories must be established. First on the list for reduction are cholesterol-raising fatty acids. These are present in animal fats (e.g., meat fats and milk fat), tropical oils and transrich fats. Low-fat meat and low-fat dairy products of reduced total caloric content can be substituted. Foods high in transfatty acids also should be avoided. Second, foods with a high content of simple sugars should be avoided. These changes alone will be sufficient to correct obesity in most persons.

The remaining sources of energy — starch and unsaturated fatty acids — gener-

526

ally will not produce obesity provided that excess cholesterol-raising fatty acids and simple sugars are sufficiently reduced. The appropriate ratio of starch to unsaturated fatty acids (especially monounsaturates) remains an issue of dispute. Some investigators favor a low total percentage of fat in the diet [19], whereas others recommend intakes of 30–40%, with most of the fatty acids being monounsaturates [20]. On the basis of their relative effects on the lipid triad, a higher percentage of monounsaturates seems preferable. However, more research will be required to define the relative effects of monounsaturates and carbohydrates on the other factors of the metabolic syndrome: blood pressure, tissue sensitivity to insulin, and coagulation tendency.

References

1. Denke MA. Cholesterol-lowering diets: a review of the evidence. Arch Int Med 1995;155: 17–26.
2. Expert Panel on Detection, Evaluation and Treatment of High Blood Cholesterol in Adults. National Cholesterol Education Program: second report of the expert panel on detection, evaluation, and treatment of high blood cholesterol in adults (Adult Treatment Panel II). Circulation 1994;89:1329–1445.
3. Lamarche B, Tchernof A, Moorjani S, Cantin B, Dagenais GR, Lupien PJ, Despres JP. Small, dense low-density lipoprotein phenotype as a predictor of the risk of ischemic heart disease in men: prospective results from the Quebec Cardiovascular Study. Circulation 1996;94:69–75.
4. Grundy SM, Denke MA. Dietary influences on serum lipids and lipoproteins. J Lipid Res 1990;31:1149–1172.
5. Zock PL, de Vries JHM, Katan MB. Impact of myristic acid vs. palmitic acid on serum lipid and lipoprotein levels in healthy women and men. Arterioscl Thromb 1994;14:567–575.
6. Denke MA, Grundy SM. Comparison of effects of lauric acid and palmitic acid on plasma lipids and lipoproteins. Am J Clin Nutr 1992;56:895–898.
7. Cater NB, Heller HJ, Denke MA. Comparison of the effects of medium-chain triacylglycerols, palm oil, and high oleic sunflower oil on plasma acylglycerol fatty acids and lipid and lipoprotein concentrations in humans. Am J Clin Nutr 1997;65:41–45.
8. Bonanome A, Grundy SM. Effect of dietary stearic acid on plasma cholesterol and lipoprotein levels. N Engl J Med 1988;318:1244–1248.
9. Katan MB, Mensink RP, Zock PL. Transfatty acids and their effect on lipoproteins in humans. Ann Rev Nutr 1995;15:473–493.
10. Mensink RP, Katan MB. Effects of dietary fatty acids on serum lipids and lipoproteins: a meta-analysis of 27 trials. Arteriosclerosis 1992;12:911–919.
11. Grundy SM. Small LDL, atherogenic dyslipidemia, and the metabolic syndrome. Circulation 1997;95:1–4.
12. Reaven GM. Insulin resistance and compensatory hyperinsulinemia: role in hypertension, dyslipidemia, and coronary heart disease. Am Heart J 1991;121:1283–1288.
13. Grundy SM. Comparison of monounsaturated fatty acids and carbohydrates for lowering plasma cholesterol. N Engl J Med 1986;314:745–748.
14. West CE, Sullivan DR, Katan MB, Halferkamps IN, van der Torre HW. Boys from populations with high-carbohydrate intake have higher fasting triglyceride levels than boys from populations with high-fat intake. Am J Epidemiol 1990;131:271–282.
15. Brinton EA, Eisenberg S, Breslow JL. A low-fat diet decreases high-density lipoprotein (HDL) cholesterol levels by decreasing HDL apolipoprotein transport rates. J Clin Invest 1990;85: 144–151.

16. Garg A. High-monounsaturated-fat diet for diabetic patients. Is it time to change the current dietary recommendations? Diabet Care 1994;17:242—246.

17. Parillo M, Rivellese AA, Ciardullo AV, Capaldo B, Giacco A, Genovese S, Riccardi G. A high-monounsaturated fat/low-carbohydrate diet improves peripheral insulin sensitivity in non-insulin-dependent diabetic patients. Metabolism 1992;41:1373—1378.

18. Miller GJ, Martin JC, Webster J, Wilkes H, Miller NE, Wilkinson WH, Meade TW. Association between dietary fat intake and plasma factor VII coagulant activity — a predictor of cardiovascular mortality. Atherosclerosis 1986;60:269—277.

19. Connor WE, Connor SL. The case for a low-fat, high-carbohydrate diet. N Engl J Med 1997;337:562—563.

20. Katan MB, Grundy SM, Willett WC. Beyond low-fat diets. N Engl J Med 1997;337:563—566.

Atherosclerosis XI.
B. Jacotot, D. Mathé and J.-C. Fruchart, editors.

The effects of the Mediterranean diet on glucose metabolism and insulin sensitivity

M. Mancini, M. Parillo and A.A. Rivellese
Department of Clinical and Experimental Medicine, Federico II University Medical School, Naples, Italy

Keywords: glucose metabolism, insulin sensitivity, lipid metabolism, Mediterranean diet.

Introduction

Several epidemiological data have demonstrated that the relation between plasma cholesterol and coronary heart disease (CHD) is continuous and graded and that a decrease in plasma cholesterol by dietary or pharmacological interventions can substantially reduce cardiovascular events. Studies performed mainly in hypercholesterolemic individuals demonstrated that the reduction in dietary fat and cholesterol is the most effective dietary modification for decreasing plasma cholesterol (Oslo Study) [1—4]. Therefore, national and international medical societies advise a low-fat diet not only for hypercholesterolemic patients, but also for other individuals at high risk for CHD (i.e., diabetic and hypertensive patients) and to the general population as well.

Mortality from CHD as well as mean plasma cholesterol concentrations are different among populations. This was first indicated by Ancel Keys in the Seven Countries Study. The 15-year follow-up of this famous study revealed a lower mortality rate not only for CHD but also for all causes in the Mediterranean region (Italy, Greece) compared to non-Mediterranean ones (Finland, The Netherlands) [1]. Again, this is an observation in great favor of the Mediterranean way of eating.

By using food consumption data from FAO Food Balance Sheets, we have recently shown that the common characteristics of the diet consumed in the various Mediterranean countries are the low intake of saturated fats and the high intake of unsaturated fats and carbohydrates due to the daily consumption of olive oil, cereals, green vegetables and fresh fruit.

In this report we will indicate that monounsaturated fat, complex carbohydrates and fiber (the principal components of Mediterranean diet) affect not only lipid metabolism but also glucose metabolism and insulin sensitivity.

Address for correspondence: Prof Mario Mancini, Department of Clinical and Experimental Medicine, Federico II University Medical School, via S. Pansini 5, 80131 Naples, Italy. Tel.: +39-81-7462011. Fax: +39-81-5466152. E-mail: nmcd@unina.it

Fat-modified vs. low-fat/high-CHO diet

In the fat-modified diet, foods rich in saturated fat and cholesterol are replaced by either polyunsaturated or monounsaturated fat.

All the studies that have compared the fat-modified vs. the low-fat diet have demonstrated that the effects of the two diets on plasma cholesterol are similar [5—8]. Therefore, in individuals in whom hypercholesterolemia is the single cardiovascular risk factor, both regimes can be advised.

The majority of individuals prone to CHD show either high plasma LDL cholesterol or a clustering of cardiovascular risk factors, i.e., obesity, hypertriglyceridemia, low HDL, hypertension, abnormalities of glucose metabolism, hyperinsulinemia and insulin resistance (the plurimetabolic syndrome or Syndrome X) [8]. For the best possible control of these complex metabolic abnormalities, a comparison between the low-fat/high-carbohydrate diet and the fat-modified diet is to be evaluated.

In fact, in patients with essential hypertension, the low-fat diet as compared with the fat-modified diet, leads to a lower total- and LDL-plasma cholesterol, but causes an increase in daily plasma glucose and insulin profile [9]. The same effects have been obtained in patients with hypertriglyceridemia [10].

More data have been published on NIDDM, the most common disease characterized by insulin resistance. A few years ago some studies (partly criticized) showed an improvement in glucose metabolism with the low-fat diet [11—14] but recently the comparison between the low-fat and the fat-modified diet in diabetic patients has been carefully attempted by our group.

In fact, we have compared the effects of a fat-modified (high in monounsaturated fat) and a low-fat diet in 10 NIDDM patients treated with diet or diet plus glibenclamide. Each diet was composed exclusively of natural foods (olive oil as the main source of MUFA and bread, rice, potatoes and pasta as the main sources of carbohydrates) and was administered for 15 days in the metabolic ward [15]. The results of this study show a significant increase in postprandial plasma glucose, insulin and in fasting plasma triglyceride after the low-fat diet (Table 1). The effects on plasma cholesterol and HDL were similar after the two diets. Therefore, for individuals in whom hypercholesterolemia is not the single or predominant cardiovascular risk factor, the low-fat/high-CHO diet induces a deterioration of some other metabolic aspects and therefore, may increase the

Table 1. Effects of a fat-modified (high MUFA) and a low-fat diet on glucose metabolism (M ± SE) in patients with NIDDM.

	Fat-modified diet	Low-fat diet
Postprandial blood glucose (mmol/l)	8.6 ± 0.6	10.0 ± 0.8[b]
Postprandial plasma insulin (mmol/l)	195.0 ± 24.0	224.0 ± 24.0[a]
Glucose utilization (mmol/kg/min)	100.8 ± 12.6	84.6 ± 10.8[b]

[a]$p < 0.05$; [b]$p < 0.02$.

cardiovascular risk.

These results have been confirmed by other investigators [16,17]. Furthermore, Coulston et al. have demonstrated that the hyperglycemic and hypertriglyceridemic effect of the low-fat diet in NIDDM patients is not transient but persists after 6 weeks of dietary intervention [18].

In evaluating a diet for the treatment of NIDDM, its effect on insulin resistance deserves attention, since it plays an important role in the pathogenesis of this disease. Therefore, we have evaluated the influence of the low-fat/high-carbohydrate diet on insulin sensitivity, as compared with the fat-modified diet measured by the euglycemic hyperinsulinemic clamp. The low-fat diet decreased insulin sensitivity significantly, by 20% in NIDDM patients (Table 1) [15].

Our data clearly show a worsening of the cardiovascular risk factor profile after the low-fat diet in NIDDM patients. In fact with this diet there is an increase in plasma glucose, insulin and triglycerides, and a worsening of peripheral insulin sensitivity.

In conclusion, the data now available indicate that in patients in whom hypercholesterolemia is not the only metabolic abnormality (such as diabetic, hypertriglyceridemic and hypertensive patients) the use of a low-fat/high-CHO diet is questionable. In these patients, it seems rather advisable to substitute saturated fat and cholesterol in the diet with mono- or polyunsaturated fat.

Fat-modified vs. low-fat/high-fiber diet

Vegetable undigested fiber is the part of vegetable foods which is not digested in the human bowel. It can be classified as either water soluble or hydrophilic (guar, pectin, etc.) or insoluble or hydrophobic (cellulose, lignin, etc.). Acute metabolic studies have demonstrated that soluble fiber has a beneficial influence on glucose and lipid metabolism. In fact soluble fiber increases the viscosity of the intestinal content and forms a gel which slows down the absorption of glucose, lipids and bile acids.

Many clinical studies have evaluated the effects of a low-fat/high-CHO diet enriched with vegetable fiber on glucose and lipid metabolism. In particular this type of diet (in which the enrichment with fiber is due exclusively to the use of natural foods with a high content of soluble fiber, such as legumes, fresh fruit and vegetables) reduces the concentrations of plasma cholesterol in hypercholesterolemic patients (Table 2). No consistent effect of dietary fiber has been shown on plasma triglycerides and HDL cholesterol. Even more striking are the results obtained with the high-fiber diet in diabetic patients. In IDDM and NIDDM patients we have compared the fat-modified (CHO: 42%, fat: 38%, fiber 20 g) and the low-fat/high-CHO and fiber diet (CHO: 53%, fat: 30%, fiber: 54 g). The two diets were consumed for consecutive periods of 10 days in diabetic patients hospitalized in the metabolic ward. In both IDDM and NIDDM patients the low-fat/high-CHO and fiber diet produced a significant decrease in plasma postprandial glucose and insulin in comparison with the fat-modified diet. Also

532

Table 2. Effects of diets rich in soluble fiber on plasma total and lipoprotein cholesterol in patients with type II hyperlipoproteinemia.

Cholesterol (mmol/l)	Low-fiber diet	High-fiber diet
Total	7.6 ± 1.2	7.2 ± 1.4
VLDL	0.8 ± 0.5	0.9 ± 0.8
LDL	5.8 ± 1.5	5.2 ± 1.3[a]
HDL	1.0 ± 0.2	1.1 ± 0.2

[a]p < 0.05. Mean ± SE.

plasma-cholesterol levels were significantly reduced, while there were no differences in plasma triglycerides and HDL-cholesterol concentrations [19—21].

In summary, the use of fiber-rich foods in the low-fat/high-CHO diet induces a larger decrease in plasma-cholesterol levels and prevents the untoward effects of dietary carbohydrates on plasma glucose, insulin and triglyceride levels in diabetic patients. In these patients a high-CHO and fiber diet has more beneficial effects on glucose metabolism than a fat-modified diet. These data have been confirmed by other investigators.

Very few studies have evaluated the effects of dietary fiber on insulin sensitivity. In nondiabetic individuals Fugawa et al. have demonstrated that the low-fat/high-CHO and fiber diet improves insulin sensitivity [22].

The adoption of a high-fiber diet for long periods of time is considered unfeasible by many clinicians. The consumption of fiber-rich foods is usually low in Western countries and studies on dietary fiber have so far been short-term. Therefore, in order to assess the long-term feasibility of the high-fiber diet we have recently undertaken a controlled trial in mildly hyperlipidemic patients. Forty-four hyperlipidemic patients were randomly allocated to follow, for 6 months, either a fat-modified (CHO:40%, fat: 38%, fiber: 15 g) or a low-fat/high-CHO and fiber diet (CHO: 55%, fat: 25%, fiber: 30 g). Both diets were equally effective in reducing not only plasma-cholesterol levels but also plasma concentrations of triglycerides, glucose and insulin (Table 3) [23]. Also, HDL-cholesterol levels were similar after the two diets. Adherence to the diet was better with the high-fiber diet than with the fat-modified diet. This study has, in fact, demonstrated that the low-fat/high-CHO and fiber diet is feasible for a long period of time. Moreover, it has confirmed the importance of soluble fiber to prevent the untoward effects of a high-CHO diet on triglyceride and glucose metabolism in the long term. Therefore, a low-fat/high-CHO and fiber diet in comparison with a fat-modified diet seems the best approach to treat patients with abnormalities of both lipid and glucose metabolism.

Conclusions

Reducing cholesterol and saturated fat intake is advisable to prevent cardiovascular disease. The low-fat diet with high CHO (starchy food), however, is not recom-

Table 3. Long-term (6 months) effects of low-fat/high-fiber diet and of the fat-modified diet on plasma lipoproteins in type II hyperlipidemic patients.

	Low-fat/high-CHO/high-fiber diet		Fat-modified diet	
	Baseline	6 months	Baseline	6 months
Cholesterol (mmol/l)				
Total	7.44 ± 0.18	6.78 ± 0.15^{ab}	7.23 ± 0.16	6.63 ± 0.4^{ab}
VLDL	0.63 ± 0.08	0.76 ± 0.09	0.80 ± 0.15	0.65 ± 0.05
LDL	5.54 ± 0.20	4.82 ± 0.18^{ab}	5.34 ± 0.25	4.85 ± 0.21^{a}
HDL	1.16 ± 0.06	1.22 ± 0.06	1.07 ± 0.06	1.12 ± 0.04
Triglycerides (mmol/dl)				
Total	1.71 ± 0.14	1.50 ± 0.13^{a}	1.96 ± 0.26	1.57 ± 0.17^{b}
VLDL	1.07 ± 0.13	1.01 ± 0.12	1.29 ± 0.21	1.07 ± 0.17^{a}

Significance vs. baseline [a]$p < 0.05$; [b]$p < 0.001$. Mean $\pm$ SE.

mended in patients with insulin resistance, particularly diabetic, hypertensive and hypertriglyceridemic patients.

The consumption of foods rich in fiber (legumes, fresh fruits and green vegetables) counteracts the adverse effects of dietary carbohydrate on glucose and lipid metabolism. When such a diet is not acceptable, similar effects can be obtained by enriching the diet with monoene oleic acid.

References

1. Keys A et al. The diet and 15 years death rate in the Seven Country Study. Am J Epidemiol 1986;124:903–915.
2. Lipid Research Clinics Program: The Lipid Research Clinics Coronary Primary Prevention Trial Results II. The relationship of reduction in incidence of coronary heart disease to cholesterol lowering. JAMA 1984;251:365–380.
3. The MRFIT Research Group. MRFIT risk factors changes and mortality results. JAMA 1982;248:1465–1476.
4. The Oslo Study Group. Effect of diet and smoking intervention on the incidence of coronary heart disease. Lancet 1981;ii:1303–1310.
5. Riccardi G, Rivellese AA, Mancini M. The use of diet to lower plasma-cholesterol levels. Eur Heart J 1987;8(Suppl E):79–85.
6. Mancini M, Parillo M. Role of diet in the treatment of hyperlipidemias. In: Crepaldi G, Tiengo A, Enzi G (eds) Diabetes, Obesity and Hyperlipidemias. New York: Elsevier Science Publisher, 1990;91–97.
7. Grundy SM. Comparison of monounsaturated fatty acids and carbohydrates for lowering plasma cholesterol. N Engl J Med 1986;314:745–748.
8. Reaven GM. Role of insulin resistance in human disease. Diabetes 1988;37:1595–1606.
9. Parillo M et al. Effect of a low-fat diet on carbohydrate metabolism in patients with hypertension. Hypertension 1988;11:244–248.
10. Liu GC et al. Effect of high-carbohydrate low-fat diets on plasma glucose, insulin and lipid responses in hypertriglyceridemic humans. Metabolism 1983;32:750–753.
11. Brunzell JD et al. Improved glucose tolerance with high-carbohydrate feeding in mild diabetes.

N Engl J Med 1971;284:521—524.
12. Kolterman CG et al. Effect of a high-carbohydrate diet on insulin binding to adipocytes and on insulin action in vivo in man. Diabetes 1979;28:731—736.
13. Himsworth HP. Diabetic factors influencing the glucose tolerance and the activity of insulin. J Physiol (Lond) 1934;81:29—48.
14. Himsworth HP. The dietetic factor determining the glucose tolerance and sensitivity to insulin of healthy men. Clin Sci 1935;2:67—94.
15. Parillo M et al. A high monounsaturated-fat/low-CHO diet improves peripheral insulin sensitivity in non-insulin-dependent diabetic patients. Metabolism 1992;41:1371—1378.
16. Rivellese AA et al. Effects of changing amount of carbohydrate in diet on plasma lipoproteins and apolipoproteins in type II diabetic patients. Diabet Care 1990;13:446—448.
17. Carg A et al. Comparison of a high-carbohydrate diet with a high-monounsaturated-fat diet in patients with non-insulin-dependent diabetes mellitus. N Engl J Med 1988;319:829—834.
18. Coulston AM et al. Persistence of hypertriglyceridemic effect of low-fat high-carbohydrate diets in NIDDM patients. Diabet Care 1989;12:94—100.
19. Riccardi G, Rivellese AA. Effects of dietary fiber and carbohydrate on glucose and lipoprotein metabolism in diabetic patients. Diabet Care 1991;4:1115—1125.
20. Riccardi G et al. Separate influence of dietary carbohydrate and fibre on the metabolic control in diabetes. Diabetologia 1984;26:116—121.
21. Rivellese AA et al. Effect of dietary fibre on glucose control and serum lipoproteins in diabetic patients. Lancet 1980;2:447—450.
22. Fugawa NK et al. High-carbohydrate, high-fibre diets increase peripheral insulin sensitivity in healthy young and old adults. Am J Clin Nutr 1990;52:524—528.
23. Rivellese AA et al. Long-term metabolic effects of two dietary methods of treating hyperlipidemia. BMJ 1994;308:227—231.

Clinical efficacy of soy proteins and evaluation of the potential mechanisms of their cholesterol-lowering effect

Cesare R. Sirtori[1,2], Elisabetta Gianazza[1], Maria Rosa Lovati[1], Cristina Manzoni[1], Nicoletta Della Mura[2], Lorenzo Colombo[2] and Franco Pazzucconi[2]

[1]*Institute of Pharmacological Sciences; and* [2]*Center E. Grossi Paoletti, University of Milan, Milan, Italy*

A possible role for vegetable proteins in preventing arterial disease was first proposed by a Russian physician, Ignatowsky, at the beginning of this century. Since then, evidence on a possible cholesterol-lowering activity of vegetable proteins has been accumulating [1]. Proteins (the major structural components in the diet) are the most likely candidates for this effect, but in principle other components such as fibers or isoflavones might be involved as well. Among vegetable derivatives, soy proteins have been most extensively evaluated in humans as well as in animal models of hyperlipidemia.

Clinical evidence on the role of soy-protein components in regulating cholesterolemia

Anderson et al. [2] recently analyzed 38 studies, both in patients with elevated plasma cholesterol and in normolipidemic volunteers, all treated for a variable length of time with diets with partial or total substitution of animal proteins with soy proteins. The conclusions of this meta-analysis (summarized in Fig. 1) confirm that serum and LDL-cholesterol concentrations are modified according to baseline cholesterolemia, from a minimum of -3.3% in subjects with cholesterol in the normal range, up to -19.6% (LDL-cholesterol -24%) in clear-cut hypercholesterolemics. Many of these data have been gathered by us and other Italian groups [3,4].

Very recently we have also tested the possibility that the soybean-protein diet may favourably affect LDL-cholesterol levels in patients not responding to statins. Statins reduce plasma cholesterol by inhibiting biosynthesis, and then upregulating LDL-receptors; they have been shown to synergize with soy protein in the rabbit model [5]. In some patients, either statins do not bring about any significant LDL-cholesterol reduction, or some form of tolerance seems to occur after prolonged treatment [6]. A soy-protein diet might theoretically be helpful for

---

Address for correspondence: Cesare R. Sirtori, Institute of Pharmacological Sciences, University of Milano, Via Balzaretti 9, I-20133 Milano, Italy.

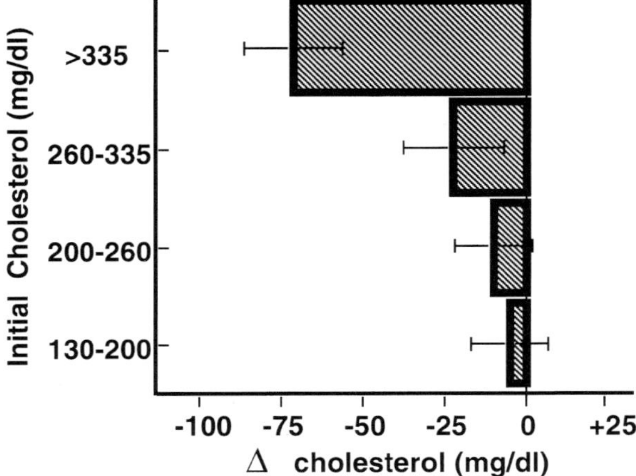

Fig. 1. Correlation between the plasma cholesterol changes and baseline cholesterolemia in the 38 studies of a recent meta-analysis [10].

such patients, acting by a different mechanism, i.e., direct LDL-receptor upregulation.

Two series of patients with an inadequate response to statins were studied. The first group was given a total substitution of animal proteins with a textured soy product, free of isoflavones: a significant LDL-cholesterol reduction was observed, most marked in patients with the highest starting levels (Table 1). In a second series, soy proteins (with isoflavones) were given to patients responding to the above criteria, added to a low-lipid diet. Soy protein was given for 4 weeks in a crossover design vs. 4 weeks of casein in a similar formulation (chocolate drink). In this controlled investigation the addition of soy protein was found to significantly reduce LDL cholesterolemia in severely hypercholesterolemic patients.

Table 1. Effect of soybean protein on nonresponders to statins.

	Initial	Final	Δ%
Total cholesterol	330 ± 59	286 ± 59	− 13.6**
LDL cholesterol	240 ± 57	204 ± 55	− 15.0**
Triglyceride	191 ± 43	183 ± 49	− 4.1
Apo C-III	7.0 ± 2.5	6.6 ± 2.3	− 6.4

Best responders
f 58 y, initial 400 mg/dl, final 304 mg/dl
m 43 y, initial 398 mg/dl, final 305 mg/dl

10 patients; age range 38–71 years; six males, four females; total cholesterol range 253–419 mg/dl. X ± SD. LDL, low-density lipoprotein; Apo-CIII, apoprotein CIII. **p < 0.01.

Definition of the soy components responsible for the plasma-cholesterol reduction in man

A potential role of fibers or fiber-like compounds (saponins) in soy preparations in lowering cholesterolemia was earlier proposed, but later ruled out by the same authors, who proved a complete lack of effect of saponins on either fecal sterol elimination or plasma cholesterol [7]. Confirmation of these findings was provided by two further studies. In the first study, we established that the cholesterol reduction can occur without any changes in fecal sterol elimination or in the plasma-cholesterol turnover, thus suggesting that cholesterol transfer to tissues (possibly followed by a slow and delayed excretion) is indeed the mechanism [8]. In the second study, Anderson et al. [9] compared a classical oat-bran diet (containing β-glucan, a water-soluble gum) with a soybean diet (with negligible cholesterol/bile acid binding properties). The authors found that both diets can reduce cholesterolemia, but only the former leads to a significant increase in fecal sterol elimination. Body cholesterol metabolism may thus be globally influenced by the soybean diet, in a way that is not different from hypocholesterolemic statins that reduce cholesterolemia, also without altering total body cholesterol content.

The 1995 meta-analysis [2] based on a recent study with monkeys [10], suggested that a large portion of the soy effect on cholesterolemia might be linked to the presence of isoflavones, i.e., genistein and daidzein and/or their conjugates. Isoflavones (compounds with a weak estrogenic/antiestrogenic activity) are believed to be responsible for the longer menstrual cycle and delayed menopause in Oriental women [11]. Some of these hypotheses were confirmed in a clinical study in healthy women [11] but not in a similar study in postmenopausal females [12]. Isoflavones are present in variable amounts in soy preparations and their absorption is highly variable, in some individuals being close to nil and highly dependent on the gut microflora.

From a biochemical point of view, if LDL-receptor activation is the mechanism of the plasma cholesterol reduction induced by soy proteins (see below), then isoflavones should have an exactly opposite effect. These products (being inhibitors of tyrosine kinase) negatively regulate LDL-receptors in cells, as clearly demonstrated in a human liver cell system [13]. At least one demonstrative animal investigation has suggested that soy isoflavones may be directly responsible for the plasma cholesterol reduction [10]. This study evaluated a soy product in which isoflavones were eliminated by ethanol extraction, thus removing not only isoflavones but possibly also small molecular-weight peptides, potentially responsible for the LDL-receptor activation [14]. A study in rats with contrasting results has been recently published [15]. Therefore, while the isoflavone hypothesis should not be totally dismissed, it would certainly need more substantial evidence.

We recently evaluated the isoflavone content of different textured products used in the clinical studies by our group and other Italian/Swiss investigators, in the past 20 years [1]. These were surprisingly found to be essentially free of isoflavones, contrary to the case of soy flour [16].

A final possibility is that soy proteins may directly reduce cholesterolemia. This notion seems reasonable in the face of evidence, some of which is very recent [17], indicating that the presence of additional components besides protein might not affect in a significant way the plasma cholesterol reduction achieved with the diet.

Experimental and clinical data lending support to the responsibility of proteins per se have come from our studies indicating that, both in laboratory animals and in man, a change from animal to vegetable protein in the diet leads to the activation of the LDL-receptor system. This occurs in the rat liver, and in man, in a cell type, circulating lymphomonocyte [18], sharing the major mechanisms of LDL-receptor regulation with hepatocytes. In order to identify the protein component/s potentially responsible for the cholesterol reduction, experiments are now being performed in a hepatoma cell line (HepG2), an in vitro model of human liver cells, highly sensitive to factors regulating LDL-receptor expression and cholesterol biosynthesis/breakdown. These studies have concluded that the 7S globulin (one of the major storage proteins of soybean) directly upregulates LDL-receptor expression by 50% or more vs. controls after prolonged incubation [19].

Experiments on the 7S soy-globulin subunits have clearly shown that the purified $\alpha+\alpha'$ subunits from 7S markedly increase uptake and degradation of ^{125}I-LDL, whereas the β chains are ineffective. Soybean varieties deficient in the α' subunits appeared to be ineffective in LDL-receptor regulation. More recently, in degradation studies, we evaluated whether 7S components may in some way provide more explicit suggestions on the final mechanism by which these products modify LDL-cholesterol activity. By incubating 7S components with HepG2 cells it appears that the $\alpha+\alpha'$ subunits may be more completely degraded, whereas most of the β chains are unaffected or barely reduced in size. In addition, by monitoring LDL-receptor mRNA level by Northern blotting, it could be clearly established that 7S globulin or subunits thereof can activate the transcription of the LDL-receptor gene into the mRNA for LDL-receptors in liver cells.

In spite of these confirmative data, the hypothesis of a direct activity of proteins on the plasma-cholesterol regulation is still open to criticism. While the pros for a direct activity of soy proteins appear to be consistent, being supported by clinical data and by in vitro and in vivo experiments, we still lack a clear understanding of the digestion pattern of soy proteins in vivo and of the possible absorption of undegraded, biologically active peptide fragments. Until these data provide satisfactory evidence for a reliable digestion pattern of soy protein, the final mechanism of cholesterol reduction, induced by this dietary addition, will remain unclear.

Conclusions

The clinical data in support of a significant cholesterol-lowering property of soy proteins confirm findings of 20 years ago in our laboratory. Collection of experimental and clinical evidence has gone together with major developments in technologies for more varied and palatable preparations of soy for human use. This has resulted in a dramatic increase in consumption of soy products in the Western world.

It was recently indicated that population approaches with hypocholesterolemic diets may be followed by a more effective prevention of coronary disease vs. a patient-based approach, e.g., with statins. In clinical hypercholesterolemia the percent reduction of cardiovascular events with the population approach may be in fact higher than 30 vs. 15—20% at most for a drug approach. A soybean-based diet may be ideally suited for this objective.

References

1. Sirtori CR, Lovati MR, Manzoni C, Monetti M, Pazzucconi F, Gatti E. Soy and cholesterol reduction: clinical experience. J Nutr 1995;125:598S—605S.
2. Anderson JW, Johnstone BJ, Cook-Newell ME. Meta-analysis of the effects of soy protein intake on serum lipids. N Engl J Med 1995;333:276—282.
3. Sirtori CR, Agradi E, Sirtori M, Conti F, Paoletti R. Soybean-protein diet in the treatment of type II hyperlipoproteinemia. Lancet 1977;i:275—278.
4. Descovich GC, Ceredi C, Gaddi A et al. Multicentre study of soybean protein diet for outpatient hyper-cholesterolaemic patients. Lancet 1980;2:709—712.
5. Giroux I, Lavigne C, Moorjani S, Jacques H. Simvastatin further enhances the hypocholesterolemic effect of soy protein in rabbits. J Am Coll Nutr 1997;16:166—174.
6. Pazzucconi F, Dorigotti F, Gianfranceschi G et al. Therapy with HMG CoA reductase inhibitors; characteristics of the long-term permanence of hypocholesterolemic activity. Atherosclerosis 1995;117:189—198.
7. Calvert GD, Blight L, Illman RJ, Topping DL, Potter JD. A trial of the effects of soyabean flour and soyabean saponins on plasma lipids, faecal bile acids and neutral sterols in hypercholesterolaemic men. Br J Nutr 1981;45:277—281.
8. Fumagalli R, Soleri L, Musanti R et al. Fecal cholesterol excretion studies in type II hypercholesterolemic patients treated with the soybean protein diet. Atherosclerosis 1982;43:341—353.
9. Anderson JW, Story L, Sieling B, Lin Chen W-J, Petro MS, Story J. Hypocholesterolemic effects of oat-bran or bean intake for hypercholesterolemic men. Am J Clin Nutr 1984;40:1146—1155.
10. Anthony MS, Clarkson TB, Hughes CL Jr, Morgan TM, Burke GL. Soybean isoflavones improve cardiovascular risk factors without affecting the reproductive system of peripubertal Rhesus Monkeys. J Nutr 1996;126:43—50.
11. Cassidy A, Bingham S, Setchell KDR. Biological effects of a diet of soy protein rich in isoflavones on the menstrual cycle of premenopausal women. Am J Clin Nutr 1994;60:333—340.
12. Baird DD, Umbach DM, Lansdell L et al. Dietary intervention study to assess estrogenicity of dietary soy among postmenopausal women. J Clin Endocrinol Metab 1995;80:1685—1690.
13. Grove RI, Mazzucco CE, Radka SF, Shoyab M, Kiener PA. Oncostatin M upregulates low-density lipoprotein receptors in HepG2 cells by a novel mechanism. J Biol Chem 1991;266:18194—18199.
14. Lovati MR, Manzoni C, Agostinelli P, Ciappellano S, Mannucci L, Sirtori CR. Studies on the mechanism of the cholesterol-lowering activity of soy protein. Soy protein extract reduces plasma cholesterol and increases liver β-VLDL receptors in mice. NMCD 1991;1:18—24.
15. Arjmandi BH, Khan DA, Juma SS, Svanborg A. The ovarian hormone deficiency-induced hypercholesterolemia is reversed by soy protein and the synthetic isoflavone, ipriflavone. Nutr

Res 1997;17:885—894.

16. Sirtori CR, Gianazza E, Manzoni C, Lovati MR, Murphy PA. Role of isoflavones in the cholesterol reduction by soy proteins in the clinic. Type II patients in the Italian studies with the soybean protein diet did not receive isoflavones. Am J Clin Nutr 1997;65:166—167.

17. Potter SM, Pertile J, Berbez-Jimenez MD. Soy protein concentrate and isolated soy protein similarly lower blood serum cholesterol but differently affect thyroid hormones in hamsters. J Nutr 1996;126:2007—2011.

18. Lovati MR, Manzoni C, Canavesi A et al. Soybean protein diet increases low-density lipoprotein receptor activity in mononuclear cells from hypercholesterolemic patients. J Clin Invest 1987; 80:125—130.

19. Lovati MR, Manzoni C, Corsini A et al. 7S globulin from soybean is metabolized in human cell cultures by a specific uptake and degradation system. J Nutr 1996;126:2831—2843.

The epidemiology of vitamin E and coronary heart disease

Meir J. Stampfer and Eric B. Rimm
Departments of Epidemiology and Nutrition, Harvard School of Public Health; Channing Laboratory, Department of Medicine, Brigham and Women's Hospital; and Harvard Medical School, Boston, Massachusetts, USA

Abstract. Vitamin E is a key lipid soluble antioxidant which may reduce atherogenesis and lower risk of coronary heart disease (CHD), presumably by reducing lipid peroxidation of low-density lipoprotein particles. Cross-cultural studies find that regions with relatively low-dietary intake tend to have higher rates of CHD, but in these studies it is difficult to account for other important cardiovascular risk factors. The evidence for a cardiovascular benefit of antioxidants is strongest for vitamin E. Three large prospective studies find that vitamin E supplement users have approximately 40% lower rates of CHD. Short durations and doses of less than 100 IU/per day (when data were available) have no significant effect. The effect of dietary vitamin E may be more modest, but is still associated with lower risk of CHD in populations where vitamin E supplementation is infrequent. In a large randomized trial a nonsignificant reduction in CHD risk was reported for 50 IU/per day, although the dose may have been insufficient. The same dose in a secondary prevention setting appeared to reduce nonfatal but not fatal outcomes. A secondary prevention trial of 400 and 800 IU/day reported a strong reduction in nonfatal myocardial infarction further supporting the large body of evidence which suggests that high doses of vitamin E reduce risk of CHD. Although the findings are not entirely consistent, emerging evidence taken together continues to support a benefit from vitamin E supplementation. Further study, and data from pending randomized trials are necessary before general public health policy recommendations to take vitamin E supplements can be justified.

Oxidation of low-density lipoprotein (LDL) appears to be important in atherogenesis. As reviewed by Steinberg et al. [1], oxidized LDL is preferentially taken up by macrophages to create foam cells. In addition, it appears to be cytotoxic to endothelial cells and decreases motility of tissue macrophages. Vitamin E is a fat-soluble antioxidant and can function as a free-radical scavenger to decrease the initiation and propagation of fatty-acid oxidation [2]. Vitamin E is predominantly carried in LDL and is particularly effective in protecting it from oxidation [3]. In addition, vitamin E can inhibit smooth muscle cell proliferation, an important component of atherogenesis [4]. Finally, vitamin E may reduce risk of cardiovascular disease through its effect on platelet adhesion [5]. Laboratory data and recent animal and epidemiologic data also support the hypothesis that vitamin E may reduce risk of cardiovascular disease [6]. This review focuses on recent epidemiological findings which have addressed the role of vitamin E in the prevention of CHD.

Address for correspondence: Meir Stampfer MD, Channing Laboratory, 181 Longwood Avenue, Boston, MA 02115, USA. Tel.: +1-617-525-2747. Fax: +1-617-525-2008.

In a cross-cultural study, Gey et al. [7] found a remarkable inverse correlation between plasma vitamin E levels (adjusted for cholesterol) and the rates of coronary mortality, even among the 12 centers with similar distributions of classical coronary risk factors. Similarly, Kristenson et al. [8] found lower plasma vitamin E in men from Vilnius (a high-incidence region) compared to the lower risk area of Linkoping, Sweden. In contrast, in the large EURAMIC case-control study of myocardial infarction from 10 centers in Europe, adipose tissue concentrations of α-tocopherol, assayed from 683 patients with acute myocardial infarction and 727 controls, were not associated with CHD risk. Indeed, those within the lowest quintile for α-tocopherol had a slightly (and nonsignificant) lower risk of myocardial infarction, with a multivariate odds ratio of 0.83 (95% confidence interval, 0.57−1.21). In this European population it is likely that use of vitamin E supplements was very uncommon [9].

In a case-control study, Regnstrom et al. [10] found that LDL vitamin E levels were lower in cases than controls, and they observed an inverse relation between those levels and the coronary stenosis score.

Prospective designs are generally considered superior because the time sequence is clear; the exposure status is established before the diagnosis of disease. In a recent nested case-control study, Street et al. [11] assayed blood samples collected from adults in Washington County, Maryland. The individuals were all healthy at the time the blood was drawn. Vitamin E levels in serum from 123 participants who later developed myocardial infarction were compared with controls. For individuals in the lowest quintile for vitamin E (after adjustment for cholesterol), the relative risk was 1.4, but there was no consistent trend across the quintiles. In further analyses, Street et al. found a suggestion of a decreased risk of myocardial infarction among those with higher levels of serum α-tocopherol only in the group with higher levels of total cholesterol. However, that finding was not statistically significant.

In a larger study, Knekt and colleagues [12] ascertained dietary intake of vitamin E and other nutrients, in a cohort of 5,133 Finnish men and women aged 30−69, and followed them for 14 years for occurrence of new fatal coronary heart disease. When divided into tertiles of intake for vitamin E, the rates were lowest among men and women who consumed the highest amounts of vitamin E; trends were significant for both men and women. Only 3% of this population took supplements containing vitamin E or C. The analysis adjusted for age, smoking, serum cholesterol, hypertension, body-mass index, and energy intake, but not other potential dietary and lifestyle confounders.

Meyer et al. [13] followed a cohort of 2,313 individuals, and found a significant reduction in the incidence of myocardial infarction among vitamin supplement users; the impact was most pronounced among users of vitamin E supplements.

In the largest study to date, Stampfer et al. [14] have reported results from the Nurses' Health Study. In this prospective cohort study, dietary data were collected in 1980 from 87,245 US female nurses ages 34−59, who were free from diagnosed cardiovascular disease and cancer at baseline. Participants were followed for 8 years using biennial questionnaires. During 679,485 person-years of follow-up, 437 nonfatal myocardial infarctions and 115 coronary deaths were documented. After adjustment for age and smoking, women in the highest fifth of the cohort for vitamin E consumption had a relative risk of 0.66 (95% confidence interval 0.50—0.87). Further adjustment for other coronary risk factors and for dietary intake of other antioxidants had little impact. Virtually all of the effect was attributable to vitamin E from supplements, as all the women in the top 20% of vitamin E intake were users of either multivitamins or specific vitamin E supplements. Significant associations were observed only for intake of 100 IU/day or more; lower doses of vitamin E supplements had little effect. Women who used vitamin E supplements for less than 2 years had little apparent benefit, but use for 2 years or longer was associated with a 41% reduction in risk of coronary heart disease. These findings persisted after adjustment for intake of carotene and vitamin C, and use of multivitamins.

In the Health Professionals Follow-Up Study, Rimm et al. prospectively studied 39,910 men aged 40—75 in 1986 who were free of prevalent cardiovascular disease, diabetes or high cholesterol [15]. During 139,883 person-years of follow up, a total of 667 cases of fatal and nonfatal coronary disease were documented. Compared to men in the lowest fifth of vitamin E intake, men in the highest fifth had an age-adjusted relative risk of coronary disease of 0.59 (95% confidence interval 0.47, 0.75). After adjustment for age, smoking, body size, caloric intake, dietary fiber intake, average alcohol consumption, hypertension, aspirin use, physical activity, family history of heart disease, profession, and intake of other antioxidant vitamins, the relative risks were essentially unchanged (relative risk = 0.60; 95% confidence interval, 0.44, 0.81). Smoking did not modify the associations for vitamin E.

In the Health Professionals Follow-up Study, the contribution of vitamin E from foods and from supplements was examined separately. A significant reduction in risk of coronary disease was limited to those with intake of vitamin E from supplements, with only a modest inverse association between dose and coronary disease risk for doses of 100 IU/day or more. Compared to men who did not take vitamin E supplements, the maximal reduction in coronary risk was among men consuming 100—250 IU/day (relative risk = 0.54; 95% confidence interval, 0.33, 0.88). The dose-response association for vitamin E from diet alone was suggestive of an inverse association (p_{trend} 0.11). However, limited variability in intake and error in measurement due to instability of vitamin E may have obscured a stronger association.

In another recent prospective study of antioxidants and coronary heart disease among women, Kushi et al. [16] reported a strong inverse association between dietary vitamin E (RR = 0.38, 95% CI 0.18, 0.80 between extreme quintiles) and death from CHD in a subgroup limited to those who took no vitamin supplements. Overall, in the whole population, no significant trend was observed for dietary vitamin E. Unlike the Nurses' Health Study, participants who reported use of vitamin E supplements did not experience lower rates of CHD death during the 7 years of follow-up. Because no information was collected on duration of supplement use and only a small percentage of women reported taking at least 100 IU per day, results from this study cannot directly be compared with those from the Nurses' Health Study.

In the most recent observational study of vitamin E intake and risk of CHD, Losonczy et al. [17] followed 11,178 elderly persons 67—105 years of age in the EPESE study. After an average of 8.5 years of follow up a total of 1,101 coronary deaths were confirmed. Among participants reporting use of vitamin E supplements at baseline, the relative risk was 0.59 (95% CI 0.37, 0.93) for death from coronary disease compared to those not taking supplements. The risk reduction was not appreciably stronger among those taking both vitamin E and vitamin C supplements (RR = 0.52, 95% CI 0.28, 0.97).

All of the above reviewed observational studies use clinically confirmed outcomes to evaluate risk reduction associated with vitamin E. However, exploring subclinical atherosclerosis progression provides valuable insight into underlying biological mechanisms. Hodis and colleagues [18] assessed the progression of coronary-artery lesions using serial quantitative coronary angiographic methods among 162 nonsmoking men 40—59 years old. Subjects who took vitamin E supplements had significant reductions in lesion progression as compared to nonusers of supplements. The apparent benefit was limited to those taking 100 IU/day or more. In further follow-up from the same population, Azen et al. [19] reported a significant inverse association between vitamin E and early atherosclerosis as measured by high-resolution B mode ultrasound of the distal common carotid artery. Similarly, in a cross-sectional survey of 1,187 asymptomatic participants in the EVA study [20], Bonithon-Kopp et al. found that erythrocyte vitamin E was significantly and negatively associated with intima-media thickness of the common carotid artery in both men and women.

The observational studies suffer from the limitation that vitamin intake is self-selected by the study participants. Therefore, one cannot rule out the possibility that other characteristics of the health-conscious individuals who consume a healthy diet rich in antioxidant vitamins may also contribute to their reduced risk of developing coronary disease. To some extent, this potential confounding can be addressed if other coronary risk factors are ascertained. In the Nurses' and Health Professionals studies and the Iowa Women's Study, vitamin E supplement users did not differ markedly from nonusers in the prevalence of a wide array of risk factors, including diet [14—16]. Moreover, adjustment for these factors did not materially alter the risk estimates. However, one cannot adjust for unmeasured or unknown confounders. If the protective effect is due to some unknown factor, this factor would have to be very closely associated with vitamin E intake and a very powerful independent predictor of risk of coronary disease.

Further indirect evidence for a causal explanation from several of these studies is the finding that short-term use is not associated with benefit. Such a lag is consistent with the biology of the proposed mechanism, as vitamin E is thought to decrease atherosclerosis by reducing oxidation of LDL. In clinical trials of cholesterol-lowering to reduce atherosclerosis, it takes about 2 years of intervention before differences in clinical events begin to emerge. Thus, one would expect that an intervention operating through reduced atherosclerosis would take about 2 years before manifesting its benefit in terms of reduced clinical endpoints. Moreover, this 2-year lag which was observed for vitamin E also tends to refute the self-selection explanation, since self-selection pressures would operate most strongly at the time the self-selection began. Also, one would expect the same self-selection bias to operate for vitamin C supplements, but vitamin C supplement users generally do not have lower risk. The most direct way to address this issue is through randomized trials.

Several trials of vitamin E have been conducted [6], but with the notable exceptions of the Finnish and the CHAOS trials [21,22], these have been small and inconclusive. In the Alpha-Tocopherol Beta-Carotene Lung Cancer Prevention Study started in Finland in 1985 among 29,133 male smokers aged 50—69 [21], men were enrolled in a randomized double-blind trial of β-carotene (20 mg/dl) or α-tocopherol (50 mg/day) using a 2×2 factorial design. Although the primary endpoint was incidence of lung cancer, information was also collected on coronary disease. For mortality from ischemic heart disease, men assigned to vitamin E (50 mg/day) had only a very small, nonsignificant reduction in risk (crude relative risk = 0.95). In a more detailed analysis of angina from the ATBC trial, supplementation of 50 mg/day was associated with only a minor decrease in the incidence of angina pectoris [23]. Although some have interpreted these findings as disproving the vitamin E hypothesis for coronary disease, it is important to note that the results are entirely consistent with those observed in the Nurses' Health Study and the Health Professionals Follow-up Study. In those observational studies, intake of low-dose vitamin E, in the range used in the Finnish trial (50 mg/day) also was not associated with any material decrease in risk of coronary disease, as discussed earlier. In the Health Professionals Follow-up Study, men consuming vitamin E supplements with a dose of 25—99 IU/day had a nonsignificant relative risk of 0.78 (95% confidence interval, 0.59—1.08), compared to nonusers of vitamin E supplements. Hence, the Finnish trial did not provide an adequate test of the hypothesis because the dose of vitamin E was too low. In the same trial, findings for men with a prior myocardial infarction were reported separately. In those men, a significant reduction in risk was observed in the vitamin E only for nonfatal myocardial infarction (RR = 0.62, 95% CI 0.41—0.96), but for fatal CHD, a nonsignificant increase was observed (RR = 1.33, 95% CI 0.86—2.05).

As a further indication that higher doses of vitamin E may be necessary, Stephens et al. [22] found a significant reduction in cardiovascular death and nonfatal MI among men with angiographically proven atherosclerosis randomized to 400 or 800 IU per day and followed for an average of 1.5 years. In this double-blind, placebo-controlled secondary prevention trial of 2,002 patients, the 1,035 patients assigned to 400 or 800 IU/day had a relative risk (RR = 0.53, 95% CI 0.34, 0.83) of cardiovascular death and nonfatal MI similar to the rela-

546

tive risks reported for comparable doses in the Nurses' and Health Professionals Follow-up Study [14,15]. The beneficial effects on the composite endpoint were due only to a significant reduction in nonfatal MI and not death from cardiovascular disease. Indeed, in that trial, total mortality was (nonsignificantly) higher in the vitamin E group.

Several small trials have also recently been described. Steiner et al. [24] found that patients with cerebrovascular disease randomized to aspirin plus vitamin E (n = 52) had fewer recurrent events than those given aspirin alone (n = 48). In another trial, Kooyenga and colleagues [25] randomized 50 cerebrovascular patients either to vitamin E (96 IU/day) plus mixed tocotrienols or to the vehicle alone, and followed them for 2 years with carotid ultrasound. In the placebo group, 28% showed progression of lesions compared with 8% in the vitamin E group; none of the placebo group showed improvement compared with 28% in the vitamin E group.

In summary, results from observational and experimental studies support an effect of vitamin E supplementation on reducing risk of CHD with reasonable, though imperfect consistency. Evidence from the Nurses' Health Study [14], Health Professionals Follow-Up Study [15], CLAS study [18,19], CHAOS study [22], and the Finnish trial [21,23] suggest that the major effect, if any, is found at supplemental intake levels at or above 100 IU/day. If so, this could explain some of the inconsistent results for the effect of differences in plasma vitamin E levels on CHD risk in populations where supplementation is uncommon. Also, in some of the studies of vitamin E from dietary sources, part or all of the apparent benefit could derive from other nutrients in the vitamin E rich foods.

Because vitamin E has little toxicity [26,27] this research represents a promising approach to prevention of coronary heart disease. If the true magnitude of such an effect is similar to that observed in the Health Professionals Follow-Up Study, the Nurses' Health Study, the EPESE study, and the CHAOS study, then vitamin E supplementation could have a major impact on the incidence of CHD.

References

1. Steinberg D, Parthasarathy S, Carew TE, Khoo JC, Witztum JL. Beyond cholesterol: modifications of low-density lipoprotein that increase its atherogenicity. N Engl J Med 1989;320: 915–924.
2. Sies H, Stahl W. Vitamins E and C, beta-carotene, and other carotenoids as antioxidants. Am J Clin Nutr 1995;62(Suppl):1315S–1321S.
3. Princen HMG, van Poppel G, Vogelezang C, Buytenhek R, Kok FJ. Supplementation with vitamin E but not beta-carotene in vivo protects low-density lipoprotein from lipid peroxidation in vitro. Effect of cigarette smoking. Arterioscl Thromb 1992;12:554–562.
4. Boscoboinik D, Szewczyk A, Hensey C, Azzi A. Inhibition of cell proliferation by α-tocopherol: role of protein kinase C. J Biol Chem 1991;266:6188–6194.
5. Steiner M. Vitamin E enhances the benefits of aspirin in preventing or reducing the incidence of strokes. Second International Congress on Antioxidant Vitamins and Beta-Carotene in Disease Prevention, Berlin, October 10-12, 1994;22 (Abstract).
6. Stampfer MJ, Rimm EB. Epidemiologic evidence for vitamin E in the prevention of cardiovas-

cular disease. Am J Clin Nutr 1995;62(Suppl):1365S—1369S.

7. Gey KF, Moser UK, Jordan P, Stahelin HB, Eichholzer M, Ludin E. Increased risk of cardio-vascular disease at suboptimal plasma concentrations of essential antioxidants: an epidemiological update with special attention to carotene and vitamin C. Am J Clin Nutr 1993;57(Suppl): 787S—797S.

8. Kristenson M, Ziedén B, Kucinskienë Z, Elinder LS, Bergdahl B, Elwing B, Abaravicius A, Razinkovienë L, Calkauskas H, Olsson A. Antioxidant state and mortality from coronary heart disease in Lithuanian and Swedish men: concomitant cross sectional study of men aged 50. BMJ 1997;314:629—633.

9. Kardinaal AF, Kok FJ, Ringstad J, Gomez-Aracena J, Mazaev VP, Kohlmeier L, Martin BC, Aro A, Kark JD, Delgado-Rodriguez M et al. Antioxidants in adipose tissue and risk of myocardial infarction: the EURAMIC Study. Lancet 1993;342:1379—1384.

10. Regnstrom J, Nilsson J, Modeus P, Strom K, Bavenholm P, Tornvall P, Hamsten A. Inverse relation between the concentration of low-density lipoprotein vitamin E and severity of coronary artery disease. Am J Clin Nutr 1996;63:377—385.

11. Street DA, Comstock GW, Salkeld RM, Schuep W, Klag MJ. Serum antioxidants and myocardial infarction. Are low levels of carotenoids and alpha-tocopherol risk factors for myocardial infarction? Circulation 1994;90:1154—1161.

12. Knekt P, Reunanen A, Jarvinen R, Seppanen R, Heliovaara M, Aromaa A. Antioxidant vitamin intake and coronary mortality in a longitudinal population study. Am J Epidemiol 1994;139: 1180—1189.

13. Meyer F, Bairati I, Dagenais GR. Lower ischemic heart disease incidence and mortality among vitamin supplement users. Can J Cardiol 1996;12:930—34.

14. Stampfer MJ, Hennekens CH, Manson JE, Colditz GA, Rosner B, Willett WC. A prospective study of vitamin E consumption and risk of coronary disease in women. N Engl J Med 1993;328:1444—1449.

15. Rimm EB, Stampfer MJ, Ascherio A, Giovannucci E, Colditz GA, Willett WC. Vitamin E consumption and the risk of coronary heart disease in men. N Engl J Med 1993;328:1450—6.

16. Kushi LH, Folsom AR, Prineas RJ, Mink PJ, Wu Y, Bostick RM. Dietary antioxidant vitamins and death from coronary heart disease in postmenopausal women. N Engl J Med 1996;334: 1156—1162.

17. Losonczy KG, Harris TB, Havlik RJ. Vitamin E and vitamin C supplement use and risk of all-cause and coronary heart disease mortality in older persons: the established populations for epidemiologic studies of the elderly. Am J Clin Nutr 1996;64:190—196.

18. Hodis HN, Mack WJ, LaBree L, Cashin-Hemphill L, Sevanian A, Johnson R, Azen SP. Serial coronary angiographic evidence that antioxidant vitamin intake reduces progression of coronary artery atherosclerosis. J Am Med Assoc 1995;273:1849—1854.

19. Azen SP, Qian D, Mack WJ, Sevanian A, Selzer RH, Liu C-R, Liu C-H, Hodis HN. Effect of supplementary antioxidant vitamin intake on carotid arterial wall intima-media thickness in a controlled clinical trial of cholesterol lowering. Circulation 1996;94:2369—2372.

20. Bonithon-Kopp C, Coudray C, Berr C, Touboul P, Fève JM, Favier A, Ducimetière P. Combined effects of lipid peroxidation and antioxidant status on carotid atherosclerosis in a population aged 59—71: the EVA Study. Am J Clin Nutr 1997;65:121—127.

21. The Alpha-Tocopherol Beta-Carotene Cancer Prevention Study Group. The effect of vitamin E and beta carotene on the incidence of lung cancer and other cancers in male smokers. N Engl J Med 1994;330:1029—1035.

22. Stephens NJ, Parsons A, Schofield PM, Kelly F, Cheeseman K, Mitchinson MJ, Brown MJ. Randomised controlled trial of vitamin E in patients with coronary disease: Cambridge Heart Antioxidant Study (CHAOS). Lancet 1996;347:781—786.

23. Rapola JM, Virtamo J, Haukka JK, Heinonen OP, Albanes D, Taylor PR, Huttunen JK. Effect of vitamin E and beta carotene on the incidence of angina pectoris — a randomized, double-blind, controlled trial. J Am Med Assoc 1996;275:693—698.

24. Steiner M, Glantz M, Lekos A. Vitamin E plus aspirin compared with aspirin alone in patients with transient ischemic attacks. Am J Clin Nutr 1995;62(Suppl):1381S—1384S.
25. Kooyenga DK, Geller M, Watkins TR, Gapor A, Diakoumakis E, Bierenbaum ML. Palm oil antioxidant effects in patients with hyperlipidaemia and carotid stenosis — 2 year experience. Asia Pac J Clin Nutr 1997;6:72—75.
26. Meydani SN, Meydani M, Rall LC, Morrow F, Blumber JB. Assessment of the safety of high-dose, short-term supplementation with vitamin E in healthy older adults. Am J Clin Nutr 1994;60:704—709.
27. Bendich A, Machlin L. Safety of oral intake of vitamin E. Am J Clin Nutr 1988;48:612—619.

Lp(a) and athero-thrombosis

Lipoprotein(a) and the endothelium: a feedback loop in atherosclerosis

David J. Grainger[1], Jill Reckless[1], James C. Metcalfe[2], Steven D. Hughes[3], Edward M. Rubin[3] and Richard M. Lawn[4]

Departments of [1]Medicine and [2]Biochemistry, Cambridge University, Cambridge, UK; [3]Lawrence Berkeley Laboratory, Human Genome Center, Berkeley, California; and [4]Stanford University School of Medicine, Division of Cardiovascular Medicine, Stanford, California, USA

Abstract. We have previously demonstrated that the atherogenic lipoprotein Lp(a) can inhibit activation of the cytokine TGF-β in vivo [1]. TGF-β is important for the maintenance of a healthy endothelium, and hence low levels of TGF-β activity result in activation of endothelial cells and expression of proinflammatory cytokines and adhesion molecules. Since, Lp(a) is known to preferentially accumulate at sites of endothelial activation, we proposed that Lp(a) promoted atherogenesis in a positive feedback loop [2]. Here we demonstrate that when mice expressing a human apoB transgene are infected with an apo(a)-expressing adenovirus, focal accumulation of apo(a) protein into the vessel wall occurs by day 15 after infection. At these sites, TGF-β activity is depressed and the endothelium is activated, marked by expression of ICAM-1. No similar endothelial cell activation was noted in mice infected with adenoviral constructs expressing a β-galactosidase gene. Treatment of apo(a) transgenic mice with tamoxifen (1 mg/kg/day) for 3 months resulted in a 2.0-fold increase in active TGF-β ($p < 0.001$) in active TGF-β in the aortic media. This was associated with a 97% reduction ($p < 0.001$) in vessel wall accumulation of apo(a) protein. Furthermore, endothelial cell activation was suppressed by 83% ($p < 0.001$). We conclude that apo(a) promotes atherogenic changes in vessel wall structure, at least in part, by a positive feedback loop in which apo(a) decreases TGF-β activity, resulting in endothelial cells activation which in turn promotes additional apo(a) accumulation.

Introduction

An elevated plasma concentration of the lipoprotein Lp(a) represents a major independent risk factor for vascular diseases, including atherosclerosis and restenosis [3,4]. Lp(a) consists of an LDL particle, covalently associated to an additional protein termed apolipoprotein(a) (apo(a)). Plasma-derived Lp(a) accumulates in the vessel wall more readily than does LDL demonstrating the ability of its unique component, apo(a), to bind to cells and extracellular matrix in the vessel wall [5]. Lp(a) accumulates at focal sites in the vessel wall, although the reasons for the focal nature of this accumulation are not well understood. There is some evidence that Lp(a) specifically accumulates at sites of endothelial damage or dysfunction. For instance, Lp(a) localises at the site of physical injury to the endothelium in rabbits following balloon catheter injury [6]. Similarly, in humans Lp(a) accumulates at sites of microvascular inflammation, where

---

Address for correspondence: D.J. Grainger, Department of Medicine, Cambridge University, P.O. Box 157, Addenbrookes Hospital, Hills Road, Cambridge CB2 2QQ, UK.

endothelial permeability is known to be increased [7]. Following accumulation the Lp(a) may further enhance endothelial dysfunction, as evidenced by studies which demonstrate impaired endothelium-dependent vasodilation in the presence of high levels of Lp(a) before atherosclerotic lesions are detectable by angiography [8].

One mechanism by which apo(a) might promote endothelial dysfunction and ultimately atherosclerosis is inhibition of plasminogen activation, suggested by the sequence homology between apo(a) and plasminogen. Reduced plasmin activity would be expected to have at least two atherogenic consequences: reduced clot lysis resulting in an increased risk of thrombosis and reduced activation of the cytokine TGF-β. Studies of mice lacking TGF-β1 has provided strong evidence that this cytokine has protective effects on the vascular endothelium [9]. In the absence of TGF-β, the endothelium is activated to express proinflammatory cytokines and adhesion molecules. This has led to the hypothesis that Lp(a) can cause focal atherosclerotic lesions by the positive feedback mechanism illustrated in Fig. 1. Initial accumulation of Lp(a) at sites where endothelial activation had occurred would result in local depression of TGF-β activity, which in turn would lead to further activation of the endothelium avid accumulation of further Lp(a) at these sites [2,10].

In this study, we have investigated whether we observe endothelial cell activation at sites where Lp(a) accumulates in vivo, and whether elevation of TGF-β using the anticancer drug tamoxifen reduces this activation of the endothelium.

Materials and Methods

Mice

In order to examine the rapid response of the endothelium to accumulated Lp(a),

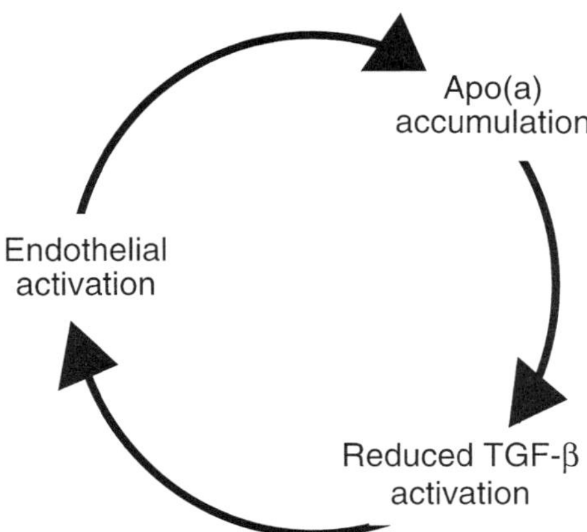

Fig. 1. Proposed positive-feedback loop mediating vascular accumulation of Lp(a).

transgenic mice overexpressing human apoB were injected with modified adenovirus particles expressing a human apo(a) minigene known to inhibit plasminogen activation in vitro, as previously described [11]. After 15 days, mice were sacrificed and the heart, lungs and aorta excised and embedded in OCT embedding medium, then frozen at $-20°C$.

We also examined the chronic response to accumulated Lp(a), as well as the effects of prolonged elevation of the cytokine TGF-β, in transgenic mice expressing human apo(a) from the liver-specific transferrin promoter, as previously described [1]. Groups of eight mice were fed either a high-cholesterol diet, or a high-cholesterol diet supplemented with 1 mg/kg body weight/day tamoxifen from the age of 12 weeks onwards. After 3 months mice in both groups were sacrificed and the heart, lungs and aorta excised and embedded as above.

Quantitative immunofluoresence

The amount of apo(a) present in the vessel wall was measured in 4 µm cryosections prepared from the aortic sinus region, using quantitative immunofluoresence protocols as previously described [1,12]. ICAM-1 (as a marker of endothelial cell activation), active TGF-β and TGF-β1 antigen were measured in adjacent cryosections using the same technique. The primary antibodies used were: for apo(a), sheep antihuman-apo(a) (immunoscientific) at 1:1,000 dilution, for ICAM-1, rat monoclonal antimouse ICAM-1 (BSA2; R&D Systems) at 10 µg/ml, for TGF-β1 antigen, chicken antihuman TGF-β1 (BDA19; R&D Systems) at 25 µg/ml and for active TGF-β, the recombinant extracellular domain of the type II TGF-β receptor (R2X; as previously described) at 1 µg/ml.

Results

Fifteen days after infection of mice expressing a human apoB transgene with apo(a) expressing adenovirus, significant levels of apo(a) protein could be detected in the blood vessel wall by quantitative immunofluoresence microscopy. The apo(a) protein was located in focal patches in the subendothelial space (Fig. 2) resembling the accumulation of apo(a) seen in the aortae of apo(a) transgenic mice. In contrast, no apo(a) staining was detected in mice injected with a control adenovirus preparation which expresses β-galactosidase. We confirmed that the adenovirus used did not locally infect endothelial cells or smooth muscle cells (by the absence of β-galactosidase staining), demonstrating that the apo(a) observed in the vessel wall had been accumulated from the circulation, rather than been locally produced.

At sites where apo(a) had accumulated we found that TGF-β activity (measured using R2X as previously described [1,13]) was decreased, but the amount of TGF-β1 antigen was unaffected (Table 1). In contrast, TGF-β activity was unaffected at sites where apo(a) protein could not be detected. Consistent with our earlier observation that TGF-β activation is suppressed by apo(a) in transgenic

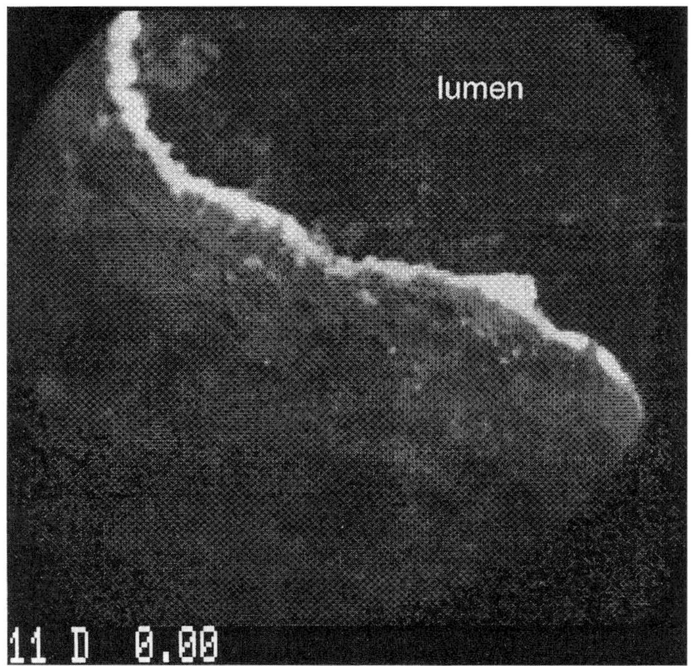

Fig. 2. Immunofluoresence micrograph of apo(a) 15 days following infection with an apo(a)-expressing adenovirus. Magnification = × 400.

Table 1.

	Apo(a)-expressing adenovirus (lesion sites)	Apo(a)-expressing adenovirus (nonlesion sites)	β-gal-expressing adenovirus
Plasma			
Apo(a) (mg/dl)	42.4 ± 2.8		< 1
Vessel wall			
Apo(a) (pixels/section)	1670 ± 220[a]	80 ± 60[a]	< 10
Active TGF-β (AU)	46 ± 2[a]	59 ± 6	62 ± 5
TGF-β1 antigen (AU)	68 ± 7	62 ± 9	65 ± 4
ICAM-1 (AU)	27 ± 4[a]	< 1	< 1

Plasma apo(a) was measured by ELISA and vessel-wall proteins by quantitative immunofluoresence (see "Materials and Methods"). AU = arbitrary units. [a]$p < 0.05$ (Mann-Whitney U test) vs. β-gal-expressing adenovirus infected group.

mice, we now find that TGF-β activation is already suppressed with 15 days of apo(a) accumulating into the vessel wall.

Since endothelial cell activation occurs when TGF-β activity is depressed in TGF-β1 null mice [9], we investigated whether the endothelium was activated, marked by ICAM-1 expression, at the sites of apo(a) accumulation. ICAM-1 staining was detectable only at sites where apo(a) was accumulated (Table 1). Thus within 15 days, apo(a) had accumulated, TGF-β activity was suppressed and ICAM-1 was expressed as a marker of endothelial cell activation.

To determine whether the depressed TGF-β activity was likely to be causative in the observed endothelial cell activation, we treated transgenic mice with tamoxifen, an agent previously reported to elevate TGF-β activity in a variety of tissues, including the blood vessel wall [2,14,15]. At 24 weeks of age in apo(a) transgenic mice which had not received tamoxifen, we observed focal apo(a) accumulation, and an associated decrease in TGF-β activity. At the sites of apo(a) accumulation, we again observed ICAM-1 expression, consistent with the data obtained from adenovirus-mediated apo(a) expression. In marked contrast, in the mice which had received tamoxifen for 3 months prior to sacrifice, the level of ICAM-1 expression was reduced by 83% (p < 0.001; Mann-Whitney U test; n = 8 per group; Table 2). We conclude that treatment with tamoxifen markedly inhibited apo(a)-induced endothelial activation, possibly mediated through increased TGF-β activity.

We next investigated whether there was any evidence to support the hypothesis that apo(a) accumulation was driven by a positive feedback loop (Fig. 1). If further apo(a) accumulation depended on apo(a)-induced endothelial activation, then tamoxifen treatment would be expected to reduce apo(a) accumulation, presumably by inhibiting endothelial activation. In contrast, if apo(a) accumulation was independent of endothelial activation, then tamoxifen would not be expected to affect apo(a) accumulation. In apo(a) transgenic mice treated with tamoxifen,

Table 2.

	Apo(a) mice untreated	Apo(a) mice TMX treated
Plasma		
Apo(a) (mg/dl)	9.3 ± 0.9	8.8 ± 0.8
Vessel wall		
Apo(a) (pixels/section)	2170 ± 380	70 ± 110[a]
Active TGF-β (AU)	25 ± 2	51 ± 6[a]
TGF-β1 antigen (AU)	47 ± 7	60 ± 7[a]
ICAM-1 (AU)	51 ± 11	9 ± 3[a]

Plasma apo(a) was measured by ELISA and vessel wall proteins by quantitative immunofluoresence (see "Materials and Methods"). AU = arbitrary units. [a]p < 0.05 (Mann-Whitney U test) vs. untreated group.

apo(a) accumulation into the vessel wall was reduced by 97% (p < 0.0001; Mann-Whitney U test; Table 2). This is consistent with the hypothesis that focal accumulation of apo(a) into the vessel wall depends on a positive feedback loop.

Discussion

We have demonstrated here that when apo(a) accumulates in the vessel wall, it is associated with both focal depression of TGF-β activation and local activation of the endothelium marked by ICAM-1 expression. Although our in vivo experiments cannot demonstrate a causal relationship between these events, a causal pathway in which apo(a) accumulation inhibits TGF-β activation, which in turns reduces the protective effect of TGF-β on the endothelium is consistent with the available in vitro evidence. Apo(a) has been shown to inhibit TGF-β activation in vitro, [16,17] while TGF-β inhibits ICAM-1 expression on cultured endothelial cells [18].

Our inference that apo(a) accumulation and endothelial cell activation proceed via a positive feedback loop has important implications for the pathogenesis of atherosclerosis. The atherosclerotic plaque is both progressive and focal in nature. Such a focal disruption of vessel wall architecture is itself consistent with the idea that the plaque develops as a consequence of a positive feedback loop, irrespective of the particular molecules involved. Indeed other inhibitors of TGF-β activation may also function in a similar positive feedback mechanism: PAI-1, a known inhibitor of TGF-β activation [19] is produced during inflammation as an acute phase reaction. PAI-1-mediated reduction in TGF-β activity would likely result in further inflammation, increasing further the levels of PAI-1. It is plausible but unproven, that a number of positive feedback cycles similar to the one investigated here underlie the development of atherosclerosis on diverse genetic backgrounds.

Acknowledgements

This work was supported by grants from the Wellcome Trust, British Heart Foundation and National Institutes of Health. D.J. Grainger is a Royal Society University Research Fellow.

References

1. Grainger DJ, Kemp PR, Liu AC, Lawn RM, Metcalfe JC. Activation of TGF-β is inhibited in apolipoprotein(a) mice. Nature 1995;370:460–462.
2. Lawn RM, Pearle AD, Kunz LL, Rubin EM, Reckless J, Metcalfe JC, Grainger DJ. Feedback mechanism of focal vascular lesion formation in transgenic apolipoprotein(a) mice. J Biol Chem 1996;271:31367–31371.
3. Bostom AG, Cupples LA, Jenner JL, Ordovas JM, Seman LJ, Wilson PWF, Schaefer EJ, Castelli WP. Elevated plasma lipoprotein(a) and coronary heart disease in men aged 55 years and younger — a prospective study. JAMA 1996;276:544–548.

4. Jurgens G, Taddei-Peters WC, Koltringer P, Petek W, Chen Q, Greilberger J, Macomber PF, Butman BT, Stead AG, Ransom JH. Lipoprotein(a) serum concentration and apo(a) phenotype correlate with severity and presence of ischemic cerebrovascular disease. Stroke 1995;26: 1841–1848.

5. Cushing GL, Gaubatz JW, Nava ML, Burdick BJ, Bocan TMA, Guyton JR, Weilbaecher D, Debakey ME, Lawrie GM, Morrisett JD. Quantitation and localization of apolipoprotein(a) and B in coronary artery bypass vein grafts resected at reoperation. Arteriosclerosis 1989;9: 593–603.

6. Nielsen LB, Stender S, Kjeldsen K, Nordestgaard BG. Specific accumulation of lipoprotein(a) in balloon-injured rabbit aorta in vivo. Circ Res 1996;78:615–626.

7. Nachman RL. Thrombosis and atherogenesis — molecular connections. Blood 1992;79: 1897–1906.

8. Sorensen KE, Celermajer DS, Georgakopoulos D, Hatcher G, Betteridge DJ, Deanfield JE. Impairment of endothelium-dependent dilatation is an early event in children with familial hypercholesterolemia and is related to the lipoprotein(a) level. J Clin Invest 1994;93:50–55.

9. Shull MM, Ormsby I, Kier AB, Pawlowski S, Diebold RJ, Yin MY, Allen R, Sidman C, Proetzel G, Calvin D, Annunziata N, Doetschman T. Targeted disruption of the mouse TGF-β1 gene results in multifocal inflammatory disease. Nature 1992;359:693–699.

10. Grainger DJ, Metcalfe JC. A pivotal role for TGF-β in atherogenesis? Biol Rev 1995;70: 571–596.

11. Hughes SD, Ighani S, Verstuyft J, Grainger DJ, Lou XJ, Lawn RM, Rubin EM. Lipoprotein(a) vascular accumulation in mice: in vivo analysis of the role of lysine binding sites using recombinant adenovirus. J Clin Invest;(In press).

12. Mosedale DE, Metcalfe JC, Grainger DJ. Optimisation of immunofluoresence methods by quantitative image analysis. J Histochem Cytochem 1996;44:1043–1050.

13. Grainger DJ, Mosedale DE, Metcalfe JC, Weissberg PL, Kemp PR. Active and acid-activatable TGF-β in human sera, platelets and plasma. Clin Chim Acta 1995;235:11–31.

14. Colletta AA, Wakefield LM, Howell FV, Van Roozendaal KEP, Danielpour D, Ebbs SR, Sporn MB, Baum M. Antiestrogens induce the secretion of active TGF-β from human fetal fibroblasts. Br J Cancer 1990;62:405–409.

15. Grainger DJ, Witchell CM, Metcalfe JC. Tamoxifen elevates TGF-β and suppresses diet-induced formation of lipid lesions in mouse aorta. Nature Med 1995;1:1067–1072.

16. Kojima S, Harpel PC, Rifkin DB. Lipoprotein(a) inhibits the generation of TGF-β: an endogenous inhibitor of smooth muscle cell migration. J Cell Biol 1991;113:1439–1445.

17. Grainger DJ, Kirschenlohr HL, Metcalfe JC, Weissberg PL, Wade DP, Lawn RM. Proliferation of human smooth muscle cells promoted by lipoprotein(a). Science 1993;260:1655–1658.

18. Gamble JR, Khew-Goodall Y, Vadas MA. TGF-β inhibits E-selectin expression on human endothelial cells. J Immunol 1993;150:4494–4503.

19. Lyons RM, Gentry LE, Purchio AF, Moses HL. Mechanism of activation of latent recombinant TGF-β1 by plasmin. J Cell Biol 1990;119:1361–1367.

The human very low density lipoprotein receptor mediates the uptake and degradation of lipoprotein(a)

Kelley McTigue Argraves[1], Karen F. Kozarsky[2], John T. Fallon[3], Peter C. Harpel[4] and Dudley K. Strickland[1]

[1]*Department of Biochemistry, American Red Cross, Rockville, Maryland;* [2]*Institute of Human Gene Therapy and Department of Molecular and Cellular Engineering, University of Pennsylvania, Philadelphia, Pennsylvania;* [3]*Cardiovascular Institute and Departments of Pathology and Medicine; and* [4]*Division of Hematology, The Mount Sinai School of Medicine, New York, New York, USA*

Abstract. *Background.* Lp(a) is an important risk factor for premature atherosclerosis. The mechanisms for Lp(a) atherogenicity most likely involve both its capacity to influence plasminogen activation as well as its atherogenic potential as a lipoprotein particle following receptor-mediated uptake. The mechanisms responsible for the cellular catabolism of Lp(a) are currently a topic of debate.

Methods and Results. We demonstrate that fibroblasts expressing the human VLDL receptor can mediate the endocytosis of Lp(a) leading to its degradation within lysosomes. In contrast, fibroblasts deficient in this receptor are not effective in catabolizing Lp(a). Lp(a) degradation was prevented by antibodies against the VLDL receptor and by RAP, an antagonist of ligand binding. The catabolism of Lp(a) was also inhibited by apolipoprotein(a), indicating the apolipoprotein(a) mediates the binding of Lp(a) to this receptor. The removal of Lp(a) from the mouse circulation was delayed in mice deficient in the VLDL receptor when compared to control mice, indicating that the VLDL receptor may be important in in vivo Lp(a) catabolism. We also demonstrate the expression of the VLDL receptor in macrophages present in human atherosclerotic lesions.

Conclusion. The ability of the VLDL receptor to mediate endocytosis of Lp(a) could lead to cellular accumulation of lipid within macrophages, and may represent a molecular basis for the atherogenic effects of Lp(a).

Keywords: atherogenesis, catabolism, lipoprotein(a), Lp(a).

The pathways for the catabolism of lipoprotein Lp(a) remain elusive. Overexpression of the LDL receptors in the liver of transgenic mice causes increased clearance of injected Lp(a) [1]. Other studies do not support the role of the LDL receptor in Lp(a) clearance. Drugs that lower LDL by stimulating LDL receptors do not lower blood levels of Lp(a) [2]. Further, the turnover of labeled Lp(a) is similar in patients with homozygous familial hypercholesterolemia who have decreased LDL receptors [3]. A recent report demonstrates that cholesterol loading of macrophages increases Lp(a) internalization and degradation by means of a receptor different from the scavenger or LDL receptor [4]. Other members of the LDL receptor family are candidate Lp(a) receptors and include the very low density lipoprotein (VLDL) receptor and the large cell surface receptors, gp330

Address for correspondence: Peter C. Harpel MD, Box 1079, The Mount Sinai Medical Center, 1 Levy Place, New York, NY 10029, USA.

and LRP. This family participates in the catabolism of lipoproteins, proteinases and proteinase-inhibitor complexes. The LDL receptor is involved in the catabolism of apolipoprotein B and apolipoprotein E containing lipoproteins and is critical to cholesterol homeostasis [5]. LRP plays a role in the catabolism of proteinases, proteinase-inhibitor complexes and certain apoE- and lipoprotein lipase-enriched lipoproteins [6]. LRP has been reported to bind to a high molecular weight isoform of Lp(a) [7]. The biologic function of gp330 is not clear, however, it may bind many of the ligands that interact with LRP [8,9]. Its location on a restricted group of epithelial cells [10] suggests that it has an organ-specific role. The newest member of the LDL receptor family is the VLDL receptor whose physiologic role is not known [11]. The initial studies suggested that it reacts with apoE-containing proteins including VLDL, β-VLDL and IDL [11]. Our present study indicates that the VLDL receptor plays an important role in Lp(a) catabolism.

Methods and Results

Fibroblasts expressing the VLDL receptor internalize and degrade Lp(a)

Human VLDL receptor cDNA was introduced into mouse embryonic fibroblasts genetically deficient in LRP (PEA13 fibroblasts [12]) using an adenoviral vector (Ad-VLDLR). Alternatively, these cells were infected with Ad-LacZ containing LacZ cDNA as a control. In addition, mouse embryonic fibroblasts expressing LRP (MEF) were studied. These two cell lines also express the LDL receptor but not gp330. Immunoblot analysis documented that the PEA13 fibroblasts infected with Ad-VLDLR expressed the VLDL receptor, but the controls with Ad-LacZ and MEF did not. Immunoblotting studies confirmed that the infected cell lines did not express LRP whereas MEF did. All three cell lines expressed similar levels of the LDL receptor. To examine cellular uptake, ^{125}I-Lp(a) was incubated with the cells at 37°C. At varying times, the medium was removed and the amount of radiolabeled Lp(a) degraded to acid soluble material quantified. The cells were then incubated with proteinases to release surface-bound radioactivity. The radioactivity that resisted this treatment was considered to be intracellular. Our findings show that ^{125}I-Lp(a) was internalized by the cells expressing the VLDL receptor and reached a steady state with time (Fig. 1A). The internalized was degraded as shown by the appearance of acid soluble radioactive material secreted into the medium (Fig. 1B). The receptor associated protein, RAP, a molecule that inhibits ligand binding to the VLDL receptor [13], inhibited both internalization and intracellular degradation of Lp(a) indicating the specificity of the interaction. In contrast to these findings, the cells deficient in the VLDL receptor (PEA-13 fibroblasts infected with Ad-LacZ, and MEF cells) did not internalize or degrade Lp(a). Further evidence that the VLDL receptor was responsible for the binding of Lp(a) was provided using a rabbit polyclonal IgG anti-VLDL receptor. This antibody inhibited the internalization

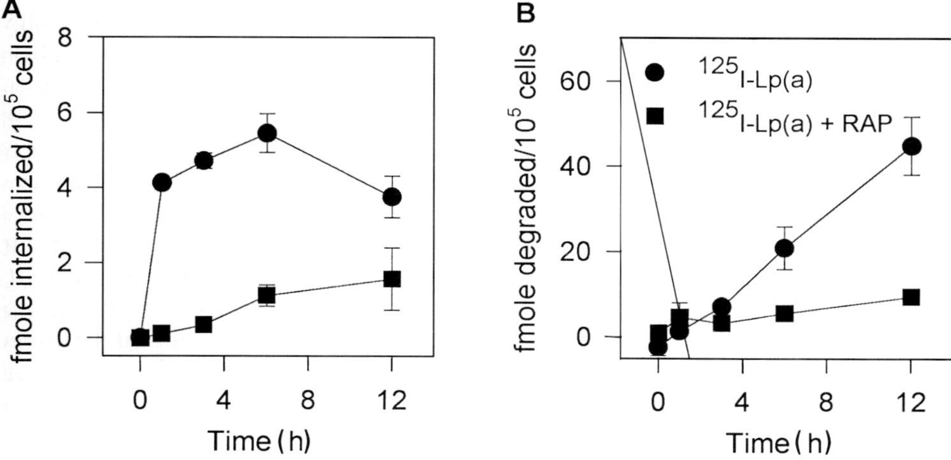

Fig. 1. Fibroblasts expressing the human VLDL receptor internalize and degrade Lp(a). PEA 13 fibroblasts infected with Ad-VLDLR were plated into wells (1×10^5 cells/well) and 10 nM ^{125}I-labeled Lp(a) (closed circles) or ^{125}I-labeled Lp(a) with 1 µM RAP included (closed squares) were added to each well. At the times indicated, the internalization (**A**) and degradation (**B**) were measured. Each data point represents the average of duplicate determinations. Figure adapted from Fig. 2 in [21].

and degradation of ^{125}I-Lp(a) by the Ad-VLDLR cells. To address the possible participation of gp330 mouse F9 tetratocarcinoma, cells were treated with retinoic acid and dibutyryl cyclic AMP, a procedure that increases expression of pg330 50-fold [14]. These cells did not internalize or degrade Lp(a).

VLDL receptor binds Lp(a) by ligand blotting studies

Purified VLDL receptor and LRP were separated by SDS-PAGE, electrotransferred to nitrocellulose membranes and incubated with Lp(a) or with uPA:PAI-1 complexes, a ligand for both the VLDL receptor and LRP. Antibodies were used to detect binding. Lp(a) bound to the VLDL receptor but not to LRP. uPA:PAI-1 complex bound to both receptors indicating that their binding capacity was relatively intact. The receptor-related protein, RAP, inhibited binding of Lp(a) to the VLDL receptor again indicating the specificity of the reaction.

Comparison of the degradation of Lp(a) by the VLDL and LDL receptors

Since it has been previously shown that overexpression of the human LDL receptor in transgenic mice enhances Lp(a) catabolism [1], we have compared the degradation of Lp(a) by PEA-13 fibroblasts infected with either Ad-VLDLR, Ad-LDLR or Ad-LacZ as control. Our data indicated that the cells infected with either receptor were effective in degrading Lp(a). RAP completely inhibited degradation of Lp(a) in cells containing the VLDL receptor whereas it only partially inhibited the uptake of Lp(a) in the LDL receptor expressing cells probably due to the relatively low affinity of RAP for the LDL receptor [15]. Comparison of the degradation of Lp(a) by the two different receptors indicated a similar profile, and the dose-response curve indicated that uptake and degradation of Lp(a) by both receptors occurred at concentrations of Lp(a) above 30 mg/dl (83 nM); concentrations of Lp(a) considered to represent an increased risk for arterial vascular disease. We have assessed the effect of increasing concentrations of LDL on the uptake of Lp(a) by the fibroblasts infected with either Ad-VLDLR or Ad-LDLR. We found that LDL inhibited the catabolism of Lp(a) by the LDL receptor, but had a much lower effect in inhibiting the uptake of Lp(a) by the VLDL receptor. These results are explained by the higher affinity of LDL for the LDL receptor as compared to Lp(a) and conversely, the greater affinity of Lp(a) for the VLDL receptor.

Structural requirements for the uptake of Lp(a) by the VLDL receptor

A monoclonal antibody, 4G3, that blocks catabolism of LDL [16] and which reacts against apolipoprotein B-100 did not inhibit the degradation of Lp(a) by the VLDL receptor containing cells. In contrast, the uptake of LDL was completely inhibited. This finding suggests that the apolipoprotein(a) portion of Lp(a) contained the VLDL receptor binding site. This was directly demonstrated by the finding that a 50-fold molar excess of apolipoprotein(a) purified from the Lp(a) used in these studies effectively blocked degradation of Lp(a). In addition, uPA:PAI-1 complexes, another ligand for the VLDL receptor, also competed for the internalization and degradation of Lp(a).

Recognition of Lp(a) isoforms by the VLDL receptor

Five different isoforms of Lp(a) were purified and tested for internalization and degradation by incubating with cells infected with Ad-VLVLR, Ad-LDLR, or Ad-LacZ. Four of the five Lp(a) isoforms tested were internalized and degraded by the cells expressing the VLDL receptor. The extent of degradation appeared to be dependent on the particular apolipoprotein(a) isoform with the lower molecular weight isoforms being internalized to a greater extent that the higher molecular weight isoforms. In contrast, the cells expressing the LDL receptor internalized the different Lp(a) isoforms similarly. These data support our observations that the VLDL receptor interacts with the apolipoprotein(a) portion of Lp(a), and not with apolipoprotein B-100.

Mice deficient in the VLDL receptor have a delayed removal of Lp(a) antigen from the circulation

Mice do not possess Lp(a), however, they express the VLDL receptor that has a high degree of homology with the human receptor [17]. We have tested the role of the VLDL receptor in vivo by injecting human Lp(a) intravenously into VLDL receptor deficient and control mice. Lp(a) concentration was quantified at intervals by immunoblot analysis. The clearance of Lp(a) was significantly slower in the VLDL receptor deficient mice (Fig. 2). It is important to note that Lp(a) is eventually cleared in the VLDL receptor deficient mice confirming that an additional mechanism must exist, most likely involving the LDL receptor.

Vascular localization of the VLDL receptor

Immunohistochemical study of normal and atherosclerotic vessels showed VLDL receptor antigen in vascular endothelial cells, as has been previously reported [18,19]. Double staining showed that in coronary atherectory specimen, the VLDL receptor antigen was present in most of plaque KP-1 positive macro-

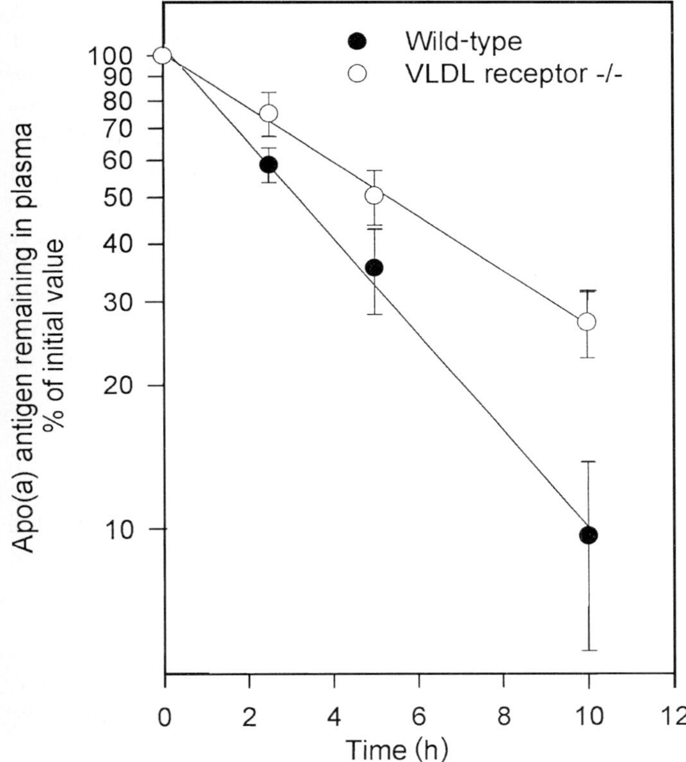

Fig. 2. VLDL receptor deficient mice demonstrate delayed intravascular clearance of Lp(a). Wild-type mice (closed circles) (n = 5) and VLDL receptor-deficient mice (open circles) (n = 4) were injected intravenously with 100 µg Lp(a). Blood was drawn at various time intervals and aliquots analyzed by SDS-PAGE followed by transfer to nitrocellulose. The apolipoprotein(a) antigen was detected and quantified using monoclonal antibody against apolipoprotein(a). Reprinted with permission from [21].

phages and foam cells, however, the majority of α-actin positive smooth muscle cells did not stain for the VLDL receptor antigen. Of interest, VLDL receptor staining appeared in extracellular matrix-rich areas of the plaque, perhaps reflecting receptor shed from the cell surface.

Discussion

These studies show that the VLDL receptor may be important in the catabolism of Lp(a). We have shown that Lp(a) is internalized and degraded in fibroblasts that express the VLDL receptor but not in the control cells. Lp(a) also binds to the purified receptor by ligand blotting studies. The apolipoprotein(a) portion of Lp(a) appears to contain the structures responsible for receptor binding since a monoclonal antibody that prevents LDL from binding to the LDL receptor fails to inhibit the internalization of Lp(a). Further, apolipoprotein(a) competes effectively for the internalization and degradation of intact Lp(a). We have found that LDL competitively inhibits the uptake of Lp(a) by the LDL receptor, but that it is not an effective competitor of Lp(a) uptake by the VLDL receptor. This confirms clinical studies indicating that the LDL receptor is not an important participant in Lp(a) catabolism. Our preliminary studies also suggest that the Lp(a) isoform may modulate the reaction with the VLDL receptor. The VLDL receptor antigen has a wide distribution in endothelial cells and in macrophages in atherosclerotic plaques suggesting that the VLDL receptor may target Lp(a) both to the vessel wall and to vessel wall macrophages [20]. Combined with our recent findings that Lp(a) stimulates vascular endothelial cells to produce a monocyte chemoattractant activity [21], the present study incriminates the Lp(a) macrophage interaction as an important mechanism underlying the atherogenicity of Lp(a).

Acknowledgements

Supported by grants HL50787, GM42581 (to D.K.D.), HL54469 (to J.T.F. and P.C.H.) from the National Institutes of Health.

References

1. Hofmann SL, Eaton DL, Brown MS, McConathy WJ, Goldstein JL, Hammer RE. Overexpression of human low-density lipoprotein receptors leads to accelerated catabolism of Lp(a) lipoprotein in transgenic mice. J Clin Invest 1990;85:1542–1547.
2. Utermann G. The mysteries of lipoprotein(a). Science 1989;246:904–910.
3. Rader DJ, Mann WA, Cain W, Kraft H-G, Usher D, Zech LA, Hoeg JM, Davignon J, Lupien P, Grossman M, Wilson JM, Brewer HB Jr. The low-density lipoprotein receptor is not required for normal catabolism of Lp(a) in humans. J Clin Invest 1995;95:1403–1408.
4. Bottalico LA, Keesler GA, Fless GM, Tabas I. Cholesterol loading of macrophages leads to marked enhancement of native lipoprotein(a) and apoprotein(a) internalization and degradation. J Biol Chem 1993;12:8569–8573.

5. Brown MS, Goldstein JL. A receptor-mediated pathway for cholesterol homeostasis. Science 1986;232:34–47.

6. Strickland DK, Kounnas MZ, Williams SE, Argraves WS. LDL receptor-related protein (LRP): a multiligand receptor. Fibrinolysis 1994;8(Suppl 1):204–215.

7. Marz W, Beckmann A, Scharnagl H, Siekmeier R, Mondorf U, Held I, Schneider W, Preissner KT, Curtiss LK, Grob W, Huttinger M. Heterogeneous lipoprotein(a) isoforms differ by their interaction with the low-density lipoprotein receptor and the low-density lipoprotein receptor-related protein/alpha-2-macroglobulin receptor. FEBS 1993;325:271–275.

8. Kounnas MZ, Strickland DK, Argraves WS. Glycoprotein 330, a member of the LDL receptor family, binds lipoprotein lipase in vitro. J Biol Chem 1993;268:14176–14181.

9. Willnow TD, Goldstein JL, Orth K, Brown MS, Herz J. LDL receptor-related protein and gp330 bind similar ligands, including plasminogen activator-inhibitor complexes and lactoferrin, an inhibitor of chylomicron remnant clearance. J Biol Chem 1992;267:26172–26180.

10. Zheng G, Bachinsky DR, Stamenkovic I, Strickland DK, Borwn D, Andres G, McCluskey RT. Organ distribution in rats of two members of the low-density lipoprotein receptor gene family, gp330 and LRP/a2M receptor, and the receptor-associated (RAP). J Histochem Cytochem 1994;42:531–542.

11. Takahashi S, Kawarabayasi Y, Nakai T, Sakai J, Yamamoto T. Rabbit very low density lipoprotein receptor: a low-density lipoprotein receptor-like protein with distinct ligand specificity. Proc Natl Acad Sci USA 1992;89:9252–9256.

12. Willnow TE, Herz J. Genetic deficiency in low-density lipoprotein receptor-related protein confers cellular resistance to *Pseudomonas* exotoxin A: evidence that this protein is required for uptake and degradation of multiple ligands. J Cell Sci 1994;107:719–726.

13. Battey FD, Gafvels ME, FitzGerald DJ, Argraves WS, Chappell DA, Strauss III JF, Strickland DK. The 39-kDa receptor-associated protein regulates ligand binding by the very low density lipoprotein receptor. J Biol Chem 1994;37:23268–23273.

14. Stefansson S, Chappell DA, Argraves KM, Strickland DK, Argraves WS. Glycoprotein 330/low-density lipoprotein receptor-related protein-2 mediates endocytosis of low-density lipoproteins via interaction with apolipoprotein B 100. J Biol Chem 1995;270:19417–19412.

15. Medh JD, Fry GL, Bowen SL, Pladet MW, Strickland DK, Chappell DA. The 39 kDa receptor-associated protein modulates lipoprotein catabolism by binding to LDL receptors. J Biol Chem 1995;270:536–540.

16. Milne RW, Theolis RJ, Verdery RB, Marcel YL. Characterization of monoclonal antibodies against human low-density lipoprotein. Arteriosclerosis 1983;3:23–30.

17. Gafvels ME, Paavola LG, Boyd CO, Nolan PM, Wittmaack F, Chawla A, Lazar MA, Bucan M, Angelin B, Strauss III JF. Cloning of a complementary deoxyribonucleic acid encoding the muring homolog of the very low density lipoprotein/apolipoprotein-E receptor: expression pattern and assignment of the gene to mouse chromosome 19. Endocrinology 1994;135:387–394.

18. Wyne KL, Pathak RK, Seabra MC, Hobbs HH. Expression of the VLDL receptor in endothelial cells. Arterioscl Thromb Vasc Biol 1996;16:407–415.

19. Multhaupt HAB, Gafvels ME, Kariko K, Jin H, Arenas-Elliot C, Goldman BI, Strauss JFI, Angelin B, Warhol MJ, McCrae KR. Expression of very low density lipoprotein receptor in the vascular wall: analysis of human tissues by in situ hybridization and immunohistochemistry. Am J Path 1996;148:1985–1997.

20. Argraves KM, Kozarsky KF, Fallon JT, Harpel PC, Strickland DK. The atherogenic lipoprotein, Lp(a), is internalized and degraded in a process mediated by the VLDL receptor. J Clin Invest 1997;100:2170–2181.

21. Poon M, Zhang X, Dunsky K, Taubman MB, Harpel PC. Apolipoprotein(a) induces monocyte chemotactic activity in human vascular endothelial cells. Circulation 1997;96:2514–2519.

Assembly and catabolism of lipoprotein(a)

Wo Xingde[3], Karam Kostner[2], Sasa Frank[1] and Gert M. Kostner[1]

[1]*Institute of Medical Biochemistry, Karl-Franzens University of Graz, Graz;* [2]*Department of Cardiology, University of Vienna, Austria; and* [3]*Molecular Med. Institute, Hangzhou, China*

Abstract. *Background.* The function and catabolism of Lp(a), one of the most atherogenic lipoproteins is virtually unknown. In order to study this, the assembly, in vivo catabolism and the excretion of apo(a) fragments were investigated.

Methods. ^{131}I-Tyr-cellobiose labelled lipoproteins were injected into hedgehogs and the differential uptake into various organs was studied. Urinary apo(a) was characterised by W-blotting and an adapted immunochemical method, DELFIA. 116 male patients suffering from CHD were studied for plasma lipids and lipoproteins as well as urinary (u-) apo(a) excretion. The discriminatory power of u-apo(a) in comparison to plasma Lp(a) was calculated.

Results. Native Lp(a) is hardly recognised by the LDL receptor, yet the organ distribution of radiolabelled Lp(a) in hedgehogs was very similar to that of LDL. Only the kidney appeared to catabolise more Lp(a) than LDL. The kidney also secretes relatively large apo(a) fragments with 35—160 kD and the urinary apo(a) concentration correlated significantly with plasma Lp(a) levels. Studies in patients suffering from CAD revealed that u-apo(a) was a better discriminator than plasma Lp(a).

Conclusion. There is still a large amount of work needed to understand the metabolism and function of Lp(a). In this respect, the role of the kidney appears to be worth pursuing further.

Keywords: CAD, hedgehog, metabolism, urinary excretion.

Introduction

There are numerous reports in the literature that elevated plasma Lp(a) levels contribute significantly to the risk of atherosclerosis and related diseases such as myocardial infarction and stroke [1,2]. Over the last 30 years, intensive research in Lp(a) metabolism and its possible function have been conducted, yet there are still numerous open questions primarily related to the site of Lp(a) catabolism and physiological significance. Concerning Lp(a) biosynthesis and assembly, it has now been demonstrated by several laboratories that apo(a) is synthesized and secreted by the liver and reacts with mature LDL outside the cell forming a covalently linked complex [3—6]. Of considerable importance, however, is the site and mode of Lp(a) catabolism which not only may have some implications for its function, but certainly also may help to design specific drugs to interfere with increased plasma Lp(a) levels.

Address for correspondence: Prof Dr G.M. Kostner, Institute of Medical Biochemistry, Karl-Franzens University of Graz, Harrachgasse 21/3, 8010 Graz, Austria. Tel.: +43-316-380-4200. Fax: +43-316-380-9615.

Another point which needs to be studied in more detail is the actual patho-physiological role of Lp(a) in atherogenesis. The concepts discussed today range from binding of Lp(a) to extracellular matrix substances, interaction of apo(a) with fibrinolysis by competitively inhibiting plasminogen binding [7—9] or even other pathways in the coagulation system, up to the interference with TGF-β activation [10] and others. Unfortunately none of these theories have been convincingly proven in vivo. It is also unknown whether apo(a) isoforms with large and small molecular masses on a molar basis are equally atherogenic. In this respect, it has to be kept in mind that apo(a)'s with varying size differ by the number of repetitive kringle-4's (K-IV), the latter being completely identical and showing a rather low-binding affinity to lysine (Lys). On the other hand, unique K-IV's (mainly those involved in Lp(a) assembly) exhibit high-affinity Lys binding [3]. The role of Lys binding with respect to atherogenesis has recently been addressed by Boonmark et al. [11] in a transgenic mouse model where it was found that its destruction in kringle-IV (K-IV) type 10 (T-10) leads to a grossly reduced athero-genicity.

In this report we focus mainly on the catabolism of Lp(a) and the possible role of kidney in Lp(a) metabolism.

Material and Methods

Organ-specific uptake of Lp(a) in hedgehogs

The organ specificity of Lp(a) catabolism was investigated in Asian hedgehogs: 3—5-year-old male and female hedgehogs (*Erinaceidae dealbatus swinhoe*) from the area of Hangzhou, China were studied during summertime. For this purpose, Lp(a) and LDL were labelled with an undegradable marker, ^{125}I-tyramin cello-biose [12] labelled lipoproteins with specific activities of 20—500 μCi per mg protein were injected intravenously into the animals and the decay of radioactivity in blood was followed over time. The animals were sacrificed at various time points after injection, the organs were perfused PBS containing 10 mmol/l of EDTA, homogenized by an Ultraturrax and the radioactivity was counted in a γ-counter.

Quantification of apo(a) fragments

For this purpose, the in-house apo(a) DELFIA using polyclonal rabbit antiapo(a) for capture and detection was adapted for urinary samples [3,13,14]. This assay was linear over a wide-concentration range and yielded parallel-dilution curves in comparison to the standard. The apo(a) fragments in urine were also studied by SDS-PAGE in 15% gels followed by Western blotting in the presence of mo-lecular-weight standards as described [14].

Urinary apo (a) excretion in CAD patients and controls

116 male and female patients suffering from single or multiple vessel disease were studied. Seventy-three of them had a previous history of myocardial infarction and 59 suffered from hypertension. Except for antihypertensive drugs, the patients did not receive medication. The control group consisted of clinically healthy volunteers participating in a health-survey programme. Controls were matched for age, gender, smoking behaviour and socioeconomic status. Blood and urinary samples were collected upon admission to the clinic prior to coronary angiography in the morning after an overnight fasting period. In addition to Lp(a), all major plasma lipids, lipoproteins and related parameters were analysed using conventional laboratory methods. In urine, apo(a) fragments were studied qualitatively by Western blotting and quantitatively by DELFIA.

Results

Lp(a) assembly

There are no indications whatsoever that the assembly of Lp(a) from apo(a) and apoB containing particles might occur inside the cells. All experiments carried out in our laboratory are compatible with the concept that Lp(a) is assembled from circulating LDL and from apo(a) which is biosynthesized in the liver [3,13,15]. There is, however, the possibility that apo(a) is bound on cell surfaces or extracellular matrices upon secretion. As LDL passes by it associates with apo(a) forming Lp(a) [6]. It is known from work of Boerwinkle et al. [16] that the plasma Lp(a) concentration is approximately 90% genetically determined and correlates negatively with the apo(a) size. Experiments with primary cultures of liver cells established that large apo(a) isoforms are not only biosynthesized more slowly, but are also in part retained in the cell and degraded to a much greater extent than small isoforms [6].

The assembly of Lp(a) proceeds in two steps. In the first step, a loose complex between LDL and apo(a) is formed. This LDL:apo(a) complex dissociates upon addition of Lys, ε-amino hexoic acid (ε-AHA) or similar compounds. In a second step, a covalent-disulfide bridge is formed between LDL and apo(a). Results from previous works show that almost 100% assembly could be obtained only if the full sequence of K-IV T5—T10 were present. The results also highlighted the importance of K-IV T6 and T7 for the first step of assembly. The addition of 50 mM ε-AHA after the association between apo(a) and apoB took place dissociated part of the complexes. From this the fraction of covalently linked apo(a): apoB complexes was calculated and found to be different between various apo(a) fragments ranging from 55—97%. It appeared that K-IV T5 and/or T2 increased the efficiency of forming stable Lp(a) complexes.

570

Lp(a) catabolism in vivo

We studied the catabolism of human Lp(a) and LDL previously in normal and in LDL-receptor-deficient WHHL rabbits [17,18] and found that the fractional catabolic rate (FCR) of Lp(a) in normal rabbits is 2,00 pools per day and is significantly lower than that of LDL (2.85 pools/d). WHHL rabbits on the other hand exhibit a higher FCR for Lp(a) as compared to LDL (1.35 vs. 1.27 pools/ day). In addition, 2 days after lipoprotein injection, the specific-organ uptake of Lp(a) and LDL was studied. Looking at whole organs, the liver was by far the most important organ of Lp(a) catabolism. Since rabbits lack Lp(a) in their plasma we subsequently decided to perform further metabolic studies in hedgehogs.

Organ-specific uptake of Lp(a) in hedgehogs in comparison to LDL

For these experiments several hedgehogs were infused with LDL or Lp(a) marked with the undegradable label ^{125}I tyramine-cellobiose, blood was drawn at various time intervals and the biological half-life was calculated from the decay of specific radioactivity. T/2 of Lp(a) and LDL on average amounted to 44 and 16 h, respectively. The corresponding values for humans are 3.8 and 2.9 days.

The animals were sacrificed 12 h after lipoprotein injection and the accumulation of Lp(a) or LDL in different organs was determined. Significant amounts of radiolabel occurred in liver, spleen, kidney adrenals and bile. The other investigated organs (heart, lung, and pancreas) accumulated many less lipoproteins and will not be considered here. It can be assumed, that the radioactivity occurring in bile might reflect a sink of radiolabel not only derived from lipoprotein uptake into the liver but also of degradation products from other organs. The spleen on the other hand is known to take up aggregated or degraded material and might not be so relevant for our considerations.

Considering the remaining organs, the adrenals on a gram-organ basis took up the major amount of LDL, followed by kidney and liver (Fig. 1**A**). Concerning Lp(a), the kidney was the major organ of lipoprotein uptake followed by the two other organs. Looking at the lipoprotein catabolism by the whole organs (Fig. 1B) the dominant role of the liver becomes obvious, accounting for approximately 70% of LDL catabolism and 60% Lp(a) catabolism. Kidney took up 6.6% of Lp(a) and 5.2% LDL. The adrenals were neither important for LDL nor for Lp(a) uptake. These results in fact are in line with those of previous studies of our laboratory where lipoproteins directly labelled with iodine were injected into rabbits [18].

Secretion of apo(a) fragments into urine

The secretion of apo(a) into urine has been studied mainly by ourselves and one other research group [14,19]. It was demonstrated that neither intact Lp(a) nor LDL or apo(a) are found in urine of healthy persons, but very distinct apo(a)

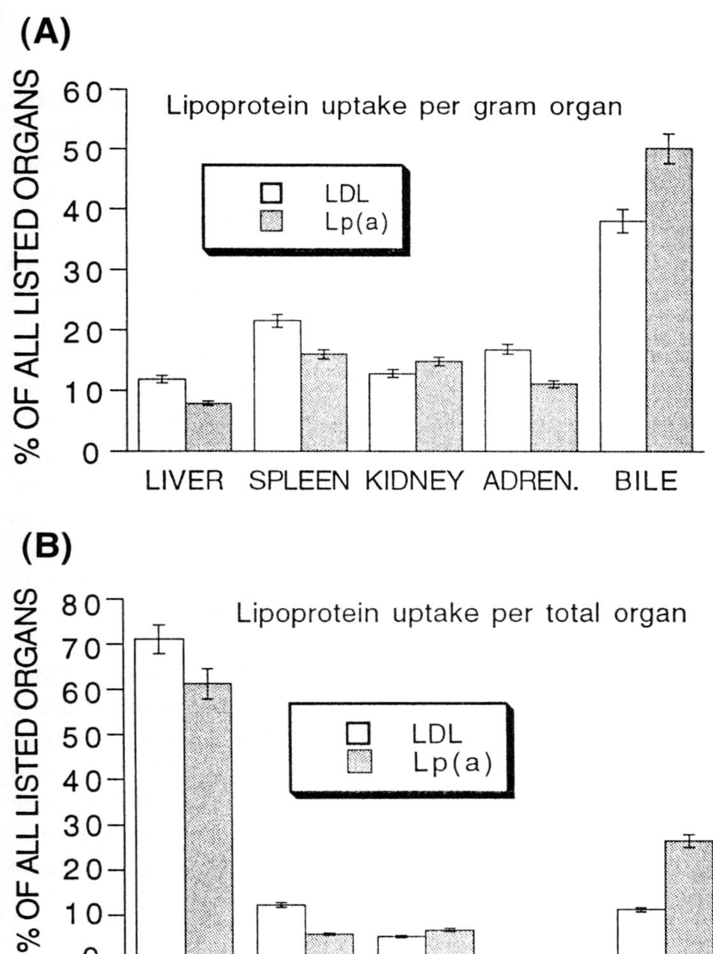

Fig. 1. Uptake of [131]I Tyr-cellobiose labelled lipoproteins into various organs of hedgehogs (mean ± SD of triplicate experiments).

fragments with molecular masses ranging from 35—160 kD. Urinary fragments represent the N-terminal portion of apo(a) of variable size. Remarkably, the size of these fragments seems to be equal in probands with large or small apo(a) isoforms [14]. We also quantitated the fraction of apo(a) secreted into urine and found that approximately 0.1% of the daily amount of catabolized Lp(a) appears to be cleared through the kidney in the form of N-terminal apo(a) fragments. In a recent report by Mooser et al. [19] it was postulated that these urinary apo(a) fragments are present already in the blood and may be cleared by a yet unknown mechanism.

572

Urinary apo (a) fragments as a discriminator for the atherosclerosis risk

As a result of the highly significant correlation between plasma Lp(a) and urinary apo(a) (u-apo(a)) concentrations [14] we tested this latter parameter for its suitability to discriminate patients with coronary artery disease (CAD) from healthy persons. Details of the collectives are given in the "Methods" section. The patients had significantly higher plasma triglyceride, cholesterol and LDL-C and lower HDL-C values as compared to controls (Table 1). In patients, median plasma Lp(a) levels were 1.52-fold higher whereas u-apo(a) excretion was 2.1-fold higher as compared to controls and had a higher power of discrimination. Figure 2 exhibits a receiver-operating-characteristic (ROC) plot comparing plasma Lp(a) with urinary apo(a) where it can be seen that mainly at lower cutoff levels u-apo(a) is superior to plasma Lp(a) (i.e., the u-apo(a) curve deviates more from the 45° regression line than plasma Lp(a)). At cutoff levels of 30 mg/dl for plasma Lp(a) and 10 µg/dl of u-apo(a) the sensitivities were comparable (34 vs. 27%); yet the specificity (76 vs. 92%) and the positive predictive value (60 vs. 76%) were significantly higher for u-apo(a).

Discussion

Despite the intensive work over the past 20 years in numerous laboratories there is still little known about the physiological role of Lp(a) and the mode and site of catabolism. We expected from our hedgehog experiments that a specific organ other than liver might accumulate the majority of injected Lp(a); yet this was unfortunately not the case. As suggested previously, kidney accumulated more Lp(a) as compared to LDL and thus it seems possible that the physiological function might be found in this organ. In this respect, it is noteworthy that in patients suffering from kidney disease plasma Lp(a) levels increase up to 3- to 4-fold. Another point which needs further study is the elucidation of the pathophysiology of Lp(a) related to atherogenesis. Although many mechanisms have been discussed which add to the atherosclerosis risk, Lp(a) may have also some protective properties, as we demonstrated that apo(a) interferes with the collagen-induced platelet aggregation [20]; Lp(a) is also less prone to oxidation than LDL. It is hoped that within the next few years these open questions may be resolved.

Table 1. Lipid and lipoprotein concentrations from 116 CHD patients and 109 matched controls.

	Triglycerides	Cholesterol	LDL-C	HDL-C	P-lp(a)	U-apo(a)
CHD-patients	192.2 ± 89.2	219.8 ± 47.6	148.5 ± 38.2	34.7 ± 11.8	18.0 (10.0/49.5)	5.7 (3.3/10.4)
Controls	106.9 ± 53.6	189.8 ± 43.3	124.7 ± 33.4	46.6 ± 14.6	11.8 (5.7/27.5)	2.6 (1.4/ 3.5)
p-value	0.0001	0.0001	0.0001	0.0001	0.003	0.0005

The values for plasma are given in mg/dl and are mean ± SD except for Lp(a) (which is given as median and 25/75 percentile). Urinary apo(a) (u-apo(a)) is given in µg/dl normalized to 100 mg/dl creatinine.

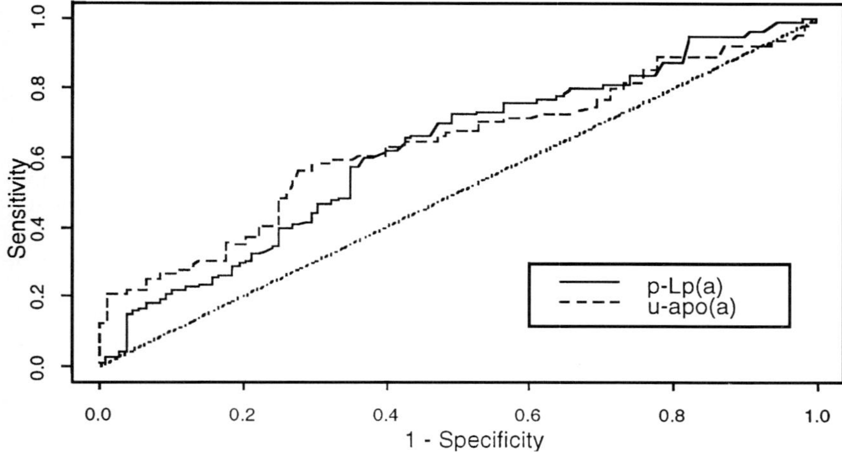

Fig. 2. Receiver-operating characteristic plot of plasma (p)-Lp(a) and urinary (u-) apo(a) in a case control study: CHD vs. controls.

Acknowledgements

This work was supported by grants from the Austrian Research Foundation P11691, Biomembrane Research Centre SFB 702, Austrian National Bank ÖNB 5956, Austrian Heart Foundation and the Franz-Lanyar Foundation.

References

1. Kostner GM, Avogaro P, Cazzolato G, Marth E, Bittolo Bon G. Lipoprotein Lp(a) and the risk for myocardial infarction. Atherosclerosis 1981;38:51—61.
2. Bostom AG, Cupples LA, Jenner JL, Ordovas JM, Seman LL, Wilson PWF, Schaefer EJ, Castelli WP. Elevated plasma lipoprotein(a) and premature coronary heart disease in Framingham men: a prospective study. JAMA 1996;276:544—548.
3. Frank S, Kostner GM. The role of apo(a) kringle-IV's in the assembly of lipoprotein(a). Protein (Eng) 1997;10:291—298.
4. Koschinsky ML, Coté GP, Gabel B, van der Hoek YY. Identification of the cysteine residue in apolipoprotein(a) that mediates extracellular coupling with apolipoprotein B-100. J Biol Chem 1993;268:19819—19825.
5. Trieu VN, McConathy WJ. A two-step model for lipoprotein(a) formation. J Biol Chem 1995; 270:15471—15474.
6. White AL, Lanford RE. Biosynthesis and metabolism of lipoprotein(a). Curr Opin Lipid 1995; 6:75—80.
7. Harpel PC, Chang VT, Borth W. Homocysteine and other sulfhydryl compounds enhance the binding of lipoprotein(a) to fibrin: a potential biochemical link between thrombosis, atherogenesis, and sulfhydryl compound metabolism. Proc Natl Acad Sci USA 1992;89:10193—10197.
8. Rouy D, Grailhe P, Nigon F, Chapman J, Anglés-Cano E. Lipoprotein(a) impairs generation of plasmin by fibrin-bound tissue-type plasminogen activator: in vitro studies in a plasma milieu. Arterioscl Thromb 1991;11:629—638.
9. Miles LA, Fless GM, Levin EG, Scanu AM, Plow EF. A potential basis for the thrombotic risks

associated with lipoprotein(a). Nature 1989;339:301–303.

10. Grainger DJ, Kemp PR, Liu AC, Lawn RM, Metcalfe JC. Activation of transforming growth factor-β is inhibited in transgenic apolipoprotein(a) mice. Nature 1994;370:460–462.

11. Boonmark NW, Lou XJ, Yang ZJ, Schwartz K, Zhang J-L, Rubin EM. Modification of apolipoprotein(a) lysine binding site reduces atherosclerosis in transgenic mice. J Clin Invest 1997; 100:558–564.

12. Pittman RC, Carew TE, Glass CK, Green SR, Taylor Jr CA, Attie AD. A radioiodinated, intracellularly trapped ligand for determining the sites of plasma protein degradation in vivo. Biochem J 1983;212:791–800.

13. Frank S, Durovic S, Kostner GM. Structural requirements of apo-a for the lipoprotein-a assembly. Biochem J 1994;304:27–30.

14. Kostner KM, Maurer G, Huber K, Stefenelli T, Dieplinger H, Steyrer E, Kostner GM. Urinary excretion of apo(a) fragments: role in apo(a) catabolism. Arteroscl Thromb Vasc Biol 1996;16: 905–911.

15. Frank S, Durovic S, Kostner GM. The assembly of lipoprotein Lp(a). Eur J Clin Invest 1996; 26:109–114.

16. Boerwinkle E, Leffert CC, Lin J, Lackner C, Chiesa G, Hobbs HH. Apolipoprotein(a) gene accounts for greater than 90% of the variation in plasma lipoprotein(a) concentrations. J Clin Invest 1992;90:52–60.

17. Kostner GM. The physiological role of Lp(a). In: Scanu AM (ed) Lipoprotein(a). San Diego, New York, Boston: Academic Press, 1990;183–204.

18. Liu R, Saku K, Kostner GM, Hirat K, Zhang B, Shiomi M, Arakawa K. In vivo kinetics of lipoprotein(a) in homozygous Watanabe heritable hyperlipidemic rabbits. Eur J Clin Invest 1993;23:561–565.

19. Mooser V, Marcovina SM, White AL, Hobbs HH. Kringle-containing fragments of apolipoprotein(a) circulate in human plasma and are excreted into the urine. J Clin Invest 1996;98: 2414–2424.

20. Gries A, Gries M, Wurm H, Kenner T, Ijsseldijk M, Sixma JJ, Kostner GM. Lp(a) inhibits collagen-induced aggregation of thrombocytes. Arterioscl Thromb Vasc Biol 1996;16:648–655.

Function and evolution of Lp(a)

Richard M. Lawn

Falk Cardiovascular Research Center, Stanford University School of Medicine, California, USA

Abstract. Apolipoprotein(a) is the distinguishing protein component of the Lp(a) lipoprotein particle. Although it represents one of the major inherited risk factors for atherosclerosis, its function remains obscure. Apolipoprotein(a) evolved from a duplicated plasminogen gene during primate evolution, although a similar gene arose independently in the lineage leading to current insectivores. In vitro and transgenic-mouse data indicate that apolipoprotein(a) contributes to atherosclerosis by inhibiting the activation of the homologous plasminogen protein. Mutagenesis implies that the ability of apolipoprotein(a) to bind to fibrin and compete for plasminogen binding to this substrate is essential for its pathogenic activity.

Keywords: apolipoprotein(a), atherosclerosis, fibrin, lipoprotein(a), plasminogen.

Structure and function of Lp(a)

High-plasma concentration of lipoprotein(a) (Lp(a)) is one of the major inherited risk factors for atherosclerosis and related disease states including myocardial infarction, cerebral stroke, peripheral vascular disease and restenosis [1,2]. Most of the published prospective studies conclude that elevated Lp(a) levels predict the development of cardiovascular disease ([3,4] and references therein). Lp(a) is comprised of a low-density lipoprotein (LDL) particle to which has been covalently attached the distinguishing feature, apolipoprotein(a) (apo(a)). DNA sequence analysis revealed that apo(a) is closely related to plasminogen, containing multiple domains resembling plasminogen kringle 4, plus a single kringle 5-like domain and an inactive protease-like domain [5].

Several hypotheses have been proposed to explain the association of plasma Lp(a) concentration to atherosclerosis, due to it containing an inactive homolog of plasminogen [1,2]. Apo(a) has been shown to compete for the binding of plasminogen to fibrin and other substrates and reduces the generation of active plasmin [6—9]. In vivo evidence that Lp(a) reduces fibrinolysis has come from studies in primates [10], human [11,12] and transgenic mice [13,14]. The decreased fibrinolysis in vessel walls might account for much of the atherogenic potential of apo(a), since the persistence of mural thrombi may stimulate repair processes that lead to the local thickening of vessel wall.

An additional substrate of plasmin is latent transforming growth factor-β

Address for correspondence: R.M. Lawn, Falk Cardiovascular Research Center, Stanford University School of Medecine, 300 Pasteur Drive, Stanford, CA 94305-5246, USA. Tel.: +1-415-725-4494. Fax: +1-415-725-1599. E-mail: richard.lawn@forsythe.stanford.edu

(TGF-β). By interfering with plasmingoen activation, apo(a) can thus also suppress the activation of TGF-β. Since TGF-β suppresses the proliferation and migration of smooth muscle cells, apo(a) could stimulate these atherogenic activities. This pathway was first shown to be operative in cultured vascular smooth muscle cells [15,16]. We subsequently used transgenic mice expressing human apo(a) (which is lacking in normal mice) to explore this process in vivo. These animals developed sites of very high focal accumulation of apo(a), mainly near the luminal surface of the assayed vessels (proximal aorta). At these sites, activation of TGF-β was inhibited, and there was greatly enhanced expression of osteopontin, an in vitro protein marker of smooth muscle cell activation [14]. When fed an atherogenic diet, lipid lesions occur at sites of apo(a) accumulation. This is consistent with the observations that proliferating activated smooth muscle cells take up cholesterol more readily than quiescent smooth muscle cells, resulting from upregulation of oxidized low-density lipoprotein receptors [17,18]. Reduction of TGF-β has also been associated with inflammatory damage to the endothelium and increased adhesiveness to leukocytes. We have proposed the existence of a positive feedback loop by which apo(a) initially accumulates at sites where integrity or function of the endothelium has been compromised, causing a local reduction of active plasmin and TGF-β. This leads to further endothelial dysfunction and access of lipoproteins such as Lp(a) to the subendothelial space. In support of this pathway in the mouse model was the observation that preventing lesion development in apo(a) transgenic mice by two independent mechanisms also inhibited the "upstream" event, the vascular accumulation of apo(a) [19].

A common feature of these mechanisms is the shared activity of apo(a) and plasminogen to bind fibrin and other substrates through its kringle lysine binding site. Sequence analysis of human apo(a) cDNA [5] and studies of human mutations [20,21], provided evidence that the major functional lysine binding site of apo(a) is located in its 37th kringle 4-like domain. In vitro experiments with recombinant apo(a) altered by mutagenesis have supported the hypothesis [22–24], although other studies [25] caution that additional fibrin binding capacity is distinct from the lysine binding site(s). In order to study this activity in vivo, we constructed an apo(a) expression plasmid in which the lysine binding site in kringle 4-37 was destroyed by changing the two key anionic residues of the lysine binding pocket to alanine. Transgenic mice overexpressing this mutated apo(a) as well as the wild-type apo(a) were generated and used to study its effect on atherosclerosis. When fed on a high-fat diet, the mutated apo(a) transgenic mice have a 5-fold reduction in fatty streak lesions in the aorta compared to the wild-type transgenic mice [26]. This result implies that the lysine-binding site of apo(a) is associated with the pathogenesis of Lp(a).

The intriguing evolution of Lp(a)

Until several years ago, Lp(a) was thought to be confined to a subset of primates, having only been detected in Old World monkeys, apes and humans ([27] and references therein). This agrees with the hypothesis that the apo(a) gene arose from a duplicated copy of the plasminogen gene during primate evolution. The report of an Lp(a)-like particle in hedgehogs (an insectivore) caused some consternation [28]. Cloning and sequencing of hedgehog apo(a) cDNA demonstrated a remarkable example of parallel gene evolution [27]. The sequenced hedgehog apo(a) cDNA contains 31 repeats that contain approximately 80% identity to hedgehog kringle 3, and no kringle 4-like, 5-like or protease domains whatsoever. Despite being built up from repeats of a different domain of plasminogen than the primate apo(a) gene, hedgehog apo(a) has a number of striking similarities. Not only does it contain more than a dozen repeated kringles, only one of the kringles contains a seventh cysteine residue (in a location distinct from the human form) and forms a covalent linkage to apoB-100, allowing it to circulate as a lipoprotein particle. Hedgehog apo(a) also retains the amino acids which constitute the plasminogen lysine binding site and binds to lysine and fibrin. In the human gene, point mutations have inactivated the protease domain, while in hedgehog apo(a) it is completely absent. Thus, by independent remodeling of a plasminogen-like gene, hedgehog and human ancestors independently evolved an apo(a) protein with multiple-kringle domains that covalently links to apoB-containing lipoproteins, binds fibrin, lacks proteolytic activity and competitively inhibits plasminogen activation [27]. By a number of analytical procedures, it appears that the "invention" of the hedgehog apo(a) gene began with a relatively ancient split from the plasminogen gene, approximately 80 million years ago, while human apo(a) derived from a duplication of the plasminogen gene during primate evolution, within the last 40 million years [29] (Fig. 1).

It is intriguing to note that, despite its recurrent evolution, we do not as yet know the adaptive function of apo(a). The fact that an apo(a)-like gene with shared properties has evolved twice, in addition to the fact that it has retained intact an extremely long open reading frame, argue that it is not simply the resi-

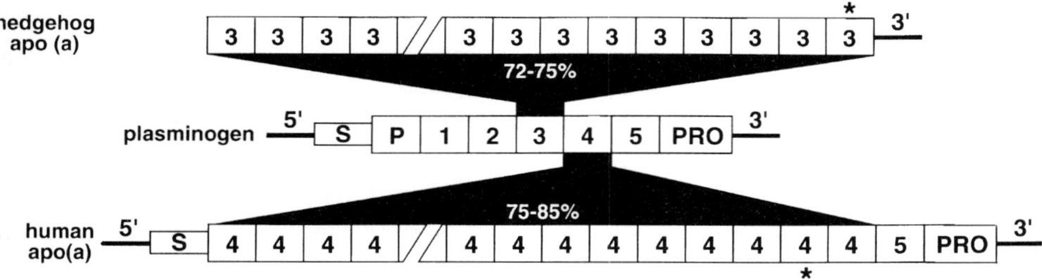

Fig. 1. The sequences of plasminogen and hedgehog and human apo(a) cDNA are compared, with the percentage of nucleotide identity shown between the corresponding multiple-kringle domains of hedgehog apo(a) and hedgehog plasminogen and between human apo(a) and human plasminogen. The one unpaired cysteine (indicated by *) is responsible for the binding of human apo(a) to apo B-100 and is postulated to be the case for the hedgehog protein. Reprinted from Lawn et al. [27] with permission of the Journal of Biological Chemistry.

due of a random duplication of DNA that has not been extinguished. Although its pathogenic activity has been well-documented, its positive functions remain unknown. It has been proposed that Lp(a) might play a role in wound healing or in angiogenesis. Although this is consistent with the immunolocalization of Lp(a) in wounded tissues, there is as yet no experimental confirmation of the efficacy of Lp(a) in wound healing models. Although a kringle containing fragment of plasminogen, called angiostatin, is an inhibitor of angiogenesis [30], we found that apo(a) fails to modulate angiogenesis in an in vivo model system [31]. We are now testing the idea that apo(a) might play an adaptive role in protection against certain infectious diseases, based on the observation that a number of invasive pathogens express plasminogen activators or receptors, which may aid in the dissolution of extracellular barriers to their migration from the site of entry to the bloodstream. Many challenges remain before we gain a full understanding of the curious Lp(a) lipoprotein, let alone learn how to control its pathogenic consequences.

References

1. Scanu AM, Fless GM. Lipoprotein(a): heterogeneity and biological relevance. J Clin Invest 1990;85:1709—1715.
2. Utermann G. The mysteries of lipoprotein(a). Science 1989;246:904—910.
3. Bostom AG, Cupples LA, Jenner JL, Ordovas JM, Seman LL, Wilson PWF, Schaefer EJ, Castelli WP. Elevated plasma lipoprotein(a) and premature coronary heart disease in Framingham men: a prospective study. JAMA 1996;276:544—548.
4. Assmann G, Schulte H, von Eckardstein A. Hypertriglyceridemia and elevated lipoprotein(a) are risk factors for major coronary events in middle-aged men. Am J Cardiol 1996;77:1179—1184.
5. McLean JW, Tomlinson JE, Kuang WJ, Eaton DL, Chen EY, Fless GM, Scanu AM, Lawn RM. cDNA sequence of human apolipoprotein(a) is homologous to plasminogen. Nature 1987;330:132—137.
6. Harpel PC, Gordon BR, Parker TS. Plasmin catalyzes binding of lipoprotein(a) to immobilized fibrinogen and fibrin. Proc Natl Acad Sci USA 1989;86:3847—3851.
7. Miles LA, Fless GM, Levin EG, Scanu AM, Plow EF. A potential basis for the thrombosis risks associated with lipoprotein(a). Nature 1989;339:301—303.
8. Hajjar KA, Gavish D, Breslow JL, Nachman RL. Lipoprotein(a) modulation of endothelial cell surface fibrinolysis and its potential role in atherosclerosis. Nature 1989;339:303—305.
9. Edelberg JM, Gonzalez-Gronow M, Pizzo SV. Lipoprotein(a) inhibition of plasminogen activation by tissue-type plasminogen activator. Thromb Res 1990;57:155—162.
10. Williams JK, Bellinger DA, Nichols TC, Griggs TR, Bumol TF, Fouts RL, Clarkson TB. Occlusive arterial thrombosis in cynomolgus monkeys with varying plasma concentrations of lipoprotein(a). Arterioscl Thromb 1993;13:548—554.
11. Moliterno DJ, Lange RA, Meidell RS, Willard JE, Leffert CC, Gerard RD, Boerwinkle E, Hobbs HH, Hillis LD. Relation of plasma lipoprotein(a) to infarct artery patency in survivors of myocardial infarction. Circulation 1993;88:935—940.
12. Grainger DJ, Kemp PR, Metcalfe JC, Liu AC, Lawn RM, Williams NR, Grace AA, Schofield PM, Chauhan A. The serum concentration of active transforming growth factor-β is severely depressed in advanced atherosclerosis. Nature 1995;1:74—79.
13. Palabrica TM, Liu AC, Aronovitz MJ, Furie B, Lawn RM, Furie BC. Human apolipoprotein(a)

transgenic mice are resistant to thrombolysis. Nature 1995;1:256—259.

14. Grainger DJ, Kemp PR, Liu AC, Lawn RM, Metcalfe JC. Activation of transforming growth factor-β is inhibited in apolipoprotein(a) transgenic mice. Nature 1994;370:460—462.

15. Kojima S, Harpel PC, Rifkin DB. Lipoprotein(a) inhibits the generation of transforming growth factor-β: an endogenous inhibitor of smooth muscle cell migration. J Cell Biol 1991;113:1439—1445.

16. Grainger DJ, Kirschenlohr HL, Metcalfe JC, Weissberg PL, Wade DP, Lawn RM. Proliferation of human smooth muscle cells promoted by lipoprotein(a). Science 1993;260:1655—1658.

17. Campbell JH, Reardon MF, Campbell GR, Nestel PJ. Metabolism of atherogenic lipoproteins by smooth muscle cells of different phenotype in culture. Arteriosclerosis 1985;5:318—328.

18. Li HM, Freeman MW, Libby P. Regulation of smooth muscle cell scavenger receptor expression in vivo by atherogenic diets and in vitro by cytokines. J Clin Invest 1995;95:122—133.

19. Lawn RM, Pearle AD, Kunz LL, Rubin EM, Reckless J, Metcalfe JC, Grainger DJ. Feedback mechanism of focal vascular lesion formation in transgenic apolipoprotein(a) mice. J Biol Chem 1996;271:31367—31371.

20. Scanu AM, Pfaffinger D, Lee JC, Hinman J. A single point mutation (Trp72 → Arg) in human apo(a) kringle 4-37 associated with a lysine binding defect in Lp(a). Biochim Biophys Acta 1994;1227:41—45.

21. Scanu AM, Edelstein C. Kringle-dependent structural and functional polymorphism of apolipoprotein(a). Biochim Biophys Acta 1995;1256:1—12.

22. LoGrasso PV, Cornell-Kennon S, Boettcher BR. Cloning, expression and characterization of human apolipoprotein(a) kringle IV-37. J Biol Chem 1994;269:21820—21827.

23. Ernst A, Helmhold M, Brunner C, Petho-Schramm A, Armstrong VW, Müller HJ. Identification of two functionally distinct lysine-binding sites in kringle 37 and in kringles 32—36 of human apolipoprotein(a). J Biol Chem 1995;270:6227—6234.

24. Hoover-Plow JL, Boonmark N, Skocir P, Lawn R, Plow EF. A quantitative immunoassay for the lysine-binding function of lipoprotein(a): application to recombinant apo(a) and lipoprotein(a) in plasma. Arterioscl Thromb Vasc Biol 1996;16:656—664.

25. Klezowitch L, Edelstein C, Scanu AM. Evidence that the fibrinogen binding domain of apo(a) is outside the lysine binding site of kringle IV-10. J Clin Invest 1996;98:185—191.

26. Boonmark NW, Lou JX, Yang ZJ, Schwartz K, Zhang J-L, Rubin EM, Lawn RM. Modification of apolipoprotein (a) lysine binding site reduces atherosclerosis in transgenic mice. J Clin Invest 1997;(In press).

27. Lawn RM, Boonmark NW, Schwartz K, Lindahl GE, Wade DP, Byrne CD, Fong KJ, Meer K, Patthy L. The recurring evolution of lipoprotein(a). J Biol Chem 1995;270:24004—24009.

28. Laplaud PM, Beaubatie L, Rall SJ, Luc G, Saboureau MJ. Lipoprotein(a) is the major apoB-containing lipoprotein in the plasma of a hibernator, the hedgehog (Erinaceus europaeus). J Lipid Res 1988;29:1157—1170.

29. Lawn RM, Schwartz K, Patthy L. Convergent evolution of apolipoprotein(a) in primates and hedgehog. Proc Natl Acad Sci USA 1997;(In press).

30. O'Reilly MS, Holmgren L, Shing Y, Chen C, Rosenthal RA, Moses M, Lane W, Cao Y, Sage EH, Folkman J. Angiostatin: a novel angiogenesis inhibitor that mediates the supression of metastases by a Lewis lung carcinoma. Cell 1994;79:315—328.

31. Lou XJ, Kwan H, Prionas SD, Yang ZJ, Lawn RM, Fajardo LF. Apolipoprotein(a) does not affect angiogenesis in vivo. Circulation 1997;(In press).

Comparative effects of Desogen® and Lo/Ovral™ contraceptive hormones on lipoprotein(a)

Joel D. Morrisett[1], Karima Ghazzaly[1], Marianne Reilly[2], Michael C. Snabes[2] and Ronald L. Young[2]

Departments of [1]Medicine and [2]Obstetrics/Gynecology, Baylor College of Medicine, Houston, Texas, USA

Abstract. *Objective.* This study was designed to compare the effect of two oral contraceptive formulations, Desogen® and Lo/Ovral™, on the lipid and lipoprotein profiles of premenopausal women.

Methods. 100 premenopausal women were randomized to one of two parallel treatment groups that received either Desogen® or Lo/Ovral™ for a 6-month treatment period. Fasting plasma lipids and lipoproteins were measured at 0, 3, and 6 months by standardized methodologies.

Results. Desogen® caused some significant changes in the lipid and lipoprotein profile: +10% in HDL cholesterol (p = 0.015) and +16% in apoA-I (p < 0.001). Lp(a) levels were decreased by 38% (p = 0.05) over 3 months, but this change was partially reversed after 6 months. Other changes include +34% in triglyceride (p < 0.001); +30% in apoB (p < 0.001); and −15% in apoE (p < 0.001). By contrast, Lo/Ovral™ significantly changed only two lipid analytes: HDL cholesterol by −8% (p = 0.05) and apoB by +29% (p = 0.01).

Conclusions. Desogen® induced multiple changes in the lipid and lipoprotein profile of premenopausal women; some changes are associated with decreased cardiovascular risk and others with increased risk. Lo/Ovral™ induced a single small change associated with lower risk and a single larger change associated with higher risk. However, in no case did either oral contraceptive formulation alter a lipid or lipoprotein level so as to place it outside normal limits.

Keywords: Desogen®, lipids, lipoproteins, Lo/Ovral™, lp(a), oral contraceptives.

Introduction

Exogenous steroid hormones can have a profound effect on lipid metabolism. Oral estrogens cause a reduction in hepatic triglyceride lipase, which typically degrades HDL [1,2]. Estrogens also enhance HDL-cholesterol production and hepatic synthesis of apoA-I. However, it is possible that the increase in HDL cholesterol accompanying estrogen treatment is not a pure effect, but is partly due to estrogen-stimulated removal of cholesterol from the systemic circulation, resulting in enhanced reverse-cholesterol transport. Reduction in LDL cholesterol is another beneficial effect of estrogen treatment. This change is probably due to both hepatic and nonhepatic effects. Although estrogens increase VLDL and triglycerides through direct enhancement of their synthesis and secretion, the ca-

Address for correspondence: Dr Joel Morrisett, The Methodist Hospital, MS 601-A, 6565 Fannin Street, Houston, TX 77030, USA. Tel.: +1-713-798-4164. Fax: +1-713-798-4121. E-mail: morriset@bcm.tmc.edu

582

tabolism of VLDL to LDL is actually decreased, probably due to enhanced uptake of VLDL by the liver [3]. Furthermore, kinetic measurements have shown that the rate of LDL removal is increased by estrogens, an effect probably resulting from the upregulation of LDL receptors both in the liver and in peripheral tissues. In contrast to estrogens, progestins induce hepatic lipase activity, resulting in increased degradation of HDL [1]. This effect appears to be related not only to the progestin dose but also to its androgenic potency. Although the estrogen-stimulated increase in HDL_2 is attenuated by progestin, HDL-cholesterol levels remain above base line and then increase again after discontinuation of the progestin. Progestins also lead to reduced total triglyceride levels. Consequently, the elevation of triglycerides with estrogen is mostly eliminated during progestin treatment.

3-keto desogestrel is the principal metabolite of desogestrel [4,5]. This active metabolite has shown relatively strong progestational activity and minimal intrinsic androgenicity. Metabolic studies have indicated a greater dissociation of the desired progestagenic effects from the undesired androgenic effects of desogestrel than was observed with norgestrel and norethindrone [6,7]. Desogen® is a monophasic oral contraceptive tablet, which contains 150 μg desogestrel and 30 μg ethinyl estradiol, whereas Lo/Ovral™ (also a monophasic contraceptive) contains 300 μg norgestrel and 30 μg ethinyl estradiol. Accordingly, undesirable changes in the lipid profile that might be induced by these contraceptives were anticipated to be significantly less with Desogen® than with Lo/Ovral™. The objective of this study was to compare the effect of these two different contraceptive formulations on the levels of lipoproteins in premenopausal women, especially Lp(a), which is now widely accepted as a risk factor for cardiovascular disease in women as well as men.

Materials, Methods and Patients

This was a randomized, open-label, single-center study in which 100 women were assigned to one of two parallel active treatment groups that received either Desogen® or Lo/Ovral™ during a 6-month treatment period. Fasting blood samples were drawn at 0, 3, and 6 months for analysis. The details of patient selection, analytical methodologies, and statistical methods have been described in a preliminary report [8].

Results

The mean total cholesterol concentration in the women on Desogen® rose from 179 to 189 mg/dl (+6%) during the initial 3 months of the study, but this change was partially reversed by 6 months, making it insignificant. In subjects on Lo/Ovral™, the total cholesterol did not change significantly during the study period (Tables 1 and 2). HDL cholesterol rose from 60 to 66 mg/dl (+10%) in subjects on Desogen®, a significant change sustained over 3—6 months; but HDL-C

Table 1. Effect of Desogen® on lipid and apoprotein levels (mg/dl) in premenopausal women.

	0 month (n = 50)	3 months (n = 46)	6 months (n = 38)
Total-Chol			
Median	174	190	184
Mean ± SD	179 ± 30	189 ± 30	185 ± 30
p		0.001	NS
HDL-C			
Median	59	66	66
Mean ± SD	60 ± 16	66 ± 14	66 ± 15
p		0.004	0.015
HDL2-C			
Median	21	24	24
Mean ± SD	23 ± 9	26 ± 10	24 ± 8
p		NS	NS
HDL3-C			
Median	38	40	42
Mean ± SD	37 ± 9	40 ± 9	41 ± 9
p		0.03	0.004
LDL-C			
Median	100	98	98
Mean ± SD	103 ± 30	101 ± 31	98 ± 29
p		NS	NS
Trig			
Median	75	105	104
Mean ± SD	79 ± 30	113 ± 42	106 ± 39
p		0.0001	0.0001
ApoA-I			
Median	128	154	150
Mean ± SD	129 ± 20	155 ± 21	150 ± 18
p		0.0001	0.0001
ApoB			
Median	76	87	99
Mean ± SD	79 ± 18	88 ± 22	103 ± 23
p		0.002	0.0001
ApoE			
Median	7.7	6.4	6.7
Mean ± SD	8.0 ± 2.2	7.0 ± 1.8	6.8 ± 1.8
p		0.001	0.0005
Lp(a) protein			
Median	6.0	3.7	4.6
Mean ± SD	10.1 ± 11.2	9.0 ± 12.5	10.2 ± 15.6
p		0.05	NS

Note: p values refer to paired comparisons of 3- or 6-month data to 0-month data; NS= not significant.

decreased from 61 to 56 mg/dl (-8%) in subjects on Lo/Ovral™ — although this latter change was statistically significant only at 6 months. These diverging effects are strikingly apparent in Fig. 1B. For women on Desogen®, this favorable

584

Table 2. Effect of Lo/Ovral™ on lipid and apoprotein levels (mg/dl) in premenopausal women.

	0 month (n = 50)	3 months (n = 36)	6 months (n = 28)
Total-Chol			
Median	181	188	188
Mean ± SD	187 ± 33	189 ± 37	193 ± 20
p		NS	NS
HDL-C			
Median	56	54	55
Mean ± SD	61 ± 18	56 ± 16	56 ± 16
p		NS	NS
HDL2-C			
Median	20	18	17
Mean ± SD	23 ± 10	19 ± 10	18 ± 10
p		NS	NS
HDL3-C			
Median	38	37	39
Mean ± SD	38 ± 10	37 ± 9	38 ± 9
p		NS	NS
LDL-C			
Median	100	113	113
Mean ± SD	109 ± 31	114 ± 41	116 ± 38
p		NS	NS
Trig			
Median	76	90	80
Mean ± SD	89 ± 50	102 ± 59	103 ± 64
p		NS	NS
ApoA-I			
Median	128	126	127
Mean ± SD	134 ± 29	130 ± 26	127 ± 24
p		NS	NS
ApoB			
Median	82	91	110
Mean ± SD	82 ± 21	93 ± 23	106 ± 29
p		0.01	0.01
ApoE			
Median	7.2	7.2	7.5
Mean ± SD	8.4 ± 4.4	8.0 ± 4.2	7.8 ± 2.6
p		0.05	NS
Lp(a) protein			
Median	8.1	6.0	5.6
Mean ± SD	12.9 ± 13.1	10.5 ± 10.5	11.3 ± 11.3
p		NS	NS

Note: p values refer to paired comparisons of 3- or 6-month data with 0-month data.

change in HDL-C was reflected in a 13% increase in the mean levels of HDL$_2$-C (not significant) and an 8% increase in HDL$_3$-C (significant). In contrast, women on Lo/Ovral™ experienced a 17% decrease in HDL$_2$-C and a 3% decrease in HDL$_3$-C — although these changes did not reach statistical significance. The

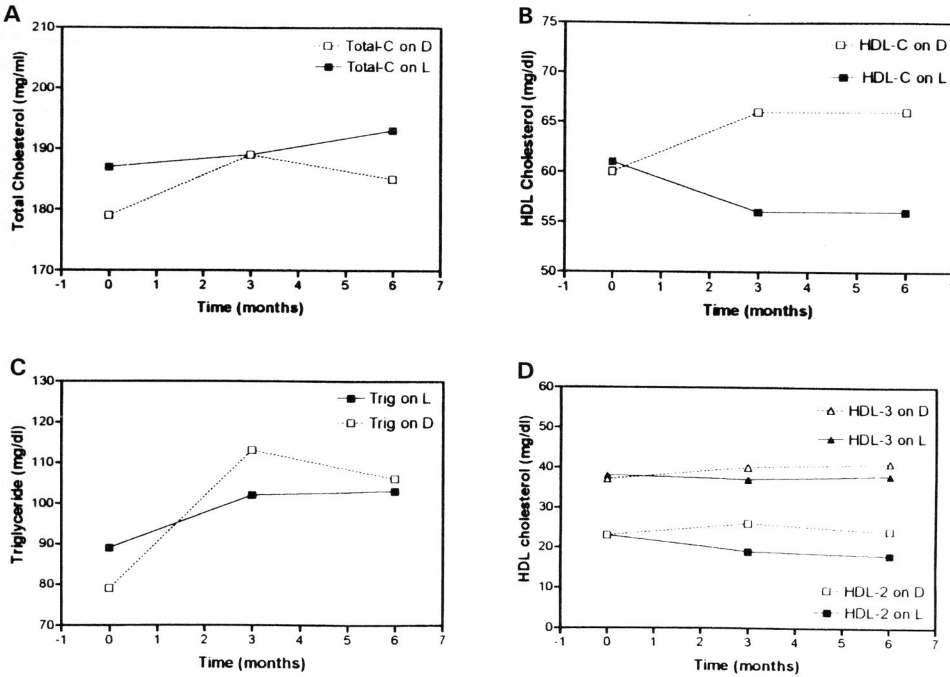

Fig. 1. Effect of Desogen® and Lo/Ovral™ on mean plasma levels of total cholesterol (**A**), HDL cholesterol (**B**), triglyceride (**C**), and HDL-2 and HDL-3 (**D**) cholesterol in premenopausal women over a 6-month period.

above significant increase in HDL_3-C in women on Desogen® is also reflected in a very significant rise of 20% in the levels of their apoA-I, an effect that was sustained out to 6 months. ApoA-I in subjects on Lo/Ovral™ did not change significantly during the entire study (Table 2 and Fig. 2A). Some of the largest changes observed in lipid analytes occurred in the triglycerides. For subjects on Desogen®, the mean triglyceride level rose significantly from 79 to 113 mg/dl (+43%) over the initial 3-month period, an effect that persisted at 6 months (Table 1 and Fig. 1C). In subjects on Lo/Ovral™, the mean triglyceride level rose from 89 to 102 mg/dl (+13%, not significant) and had not changed by 6 months. The increase in triglyceride observed in both groups over the initial 3-month period was attended by a significant 12% decrease for ApoE in subjects on Desogen® (persisting over 6 months) and by a significant 13% decrease in subjects on Lo/Ovral™ (not persisting over 6 months). LDL cholesterol showed no significant change in subjects on Desogen® and a 5–6% increase in subjects on Lo/Ovral™ during the first and latter 3 months. Nevertheless, both groups of subjects experienced significant increases in mean apoB levels during the initial 3 months and further increases in the second 3 months. The large difference

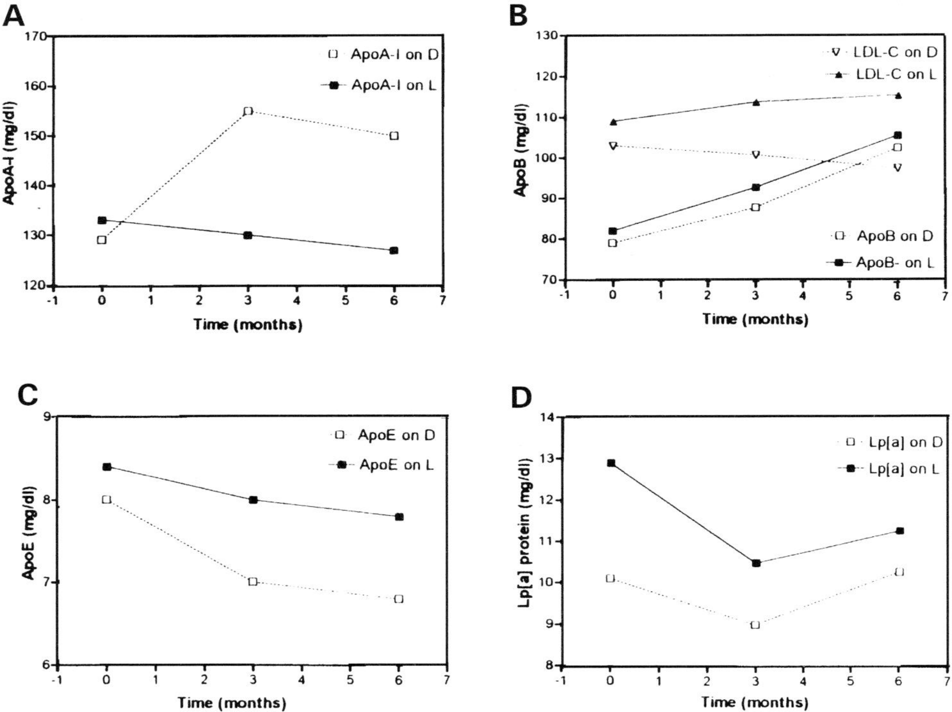

Fig. 2. Effect of Desogen® and Lo/Ovral™ on mean plasma levels of ApoA-I (**A**), ApoB-100 (**B**), ApoE (**C**) and Lp(a) (**D**) protein in premenopausal women over a 6-month period.

between the median and mean values of Lp(a) in subjects on Desogen® or Lo/Ovral™ indicates the nonnormal distribution of Lp(a) protein levels in both groups. In the Desogen® group, the median level decreased significantly from 6.0 to 3.7 mg/dl (−38%) and the mean level from 10.1 to 9.0 mg/dl (−11%), but these changes did not persist out to 6 months. In the Lo/Ovral™ group, the median level decreased by 26% and the mean by 23% (Tables 1 and 2) at 3 months, but these decrements were not significant.

Discussion

The observed decrease in Lp(a) caused by OC may have a significant linkage to the concomitant large elevation in triglyceride. Several laboratories have now observed a reciprocal relation between these two species [9–11]. The synchronous perturbation of their levels by estrogen may allow us to gain new insight into their metabolic relation. Estrogen stimulates both the secretion of VLDL and an increased uptake of VLDL remnants by hepatic receptors [3]. Lp(a) is known to associate noncovalently with other apoB100-containing lipoproteins

[12]. Hence, elevation of VLDL increases the probability of their association with Lp(a) and the formation of a VLDL-Lp(a) complex. An increased uptake of the complex would cause a net decrease in plasma Lp(a) [13]. An additional or alternative mechanism may also be operating; the increased synthesis and secretion of VLDL (which requires apoB-100) may deplete the pool of apoB, thereby making it less available for the production of Lp(a). The latter mechanism is consistent with our recent observation that Lp(a) is about 2-fold higher in type IIa than in type IIb hyperlipoproteinemic subjects and with the observation that fibrate-induced lowering of triglycerides in type IIb subjects leads to significant elevation of Lp(a) [14].

Acknowledgements

The authors thank John Gaubatz, Mauro Nava, and Charles Etta Rhodes for their technical help and Renee Wells for editorial assistance. This study was supported in part by Organon, Inc. and the Women's Fund for Health Education and Research, Houston, Texas (TTGA).

References

1. Lobo RA. Clinical review 27: Effects of hormonal replacement on lipids and lipoproteins in postmenopausal women. J Clin Endocrin Metab 1991;73(5):925—930.
2. Colvin PL, Auerbach BJ, Case DL et al. A dose-response relationship between sex hormone-induced change in hepatic triglyceride lipase and high-density lipoprotein cholesterol in postmenopausal women. Metabolism 1991;40(10):1052—1056.
3. Walsh BW, Schiff I, Rosner B et al. Effects of postmenopausal estrogen replacement on the concentrations and metabolism of plasma lipoproteins. N Engl J Med 1991;325:1196—204.
4. Virnikka L, Ylikorkala O, Vikro R et al. Metabolism of a new synthetic progestogen org 2969 (13 ethyl-11-methylene-18,19-di nor-17-alpha-pregn-4-In-20 yn-17 ol) in female volunteers: distribution and excretion of radioactivity after an oral dose of labeled drug. Acta Endocrin 1980; 93(3):375—379.
5. Hasenack HG, Bosch AMG, Kaar K. Serum levels of 3-ketodesogestrel after oral administration of desogestrel and 3-ketodesogestrel. Contraception 1986;33(6):591—596.
6. Elger W, Beier S. Aktuelle Aspekte der hormonalen Kontrazeption (Actual Aspects of Hormonal Contraception). Amsterdam-Oxford-Princeton: Excerpta Medica, 1982;9—26.
7. Bergink EW, Meel F van, Turpijn EW et al. Binding of progestogens to receptor proteins in MCG-7 cells. J Steroid Biochem 1983;19:1563—1570.
8. Morisett JD, Nava ML, Reilly M, Snabes MC, Young RL. Effect of oral contraceptive hormones on lipoprotein(a) and other lipoproteins in premenopausal women. In: Forte TM (ed) Hormonal, Metabolic and Cellular Influences on Cardiovascular Disease in Women. Armonk, NY: Futura Publishing Co. Inc., 1997;289—302.
9. Kostner GM. Interrelation of Lp(a) with plasma triglycerides. Atherosclerosis 1991;22: 131—135.
10. Bartens W, Rader DJ, Talley G et al. Decreased plasma levels of lipoprotein(a) in patients with hypertriglyceridemia. Atherosclerosis 1994;108:149—157.
11. Walek T, von Eckardstein A, Schulte H et al. Effect of hypertriglyceridemia on lipoprotein(a) serum concentrations. Eur J Clin Invest 1995;25:311—316.
12. McConathy WJ, Trieu VN, Koren E et al. Triglyceride-rich lipoprotein interactions with Lp(a).

Chem Phys Lipids 1994;67–68:105–114.

13. Marcovina SM, Morrisett JD. Structure and metabolism of lipoprotein(a). Curr Opin Lipid 1995;6:136–145.

14. Jones PH, Pownall HJ, Patsch W et al. Effect of gemfibrozil on fasting and postprandial levels of Lp(a) in type II hyperlipoproteinemic subjects. J Lipid Res 1996;37:1298–1308.

Triglycerides are an independent risk factor for coronary heart disease — a debate

Atherosclerosis XI.
B. Jacotot, D. Mathé and J.-C. Fruchart, editors.

The epidemiologic case for triglyceride as a risk factor for cardiovascular disease

Melissa A. Austin[1] and John E. Hokanson[2]

[1]*Department of Epidemiology, School of Public Health and Community Medicine; and* [2]*Division of Metabolism, Endocrinology and Nutrition, University of Washington, Seattle, Washington, USA*

Keywords: low-density lipoprotein, meta-analysis, triglyceride.

Introduction

Elevated levels of plasma triglyceride have long been associated with increased risk of cardiovascular disease (CVD). In 1959, a case-control study by Albrink and Man [1] showed that fasting triglyceride levels were increased among coronary heart disease (CHD) cases compared to control subjects. The earliest prospective study of triglyceride and ischemic heart disease (IHD) demonstrated an increased incidence of IHD among men in the cohort with elevated triglyceride levels at baseline, compared with men with lower levels [2]. However, even in this early study, the authors speculated that the triglyceride association may not have been independent of other plasma lipid levels.

In the decades following these studies, an extensive literature developed examining the role of triglyceride as a risk factor for cardiovascular disease. In a review of these studies, Austin noted that most studies showed a relationship between triglyceride and CHD [3]. However, a number of studies found that this association did not remain statistically significant after controlling for other lipid risk factors, especially high-density lipoprotein (HDL) cholesterol. In reviewing this and other evidence, the National Institutes of Health Consensus Development Panel on Triglyceride, HDL and Coronary Heart Disease concluded that, "For triglyceride, the data are mixed, although strong associations are found in some studies, the evidence for a causal relationship (with CHD) is still incomplete" [4]. Similarly, data from the Lipid Research Clinics (LRC) follow-up study demonstrated that triglyceride was related to 12-year CHD mortality in both men and women [5], but this relationship was no longer statistically significant after adjustment for covariates. Thus, the role of triglyceride as a risk factor for CHD remains to be fully elucidated.

This report will focus on the relationship between triglyceride and cardiovascular disease. In order to estimate the strength of this association in the general

---

Address for correspondence: Melissa A. Austin PhD, Department of Epidemiology, Box 357236, 1959 NE Pacific Avenue, Room HSB F261B, University of Washington, Seattle, WA 98195-7236, USA. Tel.: +1-206-685-9384. Fax: +1-206-685-3407.

592

population and to evaluate the effect of other risk factors (especially HDL cholesterol), a meta-analysis of population-based, prospective studies of triglyceride and CVD is described [6,7] and another recent prospective study is summarized.

Meta-analysis of triglyceride and cardiovascular disease

Published studies from the literature were selected for the meta-analysis based on several criteria [6]. First, only studies using a prospective study design were selected, ensuring that elevations in plasma triglyceride preceded the onset of disease. Second, only studies using population-based samples of study subjects were selected, so that relative risk estimates are as applicable as possible to the general population. Because the results from the LRC follow-up study [5] were based on a sample enriched with hyperlipidemic subjects, the relative risks for this analysis were adjusted for ascertainment (hyperlipidemic vs. random sample) based on results kindly provided by Dr M. H. Criqui (personal communication). To exclude the possibility of postprandial effects, only studies evaluating fasting triglyceride levels were included. Each study cohort was included only once in the analysis, using the publication reporting the longest follow time. Both fatal and nonfatal cardiovascular endpoints were included, although most studies focused on myocardial infarction or CHD death. Finally, only Caucasian study subjects were included in the analysis, since little data was available on other ethnic groups.

A total of 18 studies conforming to these selection criteria were identified [2,5,8–25], including 17 studies representing 2,620 events among 46,619 men followed for an average of 8.6 years, and five studies representing 439 events among 10,864 women followed for an average 11.4 years. Study subjects ranged in age from 15 to 81 years old in all the studies. Among men, seven studies were from North America, six from Scandinavian countries, and one each from France, Germany, Italy and the UK. Among women, three studies were from the USA, and two from Scandinavia.

The meta-analysis was performed separately for men and women using the techniques described by Greenland [7]. Briefly, relative risk (RR) estimates are determined for each individual study by calculating β, the estimated slope from logistic regression analysis, standardized to a 1 mmol/l increase in triglyceride. To determine the statistical significance of the association and to calculate confidence intervals (CI), the variance of β is next computed. The β value for each study is then weighted by the inverse of the variance, reflecting both the sample size and follow-up time of study. Finally, the weighted β values are averaged and converted to the summary RR value, so that the larger the study and the longer the follow-up time, the greater its contribution to the summary RR. These procedures result in the univariate summary RR for the association between triglyceride and CVD. To determine the effect of covariates on this estimate, the same procedures were used to estimate the multivariate summary RR using the seven studies that included HDL cholesterol as a covariate [5,8,16,20,22,23,25]. Of these studies, five also included adjustment for age, six for total or LDL cholesterol, five for smoking, six for body mass index, five for blood pressure, and one for both LDL size and apolipoprotein B levels. To maximize the potential effects on the multivariate summary RR, all these covariate adjustments were included in the analysis.

As shown in Fig. 1, univariate RR estimates for cardiovascular disease associated with a 1 mmol/l increase in triglyceride ranged from 1.07 to 1.98 for men with a summary RR of 1.31 (95% confidence interval (CI) 1.25—1.38). This indicates a 31% increase in disease risk associated with triglyceride. Among the five prospective studies in women, individual RR estimates for triglyceride ranged from 1.69 to 2.05 (Fig. 1), all of which were statistically significant. The summary univariate RR was higher for women than men, 1.76 (95% CI 1.50—2.07), although the confidence interval is somewhat wider due to the smaller sample size (approximately 10,800 women). Thus, a 1 mmol/l increase in triglyceride was associated with a 76% increase in risk of incident cardiovascular disease in women. Because only population-based studies were included, the summary relative risk estimates derived from this analysis provide the best available overall estimates for relationship between triglyceride and CVD.

As expected, multivariate RR estimates with adjustment for HDL cholesterol were attenuated (Fig. 2). For men, the multivariate RRs for triglyceride ranged from 0.98 to 1.39 with the summary RR of 1.15 being statistically significant (95% CI 1.09—1.21). In women, the summary multivariate RR was higher than for men, with a value of 1.37 (95% CI 1.13—1.66). Thus, even after adjustment for HDL cholesterol, a statistically significant increase in risk of incident cardiovascular disease was associated with triglyceride for both men and women. Importantly, studies conducted in Scandinavia in which univariate RRs are highest, are not included in these multivariate RRs since HDL-cholesterol adjustments were not reported. Thus, the multivariate RRs reported here for triglyceride are likely to be conservative. Furthermore, when an external adjustment procedure is used to evaluate the confounding effect of HDL cholesterol among those not reporting adjustment for this variable [7], the multivariate summary RR was 1.22 for men and 1.44 in women.

To summarize, based on all the available data from population-based, prospective studies, meta-analysis shows that increases in plasma triglyceride are associated with a significant increase in risk of incident cardiovascular disease among both men and women. In men, an increase of 1 mmol/l was associated with a 31% increase in risk of disease. A higher increased risk of 76% was found in women. Based on data from studies that reported adjustment for HDL cholesterol and other risk factors, multivariate RR estimates were attenuated, but were still statistically significant, representing a 15% increase in risk for men and a 37% increase in risk for women. Importantly, because only population-based studies were included in the analysis, these results provide the best available estimates of triglyceride risk in the general population. Therefore, triglyceride is a risk factor for cardiovascular disease, independent of HDL cholesterol.

594

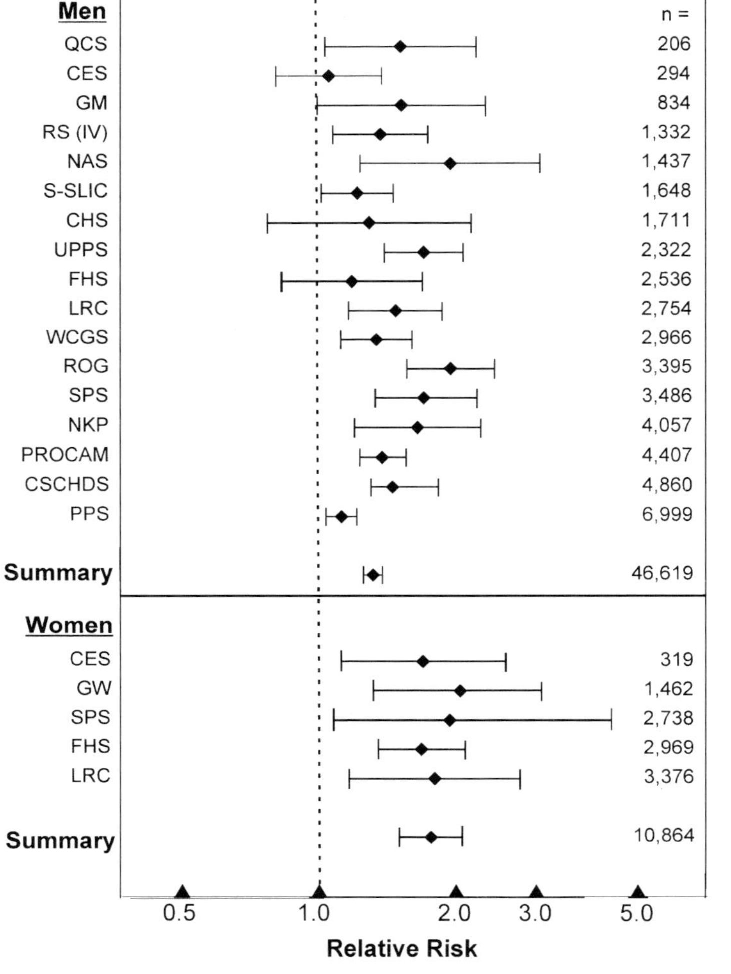

Fig. 1. Univariate relative risk estimates and 95% confidence intervals for the association between incident cardiovascular disease and a 1 mmol/l increase in triglyceride, by gender. Relative risk values are given on the X-axis on a natural logarithm scale. The Y-axis lists each study included in the meta-analysis and reference numbers, ordered by sample size and the summary relative risk. A relative risk of 1.0 (vertical dotted line) represents no association, and confidence intervals that do not cover 1.0 indicate relative risks that are statistically significant at the p = 0.05 level. Study abbreviations: CHS, Cardiovascular Health Center [2]; LRC, Lipid Research Clinics Follow-up Study [5]; WCGS, Western Collaborative Health Study [8,9]; SPS, Stockholm Prospective Study [10]; GM, Men Born in 1913 Study [11]; S-SLIC, Suomi-Salama Life Insurance Cohort [12]; PPS, Paris Prospective Study [13]; GW, Study of Women in Gothenburg [14]; UPPS, Uppsala Primary Preventive Study [15]; FHS, Framingham Heart Study [16]; NKP, North Karelia Project [17]; CES, Cardiovascular Epidemiology Study [18]; NAS, Normative Aging Study [19]; CSCHDS, Caerphilly and Speedwell Collaborative Heart Disease Studies [20]; RS(IV), Reykjavik Study, Stage IV [21]; PROCAM, Prospective Cardiovascular Münster Study [22]; ROG, Rome Occupational Groups [23,24]; QCS, Québec Cardiovascular Study [25]. Figure adapted from [6].

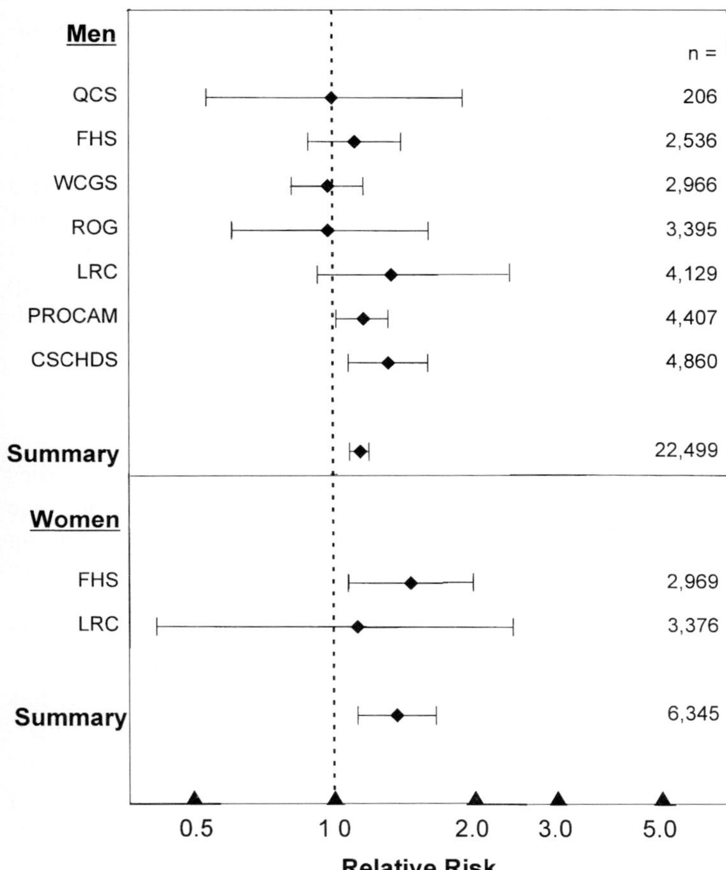

Fig. 2. Multivariate-adjusted relative risk estimates and 95% confidence intervals for the association between incident cardiovascular disease and a 1 mmol/l increase in triglyceride, by gender, for those studies that adjusted for HDL cholesterol. Relative risk values are given on the X-axis on a natural logarithm scale. The Y-axis lists each study included in the meta-analysis and reference numbers, ordered by sample size, and the summary relative risk. Note that a relative risk of 1.0 (vertical dotted line) represents no association, and confidence intervals that do not cover 1.0 indicate relative risks that are statistically significant at the p = 0.05 level. See Fig. 1 for study abbreviations. Figure adapted from [6].

Physician's Health Study

Although the findings from the Physicians' Health Study were based on study participants who were "not specifically instructed to provide fasting specimens," this recent analysis also provides important insights into triglyceride as a risk factor. The results were based on a 7-year follow-up of 266 men with incident non-fatal MI or fatal CHD. Controls were matched for age, smoking and time of randomization [26]. In this study, mean baseline triglyceride values were higher in cases compared to controls (2.29 vs. 1.75 mmol/l, respectively, p = 0.001). Similarly, LDL diameter values were smaller in cases compared with controls (256 vs. 259Å, respectively, p < 0.001). The RR for triglyceride was 1.43 for a 1.13 mmol/l increase in triglyceride (p < 0.01, 95% CI 1.22—1.68) and the RR for LDL size was 1.38 for an 8Å decrease in size (p < 0.001, 95% CI 1.18—1.62). Thus, both triglyceride and LDL size were significant predictors of future CHD in this study. However, the triglyceride association was independent of other lipids (RR = 1.33, p = 0.009) while the LDL size association was not (RR = 1.09, p = 0.46). This is due, at least in part, to the strong inverse relationship between triglyceride and LDL size, with an estimated Spearman correlation coefficient in this study of − 0.71.

Summary

In summary, meta-analysis of data from population-based prospective studies demonstrates that increased plasma triglyceride is associated with a 31% increase in risk of cardiovascular disease in men and a 76% increase in risk among women. After adjustment for HDL cholesterol and other risk factors, these risks were reduced to 15% in men and a 37% increase in women, but remained statistically significant. These results (based on more than 46,000 men and 10,800 women) show that plasma triglyceride is an independent risk factor for cardiovascular disease. Recent prospective data from the Physicians' Health Study has also shown that plasma triglyceride and LDL-particle size, two highly interrelated risk factors, predict subsequent coronary heart disease. These results demonstrate the growing recognition of the importance of triglyceride as a risk factor for cardiovascular disease and the urgent need for clinical trials to determine whether lowering plasma triglyceride levels will decrease disease risk.

Acknowledgements

This work was supported by NIH R01 Grant HL45913, and was performed during Dr Austin's tenure as an Established Investigator of the American Heart Association.

References

1. Albrink MJ, Man EB. Serum triglycerides in coronary artery disease. Arch Int Med 1959; 103:4—8.
2. Brown DF, Kinch SH, Doyle JT. Serum triglycerides in health and in ischemic heart disease. N Engl J Med 1965;273:947—952.
3. Austin MA. Plasma triglyceride and coronary heart disease. Arterioscl Thromb 1991;11:2—14.
4. NIH Consensus Development Panel on Triglyceride, High-Density Lipoprotein, and Coronary Heart Disease. Triglyceride, high-density lipoprotein and coronary heart disease. JAMA 1993; 269:505—510.
5. Criqui MH, Heiss G, Cohn R et al. Plasma triglyceride level and mortality from coronary heart

disease. N Engl J Med 1993;328:1220–1225.

6. Hokanson JE, Austin MA. Plasma triglyceride is a risk factor for cardiovascular disease independent of high-density lipoprotein cholesterol. A meta-analysis of population-based prospective studies. J Cardiovasc Risk 1996;3:2143–2219.

7. Greenland S. Quantitative methods in the review of epidemiologic literature. Epidemiol Rev 1987;9:1–30.

8. Hulley SB, Rosenman RH, Bawol RD, Brand RJ. Epidemiology as a guide to clinical decisions. The association between triglyceride and coronary heart disease. N Engl J Med 1980;302:1383–1389.

9. Rosenman RH, Brand RJ, Jenkins CD, Friedman M, Straus R, Wurm M. Coronary heart disease in the Western Collaborative Group Study. Final follow-up experience of 8 1/2 years. JAMA 1975;233:872–877.

10. Bottinger LE, Carlson LA. Risk factors for death for males and females. A study of death pattern in the Stockholm Prospective Study. Acta Med Scan 1982;211:437–442.

11. Wilhelmsen L, Wedel H, Tibblin G. Multivariate analysis of risk factors for coronary heart disease. Circulation 1973;XLVIII:950–958.

12. Pelkonen R, Nikkilä EA, Koskinen S, Penttinen K, Sarna S. Association of serum lipids and obesity with cardiovascular mortality. BMJ 1977;2:1185–1187.

13. Cambien F, Jacqueson A, Richard JL, Warnet JM, Ducimetière P, Claude JR. Is the level of serum triglyceride a significant predictor of coronary death in "normocholesterolemic" subjects? The Paris Prospective Study. Am J Epidemiol 1986;124:624–632.

14. Bengtsson C, Bjorkelund C, Lapidus L, Lissner L. Association of serum lipid concentrations and obesity with mortality in women: 20 year follow-up of participants in prospective population study in Gothenburg, Sweden. BMJ 1993;307:1385–1388.

15. Åberg H, Lithell H, Selinus I, Hedstrand H. Serum triglycerides are a risk factor for myocardial infarction but not for angina pectoris. Results from a 10-year follow-up of Uppsala Primary Preventive Study. Atherosclerosis 1985;54:89–97.

16. Wilson P, Larson G, Castelli W. Triglycerides, HDL-cholesterol and coronary artery disease: a Framingham update on the interactions. Can J Cardiol 1994;10(Suppl B):5B–9B.

17. Salonen JT, Puska P. Relation of serum cholesterol and triglycerides to the risk of acute myocardial infarction, cerebral stroke and death in eastern Finnish male population. Int J Epidemiol 1983;12:26–31.

18. Heyden S, Heiss G, Hames CG, Bartel AG. Fasting triglycerides as predictors of total and CHD mortality in Evans County, Georgia. J Chron Dis 1980;33:275–282.

19. Glynn RJ, Rosner B, Silbert JE. Changes in cholesterol and triglyceride as predictors of ischemic heart disease. Circulation 1982;66:724–731.

20. Bainton D, Miller NE, Bolton CH, Yarnell JWG, Sweetnam PM, Baker IA, Lewis B, Elwood PC. Plasma triglyceride and high-density lipoproteins cholesterol as predictors of ischaemic heart disease in British men. The Caerphilly and Speedwell Collaborative Heart Disease Studies. Br Heart J 1992;68:60–66.

21. Sigurdsson G, Baldursdottir, Sigvaldason H, Agnarsson U, Thorgeirsson G, Sigfusson N. Predictive value of apolipoproteins in a prospective survey of coronary artery disease in men. Am J Cardiol 1992;69:1251–1254.

22. Assmann G, Schulte H, von Eckardstein A. Hypertriglyceridemia and elevated lipoprotein(a) are risk factors for major coronary events in middle-aged men. Am J Cardiol 1996;77:1179–1184.

23. Menotti A, Spagnolo A, Scanga M, Dima F. Multivariate prediction of coronary disease deaths in a 10-year follow-up of an Italian occupational male cohort. Acta Cardiol 1992;XLVII:311–320.

24. Menotti A, Scanga M, Morisi G. Serum triglycerides in the prediction of coronary artery disease (an Italian experience). Am J Cardiol 1994;73:29–32.

25. Lamarche B, Tchernof A, Moorjani S, Catin B, Dagenais GR, Lupien PJ, Després J-P. Small,

dense low-density lipoprotein particles as a predictor of the risk of ischemic heart disease in men. Circulation 1997;95:69–75.
26. Stampfer MJ, Krauss RM, Ma J, Blanche PJ, Holl LG, Sacks FM, Hennekens CH. A prospective study of triglyceride level, low-density lipoprotein particle diameter and risk of myocardial infarction. JAMA 1996;276:882–888.

The clinical case for triglyceride-rich lipoproteins

Gilbert R. Thompson
MRC Lipoprotein Team, Clinical Sciences Centre, Hammersmith Hospital, London, UK

Abstract. There is increasing evidence that triglyceride-rich lipoproteins are atherogenic. Angiographic studies suggest that this applies particularly to coronary lesions of mild to moderate severity, which often progress despite marked lowering of LDL cholesterol by statins. In a recent trial both angiographic and clinical benefit accompanied triglyceride reduction by a fibrate independently of any change in LDL. Further studies are needed to assess more fully the role of triglyceride-lowering therapy in the prevention of coronary heart disease.

Keywords: coronary artery disease, fibrates, prevention statins, triglyceride-rich lipoproteins.

As has been reviewed recently [1], evidence relating triglycerides and coronary heart disease (CHD) is complex and often regarded as inconclusive. One reason for this complexity is that hypertriglyceridaemia is a heterogeneous entity, reflecting the involvement of several lipoprotein species in the carriage of triglyceride in plasma. Exogenous or dietary triglyceride is transported almost exclusively in chylomicrons and their remnants (under normal circumstances) are only found postprandially. In contrast, endogenous triglyceride, mainly of hepatic origin, is transported in the form of VLDL (and its remnants, often termed IDL) and has a circadian presence in plasma.

The concentration of endogenous triglyceride in plasma is determined by the balance between production and removal rates, the latter process involving enzymatic lipolysis and subsequent receptor-mediated uptake of the resultant remnant particles. Various markers which have been used to reflect endogenous triglyceride metabolism include measuring the triglyceride content of whole plasma and of VLDL and IDL. Alternatively VLDL and IDL can be quantified by analytical ultracentrifugation, the results being expressed as the concentration of particles with S_f 20—400 and 12—20, respectively. Another marker is the concentration of apoC-III in the heparin-manganese precipitate of plasma, i.e., non-HDL apoC-III which reflects both VLDL and IDL.

Exogenous triglyceride metabolism is less easily assessed and involves measuring postprandial levels of $apoB_{48}$ or retinyl palmitate after an oral fat load. Chylomicrons are separated from their remnants by brief ultracentrifugation at d 1.006 prior to these assays.

Address for correspondence: Prof G.R. Thompson, MRC Lipoprotein Team, Clinical Sciences Centre, Imperial College School of Medicine, Du Cane Road, London W12 ONN, UK.

Evidence that triglyceride-rich lipoproteins are a risk factor for CHD

Criteria which must be met before a marker of risk can be accepted as a risk factor include the demonstration of an independent relationship with the disease in question, a plausible causal mechanism and reversibility of the risk. The first of these criteria has already been met by Austin [2] in her analysis of the epidemiology of triglycerides in relation to CHD. Hence this presentation will focus initially on the second criterion, namely the evidence that the association between triglyceride-rich lipoproteins and CHD is causal. The case for this is based mainly upon angiographic data which suggest that triglyceride-rich lipoproteins are atherogenic.

As shown in Table 1, a number of studies have shown associations between the presence or severity of coronary artery disease (CAD) on coronary angiography and increased concentrations of triglyceride-rich lipoproteins of endogenous origin [3—5]. In the case-control study by Barbir et al. [5] fasting serum triglyceride was the strongest independent correlate of CAD on multivariate analysis.

The last two studies listed in Table 1 both show an association between decreased clearance of chylomicron remnants and the progression [6] and presence of CAD [7], respectively. The hypothesis that postprandial triglyceride-rich lipoproteins are atherogenic was first suggested by Zilversmit [8], who cited the increased risk of coronary and peripheral vascular disease observed in patients with familial type III hyperlipoproteinaemia. In this disorder, mutations of apoE, commonly homozygous inheritance of $apoE_2$, result in impaired uptake of chylomicron remnants and IDL by hepatic receptors as well as decreased conversion of VLDL to LDL. Despite their low-LDL levels type III patients are prone to the premature development of atherosclerosis, thereby implicating remnant particles in the atherogenic process.

Table 2 shows an association between triglyceride-rich lipoproteins of endogenous origin and angiographic progression of CAD in several intervention trials. In the type II trial of cholestyramine low concentrations of IDL were associated with decreased progression of CAD [9], whereas in the other trials increased levels of IDL [10,11] and of non-HDL apoC-III and small VLDL [12,13] were

Table 1. Association between triglyeride-rich lipoproteins and presence or severity of CAD on angiography.

Reference	Date	No. of cases	TG-rich lipoprotein	CAD
Jenkins et al. [3]	1978	41	VLDL-TG ↑	Severity ↑
Tatami et al. [4]	1981	182	IDL-chol. ↑	Severity ↑ (males)
Barbir et al. [5]	1988	174	Fasting TG ↑	Presence ↑
Karpe et al. [6]	1994	32 (post-MI)	Chylo remnant clearance ($apoB_{48}$) ↓	Progression ↑
Weintraub et al. [7]	1996	85 (normolipidaemic)	Chylo remnant clearance (vit. A) ↓	Presence ↑

Table 2. Correlation of triglyceride-rich lipoproteins with progression of CAD in serial angiographic studies.

Reference	Date	Trial	TG-rich lipoprotein	CAD
Krauss et al. [9]	1987	Type II	IDL (S_f 12—20) ↓	Nonprogression
Watts et al. [10]	1993	STARS	IDL chol. ↑	Progression ↑
Phillips et al. [11]	1993	Nicardipine	VLDL remnant + IDL chol. ↑	Progression ↑
Hodis et al. [12]	1994	MARS	Fasting TG & non-HDL apoC-III ↑	Progression of lesions < 50% DS ↑
Mack et al. [13]	1996	MARS	Small VLDL (S_f 20—60) ↑	Progression of lesions < 50% DS ↑

all associated with increased progression. These longitudinal findings provide further support for the concept that triglyceride-rich lipoproteins are atherogenic.

Reversibility of risk

Evidence for the third and most important criterion for acceptance of triglyceride-rich lipoproteins as a risk factor, namely reversibility, is relatively sparse at present. However (as shown in Table 3), three trials have shown a reduction in CHD in subjects treated with triglyceride-lowering drugs. In the Stockholm Trial of Secondary Prevention [14] significant decreases in both total and CHD mortality occurred after 5 years of combined therapy with clofibrate and nicotinic acid, whereas in the Helsinki Heart Study (a primary prevention trial) subgroup analysis showed that the reduction in CHD events by gemfibrozil was most marked in subjects with hypertriglyceridaemia and an increased ratio of LDL:HDL [15].

The third study, BECAIT, was an angiographic trial where the reduction in clinical events was incidental to the primary objective, which was to monitor the effect of bezafibrate on CAD by serial angiography [16]. The results showed that the decrease in minimum lumen diameter over 5 years was 0.13 mm less in the treatment than in the placebo group. This was despite the fact that LDL cholesterol decreased by only 2% on bezafibrate. The authors contrasted their results with those of the Multicentre Antiatherosclerosis Study (MAAS) where the treat-

Table 3. Reduction in clinical events during triglyceride-lowering drug therapy.

Reference	Date	Trial	Δ TG	Outcome
Carlson and Rosenhamer [14]	1988	Stockholm 2yr. prev.	− 19%	CHD mort. ↓ 36% Total mort. ↓ 26%
Manninen et al. [15]	1992	HHS sub-group[a]	− 34%	CHD events ↓ 71%
Ericsson et al. [16]	1996	BECAIT	− 31%	CHD events ↓ 73%

[a]TG > 2.3 mmol/l, LDL:HDL > 5.

ment effect of simvastatin was less marked (0.08 mm) despite a 31% reduction in LDL cholesterol [17].

Analysis of regression trials has revealed that triglyceride-rich lipoproteins are especially associated with mildly to moderately severe coronary lesions, which progress despite the 25—35% reductions in LDL cholesterol achieved by statins [1]. Such lesions often give rise to clinical events, which may explain why the reduction in CHD in three large prevention trials of statin therapy (4S, WOS-COPS and CARE) was only partial. It remains to be shown whether a greater decrease in LDL will result in a greater reduction in clinical events or whether concomitant reduction in triglyceride-rich lipoproteins is necessary for this objective to be achieved.

References

1. Hodis HN, Mack WJ. Triglyceride-rich lipoproteins and the progression of coronary artery disease. Curr Opin Lipid 1995;6:209—214.
2. Austin M, Hokanson JE. The epidemiologic case for triglyceride as a risk factor for cardiovascular disease. In: Jacotot B, Mathé D, Fruchart J-C (eds) Atherosclerosis XI. Singapore: Elsevier Science Pte Ltd, 1998;591—598 (this volume).
3. Jenkins PJ, Harper RW, Nestel PJ. Severity of coronary atherosclerosis related to lipoprotein concentration. Br Med J 1978;2:388—391.
4. Tatami R, Mabuchi H, Ueda K, Ueda R, Haba T, Kametani T, Ito S, Koizumi J, Ohta M, Miyamoto S, Nakayama A, Kanaya H, Oiwake H, Genda A, Takeda, R. Intermediate density lipoprotein and cholesterol-rich very low-density lipoprotein in angiographically determined coronary artery disease. Circulation 1981;64:1174—1184.
5. Barbir M, Wile D, Trayner I, Aber VR, Thompson GR. High prevalence of hypertriglyceridaemia and apolipoprotein abnormalities in coronary artery disease. Br Heart J 1988;60:397—403.
6. Karpe F, Steiner G, Uffelman K, Olivecrona T, Hamsten A. Postprandial lipoproteins and progression of coronary atherosclerosis. Atherosclerosis 1994;106:83—97.
7. Weintraub MS, Grosskopf I, Rassin T, Miller H, Charach G, Rotmensch HH, Liron M, Rubinstein A, Iaina A. Clearance of chylomicron remnants in normolipidaemic patients with coronary artery disease: case control study over three years. Br Med J 1996;312:935—939.
8. Zilversmit DB. Atherogenesis: a postprandial phenomenon. Circulation 1979;60:473—485.
9. Krauss RM, Lindgren FT, Williams PT, Kelsey SF, Brensike J, Vranizan K, Detre KM, Levy RI. Intermediate-density lipoproteins and progression of coronary artery disease in hypercholesterolaemic men. Lancet 1987;2:62—66.
10. Watts GF, Mandalia S, Brunt JNH, Slavin BM, Coltart DJ, Lewis B. Independent associations between plasma lipoprotein subfraction levels and the course of coronary artery disease in the St. Thomas' Atherosclerosis Regression Study (STARS). Metabolism 1993;42:1461—1467.
11. Phillips NR, Waters D, Havel RJ. Plasma lipoproteins and progression of coronary artery disease evaluated by angiography and clinical events. Circulation 1993;88:2762—2770.
12. Hodis HN, Mack WJ, Azen SP, Alaupovic P, Pogoda JM, LaBree L, Hemphill LC, Kramsch DM, Blankenhorn DH. Triglyceride- and cholesterol-rich lipoproteins have a differential effect on mild/moderate and severe lesion progression as assessed by quantitative coronary angiography in a controlled trial of lovastatin. Circulation 1994;90:42—49.
13. Mack WJ, Krauss RM, Hodis HN. Lipoprotein subclasses in the monitored atherosclerosis regression study (MARS). Arterioscl Thromb Vasc Biol 1996;16:697—704.
14. Carlson LA, Rosenhamer G. Reduction of mortality in the Stockholm Ischaemic Heart Disease Secondary Prevention Study by combined treatment with clofibrate and nicotinic acid. Acta

Med Scan 1988;223:405—418.
15. Manninen V, Tenkanen L, Koskinen P, Huttunen JK, Mänttäri M, Heinonen OP, Frick MH. Joint effects of serum triglyceride and LDL cholesterol and HDL cholesterol concentrations on coronary heart disease risk in the Helsinki Heart Study. Circulation 1992;85:37—45.
16. Ericsson C-G, Hamsten A, Nilsson J, Grip L, Svane B, de Faire U. Angiographic assessment of effects of bezafibrate on progression of coronary artery disease in young male postinfarction patients. Lancet 1996;347:849—853.
17. MAAS Investigators. Effect of simvastatin on coronary atheroma: the Multicentre Antiatheroma Study (MAAS). Lancet 1994;344:633—638.

The relationship of triglycerides and LDL cholesterol to coronary heart disease

Ole Faergeman
Aarhus Amtssygehus University Hospital, Aarhus, Denmark

The idea that high concentrations of low-density lipoproteins in blood plasma cause atherosclerosis has survived many attempts to disprove it and is widely accepted as an approximation of the truth. In contrast, the idea that high concentrations of triglycerides in plasma cause atherosclerosis has been inconsistent with the results of many experiments, and it has therefore been debated for a long time [1].

Mainly an epidemiological question in the beginning, it has re-emerged as an issue because of the recently developed importance of the market for lipid-lowering drugs. The fibrate group of drugs are potent triglyceride lowering agents and the same claim is made concerning one of the statin drugs, atorvastatin. The relationship of triglycerides to atherosclerosis is confusing to clinicians for several reasons, and I would like to address two of them.

The first has to do with the form in which triglycerides are present in plasma. Triglycerides, like cholesteryl ester, unesterified cholesterol and various phospholipids are transported in plasma as components of lipoproteins. In clinical chemistry, concentrations of lipoproteins are not measured directly. Rather, a component of the lipoprotein class in question is measured. An example is low-density lipoprotein cholesterol (LDL cholesterol).

All lipoproteins contain triglyceride. The most triglyceride-rich lipoproteins are chylomicrons, synthesized by the mucosa of the small intestine, and very low-density lipoproteins (VLDL), synthesized in the liver. LDL and high-density lipoproteins (HDL) also contain small amounts of triglyceride.

Concentrations of plasma triglyceride and LDL cholesterol are, therefore, not commensurate entities. One — triglycerides, is a measurement of all triglycerides in several different classes of lipoproteins. The other — LDL cholesterol, is a measurement of the cholesterol component of only one class of lipoproteins. These relationships are apparent from the data given in Table 1 [2].

Chylomicrons and large forms of VLDL can cause pancreatitis. They are not atherogenic, however, because they are too large to enter into the arterial wall. In contrast, small forms of VLDL as well as intermediate-density lipoproteins

---

Address for correspondence: Prof O. Faergeman, Aarhus Amtssygehus University Hospital, Gade 2, DK-8000 Aarhus, Denmark.

Table 1. Composition of plasma lipoproteins (% of mass).

	CM	VLDL	IDL	LDL	HDL
Triglyceride	86	55	23	6	4
Cholesteryl ester	3	12	29	42	14
Cholesterol	2	7	9	8	4
Phospholipid	7	18	19	22	34
Protein	2	8	19	22	45

Abbreviation not given in text; CM: chylomicrons.

(IDL) and LDL are atherogenic. Hypertriglyceridemia due to high concentrations in plasma of small VLDL and IDL, therefore, identifies a patient at risk of coronary artery disease.

A second reason for confusion has to do with how closely triglycerides are related to genesis of disease. Let us contrast what is known about the role of triglycerides in two of the diseases associated with hypertriglyceridemia.

Hypertriglyceridemia causes pancreatitis probably by participation in a vicious circle of some sort of damage to pancreatic cells, release of cellular lipase into the blood and hydrolysis of triglycerides to glycerol and fatty acids. The fatty acids are toxic to cells and cause them to release more lipase [3]. Triglycerides are thus central to the pathogenesis of pancreatitis.

In atherogenesis, small VLDL, IDL and LDL penetrate into the arterial wall. HDL can also enter the arterial wall, but they are not retained there. Small VLDL, IDL and LDL can be retained, especially if they have been chemically modified, for example by oxidation. Small VLDL and IDL are in fact more likely to be retained in the arterial wall than LDL, because they are larger [4]. Whereas the cholesterol of small VLDL, IDL and LDL is intimately involved in the development of the atherosclerotic lesion [5], the triglycerides probably do not participate at all [1].

These relationships are consistent with the results of clinical trials using both statin and fibrates. In the 4S trial of 4,444 patients [6], plasma triglycerides were a good indicator of risk of recurrence of coronary heart disease in the placebo group, consistent with the concept that small VLDL (which still contain substantial amounts of triglyceride) contributed to the continued progression of the disease. In the group of patients given simvastatin, triglycerides were reduced, and they lost their power to predict recurrence of disease (unpublished data). This finding is consistent with data indicating that simvastatin preferentially removes LDL and smaller species of VLDL from plasma, whereas larger VLDL are unaffected [7].

In the BECAIT trial of 92 patients [8], LDL cholesterol was unaffected and angiographic and clinical benefit seemed to be related to reductions in VLDL and fibrinogen, and elevations of HDL. Bezafibrate reduced VLDL triglycerides (and total triglycerides) by 26% but reduced VLDL cholesterol by 36% (Table 2). These findings are also consistent with preferential removal from plasma of

Table 2. Selected results from the Bezafibrate Coronary Atherosclerosis Intervention Trial (BECAIT) [7].

	Placebo (n = 45)	Bezafibrate (n = 47)
Decrease MMLD	0.17 mm	0.06 mm
CHD events	11/45	3/47
Change in TG	− 26%	3%
Change in VLDL TG	− 26%	8%
Change in VLDL C	− 36%	2%

Abbreviations not given in the text: MMLD, mean minimum lumen diameter; CHD, coronary heart disease; TG, triglyceride.

the smaller species of VLDL and IDL, which contain relatively more cholesterol and relatively less triglyceride than larger species of VLDL (Table 1).

In conclusion, plasma triglycerides can be dangerous in high concentrations because they can cause pancreatitis. Much of plasma triglyceride is in nonatherogenic lipoproteins, but some of the atherogenic lipoproteins of plasma do carry fairly large amounts of triglyceride. Triglycerides, therefore, become inconsistently associated with atherosclerotic disease. Triglycerides as such have little or nothing to do with atherosclerosis.

References

1. NIH Consensus Development Panel. Triglyceride, high-density lipoprotein and coronary heart disease. JAMA 1993;269:505−510.
2. Kane JP. Structure and function of the plasma lipoproteins and their receptors. In: Fuster V, Ross R, Topol EJ (eds) Atherosclerosis and Coronary Artery Disease. Philadelphia: Lippincott-Raven, 1996;89−103.
3. Havel RJ. Pathogenesis, differentiation and management of hypertriglyceridemia. Adv Int Med 1969;15:117.
4. Nordestgaard BG. The vascular endothelial barrier − selective retention of lipoproteins. Curr Opin Lipid 1996;7:269−273.
5. Kruth H. The fate of lipoprotein cholesterol entering the arterial wall. Curr Opin Lipid 1997; 8:246−252.
6. The Scandinavian Simvastatin Survival Study Group. Randomised trial of cholesterol lowering in 4,444 patients with coronary heart disease: the Scandinavian Simvastatin Survival Study (4S). Lancet 1994;344:1383−1389.
7. Gaw A, Packard CJ, Murray EF, Lindsay GM, Griffin BA, Caslake MJ, Vallance BD, Lorimer AR, Shepherd J. Effects of simvastatin on apoB metabolism and LDL subraction distribution. Arterioscl Thromb 1993;13:170−189.
8. Ericsson C-G, Hamsten A, Nilsson J, Grip L, Svane B, de Faire U. Angiographic assessment of effects of bezafibrate on progression of coronary artery disease in young male postinfarction patients. Lancet 1996;347:849−853.

Growth factors, cytokines and vasoactive peptides

Regulation of apoptosis in vascular smooth muscle cells

Martin R. Bennett
Department of Medicine, Addenbrooke's Hospital, Cambridge, UK

Abstract. Apoptosis or programmed cell death has recently been shown to occur in physiological and pathological remodelling of the vessel wall, and in disease states such as atherosclerosis. Apoptosis of vascular smooth muscle cells is regulated by the interaction between local cytokine signals, cell-cell contact and the expression of specific proapoptotic and antiapoptotic genes. However, the precise role of apoptosis in vessel wall homeostasis is still unclear.

Keywords: apoptosis, atherosclerosis, remodelling.

Apoptosis of vascular smooth muscle cells in vivo

Cell death has long been recognised within the vessel wall, in particular in disease states such as atherosclerosis [1,2]. High rates of cell death are also evident in animal models of atherosclerosis, such as balloon catheter injury to arteries of pigs fed a cholesterol-rich diet [3,4]. Traditionally, cell death has been considered to be due to a toxic insult. However, more recently, death in cells of the vessel wall has been shown to occur by apoptosis [5—9], a mode of death considered to be more highly regulated or programmed.

Apoptosis defines a type of cell death distinct from necrosis on the basis of characteristic morphological features. Specifically, these features are condensation of nuclear chromatin around the inner face of the nuclear membrane, loss of cell-cell contact with cell shrinkage and fragmentation of the cell with formation of membrane-bound processes and vesicles containing nuclear material or organelles (apoptotic bodies), which may be phagocytosed by adjacent cells. Apoptosis occurs with minimal disruption of membrane integrity, or release of lysosomal enzymes, with consequently little inflammatory reaction. In addition, organelle structure and function is maintained until late into the process.

Regulators of apoptosis

The regulation of apoptosis occurs in two distinct phases. First, there is integration of the many proapoptotic and antiapoptotic signals arising from the cell surface, which are transmitted by specific second-messenger pathways. This is the

---

Address for correspondence: Dr M. Bennet PhD, Department of Medicine, Box 157, Addenbrooke's Hospital, Cambridge CB2 2QQ, UK. Tel.: +44-1223-331504. Fax: +44-1223-331505. E-mail: mrb@mole.bio.cam.ac.uk

612

"decision" phase, and includes expression of specific proapoptotic and antiapoptotic gene products, such as proto-oncogenes, tumour suppressor genes, etc. If the summation of these signals is to induce apoptosis, there is an irreversible activation of a cascade of cysteine proteases (Caspases) which orchestrate the actual cell disintegration, by cleavage of nuclear lamins and destruction of the cytoskeleton, for instance. This is the "execution" phase. Whilst the signals which promote or protect against apoptosis may be specific to one particular cell type, the proteases mediating cell destruction are conserved in virtually all cells.

The regulators of VSMCs in atherosclerotic plaques has been difficult to establish as many stimuli have been identified in plaques which induce VSMC apoptosis. Macrophage cytokines such as TNF-α, and IL-1 and T-lymphocyte cytokines such as IFN-γ can all induce apoptosis of VSMCs [10]. T-lymphocytes can also induce apoptosis via release of perforin, a pore-forming protein, and Granzyme B. Both endothelial cells and VSMCs express Fas and endothelial cells also express Fas ligand, suggesting that Fas-mediated apoptosis of VSMCs may also occur. Indeed, nitric oxide released by endothelial cells can induce apoptosis [11], possibly by upregulating Fas on the surface of VSMCs [12]. In contrast, angiotensin II appears to protect VSMCs from apoptosis [11]. Extracellular matrix and cell-cell interactions can also promote survival of VSMCs, as can the presence of soluble cytokines such as IGF-1. These cytokines or receptors converge on second-messenger pathways to mediate apoptosis in a manner similar to those signalling cell proliferation, and frequently the same signalling pathways signal both processes. Similarly, many of the downstream gene products which regulate apoptosis, such as proto-oncogenes and tumour suppressor genes, are mediators of both apoptosis and cell proliferation (see [13,14] for reviews). Although most of the signalling pathways leading to apoptosis are not yet characterised, some of the mediators of apoptosis of VSMCs are known, at least in vitro.

Genes regulating apoptosis of VSMCs

Apoptosis of VSMCs can be promoted by deregulated expression of the proto-oncogene c-myc [5,15], via a pathway which can be regulated by expression of the tumour suppressor gene p53 [15]. p53 expression can also induce apoptosis of human VSMCs [16] (and plaque VSMCs are particularly sensitive [17]) via a mechanism which is distinct from that inducing growth arrest. C-myc-induced death can also be blocked by coexpression of the proto-oncogene bcl-2, which can also prevent apoptosis of normal VSMCs in low serum, both human and rat [6,15]. Whether bcl-2, or bcl-2 family members (of which there are an increasing number) regulate apoptosis of VSMCs in vivo is more debatable. VSMCs express low levels of bcl-2 in vitro and in vivo [6,15,18], although this is not universally found [7,19], but only when bcl-2 was overexpressed could effects on VSMC apoptosis be demonstrated [6,15].

Survival cytokines

Another key regulator of apoptosis of VSMCs appears to be the presence of survival cytokines. VSMCs cultured in low serum undergo apoptosis, which can be partially prevented by the presence of IGF-1 and bFGF and to a lesser extent, PDGF [6,20,21]. These agents do not act as mitogens under these circumstances, arguing that different signalling pathways exist for each agent to induce proliferation or protect against cell death. Although both IGF-1 and PDGF are present in the normal vessel wall and the atherosclerotic plaque, low concentrations of survival factors may induce apoptosis in the deeper regions of the plaque.

Consequences of apoptosis in the vessel wall

The role of apoptosis in vivo in the vessel is only speculative although there is increasing evidence that apoptosis may regulate VSMC numbers physiologically. The identification that different mediators may regulate both proliferation and apoptosis simultaneously (and also differentially regulate both processes independently), however, suggests a mechanism by which vessel-wall mass can be maintained. Indeed, regulation of apoptosis per se may be responsible for changes in vessel-wall mass irrespective of changes in rate of cell proliferation. Examples include closure of the ductus arteriosus [22] and physiological remodelling of umbilical arteries and aorta after birth [23]. Furthermore, remodelling during atherogenesis or in hypertension may also be mediated by coordinated action of cell proliferation and apoptotic cell death [24].

The role of apoptosis in the response to vessel injury, or in atherogenesis, is also unknown. So far, apoptotic VSMCs have been demonstrated in the ballooned rat and mouse carotid arteries after injury, particularly after 7–15 days, but is no longer present after re-endothelialisation [9,25]. Similarly, atherectomy specimens from human coronary and peripheral plaques demonstrate apoptotic VSMCs and macrophages, with a higher incidence of apoptosis in specimens from restenotic tissues [7–9]. It may be that apoptosis of VSMCs in critical regions of the plaque predisposes to plaque rupture and thus subsequent thrombosis, or that apoptosis of macrophages removes potentially damaging cells from the plaque, promoting plaque stability. Apoptotic VSMCs can also promote thrombosis directly, by exposure of phosphatidylserine on their surface which can generate thrombin [26]. In addition, apoptosis of VSMCs may occur in the profound changes in arterial calibre observed during atherogenesis, or in the atrophy of the media below a plaque. At present, we lack information on the location, frequency and time-course of apoptosis in any of these pathological entities. However, apoptosis of VSMCs represents a valuable new mechanism for regulating vessel-wall mass.

614

Acknowledgements

MRB is supported by a British Heart Foundation Senior Research Fellowship.

References

1. Garratt KN, Edwards WD, Kaufmann UP, Vlietstra RE, Holmes DRJ. Differential histopathology of primary atherosclerotic and restenotic lesions in coronary arteries and saphenous vein bypass grafts: analysis of tissue obtained from 73 patients by directional atherectomy. J Am Coll Cardiol 1991;17:442–448.
2. Arbustini E, Grasso M, Diegoli M, Pucci A, Bramerio M, Ardissino D, Angoli L, de Seriv S, Bramucci E, Mussini A, Minizioni G, Vigano M, Specchia G. Coronary atherosclerotic plaques with and without thrombus in ischemic heart syndromes: a morphologic, immunohistochemical, and biochemical study. Am J Cardiol 1991;68:36B–50B.
3. Thomas WA, Reiner JM, Florentin FA, Lee KT, Lee WM. Population dynamics of arterial smooth muscle cells. V. Cell proliferation and cell death during initial 3 months in atherosclerotic lesions induced in swine by hypercholesterolemic diet and intimal trauma. Exp Mol Pathol 1976;24:360–374.
4. Thomas W, Kim D, Lee K, Reiner J, Schmee J. Population dynamics of arterial cells during atherogenesis. XIII. Mitogenic and cytotoxic effects of a hyperlipidaemic (HL) diet on cells in advanced lesions in the abdominal aortas of swine fed an HL diet for 270–345 days. Exp Mol Pathol 1983;39:257–270.
5. Bennett MR, Evan GI, Newby AC. Deregulated c-myc oncogene expression blocks vascular smooth muscle cell inhibition mediated by heparin, interferon-γ, mitogen depletion and cyclic nucleotide analogues and induces apoptotic cell death. Circ Res 1994;74:525–536.
6. Bennett MR, Evan GI, Schwartz SM. Apoptosis of human vascular smooth muscle cells derived from normal vessels and coronary atherosclerotic plaques. J Clin Invest 1995;95:2266–2274.
7. Isner J, Kearney M, Bortman S, Passeri J. Apoptosis in human atherosclerosis and restenosis. Circulation 1995;91:2703–2711.
8. Geng Y, Libby P. Evidence for apoptosis in advanced human atheroma: colocalization with interleukin-1β converting enzyme. Am J Pathol 1995;147:251–266.
9. Han D, Haudenschild C, Hong M, Tinkle B, Leon M, Liau G. Evidence for apoptosis in human atherosclerosis and in a rat vascular injury model. Am J Pathol 1995;147:267–277.
10. Geng Y, Wu Q, Muszynski M, Hansson G, Libby P. Apoptosis of vascular smooth-muscle cells induced by in vitro stimulation with interferon-gamma, tumor necrosis factor-alpha, and interleukin-1-beta. Arterscl Thromb 1996;16:19–27.
11. Pollman M, Yamada T, Horiuchi M, Gibbons G. Vasoactive substances regulate vascular smooth muscle cell apoptosis — countervailing influences of nitric oxide and angiotensin II. Circ Res 1996;79:748–756.
12. Fukuo K, Hata S, Suhara T, Nakahashi T, Shinto Y, Tsujimoto Y, Morimoto S, Ogihara T. Nitric oxide induces upregulation of fas and apoptosis in vascular smooth muscle. Hypertension 1996;27:823–826.
13. Bennett MR, Evan GI. The molecular basis of apoptosis. Heart Failure 1994;9:199–212.
14. Whyte M, Evan G. The last cut is the deepest. Nature 1995;376:17–18.
15. Bennett MR, Evan GI, Schwartz SM. Apoptosis of rat vascular smooth muscle cells is regulated by p53 dependent and independent pathways. Circ Res 1995;77:266–273.
16. Katayose D, Wersto R, Cowan K, Seth P. Consequences of p53 gene-expression by adenovirus vector on cell-cycle arrest and apoptosis in human aortic vascular smooth-muscle cells. Biochem Biophys Res Comm 1995;215:446–451.
17. Bennett M, Littlewood T, Schwartz S, Weissberg P. Increased sensitivity of human atherosclerotic plaque vascular smooth muscle cells to p53-induced apoptosis. Circ Res 1997;(In press).

18. Hockenbery DM, Zutter M, Hickey W, Nahm M, Korsmeyer SJ. BCL2 protein is topographically restricted in tissues characterized by apoptotic cell death. Proc Natl Acad Sci USA 1991;88:6961—6965.
19. Leszczynski D, Zhao Y, Luokkamaki M, Foegh ML. Apoptosis of vascular smooth muscle cells. Protein kinase C and oncoprotein Bcl-2 are involved in regulation of apoptosis in nontransformed rat vascular smooth muscle cells. Am J Pathol 1994;145:1265—70.
20. Harrington EA, Bennett MR, Fanidi A, Evan GI. c-Myc induced apoptosis in fibroblasts is inhibited by specific cytokines. EMBO J 1994;13:3286—3295.
21. Fox J, Shanley J. Antisense inhibition of basic fibroblast growth factor induces apoptosis in vascular smooth muscle cells. J Biol Chem 1996;271:12578—12584.
22. Slomp J, Gittenberger de Groot AC, Glkhova MA, van Munsteren JC, Kockx MM, Schwartz SM, Koteliansky VE. Differentiation, dedifferentiation, and apoptosis of smooth muscle cells during the development of the human ductus arteriosus. Arterioscl Thromb Vasc Biol 1997;17:1003—1009.
23. Cho A, Courtman D, Langille L. Apoptosis (programmed cell death) in arteries of the neonatal lamb. Circ Res 1995;76:168—175.
24. Hamet P, Richard L, Dam T, Teiger E, Orlov S, Gaboury L, Gossard F, Tremblay J. Apoptosis in target organs of hypertension. Hypertension 1995;26:642—648.
25. Bochatonpiallat M, Gabbiani F, Redard M, Desmoulière A, Gabbiani G. Apoptosis participates in cellularity regulation during rat aortic intimal thickening. Am J Pathol 1995;146:1059—1064.
26. Flynn P, Byrne C, Baglin T, Weissberg P, Bennett M. Thrombin generation by apoptotic vascular smooth muscle cells. Blood 1997;89:4373—4384.

Potential roles of extracellular nucleotides in atherosclerosis and restenosis

Alain-Pierre Gadeau, Cheikh Ibra Seye, Xavier Pillois, Marie-Line Peyot,
Rabé Malam-Souley and Claude Desgranges
Unité 441 d'Athérosclérose de l'INSERM, Pessac, France

Abstract. The recent cloning of several P2 receptor subtypes has enabled progress in the molecular characterization of the P2 nucleotide receptors that mediate the vasoreactivity induced by the extracellular nucleotides ATP, ADP and UTP. The metabotropic receptors $P2Y_1$ and $P2Y_2$, which mediate nucleotide-induced vasorelaxation, are also found in smooth muscle cells (SMCs) in which the ionotopic $P2X_1$ receptor is also expressed. SMC $P2Y_2$ and $P2X_1$ receptors are involved in nucleotide-induced vasoconstriction.

In addition to their vasoactive role, extracellular nucleotides could also modulate several other processes such as cell migration and proliferation of SMCs, which are known to be involved in intimal hyperplasia. Indeed, extracellular ATP and UTP induce mitogenic activation of cultured arterial SMCs and act synergistically with other factors to induce SMC proliferation. Moreover, extracellular nucleotides favour blood-cell adhesion on ECs and induce the SMC expression of chemoattractant proteins for both SMCs and monocytes. The $P2Y_2$ receptor appears particularly involved in these nucleotide-mediated responses. The in vivo role of extracellular nucleotides and of the $P2Y_2$ receptor in intimal cell recruitment is also suggested by the high expression of this receptor found in intimal thickenings.

Therefore, modulation of arterial P2 receptor subtypes, associated with an increase in local nucleotide concentration, could be involved in intimal hyperplasia and alterations of vasoreactivity observed in atherosclerotic and restenotic processes.

Keywords: arterial remodeling, atherosclerosis, extracellular nucleotides, P2 receptors, restenosis.

Introduction

The development of atherosclerotic lesions involves the intimal recruitment not only of arterial smooth muscle cells (SMCs) but also of blood-derived cells, macrophages and T-lymphocytes [1]. This process necessitates the migration of SMCs from the underlying media, their intimal proliferation and the endothelial adhesion of leukocytes, their infiltration and their eventual proliferation into the subendothelium. A similar intimal SMC accumulation also takes place during the postangioplasty restenotic process. However, the factors involved in intimal cell recruitment are not clearly identified, although various molecules have been involved according to experimental studies. Extracellular nucleotides (and particularly ATP) have been demonstrated to induce not only the proliferation of

---

Address for correspondence: C. Desgranges, Unité 441 d'Athérosclérose de l'INSERM, Avenue du Haut-Lévêque, 33600 Pessac, France.

various cell types but also cell apoptosis [2], a process involved in intimal plaque evolution [3]. Moreover, it has been demonstrated that extracellular nucleotides mediate both vasorelaxation and vasoconstriction; a dysfunctioning in this system may be involved in the chronic constriction of injured arteries often observed in postangioplasty restenosis [4].

Since extracellular nucleotides might be released from arterial and blood cells during pathological and traumatical events [5], they could play an important role in intimal cell recruitment or apoptosis, and consequently play a role in the vascular remodeling accompanying atherosclerosis and postangioplasty restenosis.

To demonstrate nucleotide involvement in arterial pathologies, it is necessary to define their role in intimal recruitment processes and to characterize the P2 nucleotide receptors mediating their effects both in normal and pathological arteries.

P2 nucleotide receptors of arterial and blood cells

Classification of P2 nucleotide receptors

Extracellular nucleotides bind to cell surface receptors, known as P2 purinoceptors or nucleotide receptors, which are present in many tissues. Functional studies using selective agonists have been used to identify various P2 receptor subtypes. The original classification proposed by Burnstock has been recently modified after the cloning of several P2 receptors [6]. To date, these receptors have been classified into two main families: the P2X receptor subtypes are intrinsic ion channels and pores that mediate the influx of calcium, whereas the P2Y receptor subtypes are coupled through G proteins to mobilize intracellular calcium.

P2 nucleotide receptors of arterial cells

Extracellular nucleotides are involved in the regulation of vascular tone with two opposing effects: a vasorelaxant effect which is essentially mediated by ECs, but which may be in part mediated by vascular SMCs in some vascular beds, and a vasoconstrictor effect which is directly mediated by vascular SMCs. These different responses are the consequence of the binding of nucleotides on P2 receptors located both on ECs and SMCs. Endothelium-dependent vasorelaxation has been attributed to the endothelial release of prostacyclin and NO after binding of nucleotides to metabotropic $P2Y_1$ and $P2Y_2$ (formerly P_{2y} and P_{2u}) receptors. Vasoconstrictor effects result from the action of extracellular nucleotides both on one ionotropic P2X (formerly P_{2x}) receptor and on the metabotropic $P2Y_2$ receptor. Although still incomplete, molecular biology studies have confirmed the expression of $P2Y_2$ and $P2Y_1$ receptors in ECs and SMCs in vitro and in situ [7,8]. Moreover, the expression of the $P2Y_6$ receptor has also been detected in rat aortic SMCs [9]. Our recent studies indicate that the $P2X_1$ receptor is expressed in medial SMCs.

P2 receptors of blood and blood-derived cells

An ionotropic receptor bearing the properties of a pore, the P_{2z} receptor (which was recently identified as the $P2X_7$ receptor) has been described both in macrophages and T lymphocytes [10]. Recently, we demonstrated the presence of $P2Y_2$ receptor mRNA in cultured and resident macrophages. The hypothetical platelet P_{2t} receptor mediating platelet aggregation and combining properties of both ionotropic and metabotropic receptors, could be in fact due to the coexpression of $P2X_1$ and $P2Y_1$ receptors [11]. However, it is still unknown whether other P2 subtypes of this family are present in these cells.

Nucleotides and mechanisms of intimal cell recruitment

Intimal hyperplasia results from the accumulation of SMCs, macrophages and T lymphocytes, requiring blood cell adhesion to ECs, migration and proliferation of both blood-derived cells and arterial SMCs. Various experimental studies suggest that extracellular nucleotides may modulate these processes, and consequently intervene in the development and evolution of atherosclerotic and restenotic lesions.

Extracellular nucleotides and cell proliferation

SMC proliferation
Extracellular nucleotides affect the mitosis of a number of different cell types in culture, ranging from various tumor cell lines to epithelial cells [2]. Wang et al. [12] were the first to describe ATP-induced proliferation of cultured porcine aortic SMCs and to suggest that this response was mediated via P2Y receptors. Later on, this observation was extended to rat aortic SMCs [7,8,13—15], human [16] and bovine [17] arterial SMCs.

In our studies, we have demonstrated that stimulation of quiescent SMCs by extracellular ATP induces a limited progression through the G_1-phase of the cell cycle, characterized by the chronological activation of immediate-early and of delayed-early cell cycle-dependent genes [18], which are usually expressed after a mitogenic activation. In contrast, ATP induces only a faint and belated expression of genes normally induced during S-phase entry, suggesting that extracellular nucleotides are faint mitogenic factors and that the ATP-induced mitogenic action could be mediated by an autocrine production of complementary factors. In fact, nucleotide ATP-induced proliferation is often low and needs the occurrence and presence of small amounts of seric factors. Moreover, extracellular nucleotides act in complement, and often in synergy with various factors such as PDGF, EGF, angiotensin II, some of them being inefficient by themselves [12—17]. More-

620

over, a 1 h transitory ATP activation is sufficient to induce mitogenic. So, extracellular nucleotides may be considered as a competence factor for SMCs.

P2 receptors involved in SMC proliferation
In addition to ATP, ADP and 2-methylthio ATP, a preferential $P2Y_1$ agonist also induces SMC cell cycle progression. In contrast, the preferential P2X receptor agonist $\alpha\beta$-methylene ATP and adenosine are ineffective. UTP, a preferential agonist of $P2Y_2$ receptors induces a response at least equivalent to that induced by an equimolar concentration of ATP. Furthermore, ATP and UTP induce delayed-early genes which are not induced by 2-methylthio ATP. Taken together, these results [7,8,18] indicate:
1) that cell cycle activation by extracellular nucleotides is mediated by P2 nucleotide receptors but not by P1 nucleoside receptors;
2) that this response is due to P2Y and not to P2X receptors; and
3) that at least the $P2Y_1$ and $P2Y_2$ receptors are involved in this activation.
Studies to date have shown that several P2 receptors could be potentially involved in the induction of nucleotide-mediated SMC proliferation. However, among them, it seems that the nucleotide $P2Y_2$ receptor is particularly involved in this process [7,8,13,14]. The role of $P2Y_2$ in nucleotide-induced proliferation is partially confirmed by the fact that A10 aortic SMCs (which lack $P2Y_2$ receptor expression) do not respond to UTP mitogenic stimulation [8]. However, in addition to the $P2Y_2$ receptor, it may be possible that other P2 receptors that are also expressed in SMCs may be involved in nucleotide-induced proliferation.

Production of SMC mitogenic factors
Nucleotides could also be involved in both autocrine and paracrine regulation of SMC growth by stimulating the production of trophic substances by SMCs themselves, or by other target cells of the arterial wall. Indeed, macrophages and platelets can release SMC mitogenic factors under nucleotide stimulation [19].

Proliferation of other cells
In contrast to their action on SMC, extracellular nucleotides do not induce EC proliferation [20]. However, they could be involved in proliferation of intimal T-lymphocytes [21] since they induce mitosis of these cells in culture [22].

Extracellular nucleotides and cell adhesion/migration

In addition to their mitogenic effects, extracellular nucleotides may also intervene in cell recruitment by inducing lymphocyte and macrophage adhesion to endothelial cells as demonstrated in vitro [23]. They could also modulate SMC adhesion and migration by increasing the SMC expression of OPN [7], a protein involved in these two processes. Moreover, extracellular nucleotides could play a role in the intra-arterial attraction of monocytes by inducing an increased expression of monocyte-chemoattractant protein-1 by arterial SMCs [7].

Nucleotides and cell death

Apoptosis has been described in human atherosclerotic lesions where it could induce deleterious events leading to plaque rupture [3]. Both arterial SMCs and macrophages are affected by this process. Several studies indicate that extracellular ATP and its nucleoside counterpart adenosine may induce apoptosis of various cell types [2]. This particularly concerns lymphocytes and macrophages which undergo apoptosis under ATP stimulation [24]. The P2X$_7$ receptor controlling pore opening is involved in this process [25]. Influence of extracellular nucleotides on SMC- or EC-death has not been clearly established. The cytotoxic effects of high-ATP concentrations [16] may be related not only to the activation of specific membrane P2 receptors, but also to the rapid hydrolysis and breakdown of the nucleotide to adenosine in the extracellular space. Indeed, adenosine has been shown not only to inhibit arterial SMC proliferation, but also to induce apoptosis of these cells in culture.

Conclusion

So, in normal conditions, released nucleotides may be used to assume the normal physiological functions of the arterial wall. In contrast, under pathological conditions and traumatic arterial events, the local increase in nucleotide release may (in synergy with other locally present factors) initiate several stimuli leading to arterial remodeling, i.e., adhesion, migration, proliferation, apoptosis of SMCs, macrophages and T lymphocytes. The concentrations required for stimulating these processes (higher than 1 μM) may appear high in comparison with reported circulating concentrations. However, such concentrations might be locally generated in vivo under conditions such as platelet aggregation, vascular cell release and particularly cell lysis, occurring during transluminal angioplasty.

In most cases, these nucleotide effects are mediated by P2 nucleotide receptors, and P2Y$_2$ and P2X$_7$ receptors particularly seem to be involved. Consequently, it appears necessary to confirm by in vivo experiments the role of extracellular nucleotides in initiating events leading to the development of intimal lesions or to atherosclerotic plaque complications. If so, particular efforts must be made to develop therapeutic strategies for limiting both nucleotide release and their effects at the arterial level.

References

1. Ross R. The pathogenesis of atherosclerosis: a perspective for the 1990s. Nature 1993;362: 801–809.
2. Abbrachio MP. P1 and P2 receptors in cell growth and differentiation. Drug Devel Res 1996; 39:393–406.
3. Isner JM, Kearney M, Bortman S, Passeri J. Apoptosis in human atherosclerosis and restenosis. Circulation 1995;91:2703–2711.
4. Lafont A, Guzman LA, Whitlow PL, Goormastic M, Cornhill JF, Chisolm GM. Restenosis

after experimental angioplasty. Intimal, medial, and adventitial changes associated with constrictive remodeling. Circ Res 1995;76:996–1002.

5. Gordon JL. Extracellular ATP: effects, sources and fate. Biochem J 1986;233:309–319.

6. Fredholm BB, Abbracchio MP, Burnstock G, Dubyak GR, Harden TK, Jacobson KA, Schwabe U, Williams M. Towards a revised nomenclature for P1 and P2 receptors. Trends Pharmacol Sci 1997;18:79–82.

7. Malam-Souley R, Seye C, Gadeau A-P, Loirand G, Pillois X, Campan M, Pacaud P, Desgranges C. Nucleotide receptor P2u partially mediates ATP-induced cell cycle progression of aortic smooth muscle cells. J Cell Physiol 1996;166:57–65.

8. Seye S, Gadeau AP, Daret D, Dupuch F, Alzieu P, Capron L, Desgranges C. Overexpression of the $P2Y_2$ purinoceptor in intimal lesions of the rat aorta. Arterioscl Thromb Vasc Biol (In press).

9. Chang K, Hanaoka K, Kumada M, Takuwa Y. Molecular cloning and functional analysis of a novel P2 nucleotide receptor. J Biol Chem 1995;44:26152–26158.

10. Falzoni S, Munerati M, Ferrari D, Spinani S, Moretti S, Di Virgilio F. The purinergic P_{2z} receptor of human macrophages cells. J Clin Invest 1995;95:1207–1216.

11. Léon C, Hechler B, Vial C, Leray C, Cazenave JP, Gachet C. The $P2Y_1$ receptor is an ADP receptor antagonized by ATP and expressed in platelets and megakaryoblastic cells. FEBS Lett 1997;403:26–30.

12. Wang DJI, Huang NN, Heppel LA. Extracellular ATP and ADP stimulate proliferation of porcine aortic smooth muscle cells. J Cell Physiol 1992;153:221–233.

13. Erlinge D, You J, Wahlestedt C, Edvinsson L. Characterisation of an ATP receptor mediating mitogenesis in vascular smooth muscle cells. Eur J Pharmacol 1995;289:135–149.

14. Miyagi Y, Kobayashi S, Ahmed A, Nishimura J, Fukui M, Kanaide H. P-2U purinergic activation leads to the cell cycle progression from the G(1) to the S and M phases but not from the G(0) to G(1) phase in vascular smooth muscle cells in primary culture. Biochem Biophys Res Commun 1996;222:652–658.

15. Yu SM, Chen SF, Lau YT, Yang GM, Chen JC. Mechanism of extracellular ATP-induced proliferation of vascular smooth muscle cells. Molec Pharmacol 1996;50:1000–1009.

16. Erlinge D, Brunkwall J, Edvinsson L. Neuropeptide Y stimulates proliferation of human vascular smooth muscle cells: cooperation with noradrenaline and ATP. Reg Peptides 1994;50:259–265.

17. Crowley ST, Dempsey EC, Horwitz KB, Horwitz LD. Platelet-induced vascular smooth muscle cell proliferation is modulated by the growth amplification factors serotonin and adenosine diphosphate. Circulation 1994;90:1908–1918.

18. Malam-Souley R, Campan M, Gadeau A-P, Desgranges C. Exogenous ATP induces a limited cell cycle progression of arterial smooth muscle cells. Am J Physiol 1993;33:C783–C788.

19. Griffiths RJ, Stam, EJ, Downs JT, Otterness IG. ATP induces the release of IL-1 from LPS-primed cells in vivo. J Immunol 1995;154:2821–2828.

20. Van Daele P, Van Coeverden A, Roger PP, Boeynaems JM. Effects of adenine nucleotides on the proliferation of aortic endothelial cells. Circ Res 1992;70:82–90.

21. Rekhter MD, Gordon D. Active proliferation of different cell types, including lymphocytes, in human atherosclerotic plaque. Am J Pathol 1995;147:668–677.

22. Baricordi OR, Ferrari D, Melchiorri L, Chiozzi P, Hanau S, Chiari E, Rubini M, Di Virgilio F. An ATP-activated channel is involved in mitogenic stimulation of human T lymphocytes. Blood 1996;87:682–690.

23. Parker AL, Likar LL, Dawicki DD, Rounds S. Mechanism of ATP-induced leukocyte adherence to cultured pulmonary artery endothelial cells. Am J Physiol 1996;270:L695–L703.

24. Di Virgilio F. The P2Z purinoceptor: an intriguing role in immunity, inflammation and cell death. Immunol Today 1995;16:254–258.

25. Surprenant A, Rassendren F, Kawashima E, North RA, Buell G. The cytolytic P_{2z} receptor for extracellular ATP identified as a P_{2X} receptor (P2X7). Science 1996;272:735–738.

Atherosclerosis XI.
B. Jacotot, D. Mathé and J.-C. Fruchart, editors.

PDGF and arterial smooth muscle hyperplasia. Possible modulation by thrombin

Gunnar Fager, Alexandra Krettek, Cecilia Bondjers, Carolina Simonson, Gunnel Östergren-Lundén and Florentyna Lustig
Wallenberg Laboratory for Cardiovascular Research, Sahlgrenska University Hospital, Gothenburg, Sweden

Abstract. Intimal accumulation of arterial smooth muscle cells (ASMC) is a prominent feature of atherosclerotic lesions. Growth factors (GF) such as platelet-derived (PDGF) and fibroblast (FGF) GFs have been implicated in ASMC dedifferentiation, migration and proliferation. Apart from its role in coagulation and platelet activation, several studies have suggested that α-thrombin promotes ASMC proliferation via specific receptors. However, the signaling events after α-thrombin stimulation are partly different and delayed compared to those after GF stimulation. The most distinguishing property of α-thrombin compared to these GFs is the late induction of c-myc and cell division. The delay is compatible with the hypothesis that α-thrombin induces expression of the GF(s), which in turn are the direct stimuli to auto- and/or paracrine mitogenic response(s). Indeed, it has been shown that α-thrombin stimulates expression and release of both GFs in several relevant arterial cell types. The delay in GF release is compatible with that in c-myc expression. Both GFs rapidly induce c-fos and c-myc. α-thrombin inhibitors (PPACK and hirudin) or antibodies to PDGF or FGF inhibit α-thrombin-induced mitotic processes in ASMC in vitro. Consequently, α-thrombin can be viewed as a friend by preventing bleeding and promoting wound healing but it may also be regarded as a foe by contributing to ASMC proliferation and arterial and venous thromboses.

Keywords: arterial smooth muscle cell, atherosclerosis, platelet-derived growth factor, restenosis, thrombin.

Introduction

Thrombus formation at sites of atherosclerotic plaques precipitates events in occlusive arterial disease such as acute coronary heart disease (CHD) syndromes and ischaemic stroke. Active thrombin (α-thrombin) has three key functions in these processes. First, α-thrombin activates platelets via thrombin receptors to form aggregates and release a number of cytokines and procoagulatory substances (references in [1]). Second, α-thrombin regulates the final common pathway in the complicated coagulation cascade; the enzymatic hydrolysis of fibrinogen to fibrin monomers, which immediately polymerise into the fibrin network of the growing thrombus. Third, α-thrombin promotes proliferation of mesenchymal cells including the arterial smooth muscle cells (ASMC).

Address for correspondence: Gunner Fager, Wallenberg Laboratory for Cardiovascular Research, Sahlgrenska University Hospital, S-413 45 Gothenburg, Sweden. Tel.: +46-31-602950. Fax: +46-31-823762.

The aim of this paper was to review the literature on relationships between α-thrombin and ASMC hyperplasia in atherosclerosis with focus on studies in human material or in human cell systems.

The atherosclerotic plaque

Atherosclerotic plaques develop over decades in the arterial intima from the accumulation of arterial smooth muscle cells (ASMC), ASMC-derived intercellular matrix and lipids in varying proportions [2,3]. Intervention trials predict that, at best, cholesterol-lowering therapy can reduce the CHD incidence by 50% in hypercholesterolaemic subjects [4]. Thus, other components of atherosclerosis must be addressed to prevent arterial occlusion. At sites of arterial narrowings, a defective endothelial lining or frank rupture of atherosclerotic plaques trigger adhesion of platelets and formation of the occluding fibrin clot. Consequently, much effort is currently spent in the search for efficient inhibitors of platelet adhesion/aggregation, fibrin formation and ASMC hyperplasia. By its three main effects, α-thrombin may be a good target for such efforts.

Thrombin

Activation and inactivation of thrombin

α-thrombin is formed from its circulating precursor prothrombin through enzymatic hydrolysis by factor Xa [5]. α-thrombin is inactivated by proteolytic degradation to β- and γ-thrombin. Circulating antithrombin III (AT III) slowly binds α-thrombin to form the inactive TAT complex. Little or no free α-thrombin is present in normal plasma.

There are several pharmacological inhibitors of α-thrombin. One effect of heparin is to facilitate the inactivation of α-thrombin by AT III. Inhibition of α-thrombin by hirudin and hirulog involves binding to the anion-binding site by which a steric hindrance is created for cleavage of the appropriate substrates (see below). Low molecular weight inhibitors such as PPACK (phenylalanyl-prolyl-arginine chloromethyl ketone) and melagatran (ASTRA, Sweden) specifically block the catalytic site of α-thrombin.

Enzymatic effects of α-thrombin

α-thrombin belongs to the serine proteases and cleaves its target peptides proximal to S^1 residues located immediately distal to an R residue. The catalytic site of α-thrombin contains an S-H-D motif immediately distal to the guanidine side-chain pocket (Fig. 1A), which binds the guanidine side-chain of R [6]. The specificity for the appropriate substrates is governed by two flanking amino acid

---

[1]One letter codes are used for amino acids in this paper.

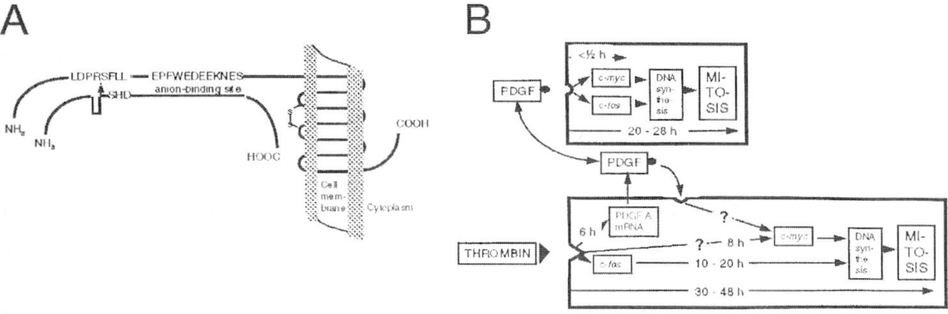

Fig. 1. Schematic showing; **A**: α-thrombin and its receptor; **B**: similarities and differences between α-thrombin and PDGF stimulation. In **A**, one letter codes are used for amino acids and arrowhead indicates cleavage site. In **B**, PDGF- (upper box) and α-thrombin- (lower box) induced cell stimulation is shown with temporal events horizontally and cellular events vertically. Modified from [1] with permission.

motifs. Proximal to the catalytic site is an apolar-binding site and distal is an anion-binding site. This allows selective binding to the fibrinogen molecule and to the thrombin receptor and specific cleavage of target R-S bonds.

The thrombin receptor

The presence of a cell-surface receptor for thrombin was deduced from the many cellular effects of α-thrombin (references in [1]). Vu et al. [7] used a cDNA library from megakaryocyte-like cells to clone and express a functional human thrombin receptor. The deduced 425 amino acids long peptide contained seven repeats of hydrophobic domains (Fig. 1B) indicating a new member of the 7-transmembrane domain family of receptors [8].

Transcripts for the human thrombin receptor have been found in human endothelial cells, platelets, macrophages and alveolar monocytes (references in [1]). In normal human arterial specimens, receptor protein and mRNA were found only in endothelial cells, whereas in atherosclerotic specimens, macrophages and intimal (not medial) ASMC also showed positive signals for receptor protein and mRNA by immunohistochemistry and in situ hybridisation [9].

The regulation of thrombin receptor expression in human cells has not been studied in detail. Growth-stimulated (basic FGF) but not growth-arrested (no FGF) rat vascular SMC express thrombin receptor mRNA in vitro [10]. Antibodies to basic FGF abrogated the proliferative response of rat SMC to α-thrombin but not to PDGF stimulation [11]. This is consistent with the finding that thrombin receptors are expressed in growth-stimulated but not quiescent ASMC in human atherosclerotic lesions [9]. Consequently, the expression of thrombin receptors is probably regulated and determines the proliferative response to stimulation by α-thrombin not only in rat ASMC.

Stimulation of the thrombin receptor

α-thrombin binds via its anionic binding site to an acidic sequence in the thrombin receptor and causes a specific cleavage between R^{41} and S^{42} in the intrinsic receptor ligand sequence (-L-D-P-R^{41}-S^{42}-F-L-L-, Fig. 1A) [7]. Substitution of R^{41} or S^{42} renders the mutant receptors resistant to thrombin stimulation. Synthetic oligopeptides with H_3N-S-F-L-L-$(X)^n$ ($n \geqslant 1$) are able to stimulate the wild-type as well as thrombin-resistant mutant receptors. Successful cleavage by α-thrombin liberates the "tethered" ligand sequence (NH_3-S-F-L-L-), which folds to activate the receptor in a self-stimulatory or intrinsic manner. This change is irreversible and explains the observed desensitisation of cells to repeated thrombin challenges (references in [1]).

Thrombin-mediated cell proliferation

The subcellular signalling events of α-thrombin are partially different from those of PDGF and FGF, which also show distinct discrepancies between them (references in [1]). A major difference seems to be that the GFs induce c-fos and c-myc within minutes, whereas the induction of c-myc is delayed by about 8 h after thrombin stimulation in hASMC [12]. Since expression of both c-fos and c-myc is necessary for mitosis, this correlates with the finding that DNA synthesis begins after 20 h of PDGF stimulation, but only after 30 h of thrombin stimulation (Fig. 1B). One explanation might be that α-thrombin induces expression of GF(s), which in turn induce c-myc and mitosis in an auto- or paracrine manner (Fig. 1B). Indeed, there is a transcriptionally regulated [12,13] secretion of PDGF A-chains in hASMC after 6 h of stimulation [13] and the ensuing DNA synthesis is abrogated by antibodies to PDGF [14].

Thrombin inhibitors and cell proliferation

PDGF is a dimer of A- and/or B-chains of which the A-chain occurs in two forms (long and short) due to alternative usage of exon 6 (references in [23]). The thrombin inhibitor PPACK inhibited α-thrombin-induced upregulation of PDGF A-chains and proliferation in baboon ASMC in vitro and in vivo [15]. We exposed growth-arrested (serum-free medium) hASMC to α-thrombin (Sigma, St. Louis, MO) or no thrombin, with or without melagatran for 24 h in serum-free medium. Melagatran is a selective, potent ($K_i \approx 2$ nM) and low molecular weight (MW 430) thrombin inhibitor in the clinical phase of development (ASTRA, Sweden). α-thrombin induced a transient increase in PDGF A-chain mRNA at 6 h ($p < 0.05$) but not 24 h (Fig. 2). It had no effect on PDGF B-chain mRNA or the ratio of short/long A-chain mRNA. The increase in A-chain transcripts was prevented by melagatran. This suggested that α-thrombin-induced receptor activation significantly increases transcription of the PDGF A-chain gene, but only by a factor of two. However, in studies in vivo, PPACK or hirudin

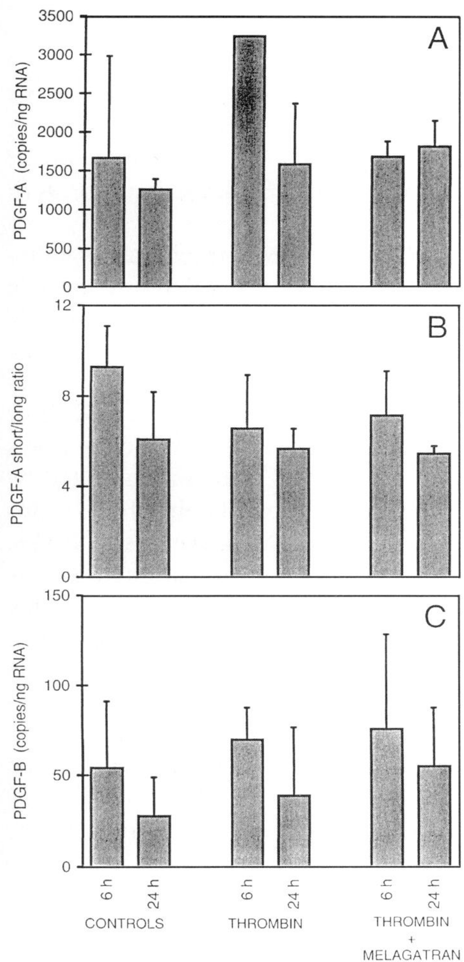

Fig. 2. Expression of PDGF isoform mRNA in hASMC in vitro. Secondary cultures of hASMC [19] were growth-arrested for 4 days in serum-free medium and then supplied with serum-free medium with 3 U/ml or without α-thrombin. Thrombin-stimulated cultures were incubated with 0.3 μM or without the thrombin inhibitor melagatran. Transcript levels of PDGF A- and B-chain mRNA (**A,C**) were determined using a quantitative RT-PCR and the ratio of short/long A-chain transcripts (**B**) using a semiquantitative RT-PCR method after 6 and 24 h of stimulation as described elsewhere [23]. Bars indicate mean values and their 95% confidence intervals.

inhibited ASMC hyperplasia in experimental atherosclerosis in animals, and this indicates a biological significance as well as a pharmacologic possibility [15—17]. Consequently, activation of the thrombin receptor is involved in thrombin-induced expression of PDGF but it is still unclear if endogenous PDGF, α-thrombin, or both explain the late expression of c-myc and the subsequent mitosis.

PDGF and hASMC proliferation

The invasion of the intima by ASMC requires a migration from the media across the internal elastic layer. PDGF (but not FGF) is a potent chemoattractant for ASMC, which migrate towards a gradient of PDGF in vitro depending on the presence of PDGF receptors ([18] and references in [2]). Both FGF and PDGF are major mitogens for ASMC.

In the presence of soluble mitogens such as PDGF, hASMC proliferate, synthesise DNA and then express a nuclear antigen specific for proliferating cells in vitro [19—21]. At the same time, the cells loose their contractile fibres with SMC-specific α-actin and myosin and develop an abundance of synthetic organelles suggesting a dedifferentiation in vitro. In plasma-derived (PDGF-free) serum or in the complete absence of serum or PDGF, hASMC become reversibly growth arrested and redifferentiate to express SMC-specific contractile fibres [19,21]. This suggests a pivotal role of PDGF for hASMC, which is inhibited by antibodies to PDGF. In PDGF-free serum [21], the addition of either PDGF isoform to hASMC causes a dose-dependent increase in DNA synthesis [22,23]. The change in apparent phenotype is fully reversible in both directions within a week depending on the presence or absence of mitogens. It is conceivable that these reciprocal changes in vitro reflect what happens in the atherosclerotic intima during ASMC hyperplasia and explain the mixture of mesenchymal cells with and without SMC-specific contractile fibres [24]. Consequently, it is conceivable that α-thrombin-induced endogenous production of PDGF may contribute by an auto- or paracrine stimulus to ASMC hyperplasia in atherosclerotic plaques.

References

1. Fager G. Thrombin and proliferation of vascular smooth muscle cells. Circ Res 1995;77:645.
2. Bobik A, Campbell JH. Vascular-derived growth factors: cell biology, pathophysiology, and pharmacology. Pharmacol Rev 1993;45:1.
3. Ross R. The pathogenesis of atherosclerosis: a perspective for the 1990s. Nature 1993;362:801.
4. Fager G, Wiklund O. Cholesterol reduction and clinical benefit. Are there limits to our expectations? Arteroscl Thromb Vasc Biol 1997;(In press).
5. Hemker HC, Kessels H. Feedback mechanisms in coagulation. Haemostasis 1991;21:189.
6. Stubbs MT, Bode W. A player of many parts: the spotlight on thrombin's structure. Thromb Res 1993;69:1.
7. Vu T-K, Hung DT, Wheaton VI, Coughlin SR. Molecular cloning of a functional thrombin receptor reveals a novel proteolytic mechanism of receptor activation. Cell 1991;64:1057.
8. Coughlin SR. Thrombin receptor structure and function. Thromb Haemost 1993;66:184.
9. Nelken NA, Soifer SJ, O'Keefe J, Vu T-K, Charo IF, Coughlin SR. Thrombin receptor expression in normal and atherosclerotic human arteries. J Clin Invest 1992;90:1614.
10. Zhong C, Hayzer DJ, Corson MA, Runge MS. Molecular cloning of the rat vascular smooth muscle thrombin receptor: evidence for in vitro regulation by basic fibroblast growth factor. J Biol Chem 1992;267:16975.
11. Weiss RH, Maduri M. The mitogenic effect of thrombin in vascular smooth muscle cells is largely due to basic fibroblast growth factor. J Biol Chem 1993;268:5724.

12. Kanthou C, Parry G, Wijelath E, Kakkar VV, Demoliou-Mason C. Thrombin-induced proliferation and expression of platelet-derived growth factor-A chain gene in human vascular smooth muscle cells. FEBS Lett 1992;314:143.
13. Nakano T, Raines EW, Abraham JA, Wenzel FG IV, Higashiyama S, Klagsbrun M, Ross R. Glucocorticoid inhibits thrombin-induced expression of platelet-derived growth factor A-chain and heparin-binding epidermal growth factor-like growth factor in human aortic smooth muscle cells. J Biol Chem 1993;268:22941.
14. Wilson E, Mai Q, Sudhir K, Weiss RH, Ives HE. Mechanical strain induces growth of vascular smooth muscle cells via autocrine action of PDGF. J Biol Chem 1993;123:741.
15. Okasaki H, Majesky MW, Harker LA, Schwartz SM. Regulation of platelet-derived growth factor ligand and receptor gene expression by α-thrombin in vascular smooth muscle cells. Circ Res 1992;71:1285.
16. Sarembock IJ, Gertz SD, Gimple LW, Owen RM, Powers E, Roberts WC. Effectiveness of recombinant desulphatohirudin reducing restenosis after balloon angioplasty of atherosclerotic femoral arteries in rabbits. Circulation 1991;84:232.
17. Abendschein DR, Recchia D, Meng YY, Oltrona L, Wickline SA, Eisenberg PR. Inhibition of thrombin attenuates stenosis after arterial injury in minipigs. J Am Coll Cardiol 1996;28:1849.
18. Koyama N, Hart CE, Clowes AW. Different functions of the platelet-derived growth factor-α and -β receptors for the migration and proliferation of cultured baboon smooth muscle cells. Circ Res 1994;75:682.
19. Fager G, Hansson GK, Ottosson P, Dahllöf B, Bondjers G. Human arterial smooth muscle cells in culture. Effects of platelet-derived growth factor and heparin on growth in vitro. Exp Cell Res 1988;176:319.
20. Fager G, Hansson GK, Gown AM, Larson DM, Skalli O, Bondjers G. Human arterial smooth muscle cells in culture. Inverse relationship between proliferation and expression of contractile proteins. In vitro Cell Devel Biol 1989;25:511.
21. Fager G, Camejo G, Rödholm M, Bondjers G. Heparin-like glycosaminoglycans influence growth and phenotype of human arterial smooth muscle cells in vitro. I. Evidence for reversible binding and inactivation of the platelet-derived growth factor by heparin. In vitro Cell Devel Biol 1992;28A:168.
22. Hosang M, Rouge M. Human vascular smooth muscle cells have at least two distinct PDGF receptors and can secrete PDGF-AA. J Cardiovasc Pharmacol 1989;14:S22.
23. Krettek A, Fager G, Lindmark H, Simonson C, Lustig F. Effect of phenotype on the transcription of the genes for platelet-derived growth factor (PDGF) isoforms in human smooth muscle cells, monocyte-derived macrophages and endothelial cells in vitro. Arterioscl Thromb Vasc Biol 1997;(In press).
24. Gown AM, Tsukada T, Ross R. Human atherosclerosis. II. Immunocytochemical analysis of the cellular composition of human atherosclerotic lesions. Am J Pathol 1986;125:191.

Retinoids and arterial smooth muscle cells

Pascal Neuville and Giulio Gabbiani
Department of Pathology, University of Geneva-CMU, Geneva, Switzerland

Keywords: α-smooth muscle actin, atheromatous, myofibroblast, retinoic acid, TGF-β.

Retinoic acid (RA), the active metabolite of vitamin A, is a crucial signaling molecule during vertebrate development and plays key roles in cellular proliferation and differentiation [1]. RA has been shown to influence the expression of many genes [2] through interactions between RA receptors and RA response element (RARE) sequences in the promoter region of target genes [3]. RA receptors (the transducers of the RA signal at the gene expression level) are members of the nuclear receptor superfamily. Essentially two subfamilies of nuclear receptors are known to function as RA-dependent transcription factors: the retinoic acid receptors (RAR) and the retinoid X receptors (RXR). For each subfamily three different genes (RAR-α, -β and -γ; RXR-α, -β, and -γ) generate multiple isoforms with specific pattern of expression both in embryo and adult, suggesting that they perform specific functions in the control of RA target genes. A second class of proteins mediates the action of retinoids: the cytoplasmic retinoid-binding proteins that include the cellular retinol-binding proteins (CRBP I and CRBP II) and the cellular retinoic acid-binding proteins (CRABP I and CRABP II). Unlike RA receptors, retinoid-binding proteins modulate the effect of RA by regulating its intracellular level. Several lines of evidence indicate that CRBPs and CRABPs have distinctive physiologic roles. CRBPs bound to retinol provide the substrate for RA biosynthesis [4], whereas CRABPs bound to RA are substrates for RA catabolism [5]. Despite their well-known antiproliferative action, retinoids have not been extensively studied with regard to smooth muscle cell (SMC) biology. However, several aspects of their potential role in SMC lineage, SMC gene expression, and SMC behavior have been reported. This review summarizes some of these advances.

Retinoic acid and smooth muscle cell lineage

RA has a teratogenic effect when applied during critical stages of embryonal development [6]. Many embryonic systems are affected by both lack and excess

---

Address for correspondence: Prof Giulio Gabbiani, Department of Pathology, University of Geneva-CMU, 1 Rue Michel Servet, 1211 Geneva 4, Switzerland. Tel.: +41-22-702-5742. Fax: +41-22-702-5746. E-mail: Giulio.Gabbiani@medecine.unige.ch

632

of RA including the cardiovascular system [7]. RA treatment induces cardiac malformations [8,9] sharing similarities with those obtained by neural crest ablation [10]. The neural crest is a transient structure in the vertebrate embryo, containing cells that develop into various cell lineages. For instance, members of the TGF-β superfamily may promote differentiation of neural crest cells into SMC [11]. These SMC, ectodermal in origin, contribute to the development of the large arteries [12] in combination with SMC originating from lateral mesoderm-derived mesenchyme [13]. The presence in the same vessel of at least two subtypes of SMC with different embryologic origin may explain the morphological and functional SMC heterogeneity described in different compartments of the vessel wall [14,15]. It is, therefore, of particular interest to investigate the intrinsic properties and the potential regulators of these SMC subtypes. The analysis of SMC differentiation markers (e.g., SM-22α, α-SM actin, desmin, calponin) in both cell types reveals identical expression levels [16]. A characteristic of neural crest-derived SMC may be their ability to be influenced by RA, since RA modulates differentiation of cardiac neural crest cells [17], and as the latter express RA receptors and binding proteins [18,19]. Evidence suggesting interactions between RA and SMC lineage have arisen from studies on the differentiation of embryonal carcinoma (EC) cells. EC cells can be induced to differentiate in vitro into a variety of cell types by treatment with different concentrations of RA [20]. At low RA concentrations they differentiate into fibroblast-like cells [20] which express high levels of α-SM actin and SM myosin heavy chain, suggesting that these cells resemble vascular SMC [21]. During RA-induced differentiation of P19 EC cells, α-SM actin and CRBP appear rapidly [22]. This CRBP induction occurs at RA concentrations that support EC cell differentiation into SMC. Increased levels of CRBP are also observed during F9 EC cell differentiation induced by RA [23]. Another cell line (9E11G) derived from RA-treated P19s stably expresses multiple properties and characteristics of differentiated SMC including functional responses to contractile agonists, α-SM actin and SM myosin heavy chain expression [24]. More generally, it seems that induction of RA-responsive genes is a prerequisite for proper EC cell differentiation, since a mutation affecting the RARα gene of the P19 mutant clone RAC65 blocks the induction of RA-responsive genes as well as RA-induced differentiation [25,26]. The fact that a number of genes characteristic of differentiated SMC appear after RA treatment argues in favor of the assumption that RA is a key molecule in SM differentiation.

Retinoic acid and SMC gene expression

RA influences the expression of many genes including those associated with cell growth and differentiation [2]. RA may activate the transcription of target genes or may repress other genes by antagonizing the function of the Activator Protein-1 (AP-1) transcription factor [27]. AP-1 is an heterodimer of Fos and Jun which binds to AP-1 consensus sequences and activates genes related to cell proliferation, migration, apoptosis, and extracellular matrix production. These four processes have been shown to play key roles in the progression of atherosclerosis and restenosis. Many of the positively or negatively RA-regulated genes are involved in the development of atherosclerotic lesions or in the formation of the arterial intima. For instance, c-fos and c-jun are rapidly induced by arterial injury leading to the formation of AP-1 and to the activation of AP-1-regulated genes [28] such as FGF, TGF-β1, c-myc, endothelin-1, stromelysin, collagenase or the precursor of the matrix metalloproteinase-1 (proMMP-1) [29–31]. RA can inhibit the expression of some of these genes such as those for collagenase [32], stromelysin [33] and proMMP-1 [31]. The RA-induced inhibition of metalloproteinases is generally accompanied by a RA-mediated activation of gene encoding components of the extracellular matrix such as fibronectin, laminin and collagen IV [34,35]. Thus, RA modifies the SMC genetic program to favor the formation of extracellular matrix which may consequently decrease the migration and maintain the differentiation [36,37]. In relation to cardiovascular diseases, the action of RA as a negative regulator of AP-1 responsive genes may be considered as beneficial. On the other hand, arterial injury results in an increase of PDGF, PDGF receptors, and TGF-β1 [38,39] that are responsible for the induction of SMC migration and proliferation and that are also potential target genes for RA [40,41]. Moreover, some of the actions of RA are considered to be mediated by induction of TGF-β1. These observations suggest that RA enhances the effects of atherogenic growth factors. Thus, it appears that the role of RA in SMC behavior and vascular diseases largely depends on the pattern of genes that are modulated. It will be interesting to analyze how RA controls SMC gene expression, in order to appreciate its potential role in vascular disorders.

Retinoic acid and SMC behavior

In an attempt to identify proteins differentially expressed between different SMC phenotypes, we have observed that CRBP expression is restricted to rat aortic SMC cultured from the intimal thickening 15 days after endothelial injury (IT15), displaying an epithelioid phenotype and epithelioid clones derived from both the normal media and the IT15 [42,43]. Moreover, CRBP is transiently expressed by proliferating SMC during neointima formation. CRBP positive cells proliferate and undergo apoptosis [43], suggesting that a modulation of the retinoid content may be required for both processes. It has been reported that RA increases [44], decreases [45] or has no effect [43] on serum-stimulated SMC proliferation. It is clearly established, however, that RA decreases PDGF-stimulated SMC proliferation [31,45] and we have observed a 30% reduction in the size of the neointima following RA treatment in the rat balloon injury model (Neuville and Gabbiani, in preparation). RA modulates SMC morphology and CRBP expression at the same time. These effects are part of a true phenotypic modulation since a morphological change is accompanied by a modulation of gene expression. CRBP upregulation is a direct transcriptional effect of RA, mediated through the binding of RARα-RXRα heterodimer to the RARE of the CRBP promoter [46]. In SMC, the pattern of expression of the three RAR and RXR genes has been studied [45]. Five of the six receptors are expressed in rat SMC in vitro and in vivo: only the RXR-γ is undetectable. The presence of these receptors indicates that SMC can respond to RA. Since different SMC phenotypes are engaged in different genetic programs, it will be of great interest to investigate a possible differential expression of the five receptors, or of the isoforms corresponding to a given RA receptor subtype. In this respect, in order to identify which RA receptor may have a differential effect on the differentiated or the proliferating SMC phenotype, we have used RA agonists specific to each receptor. An inhibition of α-SM actin expression restricted to proliferating SMC is observed when epithelioid cells are treated with RA or with RAR-α agonists (Neuville and Gabbiani, in preparation). Thus, RA may specifically influence the SMC phenotype responsible for the formation of the neointima through a RAR-α-dependent signaling pathway. Our data show that RA downregulates or at least does not affect α-SM actin expression depending on the SMC phenotype studied [43] (Neuville and Gabbiani in preparation), but this is not consistent with Haller et al. who report a differentiating effect of RA on SMC, based on an increased expression of α-SM actin mediated by an increase in PKC activity [47]. PKC activation, however, is considered to be a SMC growth transducing mechanism [48]. Taken together, these data suggest that RA specifically influences a subpopulation of SMC prone to migrate and proliferate. This RA responsiveness may be correlated to a particular embryologic origin. During the vascular healing process the action of RA is certainly beneficial since it antagonizes AP-1 [45]. The presence of CRBP in proliferating and apoptotic cells is probably necessary to maintain a low level of RA and to counteract its differentiating and antiproliferative effects. Finally, it has been recently suggested that adventitial fibroblasts may be responsible for the remodeling of arteries and also may participate in the formation of the neointima following angioplasty (for review see [49]). These fibroblasts modulate into myofibroblasts expressing α-SM actin under TGF-β stimulation. We have observed that during rat skin wound healing myofibroblasts express CRBP during the proliferation phase and when they disappear through apoptosis [50]. These observations are compatible with the possibilities that CRBP expression and RA modulation are common features of repair processes. Thus, we suggest that RA may be potentially useful in vascular diseases involving neointima formation.

Acknowledgements

Supported in part by the Swiss National Science Foundation (Grant no. 3100.50568-97). We thank Mrs M. Vitali for typing the manuscript.

References

1. Blomhoff RB. Vitamin A in Health and Disease. New York: Marcel Dekker, 1994;1–37.
2. Chytil F, Haq R. Vitamin A mediated gene expression. Crit Rev Eucaryot Gene Exp 1990;1: 61–73.
3. Giguère V. Retinoic acid receptors and cellular retinoid binding proteins: complex interplay in retinoid signaling. Endocrine Rev 1994;15:61–79.
4. Boerman MH, Napoli JL. Cellular retinol-binding protein-supported retinoic acid synthesis. Relative roles of microsomes and cytosol. J Biol Chem 1996;271:5610–5616.
5. Napoli JL, Posch KP, Fiorella PD, Boerman MH. Physiological occurrence, biosynthesis and metabolism of retinoic acid: evidence for roles of cellular retinol binding protein (CRBP) and cellular retinoic acid binding protein (CRABP) in the pathway of retinoic acid homeostasis. Biomed Pharmacother 1991;45:131–143.
6. Kochhar DM. Limb development in mouse embryos. I. Analysis of teratogenic effects of retinoic acid. Teratology 1973;7:289–298.
7. Morriss-Kay G. Retinoic acid and development. Pathobiology 1992;60:264–270.
8. Taylor IM. The effect of retinoic acid on the developing hamster heart – an ultrastructural and morphological study. In: Persaud TVN (ed) Advances in the Study of Birth Defects III. Lancaster: M.T.P. Press, 1979;119–134.
9. Heine UI, Roberts AB, Munoz NS, Roche NS, Sporn MB. Effects of retinoid deficiency on the heart and vascular system of the quail embryo. Virchows Arch 1985;50:135–152.
10. Hart RC, McCue PA, Ragland WL, Winn KJ, Unger ER. Avian model for 13-cis-retinoic acid embryopathy: demonstration of neural crest related defects. Teratology 1990;41:463–472.
11. Shah NM, Groves AK, Anderson DJ. Alternative neural crest cell fates are instructively promoted by TGFβ superfamily members. Cell 1996;85:331–343.
12. Kirby ML, Waldo KL. Role of neural crest in congenital heart disease. Circulation 1990; 86:332–340.
13. Le Lievre C, Le Douarin N. Mesenchymal derivatives of the neural crest: analysis of chimeric quail and chick embryos. J Embryol Exp Morphol 1975;34:125–154.
14. Orlandi A, Ehrlich H, Ropraz P, Spagnoli L, Gabbiani G. Rat aortic smooth muscle cells isolated from different layers and at different times after endothelial denudation show distinct biological features in vitro. Arterioscl Thromb 1994;14:982–989.
15. Villaschi S, Nicosia RF, Smith MR. Isolation of a morphologically and functionally distinct smooth muscle cell type from the intimal aspect of the normal rat aorta. Evidence for smooth muscle cell heterogeneity. In Vitro Cell Devel Biol Anim 1994;30A:589–595.
16. Topouzis S, Majesky MW. Smooth muscle lineage diversity in the chick embryo. Devel Biol 1996; 178:430–445.
17. Ito K, Morita T. Role of retinoic acid in mouse neural crest cell development in vitro. Devel Dyn 1995;204:211–218.
18. Smith SM. Retinoic acid receptor isoform beta 2 is an early marker for alimentary tract and central nervous system positional specification in the chicken. Devel Dyn 1994;200:14–25.
19. Maden M, Hunt P, Erikson U, Kuriowa A, Krumlauf R, Summerbell D. Retinoic acid binding protein, rhombomeres and the neural crest. Development 1991;111:35–44.
20. Edwards MKS, McBurney MW. The concentration of retinoic acid determines the differentiated cell types formed by a teratocarcinoma cell line. Devel Biol 1983;98:187–191.
21. Rudnicki MA, Sawtell NM, Reuhl KR, Berg R, Craig JC, Jardine K, Lessard JL, McBurney MW. Smooth muscle actin expression during P19 embryonal carcinoma differentiation in cell culture. J Cell Physiol 1990;142:89–98.
22. Wei LN, Blaner WS, Goodman DWS, Nguyen-Huu MC. Regulation of the cellular retinoid-binding proteins and their messenger ribonucleic acids during P19 embryonal carcinoma cell differentiation induced by retinoic acid. Molec Endocrinol 1989;3:454–463.
23. Eriksson U, Hansson E, Nilsson M, Jonsson KH, Sundelin J, Peterson PA. Increased levels of

several retinoid binding proteins resulting from retinoic acid-induced differentiation of F9 cells. Cancer Res 1986;56:717−722.

24. Blank RS, Swartz EA, Thompson MM, Olson EN, Owens GK. A retinoic acid-induced clonal cell line derived from multipotential P19 embryonal carcinoma cells expresses smooth muscle characteristics. Circ Res 1995;76:742−749.

25. Pratt MAC, Kralova J, McBurney MW. A dominant negative mutation of the alpha retinoic acid receptor gene in a retinoic acid-nonresponsive embryonal carcinoma cell. Molec Cell Biol 1990;10:6445−6453.

26. Costa SL, McBurney MW. Dominant negative mutant of retinoic acid receptor inhibits retinoic acid-induced P19 cell differentiation by binding to DNA. Exp Cell Res 1996;225:35−43.

27. Schüle R, Rangarajan P, Yang N, Kliever S, Ransone LJ, Bolado J, Verma IM, Evans RM. Retinoic acid is a negative regulator of AP-1 responsive genes. Proc Natl Acad Sci 1991;88: 6092−6096.

28. Miano JM, Vlasic N, Tota RR, Stemerman MB. Smooth muscle cell immediate early gene and growth factor activation follows vascular injury. Arterioscl Thromb 1993;13:211−219.

29. Griendling KK, Alexander RW. Endothelial control of the cardiovascular system: recent advances. FASEB J 1996;10:283−292.

30. Bennett MR, Anglin S, McEwan JR, Jagoe R, Newby AC, Evan GI. Inhibition of vascular smooth muscle cell proliferation in vitro and in vivo by c-myc antisense oligodeoxynucleotides. J Clin Invest 1994;93:820−828.

31. Kato S, Sasaguri Y, Morimatsu M. Down regulation in the production of matrix metalloproteinase 1 by human aortic intimal smooth muscle cells. Biochem Mol Biol Int 1993;31: 239−248.

32. Lafyatis R, Kim SJ, Angel P, Roberts AB, Sporn MB, Karin M, Wilder RL. Interleukin-1 stimulates and all-trans retinoic acid inhibits collagenase gene expression through its 5′ activator protein-1-binding site. Mol Endocrinol 1990;4:973−980.

33. Nicholson RC, Mader S, Nagpal S, Leid M, Rochette-Egly C, Chambon P. Negative regulation of the rat stromelysin gene promoter by retinoic acid is mediated by an AP-1 binding site. EMBO J 1990;9:4443−4454.

34. Varani J, Mitra RS, Gibbs D, Phan SH, Dixit VM, Mitra R Jr, Wang T, Siebert KJ, Nickoloff BJ, Voorhees JJ. All-trans retinoic acid stimulates growth and extracellular matrix production in growth-inhibited cultured human skin fibroblasts. J Invest Dermatol 1990;94:717−723.

35. Wang SY, LaRosa GJ, Gudas LJ. Molecular cloning of gene sequences transcriptionally regulated by retinoic acid and dibutyryl cyclic AMP in cultured mouse teratocarcinoma cells. Devel Biol 1985;107:75−86.

36. Bendeck M, Irvin C, Reidy MA. Inhibition of matrix metalloproteinase activity inhibits smooth muscle cell migration but not neointimal thickening after arterial injury. Circ Res 1996;78: 38−43.

37. Hayward IP, Bridle KR, Campbell GR, Underwood PA, Campbell JH. Effect of extracellular matrix proteins on vascular smooth muscle cell phenotype. Cell Biol Int 1995;19:727−734.

38. Ross R. The pathogenesis of atherosclerosis: a perspective for the 1990s. Nature 1990;362: 801−809.

39. Schwartz SM, deBlois D, O'Brien ERM. The intima: soil for atherosclerosis and restenosis. Circ Res 1995;77:445−465.

40. Mercola M, Wang CY, Kelly J, Brownlee C, Jackson-Grusby L, Stiles C, Bowen-Pope D. Selective expression of PDGF A and its receptor during early mouse embryogenesis. Devel Biol 1990;138:114−122.

41. Roberts AB, Sporn MB. Mechanistic interrelationships between two superfamilies: the steroid/ retinoid receptors and transforming growth factor-beta. Cancer Surv 1992;14:205−220.

42. Cremona O, Muda M, Appel RD, Frutiger S, Hughes GJ, Hochstrasser DF, Geinoz A, Gabbiani G. Differential protein expression in aortic smooth muscle cells cultured from newborn and aged rats. Exp Cell Res 1995;217:280−287.

43. Neuville P, Geinoz A, Benzonana G, Redard M, Gabbiani F, Ropraz P, Gabbiani G. Cellular retinol-binding protein-1 is expressed by distinct subsets of rat arterial smooth muscle cells in vitro and in vivo. Am J Pathol 1997;150:509–521.
44. Peclo MM, Printseva OY. Retinoic acid enhances the proliferation of smooth muscle cells. Experientia 1987;43:196–198.
45. Miano JM, Topouzis S, Majesky MW, Olson EN. Retinoid receptor expression and all-trans retinoic acid-mediated growth inhibition in vascular smooth muscle cells. Circ Res 1996;93:1886–1895.
46. Husmann M, Hoffmann B, Stump DG, Chytil F, Pfahl M. A retinoic acid response element from the rat CRBP1 promoter is activated by a RAR/RXR heterodimer. Biochem Biophys Res Commun 1992;187:1558–1564.
47. Haller H, Lindschau C, Quass P, Distler A, Luft FC. Differentiation of vascular smooth muscle cells and the regulation of protein kinase C-α. Circ Res 1995;76:21–29.
48. Newby AC, Lim K, Evans MA, Brindle NPJ, Booth RFG. Inhibition of rabbit aortic smooth muscle cell proliferation by selective inhibitors of protein kinase C. Br J Pharmacol 1995;114:1652–1656.
49. Zalewski A, Shi Y. Vascular myofibroblasts. Lessons from coronary repair and remodeling. Arterioscl Thromb Vasc Biol 1997;17:417–422.
50. Xu G, Redard M, Gabbiani G, Neuville P. Cellular retinol-binding protein-1 is transiently expressed in granulation tissue fibroblasts and differentially expressed in fibroblasts cultured from different organs. Am J Pathol 1997;151:1741–1749.

Epidemiology: geographical variations of cardiovascular incidence and risk factors

Geographical variation of cardiovascular incidence and risk factors: a comparison of the data of an Asian (Singapore) and a European (PROCAM) Study

Q.W. Yong, S. Tavintharan and L.S. Chew
Department of Medicine, Alexandra Hospital, Singapore

Abstract. Singapore is a tropical island with three main ethnic groups. The Chinese constitute the majority at 77.4%, followed by Malays at 14.2% and Indians (mainly Tamil) at 7.2%. A comparison of the lipid levels of two population surveys, the Thyroid Heart Study (THS) conducted in 1986 and the National Health Survey (NHS) conducted in 1992, show that there has been a 10.5% fall in total serum cholesterol from 5.80 to 5.19 mmol/l. This is associated with a fall in the incidence rate of acute myocardial infarction (MI) events in the Indians by 20.1, Malays by 10.0% but this fall is not seen in the Chinese. In spite of this fall, the incidence rate of acute MI events is still highest amongst the Indians, who make up only 7.2% of the population. The prevalence of diabetes amongst these ethnic groups is on the rise. The highest current prevalence is amongst the Indians. It is speculated that the high-incidence rate of acute myocardial infarction (MI) events amongst the Indians is due to a higher prevalence of diabetes mellitus amongst them, and that the lack of a fall in the incidence rate of acute myocardial infarction (MI) events amongst the Chinese is due to a rising prevalence of diabetes mellitus in this ethnic group. A comparison of the levels and prevalence of diabetes mellitus of the Singapore population and patients (377 who were admitted for acute myocardial infarction) is made with that of the PROCAM population. It shows that the Singapore population and the patients admitted with acute myocardial infarction have lower total cholesterol levels but higher prevalence of diabetes mellitus.

The emergence of Singapore as an economic "tiger" is contributed to, in no small measure by its strategic location at the crossroads between the Western and the Eastern halves of the world. A small island of 26 square miles, it has a resident population of 2.99 million people made up of three main ethnic groups. The Chinese constitute the majority at 77.4, followed by Malays at 14.2 and Indians (mainly Tamils) at 7.2%. The mean age of the population is 31.8 years, with the proportion of elderly (aged 65 years and above) at 6.8% [1].

The number of deaths in 1995 was 15,569. The crude death rate remained low at 4.8 deaths per 1,000 resident population. The leading causes of death are cancer (25%), ischaemic and other heart disease (23.6%), pneumonias (13.0%), cerebrovascular disease (10.9%), injuries (7.2%) with diabetes mellitus (1.7%) as the sixth major cause of death. The promotion of good health through preventive health care, health education and personal responsibility (through changes towards a healthy lifestyle) remains the main thrust of reducing these main causes

---

Address for correspondence: L.S. Chew, Department of Medicine, Alexandra Hospital, Alexandra Road, Singapore 159964.

642

of death [1].

The choice of meat, prepared with spices, varies with the religious beliefs of the ethnic groups. Together with vegetables, meats are a supplement to rice as the staple diet. There is anxiety that this Eastern diet could be replaced with the advent of Western fast foods and a higher intake of meat, fats and oils. A rise in the prevalence of obesity — already 5% of the population have a BMI > 30 — could contribute to an increase in chronic disease states of hypertension (currently at 13.6%), diabetes mellitus and coronary atherosclerotic heart disease [2].

Lipid levels were estimated in two studies: the Thyroid Heart Study (THS) 1986 [3] and the National Health Survey (NHS) 1992 [2]. These studies highlight several features (Table 1).

1. The lipids levels of the three ethnic groups in both the studies are low, when compared to the lipid guidelines recommended by the European Atherosclerosis Society for a Western population [4]. The exception was a lower HDL-C level seen in the Indian male (0.69 mmol/l) in the Thyroid Heart Study. The Indian female had an HDL-C level of 0.94 mmol/l.
2. The similarity of lipid levels in the three ethnic groups may be accounted for by their similarity of diet with mainly rice as the staple.
3. Total serum cholesterol has fallen by 10.5% from 5.80 (1986) to 5.19 mmol/l in 1992.

Our preliminary study of patients admitted to intensive care in Alexandra Hospital with myocardial infarction (MI) indicate that they have a mean serum-cholesterol level of 5.80 (1.20) mmol/l. All the lipid parameters, fasting blood glucose, HbA_1C and serum insulin were measured at admission or within 24 h of admission. Our MI patients have serum-cholesterol levels similar to that of the PROCAM [5] population without CHD (Table 2). The PROCAM study patients who have had an MI have total serum cholesterol levels average 6.51 (1.22) mmol/l.

The fasting glucose amongst our MI patients are higher than those in the PROCAM CHD+ population, 7.98 (4.52) vs. 6.01 (1.87) and the HbA_1C is high 7.32% (2.63). Unfortunately, there is no HbA_1C estimation in the PROCAM study for comparison (Table 3).

The falls in the total serum cholesterol in the Singapore studies over the years

Table 1. A comparison of the mean lipid levels in two Singapore surveys; the Thyroid Heart Study (THS 1986) and the National Health Survey (NHS 1992).

Age range	18—69				18—64			
Number surveyed	2046	1343	406	297	2771	1807	515	449
Ethnic	Overall	Chinese	Malay	Indian	Overall	Chinese	Malay	Indian
T. cholesterol (mmol/l)	5.80	5.81	5.85	5.71	5.19	5.13	5.34	5.24
Triglyceride (mmol/l)	1.24	1.22	1.27	1.26	1.26	1.25	1.27	1.30
HDL (mmol/l)	0.92	0.95	0.92	0.80	1.28	1.33	1.25	1.13
LDL (mmol/l)	4.28	4.28	4.31	4.26	3.35	3.25	3.52	3.53

Table 2. A comparison of the lipid levels in the PROCAM study, the National Health Survey (NHS) 1992 and the Alexandra Hospital MI Patient Study (CHD + AH).

Study	PROCAM study			Singapore study		
				Alexandra Hospital	NHS 1992	
	CHD+	CHD−	p value	CHD+ AH	Population study	
Number surveyed	186	4221		377	2720	
T. cholesterol (mmol/l)	6.51 (1.22)	5.76 (1.06)	<0.001	5.80 (1.20)	5.19 (1.80)	<0.001
Triglyceride (mmol/l)	1.80	1.51	<0.001	1.82	1.26	<0.001
HLD-C (mmol/l)	1.02 (0.27)	1.16 (0.3)	<0.001	1.11 (0.29)	1.28 (0.59)	<0.001
LDL-C (mmol/l)	4.55 (1.02)	3.80 (0.93)	<0.001	3.90 (1.12)	3.35 (1.71)	<0.001

1986–1992 have been translated into a fall in the incidence rate of acute MI events in the ethnic Indians and Malays, for patients aged 20–65 years. This difference in incidence rates of acute MI events is best illustrated between the years 1994 and 1995 where the ethnic Malays showed a 10.0% fall from 100.5 to 90.1, and the Indians showed a 20.1% fall from 205.1 to 166.4. Only the ethnic Chinese do not show any fall in the incidence rate of acute MI events (Table 4).

There is a need to explain changes in incidence rate of acute MI events amongst the Singapore population who have lower lipid levels when compared to that of the PROCAM subjects. Although there has been a fall in the incidence rate of acute MI events amongst the ethnic Indians and Malays, the incidence rate remains high amongst the Indians who make up only 7.2% of the population. The causative factor is the high prevalence of diabetes amongst the Indians. The three diabetes surveys conducted in Singapore (1974 [6], 1986 and 1992) have shown a progressive rise in diabetes prevalence in all ethnic groups (Table 5). The prevalence of diabetes in the NHS 1992 study shows that amongst the ethnic Chinese the prevalence is 8.0%, amongst the ethnic Malay 9.3% and amongst the ethnic Indians it is 12.9%. Type II diabetes is the most common type of diabetes. The NHS 1992 study also shows that 97.5% of the prevalence of diabetes

Table 3. A comparison of various indices, BMI, fasting blood, HbA$_1$C, DM%, IGT% in the population of the PROCAM study, National Health Survey (NHS) 1992 and the Alexandra MI Study (CHD+ AH).

	CHD+	CHD−	CHD+ (AH)	NHS 1992
Number surveyed	186	4221	377	2720
BMI (kg/m^2)	26.7 (29)	26.3 (3.0)	25.5 (4.92)	
Fasting glucose (mmol/l)	6.01 (1.87)	5.67 (1.17)	7.98 (4.52)	5.29 (0.84)
HbA$_1$C (%)			7.32 (2.63)	
DM	5.9%	3.2%	34.0%	8.4%
IGT	8.1%	4.9%	11.6%	14.0%

Table 4. Incidence rate of AMI events (per 100,000 of resident population) by ethnic group for patients aged 20—64 years 1988, 1990, 1993, 1994 and 1995. Source: Singapore Myocardial Infarct Registry, Ministry of Health, Singapore.

Year	Chinese	Malay	Indian	Total
1988	54.7	116.6	218.6	76.0
1990	52.4	102.6	209.3	71.6
1993	58.3	105.8	193.4	75.5
1994	53.3	100.5	205.1	70.9
1995	53.0	90.1	166.4	66.1

occurs in the adult population (40—69 years) with only 2.5% prevalence in those below 40 years. The PROCAM population has a diabetes prevalence of 3.2%.

Diabetics have a 3—4 times greater incidence of myocardial infarction than nondiabetics [7]. The National Health Survey recorded that 56.0% of those found to be diabetic did not know that they had the disease. The prevalence of those with impaired glucose tolerance (IGT) was 14.0%. Our preliminary study of the diabetic status of our patients admitted with acute myocardial infarction was based on HbA_1C levels. Of those who were presented with acute myocardial infarction 34.0% were considered diabetic (i.e., they had HbA_1C levels $> 8.0\%$). 11.6% had impaired glucose tolerance ($HbA_1C > 6.0$ to < 8.0). 10.0% of the patients had $HbA_1C < 6.0\%$ (HbA_1C of $< 6.0\%$ was considered normal). This 10% of patients had fasting serum insulin levels that were greater than 11.1 mU/l, and they were considered to be hyperinsulinaemic in our study. The fasting serum insulin level of the National Lifestyle population survey was 6.37 ± 4.82 mU/l.

In spite of the rise in prevalence of diabetes there has been a gradual fall in the incidence rate of acute MI events especially in the ethnic Malays (10.0%) and the ethnic Indians (20.1%) but not in the ethnic Chinese (0%). A plausible explanation for this fall in the incidence rate of acute MI events is the fall in the lipids from more adverse levels to more favourable lower levels as seen in the NHS 1992. Another survey in diabetes at the turn of the century will indicate whether the diabetes prevalence in the ethnic Chinese has increased and that of the ethnic Malays and Indians has "matured" or reached a plateau.

Table 5. The rising prevalence of diabetes mellitus in Singapore. Results from three surveys: Diabetes mellitus in Singapore 1974, Thyroid Heart Study 1985 and National Health Survey 1992.

Year of survey	Overall prevalence (%)	Ethnic prevalence (%)		
		Chinese	Malay	Indian
1974	2.0	1.6	2.4	6.1
1985	4.7	4.0	7.6	8.9
1992	8.6	8.0	9.3	12.9

Conclusion

Compared to a Western study (the PROCAM study) the lipid levels are low in both surveys of the population of Singapore in 1986 and 1992 including those who have suffered an acute MI event. Even those who have suffered a myocardial infarction have lipid levels that by European guidelines would only require dietary counselling [4]. Our preliminary study shows that the "insulin resistance syndrome" (diabetes mellitus, impaired glucose tolerance and hyperinsulinaemia) is the main contributor to the incidence of myocardial infarction. This is best illustrated in the Indians who have both a high incidence of myocardial infarction and a higher prevalence of diabetes mellitus when compared to the other ethnic groups in Singapore (Malays and Chinese).

The recent falls in the incidence rates of acute myocardial infarction events amongst the Singapore Indians and Singapore Malays may be attributed to the fall in total serum cholesterol, LDL-C and the rise of HDL-C. There is, however, no similar fall in the incidence of acute MI events in the Singapore Chinese. Diabetics are known to have a higher incidence of myocardial infarction than non-diabetics. This fall in the incidence rate of acute myocardial infarction events that we see, is most likely due to the fall in total cholesterol, and due to the possibility that the prevalence of diabetes in both the Indians and Malays has reached a plateau. However, in the Singapore Chinese, the prevalence of diabetics is set to rise to a higher level. Hence we see no fall in the incidence rate of acute myocardial infarction events in this ethnic group.

Another survey of the prevalence of diabetes mellitus in the Singapore population will increasingly highlight the contributions of diabetes and changes in lipid levels to the incidence rate of acute myocardial infarction events in Singapore. This data contribution will be seen in the next prevalence survey of diabetes at the end of this century.

References

1. Ministry of Health, Singapore, Annual Report 1995.
2. National Health Survey 1992, Highlights of Main Survey Findings Research and Evaluation Department, Ministry of Health (HQ), January 1993.
3. Hughes K, Yeo PPB, Lim KC, Thai AC, Sothy SP, Wang KW, Cheah JS, Phoon WO, Lim P. Cardiovascular disease in Chinese, Malays and Indians in Singapore. II. Differences in risk factor levels. J Epidemiol Commun Health 1990;44:29–35.
4. International task force for prevention coronary heart disease. Prevention of coronary heart disease: scientific background and new guidelines. Recommendations of the European Atherosclerosis Society. Nutr Metab Cardiovasc Dis 1992;2:113–156.
5. Assman G, Schulte H. The prospective cardiovascular Munster (PROCAM) study: prevalence of hyperlipidaemia in persons with hypertension and/or diabetes mellitus and the relationship to coronary artery disease. Am Heart J 1988;116:1713–1724.
6. Cheah JS, Lui KF, Yeo PPB, Tan BY, Tan YT, Ng YK. Diabetes mellitus in Singapore: results of a country wide population survey. In: Cheah JS et al. (eds) Proc. 6 Asia and Oceania Congress of Endocrinology Singapore, vol 1. Singapore: Stamford College Press, 1978;227–238.

7. Wilson PWF, Kannel WB. Epidemiology of hyperglycaemia and atherosclerosis. In: Rudepman N, Wilson J, Brown Lee M (eds) Hyperglycaemia, Diabetes and Vascular Disease. New York, NY: Oxford University Press, 1992;2:21–29.

Association of westernized lifestyle and coronary risk factors in the Japanese

Genshi Egusa and Michio Yamakido
Second Department of Internal Medicine, Hiroshima University School of Medicine, Hiroshima, Japan

Abstract. The risk factors of coronary heart disease (CHD) have been altered through a westerniza-tion of lifestyle, with the degree and duration of lifestyle westernization resulting in an increased risk of CHD among Japanese. Japanese residing in Hiroshima (JH) and Kitaaiki (JK), as well as first-generation Japanese-Americans (JAI) and second- and later-generation Japanese-Americans (JAII) originally from Hiroshima underwent this medical survey between 1986 and 1996.

The consumption of animal fat and simple carbohydrates increased in the following order: JH < JAI < JAII. The consumption of complex carbohydrates decreased as follows: JH > JAI > JAII. Waist-hip ratio in males and females increased relation to fat consumption: JH < JAI < JAII. Age- and sex-adjusted means of serum cholesterol, triglyceride (TG), fasting IRI, prevalence of hyperten-sion,and prevalence of LDL subpattern B also increased in order of JH, JAI, and JAII. Age- and sex-adjusted prevalence of abnormal Q on ECG and death rate due to CHD increased in the same order.

Serum TG were highest in JA, followed by JK, a depopulated mountain village which has under-gone rapid westernization of the diet in recent years, followed by JH. However, the IRI levels in the 75 g GTT were higher in JA, followed by JH and JK, respectively.

Thus, with a greater degree of westernization in Japanese lifestyle, the risks of developing CHD increase, and the more prevalent it will become. It is suggested that the westernization of the diet first affected serum lipids, followed by insulin resistance in this population.

Keywords: eating habit, insulin resistance, Japanese-American.

Introduction

In Japan, mortality due to coronary heart disease (CHD) is lower than that in the West, though mortality due to cerebrovascular disease tends to be higher. Serum cholesterol levels in the Japanese population have increased with the progressive westernization of the lifestyle, especially the diet, though CHD mortality in Japan has shown no significant increase over the past 20 years [1].

To assess the possibility of a future increase of CHD in Japan, this study exam-ined the change in CHD risk factors resulting from lifestyle westernization, and how the degree and duration of this westernization have influenced the appear-ance of CHD risk factors, especially hyperlipidemia and insulin resistance.

Address for correspondence: Genshi Egusa MD, Second Department of Internal Medicine, Hiroshima University School of Medicine, 1-2-3 Kasumi, Minami-ku, Hiroshima 734, Japan.

648

Materials and Methods

The subjects were Japanese residents of Hiroshima (JH, n = 962), Kitaaiki (JK, n = 328) and Japanese immigrants who moved from Hiroshima to the USA, as well as their descendants, i.e., Japanese-Americans. Hiroshima is a typical urban area where westernization of lifestyle has progressed gradually since World War II. Kitaaiki is a depopulated mountain village, which has only recently experienced rapid westernization of the diet. Japanese-Americans were divided into first-generation immigrants who had been born in Japan (JAI, n = 765), and second- and later-generations born in the USA (JAII, n = 875).

All subjects underwent a nutritional survey, a physical-activity survey, physical measurements, a 75 g oral glucose tolerance test (GTT), measurement of serum lipids and lipoproteins, and determination of LDL particle size. Diabetics according to WHO criteria were excluded from the sample.

Results

There were no differences in the total energy intake of both males and females among JH, JAI and JAII. However, the intakes of animal fat and simple carbohydrates for both genders increased in that order, while the intake of complex carbohydrates decreased in the same order. The percentage of subjects engaging in strenuous physical activity was observed to be the highest in JH, followed by JAI and JAII, for both males and females. The mean body mass index (BMI: kg/m^2) increased in males as follows: JH < JAI < JAII. Similarly in both males and females the ratio of waist-hip circumference increased in the same order, i.e., JH < JAI < JAII.

The age- and sex-adjusted mean serum cholesterol (TC), triglyceride (TG) and LDL-cholesterol levels showed stepwise increases in the following order: JH < JAI < JAII. Fasting insulin (IRI) (5.1, 6.0, 8.1 µu/ml, respectively), prevalence of hypertension (29, 32 and 38%, respectively) and LDL subpattern B (16.9, 20.4 and 26.2%, respectively) tended to increase in the same order. In the three groups, fasting IRI correlated positively with TG and inversely with HDL-C, with the correlations becoming stronger in the order of JH < JA1 < JAII. The age- and sex-adjusted prevalence of abnormal Q waves on resting ECG was 3.8% for JAI and 4.7% for JAII, both of which were higher than the value of 0.8% for JH. Crude death rate due to CHD in the entire Japanese population (based on annual Health Statistics for Japan 1996) was 6.7 for JH, 21.0 for JAI and 31.6% for JAII (based on results obtained from the Public Health Bureau in the state of Hawaii).

Data obtained from Japanese residents of Kitaaiki (JK), and Hiroshima (JH), as well as Japanese-Americans residing in Hawaii (JA) were compared to investigate the influence of the degree and duration of lifestyle westernization on the presence of CHD risk factors.

Both males and females in Kitaaiki had significantly higher total daily energy intakes than those in the other two groups. The percentage of the energy intake in residents of Hawaii was higher for animal fat and simple carbohydrates, but lower for complex carbohydrates than they were in the other two groups. However, the total dietary intake of protein, fat and complex carbohydrates was higher in Kitaaiki than in Hiroshima. Though there were no differences in the BMI of females residing in the three districts, there were differences among the males, whose BMI increased as follows: JK < JH < JA. Japanese-Americans had the highest value of TC for all ages. There were no differences between females from Hiroshima and Kitaaiki, but males in their 50s and 60s from Hiroshima had higher serum cholesterol levels than those of Kitaaiki. However, males in their 40s from Kitaaiki showed significantly higher values than those from Hiroshima. The mean triglyceride levels were also significantly higher in residents of Hawaii than in members of the other two groups, though subjects in Kitaaiki had higher TG levels than those in Hiroshima. The mean HDL-cholesterol levels were not significantly different among the three groups, while hypertension was more prevalent in Kitaaiki than in the other two districts. The age- and sex-adjusted mean value of IRI was significantly higher both before and after the 75 g GTT in Hawaii, followed by Hiroshima and Kitaaiki, respectively.

Discussion

The suggestion that the changes of lifestyle imposed by "westernization" are associated with the development of CHD has been confirmed by migrant studies [2]. The lifestyles and risk factors of CHD for Japanese in Japan and the USA were compared. Since the genetic backgrounds of the subjects were almost identical, the differences observed were attributed to environmental influences.

In this study, a westernized lifestyle was associated with an increased intake of animal fat and simple carbohydrates without an accompanying increase in total energy intake, as well as a reduction in physical activity.

It was observed that the risk factors of CHD (such as upper-body obesity, hyperlipidemia, insulin resistance, prevalence of LDL subpattern B, and hypertension) all increase relative to the increasing degree to which the Japanese lifestyle becomes westernized. The prevalence of CHD in accordance with the degree of westernization of Japanese lifestyle has been shown in epidemiological studies which indicate that the change of lifestyle resulting from emigration is associated with increased CHD mortality among South Asians [3]. Thus, a westernized lifestyle may increase the risk of developing atherosclerosis and accelerate the development of CHD in Japanese, as well as in other Asian peoples.

Mckeigue et al. [4] reported that metabolic disturbances associated with central obesity and insulin resistance might contribute to the higher rates of CHD in South Asian people. Results from the present study show stepwise increases in the waist-hip ratio and fasting IRI, which correlate directly to the degree of westernization of lifestyle. Furthermore, positive correlation of fasting IRI with TG and inverse correlation with HDL showed a stepwise increase in order of JH,

650

JAI and JAII. Fujimoto et al. [5] also pointed out the close relationship between visceral fat accumulation, insulin resistance and metabolic abnormalities in second-generation Japanese-American men in Seattle. An increase in upper-body obesity is, therefore, a key component linking increased risk of CHD with westernization of lifestyle in Asian peoples.

It has been suggested that the rapid westernization of the Japanese diet resulted in an initial increase in serum lipids, followed by an increased insulin resistance. As the duration of lifestyle westernization lengthened, the risk of CHD appeared to increase even more, due to the synergy of abnormal lipid metabolism and insulin resistance, as represented by the results obtained from Japanese-Americans. Haffner et al. [6] found that insulin resistance preceded the development of metabolic disorders, including hypertriglyceridemia. Further studies are necessary to elucidate whether a rapid change of lifestyle influences lipid metabolism or insulin resistance first.

In conclusion, it appears likely that risk factors of CHD are greatly modified by changes in environment and lifestyle. Thus lifestyle intervention may be extremely important as a strategy for prevention of CHD.

References

1. Research committee on serum lipid level survey 1990 in Japan. Current state of and recent trends in serum lipid levels in the general Japanese population. Atheroscl Thromb 1996;2: 122–132.
2. Pedoe HT et al. Coronary heart attacks in east London. Lancet 1975;II:833–838.
3. Mckeigue PM et al. Association of early-onset coronary heart disease in South Asia men with glucose intolerance and hyperinsulinemia. Circulation 1993;87:152–161.
4. Mckeigue PM et al. Relation of central obesity and insulin resistance with high diabetes prevalence and cardiovascular risk in South Asians. Lancet 1991;337:382–386.
5. Fujimoto WY et al. Metabolic basis for coronary heart disease risk in central obesity and glucose intolerance. In: Yamamoto A (eds) Multiple Risk Factors in Cardiovascular Disease. Takyo, Osaka. Edinburgh, London, Madrid, Melbourne, Milan, New York: Churchill Livingstone, 1994; 189–192.
6. Haffner SM et al. Prospective analysis of the insulin-resistance syndrome (Syndrome X). Diabetes 1992;41:715–722.

Geographic variation and time trends in stroke occurrence

Cinzia Sarti and Jaakko Tuomilehto
National Public Health Institute, Department of Epidemiology and Health Promotion, Helsinki, Finland

Abstract. *Background.* Trends in stroke mortality and incidence have shown considerable variations between countries. Here we present a summary of trends in stroke occurrence in several countries during the 1970s and 1980s from databases of the World Health Organization.

Methods. Two main sources of data were used: stroke mortality from the WHO data bank, both previously published and updated by the authors, and the trends in stroke mortality and attack rates from the WHO MONICA Project.

Results. The different sources showed a consistent decline in stroke mortality in almost all countries, excluding Eastern Europe where trends were either increasing or flat. A decline could also be observed for the attack rates of stroke in most countries, although usually smaller than that observed for stroke mortality. Again, in Eastern Europe the trends in attack rate of stroke were mostly increasing or flat.

Conclusions. The declining trends in stroke mortality observed in most countries were associated with a lesser decline in stroke attack rate, indicating both improvement in survival and in primary prevention of stroke in these countries. Conversely, the increase in stroke mortality and attack rates in some Eastern European countries suggests worsening in cerebrovascular risk factor levels.

Keywords: cerebrovascular disease, epidemiology.

Introduction

Stroke mortality varies considerably within countries but often also between countries [1—6]. While data from many industrialised countries indicate that stroke mortality has been on the decline during the past several decades, there are also countries where stroke mortality has not declined, or has even increased [1,2,6—8]. These trends have been mostly parallel to trends in coronary heart disease mortality [1]. Data on stroke incidence also show large geographic variation, both between and within countries [9—14].

The trends in stroke incidence, in addition, do not always parallel the trends in stroke mortality: there are populations with a clearly documented decrease in stroke mortality which have reported flat or even increasing trends in stroke incidence [12—16]. In this paper we present currently available data on trends in stroke mortality and incidence, concentrating on international comparisons from databases of the World Health Organization (WHO).

Address for correspondence: Cinzia Sarti MD, PhD, National Public Health Institute, Department of Epidemiology and Health Promotion, Mannerheimintie 166, FIN—00300 Helsinki, Finland. Tel.: +358-9-622-5338. Fax: +358-9-629-518. E-mail: cinzia.sarti@ktl.fi

Materials and Methods

Two main sources of data are presented here. Firstly, international trends in stroke mortality were published in 1990 by Bonita et al. [2]. The authors presented trends calculated from the WHO data bank for the years 1970–1985, in the age group of 40–69 years. This paper also presents original calculations of stroke mortality from an updated version of the WHO stroke data bank, which includes fatal stroke events from 1968–1971 to 1991–1993 (depending on the country, although for most countries data for the whole period were available), and for a wider age range, from 35 to 84 years. A logarithmic regression model, assessing percentage changes in the rates, was applied both in the present analyses and in the Bonita model.

The other sources of information used here are the trends in stroke mortality and attack rate, the latter including both first and recurrent strokes, recently published by the WHO MONICA Stroke Study [17], part of the WHO MONICA project. This is a multinational study started in the first half of the 1980s, whose primary objective was to continuously register the occurrence of myocardial infarction and stroke in many populations, to monitor the risk-factor levels in these populations, and to analyse the relationship between temporal trends in morbidity and mortality rates and changes over time in major cardiovascular risk factors [3]. MONICA Collaborating Centres (MCCs) were established and data collection was started between 1982 and 1985.

Table 1. Age-standardized stroke mortality rates per 100,000 in 1985 and annual percentage change in stroke mortality in selected countries during 1970–1985 by sex, age group 40–69 years[a].

Country	Men		Women	
	Rate	Change (%) per year	Rate	Change (%) per year
Hungary	229.4	+3.9	130.4	+2.1
Poland	95.8	+2.9	62.5	+1.7
Bulgaria	249.2	+2.2	155.8	−0.5
Yugoslavia (1984)	145.1	+0.7	101.2	−0.3
Austria	89.9	−2.3	48.5	−3.3
Sweden	48.1	−2.7	30.5	−4.0
Singapore	136.0	−2.8	92.0	−2.6
Netherlands	47.0	−3.1	31.1	−4.0
Finland	98.1	−3.6	62.5	−5.0
Ireland	72.2	−3.7	58.6	−4.7
Northern Ireland	84.4	−3.8	66.8	−3.6
New Zealand	62.0	−3.8	49.9	−4.7
Canada	39.1	−4.6	28.3	−4.8
Australia	60.3	−5.4	44.7	−6.5
USA	45.4	−5.7	35.1	−5.2
Japan	106.9	−7.1	60.4	−7.0

[a]Adapted from [2].

WHO defines stroke as rapidly developing signs of focal (or global) disturbance of cerebral function lasting more than 24 h (unless interrupted by surgery or death), with no apparent nonvascular cause; this definition included patients presenting with clinical signs and symptoms suggestive of subarachnoid hemorrhage, intracerebral hemorrhage, or cerebral infarction [3]. Hence, the study is based on clinical diagnoses, which have been shown to be reliable [18,19].

Stroke incidence, recurrent rates, and mortality were registered in several populations using standard study procedures and diagnostic criteria [18,19]. We compare here data from a recent publication [17] reporting 5-year trends in stroke mortality and stroke attack rate, the latter including both first in a lifetime events (incidence) and recurrent events. From previously published data we know that about 80% of all strokes in the MONICA stroke study were a first in a lifetime event, ranging from 92% in Gothenburg to 71% in Beijing [9].

Results

Stroke mortality

The paper published in 1990 reported that stroke mortality declined in 23 out of

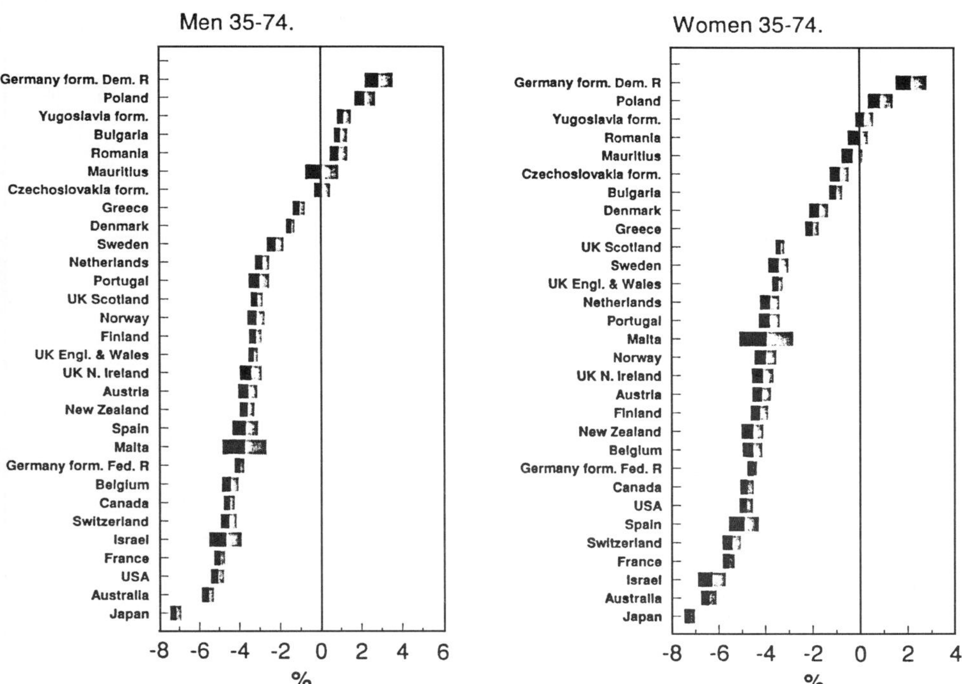

Fig. 1. Trends in stroke mortality (% per year) in selected countries during 1968—1993 by sex, age group 35—74 years. Source: WHO stroke data bank.

27 countries, the largest decline being found in Japan, USA, Australia and Canada, and no decline or increase in Hungary, Poland, Bulgaria and Yugoslavia (Table 1). Mortality from stroke also declined, albeit not so steeply, in Hong Kong, Singapore, New Zealand and in most of Western Europe.

Our analyses (Figs. 1 and 2) produced trends substantially similar to those reported by Bonita et al. Between 1968 and 1993, stroke mortality declined in most countries in people aged 35—74 years old. In addition, we found that the trends in stroke mortality in the age group 75—84 years are substantially similar within each country to that observed in the younger age group.

The published mortality data from the MONICA stroke registers included the population aged 35—64 years and are summarised in Tables 2 and 3. Although the trends in stroke mortality were calculated in a different way from our calculations (using linear regression), the results substantially corroborate the above findings: declining trends were observed in 10 out of 17 populations among men, and in 14 out of 17 populations among women.

Stroke attack rate

The average annual attack rates for all stroke events reported from the WHO

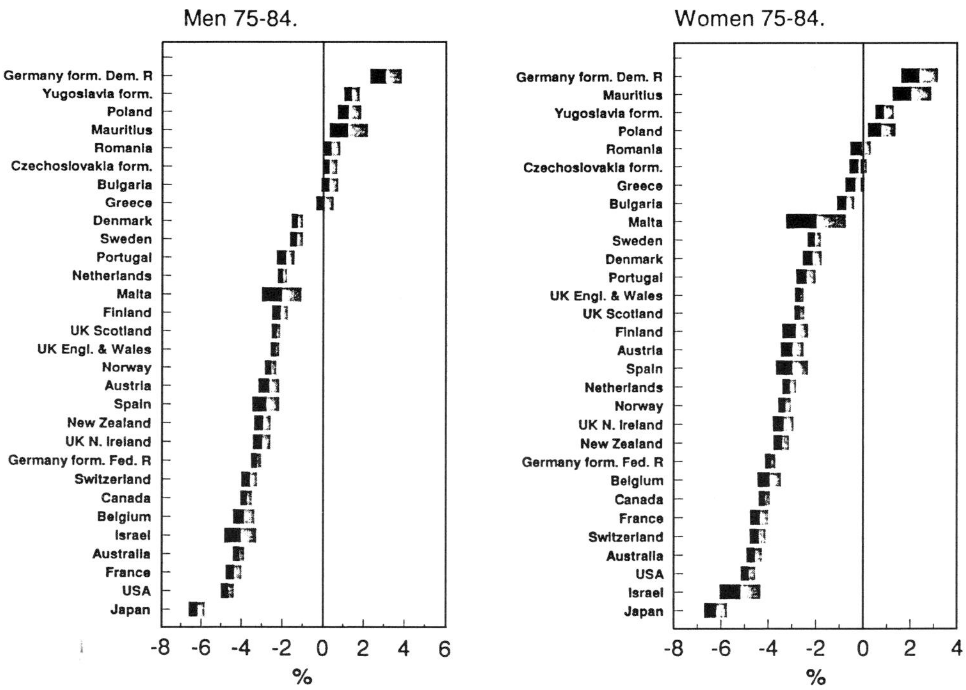

Fig. 2. Trends in stroke mortality (% per year) in selected countries during 1968—1993 by sex, age group 75—84 years. Source: WHO stroke data bank.

Table 2. Age-standardized stroke mortality rates per 100,000 and their trends by sex, age group 35–64 years[a].

Country	Men		Women	
	Rate	Change (%)	Rate	Change (%)
Finland — North Karelia	70.0	− 10.6[c]	30.8	− 18.7[c]
Denmark — Glostrup	32.7	− 8.6	20.9	− 2.5
Germany — rest of DDR-MONICA[b]	41.5	− 7.1	27.4	− 1.7
Sweden — Northern Sweden	31.0	− 6.6	22.9	− 4.3
Italy — Friuli	41.9	− 5.7	23.6	− 7.5[c]
Germany — Halle County[b]	53.4	− 5.2	31.5	− 4.1
Finland — Turku/Loimaa	50.2	− 3.6	24.9	+2.3
Russian Fed. — Novosibirsk i.	113.0	− 2.9	76.1	− 10.4
Germany — Karl-Marx-Stadt County[b]	54.7	− 2.5	31.5	− 10.9[c]
Poland — Warsaw	79.4	− 1.1	47.2	− 1.2
Finland — Kuopio	64.7	− 0.0	30.2	− 13.4
China — Beijing	66.7	+0.1	58.0	− 7.3
Yugoslavia — Novi Sad	72.3	+1.1	47.2	− 3.2
Russian Fed. — Moscow i.	95.5	+1.6	51.4	+0.5
Russian Fed. — Moscow c.	95.8	+5.1	44.5	− 14.8
Sweden — Gothenburg	28.6	+9.1	16.1	− 21.3
Lithuania — Kaunas	80.0	+10.0	39.3	+7.5

[a]Adapted from [17]; [b]former German Democratic Republic; [c]$p < 0.05$.

MONICA Stroke study are shown in Table 3. The attack rate of stroke declined in 13 out of 17 populations among men and 15 out of 17 populations among women. Due to lack of statistical power, the declining trends in stroke in stroke attack rate were statistically significant only in two populations among men and in three populations among women. The lowest rates among men and women in the MONICA populations were found in Friuli (Italy) and the highest rates in Novosibirsk (Russian Federation). Stroke incidence rates varied 3-fold among men and 5-fold among women in the populations studied. For both men and women, stroke incidence was higher in the MONICA populations in Finland, Lithuania, the Russian Federation and China than in those in the Scandinavian and Western and Central European countries. Overall, stroke was almost twice as frequent for men aged 35–64 years than for women of the same age.

Discussion

Although mostly declining trends were observed in the attack rate of stroke (which reflect closely the correspondent incidence rate for any given), the patterns are not as consistent as those observed in stroke mortality. In fact, a decline in the attack rate of stroke has been found only in some Western European countries while in others no decline, or even an increase in the attack rate of stroke was

Table 3. Age-standardized stroke attack rates per 100,000 and their trends, by sex, age group 35—64 years[a].

Country	Men		Women	
	Rate	Change (%)	Rate	Change (%)
Russian Fed. — Novosibirsk i.	338	− 6.5	312	− 4.6
Denmark — Glostrup	173	− 4.6[c]	92	− 3.3
Sweden — Northern Sweden	207	− 3.6[c]	111	− 3.5
Germany — Halle County[b]	151	− 3.1	86	− 8.3
Finland — Turku/Loimaa	247	− 3.0	105	− 0.4
Finland — North Karelia	280	− 2.3	123	− 1.6
Finland — Kuopio	351	− 2.9	173	− 9.4[c]
Yugoslavia — Novi Sad	228	− 2.4	107	− 3.2
Russian Fed. — Moscow i.	241	− 2.2	126	− 3.7[c]
Russian Fed. — Moscow c.	257	− 2.2	121	− 13.8[c]
Italy — Friuli	124	− 1.9	61	− 1.7
Germany — rest of DDR-MONICA[b]	141	− 1.3	74	− 3.6
Germany — Karl-Marx-Stadt County[b]	176	− 0.4	104	− 3.3
Lithuania — Kaunas	308	+0.6	159	+2.0
China — Beijing	247	+1.9	175	− 0.3
Sweden — Gothenburg	137	+3.5	69	− 5.0
Poland — Warsaw	184	+6.8[c]	90	+4.5

[a]Adapted from [17]; [b]former German Democratic Republic; [c]$p < 0.05$.

already observed in the 1980s (Table 3). In general, a decline in the incidence of stroke can also be observed in more recent years in those European countries which started out with higher incidence levels, for example in Finland [20], even though a levelling off of the decline is probably taking place also in this country [21]. In the USA, while a general decline in the incidence of stroke had been seen during the 1970s and 1980s, there are indications that in the 1990s this decline is levelling off [5,22,23]. Mostly increasing or flat trends can be observed in the Eastern European countries, similar to the mortality trends observed in these countries.

Declining trends in stroke mortality have been observed over recent decades in almost all of Western Europe, North America, Australia and New Zealand, excluding most of Eastern European countries, where stroke mortality has been increasing since the 1970s. The present results indicate that stroke mortality declined in most of the populations studied, corroborating the findings of the studies above. The results also show that declining stroke mortality rates were not only due to improved survival, but also attributable in part to a concomitant incidence decline. There are some indications that this declining trend in stroke mortality may be slowing down, at least in the USA [22—24], but it is too early to say whether this is related to a levelling off in the incidence of stroke.

Changing stroke rates should be analysed in relation to changes in cardiovascular risk factors in the population. Declining stroke rates have been attributed in part to improved hypertension control [23,25], and increasing stroke incidence has been considered partly an effect of deteriorating lifestyle factors in the population [26]. As the ultimate goal of stroke epidemiology is the prevention of stroke, continuing research is needed to facilitate efforts toward stroke prevention. The WHO MONICA collaborative study on stroke, coronary heart disease and cardiovascular risk factors has the potential to add a significant contribution to current knowledge in the field of cardiovascular epidemiology.

References

1. Uemura K, Pisa Z. Trends in cardiovascular disease mortality in industrialized countries since 1950. World Health Stat Q 1988;41:155—168.
2. Bonita R, Stewart A, Beaglehole R. International trends in stroke mortality: 1970—1985. Stroke 1990;21:989—992.
3. Tuomilehto J, Kuulasmaa K, Torppa J, for the World Health Organization MONICA Project. Geographic variation in mortality from cardiovascular diseases: WHO MONICA Project Principal Investigators. World Health Stat Q 1987;40:171—184.
4. Thom JT. Stroke mortality trends: and international perspective. Ann Epidemiol 1993;3: 509—518.
5. Lanska DJ, Peterson PM. Geographic variation in the decline of stroke mortality in the United States. Stroke 1995;26:1159—1165.
6. Tuomilehto J, Geboers J, Joossens JV, Wolf E. Trends in stomach cancer in Austria compared to selected Eastern and Western European Countries. Cancer Detect Prev 1987;10:311—319.
7. Rastenyte D, Tuomilehto J, Sarti C, Cepaitis Z, Bluzhas J. Trends in the incidence and mortality of stroke in Kaunas, Lithuania, 1986—1993. Cerebrovasc Dis 1996;6:13—20.
8. Vlajinac HD, Adanja BJ, Jarebinski MS, Sipetic SB. Cardiovascular disease mortality in Belgrade: trends from 1975—79. J Epidemiol Commun Health 1994;48:254—257.
9. Thorvaldsen P, Asplund K, Kuulasmaa K, Rajakangas AM, Schroll M, for the WHO MONICA Project. Stroke incidence, case fatality, and mortality in the WHO MONICA Project. Stroke 1995;26:361—367.
10. Aho K, Harmsen P, Hatano S, Marquardsen J, Smirnov VE, Strasser T. Cerebrovascular disease in the community; results of a WHO collaborative study. Bull WHO 1980;58:113—130.
11. Malmgren R, Warlow C, Bamford J, Sandercock P. Geographical and secular trends in stroke incidence. Lancet 1987;2:8569:1196—1200.
12. Terent A. Increasing incidence of stroke in Swedish women. Stroke 1988;19:598—603.
13. Harmsen P, Tsipogianni A, Wilhelmsen L. Stroke incidence rates were unchanged, while fatality rates declined during 1971—1987 in Göteborg, Sweden. Stroke 1992;23:1410—1415.
14. Wolfe CDA, Taub NA, Woodrow J, Richardson E, Warburton FG, Burney PGJ. Does the incidence, severity, or case-fatality of stroke vary in southern England? J Epidemiol Commun Health 1993;47:139—143.
15. Stegmayr B, Asplund K, Wester PO. Trends in incidence, case fatality rate, and severity of stroke in northern Sweden, 1985—1991. Stroke 1994;25:1738—1745.
16. Jørgensen HS, Plesner A-M, Hübbe P, Larsen K. Marked increase of stroke incidence in men between 1972 and 1990 in Frederiksberg, Denmark. Stroke 1992;23:1701—1704.
17. Thorvaldsen P, Kuulasmaa K, Rajakangas A-M, Rastenyte D, Sarti C, Wilhemsen L, for the WHO MONICA Project. Stroke Trends in the WHO MONICA Project. Stroke 1997;28:

500—506.
18. Asplund K, Tuomilehto J, Stegmayr B, Wester PO, Tunstall-Pedoe H. Diagnostic criteria and quality control of the registration of stroke events in the MONICA project. Acta Med Scand 1988;728(Suppl):26—39.
19. Asplund K, Bonita R, Kuulasmaa K, Rajakangas A-M, Feigin V, Schaedlich H, Suzuki K, Thorvaldsen P, Tuomilehto J, for the WHO MONICA Project. Multinational comparisons of stroke epidemiology: evaluation of case ascertainment in the WHO MONICA Stroke Study. Stroke 1995;26:355—360.
20. Tuomilehto J, Rastenyte D, Sivenius J, Sarti C, Immonen-Rähiä P, Kaarsalo E, Kuulasmaa K, Narva EV, Salomaa V, Salmi K, Torppa J. Ten year trends in stroke and mortality in the FINMONICA Stroke Study. Stroke 1996;27:825—832.
21. Numminen H, Kotila M, Waltimo O, Aho K, Kaste M. Declining incidence and mortality rates of stroke in Finland from 1972 to 1991. Results of three population-based registers. Stroke 1996;27:1487—1491.
22. Gillum RF, Sempos CT. The end of the long-term decline in stroke mortality in the United States? Stroke 1997;28:1527—1529.
23. McGovern P, Burke GL, Sprafka M, Xue S, Folsom AR, Blackburn H. Trends in mortality, morbidity, and risk-factor levels for stroke from 1960 through 1990. The Minnesota Heart Survey. JAMA 1992;268:753—759.
24. Shahar E, McGovern P, Pankow JS, Doliszny KM, Smith M, Blackburn H, Luepker RV. Stroke rates during the 1980s. The Minnesota Stroke Survey. Stroke 1997;28;275—279.
25. Vartiainen E, Sarti C, Tuomilehto J, Kuulasmaa K. Do changes in cardiovascular risk factors explain changes in mortality from stroke in Finland. Br Med J 1995;310:901—904.
26. Stegmayr B, Asplund K, Kuulasmaa K, Rajakangas AM, Thorvaldsen P, Tuomilehto J, for the WHO MONICA Project. Stroke incidence and mortality correlated to stroke risk factors in the WHO MONICA Project. An ecological study of 18 populations. Stroke 1997;28:1367—1374.

Secular trends in cardiovascular risk factor levels: a Framingham perspective

Peter W.F. Wilson[1], Ralph B. D'Agostino[2] and William B. Kannel[3]

[1]*Framingham Heart Study, National Heart Lung and Blood Institute, Framingham, Massachusetts;* [2]*Boston University, Boston; and* [3]*Boston University School of Medicine, Framingham, Massachusetts, USA*

Abstract. The purpose of this brief summary is to provide comparisons of risk-factor levels determined in 1966–1969 (original Framingham cohort) with levels measured in 1984–1988 (second generation Framingham offspring). Mean systolic pressure levels were lower in the second generation, diastolic-pressure levels were similar in each sample, and the proportion of persons on blood pressure therapy increased in both sexes. The fraction of persons reporting current cigarette smoking decreased and physical activity index was slightly higher, but mean body mass index levels were generally greater and a tendency toward overweight and severe overweight was very evident in men and women from the offspring sample. Total and LDL cholesterol levels were generally lower in the offspring, but there were no significant differences in mean triglycerides and HDL cholesterol compared to the cohort. Although coronary death rates have declined greatly in Framingham and the USA since 1970, evidence for a commensurate decrease in levels of coronary risk factors is less apparent, and differences in risk-factor levels account for only part of the decrease in coronary mortality.

Keywords: blood pressure, cholesterol, coronary heart disease, obesity, smoking.

Introduction

A decline of 40% or more in coronary heart disease (CHD) mortality has occurred in developed areas such as the USA, Canada, Australia and Western Europe over the past 25 years [1]. A commensurate decline in CHD morbidity, manifested as angina pectoris and myocardial infarction, has not occurred [2]. Over this interval there have been a variety of reports concerning trends in blood pressure and cholesterol levels [3], but studies of coronary risk factor levels from long-term studies have been less common.

This brief review provides estimates of risk factors from the Framingham Heart Study participants, drawing on the experience of the original and offspring cohort samples. It provides information on blood pressure, cholesterol and its subfractions, obesity and cigarette smoking.

Address for correspondence: Peter W.F. Wilson MD, Framingham Heart Study, NHLBI, 5 Thurber Street, Framingham, MA 01701, USA. Tel.: +1-508-935-3452, voice +1-508-626-1262. E-mail: peter@fram.nhlbi.nih.gov

660

Methods

The original cohort of the Framingham Heart Study has been examined every 2 years since the inception of the study in 1948. The study included 5,209 men and women who were residents of Framingham, Massachusetts, ranging in age from 30 to 62 years at the time of their initial examination. A second cohort, representing the children of the original cohort and their spouses, were examined initially in 1971 and have undergone examinations on a regular basis, typically at 4-year intervals since that time.

Clinical examinations included a cardiac history and a physical examination. Persons reporting regular cigarette smoking during the year prior to the clinic examination were considered smokers. Body mass index (BMI) (a measure of obesity) was calculated by dividing a subject's weight expressed in kilograms by height in meters squared. "Overweight" was present if the body mass index exceeded the 85th percentile for persons 20–29 years old in the second National Health and Nutrition Examination Survey (BMI $\geqslant$ 27.8 for men and $\geqslant$ 27.3 for women) [4]. Similarly, the criteria for "severe overweight" were the 95th percentile levels (BMI $\geqslant$ 31.1 for men and $\geqslant$ 32.2 for women). Blood pressure was determined in the sitting position with a mercury sphygmomanometer. Treated hypertension was considered present if the subject reported use of any antihypertensive medication. A physical-activity index (the weighted average of hours spent daily at various levels of exercise intensity) was calculated from the reported number of hours spent regularly at rest, sedentary, or at higher levels of exertion using previously published methods [5]. Cholesterol, HDL-cholesterol and triglyceride levels were determined from nonfasting specimens in 1957–1960 and fasting at later examinations. Established, previously published methods were employed and low-density lipoprotein cholesterol was estimated in persons with triglycerides less than 4 mmol/l using the Friedewald equation [6,7]. Data from the 1950s (original cohort exam 5), 1960s (original cohort exam 10) and 1980s (offspring cohort exam 3) were used in the comparisons, and comparisons were made after age adjustment using analysis of covariance techniques for continuous measures. The Mantel-Haenszel test of homogeneity was used to test for differences in categorical variables over time.

Results

Data from three time periods in men and two time periods in women were available for comparisons, and age adjusted mean values appear in Tables 1 and 2 for men and women, respectively. A significant downward trend in mean systolic pressure was observed in both sexes, but a similar decline in mean diastolic pressure was evident for women only. In addition, hypertension treatment was much more frequent at later time periods, and approximately 20% of the middle-aged offspring sample were taking hypertensive medications in the mid-1980s.

Cigarette smoking declined in both sexes from the 1950s to the 1980s, and

Table 1. Secular trends in age-adjusted mean risk factor levels: Framingham Heart Study. Men.

Risk factor	1957—1960 (aged 37—70, n = 435)	1966—1969 (aged 47—65, n = 865)	1984—1988 (aged 37—70, n = 1602)
Age (year)	50.7	55.9	50.7[****]
Systolic BP (mmHg)	131.2	134.2	129.3[****]
Diastolic BP (mmHg)	82.1	82.3	82.3
Treated hypertension (%)	0.9	5.8	21.5[****]
Cigarette smoking (%)	57.1	40.7	27.3[****]
Body mass index (kg/m^2)	25.8	26.9	27.4[****]
Overweight (%)	25.3	33.7	40.2[****]
Severe overweight (%)	5.4	10.3	14.8[****]
Physical activity (units)	32.3	34.3	35.4[***]
Total cholesterol (mmol/l)	5.94	5.71	5.57[****]
HDL cholesterol (mmol/l)	NA	1.17	1.14
LDL cholesterol (mmol/l)	NA	3.71	3.59[***]
Triglycerides (mmol/l)	NA	1.58	1.72

NA denotes not available. [****]p < 0.0001; [***]p < 0.001; [**]p < 0.01; [*]p < 0.05. (An increasing number of asterisks was used to denote greater statistical significance.)

mean body mass index tended to increase in both men and women. "Overweight" and "severe overweight" were also much more common conditions at the later study periods, despite a mild increase in the mean level of the physical activity index.

Mean cholesterol levels declined from 5.94 to 5.57 mmol/l, or approximately 6%, in men, and from 6.18 to 4.59, or 11%, in women over the study interval. The earlier determinations were made on plasma specimens and the later values were based on serum; as much as 4% of the decrease may be accounted for my

Table 2. Secular trends in age-adjusted mean risk factor levels: Framingham Heart Study. Women.

Risk factor	1957—1960 (aged 37—70, n = 473)	1984—1988 (aged 37—70, n = 1704)
Age (year)	50.4	50.2
Systolic BP (mmHg)	130.9	124.1[****]
Diastolic BP (mmHg)	80.6	78.3[****]
Treated hypertension (%)	6.1	19.1[****]
Cigarette smoking (%)	44.3	28.4[****]
Body mass index (kg/m^2)	24.9	25.7[***]
Overweight (%)	24.9	29.0
Severe overweight (%)	4.5	11.1[****]
Physical activity (units)	30.9	33.7[***]
Total cholesterol (mmol/l)	6.18	5.49[****]
HDL cholesterol (mmol/l)	NA	1.47
LDL cholesterol (mmol/l)	NA	3.47
Triglycerides (mmol/l)	NA	1.32

NA denotes not available. [****]p < 0.0001; [***]p < 0.001; [**]p < 0.01; [*]p < 0.05. (An increasing number of asterisks was used to denote greater statistical significance.)

changes in methodology [8]. Even after such considerations, there appear to be mild to moderate decreases in total cholesterol levels from the late 1950s to the mid 1980s. Although data were relatively scant for the lipoprotein cholesterol fractions, it appeared that the decline appeared to be greatest for the low-density lipoprotein (LDL) cholesterol component.

Discussion

In an investigation restricted to Framingham men and women of 50—59 years during the 1950s, 1960s and 1970s, a 51% decline in coronary heart disease mortality and a 20% decline in coronary heart disease morbidity were reported [9]. Data from the current article and other information published previously [10], demonstrate that the recent decline in coronary disease has been generally accompanied by lower blood pressure and more treatment for hypertension. Corroborative data are available from longitudinal studies in Minnesota and US national survey data [3,11—13].

Trends have also been generally downward for mean cholesterol levels among middle-aged adults in Framingham and other locations in the USA [3,12]. A comprehensive national survey detected little change in HDL and VLDL cholesterol from 1960 to 1991, and the authors concluded the decrease in total cholesterol levels was largely due to a decline in LDL cholesterol [14].

Cigarette smoking appears to be less common in Framingham men and women in recent times, and similar tendencies have been described in longitudinal data from the Minnesota Heart Survey, where they compared trends in smoking habits from the early 1980s to the mid-1980s, spanning an interval of approximately 5 years. In the Minnesota experience the prevalence of cigarette smoking declined from 42.1 to 36.3% in men and from 38.8 to 35.6% in women. On the other hand, the daily consumption of cigarettes by smokers remained constant in men, but actually increased in women [12].

In more recent times, obesity has become more common and this undesirable tendency counterbalances favorable trends observed for other risk factors. A general increase in obesity in the middle-aged American population is apparent from several different perspectives, including greater mean levels for body mass index, more persons "overweight" and more persons "severely overweight". In the USA these trends appear to translate into more diabetes mellitus, impaired glucose tolerance, hypertension and dyslipidemia in the population, especially among the middle-aged and elderly [15—18].

It is now possible, with the use of modern blood pressure and lipid-lowering therapies, to produce substantial improvements in the risk factor profile in persons at high risk of coronary heart disease. Short-term trials to date have effected only trivial reductions in the bulk of atherosclerotic lesions, but they have shown impressive slowing of the rate of progression of lesions, and even more impressive reduction in clinical events. This disproportionate reduction in clinical events suggests that medications, particularly the newer statins, may stabilize plaques and reduce the vulnerability to myocardial infarction.

Diet therapy alone has often been unable to achieve the lipid reductions recommended by the National Cholesterol Education Program. However, epidemiologic data indicate that the national diet is the chief determinant of the population level of blood lipids, and the main factors appear to be total fat intake, particularly saturated fat [10,19,20]. The decline in blood cholesterol among middle-aged persons in Framingham and other Western populations is no doubt linked to favorable dietary changes. On the other hand, dyslipidemia is worsening and CHD incidence is rising in several areas where CHD incidence rates have historically been low [1].

In the long run, the change in national diet has the greatest potential to produce a substantial reduction in dyslipidemia and CHD risk [21]. Although clinical practice stresses the identification of high-risk individuals, we must also take a public health view and emphasize that "sick populations" account for a heavy burden of chronic disease [22]. Even minor changes in risk-factor levels in a population setting may lead to less coronary heart disease morbidity and mortality.

References

1. Beaglehole R. International trends in coronary heart disease mortality, morbidity, and risk factors. Epid Rev 1990;12:1—15.
2. McGovern PG, Pankow JS, Shahar E, Doliszny KM, Folsom AR, Blackburn H, Luepker RV. Recent trends in acute coronary heart disease — mortality, morbidity, medical care, and risk factors. The Minnesota Heart Survey Investigators. N Engl J Med 1996;334:884—890.
3. Sempos CT, Cleeman JI, Carroll MD, Johnson CL, Bachorik PS, Gordon DJ, Burt VL, Briefel RR, Brown CD, Lippel K, Rifkind BM. Prevalence of high blood cholesterol among US adults: an update based on guidelines from the second report of the National Cholesterol Education Program Adult Treatment Panel. JAMA 1993;269:3009—3014.
4. Van Itallie TB. Health implications of overweight and obesity in the United States. Ann Int Med 1985;103:983—988.
5. Kannel WB, Sorlie PD. Some health benefits of physical activity: the Framingham Study. Arch Int Med 1979;139:857—861.
6. Lipid Research Clinics Program. Manual of Laboratory Operation. Bethesda: NIH, 1974; 75—628.
7. Friedewald WT, Levy RI, Fredrickson DS. Estimation of the concentration of low-density lipoprotein cholesterol in plasma, without the use of the preparative ultracentrifuge. Clin Chem 1972;18:499—502.
8. Cloey T, Bachorik PS, Becker D, Finney C, Lowry D, Sigmund W. Reevaluation of serum-plasma differences in total cholesterol concentration. JAMA 1990;263:2788—2789.
9. Sytkowski PA, D'Agostino RB, Belanger A, Kannel WB. Sex and time trends in cardiovascular disease incidence and mortality: the Framingham Heart Study, 1950—1989. Am J Epidemiol 1996;143:338—350.
10. Posner BM, Franz MM, Quatromoni PA, Gagnon DR, Sytkowski PA, D'Agostino RB, Cupples LA. Secular trends in diet and risk factors for cardiovascular disease: the Framingham Study. J Am Diet Assoc 1995;95:171—179.
11. Sytkowski PA, D'Agostino RB, Belanger AJ, Kannel WB. Secular trends in long-term sustained hypertension, long-term treatment and cardiovascular mortality. The Framingham Heart Study

1950 to 1990. Circulation 1996;93:697—703.

12. Luepker RV, Jacobs DR Jr, Folsom AR, Gillum RF, Frantz ID Jr, Gomez O, Blackburn H. Cardiovascular risk factor change — 1973—74 to 1980—82: the Minnesota Heart Survey. J Clin Epidemiol 1988;41:825—833.

13. Burke GL, Sprafka JL, Folsom AR, Hahn LP, Luepker RV, Blackburn H. Trends in serum cholesterol levels from 1980 to 1987 — The Minnesota Heart Survey. N Engl J Med 1991;324:941—946.

14. Johnson CL, Rifkind BM, Sempos CT, Carroll MD, Bachorik PS, Briefel RR, Gordon DJ, Burt VL, Brown CD, Lippel K, Cleeman JI. Declining serum total cholesterol levels among US adults: the National Health and Nutrition Examination Surveys. JAMA 1993;269:3002—3008.

15. Harris MI, Hadden WC, Knowler WC, Bennett PH. Prevalence of diabetes and impaired glucose tolerance and plasma glucose levels in US population aged 20—74 yrs. Diabetes 1987;36:523—534.

16. Kannel WB, Garrison RJ, Dannenberg AL. Secular blood pressure trends in normotensive persons: the Framingham Study. Am Heart J 1993;125:1154—1158.

17. Garrison RJ, Kannel WB, Stokes J, Castelli WP. Incidence and precursors of hypertension in young adults: the Framingham Offspring Study. Prev Med 1987;16:235—251.

18. Anderson KM, Wilson PWF, Garrison RJ, Castelli WP. Longitudinal and secular trends in lipoprotein cholesterol measurements in a general population sample: the Framingham Offspring Study. Atherosclerosis 1987;68:59—66.

19. Lee-Han H, McGuire V, Boyd NF. A review of the methods used by studies of dietary measurement. J Clin Epidemiol 1989;42:269—279.

20. Gotto AM Jr, LaRosa JC, Hunninghake D, Grundy SM, Wilson PWF, Clarkson TB, Hay JW. The cholesterol facts: a summary of the evidence relating dietary fats, serum cholesterol and coronary heart disease: a joint statement by the American Heart Association and the National Heart, Lung and Blood Institute. Circulation 1990;81:1721—1733.

21. Gotto AM. Cholesterol levels in young adults: screen and intervene? Hosp Pract (Off Ed) 1994;29:109—116.

22. Rose G. Sick individuals and sick populations. Int J Epidemiol 1985;14:32—38.

Gene therapy of atherosclerosis and restenosis

Novel approach to somatic gene therapy for dyslipidemia

Lawrence Chan, Kunihisa Kobayashi and Kazuhiro Oka
Departments of Cell Biology and Medicine, Baylor College of Medicine, Houston, Texas, USA

Abstract. Hyperlipoproteinemia involving very low density lipoproteins (VLDL), intermediate density lipoproteins (IDL), low-density lipoproteins (LDL) or lipoprotein(a) (lp(a)), is a major risk factor in atherosclerosis development. For patients with hyperlipidemia who do not respond adequately to other therapeutic interventions, somatic gene therapy is being explored as a treatment option. We have examined the therapeutic potential of the VLDL receptor (VLDLR) gene in experimental animals with LDL receptor (LDLR) deficiency. We found that adenovirus-mediated gene transfer of the VLDLR completely reverses the dyslipidemia of LDLR-knockout mice. The action of the VLDLR transgene is much more prolonged than that of the LDLR gene delivered by the same method, probably because cytotoxic T-lymphocyte response is induced only with LDLR (but not with VLDLR) expression in LDLR-deficient mice. Transgenic mice with hepatic expression of VLDLR are healthy, and VLDLR transgene expression in an LDLR-deficient background partially attenuates the associated hypercholesterolemia. VLDLR is a promising therapeutic gene in the treatment of hypercholesterolemia associated with LDLR deficiency.

Keywords: adenovirus, apolipoprotein E, hyperlipidemia, VLDL receptor.

Introduction

Hyperlipoproteinemia involving the atherogenic lipoproteins (VLDL, IDL, LDL and lp(a)) is a major risk factor in the development of atherosclerosis. In a non-diabetic patient presenting with high serum lipids, a number of therapeutic options are available [1]. The first step is to get the individual to adopt a more healthy lifestyle; such as proper diet and weight loss for those that are over their ideal body weight, to commit to an exercise program and to stop smoking (for smokers). If the diet (and weight loss) do not result in an acceptable plasma cholesterol level, a lipid-lowering agent will be the next line of defense. With the development of potent lipid-lowering drugs, especially the HMGCoA reductase inhibitor class of drugs (which are relatively free of side effects) and the emerging evidence that primary prevention may forestall an acute myocardial infarction, the use of such agents is now becoming an accepted form of treatment by many physicians. The majority of patients respond to lifestyle changes plus the latest generation of lipid-lowering drugs and do not need any other therapeutic inter-

Address for correspondence: Dr Lawrence Chan, Departments of Cell Biology and Medicine, Baylor College of Medicine, One Baylor Plaza, Houston, TX 77030, USA. Tel.: +1-713-798-4478. Fax: +1-713-798-8764.

vention. However, a sizeable minority do not show an adequate response and are candidates for more drastic or experimental forms of treatment.

Some of these forms of treatment are of historical interest. Portacaval shunts were serendipitously found to be associated with substantial lowering of serum cholesterol [2]. However, the operation has never been considered seriously as a form of treatment because of major side effects. Similarly in a clinical trial, partial ileal bypass was found to result in a marked reduction in plasma cholesterol and mortality from coronary artery disease [3]. The trial was initiated before the availability of the potent lipid-lowering drugs developed in the last two decades. Nowadays, this study is largely of historical interest. The requirement for a major surgical operation and the associated side effects make it unacceptable as a form of treatment for hypercholesterolemia.

Two other drastic forms of treatment, liver transplantation and extracorporeal LDL removal, are still used under unusual circumstances. Combined heart-liver transplantation in patients with homozygous familial hypercholesterolemia (FH) has been found to be effective in replacing a heart damaged by coronary artery disease and supplying the body with normal LDLR function in the transplanted liver [4]. Such a drastic surgical operation should be considered in FH patients who have sustained irreparable cardiac damage. Transplantation of the liver only can probably be justified for some other FH patients with limited coronary heart disease but marked hypercholesterolemia who do not respond to drugs. For others, extracorporeal LDL removal is a procedure that effectively lowers plasma LDL [5]. Unfortunately, since the basic pathology is not altered, there is rapid reaccumulation of plasma LDL and the procedure is only a temporizing measure that must be repeated usually every 2 weeks.

Thus, since liver transplantation is such a major surgical operation and extracorporeal LDL removal is not a true "cure", new forms of treatment for hyperlipoproteinemia are clearly needed. Somatic gene therapy is an experimental solution to this problem that may represent a paradigm shift in our approach to hyperlipidemia in the future.

VLDL receptor

The VLDLR is a member of the expanding mammalian LDLR gene family that also includes LDLR, LDLR-related protein, glycoprotein 330 (for review see [6,7]), apolipoprotein (apo) receptor 2 [8], LR8B [9] and LR11 [10]. All members are characterized by common structural features, including:
1) cysteine-rich repeats consisting of ~ 40 amino acid residues in the ligand binding domain or in complement-type domain;
2) epidermal growth factor precursor-type repeats;
3) module of ~ 50 amino acid residues with a consensus tetrapeptide, YWTD;
4) a single transmembrane domain; and
5) a cytoplasmic domain containing an NPXY sequence required for clustering of the receptor into coated pits.

The VLDLR is structurally closely related to LDLR, except that it contains an 8-fold repeat in the ligand-binding domain instead of a 7-fold repeat in LDLR. The VLDLR is expressed in muscle, heart, adipose tissue and numerous other tissues except liver. The natural ligand for the VLDLR is unknown. In vitro, it binds to apoE-containing lipoproteins [6,7].

Use of the VLDLR as a therapeutic gene

The VLDLR has been tested as a therapeutic gene in LDLR-deficient mice in two laboratories [11,12]. LDLR-knockout mice developed significant hypercholesterolemia (up to about 400 mg/dl in our study) when they were fed a high-fat high-cholesterol diet. We treated the hypercholesterolemic mice intravenously with a replication-defective adenoviral vector containing the mouse VLDLR gene (AdmVLDLR) or a control gene, β-galactosidase (AdLacZ), (both at 3×10^9 pfu per animal) or with a similar volume of phosphate-buffered saline (Mock). In the AdmVLDLR-treated mice, there was a 50—60% drop in plasma cholesterol on day 4 and 9. AdLacZ- and Mock-treated controls did not display any change in cholesterol. By day 21 the plasma cholesterol started returning toward control levels. During this 3-week period, there was no difference in plasma triglyceride among the three groups. We analyzed the plasma lipoproteins on day 4 of treatment. Mock- and AdLacZ-treated mice had markedly elevated cholesterol in the IDL/LDL fraction. In AdmVLDLR-treated animals, the marked hypolipidemic response was almost exclusively confined to this fraction, which went down by >80%. We next measured the disappearance rate of ^{125}I-lipoproteins in AdmVLDLR and AdLacZ animals 4 days after treatment. The rate was 5- to 10-fold faster in AdmLDLR mice compared to the AdLacZ mice. Therefore, induced hepatic expression of VLDLR resulted in an accelerated removal of IDL in the circulation, which in turn reduced the plasma concentration of LDL, its metabolic product.

We further compared the hypolipidemic response of VLDLR and LDLR delivered by the respective adenoviruses. We found that the VLDLR response lasted about 3-fold longer than the LDLR response. This finding corroborates that of Kozarsky et al. [12]. The substantially attenuated response to LDLR appears to be the result of a cytotoxic T-lymphocyte response elicited by LDLR but not by VLDLR [12]. In LDLR-deficient mice, the appearance of normal LDLR is recognized as a foreign protein and the body mounts a cytotoxic T-lymphocyte response to the protein, destroying cells carrying the protein in the process. In contrast, the VLDLR is a cellular protein normally present in various nonhepatic tissues of LDLR-deficient mice, and is not treated as a foreign protein when it is expressed ectopically in the liver. In this respect the VLDLR may be superior to LDLR as a therapeutic gene in the treatment of FH.

Other considerations for the future

We and others have shown that the VLDLR is an effective hypolipidemic gene in animal models of FH [11,12]. It is likely that it can be applied to other non-FH hyperlipidemic states, as long as elevation of IDL/LDL is a major abnormality. Furthermore, since the VLDLR appears to require apoE as a ligand, the coexpression of an apoE adenoviral vector in the liver might enhance the hypolipidemic response of VLDLR.

Despite the lack of a cytotoxic T-lymphocyte response, AdmVLDLR-treated animals display only a transient hypolipidemic response, because the early generation adenoviral vectors can effect only transient transgene expression. In the past year, novel adenoviral vectors that have all their endogenous viral protein genes deleted have become available [13] and an efficient helper virus-dependent vector production system has been developed [14]. Use of these adenoviral vectors should produce a therapeutic response that lasts many months or longer. Transient immunosuppression should also allow the effective readministration of the vector [15]. Application of such a strategy should enhance the usefulness of the VLDLR gene in the treatment of hyperlipidemia.

Finally, it is not clear if the ectopic expression of the VLDLR in the liver is associated with any abnormalities in liver function. We have generated transgenic mice with hepatic expression of VLDLR. These animals appear healthy; they are partially protected against the hyperlipidemia associated with LDLR deficiency when they are bred into an $LDLR^{-/-}$ background. However, an in-depth investigation into the pathophysiology of hepatic VLDLR expression must be undertaken before we can conclude that the hepatic expression of VLDLR is completely innocuous. Further experimentation with this animal model is clearly indicated.

Acknowledgements

The work described in this manuscript performed in the authors' laboratory was supported by grants HL-16512 and HL-59314 from the US National Institutes of Health.

References

1. Chan L, Boerwinkle E. Gene-environment interactions and gene therapy in atherosclerosis. Cardiol Rev 1994;2:130–137.
2. Starzl TE, Putnam CW, Chase HP, Porter KA. Portacaval shunt in hyperlipoproteinemia. Lancet 1973;2:940–944.
3. Buchwald H, Varco RL, Matts JP. Effect of partial ileal bypass surgery on mortality and morbidity from coronary heart disease in patients with hypercholesterolemia. N Engl J Med 1990; 323:946–955.
4. Bilheimer DW, Goldstein JL, Grundy SM, Starzl TE, Brown MS. Liver transplantation to provide low-density lipoprotein receptors and lower plasma cholesterol in a child with homozygous

familial hypercholesterolemia. N Engl J Med 1984;311:1658—1664.

5. Gordon BR, Saal SD. Advances in LDL-apheresis for the treatment of severe hypercholesterolemia. Curr Opin Lipid 1994;5:69—73.

6. Jingami H, Yamamoto T. The VLDL receptor: wayward brother of the LDL receptor. Curr Opin Lipid 1995;6:104—108.

7. Strickland DK, Kounnas MZ, Argraves WS. LDL receptor-related protein: a multiligand receptor for lipoprotein and proteinase catabolism. FASEB J 1995;9:890—898.

8. Multhaupt HAB, Gafvels ME, Hariko K, Jin H, Arenas-Elliott C, Goldman BI et al. Expression of very low density lipoprotein receptor in the vascular wall. Analysis of human tissues by in situ hybridization and immunohistochemistry. Am J Pathol 1996;148:1985—1997.

9. Novak S, Hiesberger T, Schneider WJ, Nimpf J. A new low-density lipoprotein homologue with 8 ligand binding repeats in brain of chicken and mouse. J Biol Chem 1996;271:11732—11736.

10. Yamazaki H, Bujo H, Kusunoki J, Seimiya K, Kanaki T, Morisaki N et al. Elements of neural adhesion molecules and a yeast vacuolar protein sorting receptor are present in a novel mammalian low-density lipoprotein receptor family member. J Biol Chem 1996;271:24761—24768.

11. Kobayashi K, Oka K, Forte T, Ishida BY, Teng B-B, Ishimura-Oka K et al. Reversal of hypercholesterolemia in low-density lipoprotein receptor knockout mice by adenovirus-mediated gene transfer of the very low density lipoprotein receptor. J Biol Chem 1996;271:6851—6860.

12. Kozarsky KF, Jooss K, Donahee M, Strauss III JF, Wilson JM. Effective treatment of familial hypercholesterolaemia in the mouse model using adenovirus-mediated transfer of the VLDL receptor gene. Nature Genet 1996;13:54—62.

13. Kochanek S, Clemens PR, Mitani K, Chen H-H, Chan S, Caskey CT. A new adenoviral vector: replacement of all viral coding sequences with 28kb of DNA independently expressing both full-length dystrophin and β-galactosidase. Proc Natl Acad Sci USA 1996;93:5731—5736.

14. Parks RJ, Chen L, Anton M, Sankar U, Rudnicki MA, Graham FL. A helper-dependent adenovirus vector system: removal of helper virus by Cre-mediated excision of the viral packaging signal. Proc Natl Acad Sci USA 1996;93:13565—13570.

15. Kay MA, Holterman A-X, Meuse L, Gown A, Ochs HD, Linsley PS et al. Long-term hepatic adenovirus-mediated gene expression in mice following CTLA4Ig administration. Nature Genet 1995;11:191—197.

Gene therapy of vascular disorders. Use of gax gene transfer as a molecular strategy to prevent postangioplasty restenosis

Aude Le Roux[1], Luc Maillard[2], Valérie Conard[1], Nathalie Ratet[1], Harris Perlman[2], Abderrahim Mahfoudi[1], Jeffrey M. Isner[2], Kenneth Walsh[2] and Didier Branellec[1]

[1]*Rhône-Poulenc Rorer Gencell, Centre de recherche de Vitry-Alfortville, Vitry sur Seine, France; and* [2]*Division of Cardiovascular Research, St. Elizabeth's Medical Center and Tufts University School of Medicine, Boston, Massachusetts, USA*

Introduction

The excessive proliferation of vascular smooth muscle cells (V-SMCs) is a key event for coronary restenosis that occurs in 30—50% of patients undergoing balloon angioplasty and is the major cause of in-stent restenosis [1,2]. In the neointima lesion V-SMCs exhibit a synthetic or embryonic phenotype which is characterized by enhanced growth activities, reorganization of the cytoskeleton and suppressed contractile activities.

Until now the interaction between cell growth regulation and transcription factors involved in proliferation and differentiation of V-SMCs has not been well-understood. The homeobox containing transcription factors have been implicated in cell differentiation and migration, and abnormal expression of some of these factors is associated with deregulation of cell growth. Recently a growth-arrest homeobox gene (gax) has been cloned [3,4]. Its expression is rapidly downregulated in V-SMCs after mitogen stimulation in vitro, or after vascular injury in vivo. The downregulation in response to mitogen stimulation is dose-dependent and correlates with enhanced DNA synthesis. On the contrary, in conditions that favor differentiation or cell-cycle arrest the expression of gax is upregulated [5]. In adults, rat gax expression is restricted to cardiovascular tissues (including the V-SMCs), thus suggesting a possible role of gax in the control of V-SMCs growth and differentiation. In fact, we previously showed that overexpression of gax increases the expression of the cdk inhibitor p21$^{\text{CIP1}}$ in rat V-SMCs and inhibits the neointima formation in a model of rat carotid injury [5]. Here, we examine the growth-regulatory properties of gax homeoprotein in vitro towards rabbit primary V-SMC as well as in a rabbit model in vivo of arterial stenosis. Primary smooth muscle cells, like other cell types are known to be relatively refractory to recombinant adenoviral infection because of a low level of adenovirus receptor [6,7]. We previously developed a new method based on noncovalent

Address for correspondence: Aude Le Roux, Rhône-Poulenc Rorer Gencell, Centre de recherche de Vitry-Alfortville, 94003 Vitry sur Seine, France.

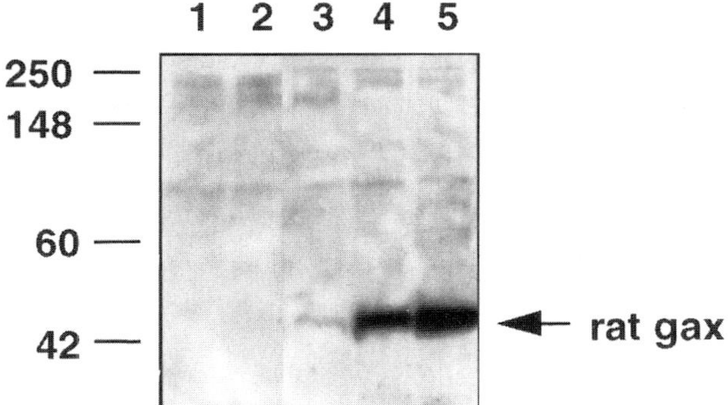

Fig. 1. Immunoblot analysis of gax expression in rabbit V-SMCs. Cells were infected at MOI 10^3, 3 10^3 and 10^4 VP/cell with $AV_{1.0}$CMVrGax (3–5) or with $AV_{1.0}$CMVβGal at 3 10^3 VP/cell (1) and 10^4 VP/cell (2). Whole cell extracts were prepared 24 h postinfection. gax protein was detected using polyclonal antibodies raised against gax.

association of cationic lipids with recombinant adenovirus to transduce V-SMC (manuscript in preparation). Here, we used the process cationic lipid-associated adenoviral transduction (referred to as CLAAT) and showed that it is also useful to study cytotoxic gene activity in vitro.

Several cytostatic gene-based approaches are designed to target specific cell cycle regulatory pathways thereby inhibiting SMC proliferation in vivo. Most of these approaches used recombinant viruses encoding tumor-suppressor genes like the retinoblastoma gene product [8,9], p53, or cell cycle inhibitors such as the cyclin-dependent kinase inhibitor p21/waf1/cip1 [10]. However, expression of these genes has not been shown to be dramatically modified during smooth muscle cell proliferation. Albeit using recombinant adenovirus-mediated overexpression, gax-gene replacement in proliferating SMCs is likely to approach a physiological growth arrest of this cell type. Here, we reported preclinical data supporting the potential use of the homeoprotein gax to modulate vascular lesion formation in a rabbit model.

Materials and Methods

Cell culture

Rabbit primary V-SMCs were obtained by enzymatic digestion of the media from iliac arteries of New Zealand White rabbit according to the method of Mader and used before passage 10 in DMEM with penicillin/streptomycin, glutamin and FBS [11].

Replication-defective adenovirus preparation

The adenoviral vector encoding gax used in this study has been described previously (Roy Smith, 1997 [9]). $AV_{1.0}CMV$ and $AV_{1.0}CMV\beta Gal$ were constructed using homologous recombination in *Escherichia coli* as described by Crouzet et al. [12]. $AV_{1.0}CMV$ contains the CMV promoter and SV40 late polyA in place of E1 adenovirus sequences but encodes no transgene. Viral preparations were purified by two CsCl gradient centrifugation, desalted on PD10 columns (Pharmacia), eluted in PBS and stored at $-70°C$ in PBS-10% glycerol. The titer in VP/cell was determined by HPLC. Titration by plaque assay on 293 cells was also performed to determine the number of plaque forming units per ml (pfu/ml) as previously described [13].

Adenovirus infection in vitro and cell proliferation assay

Cells were plated at 75% confluence in 48-well tissue culture dishes in DMEM with 10% FBS overnight. Adenovirus infection was carried out at different MOIs in DMEM with 0.5% FBS 1 h at 37°C. The virus-containing medium was removed and cells were incubated in DMEM with 0.5% FBS for 24 h. The culture medium was then changed to DMEM 10% FBS and cells incubated at 37°C for 48 h to allow cell-cycle progression. Cell viability was determined using Alamar blue assay according to the instructions of the manufacturer (Biosource).

Western blot analysis

Polyclonal antibodies to the gax protein were generated by immunizing rabbits against peptide encoded for in the C-terminus of gax protein (GTLLPSELSGI-GAATLQQTG) which is conserved between rat and human gax protein.

Whole cell extracts were harvested from infected V-SMC 24 h postinfection. The extracts corresponding to 10^4 viable cells were analyzed by SDS-Page on a 10% polyacrylamide gel (Novex) and transferred to nitrocellulose (Amersham) by semidry blotting. Filters were soaked 15 min at room temperature in phosphate-buffered saline (PBS)/0.2% tween 20/5% nonfat dry milk (blocking solution). They were then incubated with the polyclonal antigax antibody 154 diluted to 0.1 μg/ml in blocking solution. Filters were washed with the blocking solution and then incubated in a 1/2,000 dilution of horseradish peroxidase-coupled goat polyclonal antibodies raised against rabbit IgGs (Nordic immunology). Immune complexes were visualized by Enhanced Chemiluminescence kit (Amersham).

Immunostaining

Rabbit V-SMCs were plated at five 10^4 cells/well in growth medium in 4 chambers slides (Labtek). Adenovirus infection was carried out in low serum medium for 1 h after which the virus solution was removed and replaced by DMEM 10% FBS. 24 h postinfection, cells were fixed 5 min with PBS 4% formaldehyde and permeabilized with PBS 0.2% Triton X-100. Cells were incubated for 30 min in the blocking solution (PBS 0.5% FBS) with the polyclonal antigax antibody 154 used at a final concentration of 10 μg/ml. Antibodies were removed by washes with PBS and then cells were incubated for 30 min in FITC- or TRITC-conjugated goat IgGs raised against rabbit IgGs (working dilution 1/50, Sigma). Cells were rinsed with PBS and incubated 15 min in PBS/DAPI (0.2 μg/ml). Slides were mounted and visualized by fluorescent microscopy. TUNEL labeling was performed according to in situ apoptosis detection kit (ONCOR: Apoptag Direct).

Cationic lipid-associated adenoviral transduction (CLAAT)

Cells were plated at five 10^4 cells per well in 48-well tissue culture plates in DMEM with 10% FBS overnight. Dilutions of adenovirus were mixed with 60 ng per well of lipofectamine (Gibco BRL) and the final volume was adjusted to 25 μl with PBS. This solution was incubated 30 min at room temperature. Growth medium was replaced by 175 μl of serum-free DMEM and the adeno-virus-lipofectamine mix was added to the cells. The virus-containing medium was removed and cells incubated in DMEM 0.5% FBS for 24 h. Cell proliferation was then triggered by adding high-serum medium. Cell viability was evaluated 72 h postinfection using the Alamar blue assay.

Percutaneous arterial gene transfer and balloon angioplasty in vivo

Local gene delivery was performed using a channel balloon catheter introduced via the right common carotid and then advanced into the external iliac artery immediately distal to the origin of the internal iliac artery. Each animal received four 10^9 pfu (plaque forming unit) of $AV_{1.0}$CMVrGax in the iliac artery and the same dose of $AV_{1.0}$CMVβGal in the contralateral artery. Control animals were treated with the same dose of $AV_{1.0}$CMVβGal and PBS using the same model of bilateral delivery. The effect of gax overexpression vs. β-galactosidase was evaluated 1 month after gene transfer by light microscopic examination and quantitative morphometric analysis on longitudinal section.

Results

Expression of gax following infection of rabbit V-SMCs by a replication defective adenovirus encoding gax

To examine the effects of gax on primary rabbit V-SMCs, a replication defective adenovirus encoding the full length rat gax c-DNA was constructed. The resulting adenovirus referred to as $AV_{1.0}$CMVrGax, contains the amino-terminal peptide sequence to the influenza hemagglutinin epitope (HA) fused in frame to rat gax and its expression is under control of the cytomegalovirus (CMV) promoter (Smith et al. 1997 [9]). The growth properties of gax were compared to those of control adenoviruses containing no transgene ($AV_{1.0}CMV$) or encoding the gene of the β-galactosidase under the control of the CMV promoter ($AV_{1.0}CMV\beta$ Gal).

The expression level of gax after infection of rabbit V-SMCs with $AV_{1.0}CMVr$-Gax at multiplicities of infection (MOIs) between 1,000 and 10,000 viral particles (VP)/cell was determined by Western blotting analysis. Whole cell extracts were harvested 24 h postinfection. We observed expression of a 42 kD protein corresponding to the HA tagged rat gax protein in the $AV_{1.0}CMVrGax$ infected V-SMCs compared to uninfected cells or $AV_{1.0}CMV\beta Gal$ infected cells (Fig. 1). The level of gax protein expression correlated with the MOI used to infect rabbit V-SMCs. The endogenous gax protein was not detectable in these culture and assay conditions.

To determine the number of V-SMCs expressing the transgene, immunostaining was performed on cells infected by $AV_{1.0}CMVrGax$ at different MOIs using the same rabbit polyclonal antigax antibodies. 100% of the $AV_{1.0}CMVrGax$ infected cells expressed the gax protein at MOIs equal or superior to 10^4 VP/cell. The protein was uniformly distributed in the nucleus (data not shown).

Inhibition of cell proliferation by overexpression of gax using a replication defective adenovirus

$AV_{1.0}CMVrGax$ was used to examine the effects of gax overexpression on primary rabbit V-SMCs growth. Cells were infected at MOIs between 10^3 VP/cell

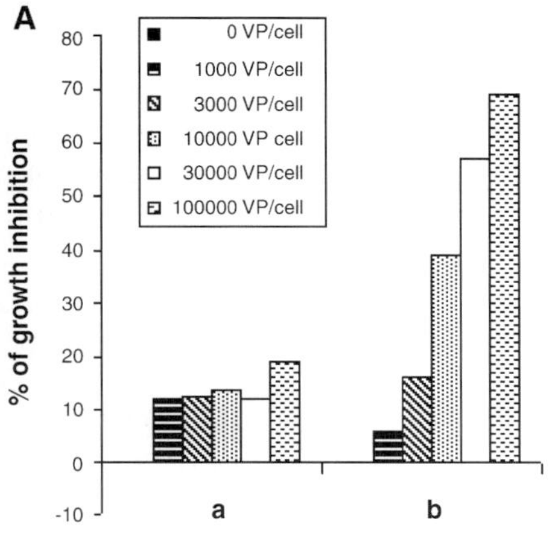

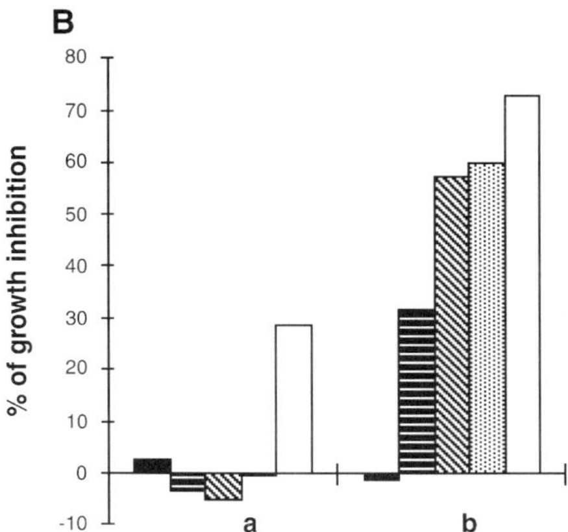

Fig. 2. Inhibition of rabbit V-SMCs proliferation by overexpression of gax using adenovirus alone (**A**) or CLAAT (**B**). Cells were infected at MOI 0 to 10^5 VP/cell with $AV_{1.0}CMV$ (**a**) or with $AV_{1.0}CMVr$-Gax (**b**) or using CLAAT at MOI between 0 and 3 10^4 VP/cell. After infection cells were incubated in low serum medium for 24 h. Cell cycle progression was then triggered by adding high serum containing medium. Forty-eight hours postserum stimulation, cell viability was determined by Alamar blue assay.

and 10^5 VP/cell. After infection cells were incubated in low-serum medium for 24 h. Growth medium was then added for 48 h to allow cell-cycle progression. Cell viability was determined using Alamar blue assay. A 50% decrease in cell viability at 48 h postserum stimulation was observed in the $AV_{1.0}$CMVrGax infected cells compared to the quiescent control cells (i.e., cells infected with $AV_{1.0}$CMVrGax and maintained in low-serum medium) when the MOIs used ranged between 10^3 and three 10^4 PV/cell (Fig. 2A). The viability of cells infected at higher MOIs was slightly affected in low serum-containing medium. Following these 48 h of serum stimulation, a 4-fold increase in cell number was recorded in noninfected cells.

Cationic lipids improve replication defective adenovirus transduction of primary smooth muscle cells

Rabbit SMCs are known to exhibit moderate levels of the fiber receptor [7]. Therefore, the MOIs required to transduce 100% rabbit SMCs are very high, ranging from 1 to 3 10^4 PV/cell. To bypass the fiber receptor deficiency, we have mixed first generation recombinant adenovirus encoding either the *E. coli* β-galactosidase gene or the luciferase gene with the commercial cationic liposome Lipofectamine (GIBCO-BRL). We observed an increase of adenovirus uptake and transgene expression up to 10-fold in rabbit SMCs (manuscript in preparation). To further extend these data from a marker to a therapeutic gene, rabbit SMCs were infected by $AV_{1.0}$CMVrGax at different MOIs using CLAAT. After infection, cells were maintained in low serum containing medium. 24 h postinfection, cell growth was triggered by adding fresh medium containing 10% serum. Cell viability was assessed 48 h later using Alamar blue assay (Fig. 2B). Our results clearly show that lipofectamine alone has no effect on cell viability. Interestingly, the MOI necessary to obtain 50% of growth inhibition is 10-fold lower than the MOI used with $AV_{1.0}$CMVrGax alone. This effect is correlated with a 10-fold increase of gax expression when CLAAT is used to transduce rabbit SMCs (data not shown). There is an increase in the same range of $AV_{1.0}$CMVrGax toxicity and the nonspecific effect of $AV_{1.0}$CMV (which contains no transgene) which is probably due to the overall improvement of adenovirus uptake. Thus CLAAT, although not improving the differential of cell toxicity between $AV_{1.0}$CMVrGax and control viruses, allows the use of lower MOIs.

Gax overexpression induces apoptosis in rabbit vascular smooth muscle cells

Apoptosis is a noninflammatory mechanism of cell death and is characterized by cellular and cytoplasmic shrinkage, maintenance of membrane integrity and by DNA fragmentation and condensation. Fragmentation of DNA can be visualized on a single-cell level by fluorescent labelling of DNA ends using a terminal transferase (TdT). The widely used TUNEL method (TdT mediated dUTP-fluorescein nick-ends labeling) is based on the specific binding of TdT enzyme to the exposed 3'-OH of fragmented DNA and the terminal addition of labelled deoxynucleotide molecules. After infection of rabbit V-SMCs, we showed that in individual cells transduced with $AV_{1.0}CMVrGax$, gax immunolabelling cosegregates with genomic DNA nicks revealed by the TUNEL method. Same results have been obtained after transduction of rat or human V-SMC and were obtained in transient transfection of rabbit V-SMCs using an gax expression vector, this precluding a nonspecific apoptotic effect due to adenovirus per se (Fig. 3).

Percutaneous delivery of gax inhibits neointimal formation in a rabbit model of balloon angioplasty

Data depicted above clearly show that $AV_{1.0}CMVrGax$ encoding rat gax efficiently blocks proliferation of serum-stimulated rabbit V-SMCs. We previously demonstrated that $AV_{1.0}CMVrGax$ can inhibit luminal narrowing and neointimal formation when transferred locally into balloon-injured rat carotid. The goal of our study was to test whether these data could be extended in a rabbit model of percutaneous gene transfer. Local gene delivery was performed using a channel balloon catheter into the external iliac artery and each animal received four 10^9 pfu of $AV_{1.0}CMVrGax$ and the same dose of $AV_{1.0}CMV\beta Gal$ using a model of bilateral delivery described in "Material and Methods". The effect of gax overexpression vs. βgalactosidase was evaluated 1 month after gene transfer by light microscopic examination and quantitative morphometric analysis on longitudinal section. In $AV_{1.0}CMVrGax$ treated arteries, the area of the intima to that of the

DAPI   **TUNEL**   **ANTI-GAX**

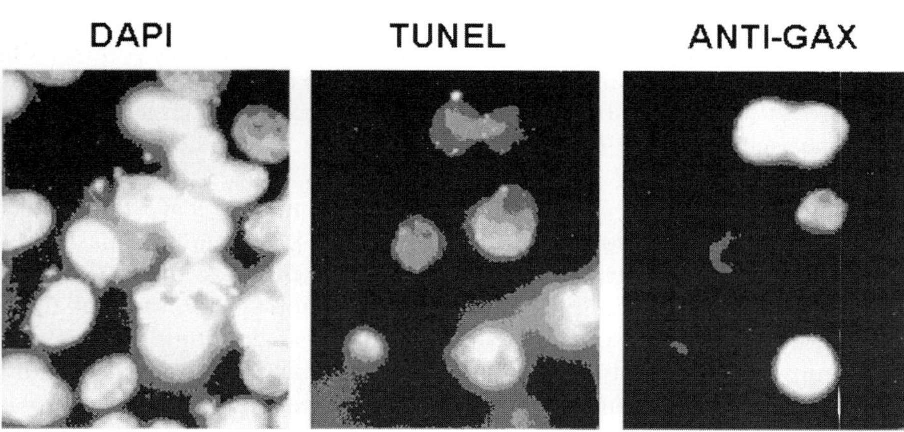

Fig. 3. Gax and TUNEL signals are colocalized in transiently transfected SMC. Rabbit SMCs were transiently transfected with a plasmid encoding human gax under the control of the CMV promoter. Twenty-four hours following the transfection, SMCs were processed for immunofluorescence. Cell nuclei were stained for DNA using DAPI. TUNEL (Terminal transferase dUTP-Fluorescein nick-end labeling) was used to visualize apoptotic cells. Human gax was detected by indirect immunofluorescence using polyclonal antibodies raised against gax. Note that gax exhibits a nuclear localization and cosegregates with TUNEL positive nuclei.

680

media (I/M ratio) was 56% less than the I/M ratios in the contralateral $AV_{1.0}CMV\beta Gal$ treated arteries ($AV_{1.0}CMVrGax = 0.35 \pm 0.15$; $AV_{1.0}CMV\beta Gal = 0.8 \pm 0.18$; $p < 0.02$). In contrast, no significant difference between the $AV_{1.0}CMV\beta Gal$ and the contralateral PBS-treated animals was observed in the control group ($AV_{1.0}CMV\beta Gal = 0.81 \pm 0.19$; PBS $= 0.84 \pm 0.21$; p = ns). We concluded that local delivery of $AV_{1.0}CMVrGax$ in the iliac artery with conventional angioplasty balloon reduces neointima formation. Further studies on the gax transferred arteries have shown that the re-endothelialization and vasomotor reactivity were not significantly affected at the site of vessel injury, whereas lumen diameter was significantly increased in gax-treated vessels [14].

Conclusion

Percutaneous transluminal angioplasty is a noninvasive method that is widely used for debulking of occluded arteries. However, it has the disadvantage of recurrent restenosis owing to vascular constrictive remodeling and extensive migration and proliferation of the medial smooth muscle cells. Vascular remodeling has been significantly attenuated by the spreading use of intravascular stents [15]. Nonetheless, proliferation of SMCs in the vascular wall still plays a key role in vascular reocclusion following angioplasty as well as stenting.

Transition of SMC from a quiescent and contractile phenotype to migratory and proliferating cells correlates with a dramatic change in the expression of genes involved in various pathways such as cellular oncogene expression, production of extracellular and adhesion molecules. Recently, Gorski et al. have identified a growth arrest-specific homeobox gene (gax) which expression is rapidly downregulated by mitogens and is gradually upregulated by conditions that lead to growth arrest in vitro [3]. In vivo, gax expression in adults is largely confined to the cardiovascular tissues, including the resting SMC of the aorta wall and is rapidly downregulated after acute vessel wall injury [16]. Microinjection of recombinant gax protein as well as adenoviral gene transfer have been lately shown to efficiently arrest growth of cultured SMCs [5]. Moreover, Yamashita et al. reported that C-type natriuretic peptide (CNP), which can act as a rat V-SMCs growth inhibitor, increases gax mRNA expression [17]. Altogether these data suggest that; firstly, gax plays an important role in maintaining the contractile and nonmigrating phenotype of quiescent smooth muscle cells; and secondly, possesses growth inhibition properties and could mediate those of other molecules like CNP.

Our data clearly show that gax-mediated gene transfer efficiently blocks rabbit V-SMC proliferation in vitro, thus confirming our recent data in human and rat smooth muscle cell models [5]. We previously reported that adenovirus-mediated overexpression of gax led to G0/G1 cell cycle arrest in V-SMC through a p21-dependent mechanism within 24 h following addition of serum. Interestingly, at longer time points following addition of serum (48–72 h), a marked apoptosis can be observed in V-SMCs. Such a cell death could not be observed neither in V-SMCs incubated with a control adenovirus nor in quiescent V-SMCs (i.e., not exposed to high serum concentration) transduced with similar MOIs of $AV_{1.0}CMVrGax$. Taken together, our data show that gax overexpression selectively triggers apoptosis in serum-stimulated V-SMCs. However, this effect can be achieved only at high amounts of gax recombinant adenovirus.

Human adenoviruses efficiently infect a variety of cell types through a two-step process. First, the viral fiber interacts with one cell surface receptor which mediates attachment of the adenovirus particle to the surface of the target cell [18,19]. The subsequent association of the penton base RGD sequences with cell surface $\alpha_v\beta_3$ and/or $\alpha_v\beta_5$ integrins which act as coreceptors potentiates virus internalization by endocytosis [6]. The major hurdle to adenovirus-mediated gene transfer into the blood vessel wall is that the level of receptors to mediate the primary step of virus attachment via its fiber coat protein is not sufficient in both endothelial and smooth muscle cells. Several approaches have been successfully developed to circumvent this fiber receptor-mediated binding:
1) the targeting of the α_v integrins by modifying the penton RGD or by introducing a Flag epitope within the penton base; and
2) the use of bispecific monoclonal antibodies against the integrins [7].

By combining a cationic lipid with its property as a vehicle and the adenovirus with its active interaction with cell surface targets, it is possible to synergistically increase the transduction efficiency of recombinant adenoviruses (manuscript in preparation). Our data clearly show that by assisting adenoviral transduction with a cationic lipid, a maximal effect of gax on cell growth can be obtained with 10-fold less recombinant virus.

Several gene-based approaches have been reported to inhibit in vivo SMC proliferation following balloon angioplasty. Recombinant adenoviruses encoding tumor-suppressor genes like the retinoblastoma gene product [8,9] or cell cycle inhibitors such as the cyclin-dependent kinase inhibitor p21/waf1/cip1 [10] were successfully used to reduce neointima formation in the rat carotid. Delivery of the thymidine kinase (tk) gene combined with ganciclovir (GCV) was reported to inhibit neointima formation in a rat carotid model as well as in an atheromatous rabbit model [20,21]. We previously showed that gax compares favorably with Rb, p21 or tk in the injured rat-carotid model [8—10,20]. In this study, we have extended the results to a stenosis rabbit model. In fact, when recombinant adenovirus encoding gax was locally delivered in a rabbit model of vascular injury, a significant decrease in neointima formation was observed. Whether gax inhibitory effect on vascular lesion formation results in part from triggering of apoptosis needs to be further investigated. It must be outlined that V-SMC apoptosis has been described upon arterial remodeling during embryogenesis as well as in animal models of vessel wall stenosis [22,23].

These results suggest that $AV_{1.0}CMVrGax$ may be used for the treatment of proliferative vessel wall disorders including in-stent restenosis that results from extensive intimal hyperplasia. Furthermore, it will be of interest to identify the downstream gene regulatory targets of gax transcription factor and to further delineate the mechanisms by which gax overexpression inhibits vessel stenosis.

Acknowledgements

We thank Karine Berthelot for excellent technical assistance, Jean-Jacques Robert and Laurent Naudin for adenovirus construction, Jean-Marc Guillaume for adenovirus production, and Sandrine Séguret-Macé and Nathalie Aubailly for helpful discussion.

References

1. Nobuyoshi MT, Kimura T, Nosaka H, Mioka S, Ueno K, Yokoi H, Hamasaki N, Horiuchi H, Ohishi H. Restenosis after successful percutaneous transluminal coronary angioplasty: serial angiographic follow-up of 229 patients. J Am Coll Cardiol 1988;12:616—623.
2. Dussaillant G, Mintz G, Pichard A, Kent K, Satler L, Popma J, Wong S, Leon M. Small stent size and intimal hyperplasia contribute to restenosis: a volumetric intravascular ultrasound analysis. J Am Coll Cardiol 1995;26:720—724.
3. Gorski DH, LePage DF, Patel CV, Copeland NG, Jenkins NA, Walsh K. Molecular cloning of a diverged homeobox gene that is rapidly downregulated during the G0/G1 transition in vascular smooth muscle cells. Molec Cell Biol 1993;13:3722—3733.
4. LePage D, Altomare D, Testa J, Walsh K. Molecular cloning and localization of the human GAX gene to 7p21. Genomics 1994;24:535—540.
5. Smith R, Branellec D, Gorski D, Guo K, Perlman H, Dedieu J, Pastore C, Mahfoudi A, Denefle P, Isner J, Walsh K. p21CIP1-mediated inhibition of cell proliferation by overexpression of the gax homeodomain gene. Genes Dev 1997;11:1674—1689.
6. Wickham TJ, Mathias P, Cheresh DA, Nemerow GR. Integrin-alpha-v-beta-3 and Integrin-alpha-v-beta-5 promote adenovirus internalization but not virus attachment. Cell 1993;73: 309—319.
7. Wickham TJ, Segal DM, Roelvink PW, Carrion ME, Lizonova A, Lee GM, Kovesdi I. Targeted adenovirus gene transfer to endothelial and smooth muscle cells by using bispecific antibodies. J Virol 1996;70:6831—6838.
8. Chang M, Barr E, Seltzer J, Jiang Y, Nabel G, Nabel E, Parmacek M, Leiden J. Cytostatic gene therapy for vascular proliferative disorders with a constitutively active form of the retinoblastoma gene product. Science 1995;267:518—522.
9. Smith RC, Wills KN, Antelman D, Perlman H, Truong LN, Krasinski K, Walsh K. Adenoviral constructs encoding phosphorylation-competent full-length and truncated forms of the human retinoblastoma protein inhibit myocyte proliferation and neointima formation. Circulation 1997;96:1899—1905.
10. Chang M, Barr E, Lu M, Barton K, Leiden J. Adenovirus-mediated overexpression of the cyclin/cyclin-dependent kinase inhibitor, p21 inhibits vascular smooth muscle cell proliferation and neointima formation in the rat carotid artery model of balloon angioplasty. J Clin Invest 1995;96:2260—2268.
11. Mader S. Influence of animal age on the beta-adrenergic system in cultured rat aortic and mesenteric artery smooth muscle cells. J Gerontol 1992;47:B32—36.
12. Crouzet J, Naudin L, Orsini C, Vigne E, Ferrero L, Le RA, Benoit P, Latta M, Torrent C, Branellec D, Denefle P, Mayaux J, Perricaudet M, Yeh P. Recombinational construction in *Escherichia coli* of infectious adenoviral genomes. Proc Natl Acad Sci USA 1997;94:1414—1419.
13. Stratford-Perricaudet L, Levrero M, Chasse J, Perricaudet M, Briand P. Evaluation of the transfer and expression in mice of an enzyme-encoding gene using a human adenovirus vector.

Hum Gene Ther 1990;1:241—256.

14. Maillard L, Van Belle E, Smith RC, Le Roux AC, Denèfle P, Steg G, Barry JJ, Branellec D, Isner JM, Walsh K. Percutaneous delivery of the gax gene inhibits vessel stenosis in a rabbit model of balloon angioplasty. Cardiovasc Res 1997;(In press).

15. Sigwart U. Endovascular stents. Science Med 1997;(Sept/Oct):16—25.

16. Skopicki H, Lyons G, Schatteman G, Smith R, Andres V, Schirm S, Isner J, Walsh K. Embryonic expression of the Gax homeodomain protein in cardiac, smooth, and skeletal muscle (see comments). Circ Res 1997;80:452—462.

17. Yamashita J, Itoh H, Ogawa Y, Tamura Y, Takaya K, Igaki T, Doi K, Chun T, Inoue M, Masatsugu K, Nakao K. Opposite regulation of Gax homeobox expression by angiotensin II and C-type natriuretic peptide. Hypertension 1997;29:381—387.

18. Bergelson J, Cunningham J, Droguett G, Kurt-Jones E, Krithivas A, Hong J, Horwitz M, Crowell R, Finberg R. Isolation of a common receptor for Coxsackie B viruses and adenoviruses 2 and 5. Science 1997;275:1320—1323.

19. Hong S, Karayan L, Tournier J, Curiel D, Boulanger P. Adenovirus type 5 fiber knob binds to MHC class I alpha2 domain at the surface of human epithelial and B lymphoblastoid cells. EMBO J 1997;16:2294—2306.

20. Chang M, Ohno T, Gordon D, Lu M, Nabel G, Nabel E, Leiden J. Adenovirus-mediated transfer of the herpes simplex virus thymidine kinase gene inhibits vascular smooth muscle cell proliferation and neointima formation following balloon angioplasty of the rat carotid artery. Molec Med 1995;1:172—181.

21. Steg PG, Tahlil O, Aubailly N, Caillaud JM, Dedieu JF, Berthelot K, LeRoux A, Feldman L, Perricaudet M, Denefle P, Branellec D. Reduction of restenosis after angioplasty in an atheromatous rabbit model by suicide gene therapy. Circulation, 1997;96:408—411.

22. Cho A, Courtman D, Langille B. Apoptosis (programmed cell death) in arteries of the neonatal lamb. Circ Res 1995;76:168—175.

23. Perlman H, Maillard L, Krasinski K, Walsh K. Evidence for the rapid onset of apoptosis in medial smooth muscle cells after balloon injury (see comments). Circulation 1997;95:981—987.

CKIs and regulation of cell cycle in vascular cells

Felix C. Tanner[1], Zhi-Yong Yang[1,5], Hong San[1], David Gordon[4], Gary J. Nabel[1,3,5] and Elizabeth G. Nabel[1,2]
Departments of [1]Internal Medicine, [2]Physiology, [3]Biochemistry, and [4]Pathology, [5]Howard Hughes Medical Institute, University of Michigan, Ann Arbor, Michigan, USA

Smooth muscle cells normally reside in the media in a nonproliferative state. When stimulated to divide by mitogens, smooth muscle cells enter G1 phase of the cell cycle. Progression through G1 is regulated by the assembly, activation, and phosphorylation of cyclin/cyclin-dependent kinase (CDK) complexes. There are two major cyclin-CDKs which regulate G1 progression: cyclin D-CDK4/6 and cyclin E-CDK2. Activation and phosphorylation of these cyclin-CDK complexes results in phosphorylation of the retinoblastoma gene product (Rb), release of E2F and other transcription factors, and transition from G1 to S phase of the cell cycle. In S phase, DNA synthesis occurs, and G2 and M phase follow (for a review of the cell cycle, see [1—3]).

There are naturally occurring endogenous inhibitors of the G1 cyclin-CDK complexes, termed cyclin-dependent kinase inhibitors (CKIs) [4,5]. Over the past 5 years, several families of CKIs have been identified and studied for their role in cell transformation, growth regulation, and tumor biology. These include the CIP/KIP family: p21, p27 and p57 [6—9], and the INK family: p15, p16, p18 and p19 [10,11]. This paper will focus on the role of the CIP/KIP family members in regulation of cell cycle progression in vascular smooth muscle cells.

In order to determine the role of the CIP/KIP family members in vascular diseases, studies were performed in balloon injured pig arterial tissue [12]. Western blot analysis demonstrated that p21 was not expressed in normal, uninjured pig arteries. At 7 days following vascular injury, there was upregulation of p21 in injured arteries. The most abundant expression was observed at 21 days. To further pursue the cell types which expressed p21 and to correlate the expression of p21 with cell proliferation, additional immunohistochemical studies were performed. In the balloon injured pig arteries, cell proliferation in the intima began within 24 h after injury. Cell proliferation in the intima peaked at 15—18% of intimal cells at approximately 7 days, and then rapidly declined to 2% of cells by 14 days. Cell proliferation in the intima remained at this low level for at least 60

Address for correspondence: Elizabeth G. Nabel, University of Michigan, 7220 MSRB III, 1150 W. Medical Center Dr., Ann Arbor, MI 48109-0644, USA. Tel.: +1-313-763-5103. Fax: +1-313-763-4851. E-mail: enabel@umich.edu

days after injury. Thus, there was a brief initial period after vascular injury in which there is a rapid rise in cell proliferation followed by a rapid decline in cell proliferation during the latter phases of arterial repair. Immunohistochemistry studies for p21 protein were consistent with Western blot analyses. That is, p21 was not expressed in normal, uninjured blood vessels. One day after vascular injury, p21 expression was noted in $<2\%$ of medial smooth muscle cells. By 7 days after injury, p21 was detected in smooth muscle cells in the developing neointima. p21 expression increased, and by 14 days, was abundantly expressed in smooth muscle cells in the intima. Between 21 and 60 days, there was a decline in p21 expression such that at 60 days, the protein was no longer detected. Interestingly, p21 expression in the intima was localized to the lower regions, adjacent to the internal elastic lamina. In balloon injured pig arteries, this region of the neointima is also associated with procollagen expression and TGFβ expression. These data suggest that in this animal model, the expression of p21 was inversely associated with cell proliferation and potentially function to limit cell proliferation during the later phases of arterial remodeling. We hypothesize that extracellular matrix synthesized by proliferating smooth muscle cells may signal back to the smooth muscle cell via integrin receptors, resulting in upregulation of p21. Support for this hypothesis is provided by in vitro studies of human smooth muscle cell cultures [13].

To further explore the function of p21 in arterial repair, adenoviral vectors encoding for p21 were constructed and tested in vitro in pig endothelial and smooth muscle cells [12]. Overexpression of p21 in endothelial and smooth muscle cells resulted in inhibition of cell proliferation, determined by cell growth studies. These cells were arrested in G1 phase, demonstrated by FACS analysis. When the p21 adenoviral vector was introduced into balloon injured pig arteries, a decrease in intimal smooth muscle cell proliferation was noted at 7 days, determined by the BrdU labeling studies [12,14]. This decline in intimal smooth muscle cell proliferation was associated with a decrease in neointimal formation, determined by quantitative morphometry analysis.

These studies of the expression and function of p21 in arteries led us to explore other CIP/KIP family members, including p27. We first explored the expression pattern of p27 in normal and injured pig arteries [15]. There were similarities and differences compared to p21. In contrast to p21, p27 was present in medial smooth muscle cells in normal uninjured arteries. This suggested that p27 may play a role in basal inhibition of smooth muscle cell proliferation. Following balloon injury, p27 was downregulated and was not detected in intimal or medial smooth muscle cells 1 and 4 days after injury. By 7 days, however, p27 was upregulated and expressed in intimal and medial smooth muscle cells. This expression continued to 14 and 21 days. At these time points, p27 was detected in intimal smooth muscle cells in a pattern similar to p21. The protein was found in intimal smooth muscle cells adjacent to the internal elastic lamina. This expression pattern was similar to p21. At 60 days after injury, p27 was still detected in intimal smooth muscle cells, unlike p21. This data might further suggest that p27 is constitutively expressed in normal and injured arteries to limit smooth muscle cell proliferation.

Of interest, we also explored the expression pattern of INK family in balloon injured pig arteries. p16 was evaluated as a representative family member. p16 was transiently expressed in balloon injured arteries 4 days after injury [15]. By 7 days, p16 was no longer detected and was not expressed at subsequent later time points. p16 was also not detected in normal, uninjured vessels. The purpose of this transient expression of p16 is not known but is currently being explored.

We further explored the relevance of these expression patterns in balloon injured pig arteries to human atherosclerosis. Thirty-five human coronary artery specimens were analyzed [15]. These coronary arteries were retrieved from explanted hearts of patients undergoing cardiac transplantation at the University of Michigan. The 35 coronary artery samples were divided into three categories upon blinded review by an experienced cardiovascular pathologist (D.G.). Category I were nonatherosclerotic arteries with diffuse intimal hyperplasia. These patients had dilated cardiomyopathies. Category II was early atherosclerosis characterized by lipid accumulation and smooth muscle cell proliferation. Category III was late atherosclerosis characterized by regions of necrosis and calcification. There were eight samples in category I, 17 samples in category II, and 18 samples in category III. We found that p27 was expressed in smooth muscle cells and endothelial cells in seven of eight samples in patients with diffused intimal thickening. p27 was also abundantly expressed in the majority of samples with early and late atherosclerosis and was found in endothelial cells, smooth muscle cells, and macrophages. In contrast, p21 was noted in only one of the samples with diffuse intimal thickening. It colocalized to the same regions as the p27 and was not found in its absence. p21 was also detected in a small number of samples with early atherosclerosis, but its expression increased as disease severity progressed. Both p21 and p27 were not found in regions of cell proliferation, determined by double label immunohistochemistry. Interestingly, p16 was not detected in any of the 35 human coronary artery samples. These studies parallel the findings in balloon injured pig arteries. They suggest that the CIP/KIP family members p27 and p21 play a role in the regulation of vascular cell proliferation during arterial repair. In contrast, p16 played little to no role in growth regulation of vascular cells. The mechanisms accounting for the differences in expression patterns in p27 and p21 are not currently known but are being actively pursued.

These studies suggest then that the CIP/KIP cyclin-dependent kinase inhibitors, p27 and p21, function to limit vascular cell proliferation following arterial injury. Furthermore, these CKIs are expressed in human atherosclerosis, in regions in which active proliferation is not present. Whether these CKIs can be manipulated to treat abnormal cell proliferation in vascular diseases is currently being explored.

688

References

1. Sherr CJ. Mammalian G_1 cyclins. Cell 1993;73:1059–1065.
2. Hunter T. Braking the cycle. Cell 1993;75:839–841.
3. Sherr CJ. G1 phase progression: cycling on cue. Cell 1994;79:551–555.
4. Peter M, Herskowitz I. Joining the complex: cyclin-dependent kinase inhibitory proteins and the cell cycle. Cell 1994;79:181–184.
5. Sherr CJ, Roberts JM. Inhibitors of mammalian G1 cyclin-dependent kinases. Genes Dev 1995; 9:1149–1163.
6. Xiong Y, Hannon GJ, Zhang H, Casso D, Kobayashi R, Beach D. p21 is a universal inhibitor of cyclin kinases. Nature 1993;366:701–704.
7. Harper JW, Adami GR, Wei N, Keyomarsi K, Elledge SJ. The p21 Cdk-interacting protein Cip1 is a potent inhibitor of G1 cyclin-dependent kinases. Cell 1993;75:805–816.
8. Toyoshima H, Hunter T. p27, a novel inhibitor of G1 cyclin-cdk protein kinase activity, is related to p21. Cell 1994;78:67–74.
9. Polyak K, Lee MH, Erdjument-Bromage H, Koff A, Roberts JM, Tempst P, Massague J. Cloning of p27Kip1, a cyclin-dependent kinase inhibitor and a potential mediator of extracellular anti-mitogenic signals. Cell 1994;78:59–66.
10. Quelle DE, Ashmun RA, Hannon GJ, Rehberger PA, Trono D, Richter KH, Walker C, Beach D, Sherr CJ, Serrano M. Cloning and characterization of murine p16(ink4a) and p15(ink4b) genes. Oncogene 1995;11:635–645.
11. Hirai H, Roussel MF, Kato J, Ashmun RA, Sherr CJ. Novel INK4 proteins, p19 and p18, are specific inhibitors of cyclin D-dependent kinases CDK4 and CDK6. Molec Cell Biol 1995;15: 2672–2681.
12. Yang Z, Simari RD, Perkins ND, San H, Gordon D, Nabel GJ, Nabel EG. Role of the p21 cyclin-dependent kinase inhibitor in limiting intimal cell proliferation in response to arterial injury. Proc Natl Acad Sci USA 1996;93:7905–7910.
13. Koyama H, Raines EW, Bornfeldt KE, Roberts JM, Ross R. Fibrillar collagen inhibits arterial smooth muscle proliferation through regulation of Cdk2 inhibitors. Cell 1996;87:1069–1078.
14. Chang MW, Barr E, Lu M, Barton K, Leiden JM. Adenovirus-mediated overexpression of the cyclin/cyclin-dependent kinase inhibitor, p21 inhibits vascular smooth muscle cell proliferation and neointima formation in the rat cartoid artery model of balloon angioplasty. J Clin Invest 1995;96:2260–2268.
15. Tanner FC, Yang Z, Gordon D, Nabel GJ, Nabel EG. Expression of cyclin-dependent kinase inhibitors in vascular disease. Submitted.

Adventitial gene transfer to rabbit carotid arteries

Marja Laitinen and Seppo Ylä-Herttuala
A. I. Virtanen Institute and Department of Medicine, University of Kuopio, Kuopio, Finland

Introduction

Gene transfer to arterial wall can be accomplished both from lumen and adventitia [1]. Strategies for local vascular gene delivery are listed in Table 1. A major problem in the intra-arterial gene transfer is that endothelium and internal elastic lamina form physical barriers that limit penetration of gene-transfer vectors into the arterial wall [2]. In addition, plasma interferes with all gene-transfer methods and the systemic leakage of the gene transfer vector is more likely in intravascular approach. Gene-transfer efficiency using intravascular delivery of plasmid/liposome complexes and retroviruses has also been very low [3—5].

Adventitial gene delivery is an alternative to the intravascular delivery. Previously, drugs, growth factors, antisense oligonucleotides and plasmids have been delivered to the vessel wall via adventitia [6—9]. We have developed a model for arterial gene transfer via adventitia using a silastic collar installed around rabbit carotid arteries. The collar also provides a gene-delivery reservoir. Since no intraluminal manipulations are performed, endothelium remains anatomically intact throughout the procedure [10]. Adventitial delivery could be useful for vascular gene therapy during prosthesis and anastomosis surgery and bypass operations.

Gene transfer efficiency from adventitia

We have tested the efficiency of plasmid/liposome, Moloney murine leukemia virus-derived (MMLV) retroviruses, pseudotyped retroviruses and adenoviruses using the adventitial collar [10]. The following doses of gene transfer vectors were used in 600 µl gene-transfer solution applied inside the collar: 25 µg pCMV-β-galactosidase expression plasmid (Promega) complexed with Lipofectin (BRL); 5×10^5 cfu/ml pLZRNL amphotrophic β-galactosidase-containing retroviruses 5; 1×10^7 cfu/ml pseudotyped pLZRNL + G retroviruses [11] and 1×10^9 pfu/ml β-galactosidase-containing first generation E1-deleted adenoviruses [12]. It was found that mean gene transfer efficiency with the various

Address for correspondence: Seppo Ylä-Herttuala MD, PhD, A.I. Virtanen Institute, University of Kuopio, P.O. Box 1627, FIN-70211 Kuopio, Finland.

Table 1. Vascular gene delivery.

Luminal delivery

Balloon catheters: double-balloon, microporous, hydrogel-coated, channel balloons,
Iontophoresis catheters, needle catheters, nipple catheters,
Biodegradable polymers, fibrin clue, and
Coated stents.

Adventitial delivery

Direct injection, needle catheters,
Adventitial collar or other type of gene delivery reservoir,
Biodegradable polymers, fibrin clue,
Seeding of transfected cells outside the vessel, and
Microparticles.

---

gene transfer vectors was as follows: plasmid/liposomes 0.05%; MMLV retroviruses < 0.01; pseudotyped retroviruses 0.05 and adenoviruses 10% [10]. Transfected cells were located in adventitia and outer media except with adenoviruses where some transfected cells were also detected in intima and endothelium.

Adventitial delivery of vascular endothelial growth factor was tested in rabbit carotid arteries using the collar model. It was found that VEGF gene transfer reduced intimal thickening 7 days after the gene transfer [13]. Transfected VEGF mRNA was detectable in adventitia and outer media.

Conclusions

Adventitial delivery can be successfully performed using all available gene transfer vectors. When vectors are applied directly on the adventitial surface within the collar, close contact to the vessel wall is maintained. A major advantage of the adventitial delivery is that endothelial layer remains anatomically intact. Thus, the model can be used for expression in the adventitia and media of diffusible or secreted gene products, which then can act on the endothelium and elsewhere in the arterial wall.

It is concluded that the extra-arterial gene transfer can be used for the delivery of genetic material into the arterial wall. It is possible to develop biodegradable adventitial gene delivery into reservoirs for the treatment of arterial diseases during vascular surgery, such as prosthesis and anastomosis operations and bypass surgery.

Acknowledgements

This work was supported by grants from the Finnish Heart Foundation, Sigrid Juselius Foundation and Biomed grant from the European Union (PL 950329). We thank Ms Marja Poikolainen for typing the manuscript.

References

1. Ylä-Herttuala S. Vascular gene transfer. Curr Opin Lipid 1997;8:72—76.
2. Rome JJ, Shayani V, Flugelman MY, Newman KD, Farb A, Virmani R, Dichek DA. Anatomic barriers influence the distribution of in vivo gene transfer into the arterial wall. Arterioscl Thromb 1994;14:148—161.
3. Nabel EG, Nabel GJ. Complex models for the study of gene function in cardiovascular biology. Ann Rev Phys 1994;56:741—761.
4. Lim CS, Chapman GD, Gammon RS, Muhlestein JB, Bauman RP, Stack RS, Swain JL. Direct in vivo gene transfer into the coronary and peripheral vasculatures of the intact dog. Circulation 1991;83:2007—2011.
5. Ylä-Herttuala S, Luoma J, Viita H, Hiltunen T, Sisto T, Nikkari T. Transfer of 15-lipoxygenase gene into rabbit iliac arteries results in the appearance of oxidation-specific lipid-protein adducts characteristic of oxidized low-density lipoprotein. J Clin Invest 1995;95:2692—2698.
6. Edelman ER, Adams DH, Karnovsky MJ. Effect of controlled adventitial heparin delivery on smooth muscle cell proliferation following endothelial injury. Proc Natl Acad Sci USA 1990; 87:3773—3777.
7. Simons M, Edelman ER, DeKeyser J, Langer R, Rosenberg RD. Antisense c-myb oligonucleotides inhibit arterial smooth muscle cell accumulation in vivo. Nature 1992;359:67—70.
8. Villa AE, Guzman LA, Chen W, Golomb G, Levy RJ, Topol EJ. Local delivery of dexamethasone for prevention of neointimal proliferation in a rat model of balloon angioplasty. J Clin Invest 1994;93:1243—1249.
9. Rios CD, Ooboshi H, Piegors D, Davidson BL, Heistad DD. Adenovirus-mediated gene transfer to normal and atherosclerotic arteries. Arterioscl Thromb Vasc Biol 1995;15:2241—2245.
10. Laitinen M, Pakkanen T, Luoma J, Viita H, Lehtolainen P, Donetti E, Baetta R, Soma M, Miyanohara A, Friedmann T, Risau W, Martin J, Ylä-Herttuala S. Gene transfer into the carotid artery using an adventitial collar. Comparison of the effectiveness of plasmid-liposome complexes, retroviruses, pseudotyped retroviruses and adenoviruses. Hum Gene Ther 1997;8: 1657—1662.
11. Yee J-K, Miyanohara A, LaPorte P, Bouic K, Burns JC, Friedmann T. A general method for the generation of high-titer, pantropic retroviral vectors: highly efficient infection of primary hepatocytes. Proc Natl Acad Sci USA 1994;91:9564—9568.
12. Chang MW, Barr E, Seltzer J et al. Cytostatic gene therapy for vascular disorders with a constitutively active form of the retinoblastoma gene product. Science 1995;267:518—522.
13. Laitinen M, Zachary I, Breier G, Pakkanen T, Häkkinen T, Luoma J, Abedi H, Risau W, Soma M, Laakso M, Martin J, Ylä-Herttuala S. VEGF gene transfer reduces intimal thickening via increased production of nitric oxide in carotid arteries. Hum Gene Ther 1997;8:1737—1744.

Molecular genetics of monogenic disorders of lipoprotein metabolism

Atherosclerosis XI.
B. Jacotot, D. Mathé and J.-C. Fruchart, editors.

Redefining familial lipoprotein lipase deficiency in the era of molecular medicine

Pascale Benlian

Department of Molecular Biology, Hôpital Saint Antoine, Paris, France

Abstract: A decade after the cloning of the LPL cDNA, more than 60 mutations have been reported worldwide, linking genetic defects with their clinical consequences. To complement observations in French Canadians who carry only three mutations, the disease may be further defined with patients who are commonly observed with different mutations (n = 75 cases, including 18 in France). Linkage is almost exclusive between chylomicronemia with a plasma LPL activity < 10% than normal, and the LPL gene locus. Homozygotes with null alleles appear to manifest the disease earlier than carriers of missense alleles. However, the type of mutation was not a predictor of the risk of pancreatitis. Surprisingly, adult homozygotes with mutations preserving enzymatic mass in plasma may develop cardiovascular disease, despite a life-long low-fat diet. In heterozygotes, independent of the type of mutation (promoter, primary sequence), low plasma HDL/high triglycerides was a common trait of partial LPL deficiency, increasing susceptibility to atherogenic hyperlipidemias. However, conditions favouring atherosclerosis in carriers of common variants (D9N, N291S), remain to be defined. Finally, mutations located outside the catalytic site may be associated with unusual phenotypes (protective alleles?) suggesting that yet unknown functions/phenotypes remain to be identified at the LPL gene locus.

Keywords: atherosclerosis, familial chylomicronemia, founder mutation, hyperlipidemia, lipoproteins.

When Wion and colleagues first reported the cloning of the LPL cDNA in 1987 [1], they suggested that this "...will allow analysis of the defect responsible for LPL deficiency in certain subjects and facilitate elucidation of the structure and function of this vital enzyme of lipid metabolism." At that time, they did not know that this prediction would be far more than verified within a decade. Lipoprotein lipase (LPL) present at the vessels surface hydrolyses triglycerides from chylomicrons and VLDL, to release free fatty acids taken up by extrahepatic tissues (mainly muscles and adipose tissue) for energy or storage. A defective catalytic activity of LPL will result in a massive accumulation of triglyceride-rich lipoproteins in plasma, which may complicate with acute pancreatitis. LPL deficiency (classically denominated "familial chylomicronemia") is a rare (1/1 million), autosomal recessive condition usually discovered in childhood [2]. Numerous individuals have now been characterised with LPL gene mutations

---

Address for correspondence: Pascale Benlian, Laboratoire Commun de Biologie Moléculaire, Hôpital Saint Antoine, 184 rue du Faubourg Saint Antoine, 75012 Paris, France.

696

offering an opportunity to refine the clinical description of LPL deficiency, on the basis of its underlying molecular defects.

Classical description of LPL deficiency

Havel and Gordon demonstrated in 1960, that the metabolic basis of familial chylomicronemia was an impaired catalytic activity of LPL [3]. Thereafter, the disorder was distinguished from other familial hyperlipidemias on the basis of its recessive mode of inheritance, the absence of inhibitors, the detection of a functional apo C-II, and most importantly, a low LPL activity in plasma after intravenous injection of heparin [2]. LPL deficiency is observed worldwide. It manifests early in life (80% before age 20) with recurrent abdominal pain, failure to thrive in infants, fasting chylomicronemia or acute pancreatitis. Symptoms (hepatosplenomegaly, eruptive xanthomatosis and lipemia retinalis) and risk of acute pancreatitis have been shown to evolve as a function of the intensity of hypertriglyceridemia (chylomicronemia), and are strongly inducible by dietary-fat intake.

Naturally occurring mutations on the LPL gene

The LPL gene spans approximately 30 kb on the short arm of human chromosome 8 (8p22). It contains 10 exons of which exon 1 encodes mainly for the signal peptide and exon 10 encodes for the last nucleotide of the termination codon [1]. Structure-function studies have demonstrated that most of the elements required for LPL catalytic activity appear to be confined to exons 4, 5 and 6 [4,5]. Therefore, one would predict that a defective lipolysis in plasma would result from mutations located within this region. Naturally occurring mutations of the LPL gene in patients with familial LPL deficiency are summarised in Table 1. As previously observed [2−7], nonsense mutations (premature stop codon, frameshift, splice site mutations or large gene rearrangements) occur all along the gene sequence. However, 78% of missense mutations (single amino acid change) reported to cause LPL deficiency were found within exons 4, 5 or 6. Moreover, missense mutations were 2.4 times more frequent in exon 5, 1.5 times more frequent in exon 6 and 1.2 times more frequent in exon 4 than expected, if randomly distributed along the gene sequence.

Likewise, levels of plasma LPL activity appear a strong predictor of the presence of an underlying LPL gene mutation. We have investigated a series of 22 unrelated probands with chylomicronemia. Only those who exhibited < 20% normal plasma LPL activity were carriers of two defective LPL gene mutations. Reciprocally, 97% of patients presented in Table 1 had a plasma LPL activity < 10% than normal. A practical consequence is that a profound decrease in postheparin plasma LPL activity will point to a primary defect at a unique locus: the LPL gene. This strong linkage indicates that other factors (environmental or genetic) which modulate LPL activity, are not a major cause of this extreme phenotype.

Table 1. Naturally occurring mutations in subjects of different ancestries with LPL deficiency.

Allele 1	Allele 2	Ancestry	Consanguinity	Gender	Age at discovery	Triglycerides	Pancreatitis	Reference
Nonsense/LPL mass absent								
5′ splice (Int 2)	Hmz	Japan	+	M	34 y	4,928	+	2,7
3′ splice (Int 2)	Ser^{244}→Thr (6)	France	−	M	< 2 y	4,800	−	7
FS, Arg^{34} (2)	Hmz	France	−	F	1 mo	1,120	+	8
Tyr^{61}→STOP(2)	Hmz	Japan	+	F	3 mo	19,120	−	6,7
Tyr^{61}→STOP(2)	FS, Ala^{221} (5)	Japan	−	M	10 mo	4,088	nr	2
FS, Val^{69} (3)	FS, Asn^{120} (4)	France	−	F	1 mo	14,000	−	9
Gln^{106}→STOP (3)	Hmz	Germany, Poland	+	M	5 mo	2,674	−	6,7
FS, Asn^{120} (4)	Duplic Ex 6	England	−	F	3 y	6,500	−	10
FS, Ala^{221} (5)	Hmz	Japan	+	M[a]	58 y	2,028	+	2
FS, Ala^{221} (5)	Hmz	Japan	+	M[a]	59 y	1,899	+	
Cys^{239}→STOP(6)	Hmz	Japan	nr	M[a]	49 y	381	nr	11
Cys^{239}→STOP(6)	Hmz	Japan	nr	F[a]	57 y	1,187	nr	
3′ splice (Int 6)	Hmz	Austria	−	M	27 y	6,560	−	12
Trp^{382}→STOP (8)	Hmz	Japan	+	F	6 mo	6,010	−	2
Del Ex 9	Hmz	France	+	M	9 y	5,800	+	13
Missense/LPL mass present								
Val^{69}→Leu (3)	Gly^{188}→Glu (5)	Holland	−	M	> 2	1,567	+	2
Arg^{75}→Ser (3)	Tyr^{73}→STOP(3)	Germany, Ireland	−	M	< 2 y	10,000	+	4
Trp^{86}→Arg (3)	Gln^{106}→Stop(3)	England	−	M	< 1 mo	705	−	6,7
Trp^{86}→Arg (3)	His^{136}→Arg (4)	USA	−	F	19 y	1,800	nr	2,7
Thr^{101}→Ala (3)	Asp^{250}→Asn (6)	France	−	F	39 y	2,080	+	14
Gly^{139}→Ser (4)	Hmz	Spain	−	M	1 mo	1,130	−	2
Gly^{142}→Glu (4)	Hmz	USA, N. Europe	+	M[a]	< 1 mo	30,000	−	2,7
Gly^{142}→Glu (4)	Hmz	USA, N. Europe	+	F[a]	3 mo	2,000	+[b]	
Asp^{156}→Gly (5)	Hmz	Turkey	+	M[a]	1 y	4,100	+	2,7
Asp^{156}→Gly (5)	Hmz	Turkey	+	M[a]	17 y	1,460	−	
Asp^{156}→His (5)	Hmz	France	+	F[a]	< 1 mo	1,530	−	15
Asp^{156}→His (5)	Hmz	France	+	M[a]	15 y	520	+	
Asp^{156}→His (5)	Hmz	France	+	M[a]	11 y	2,200	−	
Asp^{156}→Asn (5)	Cys^{216}→Ser (5)	Italy	−	M[a]	25 y	3,400	+	2,7
Asp^{156}→Asn (5)	Cys^{216}→Ser (5)	Italy	−	M[a]	58 y	7,800	−	
Ser^{172}→Cys (5)	Hmz	India	+	F	30 y	2,464	+[b]	2
Ala^{176}→Thr (5)	Hmz	USA, Black	nr	M	21 y	2,880	+	2,7
Asp^{180}→Glu (5)	Hmz	Italy	−	F[a]	10 y	625	−	16
Asp^{180}→Glu (5)	Hmz	Italy	−	M[a]	9 y	877	−	

(cont.)

Table 1. Continued.

Missense/LPL mass present

Allele 1	Allele 2	Ancestry	Consanguinity	Gender	Age at discovery	Triglycerides	Pancreatitis	Reference
His[183]→Gln (5)	WT	Russia, Switzerland	−	F	50 y	720	−	17
Gly[188]→Arg (5)	Hmz	France	+	M[a]	29 y	3,800	−	14
Gly[188]→Arg (5)	Hmz	France	+	F[a]	22 y	4,100	+[b]	
Gly[188]→Arg (5)	Hmz	France	+	M[a]	25 y	1,600	−	
Gly[188]→Arg (5)	Hmz	France	+	F[a]	12 y	1,860	−	
Gly[188]→Arg (5)	Hmz	France	+	F[a]	22 y	580	−	
Gly[188]→Glu (5)	Hmz	Northern Europe	−	F	<2 y	2,500	−	2,7
Gly[188]→Glu (5)	Hmz	Spain	−	M	<1 mo	5,000	−	2
Gly[188]→Glu (5)	Hmz	Austria	−	M[a]	>2 y	3,980	+	2
Gly[188]→Glu (5)	Hmz	Austria	−	M[a]	>2 y	4,970	+	2
Gly[188]→Glu (5)	Hmz	Austria	−	M[a]	>2 y	2,740	−	2
Gly[188]→Glu (5)	Hmz	India	−	F[a]	27 y	5,390	nr	2
Gly[188]→Glu (5)	Hmz	India	−	M[a]	26 y	4,920	nr	2
Gly[188]→Glu (5)	Hmz	India	−	F[a]	15 y	3,760	nr	2
Gly[188]→Glu (5)	FS, Ala[17] (2)	Spain	−	M	<1 mo	nr	+	2
Gly[188]→Glu (5)	Dupl Ex6	France	−	F	16 y	6,600	+	15
Ile[194]→Thr (5)	Hmz	France, Holland	−	F	4 y	4,180	−	2
Ile[194]→Thr (5)	Hmz	Spain	−	M	25 y	2,500	−	2
Ile[194]→Thr (5)	Trp[64]→STOP(3)	USA	−	M	<1 y	20,000	−	2
Ile[194]→Thr (5)	Gly[188]→Glu (5)	USA	−	F	1 mo	17,000	−	2
Ile[194]→Thr (5)	Arg[243]→His (6)	USA	−	F	<1 mo	2,500	+	2
Gly[195]→Glu (5)	Hmz	USA, Hispanic	+	M	3 y	7,000	+	4
Asp[204]→Glu (5)	Hmz	Japan	+	F	44 y	1,528	−	2
Ile[205]→Ser (5)	Hmz	Spain	+	F	4 y	2,900	+	2
Leu[207]→Pro (5)	Gly[188]→Glu (5)	USA	−	M[a]	<1 mo	16,000	−	2,7
Leu[207]→Pro (5)	Gly[188]→Glu (5)	USA	−	M[a]	3 y	10,000	+	2
Ile[225]→Thr (5)	Arg[243]→His (6)	Holland	−	M	3 y	17,000	−	18
Arg[243]→His (6)	Hmz	Japan	+	F	<1 mo	4,794	−	2,7
Arg[243]→His (6)	Hmz	China	+	F	2 mo	26,107	−	18
Arg[243]→His (6)	Asp[250]→Asn (6)	Italy	−	F[a]	3 mo	1,520	−	2
Arg[243]→His (6)	Asp[250]→Asn (6)	Italy	−	M[a]	nr	858	−	
Arg[243]→Cys (6)	Gly[188]→Glu (5)	France	−	F	7 y	5,200	−	18
Arg[243]→Cys (6)	Pro[207]→Leu (5)	Germany	−	M	<1 mo	3,560	+	18
Asp[250]→Asn (6)	Gly[188]→Glu (5)	France	−	F	6 mo	1,929	+[b]	2,7
Leu[252]→Arg (6)	Ala[261]→Thr (6)	China	−	F	37 y	nr	+[b]	19
Ser[259]→Arg (6)	Hmz	Morocco	+	M	6 mo	6,000	+	20

(cont.)

Table 1. Continued.

Missense/LPL mass present

Allele 1	Allele 2	Ancestry	Consan-guinity	Gen-der	Age at discovery	Triglc-erides	Pancre-atitis	Refer-ence
Tyr[262]→His (6)	Hmz	USA, Black	—	M	22 y	10,200	+	21
Leu[286]→Pro (6)	FS, Ala[71] (3)	France	—	M	48 y	12,800	+	14
Ala[334]→Thr (7)	Hmz	Japan	nr	F	34 y	7,523	+[b]	4
Trp[382]→STOP (8)	WT	Caucasian		F	24 y	nr	+[b]	2
Glu[410]→Val (8)	Hmz	Egypt	—	M	2 mo	12,000	+	22

Common variants		Frequency		LPL Act	LPL Mass	HDL	TG	
G→T (−93)	Promoter	70—75% (Black)	1.6—3.4% Caucasian	↓	↓	—	↑	23
Asp[9]→Asn	exon 2		1.6—4.1%	66—92%	70—100%	↓	↑	23
			Caucasian	N	N			
Asn[291]→Ser	exon 6		1.3—6.7%	50—68%	77—100%	↓	↑	23
			Caucasian	N	N			
Ser[447]→STOP	exon 6		10—23% Caucasian	120% N	130% N	↑	↓	23

(FS): frameshift. (Hmz): homozygote. (WT): wild-type allele. Triglycerides: maximum plasma levels in mg/dl. [a]Members of a family. [b]Occurred during pregnancy. Common variants: do not cause chylomicronemia in homozygotes. References: citation of original article when not previously reviewed. (nr): not reported.

Finally, consanguinity was considered a predominant feature in LPL deficiency. Indeed, in French Canadians, LPL deficiency is explained by only three mutations in >97% cases [24]. Moreover, a founder mutation underlies LPL deficiency in Berbers from Morocco [20]. In contrast, consanguinity is not frequent (28% cases) in other populations (see Table 1). Among 15 French families, consanguinity was found only in three (20%). Except for Gly188Glu, Ile194Thr, Arg243His and Asp250Asn mutations which are found in patients of different ancestries [24], mutations usually differ from one family to the other. Therefore, the disorder has greater allelic heterogeneity than initially predicted.

Homozygous or complete LPL deficiency

Signs and symptoms are not constant; they vary in precocity and intensity in homozygotes with lipoprotein lipase deficiency [2]. Apart from the level of plasma triglyceride, predictors of the risk of acute pancreatitis are poorly defined. Mutations of the LDL receptor gene underlying familial hypercholesterolemia have been reported to be correlated with precocity and severity of the disease depending on whether the protein was detectable (missense mutations) or not (nonsense mutation) [25]. We addressed the same question depending upon whether a LPL gene mutation would preserve LPL mass in plasma or not. We analysed two groups of subjects: carriers of nonsense alleles (LPL mass absent) and carriers of missense alleles. In the latter group, 99% had lowered to normal levels of enzymatic mass, in vivo and/or in vitro (after expression of individual alleles in COS cells by site directed mutagenesis, [2–7] and Table 1). Nonsense mutations appeared to express earlier in life [9]. In 47% of carriers of nonsense mutations the disease was discovered before age two while it manifested in 37% of carriers of missense mutations at similar age. This is reminiscent of the precocity of the disease in LPL knock-out mice (animal model of null allele), in which the absence of LPL is lethal at birth, just after they begin to feed [26]. A residual ability to clear some of the circulating triglyceride-rich lipoproteins may account for this delay in disease manifestation in carriers of missense alleles. In contrast, pancreatitis had a similar prevalence in carriers of nonsense or missense mutations (42 vs. 48%), suggesting that LPL mass is not a protective factor in this case. As previously mentioned, pregnancy stood out as a risk factor for acute pancreatitis [2]. More than two out of three of LPL-deficient women were reported to suffer from their first episode of pancreatitis during the last trimesters of pregnancy. Interestingly, pregnancy may also predispose women to bouts of pancreatitis in heterozygous carriers of mutations of the LPL gene [19,27]. Remarkably, clinical findings in patients of different ancestries with different mutations, were very similar with those reported in French Canadians who are carriers of only three missense mutations (Pro207Leu, Gly188Glu and Asp250Asn [24,28]). Therefore, the loss of LPL activity in plasma seems a much stronger determinant of the severity of the disease than the loss of enzymatic mass.

However, mass assessment in conjunction with mutation identification may be useful in exploring the relationships between LPL deficiency and development of atherosclerosis. We have observed the unexpected development of peripheral atherosclerosis and of coronary artery disease, after a two-to-three decade follow-up in four patients after the age of 50 [14]. They were all carriers of missense mutations, with low to normal levels of LPL mass in plasma. Cardiovascular disease had been reported in patients with LPL deficiency aged over 50, including one French Canadian [17,28,29]. These findings appear contradictory with the classical assumption that LPL deficiency would not cause a predisposition to atherosclerosis, since these patients are lean, follow a low-fat diet and since chylomicrons are too large to penetrate the arterial wall and plasma levels of LDL cholesterol are low. However, along with profound disturbances in lipoprotein metabolism (delayed clearance of triglyceride rich particles, impaired HDL metabolism), which may in turn activate thrombogenesis and lipoprotein modification, the presence of an inactive enzyme may favour the binding and retention of lipoproteins within the arterial wall, thereby inducing foam-cell formation

[4,5]. It has been suggested that the chances were low of observing cardiovascular disease because LPL deficiency is rare and manifests during childhood. Indeed, 75% of patients in the homogeneous group of French Canadians and 70% of patients of different ancestries were discovered before age 20. Therefore, prospective studies in subjects with LPL deficiency, who may accumulate more VLDL particles and express other risk factors as they grow in age [2], would help determine if atherosclerosis is a common feature of the disease in adults.

Heterozygous or partial LPL deficiency

The existence of a phenotype in heterozygotes for LPL deficiency (who have an estimated prevalence of $1/500$ in the general population) was a long-lasting debate [2]. A low-HDL high-triglyceride trait has been found in heterozygous carriers of the same mutation in large families [30], or in homogeneous populations such as French Canadians [31]. We observed in 12 families of French ancestry (who carried different mutations of the LPL gene) that heterozygotes (n = 35) had a 49% increase in triglycerides (115 ± 73 vs. 77 ± 43 mg/dl, $p < 0.05$) and a 19% decrease in HDL cholesterol (47 ± 11 vs. 58 ± 18 mg/dl, $p < 0.05$) as compared with 26 noncarrier relatives. This trait appears as a common feature of partial LPL deficiency, more than the effect of a specific allele. Carriers of common variants which partially decrease LPL activity (see Table 1), also have a lipoprotein profile which reflects minor alterations of triglyceride or HDL cholesterol metabolism [23]. Mutations decreasing promoter activity have been recently identified as another cause of partial LPL deficiency [32]. Therefore, a partially defective lipolysis in plasma will result in a low-HDL high-triglyceride trait, the strength of its effect being a function of the level of residual LPL activity, and of other factors challenging lipoprotein metabolism.

In keeping, this trait may be worsened to frank combined hyperlipidemia or to hypertriglyceridemia in conjunction with interacting factors such as diabetes, increased BMI, apoE isoforms, high-fat diet, etc. [2,23]. Indeed prevalence of heterozygous LPL gene mutations is increased in familial-combined hyperlipidemia or in several forms of hypertriglyceridemias. An interesting link has been found between high blood pressure and the LPL gene locus by quantitative linkage mapping [33], and by a careful examination of heterozygous carriers of LPL gene mutations [34]. This may reflect, in vivo, functions of LPL at the endothelial-cell surface and in the arterial wall [4,5]. This brings up the question of the role of partial LPL deficiency in the susceptibility to atherosclerosis. So far, if the low-HDL high-triglyceride trait is common in premature coronary artery disease, the prevalence of partial mutants appears similar in patients and in their matched controls [23]. However, the Aps9Asn mutation has been shown to be more prevalent in subjects with increased progression of coronary artery disease. Thus, factors which favour the development of atherosclerosis in partial LPL deficiency need further investigation.

Other alleles and unknown phenotypes at the LPL locus?

As previously mentioned the majority of missense mutations have been found in the LPL catalytic site. This was predicted, since they were selected for a defective lipolysis in vivo. However, studies using recombinant LPL in vitro have shown that other noncatalytic domains may be involved in the interaction with cell-surface proteins and receptors on the one hand, and with lipoproteins on the other hand [4,5]. These functions may modulate cellular signalling, local endocytosis or retention of lipoproteins at the cell surface or their release in the extracellular medium. There is one example of a common mutation (Ser447Stop), which does not impair catalytic activity although a functional effect is suspected in vivo. The mutation creates a premature stop codon on the amino acid before the least of LPL primary sequence. However, LPL activity is normal in vitro and mass may be increased as compared with the wild-type allele [23]. A raising effect on plasma HDL levels, repeatedly observed in numerous individuals across different populations, has suggested a protective role for this mutation. We have investigated this hypothesis in 404 centenarians (mean age 100.5 years) and 361 younger controls (mean age 50.7 years) living in the same areas in France (Chronos 2 project, CEPH-GENSET, Paris). Interestingly, the frequency of the Ser447Stop mutation was significantly higher in centenarians (10.7 vs. 7.3%, $p < 0.025$) while the prevalence of the Asn291Ser mutation was lower (0.6 vs. 1.3%, $p < 0.001$) as compared with younger controls. Moreover, no significant effect could be detected on levels of lipoproteins which are already low in centenarians. In keeping with previous observations about apoE alleles and longevity [35], the Ser447-stop mutation is another protein variant which may determine yet unknown cellular and tissular functions and phenotypes at the LPL gene locus.

References

1. Wion KL, Kirchgessner TG, Lusis AJ, Schotz MC, Lawn RM. Human lipoprotein lipase complementary DNA sequence. Science 1987;235:1638—1641.
2. Brunzell JD. Familial lipoprotein lipase deficiency and other causes of the chylomicronemia syndrome. In: Scriver CR, Beaudet AL, Sly WS, Valle D (eds) The Metabolic Basis of Inherited Disease, 7th edn. Highstown, New Jersey: McGraw Hill, 1995;59:1913—1932.
3. Havel RJ, Gordon RS. Idiopathic hyperlipidemia: metabolic studies in an affected family. J Clin Invest 1960;39:1777.
4. Fojo SS, Dugi KA. Structure, function and role of lipoprotein lipase in lipoprotein metabolism. Curr Opin Lipid 1994;5:117—125.
5. Olivecrona G, Olivecrona T. Triglyceride lipases and atherosclerosis. Curr Opin Lipid 1995;6: 291—305.
6. Hayden MR, Ma Y, Brunzell J, Henderson HE. Genetic variants affecting human lipoprotein and hepatic lipases. Curr Opin Lipid 1991;2:104—109.
7. Lalouel JM, Wilson DE, Iverius P-H. Lipoprotein lipase and hepatic triglyceride lipase: molecular and genetic aspects. Curr Opin Lipid 1992;3:86—95.
8. Benlian P, Foubert L, Gagné E, Bernard L, De Gennes J-L, Langlois S, Robinson W, Hayden M. Complete paternal isodisomy for chromosome 8 unmasked by lipoprotein lipase deficiency.

Am J Hum Genet 1996;59:431—436.

9. Foubert L, De Gennes J-L, Benlian P, Truffert J, Miao L, Hayden MR. Compound heterozygosity for frameshift mutations in the gene for lipoprotein lipase in a patient with early-onset chylomicronemia. Hum Mutat 1997;(In press).

10. Ma Y, Liu MS, Zhang H, Forsythe IJ, Brunzell JD, Hayden MR. A 4 basepair deletion in exon 4 of the human lipoprotein lipase gene results in type I hyperlipoproteinemia. Hum Mol Genet 1993;2:1049—1050.

11. Takagi A, Ikeda Y, Mori A, Tsutsumi Z, Oida K, Nakai T, Yamamoto A. A newly identified heterozygous lipoprotein lipase gene mutation ($Cys^{239} \rightarrow Stop/TGC^{972} \rightarrow TGA$; LPL_{obama}) in a patient with primary type IV hyperlipoproteinemia. J Lipid Res 1994;35:2008—2018.

12. Hölzl B, Huber R, Paulweber B, Patsch JR, Sandhofer F. Lipoprotein lipase deficiency due to a 3′ splice site mutation in intron 6 of the lipoprotein lipase gene. J Lipid Res 1994;35:2161—2169.

13. Benlian P, Étienne J, De Gennes J-L, Noe L, Brault D. Raisonnier A, Arnault F, Hamelin J, Foubert L, Chuat JC, Tse C, Galibert F. A homozygous gene deletion of exon 9 causes lipoprotein lipase deficiency: possible intron-Alu recombination. J Lipid Res 1995;36:356—366.

14. Benlian P, De Gennes J-L, Foubert L, Zhang H, Gagné ES, Hayden M. Premature atherosclerosis in patients with familial chylomicronemia caused by mutations in the LPL gene. N Engl J Med 1996;335:848—854.

15. Foubert L, De Gennes J-L, Lagarde J-P, Ehrenborg E, Raisonnier A, Girardet J-P, Hayden MR, Benlian P. Assessment of French patients with LPL deficiency for French Canadian mutations. J Med Genet 1997;34:672—675.

16. Haubenwallner S, Hörl G, Shachter NS, Presta E, Fried SK, Höfler G, Kostner GM, Breslow JL, Zechner R. A novel missense mutation in the gene for lipoprotein lipase resulting in a highly conservative amino acid substitution ($Asp^{180} \rightarrow Glu$) causes familial hyperchylomicronemia (type I hyperlipoproteinemia). Genomics 1993;18:392—396.

17. Tenkanen H, Taskinen MR, Antikainen M, Ulmanen I, Kontula K, Ehnholm C. A novel amino acid substitution ($His183 \rightarrow Gln$) in exon 5 of the lipoprotein lipase gene results in loss of catalytic activity: phenotypic expression of the mutant gene in a heterozygous state. J Lipid Res 1994;35:220—228.

18. Ma Y, Liu MS, Chitayat D, Bruin T, Beisiegel U, Benlian P, Foubert L, De Gennes JL, Funke H, Forsythe I, Blaichman S, Papanicolaou D, Erkelens W, Kastelein J, Brunzell JD, Hayden MR. Recurrent missense mutations at the first and second base of codon ARG^{243} in human lipoprotein lipase causing chylomicronemia in patients of different ancestries. Hum Mutat 1994;3:52—58.

19. Ma Y, Ooi TC, Liu MS, Zhang H, MacPherson R, Edwards AL, Forsythe I, Frohlich J, Brunzell JD, Hayden MR. High frequency of mutations in the human lipoprotein lipase gene in pregnancy-induced chylomicronemia: possible association with apolipoprotein E2 isoform. J Lipid Res 1994;35:1066—1075.

20. Foubert L, Bruin T, De Gennes J-L, Ehrenborg E, Furioli J, Kastelein J, Benlian P, Hayden M. A single Ser259Arg mutation in the gene for lipoprotein lipase causes chylomicronemia in Moroccans of Berber ancestry. Hum Mutat 1997;(In press).

21. Rouis M, Lohse P, Dugi KA, Lohse P, Beg OU, Ronan R, Talley GD, Brunzell JD, Santamarina-Fojo S. Homozygosity for two point mutations in the lipoprotein lipase (LPL) gene in a patient with familial LPL deficiency: LPL ($Asp^9 \rightarrow Asn$, $Tyr^{262} \rightarrow His$). J Lipid Res 1996;37:651—661.

22. Previato L, Guardamagna O, Dugi KA, Ronan R, Talley GD, Santamarina-Fojo S, Brewer HB. A novel missense mutation in the C-terminal domain of lipoprotein lipase ($Glu^{410} \rightarrow Val$) leads to enzyme inactivation and familial chylomicronemia. J Lipid Res 1994;35:1552—1560.

23. Fisher RM, Humphries SE, Talmud PJ. Common variation in the lipoprotein lipase gene: effects on plasma lipids and risk of atherosclerosis. Atherosclerosis 1997;(In press).

24. Hayden MR, De Braekeleer M, Henderson HE, Kastelein J. Molecular geography of inherited disorders of lipoprotein metabolism: lipoprotein lipase deficiency and familial hypercholesterolemia. In: Lusis AJ, Rotter JI, Sparkes RS (eds) Molecular Genetics of Coronary Artery Disease.

Candidate Genes and Processes in Atherosclerosis. Basel/Switzerland: Monogr Human Genet Karger, 1992;14:350—362.

25. Hobbs HH, Brown MS, Goldstein JL. Molecular genetics of the LDL receptor gene in familial hypercholesterolemia. Hum Mutat 1992;1:445—466.

26. Weinstock PH, Bisgaier CL, Aalto-Setälä K, Radner H, Ramakrishnan R, Leva-Frank S, Essenburg AD, Zechner R, Breslow JL. Severe hypertriglyceridemia, reduced high-density lipoprotein and neonatal death in lipoprotein lipase knock out mice. J Clin Invest 1995;96: 2555—2568.

27. Keilson LM, Vary CPH, Sprecher DL, Renfrew R. Hyperlipidemia and pancreatitis during pregnancy in two sisters with a mutation in the lipoprotein lipase gene. Ann Int Med 1996;124: 425—428.

28. Gagné C, Brun DL, Julien P, Moorjani S, Lupien P-J. Primary lipoprotein lipase activity deficiency: clinical investigation of a French Canadian population. CMAJ 1989;140:405—411.

29. Hoeg JM, Osborne JC, Gregg RE, Brewer HB. Initial diagnosis of lipoprotein lipase deficiency in a 75-year-old man. Am J Med 1983;75:889—892.

30. Wilson DE, Emi M, Iverius PH, Hata A, Wu LL, Hillas E, Williams RR, Lalouel JM. Phenotypic expression of heterozygous lipoprotein lipase deficiency in the extended pedigree of a proband homozygous for a missense mutation. J Clin Invest 1990;86:735—750.

31. Bijvoet S, Gagné ES, Moorjani S, Gagné C, Henderson HE, Fruchart J-C, Dallongeville J, Alaupovic P, Prins M, Kastelein JJP, Hayden MR. Alterations in plasma lipoproteins and apolipoproteins before the age of 40 in heterozygotes for lipoprotein lipase deficiency. J Lipid Res 1996;37:640—650.

32. Yang W-S, Nevin DN, Iwasaki L, Peng R, Brown GB, Brunzell JD, Deeb SS. Regulatory mutations in the human lipoprotein lipase gene in patients with familial combined hyperlipidemia and coronary artery disease. J Lipid Res 1996;37:2627.

33. Wu D-A, Bu X, Warden CH, Shen DDC, Jeng C-Y, Sheu WHH, Fuh MMT, Katsuya T, Dzau VJ, Reaven GM, Lusis AJ, Rotter JI, Chen IYD. Quantitative trait locus mapping of human blood pressure to a genetic region at or near the lipoprotein lipase gene locus on chromosome 8p22. J Clin Invest 1996;97:2111—2118.

34. Sprecher DL, Harris BV, Stein EA, Bellet PS, Keilson LM, Simbartl LA. Higher triglycerides, lower high-density lipoprotein cholesterol, and higher systolic blood pressure in lipoprotein lipase-deficient heterozygotes. Circulation 1996;94:3239—3245.

35. Schächter F, Faure-Delanef L, Guenot F, Rouger H, Froguel P, Lesueur-Ginot L, Cohen D. Genetic associations with human longevity at the APOE and ACE loci. Nature Genet 1994;6:29—32.

Molecular genetics of familial hypercholesterolemia in Italy. Outcomes and future prospects

Sebastiano Calandra[1] and Stefano Bertolini[2]
[1]*Department of Biomedical Sciences, University of Modena; and* [2]*Department of Internal Medicine, University of Genova, Italy*

Introduction

Familial hypercholesterolemia (FH) is an autosomal codominant disorder due to defects of the LDL-receptor (LDL-R) function caused by mutations of LDL-R gene [1]. Up to now more than 200 mutations of this gene have been reported in FH subjects [1,2]. Over the last several years our group has been involved in the characterization of LDL-R gene mutations in Italian FH patients. During this survey we have characterised several novel mutations of this gene [3]. In this overview we summarize our recent findings by focusing on three topics: 1) a summary of the mutations found so far; 2) the results of the study of LDL-R gene mutations in a large group of phenotypically FH homozygotes; and 3) the identification of clusters of LDL-R gene mutations in Italy.

Results and Discussion

Selection of patients with FH and identification of the mutations in LDL-R gene

Several criteria were adopted to select the patients to be included in the study. The entry criteria were: 1) a level of plasma LDL-cholesterol (LDL-CH) in the proband above the 95th percentile value for the population; 2) the vertical transmission of hypercholesterolemia in the proband's family; 3) the bimodal distribution of cholesterol levels within the family. Validation criteria were: the presence of tendon xanthomas in the proband or in some of his/her family members; and/ or the presence of severe hypercholesterolemia in prepuberal children in the family. If validation criteria were satisfied the diagnosis of FH was made. If validation criteria were not present or family data were not available, the proband was labeled as "probable FH". By using these criteria, we selected 465 FH families and 206 "probable FH" families. The analysis of LDL-R gene has been performed in several families and it is still in progress. To date we identified a mutation of LDL-R gene in 193 families. The total number of subjects in whom a mutation has been identified is approximately 750 (3.5 mutation carriers per family). Fifty-seven mutations of LDL-R gene have been found so far: 15 major rearrangements (11 deletions and four insertions); eight minute mutations (four deletions and four insertions) and 34 point mutations (24 missense, six nonsense and four splice site mutations). Most of the point mutations can be screened by simple procedures based on selective PCR amplification of specific regions of LDL-R gene, followed by the digestion with restriction enzymes.

Study of FH-homozygotes

During the last few years we have performed DNA analysis in 39 patients with the clinical phenotype of homozygous FH; these patients have been identified in Italy over the last decade. The systematic analysis of LDL-R gene revealed that 29 patients were true homozygotes (i.e., they carried two identical mutant alleles) and 10 patients were compound heterozygotes. In homozygotes we found 13 different mutations (two major rearrangements, eight point mutations in coding sequence and three splice site mutations). In compound heterozygotes we found 12 different mutations (one major rearrangement, 10 point mutations in the coding sequence and one splice site mutation). In three compound heterozygotes we failed to identify the second mutant allele. In both groups of patients a large interindividual variability of LDL-CH levels was observed (from 11 to 26 mmol/l). The residual LDL-R activity in cultured fibroblasts ranged from < 2 to 30% of the control value. There was a significant inverse correlation between plasma LDL-CH levels and the residual LDL-R activity. The severity of coronary heart disease was more pronounced in subjects whose plasma LDL-CH levels were > 20 mmol/l.

Identification of clusters of LDL-R mutations

We identified 10 clusters of mutations located in various districts of Northern, Central and Southern Italy. These clusters include two large deletions and eight point mutations. In some clusters the number of FH-heterozygotes was sufficiently large to ascertain to what extent the type of mutation of LDL-R gene influences the elevation of plasma LDL-CH levels in FH-heterozygotes. When these clusters were grouped into a receptor negative group (which included the mutations known to abolish LDL-R function) and into a receptor defective group (which included the mutations known to reduce LDL-R function) we were able to detect differences in plasma LDL-CH levels among the clusters. Mean plasma LDL-CH levels were higher (or tended to be higher) in the clusters of the receptor negative group than in those of the receptor defective group. This indicates that, as observed in FH-homozygotes, the type of LDL-R mutation plays a role in determining LDL-CH levels in FH-heterozygotes. In all clusters, however, we observed a large interindividual variability of age adjusted plasma LDL-CH levels, a finding which suggests that other environmental and genetic factors play a role in controlling plasma LDL-CH levels in FH-heterozygotes. As the number of patients in each cluster increases, it will be possible to use these clusters of molecularly defined FH-heterozygotes to dissect the role of other genetic or environmental factors in affecting not only plasma lipoprotein levels but also other features of the phenotypic expression of FH (i.e., tendon xanthomas, premature cardiovascular disease, premature cardiac death, etc.)

References

1. Goldstein JL, Hobbs HH, Brown MS. Familial hypercholesterolemia. In: Scriver CR, Beaudet AL, Sly WS, Valle D (eds) The Metabolic and Molecular Bases of Inherited Disease. New York: McGraw-Hill, Inc., 1995;1981—2030.
2. Warrett M, Rabes JP, Collod-Beroud G, Junien C, Boileau C, Beroud C. Software and data base for the analysis of mutations in the human LDL-receptor. Nucl Acid Res 1997;25:172—180.
3. Calandra S, Bertolini S. The low density lipoprotein (LDL) receptor and familial hypercholesterolemia. In: Swallow DM, Edwards YH (eds) Protein Dysfunction and Human Genetic Disease. Oxford, UK: Bios Scientific Publishers, 1997;(In press).

Familial hypercholesterolemia: molecular genetics and clinical expression

Joep C. Defesche, Marianne E. Wittekoek and John J.P. Kastelein
Department of Vascular Medicine, Academic Medical Centre, University of Amsterdam, Amsterdam, The Netherlands

Introduction

The genetic predisposition for atherosclerotic vascular disease probably involves more than 200 genes. Their exact role in the atherosclerotic process is largely unknown, including their gene-gene and gene-environment interactions. Fortunately the molecular basis of familial hypercholesterolemia (FH) is completely elucidated and therefore, FH can serve as a model to study these interactions. We have assessed the influence of lipoprotein lipase (LPL) gene mutations (lipoprotein(a) (Lp(a)), homocysteine and apo E-genotype) on the clinical expression of FH. LPL gene mutations and elevated Lp(a) levels were associated with a higher incidence of cardiovascular disease (CVD) in patients with FH. Homocysteine and apo E-genotype did not seem to influence the clinical outcome.

FH and LDL-receptor mutations

Today, more than 300 mutations underlying FH, have been identified [1]. These mutations will result in the loss of specific functions of the low-density lipoprotein (LDL) receptor: ligand binding, intracellular transport, maturation, membrane anchoring, internalisation or recycling. Several studies have demonstrated that the mutation type (i.e., null alleles or defective receptors) can partly explain the variation in clinical expression of FH in terms of lipoprotein levels, severity of CVD or response to lipid-lowering therapy [2–4].

The role of lipoprotein lipase in FH

LPL is a key enzyme in the metabolism of triglyceride-rich lipoproteins. LPL mutations have been shown to alter lipoprotein levels in healthy controls as well as in patients with CVD [5,6]. A group of 1,045 FH patients was analysed for

---

Address for correspondence: Dr Ir J.C. Defesche, Department of Vascular Medicine, Academic Medical Centre at the University of Amsterdam, P.O. Box 22 660, NL-1100 DD Amsterdam, The Netherlands. Tel.: +31-20-566-6528 (direct) or +31-20-566-2824 (secretary). Fax: +31-20-691-6972. E-mail: defesche@pi.net

the presence of a common mutation in the LPL gene: N291S. In this group, 68 patients with FH (6.5%) were carriers of N291S [7]. Comparison of FH-N291S carriers with FH-noncarriers showed that N291S significantly reduced HDL-cholesterol levels and increased total cholesterol and triglyceride levels (Table 1).

The differences in triglycerides and HDL-cholesterol levels between FH-N291S carriers and FH-noncarriers were more evident in the middle and upper BMI tertiles (data not shown). This suggests an interaction between the N291S mutation and increasing body weight. Moreover, the incidence of CVD in FH patients carrying the N291S-mutation was higher than in noncarriers: 29.7 vs. 12.0% with an odds ratio of 3.88 (p = 0.006) [7].

Symptomatic vs. asymptomatic FH

In order to identify new risk factors for CVD, a group of FH patients with CVD was compared with a matched group of asymptomatic FH patients. The groups were matched for age, gender, BMI and blood pressure. No differences were found for levels of total-, LDL-, HDL-cholesterol, triglycerides, apo A1 and B, or homocysteine (after fasting and methionine loading) (Table 2).

The two FH patient groups were also analysed for the frequency of the $C_{677} \rightarrow T$ mutation in the methylenetetrahydrofolate reductase gene, which proved to be present in both groups in similar allele frequencies: 34.7 in the asymptomatic vs. 31.2% in the symptomatic group. Only levels of Lp(a) were significantly higher in the symptomatic FH patients. These increased Lp(a) levels were also strongly associated with the number of kringle IV repeats in the apo(a) gene (Table 2).

Intima-media thickness

The thickness of the intima-medial complex (IMT) was measured in sympto-

Table 1. Characteristics of FH patients with and without the LPL N291S mutation.

	FH-N291S carriers	FH matched controls	p-value
n	64	175	
Age (years)	39.9 ± 16.5	38.2 ± 15.0	ns
BMI (kg/m^2)	23.58 ± 3.64	23.08 ± 3.29	ns
Male/female (%)	47/53	48/52	ns
Syst BP (mmHG)	129.14 ± 16.25	129.86 ± 18.21	ns
Smoking (cig/day)	5.1	5.7	ns
Alcohol (units/day)	1.5	1.4	ns
TC (mmol/l)	8.96 ± 1.65	8.42 ± 1.60	0.02
LDL (mmol/l)	6.70 ± 1.55	6.45 ± 1.63	ns
HDL (mmol/l)	1.15 ± 0.36	1.32 ± 0.37	0.002
Trigs	1.83 ± 3.63	1.41 ± 0.64	0.004

BMI: body mass index; Syst BP: systolic blood pressure; TC: total cholesterol; LDL: LDL-cholesterol; HDL: HDL-cholesterol; Trigs: triglycerides; ns: not statistically significant.

Table 2. Characteristics of symptomatic and asymptomatic FH patients.

	Asymptomatic FH	Symptomatic FH	p-value
n	142	106	
Age (years)	48 ± 9.2	48 ± 9.2	ns
BMI (kg/m^2)	26 ± 4.1	26 ± 3.3	ns
Syst BP (mmHg)	126.6 ± 4.1	131.7 ± 16.1	ns
Diast. BP (mmHg)	81.4 ± 9.3	83.0 ± 10.0	ns
Male/female (%)	49/51	58/42	ns
TC (mmol/l)	9.79 ± 2.27	9.50 ± 2.21	ns
LDL (mmol/l)	7.69 ± 2.33	7.61 ± 2.12	ns
HDL (mmol/l)	1.18 ± 0.74	1.20 ± 0.36	ns
Trigs (mmol/l)	2.01 ± 1.08	1.68 ± 0.68	ns
ApoA1 (g/l)	1.43 ± 0.20	1.50 ± 0.32	ns
ApoB (g/l)	2.42 ± 0.74	2.51 ± 0.61	ns
Hcy-fast (μmol/l)	11.7 ± 7.13	11.9 ± 3.42	ns
Hcy-load (μmol/l)	37.9 ± 16.6	39.7 ± 12.7	ns
Lp(a) (mg/l)	403 ± 448	786 ± 719	< 0.001
Log Lp(a) (mg/l)	2.38 ± 0.45	2.65 ± 0.54	0.004
K IV < 25/ > 25 (%)	46.2/53.8	68.9/31.1	0.024

BMI: body mass index; Syst BP: systolic blood pressure; Diast. BP: diastolic blood pressure; TC: total cholesterol; LDL: LDL-cholesterol; HDL: HDL-cholesterol; Trigs: triglycerides; Apo A1 and B: apolipoprotein A1 and B; Lp(a): lipoprotein(a); Log: logarithmic transformed; Hcy: homocysteine; fast: fasting; load: after methionine loading; K IV < 25/ > 25: number of kringle IV repeats below or over 25; ns: not statistically significant.

matic and asymptomatic FH patients. The IMT of the common and internal artery, the carotid bulb and the common and superficial femoral artery was greater in the symptomatic FH patients. Especially the IMT of the common femoral artery differed significantly between the symptomatic and asymptomatic FH groups. IMT was shown to be a good predictor of cardiovascular disease (publication in preparation).

Apolipoprotein E (apoE)

The apo E-genotype is known to influence lipid levels, albeit to a small extent. Apo E2 is associated with slightly decreased cholesterol levels while for apo E4 the opposite is the case. Previous studies in FH patients and analysis of our FH patient population (data not shown) show a similar trend, but a relation between apoE genotype and clinical phenotype could not be established [8].

Conclusions

The clinical expression of FH does not seem to depend on lipid and lipoprotein levels in a given patient. In addition, homocysteine levels or mutations affecting homocysteine metabolism do not alter CVD risk in FH patients. Conversely,

Lp(a), especially the number of kringle IV repeats in the apo(a) gene, and mutations in the LPL gene do modulate the clinical expression. IMT was larger in symptomatic FH patients, but whether differences in apo(a) kringles and mutations in the LPL gene underlie these differences in IMT is still under investigation.

References

1. Varret M, Rabes JP et al. Nucl Ac Res 1997;25:172—180.
2. Jeenah M, September W, van Roggen F et al. Atherosclerosis 1993;98:51—58.
3. Gudnason V, Day INM, Humphries SE. Arterioscl Thromb 1994;14:1717—1722.
4. Sun XM, Patel DD, Bhatnagar D, Knight BL, Soutar AK. Arterioscl Thromb Vasc Biol 1995;15:219—227.
5. Pimstone SN, Gagné E, Gagné C et al. Arterioscl Thromb 1995;15:1704—1712.
6. Reymer PWA, Gagné E, Groenemeyer BE et al. Nat Genet 1995;10:28—33.
7. Wittekoek ME, Pimstone SN, Reymer PWA et al. Circulation 1997;(In press).
8. Tonsted S, Leren TP, Sivertsen M et al. Arterioscl Thromb Vasc Biol 1995;15:1009—1014.

Familial HDL deficiency syndromes

Harald Funke

Institut für Klinische Chemie und Laboratoriumsmedizin und Arbeitsgruppe Molekulare Genetik der Koronaren Herzkrankheit im Institut für Arterioskleroseforschung, Universität Münster, Germany

Abstract. Low serum concentrations of HDL cholesterol are well-established markers for a high risk of developing coronary artery disease (CAD). The absence of CAD symptoms from some individuals with familial HDL deficiency demonstrates the presence of heterogeneity in this relation and points to the important role of etiologic and modifying factors.

Introduction

Prospective epidemiological studies have identified low serum HDL-cholesterol concentrations as good predictors for clinical endpoints of coronary artery disease (CAD) [1–3]. This relation has been confirmed in numerous case control studies. Biochemical analyses have identified HDL particles as potent acceptors of excess cellular cholesterol in a pathway termed reverse cholesterol transport (RCT) [4]. Details on this pathway can be found in a recent review of the subject [5]. A concept has emerged which identifies low HDL-cholesterol levels with ineffective RCT and thus CAD risk. This interpretation has recently been challenged by the observation that complete absence of HDL-cholesterol resulting from monogenic disorders in man or from gene knockouts in mice is not in all cases related to the premature onset of CAD.

An incomplete list of the factors responsible for the variance in the clinical phenotype of complete HDL deficiency includes the gene harboring the basic defect, modifying genes, and environmental factors. While there is no doubt about the association between low HDL cholesterol and CAD risk, an assignment of causes for this observation may be premature. The rare cases of monogenic HDL deficiency are only a very minor subfraction (if present at all) within the low HDL group of epidemiologic studies (usually defined by a threshold value of 35 mg/dl, which is approx. the 17th percentile of the population distribution curve for this parameter). If there is more than one common mechanism by which low HDL is linked to increased CAD risk, the subgroups' risk has to be determined separately.

Address for correspondence: Harald Funke, Institut für Klinische Chemie und Laboratoriumsmedizin und Arbeitsgruppe Molekulare Genetik der Koronaren Herzkrankheit im Institut für Arteriosklleroseforschung, Universität Münster, Albert Schweitzer-Straße 33, 48149 Münster, Germany.

714

Table 1. Mutations in apolipoprotein A-1. Mutations causing familial absence of HDL-cholesterol.

Mutation	Frequency	Zygosity	Phenotype	References
50 kb deletion at the APOLP1 locus	1 report	Homoz.	Combined apo AI, -CIII, -AIV deficiency, low triglycerides, partial LCAT deficiency; xanthomatosis, corneal opacities, CAD	6
> 2 kb inversion between APOA1 and APOC3	1 report	Homoz.	Combined apo AI, -CIII deficiency, low triglycerides, partial LCAT deficiency; xanthomatosis, corneal opacities, CAD	7
Q-2X	1 report	Homoz.	Xanthelasmas, retinopathy, cerebellar ataxia[a], CAD[a]	8
1 bp del, C, Gln5Arg, fs 11 end	1 report	Compound heteroz. Leu141Arg	CAD[a]	9,10
1 bp ins, C, Gln5Pro, fs 34 end	Very rare	Homoz.	Low triglycerides; corneal opacities, planar xanthomas[a,b], hepatomegaly	11–13
Trp8End	1 report	Homoz.	Extremely low HDL-cholesterol, complete apo A-I deficiency; corneal opacities	14
Q32X	1 report	Homoz.	Partial LCAT deficiency; bilateral suborbital xanthelasmas	15
A37T-Q84X	1 report	Homoz.	Apo AI deficiency; normal corneas, xanthomatosis, CAD	16
Leu141Arg	1 report	Compound heteroz. 1 bp del, C, Gln5Arg, fs 11 end	CAD[a]	9,10
1 bp del, G, Thr202Thr, fs 234 end	1 report	Homoz.	HDL deficiency, hypertriglyceridemia[a], heterodimer formation with apo AII and other proteins, partial LCAT deficiency; corneal clouding	17

[a]Not an invariate finding; [b]in one report the authors of the Turkish case said CAD was present.

Table 2. Mutations in apolipoprotein A-I. Mutations causing amyloidosis.

Mutation	Frequency	Zygosity	Phenotype	References
G26R	Very rare	Heteroz.	Systemic amyloidosis, nephropathy, neuropathy[a], peptic ulcer[a], hearing loss[a], cataract[a]	18
Trp50Arg	1 report	Heteroz.	Hereditary amyloidosis	19
L60R	1 report	Heteroz.	Nonneurothathic systemic amyloidosis	20
Del 36 bp (aa 60-71) - ins 6 bp (aa 60-61; Val, Thr)	1 report	Heteroz.	Nonneuropathic amyloidosis, liver failure	21

In all reported cases the disease showed an autosomal dominant segregation pattern. [a]Not an invariate finding.

Table 3. Mutations in apolipoprotein A-I. Mutations with milder phenotypes.

Mutation	Phenotype	References
Pro3Arg	Slow propeptide cleavage	22
Pro3His	Slow propeptide cleavage	22
Pro4Arg		22
Arg10Leu		23
Asp13Tyr		24
Asp89Glu		25
Ala95Asp		26
Tyr100His		27
Asp103Asn		28
ΔLys107	Changes in lipid binding and a-helical structure, reduced LCAT cofactor activity, reduced HDL-cholesterol plasma concentrations	25,29, 30
Lys107Met		25
Trp108Arg		26
Glu110Lys		31
Glu136Lys		32,33
Glu139Gly		25
Pro143Arg		34
45 bp del (aa146-160)[a]	Reduced HDL concentration, partial LCAT deficiency; bilateral arcus senilis	35
Glu147Val		
Arg151Cys[a]	Reduced HDL cholesterol, reduced LCAT cofactor activity, partial LCAT deficiency, alterations in lipid binding, increased FCR of HDL, formation of homo- and heterodimers and of abnormal HDL particles	25 E. Bruckert et al. (In press)
Ala158Glu		36
His162Gln		27
Pro165Arg[a]	Reduced HDL cholesterol, reduced LCAT cofactor activity, diminished cholesterol efflux	22
Glu169Gln		25
Arg173Cys[a]	Reduced HDL cholesterol, reduced LCAT cofactor activity, partial LCAT deficiency, alterations in lipid binding, increased FCR of HDL, formation of homo- and heterodimers and of abnormal HDL particles	37
Arg177His		38
Glu198Lys		39
Asp213Gly		36

For the Glu136Lys has a homozygous carrier been identified; all other mutations were found in heterozygous individuals. [a]Homozygous presence of these mutations may cause familial absence of HDL.

Genetic defects causing HDL deficiency

Familial absence of HDL cholesterol is a rare metabolic disorder of which approximately 10 cases have been characterized at the molecular level (a listing of apo A-I mutations can be found in Tables 1—3). The majority of probands

Table 4. Mutations in the human lecithin: cholesterol acyltransferase (LCAT) gene.

Defect	Zygosity	Phenotype	References
IVS 4: T22C	C-het(Thr123lle)	FED	40
1 bp ins, C	Hom	Familial LCAT deficiency; inactive enzyme	41
1 bp ins, nt 937	Chet(Arg399Cys)	Familial LCAT deficiency	42
Duplic of codons −4 to +6	C-het(Gly33Arg)	LCAT deficiency (incomplete)	43
Asn%elle	Hom	Familial LCAT deficiency	64
Pro10Leu	Hom	FED	44
Pro10Gln	C-het(Arg135Gln)	FED	45
Gly30Ser	Hom	Familial LCAT deficiency; inactive enzyme	46
Gly33Arg	C-het(30bp dupl.)	LCAT deficiency (incomplete)	47
Tyr83End	Hom/het	Familial LCAT deficiency	47
	C-het(Tyr156Asn)	Familial LCAT deficiency	48
Ala93Thr, Arg158Cys	Hom	Familial LCAT deficiency	47
Thr123lle	Hom/het	FED/CAD[a]/HDL reduction	49
	C-het(Tyr144Cys)	FED/HDL reduction	50
	C-het(Thr347Met)	FED/HDL reduction	51
Asp131Ans	Hom	FED	52
Arg135Trp	C-het(376fs)/het	Familial LCAT deficiency/HDL reduction	47
Arg135Gln	C-het(Pro10Gln)	FED; mutation may cause familial LCAT deficiency	45
Arg140His	Hom	Familial LCAT deficiency	53
140(3 bp Ins)141	Hom	Familial LCAT deficiency	54
Tyr144Cys	C-het(Thr123lle)	FED?; familial LCAT deficiency?	50
Arg147Trp		Familial LCAT deficiency	55
Tyr156Asn	C-het(Tyr83End)	Familial LCAT deficiency	48
1 bp del, C, 168	C-het(Thr321Met)	Familial LCAT deficiency	56
Gly183Asp	Hom	Familial LCAT deficiency?; FED?	Funke et al., unpublished
Leu209Pro	Hom/het	Familial LCAT deficiency/HDL reduction	47
Asn228Lys	Hom	Familial LCAT deficiency	54
Met252Lys	Hom	Familial LCAT deficiency	57
1 bp del, G, Val264	Hom	Familial LCAT deficiency	58
Ille293Met	Hom	Familial LCAT deficiency	54
Thr321Met	Hom	Familial LCAT deficiency	47
	C-het(1 bp del,C,168)	Familial LCAT deficiency	56
del Leu300	Hom	FED	59
Gly344Ser	Hom	Familial LCAT deficiency	58
Tyr347Met	C-het(Thr123lle)	FED/HDL reduction	51
1 bp ins, A, Gln376Thr, fs	C-het(Arg135Trp)/het	Familial LCAT deficiency/HDL reduction	47
Arg399Cys	C-het(1bp ins,nt 937)	Familial LCAT deficiency	42

[a]Not an invariate finding.

with complete absence of HDL that we have investigated in our laboratory over the past decade either had apolipoprotein (apo) A-I deficiency or lecithin: cholesterol acyltransferase (LCAT) deficiency. The rest can be grouped into Tangier disease (familial HDL deficiency) and familial absence of HDL of unknown origin based on metabolic and clinical characteristics not seen in the other diseases.

Defects at the APOLP1 locus

Two new apo A-I mutations, one an insertion/deletion mutation [21], the other a missense mutation (Trp50Arg) [19], have been identified to cause hereditary amyloidosis (Table 2). As in the previous cases, the amyloid fibrils were composed exclusively of N-terminal fragments. The authors noted that in all four currently known cases the variant protein contained an extra positive charge in this domain. When an extra positive charge occurs very early in the apo A-I sequence, as is the case for the Pro to Arg mutations in codons three and four, amyloidosis is not observed [22].

A compound heterozygosity in the apo A-I gene was the metabolic basis for the absence of HDL in four individuals of an Italian family [9,10]. One mutation was a deletion of a cytosin from a stretch of seven consecutive cytosins encoding amino acids 3–5 of the mature plasma form of apo A-I. Two cases of cytosin insertions had previously been reported at the same location. It may thus be that the deletion and the insertion are products of the same crossing over error. The second mutation in the Italian family was a missense mutation (Leu141Arg). Thanks to its occurrence together with a null allele it was now possible to demonstrate that missense mutations in apo A-I can cause HDL deficiency.

LCAT defects

LCAT defects are usually divided into the subgroups familial LCAT deficiency (FLD) and fish eye disease (FED). The first is characterized by the absence or near absence of LCAT activity in plasma and is commonly associated with HDL deficiency, corneal opacities, proteinuria, red blood cell anomalies, and, with an onset usually before the age of 50, kidney failure. In FED the only clinical symptom is corneal clouding. The disease defining characteristic is the selective loss of enzyme activity of the mutant LCAT towards HDL particles. This is measured by a near normal endogenous cholesterol esterification rate (CER) in the absence of LCAT activity against exogenous substrates. Some LCAT defects were found to have significant residual LCAT activity. They have been classified as incomplete LCAT deficiencies.

During the review period several new LCAT gene mutations have been identified (Table 4) [42–58]. In an Australian family of British descent and in a Dutch family, carriers of the Thr123Ile mutation were detected [40,50]. This FED-causing mutation is the most frequently observed LCAT mutation. In the Dutch family it was present as part of a compound heterozygosity. The second mutation was a null allele. LCAT mass and activity in the compound heterozygotes were at the same level as previously reported for homozygous 123Ile carriers [49]. It may thus be possible that the metabolic effect of a single FED allele is sufficient to prevent kidney disease. If this hypothesis can be clearly established, the presence of at least one FED allele in an LCAT-deficient patient could be used as an advantageous prognostic marker.

Before we can use this information in the clinical management of disease, methodology will have to be developed which clearly allows to distinguish between FED mutations and those causing familial LCAT deficiency. This usually does not constitute a problem in homozygote cases. In compound heterozygosity it is difficult to assign an FED characteristic to one of the two allele products because the CER cannot be determined in an allele-specific way and cannot be measured in in vitro expression systems. Therefore, it remains unknown if the mutations in codons 144 [50] and 347 [51] are FED mutations or classical LCAT mutations.

Incorrect splicing of the LCAT gene as the direct consequence of a mutation 22 bases away from the intron/exon-boundary is the first human example to show that alterations in the Lariat branchpoint consensus sequence lead to differential gene expression [40]. An important side effect of this finding is the necessity for the inclusion of more intron sequence in mutation screening analyses.

More than 30 mutations have now been identified in the LCAT gene. From these mutations we have learned that different defects can be associated with a wide spectrum of biochemical and clinical consequences and that missense mutations from any region of the protein can cause either FLD or FED. This suggests that LCAT needs a very complex tertiary structure for proper function which can be disrupted by variation in any part of the protein. In this context it is noteworthy that, in contrast with the situation in apo A-I, no LCAT missense mutation has been reported that does not affect enzyme function.

Also, LCAT mutations have taught us that LCAT activity is a prerequisite for the presence of normal, large size HDL in plasma. As both FLD and FED cause HDL deficiency it is clear that the exogenous LCAT activity is responsible for the building of these particles. It has been suggested that this process involves a direct interaction of LCAT with HDL precursor particles which become normal size HDL particles as a consequence of this interaction. Despite the characterization of many mutations we do not know the cause of FED. Many suggestions have been made. They range from the original proposal of a specific inability of LCAT to interact with HDL to problems in the complex interaction of LCAT with substrates and transfer proteins.

Other defects

The molecular basis of Tangier disease is not known. Characteristics used for classification include a history of tonsillectomy, the presence of foam cells, hepatosplenomegaly, an increased proapo A-I-to-apo-A-I ratio, and impaired cholesterol afflux [60,61]. In the assembly of HDL particles, apo A-I serves as an essential acceptor of cholesterol and LCAT maturates the particles by providing them with cholesterol esters. It will be interesting to see if the basic defect in Tangier disease interferes with the HDL particle assembly at an even earlier stage, that is, making cellular cholesterol available for transfer [62]. A new member has been added to the heterogenous group of HDL deficiencies which is neither apo A-I or LCAT deficiency nor Tangier disease [63].

Another important subgroup of HDL deficiency, which is not usually summarized in this category, is LPL deficiency. Homozygosity for this disorder is commonly associated with HDL-cholesterol concentrations between 5 and 15 mg/dl. Arguments have been raised on whether HDL-cholesterol concentrations can be precisely measured in the presence of severe hypertriglyceridemia. Since a substantial part of HDL originates from intestinal sources, an impairment in the catalysis of chylomicrons and thus in the formation of HDL precursors justifies its listing among primary HDL deficiencies. A more detailed analysis of the role of LPL in CAD formation will appear in the August issue of Current Opinion in Lipidology.

CAD in complete HDL deficiency

From the clinical symptoms listed in Tables 1 and 4 it becomes apparent that CAD is repeatedly but not invariably associated with apo A-I deficiency and LCAT deficiency. As a consequence of the low overall case numbers it is difficult to determine if the observed CAD frequencies are typical for the underlying disorders. Underestimation may result from the relatively young age of some of the probands, while overrepresentation can be the consequence of selection bias, e.g., through a higher probability for getting an HDL cholesterol determination in CAD patients than in the general population.

LCAT-deficient patients, because they are usually seen by a physician for their kidney problems, do not have a selection bias for CAD. Is their lower CAD rate thus representative for HDL deficient individuals? The usually young age of these patients at the time of diagnosis (and report in the literature) does not allow this conclusion to be drawn. Also, the absence of CAD symptoms, a typical finding in the early reports on primary defects in the LCAT gene, is no longer a characteristic for this disorder. Recent reports on familial LCAT deficiency and FED have identified individuals with CAD [45].

In a recent paper by Miccoli et al. [10] the issue of HDL deficiency and CAD has been addressed. They found that in four HDL-deficient siblings the only one without CAD was female. It was proposed that additional risk factors present in her brothers (male sex and elevated LDL-cholesterol concentration) led to CAD formation. A generalization of this hypothesis would lead to a system in which the absence of HDL-cholesterol is not per se causing CAD. Increasingly higher concentrations of HDL cholesterol would, however, be needed to compensate for the presence of higher numbers and levels of risk factors. Marked changes in

720

LDL particles have also been observed in a Canadian family with absence of HDL and early onset CAD described by Ng et al. [8]. Other than Miccoli et al. these investigators consider this finding a pleiotropic effect of the apo A-I mutation.

The low overall number of individuals with complete absence of HDL does not allow to decide if CAD found associated with it is a consequence of this biochemical characteristic, or if it reflects the high prevalence of CAD in Western populations. Due to the fact that in only one case has an HDL-deficiency-causing mutation been found independently for a second time, it is even more difficult to judge if differences in the observed associated phenotype relate to differences in the primary defects or if they result from variation at other gene loci or in the environment.

Protective role for hyperalphalipoproteinemia?

An effect on HDL-cholesterol concentrations opposite to that resulting from mutations in apo A-I or LCAT has been observed for CETP mutations [64]. Although new cases have recently been added to the list of basic defects in familial hyperalphalipoproteinemia [65,66], their overall frequency is too low for a statistically founded analysis of a potential protection from CAD. Two mutations with a high enough frequency for statistical analyses were associated with only small changes in HDL-cholesterol. They showed a weak relation to CAD, especially in the presence of low HTGL activity [67]. Polymorphisms not known to change the encoded amino acid sequence of CETP were found to be associated with small changes in CETP concentration [68] or CETP activity [69] but not with changes in HDL-cholesterol concentration [68—70]. More insight into the role of a CETP mediated raise of HDL cholesterol and its relation to CAD can be expected from a polymorphic missense mutation which is present with a high frequency in several ethnically distinct populations and has been found to be associated with increased HDL-cholesterol concentrations [71].

Animal models in HDL research

In order to overcome the limitations related to low case numbers and ethical issues for biological studies in human HDL deficiency, animal models have been created using transgenic and knockout technology. Regarding predisposition to CAD, the knockout of the apolipoprotein A-I gene in mice was not any more conclusive than the human cases of apo A-I deficiency [72]. Cumulative evidence from several overexpression studies suggests a protective role for augmented levels of amphiphilic helical structures as they are contained in apolipoproteins. Apo A-I overexpression reduces the formation of fatty streaks in mice fed an atherosclerosis-inducing diet [73] via the induction of changes in HDL particle composition [74]. In addition, the atherosclerosis susceptibility caused by apo E deficiency was found reduced [75] in apo A-I overexpressers. Also protected from the effect of a cholesterol-rich diet were mice overexpressing human apo A-IV [76] and rabbits overexpressing human apo A-I [77]. Many-fold elevations of HDL-cholesterol concentrations following extreme overexpression of LCAT were observed in human apo A-I transgenic mice after the injection of human LCAT containing adenovirus [78] and in transgenic human LCAT rabbits [79,80]. In the latter case protection from CAD formation was reported. LCAT overexpression leads to elevated plasma HDL concentrations in a dose-dependent manner. The likely mechanism for this observation is the shift of HDL into a metabolically less active pool [80]. The role of LCAT activity as the rate-limiting step in the formation of HDL_3 and HDL_2 from smaller precursors which has been postulated from the analysis of the human deficiencies has thus been confirmed in these models.

A recent report on the overexpression of human CETP in hypertriglyceridemic mice has shown that reduced HDL-cholesterol is not always a problem. In these animals CETP expression was associated with decreased HDL cholesterol levels and at the same time with a lower atherosclerotic lesion percentage [81]. Another transfer protein, phospholipid transfer protein (PLTP), has been overexpressed in mice [82,83]. Both groups find higher HDL-cholesterol levels in the overexpressing animals than in controls. The effect was elevated in the presence of human apo A-I [82].

Atherosclerosis formation is a slow process which develops over extended periods of time as the consequence of a small imbalance between lesion-forming processes and mechanisms for their removal or prevention. It has thus been argued that in complex disorders results from transgenic models are only of limited value. Especially in rodents, most of the HDL uptake is apo E-mediated, while in humans a complex remodeling of lipoprotein particles occurs before uptake.

Differences between human and mouse proteins may also be the basis for contradicting results for the role of apo A-II in lipid metabolism. An apo A-II knockout mouse was associated with largely reduced HDL-cholesterol levels and increased remnant clearance [84]. A reduction in HDL-cholesterol was also one of the major effects of the transgenic expression of human apo A-II in mice [85]. In contrast to these observations a human apo A-II null-allele did not affect HDL-cholesterol concentration [86].

Common genetic defects associated with changes in HDL cholesterol concentration

Another strategy for assessing the relationship between genetic variation in lipoprotein metabolism and the formation of CAD has been horizontal genetics. In contrast to the complete HDL deficiencies, in these studies low case numbers were no longer the problem, but new obstacles occurred. Many of the reported positive associations between polymorphisms and CAD were not confirmed by others. To date, data from these type of studies have not reached a pragmatic value allowing its use in clinical practice.

Often, multiparametric screening studies were performed without defining a null hypothesis. Among the many factors responsible for false positive associations low case numbers are most noticeable. When factors different from the polymorphism under investigation also contribute to the tested phenotype, as is the case in CAD for several environmental factors and some genetic variants, low numbers of rare-allele carriers in the study may cause an unequal presence of these confounding factors in the case and control groups. Consequently, factors other than those under investigation might be the relevant discriminators.

Another important issue in horizontal genetics relates to the type of study. Often, results are different when data from studies in which the genotype information is used to look for associated phenotypic changes are compared with those in which genotype frequencies are determined for predefined phenotypes. A polymorphic missense mutation in codon 158 of apo E (Arg158Cys) can be used to illustrate this point. While the presence of an E2-allele (158Cys) is associated with elevated HDL-cholesterol concentrations [87] in the general population, it is associated with reduced concentrations in probands with type III hyperlipoproteinemia. The first method will only detect mutational effects when the product of its frequency and the extent of the phenotypic change is above a specific threshold value. Much more subtle changes can be detected with the second method. One should keep in mind though that an enrichment of a specific phenotype by a factor of 50,000, as is the case for type III hyperlipoproteinemics, is a rare event and is usually associated with low case numbers which, for this reason, is subject to frequent false positive results. An example of contradicting results which could be the consequence of the aforementioned difference in study design are mutations in lipoprotein lipase [88,89]. A more detailed discussion of LPL mutations will appear in the next issue of Current Opinion in Lipidology [90].

What's next?

Low HDL cholesterol is a good predictor of CAD events [1–3], and a high percentage of this association is mediated by genes [91]. The combined phenotypic effect of mutations currently known to affect this pathway explains only a minor fraction of CAD. While the other lipoprotein risk factor, low-density lipoproteins or subfractions thereof, appears to be directly involved in the metabolic cascade leading to atherosclerotic lesions, low HDL cholesterol has been proposed to be a surrogate for not yet identified gene mediated disturbances [92].

Genetic markers will only then have a place in practical medicine, if there is a benefit from their use. Currently, multiple logistic function algorithms developed from prospective data on CAD incidence allow a precise risk prediction. Genetic parameters will have to offer alternative or additional information. Apart from the possibility for genetic counseling in FH, the only current benefit from knowing ones genes is knowing.

New candidate genes

Options for the future certainly include the use of new candidate genes. Among these, the newly identified HDL-receptor (SR BI) [93] is a prime target. A precise prediction of the effect on the quantitative intermediate phenotype of mutations in the SR BI gene is a prerequisite for an enrichment of mutations in probands used for screening analysis. It is not currently known if a reduced uptake of cholesterol esters from HDL leads to an accumulation of large size HDL particles or if it causes more complex changes in lipoprotein metabolism. The latter is probably the case since it has recently been shown that this receptor is under feedback control of intracellular cholesterol stores [94] and that its expression is modified by hormones [95].

Other candidate genes include regulators of fatty acid metabolism [96,97] which have recently been shown to affect obesity [98], intracellular fatty acid transport and insulin resistance [99], all old suspects in the CAD case.

Linkage analysis

Despite the emergence of these exciting new candidates, it has been proposed that in recent decades too much of our effort has centered around lipoproteins and that candidate genes from other metabolic pathways should be considered as well as agents causative for CAD [100]. One possibility to search in an unbiased fashion for new candidate genes is linkage analysis for which new strategies have been developed to compensate for the problem of CAD's multifactorial origin [101–104]. Although the potential of sib-pair analysis has not been systematically evaluated, this method may not produce clearer results than previous association studies at candidate loci since it only leads to an enrichment of disease-causing alleles by a factor of probably a little more than two when compared with the horizontal analysis used before. The advantage of this method may lie in the use of markers which have much higher polymorphism information content (PIC) than those previously used and in its allowance for more than just candidates.

Gene-gene interactions

The majority of genetic defects known to severely affect HDL-cholesterol concentrations are very rare. More frequent variants often have an only minor effect on this quantitative intermediate phenotype for CAD. In order to become useful for individualized risk prediction, there should be an additive effect of combinations of this latter type of mutations. Initial data from our laboratory show that three common gene variants contribute in an additive manner to elevated HDL-cholesterol concentrations [105].

Gene regulation

Regulation of genes important in lipoprotein metabolism has been extensively studied in the past [106]. Dietary and hormonal regulation of genes influencing HDL metabolism have been identified [107,108]. The structural identity of adipocyte determination and differentiation-dependent factor 1 (ADD1) and sterol regulatory element binding protein 1 (SREBP1) has been shown [97] and has thereby brought together adipocyte development and cholesterol homeostasis [109]. Future research in this area will have to unravel more of the complex dependencies in the regulation of lipid metabolism. The proximal and distal CETP gene promoters provide an example of a crossroad between metabolic and dietary regulation [110]. Newly developed research tools for the precise quantification of nucleic acids (fluorescence monitoring, bDNA) and for multiparameter expression studies (high-density oligonucleotide arrays).

Conclusion

Owing to the widely used candidate gene approach, no genetically defined risk for CAD is currently known that cannot also be determined by one or more of the disease's established risk factors. A better understanding of the complex relations of genetic variation with each other and with environmental factors will be needed for the use of genetic information in the clinical management of CAD.

Roughly 17% of adult males have HDL-cholesterol concentrations below or at 35 mg/dl, the generally accepted CAD-risk threshold level for this parameter. Taken together, our knowledge on genetic parameters influencing HDL-cholesterol is rudimentary. Data shown in this report make it likely that within a short period of time the full potential of genes in the understanding the pathophysiology and for the clinical management of atherosclerotic diseases will become apparent.

Acknowledgements

Supported by Deutsche Forschungsgemeinschaft (Fu 179/1-2) and Interdisziplinäres Klinisches Forschungszentrum (A5).

References

1. Miller NE, Forde OH, Thelle DS, Mjos OD. The Tromso heart-study. High-density lipoprotein and coronary heart-diease: a prospective case-control study. Lancet 1977;I:965—968.
2. Gordon T, Kannel WB, Castelli WP, Dawber TR. Lipoproteins, cardiovascular disease and death. The Framingham Study. Arch Intern Med 1981;141:1128—1131.
3. Assmann G, Schulte H. PROCAM-Trial. Hedingen, Zürich: Panscientia Verlag,1986.
4. Glomset JA. The plasma lecithin: cholesterol acyltransferase reaction. J Lipid Res 1968;9: 155—163.
5. Von Eckardstein A. Cholesterol efflux from macrophages and other cells. Curr Opin Lipid

1996;7:308—319.
6. Ordovas JM, Cassidy DK, Civeira F, Bisgaier CL, Schaefer EJ. Familial apolipoprotein A-I, C-III, and A-IV deficiency and premature atherosclerosis due to deletion of a gene complex on chromosome 11. J Biol Chem 1989;264:16339—16342.
7. Karathanasis SK, Ferris E, Haddad IA, DNA inversion within the apolipoproteins AI/CIII/AIV-encoding gene cluster of certain patients with premature atherosclerosis. Proc Natl Acad Sci USA 1987;84:7198—7202.
8. Ng DS, Leiter LA, Vezina C, Connelly PW, Hegele RA. Apolipoprotein A-I Q(-2)X causing isolated apolipoprotein A-I deficiency in a family with analphalipoproteinemia. J Clin Invest 1994;93:223—239.
9. Navalesi R, Miccoli R, Odoguardi L, Funke H, von Eckardstein A, Wiebusch H, Assmann G. Genetically determined absence of HDL-cholesterol and coronary atherosclerosis (letter). Lancet 1995;346:708—709.
10. Miccoli R, Navalesi R, Odoguardi L, Wessling J, Funke H, Wiebusch H, von Eckardstein A, Assmann G. Compound heterozygosity for a structural apolipoprotein A-I variant, apo A-I (L141R) (Pisa), and an apolipoprotein A-I null allele in patients with absence of HDL-cholesterol, corneal opacifications, and coronary heart disease. Circulation 1996;94:1622—1628.
11. Schmitz G, Bruning T, Williamson E, Nowicka G. The role of HDL in reverse cholesterol transport and its disturbances in Tangier disease and HDL deficiency with xanthomas. Eur Heart J 1990;(Suppl E):197—211.
12. Lackner KJ, Dieplinger H, Nowicka G, Schmitz G. High-density lipoprotein deficiency with xanthomas. A defect in reverse cholesterol transport caused by a point mutation in the apolipoprotein A-I gene. J Clin Invest 1993;92:2262—2273.
13. Nakata K, Kobayashi K, Yanagi H, Shimakura Y, Tsuchiya S, Arinami T, Hamaguchi H. Autosomal dominant hypoalphalipoproteinemia due to a completely defective apolipoprotein A-I gene. Biochem Biophys Res Commun 1993;196:950—955.
14. Takata K, Saku K, Ohta T, Takata M, Bai H, Jimi S, Liu R, Sato H, Kajiyama G, Arakawa K. A new case of apoA-I deficiency showing codon 8 nonsense mutation of the apoA-I gene without evidence of coronary heart disease. Arterioscl Thromb Vasc Biol 1995;15:1866—1874.
15. Romling R, von Eckardstein A, Funke H, Motti C, Fragiacomo GC, Noseda G, Assmann G. A nonsense mutation in the apolipoprotein A-I gene is associated with high-density lipoprotein deficiency and periorbital xanthelasmas. Arterioscl Thromb 1994;14:1915—1922.
16. Matsunaga T, Hiasa Y, Yanagi H, Maeda T, Hattori N, Yamakawa K, Yamanouchi Y, Tanaka I, Obara T, Hamaguchi H. Apolipoprotein A-I deficiency due to a codon 84 nonsense mutation of the apolipoprotein A-I gene. Proc Natl Acad Sci USA 1991;88:2793—2797.
17. Funke H, von Eckardstein A, Pritchard PH, Karas M, Albers JJ, Assmann G. A frameshift mutation in the human apolipoprotein A-I gene causes high-density lipoprotein deficiency, partial lecithin: cholesterol-acyltransferase deficiency, and corneal opacities. J Clin Invest 1991;87:371—376.
18. Nichols WC, Gregg RE, Brewer HB Jr, Benson MD. A mutation in apolipoprotein A-I in the Iowa type of familial amyloidotic polyneuropathy. Genomics 1990;8:318—323.
19. Booth DR, Tan SY, Booth SE, Hsuan JJ, Totty NF, Nguyen O, Hutton T, Vigushin DM, Tennent GA, Hutchinson WL, Thomson N, Soutar AK, Hawkins PN, Pepys MB. A new apolipoprotein al variant, trp50arg, causes hereditary amyloidosis. QJM Month J Ass Phys 1995;88:695—702.
20. Soutar AK, Hawkins PN, Vigushin DM, Tennent GA, Booth SE, Hutton T, Nguyen O, Totty NF, Feest TG, Hsuan JJ et al. Apolipoprotein AI mutation Arg-60 causes autosomal dominant amyloidosis. Proc Natl Acad Sci USA 1992;89:7389—7393.
21. Booth DR, Tan SY, Booth SE, Tennent GA, Hutchinson WL, Hsuan JJ, Totty NF, Truong O, Soutar AK, Hawkins PN, Bruguera M, Caballeria J, Sole M, Campistol JM, Pepys MB. Hereditary hepatic and systemic amyloidosis caused by a new deletion/insertion mutation in the apolipoprotein al gene. J Clin Invest 1996;97:2714—2721.
22. von Eckardstein A, Funke H, Henke A, Altland K, Benninghoven A, Assmann G. Apolipo-

protein A-I variants. Naturally occurring substitutions of proline residues affect plasma concentration of apolipoprotein A-I. J Clin Invest 1989;84:1722—1730.

23. Ladias JA, Kwiterovich PO Jr, Smith HH, Karathanasis SK, Antonarakis SE. Apolipoprotein A1 Baltimore (Arg10→Leu), a new ApoA1 variant. Hum Genet 1990;84:439—445.

24. Takada Y, Sasaki J, Seki M, Ogata S, Teranishi Y, Arakawa K. Characterization of a new human apolipoprotein A-I Yame by direct sequencing of polymerase chain reaction-amplified DNA. J Lipid Res 1991;32:1275—1280.

25. von Eckardstein A, Funke H, Walter M, Altland K, Benninghoven A, Assmann G. Structural analysis of human apolipoprotein A-I variants. Amino acid substitutions are nonrandomly distributed throughout the apolipoprotein A-I primary structure. J Biol Chem 1990;265: 8610—8617.

26. Araki K, Sasaki J, Matsunaga A, Takada Y, Moriyama K, Hidaka K, Arakawa K. Characterization of two new human apolipoprotein A-I variants: apolipoprotein A-I Tsushima (Trp-108→Arg) and A-I Hita (Ala-95→Asp). Biochim Biophys Acta 1994;1214:272—278.

27. Moriyama K, Sasaki J, Matsunaga A, Takada Y, Kagimoto M, Arakawa K. Identification of two apolipoprotein variants, A-I Karatsu (Tyr 100→His) and A-I Kurume (His 162→Gln). Clin Genet 1996;49:79—84.

28. Menzel HJ, Assmann G, Rall SC Jr, Weisgraber KH, Mahley RW. Human apolipoprotein A-I polymorphism. Identification of amino acid substitutions in three electrophoretic variants of the Munster-3 type. J Biol Chem 1984;259:3070—3076.

29. Tilly Kiesi M, Zhang Q, Ehnholm S, Kahri J, Lahdenpera S, Ehnholm C, Taskinen MR. ApoA-IHelsinki (Lys107→0) associated with reduced HDL cholesterol and LpA-I:A-II deficiency. Arterioscl Thromb Vasc Biol 1995;15:1294—1306.

30. Rall SC Jr, Weisgraber KH, Mahley RW, Ogawa Y, Fielding CJ, Utermann G, Haas J, Steinmetz A, Menzel HJ, Assmann G. Abnormal lecithin: cholesterol acyltransferase activation by a human apolipoprotein A-I variant in which a single lysine residue is deleted. J Biol Chem 1984;259:10063—10070.

31. Takada Y, Sasaki J, Ogata S, Nakanishi T, Ikehara Y, Arakawa K. Isolation and characterization of human apolipoprotein A-I Fukuoka (110 Glu→Lys). A novel apolipoprotein variant. Biochim Biophys Acta 1990;1043:169—176.

32. Schamaun O, Olaisen B, Gedde Dahl T Jr, Teisberg P. Genetic studies of an apoA-I lipoprotein variant. Hum Genet 1983;64:380—383.

33. Rall SC Jr, Weisgraber KH, Mahley RW, Ehnholm C, Schamaun O, Olaisen B, Blomhoff JP, Teisberg P. Identification of homozygosity for a human apolipoprotein A-I variant. J Lipid Res 1986;27:436—441.

34. Utermann G, Haas J, Steinmetz A, Paetzold R, Rall SC Jr, Weisgraber KH, Mahley RW. Apolipoprotein A-IGiessen (Pro143→Arg). A mutant that is defective in activating lecithin:cholesterol acyltransferase. Eur J Biochem 1984;144:325—331.

35. Deeb SS, Cheung MC, Peng RL, Wolf AC, Stern R, Albers JJ, Knopp-RH. A mutation in the human apolipoprotein A-I gene. Dominant effect on the level and characteristics of plasma high-density lipoproteins. J Biol Chem 1991;266:13654—13660.

36. Mahley RW, Innerarity TL, Rall SC Jr, Weisgraber KH. Plasma lipoproteins: apolipoprotein structure and function. J Lipid Res 1984;25:1277—1294.

37. Weisgraber KH, Rall SC Jr, Bersot TP, Mahley RW, Franceschini G, Sirtori CR. Apolipoprotein A-IMilano. Detection of normal A-I in affected subjects and evidence for a cysteine for arginine substitution in the variant A-I. J Biol Chem 1983;258:2508—2513.

38. Jabs HU, Assmann G, Greifendorf D, Benninghoven A. High performance liquid chromatography and time-of-flight secondary ion mass spectrometry: a new dimension in structural analysis of apolipoproteins. J Lipid Res 1986;27:613—621.

39. Strobl W, Jabs HU, Hayde M, Holzinger T, Assmann G, Widhalm K. Apolipoprotein A-I (Glu 198→Lys): a mutant of the major apolipoprotein of high-density lipoproteins occurring in a family with dyslipoproteinemia. Pediatr Res 1988;24:222—228.

40. Kuivenhoven JA, Weibusch H, Pritchard PH, Funke H, Benne R, Assmann G, Kastelein JP. An intronic mutation in a lariat branchpoint sequence is a direct cause of an inherited human disorder (fish eye disease). J Clin Invest 1996;98:358–364.

41. Bujo H, Kusunoki J, Ogasawara M, Yamamoto T, Ohta Y, Shimada T, Saito Y, Yoshida S. Molecular defect in familial lecithin:cholesterol acyltransferase (LCAT) deficiency: a single nucleotide insertion in LCAT gene causes a complete deficient type of the disease. Biochem Biophys Res Commun 1991;181:933–940.

42. Miettinen H, Gylling H, Ulmanen I, Miettinen TA, Kontula K. Two different allelic mutations in a Finnish family with lecithin: cholesterol acyltransferase deficiency. Arterioscl Thromb Vasc Biol 1995;15:460–467.

43. Wiebusch H, Cullen P, Owen JS, Collins D, Sharp PS, Funke H, Assmann-G. Deficiency of lecithin: cholesterol acyltransferase due to compound heterozygosity of two novel mutations (Gly33Arg and 30 bp ins) in the LCAT gene. Hum Mol Genet 1995;4:143–145.

44. Skretting G, Prydz H. An amino acid exchange in exon I of the human lecithin: cholesterol acyltransferase (LCAT) gene is associated with fish eye disease. Biochem Biophys Res Commun 1992;182:583–587.

45. Kuivenhoven JA, Stalenhoef AFH, Hill JS, Demacker PNM, Errami A, Kastelein JJP, Pritchard PH. Two novel molecular defects in the LCAT gene are associated with fish eye disease. Arterioscl Thromb Vasc Biol 1996;16:294–303.

46. Owen JS, Wiebusch H, Cullen P, Watts GF, Lima VLM, Funke H, Assmann G. Complete deficiency of plasma lecithin cholesterol acyltransferase (LCAT) activity due to a novel homozygous mutation (gly 30 ser) in the LCAT gene. Hum Mutat 1996;8:79–82.

47. Funke H, von Eckardstein A, Pritchard PH, Hornby AE, Wiebusch H, Motti C, Hayden MR, Dachet C, Jacotot B, Gerdes U, Faergeman O, Albers JJ, Colleoni N, Catapano A, Frohlich J, Assmann G. Genetic and phenotypic heterogeneity in familial lecithin: cholesterol acyltransferase (LCAT) deficiency. Six newly identified defective alleles further contribute to the structural heterogeneity in this disease. J Clin Invest 1993;91:677–683.

48. Klein HG, Lohse P, Duverger N, Albers JJ, Rader DJ, Zech LA, Santamarina Fojo S, Brewer HB Jr. Two different allelic mutations in the lecithin:cholesterol acyltransferase (LCAT) gene resulting in classic LCAT deficiency: LCAT (tyr83→stop) and LCAT (tyr156→asn). J Lipid Res 1993;34:49–58.

49. Funke H, von Eckardstein A, Pritchard PH, Albers JJ, Kastelein JJ, Droste C, Assmann G. A molecular defect causing fish eye disease: an amino acid exchange in lecithin:cholesterol acyltransferase (LCAT) leads to the selective loss of alpha-LCAT activity. Proc Natl Acad Sci USA 1991;88:4855–4859.

50. Contacos C, Sullivan DR, Rye KA, Funke H, Assmann G. A new molecular defect in the lecithin cholesterol acyltransferase LCAT) gene associated with fish eye disease. J Lipid Res 1996;37:35–44.

51. Klein HG, Lohse P, Pritchard PH, Bojanovski D, Schmidt H, Brewer HB Jr. Two different allelic mutations in the lecithin:cholesterol acyltransferase gene associated with the fish eye syndrome. Lecithin:cholesterol acyltransferase (Thr123→Ile) and lecithin:cholesterol acyltransferase (Thr347→Met). J Clin Invest 1992;89:499–506.

52. Kuivenhoven JA, Voorst EJGMVT, Wiebusch H, Marcovina SM, Funke H, Assmann G, Pritchard PH, Kastelein JJP, Hill J, Adler L, Errrami AA. Unique genetic and biochemical presentation of fish eye disease. J Clin Invest 1995;96:2783–2791.

53. Steyrer E, Haubenwallner S, Horl G, Giessauf W, Kostner GM, Zechner RA. Single G to A nucleotide transition in exon IV of the lecithin:cholesterol acyltransferase (LCAT) gene results in an arg(140) to his substitution and causes LCAT deficiency. Hum Genet 1995;96:105–109.

54. Gotoda T, Yamada N, Murase T, Sakuma M, Murayama N, Shimano H, Kozaki K, Albers JJ, Yazaki Y, Akanuma Y. Differential phenotypic expression by three mutant alleles in familial lecithin:cholesterol acyltransferase deficiency. Lancet 1991;338:778–781.

55. Taramelli R, Pontoglio M, Candiani G, Ottolenghi S, Dieplinger H, Catapano A, Albers J, Ver-

gani C, McLean J. Lecithin cholesterol acyl transferase deficiency: molecular analysis of a mutated allele. Hum Genet 1990;85:195—199.

56. Miller M, Zeller K, Kwiterovich PC, Albers JJ, Feulner G. Lecithin:cholesterol acyltransferase deficiency: identification of two defective alleles in fibroblast cDNA. J Lipid Res 1995;36: 931—938.

57. Skretting G, Blomhoff JP, Solheim J, Prydz H. The genetic defect of the original Norwegian lecithin: cholesterol acyltransferase deficiency families. FEBS Lett 1992;309:307—310.

58. Moriyama K, Sasaki J, Arakawa F, Takami N, Maeda E, Matsunaga A, Takada Y, Midorikawa K, Yanase T, Yoshino G et al. Two novel point mutations in the lecithin:cholesterol acyltransferase (LCAT) gene resulting in LCAT deficiency: LCAT (G873 deletion) and LCAT (Gly344→ Ser). J Lipid Res 1995;36:2329—2343.

59. Klein HG, Santamarina Fojo S, Duverger N, Clerc M, Dumon MF, Albers JJ, Marcovina S, Brewer HB Jr. Fish eye syndrome: a molecular defect in the lecithin:cholesterol acyltransferase (LCAT) gene associated with normal alpha-LCAT-specific activity. Implications for classification and prognosis. J Clin Invest 1993;92:479—485.

60. Oram JF, Yokoyama-S. Apolipoprotein mediated removal of cellular cholesterol and phospholipids. J Lipid Res 1996;37:2473—2491.

61. Walter M, Reinecke H, Gerdes U, Nofer Jr, Hobbel G, Seedorf U, Assmann G. Defective regulation of phosphatidylcholine specific phospholipases c and d in a kindred with tangier disease: evidence for the involvement of phosphatidylcholine breakdown in hdl mediated cholesterol efflux mechanisms. J Clin Invest 1996;98:2315—2323.

62. Czarnecka-H, Yokoyama-S. Regulation of cellular cholesterol efflux by lecithin cholesterol acyltransferase reaction through nonspecific lipid exchange. J Biol Chem 1996;271:2023—2028.

63. Marcil M, Boucher B, Krimbou L, Solymoss BC, Davignon J, Frohlich J, Genest J. Severe familial HDL deficiency in French Canadian kindreds: clinical, biochemical, and molecular characterization. Arterioscl Thromb Vasc Biol 1995;15:1015—1024.

64. Brown ML, Inazu A, Hesler CB, Agellon LB, Mann C, Whitlock ME, Marcel YL, Milne RW, Koizumi J, Mabuchi H, Takeda R, Tall AR. Molecular basis of lipid transfer protein deficiency in a family with increased high-density lipoproteins. Nature 1989;342:448—451.

65. Sakai N, Santamarinafojo S, Yamashita S, Matsuzawa Y, Brewer-HB. Exon 10 skipping caused by intron 10 splice donor site mutation in cholesterol ester transfer protein gene results in abnormal downstream splice site selection. J Lipid Res 1996;37:2065—2073.

66. Arai T, Yamashita S, Sakai N, Hirano Ki, Okada S, Ishigami M, Maruyama T, Yamane M, Kobayashi H, Nozaki S, Funahashi T, Kamedatakemura K, Nakajima N, Matsuzawa Y. A novel missense mutation (G181X) in the human cholesterol ester transfer protein gene in Japanese hyperalphalipoproteinemic subjects. J Lipid Res 1996;37:2145—2154.

67. Zhong SB, Sharp DS, Grove JS, Bruce C, Yano K, Curb JD, Tall AR. Increased coronary heart disease in Japanese American men with mutation in the cholesteryl ester transfer protein gene despite increased HDL levels. J Clin Invest 1996;97:2917—2923.

68. McPerson R, Grundy SM, Guerra R, Cohen JC. Alleleic variation in the gene encoding the cholesteryl ester transfer nprotein is associated with variation in the plasma concentrations of cholesteryl ester transfer protein. J Lipid Res 1996;37:1743—1748.

69. Tamminen M, Kakko S, Kesaniemi YA, Savolainen MJ. A polymorphic site in the 3′-untranslated region of the cholesteryl ester transfer protein (CETP) gene is associated with low CETP activity. J Lipid Res 1996;124:237—247.

70. Kinishita M, Teramoto T, Shimazu N, Kaneko K, Ohta M, Koike T, Hosogaya S, Ozaki Y, Kume S, Yamanaka M. CETP is a determinant of serum LDL cholesterol but not HDL cholesterol in healthy Japanese. Atherosclerosis 1996;120:75—82.

71. Funke H, Wiebusch H, Fuer L, Muntoni S, Schulte H, Assmann G. Identification of mutations in the cholesterol ester transfer protein in Europeans with elevated high-density lipoprotein cholesterol. Circulation 1994;90(2):241(Abstract).

72. Williamson R, Lee D, Hagaman J, Maeda N. Marked reduction of high-density lipoprotein

cholesterol in mice genetically modified to lack apolipoprotein A-I. Proc Natl Acad Sci USA 1992;89:7134—7138.

73. Rubin EM, Krauss RM, Spangler EA, Verstuyft JG, Clift SM. Inhibition of early atherogenesis in transgenic mice by human apolipoprotein AI. Nature 1991;353:265—267.

74. Schultz JR, Verstuyft JG, Gong EL, Nichols AV, Rubin EM. Protein composition determines the antiatherogenic properties of HDL in transgenic mice. Nature 1993;365:762—764.

75. Paszty C, Maeda N, Verstuyft J, Rubin EM. Apolipoprotein AI transgene corrects apolipoprotein E deficiency-induced atherosclerosis in mice. J Clin Invest 1994;94:899—903.

76. Duverger N, Tremp G, Caillaud JM, Emmanuel F, Castro G, Fruchart JC, Steinmetz A, Denefle P. Protection against atherogenesis in mice mediated by human apolipoprotein A IV. Science 1996;273:966—968.

77. Duverger N, Kruth H, Viglietta C, Castro G, Tailleux A, Fievet C, Fruchart JC, Houdebine LM, Denefle P. Inhibition of atherosclerosis development in cholesterol fed human apolipoprotein A-I transgenic rabbits. Circulation 1996;94:713—717.

78. Seguretmace S, Lattamahieu M, Castro G, Luc G, Fruchart JC, Rubin E, Denefle P, Duverger N. Potential gene therapy for lecithin: cholesterol acyltransferase (LCAT) deficient and hypo-alphalipoproteinemic patients with adenovirus mediated transfer of human LCAT gene. Circulation 1996;94:2177—2184.

79. Hoeg JM, Santamarinafojo S, Berard AM, Cornhill JF, Herderick EE, Feldman SH, Haudenschild CC, Vaisman BL, Hoyt RF, Demosky SJ, Kauffman RD, Hazel CM, Marcovina SM, Brewer HB. Overexpression of lecithin, cholesterol acyltransferase in transgenic rabbits prevents diet induced atherosclerosis. Proc Natl Acad Sci USA 1996;93:11448—11453.

80. Hoeg JM, Vaisman BL, Demosky SJ, Meyn SM, Talley GD, Hoyt RF, Feldman SH, Berard AM, Sakai N, Wood D, Brousseau ME, Marcovina S, Brewer HB, Santamarinafojo S. Lecithin cholesterol acyltransferase overexpression generates hyperalphalipoproteinemia and a nonatherogenic lipoprotein pattern in transgenic rabbits. J Biol Chem 1996;271:4396—4402.

81. Hayek T, Masuccimagoulas L, Jiang X, Walsh A, Rubin E, Breslow JL, Tall AR. Decreased early atherosclerotic lesions in hypertriglyceridemic mice expressing cholesterol ester tranfer protein transgene. J Clin Invest 1995;96:2071—2074.

82. Jiang X-C, Francone OL, Bruce C, Milne R, Mar J, Walsh A, Breslow JL, Tall AR. Increased prehigh-density lipoprotein, apolipoprotein AI, and phospholipid in mice expressing the human phospholipid transfer protein and human apolipoprotein AI transgenes. J Clin Invest 1996;98:2373—2380.

83. Albers JJ, Tu AY, Paigen B, Chen H, Cheung MC, Marcovina SM. Transgenic mice expressing human phospholipid transfer protein have increased HDL non HDL cholesterol ratio. Int J Clin Lab Res 1996;26:262—267.

84. Weng W, Breslow JL. Dramatically decreased high-density lipoprotein cholesterol, increased remnant clearance, and insulin hypersensitivity in apolipoprotein AII knockout mice suggest a complex role for apolipoprotein AII in atherosclerosis susceptibility. Proc Natl Acad Sci USA 1996;93:14788—14794.

85. Marzalcascacuberta A, Blacovaca F, Ishida BY, Julvegil J, Shen JH, Calvetmarquez S, Gonzalezsastre F, Chan L. Functional lecithin:cholesterol acyltransferase deficiency in transgenic mice overexpressing human apolipoprotein A II. J Biol Chem 1996;271:6720—6728.

86. Deeb SS, Cheung MC, Peng RL, Wolf AC, Stern R, Albers JJ, Knopp RH. A mutation in the human apolipoprotein AI gene. Dominant effect on the level and characteristics of plasma high-density lipoproteins. J Biol Chem 1991;266:13654—13660.

87. Srinivasan SR, Ehnholm C, Wattigney WA, Bao WH, Berenson GS. The relation of apolipoprotein E polymorphism to multiple cardiovascular risk in children: the Bogalusa Heart Study. Atherosclerosis 1996;123:33—42.

88. Reymer PWA, Gagne E, Groenemeyer BE, Kastelein JJP, Hayden MR. A lipoprotein lipase mutation (Asn291Ser) is associated with reduced HDL cholesterol levels in premature atherosclerosis. Nature Genet 1995;10:28—34.

89. Funke H, Assmann G. The low down on lipoprotein lipase. Nature Genet 1995;10:6−7.
90. Funke H. Lipoprotein enzyme mutations and cardiovascular disease. Curr Opin Lipid 1997;(In press).
91. Hunst SC, Hasstedt SJ, Kuida H, Stults BM, Hopkins PN, Williams RR. Genetic heritability and common environmental components of resting and stressed blood pressures, lipids, and body mass index in Utah pedigrees and twins. Am J Epidemiol 1989;129:625−638.
92. Assmann G, von Eckardstein A, Funke H. High-density lipoproteins, reverse transport of cholesterol, and coronary artery disease. Insights from mutations. Circulation 1993;87(Suppl III):28−34.
93. Acton S, Rigotti A, Landschulz KT, Xu SZ, Hobbs HH, Krieger M. Identification of scavenger receptor SR BI as a high-density lipoprotein receptor. Science 1996;271:518−520.
94. Wang N, Weng W, Breslow JL, Tall AR. Scavenger receptor BI (SR BI) is up regulated in adrenal gland in apolipoprotein AI and hepatic lipase knockout mice as a response to depletion of cholesterol stores: in vivo evidence that SR BI is a functional high-density lipoprotein receptor under feedback control. J Biol Chem 1996;271:21001−21004.
95. Landschulz KT, Pathak RK, Rigotti A, Krieger M, Hobbs HH. Regulation of scavenger receptor, class B, type I, a high-density lipoprotein receptor, in liver and steroidogenic tissues of the rat. J Clin Invest 1996;98:984−995.
96. Schoonjans K, Peinadoonsurbe J, Lefebvre AM, Heyman RA, Briggs M, Deeb S, Staels B, Auwerx J. PPAR alpha and PPAR gamma activators direct a distinct tissue specific transcritional response via a PPRE in the lipoprotein lipase gene. EMBO J 1996;15:5336−5348.
97. Kim JB, Spiegelman BM. ADD1/SREBP1 promotes adipocyte differentiation and gene expression linked to fatty acid metabolism. Genes Dev 1996;10:1096−1107.
98. Hotamisligil GS, Johnson RS, Distel RJ, Ellis R, Papaioannou VE, Spiegelman BM. Uncoupling of obesity from insulin resistance through a targeted mutation in AP2, the adipocyte fatty acid binding protein. Science 1996;274:1377−1379.
99. Peraldi P, Hotamisligil GS, Buurman WA, White MF, Spiegelman BM. Tumor necrosis factor (TNF) alpha inhibits insulin signaling through stimulation of the p55 TNF receptor and activation of sphingomyelinase. J Biol Chem 1996;271:13018−13022.
100. Hamsten A. Molecular genetics as the route to understanding, prevention and treatment. Lancet 1996;348(Suppl):s17−s19.
101. Bennett ST, Todd JA. Human type I diabetes and the insulin gene: principles of mapping polygenes. Ann Rev Genet 1996;30:343−370.
102. Matise TC. Genome scanning for complex disease genes using the transmission/disequilibrium test and haplotype based haplotype relative risk. Genet Epidemiol 1995;12:641−645.
103. Mitchel BD, Kammerer CM, Blangero J, Mahaney MC, Rainwater DL, Dyke B, Hixson JE, Henkel RD, Sharp RM, Comuzzi AG, VandeBerg JL, Stern MP, MacCluer J. Genetic and environmental contributions to cardiovascular risk factors in Mexican Americans: the San Antonio Family Heart Study. Circulation 1996;94:2159−2170.
104. Risch N, Merikangas K. The future of genetic studies of complex human diseases. Science 1996;273:1516−1517.
105. Funke H, Wiebusch H, Schulte H, Assmann G. Additive cooperative effect of three common missense mutations on serum HDL-cholesterol concentrations. Circulation 1996;94(Suppl):I−343(Abstract).
106. Kardassis D, Laccotripe M, Talianidis I, Zannis V. Transcriptional regulation of the genes involved in lipoprotein transport: the role of proximal promoters and long range regulatory elements and factors in apolipoprotein gene regulation. Hypertension 1996;27:980−1008.
107. Blangero J, Williams Blangero S, Mahaney MC, Comuzzie AG, Hixson JE, Samollow PB, Sharp RM, Stern MP, MacCluer JW. Effects of a major gene for apolipoprotein AI concentration are thyroid hormone-dependent in Mexican Americans. Arterioscl Thromb Vasc Biol 1996;16:1177−1183.
108. Azrolan N, Odaka H, Breslow JL, Fisher EA. Dietary fat elevates hepatic apo AI production by

increasing the fraction of apolipoprotein AI mRNA in the translating pool. J Biol Chem 1995;270:19833—19838.

109. Bennett MK, Lopez JM, Sanchez HB, Osborne TF. Sterol regulation of fatty acid synthase promoter: coordinate feedback regulation of two major lipid pathways. J Biol Chem 1995;270: 25578—25583.

110. Oliveira HCF, Chouinard RA, Agellon LB, Bruce C, Ma LM, Walsh A, Breslow JL, Tall AR. Human cholesteryl ester transfer protein gene proximal promoter contains dietary cholesterol positive response elements and mediates expression in small intestine and periphery while predominant liver and spleen expression is controlled by 5′ distal sequences: cis acting sequences mapped in TN transgenic mice. J Biol Chem 1996;271:31831—31838.

Atherosclerosis XI.
B. Jacotot, D. Mathé and J.-C. Fruchart, editors.

Expression of γ-IFN responsive genes in monocytes is associated with xanthomatosis

Thomas Grewal[1,2], Mathieu Boudreau[1], Madeleine Roy[1], Jean Davignon[1] and Anne Minnich[1,3]

[1]*Hyperlipidemia and Atherosclerosis Group, Clinical Research Institute of Montreal, Montreal, Quebec, Canada;* [2]*Universität Hamburg, Universitätskrankenhaus Eppendorf, Medizinische Klinik, Biochemisches Stoffwechsellabor, Hamburg, Germany; and* [3]*Rhône-Poulenc Rorer, Research and Development, Collegeville, Pennsylvania, USA*

Abstract. We have recently described an inherited overexpression of the macrophage scavenger receptor (SR) in blood monocytes from members of a kindred, only two of whom displayed extensive xanthomatosis. Using mRNA differential display we demonstrated abnormally high expression of the signal transducer and activator of transcription (STAT1α) in monocytes from the proband II-2. Expression of γ-interferon inducible protein 10 (IP-10), a STAT1α-responsive gene and mediator of inflammatory response, was also abnormally expressed in the monocytes from II-2. Overexpression of both genes was restricted to monocytes from II-2 and was not observed in monocytes from the clinically unaffected family members, unlike that of SR. Concomitant expression of STAT1α and IP-10 can be induced only in γ-interferon (γ-IFN) activated macrophages. Taken together these results suggest that γ-interferon (γ-IFN) mediated cell activation is responsible for the induction of STAT1α in monocytes from II-2. Analysis of monocytes from familial hypercholesterolemic (FH) subjects, who frequently develop xanthomatosis, revealed a significant number of subjects with elevated STAT1α and IP-10 expression. Our data suggest that the inflammatory effects of γ-IFN signaling could play a role in foam cell formation and xanthomatosis.

Keywords: foam cell, γ-interferon, IP-10, macrophage activation, scavenger receptor, STAT1α, xanthoma.

Introduction

In addition to arterial foam cell formation, it is believed that foam cells developing in cutaneous xanthoma also result from the uptake of modified LDL by the macrophage scavenger receptor [1]. We have recently characterized an apparent genetic overexpression of the scavenger receptor (SR) in monocytes from one proband (II-6) and her brother (II-2) with cutaneous xanthoma in the absence of hyperlipidemia or any other detectable etiology [2]. In these subjects and other clinically unaffected members of the C-kindred, abnormally high levels of monocyte SR expression were associated with precocious maturation of monocytes

---

Address for correspondence: Thomas Grewal, Universität Hamburg, Universitätskrankenhaus Eppendorf, Medizinische Klinik, Biochemisches Stoffwechsellabor, Martinistr. 52, D-20246 Hamburg, Germany.

into foam cell-like macrophages [2].

In order to identify genes that are differentially expressed in these monocytes and might therefore be involved in foam cell formation and/or xanthomatosis we used differential mRNA display.

Methods

Subjects

A detailed description of the proband II-2 and other members of the C-kindred has been published [2]. In addition, blood samples for monocyte isolation were obtained from 10 patients attending our lipid clinic chosen on the basis of xanthomatosis and/or heterozygous FH. Nine patients (age 25—47 years; 4 M/5 F) presented with high plasma total and LDL cholesterol levels consistent with a diagnosis of FH. FH was confirmed with molecular diagnosis in seven patients. One patient had combined hyperlipidemia, multiple myeloma, and unusually extensive xanthomatosis. None were treated for hyperlipidemia at the time of sampling. Controls were laboratory or Institute personnel (aged 32—57 years; 6 M/2 F). Blood derived-monocytes were isolated as described [2,3].

RT-PCR analysis

Differential mRNA display was performed as described [4,5]. Determination of STAT1α transcript levels in human blood monocytes was performed with semi-quantitative RT-PCR analysis. 400—800 ng of total RNA was reverse transcribed. STAT1α and GAPDH cDNA fragments were PCR-amplified in separate reactions. cDNA corresponding to 40—60 ng of total RNA was determined to be optimal for both PCR reactions. One microliter of cDNA was PCR-amplified with 100 ng of each sequence-specific PCR-primers. Measurements of cycle number vs. signal demonstrated log-linearity during cycles 21 to 23. Aliquots of duplicate reactions were taken at cycles 21 and 23 and analyzed on 1% agarose gels. Relative STAT1α expression levels are expressed as the ratio to GAPDH peak area. Alternatively IP-10 [6] was coamplified with GAPDH cDNA.

Results

Differential expression of STAT1α in II-2 monocytes and THP-1 macrophages

Differential mRNA display was used to identify differentially expressed genes between day 1 monocytes from the proband II-2 who displayed xanthomatosis in the absence of hyperlipidemia, and those from his unaffected brother II-8 [2]. Because we were initially interested in studying the expression of genes which might be involved in the macrophage-like morphology of the monocytes from the proband II-2 [2] we studied differentially induced PCR amplification products that were present in II-2 monocytes, absent in II-8 monocytes and induced in PMA-treated THP-1 monocytes. Analysis of randomly amplified PCR products identified a differentially expressed transcript in day 1 monocytes from II-2 and PMA-activated THP-1 macrophages, but not in monocytes of his brother II-8 or THP-1 monocytes. Sequencing of the differentially expressed bands revealed signal transducer and activator of transcription (STAT1α) [7].

Differential expression of STAT1α in PMA-induced THP-1 macrophages was confirmed by Northern blotting with the reamplified cDNA fragment as probe. Densitometric scanning and normalization to GAPDH revealed a 9- to 10-fold induction of STAT1α mRNA expression following PMA-induced differentiation of THP-1 cells.

STAT1α overexpression is specific for day 1 monocytes of the proband II-2 within the C-kindred

As measured by RT-PCR, STAT1α expression was induced 5.2-fold after PMA-induced THP-1 promonocyte differentiation into macrophages and 7.2-fold after 24 h treatment with γ-IFN (Fig. 1A). The combination of a 24 h PMA and γ-IFN treatment increased STAT1α expression 19-fold relative to untreated cells.

Analysis of STAT1α expression in day 1 monocytes of the proband II-2 and his

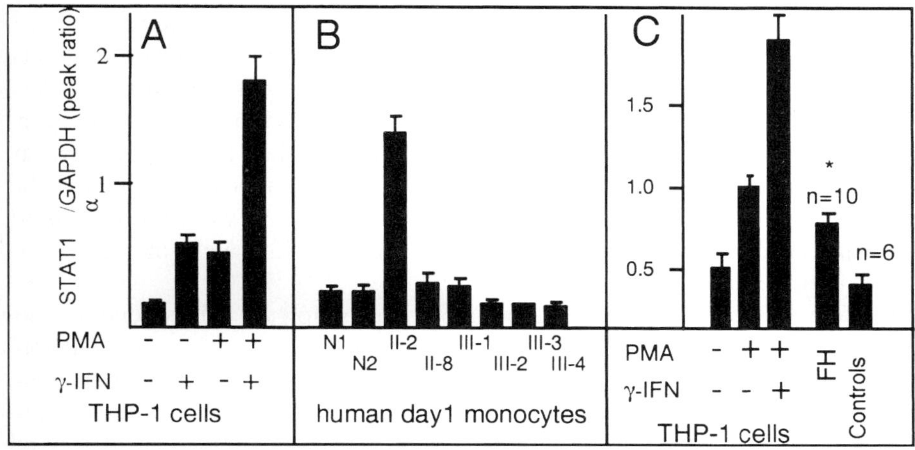

Fig. 1. Relative STAT1α expression levels in THP-1 cells (**A**) day 1 monocytes from SR-overexpressing kindred (**B**) and FH heterozygotes (**C**). **A**: 5×10^6 THP-1 monocytes (− PMA) and THP-1 macrophages (+PMA) were incubated for 24 h with or without human recombinant γ-IFN (25 ng/ml). STAT1α and GAPDH mRNA levels were determined by RT-PCR as described in "Methods". Relative STAT1α expression is calculated as the ratio of STAT1α and GAPDH peak areas. All values represent the means ± SD of three separate experiments with duplicate samples. **B/C**: 5×10^6 human blood-derived monocytes from controls (N1 and N2), the proband II-2, his unaffected brother II-8 and 4 scavenger receptor overexpressing members of the C-kindred (III-1 - III-4) or FH heterozygotes were grown for 24 h. Relative STAT1α expression was determined as in **A**. **B**: All values represent the means ± SD of two separate experiments with duplicate samples. **C**: *p < 0.004 vs. controls.

unaffected brother II-8 confirm the results of the differential display. The STAT1α/GAPDH peak area ratio in monocytes from II-2 was approximately 6-fold higher than in unaffected subjects (Fig. 1B). STAT1α expression in II-2 monocytes is of similar magnitude to that in γ-IFN activated THP-1 macrophages. In contrast, II-8 and four other members of the C-kindred exhibit low expression levels of STAT1α. These STAT1α expression levels are comparable to the STAT1α/GAPDH ratios observed in monocytes from two normal subjects (Fig. 1B).

Because PMA-induced differentiation of THP-1 cells increased STAT1α gene expression we compared STAT1α mRNA levels of the proband II-2, four other members of the C-kindred and four normals during maturation of blood-derived monocytes. Day 1 monocytes from II-2 consistently display high STAT1α/GAPDH peak ratios determined with an RNA sample taken approximately 1 year earlier. STAT1α/GAPDH ratios are reduced dramatically in day 2 monocytes and decrease during further monocyte maturation. In contrast, monocytes from all other members of the C-kindred and from control subjects show a different pattern of STAT1α expression, with relatively low STAT1α peak ratios in day 1 monocytes and peak STAT1α expression at day 4.

FH-monocytes display elevated mRNA levels of STAT1α and IP-10

FH subjects frequently develop xanthomatosis. Therefore we analyzed STAT1α and IP-10 expression in day 1 monocytes from FH subjects attending our lipid clinic (Fig. 1C). In these experiments we observed an approximately 3-fold greater average relative STAT1α expression levels in FH monocytes compared to control day 1 monocytes. Furthermore, three out of five FH-monocytes which overexpressed STAT1α also expressed IP-10. None of the day 1 monocytes from control subjects expressed detectable IP-10 mRNA.

Discussion

Macrophages play a major role in foam cell formation in atherogenesis and xanthomatosis. In order to identify factors potentially involved in foam fell formation and/or xanthomatosis we utilized differential display techniques to analyze the gene expression pattern in monocytes from a proband (II-2) with normolipidemic cutaneous xanthoma. Here we report the differential expression of STAT1α [7] in day 1 monocytes from this subject but not in his unaffected brother II-8 [2] or any other member of the kindred analyzed. Monocytes from all other family members display low STAT1α expression levels that are comparable to those in monocytes from control subjects. These results demonstrate that the high STAT1α mRNA level is restricted to the clinically affected proband II-2 within the C-kindred and does not parallel the recently described SR overexpression in monocytes from this family [2]. Although monocytes from the proband II-2 express STAT1α mRNA levels comparable to those in PMA-differentiated, γ-IFN activated THP-1 macrophages, it is unlikely that STAT1α overexpression in his monocytes reflects precocious maturation, as STAT1 levels in human blood-derived macrophages are not increased relative to those in day 1 monocytes.

Analysis of gene expression in monocytes from FH-subjects, who are at high risk of xanthomatosis, identified a significant number of FH-patients (5/10), compared to controls (0/6), with elevated STAT1α mRNA levels. Three out of these five FH subjects also expressed the STAT1-responsive gene IP-10 indicating γ-IFN induced activation of monocytes. Our data suggest that γ-IFN inducible STAT1α activity and IP-10 expression in monocytes could play a role in foam cell formation and xanthomatosis. Possibly, these circumstances reflect the involvement of a chronic inflammatory state in at least some cases of xanthomatosis.

Acknowledgements

T. Grewal was a recipient of a Quebec fellowship for excellence program from the Ministry of Education in Quebec, Canada. This work was funded by the Medical Research council of Canada (A.M.) and the MRC/Ciba-Geigy/IRCM University Industry program.

References

1. Furue M, Suzuki H, Kodama T, Hiramoto T, Sugiyama H, Tamaki K. Colocalization of scavenger receptor in CD68 positive foam cells in verruciform xanthoma. J Dermatol Sci 1995;10: 213—219.
2. Giry C, Giroux LM, Roy M, Davignon J, Minnich A. Characterization of inherited scavenger receptor overexpression and abnormal macrophage phenotype in a normolipidemic subject with planar xanthoma. J Lipid Res 1996;37:1422—1435.
3. Fogelman AM, Elahi F, Sykes K, Van Lenten BJ, Territo MC, Berliner JA. Modification of the Recalde method for the isolation of human monocytes. J Lipid Res 1988;29:1243—1247.
4. Liang P, Pardee AB. Differential display of eukaryotic messenger RNA by means of the polymerase chain reaction. Science 1992;257:967—971.
5. Liang P, Averboukh L, Pardee AB. Distribution and cloning of eukaryotic mRNAs by means of differential display: refinements and optimization. Nucl Acid Res 1993;14:3269—3275.
6. Luster AD, Ravetch JV. Genomic characterization of a gamma-IFN-inducible gene (IP-10) and identification of an IFN-inducible hypersensitive site. Molec Cell Biol 1987;10:3723—3731.
7. Schindler C, Fu XY, Improta T, Aebersold R, Darnell JE. Proteins of transcription factor ISGF-3: one gene encodes the 91- and 84 kDa ISGF-3 proteins that are activated by interferon-alpha. Proc Natl Acad Sci USA 1992;89:7836—7839.

FDB: diagnosis, laboratory and clinical findings, possibilities of treatment. Experience from homozygous and heterozygous patients

R. Češka, A. Hořínek, J. Šobra, K.H. Weisgraber, T. Innerarity and V. Šležka
IIIrd Medical Clinic, Charles University, Prague, Czech Rep., and The Gladstone Institute of Cardiovascular Disease, San Francisco, California, USA

Abstract. Familial defective apolipoprotein B-100 (FDB) is a genetic disorder caused by a glutamine for arginine substitution in position 3500 of apolipoprotein B 100.

In a group of 600 patients with hyperlipoproteinemia we identified 16 heterozygotes and one homozygote for FDB (frequency 1:32). The mean age of our patients (six males and 11 females) was 44 years. Diagnosis of FDB was based on point mutation PCR analysis of 26 exon of apo B gene. Plasma concentrations of lipid metabolism parameters in heterozygous patients were: CH: 8.26 ± 1.86, TG: 1.48 ± 1.42, HDL-CH: 1.75 ± 0.49, LDL-CH: 6.01 ± 2.01 (mmol/l), apo B: 1.66 ± 0.53, apo A1: 1.48 ± 0.09 and Lp(a): 0.17 ± 0.08. Genotype apo E 3/3 was the most frequent (11 cases), genotype E 3/4 was present in four patients and one person had E 2/3. Xanthelasma palpebrarum was present in four cases and tendon xanthomas in three (including homozygote). Premature manifestation of CHD was found in three patients. Diet treatment was used in only four patients, statins in five patients and fibrates in one case. A combination of statin and resin was used in four patients, and statin, fibrate and fibrate resin combinations were used in one patient.

Keywords: coronary artery disease, familial defective apolpiporotein B-100, familial hypercholesterolaemia, hypolipidaemic drugs, xanthomatosis.

Introduction

The primary mechanism for the homeostasis of lipoproteins is the lipoprotein receptor pathway. The initial step in this pathway is the binding of lipoproteins to receptors. Apolipoprotein B-100 (apo B-100) and apolipoprotein E (apo E) both play a crucial role in the interaction of lipoproteins with LDL receptors [1]. Apolipoprotein B is a huge protein with a molecular mass of 550,000 daltons. It is composed of 4,536 amino acids. The complete sequence and structural analysis of human apo B-100 has been already performed [2].

Familial defective apo B-100 (FDB) is a relatively recently described genetic disorder presenting with hypercholesterolemia and abnormal low-density lipoproteins (LDL) that bind poorly to LDL receptors [3—5].

Methods

Total cholesterol, triglycerides and HDL-cholesterols were measured enzymatically using sets produced by Boehringer. LDL-cholesterol was estimated by Friedewald formula. Apolipoprotein B and Lp(a) levels were measured by the rocket

Laurell method. We used antisera produced by Immuno Wien for apo. Electrophoresis of lipoproteins was performed in modification according to Rapp and Kahlke.

DNA analysis

Genomic DNA was prepared from 200 µl of frozen blood by quick 90 min method using the DNA isolation kit — ReadyAmpTMGenomic DNA Purification System (Promega, USA). Five from 200 µl of the ssDNA supernatant was used for PCR reaction.

Detection of familial defective ApoB-100

The FDB-100 mutation was determined using the PCR method and restriction enzyme isoform genotyping by ScaI (Promega, USA) restriction enzyme [6]. The change of a single nucleotide from G to A at position 10708 in exon 26 of the ApoB gene creates a ScaI restriction site. In the case of familial defective apolipoprotein B-100 the amplified DNA fragment is cut by ScaI, whereas DNA amplified from the normal allele is resistant to ScaI digestion. Considering difficulties with correct setting of the restriction enzyme digestion reaction (ScaI sensitivity to the salt concentration), we used the modified protocol with negative control [7]. A second ScaI restriction site was introduced in the upstream primer. This additional ScaI site is present in both the normal and the mutated alleles and so the restriction enzyme cleavage process can be simply controlled. DNA fragments were then divided in 2% agarose gel.

ApoE isoforms determination

ApoE determination was done by PCR and HhaI (CfoI) restriction enzyme isoform genotyping method [8] using primers published in [9]. Fragments (91, 81, 72 and 48 base pairs) were separated by horizontal electrophoresis in 4.5% DNA typing grade agarose (GIBCO).

ApoB haplotype analysis

Haplotype analysis of the ApoB gene was performed according to Ludwig and McCarthy [10] using restriction enzymes EcoRI, XbaI and MspI. Variable numbers of tandemly repeated DNA sequences (VNTR) were determined in the 3,ApoB multiallelic hypervariable region.

Results

We screened 600 patients with hyperlipoproteinemia. In this group we identified 16 heterozygotes and one homozygote for FDB. They were members of three families and the others were eight unrelated affected persons (frequency 1:32 or corrected 1:68). The mean age of the patients (six males and 11 females) was 44 years.

Lipid and lipoproteins are presented in Table 1. In the heterozygotes the following Apo E genotypes were found: E 3/3 (11 patients), E 3/4 (four) and E 2/3 (one). Homozygote had E 3/3 genotype.

The homozygote patient suffered from the first MI at the age of 34 years and the second at the age of 42 years. Due to diffuse changes on coronary angiography no revascularisation was performed. CHD was proven in two heterozygotes. One woman had angina since the age of 57 years and at the age of 63 years 4 × CABG was performed. The second woman suffered from MI at 55 years. In addition, the proband in one family (family N.) where six FDB+ patients were identified, suffered the first MI at 36 years and died at the age of 38 years from the second MI. The diagnosis of FDB in this woman has not been done since the patient died in 1986. Discussing the prevalence of CAD among FDB+ patients we should mention that seven of the patients identified as FDB+ were young (below 30 years).

Xanthelasma palpebrarum has been found in four heterozygotes and in two patients tendon xanthomas were present.

The treatment of our FDB+ patients is summarised in Table 2.

Discussion

In European and North American populations the frequency of heterozygotes for this defect is in the range of 1:500–1,700 of the general population [11]. In a recent study a much higher frequency of FDB-100 heterozygotes was shown in Switzerland. Prevalence of carriers of this metabolic defect of about 1:209 in Switzerland shows the possible origin of this mutation in this geographic region of Europe [12]. On the other hand the Finnish study proved the absence of FDB-100 in Finnish patients with hypercholesterolemia [13]. In most lipid clinics 2–5% of patients given the diagnosis of familial hypercholesterolemia had FDB and not FH [14]. Only four unrelated FDB homozygotes have been reported to

Table 1. Lipids, lipoproteins and apoproteins in FDB patients.

	Heterozygotes (n = 16)	Homozygote
Cholesterol	8.26 ± 1.86	10.2
Triglycerides	1.48 ± 1.42	1.07
HDL-chol	1.75 ± 0.49	1.17
LDL-chol	6.01 ± 2.01	8.82
(mmol/l)		
Apo B	1.66 ± 0.53	1.92
Apo A1	1.48 ± 0.09	
Lp(a)	0.17 ± 0.08	0.20

Table 2. Treatment of FDB patients.

Diet only	4
Statins	5
Fibrates	1
Statin + resin	4
Statin + fibrate	1
Resin + fibrate	1
Statin in high dose	homozygote

date. The prevalence of CAD varies in the different studies but our findings are comparable to the data of most of the authors. For the treatment of the patients we used, despite former scepsis concerning the use of statins, all available hypolipidemic drugs, respecting the guidelines of EAS and NCEP. In the treatment of homozygotes we used different treatment regimes including a combination of the three drugs. The acceptable lipid values we reached in this manner by using higher doses of simvastatin.

Conclusions

Despite the fact that our group of FDB positive patients is small we want to present the following conclusions:
1. In comparision to FH heterozygotes the plasma lipid levels of FDB+ heterozygotes were relatively lower. These findings are even more pronounced in comparision to homozygotes for both diseases.
2. FDB represents the significant risk fator for CAD.
3. Xanthomatosis is an important clinical sign not only for FH, but also for FDB patients.

Recently, it seems to be evident that the therapeutic approach is very similar or even the same for FH and FDB patients.

Acknowledgements

This publication was supported by the grants from IGA MZ CR 4041-3 and 3295-3 (Ministry of Health, Czech Rep.).

References

1. Brown MS, Goldstein JL. A receptor mediated pathway for cholesterol homeostasis. Science 1986;232:34—47.
2. Cladaras C et al. The complete sequence and structural analysis of human apolipoprotein B-100: relationship between apoB100 and apo B48. EMBO J 1986;5:3495—3507.
3. Soria LF et al. Association between a specific apolipoprotein B mutation and familial defective apolipoprotein B-100. Proc Natl Acad Sci USA 1989;86:587—591.
4. Innerarity TL et al. Familial defective apolipoprotein B-100: low density lipoproteins with abnormal receptor binding. Proc Natl Acad Sci USA 1987;84:6919—6923.

5. Weisgraber KH et al. FDB-100: enhanced binding of monoclonal antibody MB47 to abnormal low density lipoproteins. Proc Natl Acad Sci USA 1988;85:9758—9762.
6. Geisel J et al. Rapid diagnosis of familial defective apolipoprotein B-100. Eur J Clin Chem Clin Biochem 1991;29:395—399.
7. Geisel J et al. Improved detection of familial defective apolipoprotein B-100 by restriction-site-introducing polymerase chain reaction. Clin Chem 1993;39:2026—2027.
8. Hixson JE, Vernier DT. Restriction isotyping of human apolipoprotein E by gene amplification and cleavage with HhaI. J Lipid Res 1990;31:545—548.
9. Crook R, Hardy J, Duff K. Single-day apolipoprotein E genotyping. J Neuro Method 1994;53: 125—127.
10. Ludwig EH, McCarthy BJ. Haplotype analysis of the human apolipoprotein B mutation associated with familial defective apolipoprotein B-100. Am J Hum Genet 1990;47:712—720.
11. Humphries SE, Talmund PJ. Hyperlipidaemia associated with genetic variation in the apolipoprotein B gene. Curr Opin Lipid 1995;6:215—222.
12. Miserez AR et al. High prevelence of FDB 100 in Switzerland. J Lipid Res 1993;34:799—805.
13. Hamalainen T et al. Absence of familial defective apolipoprotein B-100 in Finnish patients with elevated serum cholesterol. Atherosclerosis 1990;82:177—183.
14. Myant NB. Familial defective apolipoprotein B-100: a review, including some comparison with familial hypercholesterolemia. Atherosclerosis 1993;104:1—18.

Coagulation and fibrinolysis

Thrombin interaction with vascular and nonvascular cells

Marie-Claude Guillin, Marie-Christine Bouton, Annie Bezeaud and Martine Jandrot-Perrus
Laboratoire de Recherche sur l'Hémostase et la Thrombose, Faculté Xavier Bichat, Paris, France

Abstract. Thrombin, a serine proteinase generated at sites of vascular injury, activates a number of vascular and nonvascular cells, eliciting a large variety of responses. Thrombin is the most potent physiological activator of platelets, it induces proliferation of vascular smooth muscle cells and fibroblasts, stimulates endothelial cells to produce several mediators and induces neutrophil adhesion to the endothelium. Thrombin stimulates other cell types outside the vasculature such as neuronal or tumor cells. Through its pleiotropic cellular effects, thrombin is not only involved in haemostasis and thrombosis, but is also active in various physiopathological processes such as inflammation, wound healing and atherosclerosis. Thrombin appears to elicit cellular responses mainly through proteolytically activated receptor(s) (PARs). PARs represent a subset in the larger family of seven transmembrane domains G protein-coupled receptors. A single cleavage within the N-terminal exodomain of the prototypic thrombin receptor, PAR-1, unmasks a new N-terminus that binds a specific region on the receptor to trigger activation. A second thrombin receptor belonging to the same family, PAR-3, presents both similarities and differences with PAR-1 in its mode of activation. The quantitative and qualitative differences in the responses of various cell types to thrombin could be accounted for (at least in part) by differences in tissue distribution of PAR-1 and PAR-3, or by coexpression of PAR-1 and/or PAR-3 with other thrombin binding proteins, upregulating or downregulating cell activation.

Keywords: atherosclerosis, haemostatis, healing, inflammation.

Introduction

Thrombin is a proteolytic enzyme which plays a key role in haemostasis and thrombosis. It has also been implicated as an important mediator of vascular lesion formation in atherosclerosis and restenosis, and appears to be involved in other pathophysiological processes. Thrombin is a pleiotropic enzyme which interacts with a large variety of cell types, including blood cells, cells from the vascular wall and nonvascular cells. Thrombin is the most potent physiological agonist of platelets. It also interacts with leukocytes, neutrophils, monocytes and lymphocytes. Thrombin binds and stimulates vascular cells, endothelial cells, smooth muscle cells and fibroblasts. Perhaps more surprisingly, thrombin is able to elicit responses from nonvascular cells (such as cells from neuronal origin, glomerular cells, keratinocytes, tumor cells and various other cell types). It is important to point out that the multiple actions ascribed to thrombin have been defined

Address for correspondence: Marie-Claude Guillin, Laboratoire de Recherche sur l'Hémostase et la Thrombose, Faculté Xavier Bichat, BP 416, 75870 Paris Cédex 18, France.

in cell-culture systems. At the present time, the in vivo significance of most of these activities is largely unknown.

Cellular responses to thrombin stimulation

Regulation of haemostasis

Thrombin interaction with vascular cells results in both amplification and limitation of the haemostatic process. Thrombin is the principal mediator of platelet activation, increasing platelet recruitment and therefore, the size of the platelet plug. In conjunction with collagen, thrombin causes the exposure of anionic phospholipids by platelets and formation of platelet-derived microvesicles [1], providing a catalytic surface for the assembly of enzymatic complexes which results in amplification of thrombin formation. Thrombin interaction with endothelial cells stimulates von Willebrand factor secretion [2] which contributes to platelet adhesion to the vessel wall. It also induces tissue-factor expression by the endothelium [3,4], which in turn may initiate blood clotting. Inversely, thrombin interaction with endothelial cells limits the haemostatic process by inducing nitric oxide and prostacyclin secretion. Binding to thrombomodulin at the cell surface changes thrombin specificity, promoting protein C activation and inactivation of the cofactors Va and VIIIa, which shuts off thrombin production. Lastly, glycosaminoglycans of the vessel wall catalyze the inactivation of thrombin by the serpin antithrombin III. The frontier between haemostasis and thrombosis is, therefore, as least in part dependent upon the balance between the procoagulant and anticoagulant mechanisms elicited by thrombin interaction with the blood and vascular cells.

Inflammation

Vascular inflammation is characterized by a sustained neutrophilic infiltration, due to interactions of blood cells with cytokines and adhesion molecules synthesized and expressed by vascular cells. Thrombin has been shown to be directly chemotactic for monocytes/macrophages [5]. It has also been proposed that thrombin directly elicits neutrophils chemotaxis. More probably, thrombin exerts this effect through the stimulation of cytokines production (namely IL-8) by the endothelial cell [6,7]. Thrombin induces a transient, reversible adherence of leukocytes to endothelial cells [8] by stimulating the expression of endothelial P-selectin, as well as the synthesis of platelet activating factor [9,10]. Thrombin also stimulates ICAM-1 expression which appears to mediate the prolonged neutrophil adhesion targeting leukocytes to inflammatory sites. Transmigration from the circulation to the tissues is facilitated by the increased vascular permeability, which is also directly mediated by thrombin [11].

Wound healing

Wound repair is a complex series of events, including an inflammatory response with infiltration of leukocytes, migration and proliferation of cells like endothelial cells and fibroblasts and synthesis of extracellular matrix by these cells. As discussed above, thrombin promotes the accumulation of leukocytes into the wound. Thrombin also supports the proliferation of endothelial cells and fibroblasts [12,13]. The mitogenicity of thrombin is both direct and indirect, as thrombin promotes the secretion of growth factors as well as their release from the extracellular matrix [14].

Thrombin interaction with extravascular cells

Thrombin also interacts with cells that have little to do with the clotting system. For example, evidence has accumulated for an important function for thrombin in the brain (see [15] for a review). Thrombin induces rapid changes in the morphology of various neuronal cells [16], secretion of endothelia-1 [17] and nerve growth factor [18] by astrocytes and proliferation of astrocytes. In the brain, thrombin is controlled by the serpin, protease nexin I. Both mRNA for prothrombin (the precursor of thrombin) and thrombin receptor are present in the brain, suggesting that thrombin may have an important role both in the repair process after nervous system injury and in the normal brain. Indeed, observations made after disruption of the thrombin receptor PAR-1 gene in mice [19] strongly suggest that thrombin and its receptor play an important role in embryonic development and in particular, in neural development. The observation that thrombin also stimulates mesangial cells, keratinocytes, osteoblasts, hematopoietic cells or tumor cells, underlines the ubiquitous nature of thrombin intervention and opens up a large new area for investigation.

Atherosclerosis

Early lesions of atherosclerosis are associated with endothelial cell dysfunction, characterized by increased vascular permeability, decrease in antithrombotic properties, LDL accumulation and monocyte adhesion. Within the vessel wall, infiltrating monocytes and macrophages stimulated by oxidized LDL express cell-associated procoagulant tissue factor [20]. Endothelium denudation or simply increased vascular permeability allows infiltration of blood proteins and in situ thrombin production. Within the plaque, the conjunction of thrombin production and infiltration of PDGF results in vascular smooth muscle cell proliferation in an inflammatory environment, which contributes to the development of the atherosclerotic plaque.

However, in vivo studies will be required to ascertain the direct implication of thrombin.

Structure and mode of activation of the thrombin receptor(s)

Protease-activated receptors (PARs)

Thrombin is a trypsin-like serine-protease with a restricted specificity (see [21] for a review). Most of the cellular effects of thrombin (although not all) require the proteolytic activity of the enzyme. A few years ago, three groups [22–24] simultaneously cloned the thrombin receptor PAR-1 which belongs to the ubiquitous seven transmembrane domains family of receptors. PAR-1 is the product of one of three closely related genes, the protease-activated receptors (PARs) family — a new class of receptors activated by proteolysis [25]. Interaction of thrombin with PAR-1 has been extensively characterized. A positively charged domain in thrombin referred to as anion binding exosite 1 binds a negatively charged sequence of the receptor resembling the hirudin C-terminal tail [26]. The thrombin active site undergoes a conformational change which allows docking of the receptor sequence LDPR within the catalytic site [27]. A unique cleavage at Arg41/Ser42 unmasks a new amino-terminal sequence SFLLR, which binds the remainder of the receptor within specific regions [28] located just proximal to the first transmembrane domain and in the second extracellular loop. Interactions of these regions with the tethered agonist peptide probably induce conformational changes leading to receptor activation. Once activated, responses are elicited via heterotrimeric GTP-binding proteins. The second cytoplasmic loop appears to be involved in the interactions with the G proteins [29].

Very recently, a second thrombin receptor has been cloned and designated PAR-3 [30]. The exodomain of PAR-3 contains a possible cleavage site at Lys38-Thr39 followed by a hirudin-like sequence, very similar to PAR-1. However, in contrast with PAR-1, the new N-terminus of cleaved PAR-3 does not behave as an agonist peptide, indicating that other mechanisms of proteolytic activation could operate. PAR-1 is expressed by a large variety of cells including platelets, endothelial cells, fibroblasts, smooth muscle cells, leukocytes and extravascular cells. No information on the cell-bearing PAR-3 is available to date, but PAR-3 is present in human bone marrow, kidney, intestine and lymph nodes. PAR-3 mediates platelet aggregation in mice, but other biological functions remain unknown.

Nonproteolytic cell activation

Although the majority of the cell responses are mediated by proteolysis of PAR-1, and/or perhaps PAR-3, a few number of cellular effects apparently do not require the catalytic site of thrombin. Proteolytically inactive thrombin retains chemotactic activity [31] and mitogenicity for macrophages. Monocyte chemotaxis is elicited by a cyanogen bromide fragment derived from the thrombin B-chain (residues 18–80, human thrombin B chain numbering). Macrophages chemotaxis is elicited by a fragment consisting of the insertion loop 45–57. The same fragment

(B chain 45–57) has been shown to act in synergy with the PAR-1 activating peptide SFLLR to stimulate fibroblast mitogenesis [32], indicating that thrombin can cause its cellular effect not only via the proteolytic activation of PAR-1, but also via the concurrent interaction with a distinct (yet unidentified) cell surface docking site.

Modulation of receptor-mediated cell activation by specific thrombin-binding membrane proteins

In certain cells, the effects of thrombin are modulated by specific cell membrane proteins, for example, glycoprotein Ib (GPIb) at the platelet surface or thrombomodulin at the endothelial-cell surface.

GPIb is a two subunit membrane glycoprotein, present at the platelet surface in complex with GPIX and GPV. GPIb is a binding site for von Willebrand factor and also for thrombin. When GPIb is absent and PAR-1 is present (as in platelets from patients with a Bernard-Soulier syndrome) platelets respond to thrombin stimulation but the responses are delayed and require higher concentrations of thrombin, indicating that GPIb promotes platelet activation mediated by PAR-1 proteolysis. However, in a soluble system, the extracellular domain of GPIb, glycocalicin, does not modify the rate of proteolysis of a recombinant polypeptide corresponding to the extracellular domain of PAR-1 [33]. A possibility is that the anchorage of GPIb in the cell membrane is required for a correct orientation of bound thrombin and promotion of its catalytic activity toward PAR-1. Alternatively, the binding of thrombin to GPIb could induce a signal that changes the response of PAR-1 to thrombin.

At the endothelial cell surface, both PAR-1 and thrombomodulin bind thrombin and both dock into thrombin exosite 1. In a soluble system, thrombomodulin behaves as a competitive inhibitor of thrombin-catalyzed hydrolysis of recombinant PAR-1 [33], suggesting that the density of thrombomodulin at the cell surface might modulate the responses mediated by PAR-1. Indeed, coexpression of thrombomodulin with PAR-1 on smooth muscle cells has been shown to reduce the mitogenic response to thrombin in a dose-dependent manner [34]. However, in this study, stimulation with a combination of thrombin and PAR-1 agonist peptide indicated that thrombin binding to thrombomodulin may inhibit PAR-1 mediated responses and not only thrombin binding to PAR-1. Thus, modulation of PAR-1 mediated responses by thrombomodulin could occur at least at two levels:
1) thrombomodulin may prevent PAR-1 interaction with thrombin by competition for overlapping binding sites within thrombin exosite 1; and
2) thrombin interaction with thrombomodulin may alter either the activation of PAR-1 or the response of activated PAR-1 via intracellular signaling.

Although there have been no reports that thrombin binding to thrombomodulin results in intracellular signalling, the cytoplasmic domain of thrombomodulin contains potential phosphorylation sites, which makes this pathway not unlikely.

In addition, to close the circle, it has also been reported that PAR-1 stimulation with the agonist peptide upregulates thrombomodulin expression [35].

In conclusion, several cell membrane proteins have been shown to interact with thrombin. Among them, PAR-1 and most probably PAR-3, act as true receptors which evoke intracellular signals. Other receptors activated by a nonproteolytic mechanism remain to be identified. Responses are modulated by distinct thrombin-binding membrane proteins, but the importance of the modulation and its mechanisms remain to be determined.

Acknowledgements

We thank the European Commission (Biomed 2 No BMH4-CT96-0937), the Ministère de l'Education Nationale, de l'Enseignement Supérieur et de la Recherche (ACC-SV9) and Université Paris 7 for their financial support.

References

1. Bevers EM, Comfurius P, Zwaal RF. Platelet procoagulant activity: physiological significance and mechanisms of exposure. Blood 1991;5:146–154.
2. Mayadas T, Wagner DD, Simpson PJ. Von Willebrand factor biosynthesis and partitioning between constitutive and regulated pathways of secretion after thrombin stimulation. Blood 1989;73:706–711.
3. Archipoff G, Beretz A, Freyssinet JM, Klein-Soyer C, Brisson C, Cazenave JP. Heterogeneous regulation of constitutive thrombomodulin or inducible tissue-factor activities on the surface of human saphenous-vein endothelial cells in culture following stimulation by interleukin-1, tumour necrosis factor, thrombin or phorbol ester. Biochem J 1991;273:679–684.
4. Bartha K, Brisson C, Archipoff G, De la Salle C, Lanza F, Cazenave JP, Beretz A. Thrombin regulates tissue factor and thrombomodulin mRNA levels and activities in human saphenous vein endothelial cells by distinct mechanisms. J Biol Chem 1993;268:421–429.
5. Bar-Shavit R, Kahn A, Mudd MS, Wilner GD, Mann KG, Fenton JW. Localization of a chemotactic domain in human thrombin. Biochemistry 1984;23:397–400.
6. Ueno A, Murakami K, Yamanouchi K, Watanabe M, Kondo T. Thrombin stimulates production of interleukin-8 in human umbilical vein endothelial cells. Immunology 1996;88:76–81.
7. Kaplanski G, Farigoule M, Boulay V, Dinarello CA, Bongrand P, Kaplanski S, Farnarier C. Thrombin incluces endothelial type II activation in vitro. IL-1 and TNF-α-independent IL-8 secretion and E-selectin expression. J Immunol 1997;158:5435–5441.
8. Bizios R, Lai LC, Cooper JA, Del Vecchio PJ, Malik AB. Thrombin-induced adherence of neutrophils to cultured endothelial monolayers: increased endothelial adhesiveness. J Cell Physiol 1988;134:275–280.
9. Toothill VJ, Van Mourik JA, Niewenhuis HK, Metzelaar MJ, Pearson JD. Characterization of the enhanced adhesion of neutrophil leukocytes to thrombin-stimulated endothelial cells. J Immunol 1990;145:283–291.
10. Lorant DE, Patel KD, McIntyre TM, McEver RP, Prescott SM, Zimmerman GA. Coexpression of GMP-140 and PAF by endothelium stimulated by histamine or thrombin: a juxtacrine system for adhesion and activation of neutrophils. J Cell Biol 1991;115:223–234.
11. Malik AB, Fenton JW. Thrombin-mediated increase in vascular endothelial permeability. Sem Thromb Hemostas 1992;18:193–199.
12. Belloni PN, Carney DH, Nicolson GL. Organ-derived microvessel endothelial cells exhibit differential responsiveness to thrombin and other growth factors. Microvasc Res 1992;105:

211—215.

13. Carney DH, Herbosa GJ, Stiernberg J, Bergmann JS, Gordon EA, Scott D, Fenton JW. Double signal hypothesis for thrombin initiation of cell proliferation. Sem Thromb Hemostas 1986;12: 231—240.

14. Taipale J, Koll K, Keski-Oja J. Release of transforming growth factor-β1 from the pericellular matrix of cultured fibroblasts and fibrosarcoma cells by plasmin and thrombin. J Biol Chem 1992;267:25378—25384.

15. Grand RJA, Turnell AS, Grabham PW. Cellular consequences of thrombin-receptor activation. Biochem J 1996;313:353—368.

16. Farmer L, Sommer J, Monard D. Glia-derived nexin potentials neurite extension in hippocampal pyramidal cells in vitro. Devel Neurosci 1990;12;73—80.

17. Ehrenreich H, Costa T, Clouse KA, Pluta RM, Ogino Y, Coligan JE, Burd BR. Thrombin is a regulator of astrocytic endothelia-1. Brain Res 1993;600:201—207.

18. Neveu I, Jehan F, Jandrot-Perrus M, Wion D, Brachet P. Enhancement of the synthesis and secretion of nerve growth factor in primary cultures of glial cells by proteases a possible involvement of thrombin. J Neurochem 1993;60:858—867.

19. Connolly AJ, Ishihara H, Kahn ML, Farese RV, Coughlin SR. Role of the thrombin receptor in development and evidence for a second receptor. Nature 1996;381:516—519.

20. Edwards RL, Rickles FR. The role of leukocytes in the activation of blood coagulation. Sem Hematol 1992;29:202—212.

21. Guillin MC, Bezeaud A, Bouton MC, Jandrot-Perrus M. Thrombin specificity. Thromb Haemost 1995;74:129—133.

22. Vu T-KH, Hung DT, Wheaton VI, Coughlin SR. Molecular cloning of a functional thrombin receptor reveals a novel proteolytic mechanism of receptor activation. Cell 1991;64:1057—1068.

23. Rasmussen UB, Vouret-Craviari V, Jallat S, Schlesinger Y, Pages G, Pavirani A, Lecocq JP, Pouyssegur J, Van Obberghen-Schilling E. cDNA cloning and expression of a hamster α-thrombin receptor coupled to Ca2+ mobilization. FEBS Lett 1991;288:123—128.

24. Pipili-Synetos E, Gershengorn MC, Jaffe EA. Expression of functional thrombin receptors in xenopus oocytes injected with human endothelial cell in RNA. Biochem Biophys Res Commun 1990;171:913—919.

25. Brass LF, Molino M. Protease-activated G protein coupled receptors on human platelets and endothelial cells. Thromb Haemost 1997;78:234—241.

26. Vu T-KH, Wheaton VI, Hung DT, Charo I, Coughlin SR. Domains specifying thrombin-receptor interaction. Nature 1991;353:674—677.

27. Mathews II, Padmanabhan KP, Ganesh V, Tulinsky A, Ishii M, Chen J, Turck CW, Coughlin SR, Fenton JN. Crystallographic structures of thrombin complexed with thrombin receptor peptides: existence of expected and novel binding modes. Biochem 1994;33:3266—3279.

28. Nanevicz T, Ishii M, Wang L, Chen M, Chen J, Turck CW, Cohen FE, Coughlin SR. Mechanisms of thrombin receptor agonist specificity — chimeric receptors and complementary mutations identify an agonist recognition site. J Biol Chem 1995;270:21619—21625.

29. Verrall S, Ishii M, Chen M, Wang L, Tram T, Coughlin SR. The thrombin receptor second cytoplasmic loop confers coupling to Gq-like G proteins in chimeric receptors. Additional evidence for a common transmembrane signaling and G protein coupling mechanism in G protein-coupled receptors. J Biol Chem 1997;272:6898—6902.

30. Ishihara H, Connolly AJ, Zeng D, Kahn ML, Zheng YW, Timmons C, Tram T, Coughlin SR. Protease-activated receptor 3 is a second thrombin receptor in humans. Nature 1997;386: 502—506.

31. Crago AM, Wu HF, Hoffman M, Church FC. Monocyte chemoattractant activity of Ser195→Ala active site mutant recombinant alpha-thrombin. Exp Cell Res 1995;219:650—656.

32. Hollenberg MD, Mokashi S, Leblond L, DiMaio J. Synergistic actions of a thrombin-derived synthetic peptide and a thrombin receptor-activating peptide in stimulating fibroblast mitogenesis. J Cell Physiol 1996;169:491—496.

33. Bouton MC, Jandrot-Perrus M, Moog S, Cazenave JP, Guillin MC, Lanza F. Thrombin interaction with a recombinant N-terminal extracellular domain of the thrombin receptor in an acellular system. Biochem J 1995;305:635—641.
34. Grinnell BW, Berg DT. Surface thrombomodulin modulates thrombin receptor responses on vascular smooth muscle cells. Am J Physiol 1996;270:H603—H609.
35. Ma SF, Garcia JG, Reuning U, Little SP, Bang NU, Dixon EP. Thrombin induces thrombomodulin mRNA expression via the proteolytically activated thrombin receptor in cultured bovine smooth muscle cells. J Lab Clin Med 1997;129:611—619.

Atherosclerosis XI.
B. Jacotot, D. Mathé and J.-C. Fruchart, editors.

755

Impaired fibrinolysis and the risk of coronary heart disease

Irène Juhan-Vague and Marie Christine Alessi
Laboratoire d'Hématologie, CHU Timone, Marseille, France

Keywords: genetic, insulin resistance, obesity, plasminogen activator inhibitor-1, risk factor.

Introduction

Among the list of coronary risk factors, it has recently been proposed that impairment of the fibrinolytic system detected in plasma due to increased plasminogen activator inhibitor-1 (PAI-1) levels could predict complications of atherosclerosis.

The fibrinolytic system [1] is regulated by a balance between activators and inhibitors; PAI-1, which inhibits t-PA, and u-PA, which is the main inhibitor of plasminogen activation. An increased PAI-1 concentration induces a decreased plasmin formation and leads to an accumulation of fibrin [2—4]. It also induces change in the vessel wall remodelling through activation of metalloproteinases, growth factors and degradation of the extracellular matrix [3,4]. Besides its antiprotease activity, PAI-1 also participates in the cellular adhesion and migration processes. By the mere fact that it binds to vitronectin in the same part of the molecule as vitronectin receptor or uPA receptor, it mediates release of cells from their substrate [5,6].

All of these properties indicate that PAI-1 can be involved in the risk of developing atherothrombosis.

Clinical and epidemiological studies

PAI-1 and other fibrinolytic variables have been investigated in plasma in many clinical studies. The main variables studied (PAI-1 activity and antigen and t-PA antigen, which represent mainly inactive t-PA/PAI-1 complexes) are strongly positively correlated between each other and negatively correlated with resulting fibrinolytic activity. In other words, an increased PAI-1 or t-PA antigen concentration corresponds to a decreased circulating fibrinolytic activity.

Case control studies have shown an increased plasma PAI-1 concentration in patients with coronary heart disease, or other forms of atherosclerosis, and in patients with obesity or non-insulin-dependent diabetes [7]. PAI-1 expression is

---

Address for correspondence: Prof I. Juhan-Vague, Laboratoire d'Hématologie, CHU Timone, 13385 Marseille Cedex 5, France.

756

also increased in the atherosclerotic lesions [8,9].

Fibrinolytic variables have been assayed in prospective epidemiological studies and results are in favor of a role of these parameters as predictors of coronary events [7]. The predictive capacity of fibrinolytic variables has been demonstrated in longitudinal studies including healthy subjects such as in the Northwick Park Heart Study [10] or the Physicians' Health Study [11], or including patients with coronary heart disease [7,12—17].

While clot lysis time [10] and t-PA antigen [11—13] have been shown to be predictive of cardiovascular events and mortality, conflicting results have been obtained for PAI-1 determination, PAI-1 being predictive in some reports [14,16] but not in others [13].

We have hypothesized that the discrepancy between the studies could be attributed in part to the different choice of confounding variables controlled, fibrinolytic parameters being strongly related to other coronary risk markers such as insulin-resistance parameters [18—24] and inflammation markers [25,26]. To demonstrate this we have, in the ECAT study, analyzed and compared the prognostic value of PAI-1 and t-PA antigen before and after specific adjustments for clusters of confounding variables which are potential markers of different mechanisms [17]. The ECAT study is a large prospective multicenter study of approximately 3,000 patients with angina followed up for 2 years [13]. Before adjustment, the three parameters — t-PA antigen, PAI-1 antigen and PAI-1 activity — were predictive of coronary events (p = 0.0002, 0.001 and 0.02, respectively). Adjustments were then made for the following clusters of confounding variables: insulin resistance represented by body mass index, triglyceride, HDL cholesterol and inflammation, represented by fibrinogen and C reactive protein. After adjustment with insulin resistance parameters, PAI-1 activity or PAI-1 antigen were no longer considered as risk factors, whereas adjustment for inflammation had no effect at all on PAI-1 predictive capacity. The results were different with t-PA antigen: the two different adjustments affected the prognostic value of t-PA antigen to the same extent, and when the adjustments were combined, the predictive capacity of t-PA antigen disappeared. Therefore, in patients with angina, higher levels of PAI-1 and t-PA antigen are associated with an increased risk of subsequent coronary events, plasma PAI-1 levels being mainly related to insulin resistance, whereas t-PA antigen is influenced by insulin resistance but is also a reflection of inflammatory response in patients with atherosclerosis [17].

For the identification of new risk factors, adjustments with the commonly recognized ones, such as body mass index, triglyceride and HDL cholesterol, are frequently used. These adjustments, which include insulin resistance variables, have a strong effect on PAI-1 prognostic capacity. They also modify the prognostic value of t-PA antigen which disappears when studied in a healthy population [11] and which is weaker but still persists when studied in patients with CHD and chronic inflammatory response [13].

Plasma PAI-1 and t-PA antigen levels are strongly interrelated in epidemiological studies. The reason for their association is not fully understood. We have recently proposed that t-PA-PAI-1 complex, having a delayed clearance compared to free t-PA, t-PA antigen could accumulate in the presence of a high concentration of PAI-1, as seen in insulin resistance [27].

PAI-1 and insulin resistance

Insulin resistance, also called plurimetabolic syndrome, is a largely distributed abnormality [28]. It is considered as predisposing to the development of atherosclerosis [29,30] and includes a cluster of variables such as obesity, with a repartition of the fat in the central part of the body (usually quantified by the waist on hip ratio), high blood pressure, glucose intolerance and among the biological abnormalities, fasting hyperinsulinemia, abnormalities of the lipid profile with elevated triglyceride and decreased HDL cholesterol. Increased PAI-1 and increased t-PA antigen levels must be added to the cluster of atherogenic abnormalities of this syndrome [18—25]. PAI-1 or t-PA antigen levels are very strongly correlated with all of the variables included in the metabolic syndrome and modulations of insulin resistance (by hypocaloric diet with weight loss, physical training or oral antidiabetic drugs) induce parallel changes in PAI-1 and t-PA antigen levels [18].

The mechanisms involved in PAI-1 production in the context of insulin resistance are beginning to be better understood. A production of PAI-1 by adipose tissue has attracted much attention recently. Folsom et al. [31] have shown that the reduction in PAI-1 antigen levels after weight loss was more related to the degree of weight loss than to triglyceride or insulin changes. It was also underlined that PAI-1 antigen levels were not increased in type II diabetic patients without obesity [23].

Data on PAI-1 expression by adipose tissue were first provided in rodents [32—34]. We have recently investigated PAI-1 production by human adipose tissue and its different cellular fractions [35]. As the relative degree of android (central) adiposity is better correlated with the risk of coronary heart disease than the absolute degree of fatness [36] and as the waist on hip ratio or direct measurement of visceral fat are strongly correlated with insulin resistance and plasma PAI-1 levels [21,37], we were interested in studying the capacity to produce PAI-1 of human adipose tissue from different territories. PAI-1 protein detected by immunolocalization was present at the stromal and adipocyte level whatever the territories tested (omental, mammary, gluteal). Interestingly omental tissue explants produced significantly more PAI-1 antigen than subcutaneous tissue from the same individual. These results suggest that adipose tissue, in particular visceral tissue accumulation, participates in the elevated PAI-1 levels observed in insulin-resistant patients [35]. The nature of the cells responsible for PAI-1 production in adipose tissue, as well as the mechanisms related to the insulin resistance involved, are so far an open field of investigation.

PAI-1 and genetic polymorphisms

Different polymorphisms of the PAI-1 gene have recently been described [38—40] and a contribution of genetic variation to plasma PAI-1 levels has been proposed [38,39,41—43]. An insertion-deletion on the promoter, 675 4G/5G [38,39], has been extensively studied and it was shown that subjects homozygous for the 4G allele presented higher plasma PAI-1 levels than the others. This relationship has principally been shown in patients with previous myocardial infarction [38,39,43,44]. A stronger association between triglyceride levels and plasma PAI-1 activity has been observed in diabetic patients homozygous for the 4G allele than in those homozygous for the 5G allele [42,44]. It has been proposed that the candidate site in the promoter could have a sequence involved in the binding of a transcriptional factor, whose level could be influenced by VLDL [43]. Interestingly the prevalence of the 4G allele was significantly higher in a group of 100 patients aged 35—45 years with myocardial infarction than in controls [43]. However, this relation was not confirmed in the ECTIM study of patients aged 25—64 years [41] and in the Physicians' Health Study [45].

To illustrate the relative contribution of both the insulin resistance syndrome and polymorphisms of the PAI-1 gene to plasma levels of PAI-1 in a healthy population, we have recently performed a family study involving 228 healthy nuclear families from the Stanislas cohort of Nancy (France) [46]. A gender difference was observed with fathers exhibiting higher PAI-1 levels than mothers and children. PAI-1 was, as expected, strongly correlated with insulin resistance variables, such as body mass index, waist on hip circumference ratio and insulin. They explained 48 and 28% of the variability of PAI-1 in fathers and mothers, respectively, whereas the 4G/5G polymorphism, in univariate and multivariate analysis, explained less than 5%; the effect being smaller in fathers than in mothers.

Therefore in a healthy population, plasma PAI-1 levels are primarily determined by the insulin resistance syndrome, the genetic effect being weak. The influence of a gene-environment interaction needs to be further investigated.

Conclusion

It has been shown that PAI-1 is a risk factor of CVD in the context of insulin resistance and it is produced in this context by adipose tissue, specially by fat from omentum. It could therefore be proposed that PAI-1 is a link between insulin resistance, obesity and CVD. The causal contribution of the impairment of fibrinolysis to vascular disease development has to be more extensively documented. Evaluation of a protective effect of the specific modulation of PAI-1 [47] opens up a promising field of interest.

References

1. Collen D, Lijnen HR. Basic and clinical aspects of fibrinolysis and thrombolysis. Blood 1991; 78:3114−3124.
2. Reilly CF, Fujita T, Hutzelmann JE, Mayer EJ, Shebuski RJ. Plasminogen activator inhibitor 1 suppresses endogenous fibrinolysis in a canine model of pulmonary embolism. Circulation 1991;84:287−292.
3. Erickson LA, Fici GJ, Lund JE, Boyle TP, Polites HG, Marotti KR. Development of venous occlusions in mice transgenic for the PAI-1 gene. Nature 1990;346:74−76.
4. Carmeliet P, Bouche A, De Clercq C, Janssen S, Pollefeyt S, Wyns S, Mulligan RC, Collen D. Biological effects of disruption of the tissue-type plasminogen activator, urokinase type plasminogen activator and plasminogen activator inhibitor-1 genes in mice. Ann NY Acad Sci 1995;748:367−382.
5. Stefansson S, Lawrence DA. The serpin PAI-1 inhibits cell migration by blocking integrin avb3 binding to vitronectin. Nature 1996;323:441−443.
6. Deng G, Curriden SA, Wang S, Rosenberg S, Loskutoff DJ. Is plasminogen activator inhibitor 1 the molecular switch that governs urokinase receptor-mediated cell adhesion and release? J Cell Biol 1996;134:1563−1571.
7. Juhan-Vague I, Alessi MC. Fibrinolysis and risk of coronary artery disease. Fibrinolysis 1996; 10:127−136.
8. Schneiderman J, Sawdey MS, Keeton MR, Bordin GM, Bernstein EF, Dilley RB, Loskutoff DJ. Increased type 1 plasminogen activator inhibitor gene expression in atherosclerotic human arteries. Proc Natl Acad Sci USA 1992;89:6998−7002.
9. Chomiki N, Henry M, Alessi MC, Anfosso F, Juhan-Vague I. Plasminogen activator inhibitor 1 expression in human liver and healthy or atherosclerotic vessel walls. Thromb Haemost 1994; 72:44−53.
10. Meade TW, Ruddock V, Stirling Y, Chakrabarti T, Miller GJ. Fibrinolytic activity, clotting factors and long-term incidence of ischaemic heart disease in the Northwick Park Heart Study. Lancet 1993;342:1076−1079.
11. Ridker PM, Vaughan DE, Stampfer MJ, Manson JE, Hennekens CH. Endogenous tissue type plasminogen activator and risk of myocardial infarction. Lancet 1993;341:1165−1168.
12. Jansson JH, Olofsson BO, Nilsson TK. Predictive value of tissue plasminogen activator mass concentration on long-term mortality in patients with coronary artery disease. A 7-year follow-up. Circulation 1993;88:2030−2034.
13. Thompson SG, Kienast J, Pyke SDM, Haverkate F, van de Loo JCW. Hemostatic factors and the risk of myocardial infarction or sudden death in patients with angina pectoris. N Engl J Med 1995;332:635−641.
14. Hamsten A, De Faire U, Walldius G, Dahlen G, Szamosi A, Landou C, Blombäck M, Wiman B. Plasminogen activator inhibitor in plasma: risk factor for recurrent myocardial infarction. Lancet 1987;II:3−9.
15. Munkvad S, Gram J, Jespersen J. A depression of active tissue plasminogen activator in plasma characterizes patients with unstable angina pectoris who develop myocardial infarction. Eur Heart J 1990;11:525−528.
16. Cortellaro M, Cofrancesco E, Boschetti C, Mussoni L, Donati MB, Cardillo M, Catalano M, Gabrielli L, Lombardi B, Specchia G, Tarazzi L, Tremoli E, Pozzili E, Turri M, for the PLAT Group. Increased fibrin turnover and high PAI-1 activity as predictors of ischemic events in atherosclerotic patients: a case-control study. Arterioscler Thromb 1993;13:1412−1417.
17. Juhan-Vague I, Pyke SDM, Alessi MC, Jespersen J, Haverkate F, Thompson SG. Fibrinolytic factors and the risk of myocardial infarction or sudden death in patients with angina pectoris. Circulation 1996;94:2057−2063.
18. Juhan-Vague I, Alessi MC, Vague P. Increased plasma plasminogen activator inhibitor 1 levels. A possible link between insulin resistance and atherothrombosis. Diabetologia 1991;34:457−462.

19. Juhan-Vague I, Thompson SG, Jespersen J. Involvement of the hemostatic system in the insulin resistance syndrome. A study of 1500 patients with angina pectoris. Arterioscler Thromb 1993; 13:1865—1873.

20. Potter van Loon BJ, Kluft C, Radder JK, Blankenstein MA, Meinders AE. The cardiovascular risk factor plasminogen activator inhibitor type 1 is related to insulin resistance. Metabolism 1993;42:945—949.

21. Vague P, Juhan-Vague I, Chabert V, Alessi MC, Atlan C. Fat distribution and plasminogen activator inhibitor activity in non-diabetic obese women. Metabolism 1989;38:913—915.

22. Schneider DJ, Sobel BE. Augmentation of synthesis of plasminogen activator inhibitor type 1 by insulin and insulin-like growth factor type 1: implications for vascular disease by hyperinsuline-mic states. Proc Nat Acad Sci USA 1991;88:9959—9963.

23. McGill JB, Schneider DJ, Arfken CL, Lucore CL, Sobel BE. Factors responsible for impaired fibrinolysis in obese subjects and NIDDM patients. Diabetes 1994;43:104—109.

24. Nagi DK, Hendra TJ, Ryle AJ, Cooper TM, Temple RC, Clark PMS, Schneider AE, Hales CN, Yudkin JS. The relationships of concentrations of insulin, intact proinsulin and 32-33 split proinsulin with cardiovascular risk factors in type 2 (non-insulin-dependent) diabetic subjects. Diabetologia 1990;33:532—537.

25. Juhan-Vague I, Alessi MC, Joly P, Thirion X, Vague P, Declerck PJ, Serradimigni A, Collen D. Plasma plasminogen activator inhibitor 1 in angina pectoris. Influence of plasma insulin and acute-phase response. Arteriosclerosis 1989;9:362—367.

26. Haverkate F, Thompson SG, Duckert F. Haemostasis factors in angina pectoris: relation to gender, age and acute-phase reaction. Thromb Haemost 1995;73:561—567.

27. Chandler WL, Alessi MC, Aillaud MF, Henderson P, Vague P, Juhan-Vague I. Clearance of t-PA and t-PA/PAI-1 complex: relationship to elevated t-PA antigen in patients with high PAI-1 activity levels. Circulation 1997;96:761—768.

28. Reaven GM. Banting lecture 1988. Role of insulin resistance in human disease. Diabetes 1988; 37:1595—1607.

29. Eschwege E, Richard JL, Thibult N, Ducimetière P, Warnet JM, Claude JR, Rosselin GE. Coronary heart disease mortality in relation with diabetes, blood glucose and plasma insulin levels. The Paris Prospective Study, ten years later. Horm Metab Res 1985;15:41—46.

30. Desprès JP, Lamarche B, Mauriège P, Cantin B, Dagenais GR, Moorjani S, Lupien PJ. Hyperinsulinemia as an independent risk factor for ischemic heart disease. N Engl J Med 1996; 334:952—957.

31. Folsom AR, Qamhieh HT, Wing RR, Jeffrey RW, Stinson VL, Kuller LH, Wu KK. Impact of weight loss on plasminogen activator inhibitor (PAI-1) factor VII, and other hemostatic factors in moderately overweight adults. Arterioscler Thromb 1993;13:162—169.

32. Samad F, Yamamoto K, Loskutoff DJ. Distribution and regulation of plasminogen activator inhibitor 1 in murine adipose tissue in vivo. J Clin Invest 1996;97:37—46.

33. Lundgren CH, Brown SL, Nordt TD, Sobel BE, Fujii S. Elaboration of type 1 plasminogen activator inhibitor from adipocytes. A potential pathogenetic link between obesity and cardiovascular disease. Circulation 1996;93:106—110.

34. Shimomura I, Funahashi T, Takahashi M, Maeda K, Kotani K, Nakamura T, Yamashita S, Miura M, Fukuda Y, Takemura K, Tokunaga K, Matsuzawa Y. Enhanced expression of PAI-1 in visceral fat: Possible contributor to vascular disease in obesity. Nature Med 1996;2:800—803.

35. Alessi MC, Peiretti F, Morange P, Henry M, Nalbone G, Juhan-Vague I. Production of plasminogen activator inhibitor 1 by human adipose tissue. Possible link between visceral fat accumulation and vascular disease. Diabetes 1997;46:860—867.

36. Björntorp P. "Portal" adipose tissue as a generator of risk factors for cardiovascular disease and diabetes. Arteriosclerosis 1990;10:493—496.

37. Cigolini M, Targher G, Bergamo Andreis IA, Tonoli M, Agostino G, De Sandre G. Visceral fat accumulation and its relation to plasma hemostatic factors in healthy men. Arterioscler Thromb Vasc Biol 1996;16:368—374.

38. Dawson S, Hamsten A, Wiman B, Henney A, Humphries S. Genetic variation at the plasminogen activator inhibitor-1 locus is associated with altered levels of plasma plasminogen activator inhibitor-1 activity. Arterioscler Thromb 1991;11:183−190.

39. Dawson SJ, Wiman B, Hamsten A, Green F, Hamphries S, Henney AM. The two allele sequences of a common polymorphism in the promoter of the plasminogen activator inhibitor 1 (PAI-1) gene respond differently to interleukin 1 in HepG2 cells. J Biol Chem 1993;268: 10739−10745.

40. Henry M, Chomiki N, Scarabin PY, Alessi MC, Pereitti F, Arveiler D, Ferrieres J, Evans A, Amouyel P, Poirier O, Cambien F, Juhan-Vague I. Five frequent polymorphisms of plasminogen activator inhibitor 1 gene: lack of association between genotypes, PAI activity and triglycerides levels in a healthy population. Arterioscler Thromb Vasc Biol 1997;17:851−858.

41. Ye S, Green FR, Scarabin PY, Nicaud V, Bara L, Dawson SJ, Humphries SE, Evans A, Luc G, Cambon JP, Arveiler D, Henney AM, Cambien F. The 4G/5G genetic polymorphism in the promoter of the plasminogen activator inhibitor-1(PAI-1) associated with differences in plasma PAI-1 activity but not with risk of myocardial infarction in the ECTIM study. Thromb Haemost 1995;74:837−841.

42. Panahloo A, Mohamed-Ali V, Lane A, Green F, Humphries SE, Yudkin JS. Determinants of plasminogen activator 1 activity in treated NIDDM and its relation to a polymorphism in the plasminogen activator inhibitor 1 gene. Diabetes 1995;44:37−42.

43. Eriksson P, Kallin B, van 't Hooft, Bavenholm P, Hamsten A. Allele-specific increase in basal transcription of the plasminogen-activator inhibitor 1 gene is associated with myocardial infarction. Proc Natl Acad Sci USA 1995;92:1851−1855.

44. Mansfield MW, Strickland MH, Grant PJ. Environmental and genetic factors in relation to elevated circulating levels of plasminogen activator inhibitor 1 in caucasian patients with non-insulin-dependent diabetes mellitus. Thromb Haemost 1995;74:842−848.

45. Ridker PM, Hennekens CH, Lindpaintner K, Stampfer MJ, Miletich JP. Arterial and venous thrombosis is not associated with the 4G/5G polymorphism in the promoter of the plasminogen activator inhibitor gene in a large cohort of US men. Circulation 1997;95:59−62.

46. Henry M, Tregouët DA, Alessi MC, Aillaud MF, Visvikis S, Siest G, Tiret L, Juhan-Vague I. Family study of metabolic and genetic determinants of PAI-1 activity and PAI-1 antigen plasma concentrations. The Stanislas cohort study. Thromb Haemost, XVIth ISTH Congress, Florence 1997 (Abstract).

47. Charlton PA, Faint RW, Bent F, Bryans J, Mackie I, Machin S, Bevan P. A series of low molecular weight inhibitors of plasminogen activator inhibitor (PAI-1) increase fibrinolysis and protect against thrombus formation in the rat. Thromb Haemost 1995;73:1005 (Abstract).

Does tissue factor participate in angiogenesis?

Angelika Bierhaus, Youming Zhang, Reinhard Ziegler and Peter P. Nawroth
Department of Medicine I, University of Heidelberg, Heidelberg, Germany

Abstract: Over recent decades tissue factor, the high-affinity surface receptor and cofactor for plasma factor VII/VIIa, has been generally viewed as the primary cellular initiator of the extrinsic coagulation cascade. Recent studies, however, implicate that there might be a role for tissue factor beyond hemostasis.

Introduction

Tissue factor is a 47 kd integral membrane glycoprotein, which serves as a cell-surface receptor and specific cofactor for plasma factor VII/VIIa. Since factor VII is a circulating blood component, vascular injury and/or membrane perturbation results in association of factor VIIa with tissue factor and initiation of the extrinsic coagulation cascade [1,2]. This demands for a strictly controlled tissue factor expression in cells located at the haemostatic barrier. Consistently, endothelial cells and monocytes lack detectable tissue factor expression under physiological conditions. However, constitutive tissue factor expression is present in the subendothelial layers of the vessel wall (the interstitium and throughout subcutaneous tissues) thus representing an "hemostatic envelope" [3], which can activate coagulation whenever vascular integrity has to be restored [2].

Possible roles of tissue factor apart from hemostasis

Several lines of evidence indicate that tissue factor has additional biological functions apart from hemostasis. First, tissue factor has been classified as immediate early gene product [4]. Tissue factor mRNA is rapidly induced in response to stimuli as cytokines, growth factors, endotoxin, AGEs and LDL in a variety of cells including endothelial cells and monocytes [2,5—12]. It has been demonstrated that tissue factor participates in cell proliferation, wound healing and the activation of inflammatory and immune responses. Under pathological conditions (even in the absence of vessel wall injury) aberrant tissue factor expression contributes to thrombogenesis in inflammation, septicemia, cancer, diabetes and arteriosclerosis [2,13—16].

Secondly, tissue factor expression has been demonstrated to contribute to intra-

Address for correspondence: P.P. Nawroth MD, University of Heidelberg, Department of Internal Medicine I, Bergheimer Str. 58, 69115 Heidelberg, Germany. Tel.: +49-6221-568604. Fax: +49-6221-564101.

cellular signalling. Binding of factor VIIa to tissue factor induces cytosolic Ca^{2+} signals [17]. Furthermore, the catalytic activity of the tissue factor/VIIa complex induces smooth muscle cell migration, which might promote atherogenesis and restenosis [18].

Finally, besides cells corresponding to the biological boundary layers of the organism, various cells located outside the vasculature and in particular neoplastic cells constitutively express tissue factor. Several experimental tumor models demonstrated that tissue factor expression is involved in metastasis and tumor angiogenesis [19—21] and further demand for a role for tissue factor outside of hemostasis and thrombogenesis. This view is emphasized by the detection of abundant tissue factor expression in early stages of human and mouse embryonic development, in which detectable factor VII expression is still absent [22]. In order to further define the physiological role of tissue factor, several laboratories independently constructed tissue factor "knock-out" mice with similar, but not identical results depending on the genetic background of the mouse model [23—27].

Tissue factor contributes to embryonic blood vessel development

Targeted disruption of the tissue factor gene ($TF^{-/-}$) in mice resulted in embryonic lethality beyond day 8.5. All embryos with a $129/Sv \times NIH3T3$ Black Swiss background died in utero between day 8.5 and 10.5 due to extensive hemorrhaging into the yolk sac and the loss of vascular integrity in extraembryonic tissues [25]. Similarly, $TF^{(-/-)}$ mice with a $C57BL/6 \times 129/Sv$ background exhibited defective yolk sac circulation, an abnormal fragile extraembryonic vasculature and defective vitello-embryonic connections leading to embryonic death at day 10.5 [23]. Only one out of 350 offsprings survived to gestation, although the targeted allele was inherited in a normal Mendelian inheritance [23,24]. Since differentiation of endothelial cells inside the yolk sac was normal, while the organisation of capillaries and vitello-embryonic vessels was disturbed, it is supposed that tissue factor is required rather for preserving vascular structure and integrity than for early endothelial cell differentiation [23—25]. The mechanism underlying tissue-factor-dependent early vasculogenesis has not been identified yet. One possible hypothesis is that tissue factor might directly be involved in signalling. Recent studies demonstrated that tumor-angiogenesis in Meth-A-sarcoma is at least in part dependent on tissue factor induced VEGF expression (see below) [20]. Remarkably, VEGF-deficient mice demonstrate embryonic lethality due to vasculature abnormalities of the yolk sac that in part resemble those in $TF^{(-/-)}$ mice and further implicate a connection between both genes [24]. However, it cannot be excluded that tissue factor also activates coagulation factors with cellular signalling properties as factor Xa or thrombin [23,24] has yet unknown functions that modulate cell proliferation and localisation [18,24] or contributes to local fibrin formation [24,25].

Genetic compensation of tissue factor deficiency

In contrast to the studies of Bugge et al. [25] and Carmeliet et al. [23], Toomey et al. described a small portion of TF$^{(-/-)}$ embryos with a 129/Sv × C57BL/6 background which survived into late gestation, however, the neonates died within the 1st week due to lethal hemorrhage [26,27]. They also demonstrated that TF$^{(-/-)}$ embryos with a 129/SV background uniformly died at midgestation, while in the C57BL/6 background part of the embryos survived into late gestation and died 1–2 days postpartum [27]. These data demonstrate that genetic compensation can occur and that mechanisms can become operative that adjust tissue factor deficiency for a limited time. However, the genetic compensation conferred by the C57BL/6 background only altered the time of death, but did not change the hemorrhagic phenotype [27].

Does tissue factor play a role in angiogenesis?

The close connection between tissue factor expression, neovascularisation, vasculogenesis and angiogenesis is further documented by experiments, in which Meth-A-sarcoma cells were stable transfected to overexpress or underexpress tissue factor before planted into immunodeficient mice [20]. Tumors which overexpressed tissue factor were fast growing, highly vascularized and demonstrated increased VEGF transcription. In contrast, tumors which underexpressed tissue factor due to transfection with antisense constructs were characterized by a slow growing rate, weaker vascularisation and a 50% reduced VEGF transcription compared to nontransfected control tumors [20]. VEGF transcription, however, was not completely abolished in tumors underexpressing tissue factor [20]. This might be due to the fact that transfection did not hit all cells. Furthermore, tissue factor is not the only factor involved in VEGF upregulation.

This view is emphasized by the recent observation that tumor growth, tumor frequency, morphology and vascularity of teratoma and teratocarcinoma cell lines derived from TF$^{(+/+)}$, TF$^{(+/-)}$ and TF$^{(-/-)}$ embryonic stem cells did not significantly differ [27] and implicates the existence of other factors that might induce tumor angiogenesis and vascularisation. The observation that genetic compensation under certain circumstances successfully counteracts TF$^{(-/-)}$ induced embryonic lethality further [27] supports the hypothesis that additional factors might be operative in vasculogenesis, angiogenesis and tumor vascularisation in the absence of tissue factor. Whether the genetic background of different tumors might also determine tissue factor dependent or independent angiogenesis is yet unknown.

Conclusion

Tissue factor (the principal cellular initiator of the coagulation protease cascade) is involved in a variety of nonhemostatic processes. Targeted disruption of the tissue factor gene results in embryonic lethality due to abnormal extraembryonic vessel development, disturbed vitello-embryonic circulation and massive hemorrhaging. Thus, tissue factor is required for maintaining vascular integrity in early embryonic development. A close connection between tissue factor, vascularisation and angiogenesis has also been observed in tumors, which overexpress tissue factor and thereby exhibit fast growing, increased vascularisation and VEGF transcription. On the contrary, tumors in which tissue factor expression is suppressed show retarded growth, a low grade of vascularisation and a strikingly reduced VEGF expression. Although these data point to an important role of tissue factor in vasculogenesis and angiogenesis, additional other factors are likely to be involved, since genetic compensation of tissue factor deficiency to a limited extent has been described in offsprings of tissue factor "knock-out" mice as well as in teratomas and teratocarcinomas derived from these animals.

Acknowledgements

This work was supported by a grant from the DFG (PPN). PPN performed this work as Heisenberg stipend (DFG) during the tenure of a Schilling-Stiftung professorship.

References

1. Bach R. Initiation of coagulation by tissue factor. CRC Crit Rev Biochem 1988;23:339–368.
2. Camerer E et al. Cell biology of tissue factor, the principal initiator of blood coagulation. Thromb Res 1996;81:1–41.
3. Drake TA et al. Selective cellular expression of tissue factor in human tissues. Implications for disorders of hemostasis and thrombosis. Am J Pathol 1989;134:1087–1097.
4. Hartzell S et al. A growth factor-responsive gene of murine BALB/c 3T3 cells encodes a protein homolog to human tissue factor. Molec Cell Biol 1989;9:2567–2573.
5. Mackman N. Regulation of the tissue factor gene. FASEB J 1995;9:883–889.
6. Nawroth PP, Stern DM. Modulation of endothelial cell hemostatic properties by tumor necrosis factor. J Exp Med 1986;163:740–745.
7. Bierhaus A et al. Advanced glycation endproducts (AGEs) mediated induction of tissue factor in cultured endothelial cells is dependent on RAGE. Circulation 1997;96:(In press).
8. Moll T et al. Regulation of the tissue factor promotor in endothelial cells. J Biol Chem 1995;270:3849–3857.
9. Bierhaus A et al. Mechanism of the TNFα mediated induction of endothelial tissue factor. J Biol Chem 1995;270:26419–26432.
10. Mackman N et al. Functional analysis of the human tissue factor promoter and induction by serum. Proc Natl Acad Sci USA 1990;87:2254–2258.
11. Lewis JC et al. Procoagulant activity after exposure of monocyte-derived macrophages to minimally oxidized low-density lipoprotein. Am J Pathol 1995;147:1029–1040.
12. Morissey JH, Drake TA. Tissue factor. In: Schlag G, Redl H (eds) Pathophysiology of Shock, Sepsis and Organ Failure. Berlin, New York: Springer Verlag, 1993;564–574.
13. Wilcox JN et al. Localisation of tissue factor in the normal vessel wall and in the atherosclerotic plaque. Proc Natl Acad Sci 1989;86:2839–2843.
14. Rao LV. Tissue factor as a tumor procoagulant. Cancer Metastasis Rev 1992;11:249–266.
15. Böhrer H et al. Role of NFκB in the mortality of sepsis. J Clin Invest 1997;100:974–982.

16. Drake TA et al. Expression of tissue factor, thrombomodulin and E-selectin in baboons with lethal *Escherichia coli sepsis*. Am J Pathol 1993;142:1458—1470.
17. Rottingen JA et al. Binding of human factor VIIa to tissue factor induces cytosolic Ca2+ signals in J82cells, transfected COS-1 cells, Madine-Darby canine kidney cells and in human endothelial cells induced to synthesize tissue factor. J Biol Chem 1995;270:4650—4660.
18. Sato Y et al. Tissue factor pathway inhibitor inhibits aortic smooth muscle cell migration induced by tissue factor/factor VIIa complex. Thromb Haemost 1997;78:1138—1141.
19. Bromberg E et al. Tissue factor promotes melanoma metastasis by a pathway independent of blood coagulation. Proc Natl Acad Sci USA 1995;92:8205—8209.
20. Zhang Y et al. Tissue factor controls the balance of angiogenic and antiangiogenic tumor cells in mice. J Clin Invest 1994;94:1320—1327.
21. Contrino J et al. In situ detection of tissue factor in vascular endothelial cells: Correlation with the malignant phenotype of human breast disease. Nat Med 1996;2:209—215.
22. Luther T et al. Tissue factor expression during human and mouse development. Am J Pathol 1996;149:101—113.
23. Carmeliet P et al. Role of tissue factor in embryonic blood vessel development. Nature 1996;383:73—75.
24. Carmeliet P et al. Insight in vessel development and vascular disoreder using targeted inactivation and transfer of vascular endothelial growth factor, the tissue factor receptor and the plasminogen system. Ann NY Acad Sci 1997;191—206.
25. Bugge TH et al. Fatal embryonic bleeding events in mice lacking tissue factor, the cell associated initator of blood coagulation. Proc Natl Acad Sci USA 1996;93:6258—6263.
26. Toomey JR et al. Targeted disruption of the murine tissue factor gene results in embryonic lethality. Blood 1996;88:1583—1587.
27. Toomey JR et al. Effect of tissue factor deficiency on mouse and tumor development. Proc Natl Acad Sci USA 1997;94:6922—6926.

Triglyceride-rich lipoprotein

Different approaches to the detection and quantification of triglyceride-rich lipoprotein remnants

Jeffrey S. Cohn and Jean Davignon
Hyperlipidemia and Atherosclerosis Research Group, Clinical Research Institute of Montreal, Quebec, Canada

Abstract. Both clinical and laboratory studies have implicated plasma triglyceride-rich lipoprotein (TRL) remnants in the pathogenesis of atherosclerosis and thrombosis. Remnant lipoproteins, formed through the lipolysis of intestinal chylomicrons or hepatic very low density lipoproteins (VLDL) are, however, difficult to accurately quantitate, since they exist in plasma at relatively low concentrations and are difficult to differentiate from their newly secreted precursors. A number of different biochemical techniques have been applied to the detection and quantification of TRL remnants, which recognize these lipoproteins on the basis of their density, charge, size, specific lipid components, apolipoprotein composition and/or apolipoprotein immunospecificity. No single procedure is presently considered to be the "method of choice", however, and ongoing research is devoted to the establishment of specific and clinically applicable assays which can clearly define risk of CAD associated with an elevation in plasma remnant lipoprotein concentration.

Keywords: apoE, cholesterol, coronary artery disease.

Introduction

It has been appreciated for more than 30 years that individuals with an elevated level of plasma triglyceride have an increased risk of coronary artery disease [1]. Hypertriglyceridemia in these individuals is often associated with a number of potentially atherogenic abnormalities in plasma lipoprotein metabolism, including an increase in postprandial lipemia, an increase in the concentration of triglyceride-rich lipoprotein (TRL) remnants, a decrease in low-density lipoprotein (LDL) particle size, and/or a reduction in high-density lipoprotein (HDL) cholesterol concentration [2]. The relative importance of these abnormalities in contributing to the onset and development of atherosclerosis has not been clearly defined, though their metabolic interdependence implies that they are all of pathophysiological significance. The aim of the present work is to review the different biochemical approaches that have been used to assess the plasma concentration of TRL remnants, and the evidence linking these parameters to increased risk of CAD.

Address for correspondence: Jeffrey Cohn, Clinical Research Institute of Montreal, 110 Pine Ave West, Montreal, Quebec, Canada H2W 1R7.

Detection and quantification of TRL remnants

TRL remnants are formed in the circulation when apoB-48-containing chylomicrons of intestinal origin or apoB-100-containing very low density lipoproteins (VLDL) of hepatic origin are converted by lipoprotein lipase (and to a lesser extent hepatic lipase) into smaller and more dense particles. Compared to their nascent precursors, TRL remnants are depleted of triglyceride, phospholipid, and apolipoproteins (apo) A and C, and are enriched in cholesteryl esters and apoE [3]. They have thus been identified, separated and/or quantified in plasma on the basis of their density, charge, size, specific lipid components, apolipoprotein composition and/or apolipoprotein immunospecificity. Each of these approaches has provided useful information about the structural and functional characteristics of remnant lipoproteins and has helped to define the relationship between elevated remnant lipoprotein levels and CAD (Table 1). The accurate quantification of plasma remnant lipoprotein concentration has, however, proven to be difficult, since despite their reduced size and triglyceride content, they are difficult to differentiate from their newly secreted precursors, and they exist in plasma at relatively low concentrations, i.e., under normal circumstances they are rapidly cleared from the circulation, or in the case of VLDL remnants, are efficiently converted to LDL.

TRL remnants have been separated from plasma by analytical, sequential or density gradient ultracentrifugation [4,5] within a lipoprotein fraction intermedi-

Table 1. Biochemical criteria used to separate and quantitate different remnant lipoprotein fractions in plasma and studies linking an elevated concentration of these parameters with CAD.

Criteria	Remnant fraction/ parameter	References linking remnant parameters to CAD
Density	Intermediate density lipoproteins (IDL) separated by ultracentrifugation ($1.006 < d < 1.019$ g/ml; Sf 12-20)	[6—11,17]
Density and charge	Slow pre-β- or β-migrating VLDL (d ‹ 1.006 g/ml) separated by electrophoresis	[33]
Density and lipid composition	Cholesterol/triglyceride ratio in VLDL (d < 1.006 g/ml)	[16,17]
	Following a meal containing vitamin A, retinyl ester conc. in VLDL and/or IDL	[29]
Size	"Mid-band" lipoproteins separated by polyacrylamide tube or gradient gel electrophoresis	[16]
Size and apolipoprotein concentration	Intermediate-sized lipoprotein (ISL) apoE and/or apoC-III concentration	[25,26]
Apolipoprotein	Following a fat-rich meal, plasma apoB-48 concentration	[28]
Composition	Plasma concentration of LpB:E, LpE:B and LpB:C:E and/or LpA-II:B:C:D:E	[20—24]
Apolipoprotein immunospecificity	Remnant-like particle (RLP) cholesterol concentration	[31,32]

ate in density (1.006 < d < 1.063 g/ml) between VLDL and LDL. Intermediate density lipoproteins (IDL) have been quantitated in terms of their plasma cholesterol, triglyceride and/or apoB concentration, and they have been shown in several studies to be at increased concentration in patients with CAD [6—11]. A less qualitative approach, which identifies remnants that are less dense (more triglyceride-rich) involves the separation of plasma VLDL (d < 1.006 g/ml) by agarose gel electrophoresis. In this system, VLDL normally migrate as a single band with pre-β-mobility. Smaller, less triglyceride-rich VLDL migrate with slower mobility and often appear as a diffuse smear of lipid-stained material at the trailing edge of the pre-β-migrating band. In some individuals, particularly those with combined hyperlipidemia and an apoE 3/2 or 4/2 phenotype [12], these remnants form a second distinct slow pre-β-migrating band — this characteristic being referred to as "double pre-β lipoproteinemia" [13]. In extreme cases (exemplified by patients with type III hyperlipoproteinemia) remnant lipoproteins are significantly enriched in apoE and cholesteryl ester, and they migrate (like LDL) with β-mobility (i.e., β-VLDL) [14]. The presence of slow pre-β- or β-migrating VLDL in plasma is characterized by an increased VLDL cholesterol/total triglyceride ratio [15] (or cholesterol to triglyceride ratio in VLDL), giving rise to the use of these lipid ratios as indicators of plasma remnants in individuals with and without CAD [16,17]. Polyacrylamide tube gel [18] or gradient gel electrophoresis [5] has also been used to separate remnant lipoproteins (according to size), but like agarose gel electrophoresis these systems provide a means for detecting rather than accurately quantitating remnant lipoproteins.

The association of apoE with TRL requires TRL lipolysis and subsequent change in the conformation of TRL apoB [19]. ApoE is thus a characteristic feature of remnant lipoproteins, and various assays have been applied to the measurement of TRL containing apoE [20—23], apoE associated with TRL [24], or apoE of "intermediate-sized lipoproteins" (ISL) [25,26], in normolipidemic and hyperlipidemic subjects, or in patients with and without CAD. ApoC-III has similarly been quantitated in different TRL fractions [27], though its concentration is probably more representative of triglyceride-rich rather than triglyceride-depleted particles. In the fed state, both apoB-48 [28] and retinyl esters [29] have been used to quantitate TRL remnants of intestinal origin in patients with and without CAD. Assessment of CAD risk by measuring remnant lipoprotein levels 6—8 h after meal feeding is an attractive proposition, considering that plasma triglyceride concentration at these later postprandial time points has been shown to be independently predictive of disease [30].

Recently, a more quantitative and clinically applicable assay has been established, whereby remnant-like particles (RLP) are separated from plasma using an immunoaffinity gel containing an antihuman apoA-I antibody and a specific apoB-100 monoclonal antibody, which recognizes all apoB-100-containing lipoproteins except partially lipolysed VLDL. HDL, LDL and the majority of VLDL are thus retained by the gel, and the unbound RLP fraction (which contains apoE-enriched VLDL as well as TRL containing apoB-48) is quantitated by cholesterol assay. The clinical usefulness of this assay is currently being assessed in studies which will determine the ability of RLP-cholesterol to independently predict the presence of CAD [31,32].

TRL remnants and coronary artery disease

It is significant that plasma concentration of TRL remnants is elevated in a number of disease states associated with the premature development of CAD, namely, type III hyperlipoproteinemia [33], diabetes [34], hypothyroidism [35] and renal disease [36]. This corresponds with experimental data showing that plasma remnant accumulation in cholesterol-fed [37] or transgenic animals [38,39] is associated with increased arterial atherosclerosis. The results of recent angiographic studies have also implicated remnant lipoprotein levels in the progression of CAD [23,27,28]. The relative importance of remnant lipoproteins as a risk factor for CAD still remains ill-defined, however, in large part due to shortcomings in the aforementioned methods for quantitating remnant lipoprotein concentrations. For example, the ultracentrifugal isolation of IDL provides a reproducible separation of more dense triglyceride-depleted particles, but does not account for TRL remnants in the VLDL fraction. Agarose gel electrophoresis allows for the visual assessment of remnant lipoproteins in the VLDL fraction, however, subjective judgement is required in the identification of slow pre-β-migrating lipoproteins. This approach is, therefore, difficult to standardize and is a qualitative rather than quantitative assessment of plasma remnants. Separation of "mid-band" lipoproteins by polyacrylamide gel electrophoresis has similar shortcomings. The measurement of apoE in different TRL remnant fractions is generally more accurate and precise, however, these methodologies are confined to specialized lipid laboratories. The measurement of RLP-cholesterol holds promise, although the clinical usefulness of this assay requires further evaluation. Thus, no single procedure is presently considered to be the "method of choice" for measuring plasma remnant lipoprotein concentration, and ongoing research is being carried out to establish specific and clinically applicable assays which can clearly define risk of CAD associated with elevated levels of TRL remnants.

References

1. Austin MA. Plasma triglyceride and coronary heart disease. Arterioscl Thromb 1991;11:2—14.
2. Havel RJ. McCollum Award Lecture, 1993. Triglyceride-rich lipoproteins and atherosclerosis — new perspectives. Am J Clin Nutr 1994;59:795—799.
3. Mjøs OD, Faergeman O, Hamilton RL, Havel RJ. Characterization of remnants produced during the metabolism of triglyceride-rich lipoproteins of blood plasma and intestinal lymph in the rat. J Clin Invest 1975;56:603—615.
4. Lindgren FT, Jensen LC, Hatch FT. The isolation and quantitative analysis of serum lipoproteins. In: Nelson GJ (ed) Blood Lipids and Lipoproteins. New York: John Wiley — Interscience, 1972;181—274.
5. Musliner TA, Giotas C, Krauss RM. Presence of multiple subpopulations of lipoproteins of

intermediate density in normal subjects. Arteriosclerosis 1986;6:79—87.

6. Tatami R, Mabuchi H, Ueda K, Ueda R, Haba T, Kametani T, Ito S, Koizumi J, Ohta M, Miyamoto S, Nakayama A, Kanaya H, Oiwake H, Genda A, Takeda R. Intermediate-density lipoprotein and cholesterol-rich very low density lipoprotein in angiographically determined coronary artery disease. Circulation 1981;64:1174—1184.

7. Reardon MF, Nestel PJ, Craig IH, Harper RW. Lipoprotein predictors of the severity of coronary artery disease in men and women. Circulation 1985;71:881—888.

8. Krauss RM, Williams PT, Brensike J, Detre KM, Lindgren FT, Kelsey SF, Vranizan K, Levy RI. Intermediate-density lipoproteins and progression of coronary artery disease in hypercholesterolemic men. Lancet 1987;1:62—66.

9. Steiner G, Schwartz L, Shumak S, Poapst M. The association of increased levels of intermediate-density lipoproteins with smoking and with coronary artery disease. Circulation 1987;75:124—130.

10. Mack WJ, Krauss RM, Hodis HN. Lipoprotein subclasses in the Monitored Atherosclerosis Regression Study (MARS). Treatment effects and relation to coronary angiographic progression. Arterioscl Thromb Vasc Biol 1996;16:697—704.

11. Hodis HN, Mack WJ, Dunn M, Liu C, Liu C, Selzer RH, Krauss RM. Intermediate-density lipoproteins and progression of carotid arterial wall intima-media thickness. Circulation 1997;95:2022—2026.

12. Cohn JS, Giroux L-M, Fortin L-J, Davignon J. Prevalence of double prebeta lipoproteinemia in hyperlipidemic patients is influenced by gender, menopausal status and apoE phenotype. Arterioscl Thromb Vasc Biol 1997;(In press).

13. Pagnan A, Havel RJ, Kane JP, Kotite L. Characterization of human very low density lipoproteins containing two electrophoretic populations: double prebeta lipoproteinemia and primary dysbetalipoproteinemia. J Lipid Res 1977;18:613—622.

14. Fredrickson DS, Levy RI, Lindgren FT. A comparison of heritable abnormal lipoprotein patterns as defined by two different techniques. J Clin Invest 1968;47:2446—2457.

15. Fredrickson DS, Morganroth J, Levy RI. Type III hyperlipoproteinemia: an analysis of two contemporary definitions. Ann Int Med 1975;82:150—157.

16. Kameda K, Matsuzawa Y, Kubo M, Ishikawa K, Maejima I, Yamamura T, Yamamoto A, Tarui S. Increased frequency of lipoprotein disorders similar to type III hyperlipoproteinemia in survivors of myocardial infarction in Japan. Atherosclerosis 1984;51:241—249.

17. Phillips NR, Waters D, Havel RJ. Plasma lipoproteins and progression of coronary disease evaluated by angiography and clinical events. Circulation 1993;88:2762—2770.

18. Mead MG, Dangerfield WG. The investigation of "mid-band" lipoproteins using polyacrylamide gel electrophoresis. Clin Chim Acta 1974;51:173—182.

19. Ishikawa Y, Fielding C, Fielding PE. A change in apolipoprotein B expression is required for the binding of apolipoprotein E to very low density lipoprotein. J Biol Chem 1988;263:2744—2749.

20. Genest JJ Jr, Bard JM, Fruchart J-C, Ordovas JM, Wilson PRW, Schaefer EJ. Plasma apolipoprotein A-I, A-II, B, E and C-III containing particles in men with premature coronary artery disease. Atherosclerosis 1991;90:149—157.

21. Parra HJ, Arveiler D, Evans AE, Cambou JP, Amouyel P, Bingham A, McMaster D, Schaffer P, Douste-Blazy Ph, Luc G, Richard JL, Ducimetière P, Fruchart JC, Cambien F. A case-control study of lipoprotein particles in two populations at contrasting risk for coronary heart disease. The ECTIM study. Arterioscl Thromb 1992;12:701—707.

22. Koren E, Corder C, Mueller G, Centurion H, Hallum G, Fesmire J, McConathy WD, Alaupovic P. Triglyceride enriched lipoprotein particles correlate with the severity of coronary artery disease. Atherosclerosis 1996;122:105—115.

23. Alaupovic P, Mack WJ, Knight-Gibson C, Hodis HN. The role of triglyceride-rich lipoprotein families in the progression of atherosclerotic lesions as determined by sequential coronary angiography from a controlled clinical trial. Arterioscl Thromb Vasc Biol 1997;17:715—722.

24. Luc G, Fievet C, Arveiler D, Evans AE, Bard J-M, Cambien F, Fruchart J-C, Ducimetière P.

Apolipoproteins C-III and E in apoB- and nonapoB-containing lipoproteins in two populations at contrasting risk for myocardial infarction: the ECTIM study. J Lipid Res 1996;37:508—517.

25. Cohn JS, Tremblay M, Amiot M, Bouthillier D, Roy M, Genest J Jr, Davignon J. Plasma concentration of apolipoprotein E in intermediate-sized remnant-like lipoproteins in normolipidemic and hyperlipidemic subjects. Arterioscl Thromb Vasc Biol 1996;16:149—159.

26. Fredenrich A, Giroux L-M, Tremblay M, Krimbou L, Davignon J, Cohn JS. Plasma lipoprotein distribution of apoC-III in normolipidemic and hyperlipidemic subjects: comparison of the apoC-III to apoE ratio in different lipoprotein fractions. J Lipid Res 1997;38:1421—1432.

27. Hodis HN, Mack WJ. Triglyceride-rich lipoproteins and the progression of coronary artery disease. Curr Opin Lipid 1995;6:209—214.

28. Karpe F, Steiner G, Uffelman K, Olivecrona T, Hamsten A. Postprandial lipoproteins and progression of coronary atherosclerosis. Atherosclerosis 1994;106:83—97.

29. Groot PHE, van Stiphout WAHJ, Krauss XH, Jansen H, van Tol A, van Ramshorst E, Chin-On S, Hofman A, Cresswell SR, Havekes L. Postprandial lipoprotein metabolism in normolipidemic men with and without coronary artery disease. Arterioscl Thromb 1991;11:653—662.

30. Patsch JR, Miesenböck G, Hopferwieser T, Mühlgerger V, Knapp E, Dunn JK, Gotto AM Jr, Patsch W. Relation of triglyceride metabolism and coronary artery disease. Studies in the postprandial state. Arterioscl Thromb 1992;12:1336—1345.

31. McNamara JR, Shah PK, Nelson SM, Nakajima K, Wilson PWF, Schaefer EJ. Lipoprotein remnant cholesterol and triglyceride values in coronary cases and Framingham controls. Circulation 1996;94:I—94(Abstract).

32. Devaraj S, Vega G, Grundy S, Jialal I. Evaluation of a rapid remnant lipoprotein cholesterol assay in atherosclerosis. Circulation 1996;I—704 (Abstract).

33. Morganroth J, Levy RI, Fredrickson DS. The biochemical, clinical, and genetic features of type III hyperlipoproteinemia. Ann Intern Med 1975;82:150—157.

34. James RW, Boemi M, Fumelli P, Pometta D. Lipid and lipoprotein abnormalities in non-insulin-dependent diabetes. In: Crepaldi G, Tiengo A, Manzato E (eds) Diabetes, Obesity and Hyperlipidemia: V. The Plurimetabolic Syndrome. Amsterdam: Elsevier Science Publishers, 1993;181—188.

35. Ballantyne FC, Epenetos AA, Caslake M, Forsythe S, Ballantyne D. The composition of low-density lipoprotein and very low density lipoprotein subfractions in primary hypothyroidism and the effect of hormone-replacement therapy. Clin Sci 1979;57:83—88.

36. Nestel PJ, Fidge NH, Tan MH. Increased lipoprotein-remnant formation in chronic renal failure. N Engl J Med 1982;307:329—333.

37. Mahley RW. Atherogenic hyperlipoproteinemia. The cellular and molecular biology of plasma lipoproteins altered by dietary fat and cholesterol. Med Clin N Am 1982;66:375—402.

38. Zhang SH, Reddick RL, Piedrahita JA, Maeda N. Spontaneous hypercholesterolemia and arterial lesions in mice lacking apolipoprotein E. Science 1992;258:468—472.

39. Plump AS, Smith JD, Hayek T, Aalto-Setälä K, Walsh A, Verstuyft JG, Rubin EM, Breslow JL. Severe hypercholesterolemia and atherosclerosis in apolipoprotein E-deficient mice created by homologous recombination in ES cells. Cell 1992;71:1—20.

Mechanism of the production of small dense LDL (sLDL) in hypertriglyceridemia

Yasuyuki Ikeda, Yasushi Ashida, Atsuko Takagi, Tomikazu Fukuoka, Akio Tsuru, Motoo Tsushima and Akira Yamamoto
Department of Etiology and Pathophysiology, National Cardiovascular Center Research Institute, Fujishirodai, Suita, Osaka, Japan

Keywords: cholesterol ester transfer protein, hepatic triglyceride lipase, lecithin:cholesterol acyltransferase.

Background

Human plasma low-density lipoproteins (LDL) are derived from very low density lipoproteins (VLDL) via intermediate density lipoproteins (IDL) by several intravascular enzyme actions [1]. LDLs consist of a spectrum of particles distributed across a density ranging from 1.019 to 1.063, and contain hydrophobic core lipids of cholesteryl esters (CE) and triglycerides (TG), surrounded by a polar surface of phospholipids (PL), free cholesterol (FC), and one molecule of apolipoprotein B-100 [2,3]. LDLs play an important role in transporting cholesterols from liver to peripheral tissues, and cholesterols within LDL are utilized for structural and metabolic needs by incorporating LDL particles via the LDL receptor [2]. However, hypercholesterolemia due to an accumulation of LDL particles that results from a deficiency of the LDL receptor is an independent risk factor for coronary heart disease (CHD) [4]. In addition to the abnormal quantities of LDL particles present in hypercholesterolemia, the qualitative features of LDL particles has attracted considerable interest in their metabolic behavior and atherogenic potential [5—12]. Small dense LDL (sLDL) has a mean diameter of 24.5 nm and a density of 1.040—1.065 g/ml [9,10]. It is relatively enriched in TG and less PL, FC and CE than LDL [12]. Small dense LDL is found in patients with hyperapobetalipoproteinemia [13], and frequently in those with hypertriglyceridemia [14—17]. Modifications in the size and composition of LDL are related to plasma TG levels [14—17] and become normal size in treated hypertriglyceridemic patients [15]. A preponderance of sLDL, classified as pattern B according to size estimation by nondenaturing polyacrylamide gradient gel electrophoresis (NPGGE) [9], is considered to be an elevated risk for CHD [11,12]. Its atherogenic potential has been explained as a decreased affinity for the LDL receptor

Address for correspondence: Yasuyuki Ikeda PhD, Department of Etiology and Pathophysiology, National Cardiovascular Center Research Institute, 5-7-1 Fujishirodai, Suita, Osaka 565, Japan. Tel.: +81-6-833-5012 (ext. 2476). Fax: +81-6-872-8091. E-mail: yikeda@ri.ncvc.go.jp

778

[18] and enhanced susceptibility for oxidation [19,20].

Over a decade ago, Deckelbaum et al. [21—23] reported the mechanism of sLDL production in the hypertriglyceridemic state. They demonstrated that the increased levels of triglyceride-rich lipoproteins (TGRL) such as VLDL promote cholesterol ester transfer protein (CETP)-mediated neutral lipid exchanges of TG and CE between VLDL and LDL. LDL is then remodeled to TG-rich/CE-poor particles, then TG in the remodeled LDL is hydrolyzed by lipoprotein lipase (LPL), resulting in smaller and denser LDL. However, the CETP reaction between TGRL and LDL in the first step of sLDL production is questionable, because CETP functions as a complex form with high-density lipoprotein (HDL) in the circulation [24,25]. Recent statistical studies suggest that hepatic triglyceride lipase (HTGL) is associated with generation of an LDL subpopulation [26—28]. The participation of lecithin:cholesterol acyltransferase (LCAT) should be considered in LDL remodeling, since LDL particles in patients with an LCAT deficiency are enriched in the surface lipids, PL and FC [29]. The precise mechanism of sLDL production in hypertriglyceridemia remains to be elucidated.

In the present study, we systematically investigated the mechanism of sLDL formation in hypertriglyceridemia and found that HDL particles associated with CETP and LCAT play a central role. We concluded that HDL particles are modified to TG-rich/CE-poor HDL by CETP-mediated lipid transfer between HDL and TGRL, which is elevated in hypertriglyceridemia. Thereafter, the modified HDL along with LCAT and CETP remodel LDL to TG-rich/PL-, FC- and CE-poor LDL. Finally, HTGL hydrolyzes TG in the modified LDL, which results in sLDL.

Subjects and Methods

Subjects

Three healthy male volunteers (35 ± 5 years old) with normal levels of serum triglyceride and cholesterol underwent an oral fat tolerance test. Patient TN with homozygous LPL deficiency and patient MS with homozygous HTGL deficiency were employed in this research in order to determine the size of their LDL particles. Patient TN was a 60-year-old male with type I hyperlipoproteinemia due to a homozygous deletion of G at the 916th position of exon 5 of the LPL gene [30]. Patient MS was a 50-year-old male with type IV hyperlipoproteinemia due to a homozygous missense mutation of C53G (^{230}TGC→GGC) in exon 2 of the HTGL gene [31,32].

Lipoprotein fractionation after an oral fat load and analysis of serum lipids, lipoproteins, and apolipoproteins

Serum lipoproteins were fractionated into five classes according to density by sequential flotation ultracentrifugation [33]: chylomicrons (d < 1.006 g/ml), VLDL (d < 1.006 g/ml), IDL (d = 1.006—1.019 g/ml), LDL (d = 1.019—1.063 g/ml), and HDL (d = 1.063—1.21 g/ml). Serum phospholipid, triglyceride, total and free cholesterol concentrations and those of the fractionated lipoproteins were enzymatically measured. Concentrations of apo B, apo A-I and apo A-II were determined by single radial immunodiffusion assays.

Preparation of HTGL, CETP and LCAT

HTGL was purified to homogeneity from human postheparin plasma as described by us [34] and the purified HTGL protein was quantified by the sandwich-enzyme immunoassay [35]. CETP and LCAT were partially purified from lipoprotein-free fraction of human plasma, isolated at a density of 1.21 g/ml, according to the method of Albers [36] and Tollefson [37], respectively.

Determination of LDL size and density

LDL size was determined by electrophoresis using 1.5—10% nondenaturing polyacrylamide gradient gels (4.9 × 82 × 82 mm). Electrophoresis proceeded using a GE 2/4 apparatus according to the method of Nichols et al. [38]. The diameter of LDL particles was calculated with reference to the migration of four standards: ferritin (12.2 nm), thyroglobulin (17.0 nm), α 2-macroglobulin (18.5 nm), and uniform polystyrene latex beads (35.0 nm). LDL density was determined by density gradient ultracentrifugation (d = 1.020—1.075 g/ml).

Results and Discussion

Conversion of normal-sized LDL to small-sized LDL under transient hypertriglyceridemia induced by an oral fat load

We searched for a factor that acts as a "trigger" in converting normal LDL to small LDL under transient hypertriglyceridemia induced by an oral fat load. After a 12 h fast, each participant consumed a meal consisting of 150 g of fat/ 70 kg of body weight. Blood samples were withdrawn each hour for the first 9 h and the last sample was taken 24 h after the meal. We analyzed the serum lipids, compositional lipid changes of lipoproteins, and LDL size. After fat intake, serum TG levels sharply increased from a fasting level of 135 to 400 mg/dl after 4 h due to increased concentrations of chylomicron particles. This peak level of TG was maintained until 8 h, after which it gradually decreased, returning to the fasting level after 24 h. A transient hypertriglyceridemic state during which the TG level remained above 200 mg/dl, continued for at least 10 h between 2 and 12 h after the meal.

In response to TGRL such as chylomicron particles increased by the fat load, a significant change in the lipid composition of HDL was followed by a similar

780

type of alteration in LDL. HDL became TG-rich and CE-poor and its TG/CE ratio (a maker of core-lipid changes) sharply increased from a fasting level of 0.23 to a peak of 0.70 at 6 h. After 6 h, the HDL-TG/CE ratio gradually decreased, and returned to the fasting level at 14 h. On the other hand, the LDL-TG/CE ratio was essentially unchanged during the first 1.5 h after fat intake. It thereafter gradually increased from a fasting level of 0.18 to a peak of 0.28 at 6 h, then returned to the fasting level at 14 h. During hypertriglyceridemia induced by the fat load, the magnitude of changes in the HDL-TG/CE ratio was always greater than that of LDL. Changes in LDL size were correlated with the HDL-TG/CE ratio, which was proportional to serum TG levels. During the fasting state (0 h), normal (25.94 nm) and smaller (25.7 nm) particles constituted 90 and 10%, respectively, of the LDL (Fig. 1A,B). In response to elevated HDL particles having higher TG/CE-ratio than LDL due to the TGRL levels increased by the fat load, the concentration of normal LDL particles gradually decreased with an inverse increase in that of small LDL particles. These findings indicate that normal LDL was converted to small LDL. The conversion of normal to small LDL reached a maximum at 6 h after the fat load, at an estimated distribution of 20 and 80%, respectively (Fig. 1B). The maximal reduction of LDL diameter was 0.5 nm as a consequence of the conversion (25.94–25.46 nm) (Fig. 1A). During this process, LDL particles became TG-rich and poor in PL, FC

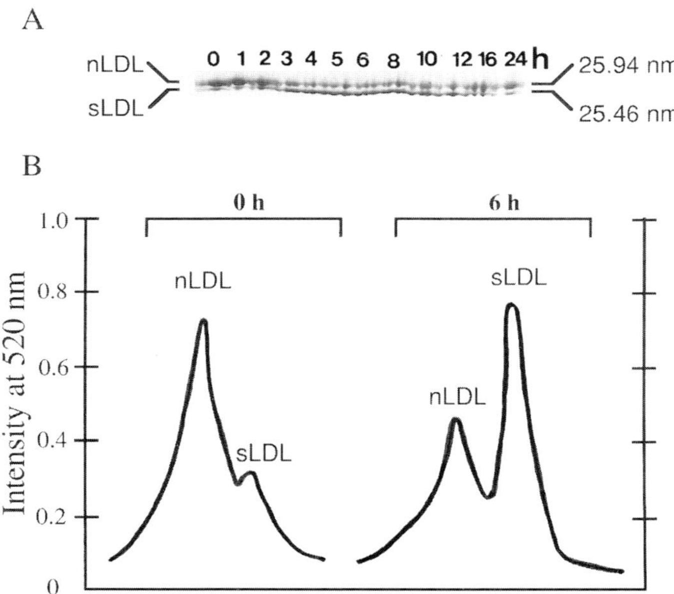

Fig. 1. Production of small-sized LDL (sLDL) from normal LDL (nLDL) during transient hypertriglyceridemic state induced by an oral fat load. LDL particle size was determined by 1.5–10% nondenaturing polyacrylamide gradient gel electrophoresis (NPGGE) at the indicated times after the oral fat load. **A:** NPGGE profile; **B:** densitometric scan of LDL at fasting (0 h), and at 6 h after fat load.

and CE. After 6 h, in response to the decreased number of HDL particles having a higher TG/CE-ratio than LDL, the amount of small LDL gradually decreased with a concomitant increase in that of normal LDL. After 24 h, the LDL distribution returned to that of the fasting level (Fig. 1A,B). These findings indicate that the conversion of normal to small LDL declines and that small LDL particles are gradually removed from the circulation by LDL receptor-mediated catabolism. Finally, normal LDL is replaced through the intravascular remodeling of VLDL to LDL.

Based on the results of the fat load experiment, we propose that the mechanism of sLDL production in hypertriglyceridemia is as follows. Core-lipid changes in LDL, particularly that of CE depletion, are mediated by the CETP reaction between LDL and TG-rich/CE-poor HDL modified by the CETP-modulated neutral lipid exchanges of TG and CE between HDL and TGRL. Furthermore, TG hydrolysis in the modified LDL by lipase results in sLDL.

CETP-mediated neutral lipid exchange between VLDL and LDL in the presence and absence of HDL

Our fat load experiments suggest that TG-rich/CE-poor HDL modified by the CETP reaction between TGRL (chylomicrons) and HDL remodels LDL to become TG-rich/CE-poor by the CETP reaction between LDL and TG-rich/CE-poor HDL. This mechanism is supported by evidence showing that CETP-HDL forms complexes that are far more stable than those of CETP-VLDL or CETP-LDL in the circulation [24]. However, this is in sharp contrast to earlier in vitro studies indicating that LDL is converted to TG-rich/CE-poor LDL by a direct CETP reaction between VLDL and LDL [22]. To clarify this discrepancy, we examined CETP-mediated lipid transfer between VLDL and LDL in the presence and absence of HDL. In the absence of HDL, ^{3}H-triolein-labeled VLDL and LDL were incubated at 37°C for 1 h with CETP, then isolated by density gradient ultracentrifugation. We then measured the ^{3}H content in the fractions. The level of ^{3}H-triolein in VLDL decreased time-dependently, and that in LDL linearly increased by ^{3}H-triolein transfer from VLDL to LDL for up to 1 h. We also examined ^{3}H-cholesteryl oleate transfer between VLDL and ^{3}H-cholesteryl oleate labeled LDL in the absence of HDL. The transfer of ^{3}H-cholesteryl oleate from LDL to VLDL was observed in the same fashion as that of ^{3}H-triolein from VLDL to LDL. As reported by Deckelbaum et al. [22], CETP-mediated neutral lipid exchanges of TG and CE between VLDL and LDL in the absence of HDL. In contrast, when ^{3}H-triolein-labeled VLDL and LDL were incubated at 37°C for 1 h with CETP in the presence of HDL, CETP-mediated neutral lipid exchange between VLDL and LDL considerably differed from that in the absence of HDL. In the presence of HDL, ^{3}H-triolein levels in LDL did not increase for the first 10 min. Thereafter, the level linearly increased for up to 1 h. On the other hand, ^{3}H-triolein levels in HDL increased in a linear fashion for up to 1 h without a time-lag. In the latter reaction, the increased ^{3}H-triolein incorporation into HDL appears to be derived from the direct transfer of ^{3}H-triolein from VLDL to HDL, but the label was not apparently transferred from VLDL to LDL. The increased amount of ^{3}H-triolein in LDL seems to be derived by transfer from HDL enriched in ^{3}H-triolein by the CETP-mediated reaction between HDL and ^{3}H-triolein-labeled VLDL. Also, CETP-mediated transfer of ^{3}H-cholesteryl oleate between VLDL and ^{3}H-cholesteryl oleate labeled LDL in the presence of HDL was essentially the same as that of ^{3}H-triolein between ^{3}H-triolein-labeled VLDL and LDL. These results indicate that CETP functions as a complex form with HDL in lipid transfer between donor and acceptor lipoproteins, instead of as a free carrier of lipids.

Effect of HDL particles having a higher TG/CE ratio than LDL, on remodeling LDL to become TG-rich/CE-poor

The fat load experiment and CETP-mediated neutral lipid exchange between VLDL and LDL in the presence of HDL indicate that HDL particles play an important role in remodeling LDL to become TG-rich/CE-poor. TGRL such as chylomicrons, increased under hypertriglyceridemic conditions, promoted CETP-mediated neutral lipid exchanges of TG and CE between TGRL and HDL, thereby converting HDL to TG-rich/CE-poor HDL having a higher TG/CE-ratio than LDL. The remodeling of LDL to become TG-rich/CE-poor was thought to be induced by CETP-mediated neutral lipid exchanges of TG and CE between LDL and TG-rich/CE-poor HDL having a higher TG/CE ratio than LDL. To evaluate this mechanism, we examined whether or not HDL with a TG/CE ratio higher than that of LDL could convert LDL to TG-rich/CE-poor LDL in vitro. First, we performed the CETP reaction between HDL and LDL having the same TG/CE-ratio. Figure 2A shows that no net mass transfers of TG and CE occurred between HDL and LDL, indicating that both lipoproteins having the same TG/CE ratio are at equilibrium for pools of TG and CE. However, when reacted with TG-rich/CE-poor HDL with a higher TG/CE ratio, LDL was converted to the TG-rich/CE-poor type by the CETP reaction as shown in Fig. 2B,C. These results indicate that CETP-mediated lipid transfer of TG and CE between LDL and HDL with a higher TG/CE ratio than LDL causes a net mass transfer of TG from HDL to LDL with a reciprocal transfer of CE from LDL to HDL, thereby remodeling LDL to become TG-rich/CE-poor.

Effect of LPL and HTGL on the hydrolysis of TG in TG-rich/CE-poor LDL during the formation of sLDL

Studies have shown that hydrolysis of TG in LDL modified by the CETP reaction between VLDL and LDL by bovine milk LPL results in sLDL [22,23]. In contrast, several reports indicate that HTGL activity is associated with a change in the size of LDL particles [26—28]. So far, it is unclear which of LPL or HTGL associates with the hydrolysis of TG in LDL to produce sLDL during hypertri-

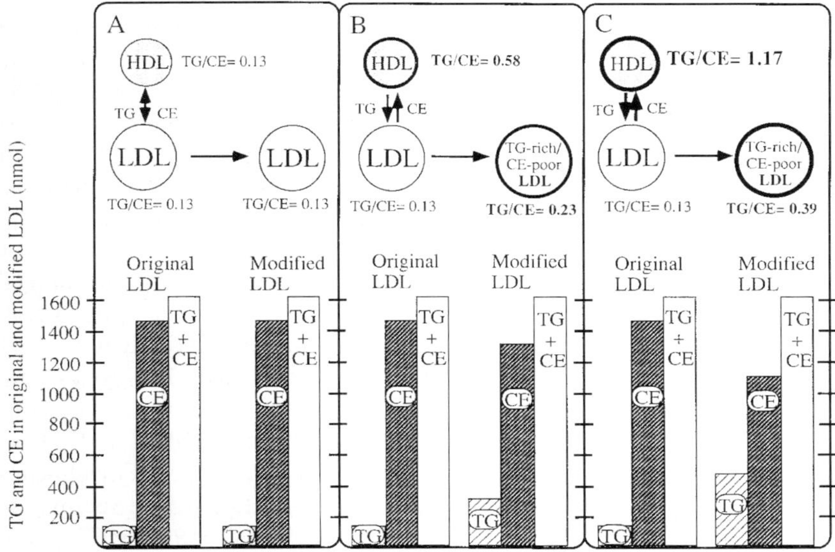

Fig. 2. Remodeling LDL to the TG-rich/CE-poor type by CETP-mediated neutral lipid transfers between LDL and HDL with a higher TG/CE-ratio than LDL. **A–C:** LDL and HDL particles having the indicated TG/CE-ratios were incubated with CETP at 37°C for 12 h. LDL and HDL were isolated by density gradient ultracentrifugation, and their lipid composition and TG/CE ratio were examined.

glyceridemia. We examined the effect of LPL and HTGL on TG hydrolysis in TG-rich/CE-poor LDL modified by CETP-mediated neutral lipid exchange between LDL and TG-rich/CE-poor HDL having a higher TG/CE ratio than LDL. Human LPL did not hydrolyze TG in TG-rich/CE-poor LDL because these particles lacked apolipoprotein C-II, which is as an essential cofactor for LPL. In contrast, HTGL hydrolyzed almost 60% of the TG in TG-rich/CE-poor LDL and the size of LDL particles was reduced. These results were supported by measuring the size of LDL particles in patients with homozygous HTGL and LPL deficiencies. In a patient with a homozygous HTGL deficiency, LDL particles were modified to become TG-rich/CE-poor in which the TG/CE-ratio was 8-fold higher than normal. However, diameter of LDL particles (26.0 nm) from the patient was the same as that (26.2 ± 0.5 nm) of normal individuals, indicating that the TG in TG-rich/CE-poor LDL was not effectively hydrolyzed by LPL action. In a patient with a homozygous LPL deficiency, small LDLs ranged from 20 to 24 nm in diameter, indicating that TG in TG-rich/CE-poor LDL was hydrolyzed by HTGL. These results show that the hydrolysis of TG in TG-rich/CE-poor LDL by HTGL results in sLDL.

Production of sLDL by synergistic effects of core and surface lipids changes in LDL in model systems containing TGRL, LDL, HDL, CETP, HTGL, and LCAT

Using three in vitro model systems, we found that sLDL formation under hypertriglyceridemic conditions can be explained as follows: 1) conversion of HDL to TG-rich/CE-poor HDL by the CETP reaction between TGRL and HDL; 2) conversion of LDL to TG-rich/CE-poor LDL by the CETP reaction between LDL and TG-rich/CE-poor HDL; and 3) formation of sLDL by TG hydrolysis in TG-rich/CE-poor LDL by HTGL. To evaluate the validity of these three step reactions in sLDL formation, we examined sLDL production by a sequential reaction using an in vitro model system. TGRL, LDL, HDL, CETP and HTGL were incubated for 16 h and HTGL was added every 6 h. The TG concentration of TGRL was adjusted to 400 mg/dl, which is about 2.5-fold of the normal TG level, to form a hypertriglyceridemic state. Concentrations of other lipoproteins and enzymes were adjusted to normal levels. TGRL, LDL and HDL were isolated by density gradient ultracentrifugation at 0, 4, 10 and 16 h. The lipid composition of these lipoproteins and the size of the LDL were examined. During the reaction, the HDL-TG/CE-ratio was always higher than that of LDL-TG/CE, indicating that LDL particles are constantly remodeled to TG-rich/CE-poor LDL by the net mass transfer of TG from HDL to LDL with a reciprocal transfer of CE from LDL to HDL. LDL was remodeled to TG-rich/CE-poor LDL and TG in the modified LDL was hydrolyzed by HTGL, but PL and FC in LDL were not affected by this reaction. At 16 h, electrophoresis showed that the diameter was maximally reduced by 0.4 nm as a consequence of remodeling the original LDL (26.2 nm) (Fig. 3, lanes 1 and 4) to small LDL (25.8 nm) (Fig. 3, lane 2). These results show that the above three steps must proceed sequentially for the production of sLDL under hypertriglyceridemic conditions.

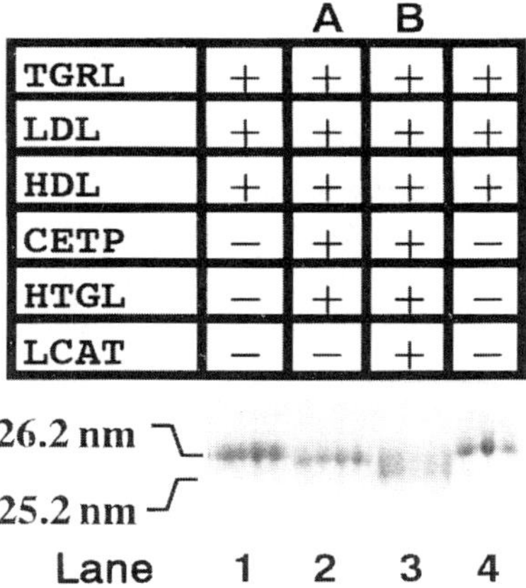

		A	B	
TGRL	+	+	+	+
LDL	+	+	+	+
HDL	+	+	+	+
CETP	−	+	+	−
HTGL	−	+	+	−
LCAT	−	−	+	−

Fig. 3. Production of sLDL due to synergistic effects of core and surface lipid changes in LDL using in vitro system. TGRL, LDL, HDL, CETP and HTGL were incubated at 37°C for 16 h in the absence (system A) and presence (system B) of LCAT. TG concentration of TGRL was adjusted to 400 mg/dl to mimic hypertriglyceridemia and other concentrations were adjusted to normal levels. After 16 h, LDL was isolated by ultracentrifugation and the size was determined by electrophoresis. Lanes 1 and 4, original LDL without enzymatic remodeling; lane 2, LDL modified by system A; lane 3, LDL modified by system B.

However, the lipid composition of sLDL modified by these reactions differed from that of the native LDL with the same size isolated from patients with hypertriglyceridemia. The amounts of PL and FC in the modified LDL were somewhat higher than those of native LDL. Thus, an additional mechanism that removes surface lipids from LDL should be considered.

Surface lipids in LDL are enriched in patients with an LCAT deficiency [29]. We therefore examined the effect of LCAT on the removal of surface lipids in LDL in terms of sLDL production under hypertriglyceridemic conditions. TGRL (400 mg of TG/ml), LDL, HDL, CETP, HTGL and LCAT were incubated for 16 h and HTGL was added every 6 h. TGRL, LDL, and HDL were isolated by density gradient ultracentrifugation at 0, 4, 10 and 16 h. The lipid composition of these lipoproteins and the size of the LDL were examined. During the reaction, HDL-TG/CE-ratio was always higher than that of LDL-TG/CE as it was in the reaction without LCAT. In the presence of LCAT, LDL was remodeled to TG-rich/CE-poor LDL and TG in the modified LDL was hydrolyzed by HTGL along with a decrease in the amount of PL and FC in LDL. Electrophoresis showed that the diameter of LDL particles was maximally reduced by 1.0 nm at 16 h due to remodeling original LDL (26.2 nm) (Fig. 3, lanes 1 and 4) to small LDL (25.2 nm) (Fig. 3, lane 3). Ultracentrifugation confirmed that the modified LDL was more dense than the original LDL. The lipid composition of sLDL produced in this reaction was almost identical to that of LDL with the same diameter isolated from patients with hypertriglyceridemia.

Conclusion

Our proposed mechanism of the production of small dense LDL (sLDL) in hypertriglyceridemia is summarized in Fig. 4. The most striking finding is that HDL particles associated with CETP and LCAT play a central role in modifying the composition of core and surface lipid of LDL during sLDL formation. Under hypertriglyceridemic conditions induced by increased levels of TGRL such as chylomicrons and VLDL, HDL particles tend to be converted to TG-rich/CE-poor HDL by the CETP-mediated lipid transfer of TG from TGRL to HDL with a reciprocal transfer of CE from HDL to TGRL. Modified TG-rich/CE-poor HDL particles have a higher TG/CE ratio than LDL. Therefore, they are capable of converting LDL to the TG-rich/CE-poor LDL by CETP-mediated lipid transfer of TG from TG-rich/CE-poor HDL to LDL with a reciprocal transfer of CE from LDL to TG-rich/CE-poor HDL. LCAT bound to HDL produces CE from FC and PL in HDL and enhances the generation of HDL particles depleted of surface lipids. Such HDL particles can remove surface PL and FC from LDL. As a consequence of these reactions, LDL is converted to TG-rich/ PL-, FC- and CE-poor LDL particles. TG in this modified LDL is hydrolyzed by HTGL, which generates sLDL.

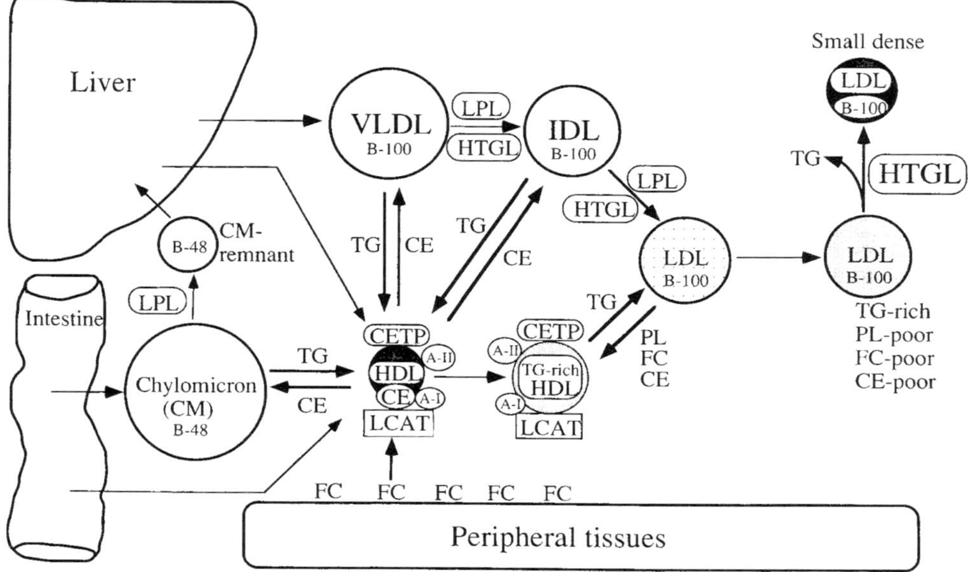

Fig. 4. Schematic illustration of mechanisms that produce sLDL under hypertriglyceridemic conditions. FC, free cholesterol; CE, cholesteryl ester; PL, phospholipid; TG, triglyceride; A-I, apolipoprotein A-I; A-II, apolipoprotein A-II; B-48, apolipoprotein B-48; B-100, apolipoprotein B-100; CETP, cholesterol ester transfer protein; LCAT, lecithin:cholesterol acyltransferase; HTGL, hepatic triglyceride lipase.

Acknowledgements

This research was supported in part by a Grant-in-Aid for Scientific Research (C) (No. 06671066) from the Ministry of Education, Science and Culture of Japan, and the Special Coordination Fund for the Promotion of Science and Technology from the Science and Technology Agency (Encouragement System of C.O.E.)

References

1. Eisenberg S, Levy RI. Lipoprotein metabolism. Adv Lipid Res 1975;13:1–89.
2. Havel RJ, Goldstein JL, Brown MS. Lipoproteins and lipid transport. In: Bondy PK, Rosenberg LE (eds) Metabolic Control and Disease. Philadelphia: W.B. Saunders, 1980;393–494.
3. Yang CY, Chen SH, Gianturco SH, Bradley WA, Sparrow JT, Tanimura M, Li WH, Sparrow DA, DeLoof H, Rosseneu M, Lee F-S, Gu Z-W, Gotto AMJ, Chan L. Sequence, structure, receptor-binding domains and internal repeats of human apolipoprotein B-100. Nature 1986; 323:738–742.
4. Goldstein JL, Brown MS. Familial hypercholesterolemia. In: Scriver CR, Beaudet AL, Sly WS, Valle D (eds) The Metabolic Basis of Inherited Disease. New York: McGraw-Hill, Inc., 1989; 1215–1250.
5. Fisher WR. Heterogeneity of plasma low density lipoproteins manifestations of the physiologic

phenomenon in man. Metabolism 1983;32:283—291.

6. Rudel LL, Parks JS, Johnson FL, Babiak J. Low density lipoproteins in atherosclerosis. J Lipid Res 1986;27:465—474.

7. Swinkels DW, Demacker PNM, Hak-Lemmers HLM, Mol MJTM, Yap SH, van 't Laar A. Some metabolic characteristics of low-density lipoprotein subfractions, LDL-1 and LDL-2: in vitro and in vivo studies. Biochim Biophys Acta 1988;960:1—9.

8. Marzetta CA, Foster DM, Brunzell JD. Relationships between LDL density and kinetic heterogeneity in subjects with normolipidemia and familial combined hyperlipoproteinemia using density gradient ultracentrifugation. J Lipid Res 1989;30:1307—1317.

9. Austin MA, Breslow JL, Hennekens CH, Buring JE, Willett WC, Krauss RM. Low-density lipoprotein subclass patterns and risk of myocardial infarction. J Am Med Assoc 1988;260:1917—1921.

10. Campos H, Blijlevens E, McNamara JR, Ordovas JM, Posner BM, Wilson PWF, Castelli WP, Schaefer EJ. LDL particle size distribution. Results from the Framingham Offspring Study. Arterioscler Thromb 1992;12:1410—1419.

11. Austin MA, Hokanson JE, Brunzell JD. Characterization of low-density lipoprotein subclasses: methodologic approaches and clinical relevance. Curr Opin Lipid 1994;5:395—403.

12. Krauss RM. Heterogeneity of plasma low-density lipoproteins and atherosclerosis risk. Curr Opin Lipid 1994;5:339—349.

13. Teng B, Thompson GR, Sniderman AD, Forte TM, Krauss RM, Kwiterovich PO Jr. Composition and distribution of low density lipoprotein fractions in hyperapobetalipoproteinemia, normolipidemia, and familial hypercholesterolemia. Proc Natl Acad Sci USA 1983;80:6662—6666.

14. Deckelbaum RJ, Granot E, Oschry Y, Rose L, Eisenberg S. Plasma triglyceride determines structure-composition in low and high density lipoproteins. Arteriosclerosis 1984;4:225—231.

15. Eisenberg S, Gavish D, Oschry Y, Fainaru M, Deckelbaum RJ. Abnormalities in very low, low and high density lipoproteins in hypertriglyceridemia. Reversal toward normal with bezafibrate treatment. J Clin Invest 1984;74:470—482.

16. McNamara JR, Jenner JL, Li Z, Wilson PW, Schaefer EJ. Change in LDL particle size is associated with change in plasma triglyceride concentration. Arterioscler Thromb 1992;12:1284—1290.

17. Coresh J, Kwiterovich PO Jr, Smith HH, Bachorik PS. Association of plasma triglyceride concentration and LDL particle diameter, density, and chemical composition with premature coronary artery disease in men and women. J Lipid Res 1993;34:1687—1697.

18. Nigon F, Lesnik P, Rouis M, Chapman MJ. Discrete subspecies of human low density lipoproteins are heterogeneous in their interaction with the cellular LDL receptor. J Lipid Res 1991;32:1741—1753.

19. de Graaf J, Hak-Lemmers HLM, Hectors MPC, Demacker PNM, Hendriks JCM, Stalenhoef AFH. Enhanced susceptibility to in vitro oxidation of the dense low density lipoprotein subfraction in healthy subjects. Arterioscler Thromb 1991;11:298—306.

20. Dejager S, Bruckert E, Chapman MJ. Dense low density lipoprotein subspecies with diminished oxidative resistance predominate in combined hyperlipidemia. J Lipid Res 1993;34:295—308.

21. Deckelbaum RJ, Eisenberg S, Fainaru M, Barenholz Y, Olivecrona T. *In vitro* production of human plasma low density lipoprotein-like particles. J Biol Chem 1979;254:6079—6087.

22. Deckelbaum RJ, Eisenberg S, Oschry Y, Butbul E, Sharon I, Olivecrona T. Reversible modification of human plasma low density lipoproteins toward triglyceride-rich precursors: a mechanism for losing excess cholesterol esters. J Biol Chem 1982;257:6509—6517.

23. Deckelbaum RJ, Olivecrona T, Eisenberg S. Plasma lipoproteins in hyperlipidemia: roles of neutral lipid exchange and lipase. In: Carlson LA, Olsson AG (eds) Treatment of Hyperlipoproteinemia. New York: Raven Press, 1984;85—93.

24. Pattnaik NM, Zilversmit DB. Interaction of cholesteryl ester exchange protein with human plasma lipoproteins and phospholipid vesicles. J Biol Chem 1979;254:2782—2786.

25. Cheung MC, Wolf AC, Lum KD, Tollefson JH, Albers JJ. Distribution and localization of

lecithin:cholesterol acyltransferase and cholesteryl ester transfer activity in A-I-containing lipoproteins. J Lipid Res 1986;27:1135—1144.

26. Karpe F, Tornvall P, Olivecrona T, Steiner G, Carlson LA, Hamsten A. Composition of human low density lipoprotein: effects of postprandial triglyceride-rich lipoproteins, lipoprotein lipase, hepatic lipase and cholesteryl ester transfer protein. Atherosclerosis 1993;98:33—49.

27. Zambon A, Austin MA, Brown BG, Hokanson JE, Brunzell JD. Effect of hepatic lipase on LDL in normal men and those with coronary artery disease. Arterioscler Thromb 1993;13:147—153.

28. Campos H, Dreon DM, Krauss RM. Associations of hepatic and lipoprotein lipase activities with changes in dietary composition and low density lipoprotein subclasses. J Lipid Res 1995; 36:462—472.

29. Glomset JA, Nichols AV, Norum KR, King W, Forte T. Plasma lipoproteins in familial lecithin: cholesterol acyltransferase deficiency. Further studies of very low and low density lipoprotein abnormalities. J Clin Invest 1973;52:1078—1092.

30. Takagi A, Ikeda Y, Tsutsumi Z, Shoji T, Yamamoto A. Molecular studies on primary lipoprotein lipase (LPL) deficiency — One base deletion (G916) in exon-5 of LPL gene causes no detectable LPL protein due to the absence of LPL messenger RNA transcript. J Clin Invest 1992;89: 581—591.

31. Ikeda Y, Takagi A, Mori A, Fukuoka T, Tsutsumi Z, Tsushima M, Yamamoto A. Molecular and metabolic studies on a patient with homozygous hepatic lipase (HL) deficiency: newly identified HLosaka allele in HL gene-exon2. Atherosclerosis 1994;109:210 (Abstract).

32. Ikeda Y, Takagi A, Tsutsumi Z, Tsuru A, Mori A, Fukuoka T, Ashida Y, Tsushima M, Yamamoto A. Physiological role of human hepatic triglyceride lipase (HTGL): HTGL regulates the multiple lipoprotein metabolism of IDL, LDL, and HDL2. In: Yamamoto A (ed) Multiple Risk Factors in Cardiovascular Disease. Tokyo: Churchill Livingstone, 1994;181—186.

33. Hatch FT, Lees RS. Practical methods for plasma lipoprotein analysis. Adv Lipid Res 1968;6: 1—68.

34. Ikeda Y, Takagi A, Yamamoto A. Purification and characterization of lipoprotein lipase and hepatic triglyceride lipase from human postheparin plasma: production of monospecific antibody to the individual lipase. Biochim Biophys Acta 1989;1003:254—269.

35. Ikeda Y, Takagi A, Ohkaru Y, Nogi K, Iwanaga T, Kurooka S, Yamamoto A. A sandwich-enzyme immunoassay for the quantification of lipoprotein lipase and hepatic triglyceride lipase in human postheparin plasma using monoclonal antibodies to the corresponding enzymes. J Lipid Res 1990;31:1911—1924.

36. Albers JJ, Chen C, Lacko AG. Isolation, characterization, and assay of lecithin-cholesterol acyltransferase. Meth Enzymol 1986;129:763—783.

37. Tollefson JH, Albers JJ. Isolation, characterization, and assay of plasma lipid transfer proteins. Meth Enzymol 1986;129:797—816.

38. Nichols AV, Krauss RM, Musliner TA. Nondenaturing polyacrylamide gradient gel electrophoresis. Meth Enzymol 1986;128:417—431.

Regulation of VLDL production in man: implications for coronary heart disease (CHD)

C.J. Packard and J. Shepherd
Institute of Biochemistry, Glasgow Royal Infirmary University NHS Trust, Alexandra Parade, Glasgow, UK

Introduction

Low-density lipoprotein (LDL), the major apoB-containing species in plasma associated with increased risk of CHD (coronary heart disease), is derived principally by the lipolysis of very low density lipoprotein (VLDL). Studies have shown LDL to be structurally heterogeneous; discrete subfractions that differ in density and size [1,2], in composition [3] and in their ability to interact with the LDL receptor [4], have been observed in the circulation of most subjects. It is clear also from turnover studies that LDL is metabolically heterogeneous. Even when isolated in a narrow density interval, the lipoprotein fraction contained particles with distinct metabolic properties with approximately 40–60% in normal subjects having a rapid fractional catabolic rate (FCR) of about 0.5 pools/d while the remainder is catabolised more slowly at about 0.2 pools/d [5]. In a series of investigations (summarised in [6]) we have provided evidence that the metabolic properties of LDL are linked to the nature of the VLDL precursor, i.e., the fate of a particle depends on its pedigree. Furthermore, the atherogenicity of LDL is likely to vary between subfractions because of their differing residence times in the circulation and susceptibility to oxidation [7]. The size of particle secreted from the liver appeared to be a major factor in determining the extent to which VLDL is converted to LDL and the size of the precursor seemed also to influence properties of the LDL product [6]. The following describes what is known about factors regulating the size and composition of VLDL released from the liver and its metabolic fate.

VLDL subfraction production in normals

Examination of the concentration of VLDL subfractions in normal subjects revealed that as plasma triglyceride rose from 0.5 to 2.5 mmol/l the concentra-

---

Address for correspondence: Prof Chris J. Packard, Department of Pathological Biochemistry, Glasgow Royal Infirmary University NHS Trust, 4th Floor Queen Elizabeth Building, Glasgow G31 2ER, UK. Tel.: +44-141-211-4979 or 4322. Fax: +44-141-553-2558.
E-mail: chrispackard@compuserve.com

tion of large VLDL (VLDL$_1$, S$_f$ 60–400) increased from 30 to 300 mg/dl while that of small VLDL (VLDL$_2$, S$_f$ 20–60) increased from 30 to 100 mg/dl [8]. Thus, across the normal range, the VLDL$_1$:VLDL$_2$ ratio changed from 1:1 to 3:1. Kinetic studies of apoB metabolism have revealed that plasma triglyceride levels are regulated by three factors, the lipolysis rate of VLDL$_1$ and VLDL$_2$, the production rate of VLDL$_1$ and the rate of VLDL$_1$ direct catabolism (Packard, Demant and Shepherd, unpublished observation). As shown in Fig. 1 the presence of an elevated plasma triglyceride (i.e., high VLDL$_1$) has been linked to the appearance of small dense LDL (LDL-III in [2,8]; pattern B in [1]) and the accumulation of slowly metabolised LDL (pool β LDL [5,6]). In this model (described in more detail in [6]), VLDL$_1$ is the source of slowly metabolised LDL while rapidly cleared LDL appears in the circulation as a result of direct secretion from the liver or by the delipidation of IDL or VLDL$_2$. In normal subjects there is a strong positive correlation between the amount of directly secreted IDL/ LDL and the LDL FCR (r = 0.65, p = 0.001, unpublished observation) and a

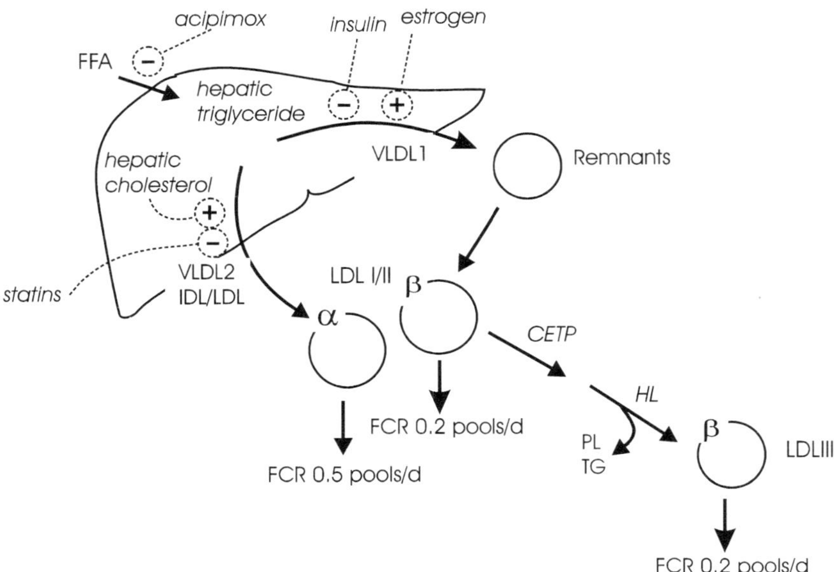

Fig. 1. In this metabolic scheme the content of potentially atherogenic lipoproteins in plasma — VLDL remnants, total LDL and small, dense LDL — is postulated to be influenced strongly by the nature of apolipoprotein B-containing lipoprotein released from the liver. The rate of production of VLDL$_1$ is governed by free fatty acid (FFA) availability and the regulatory actions of insulin and oestrogen. VLDL$_1$ once secreted, is dilipidated to remnants and eventually to a slowly metabolised LDL species (pool β). It is likely that this subfraction which has a long residence time in plasma is the substrate for the process of cholesteryl ester transfer protein (CETP) mediated lipid exchange and hepatic lipase action that gives rise to small, dense LDL (LDL-III). VLDL$_2$ secretion may be a function more of hepatic cholesterol (cholesteryl ester) than of triglyceride availability. The product of VLDL$_2$, IDL or LDL direct secretion appears to be LDL (pool) which is rapidly catabolised, probably by receptors.

negative correlation between the plasma triglyceride level and LDL FCR [5]. Thus, the nature of the lipoprotein released from the liver is of importance in determining the concentration of apoB-containing lipoproteins in plasma.

Regulation of VLDL subfraction secretion

Lipid availability in the liver is a major determinant of the rate of VLDL secretion. Cell culture studies have demonstrated that fatty acid supplementation of the medium promoted VLDL synthesis and diverted apoB from intracellular degradation towards lipoprotein production [9]. VLDL assembly appears to be a two-step process in which, at first, a small amount of lipid (triglyceride or cholesteryl ester) is added to the growing apoB polypeptide via the agency of MTP (microsomal triglyceride transfer protein) and a small nascent particle is formed in the lumen of the rough endoplasmic reticulum (ER) [10]. In the second, MTP-independent step bulk lipid is added to the nascent lipoprotein in the region of the rough ER/smooth ER junction [10]. HepG2 cells which secrete mainly IDL/LDL sized apoB-containing lipoproteins are thought to be unable to undertake this second step [11]. These cell culture findings provide a framework in which to understand human studies of the regulation of VLDL metabolism.

The complexity of the VLDL assembly process with multiple sites of addition of lipid allows for the observed independent regulation of $VLDL_1$ and $VLDL_2$ secretion. $VLDL_1$ was found to be secreted (in terms of its apoB content) at about 800 mg/d in normals [12,13] and was overproduced in hypertriglyceridaemic subjects (unpublished). Its synthesis has been shown to be influenced strongly by hormones especially insulin and oestrogen. Normal men when given an infusion of insulin exhibited a specific decrease in $VLDL_1$ production but no change in $VLDL_2$ secretion [14]. This effect was attributed partly due to the suppression of fatty acid (FFA) release from adipose tissue by the hormone. However, when insulin was given to diabetics it failed to inhibit $VLDL_1$ synthesis despite lowering the plasma FFA level by $>80\%$; a finding that indicated that the hormone might have a further, direct effect on $VLDL_1$ assembly in the liver [15]. Separate influences of insulin and FFA on VLDL production have also been documented by Lewis et al. [16]. In contrast, oestrogen has been shown to stimulate $VLDL_1$ synthesis while, again, not affecting $VLDL_2$ production [17]. This response helps explain the dramatic increase in VLDL concentration during pregnancy.

Acipimox is a nicotinic acid derivative that lowers plasma FFA profoundly. When given to normal men it was found, like insulin, to cause decreased $VLDL_1$ production but in this instance $VLDL_2$ synthesis increased, so overall, there was no change in apoB release from the liver (Malmström, Taskinen, Shepherd and Packard, unpublished observation). Thus, FFA availability is an important determinant of VLDL production but other regulatory mechanisms appear to be present in addition.

$VLDL_2$ production was increased in subjects with moderate hypercholesterolaemia and, indeed, contributed to the condition [12]. Further, across the normal range of $VLDL_2$ apoB synthesis rates (50–350 mg/d) there was a positive correlation between this parameter and LDL pool size (r = 0.55, p = 0.005). Little is known about the regulation of $VLDL_2$ secretion. It may be governed by cholesteryl ester rather than triglyceride availability [6] and may be the component of overall VLDL synthesis that is altered by statin therapy [18]. Diabetics appear to have low $VLDL_2$ production rates for reasons that are not yet clear [15].

Implications for CHD

Increased production of $VLDL_2$ by the liver contributes to the hypercholesterolaemia seen in the population at risk for CHD. The rate of release of this lipoprotein and LDL receptor activity (as reflected in the LDL-FCR) were found to be the most important determinants of the amount of LDL in the circulation. However, plasma triglyceride levels modify CHD risk at a given level of LDL. For example in a recent study in middle-aged men [19] a plasma triglyceride of 2.5 mmol/l was associated with a 2-fold higher CHD event rate than a triglyceride of 1.0 mmol/l for the same LDL cholesterol. Elevated rates of $VLDL_1$ production cause high plasma triglycerides and lead to the generation in the circulation of remnant lipoproteins (partial lipolysis products of VLDL) and slowly metabolised LDL (Fig. 1) from which small, dense LDL is likely to be formed. Large $VLDL_1$, remnants and small dense LDL are potential contributors to atherogenesis independent of the overall LDL concentration. Thus, optimal regulation of VLDL assembly in the liver is an important focus for attempts to reduce CHD risk. Drugs that control the availability of hepatic lipid pools for lipoprotein assembly or block the assembly process itself [20] are likely to have a profound effect on the spectrum of lipoprotein particles seen in the circulation and their potential atherogenicity.

Acknowledgements

The authors gratefully acknowledge the excellent secretarial assistance of Mrs Nancy Thomson in the preparation of this manuscript. The work performed in the authors' laboratory was supported by grants from the Medical Research council and the British Heart Foundation. The insulin/acipimox studies were part of a collaboration with Drs Taskinen and Malmström (Helsinki) and the normal studies were performed jointly with Dr Th. Demant (Munich).

References

1. Krauss RM, Blanche PJ. Detection and quantitation of LDL subfractions. Curr Opin Lipid 1992;3:377–383.
2. Griffin BA, Freeman DJ, Tait GW, Thomson J, Caslake MJ, Packard CJ, Shepherd J. Role of plasma triglyceride in the regulation of plasma low density lipoprotein (LDL) subfractions: relative contribution of small, dense LDL to coronary heart disease risk. Atherosclerosis 1994; 106:241–253.

3. Capell WH, Zambon A, Austin MA, Brunzell JD, Hokanson JE. Compositional differences of LDL particles in normal subjects with LDL subclass phenotype A and LDL subclass phenotype B. Arterioscler Thromb Vasc Biol 1996;16:1040—1046.

4. Nigon F, Lesnik P, Rouis M, Chapman MJ. Discrete subspecies of human low density lipoproteins are heterogeneous in their interaction with cellular LDL receptor. J Lipid Res 1991;32: 1741—1753.

5. Caslake MJ, Packard CJ, Series JJ, Yip B, Dagen MM, Shepherd J. Plasma triglyceride and low density lipoprotein metabolism. Eur J Clin Invest 1992;22:96—104.

6. Packard CJ, Shepherd J. Lipoprotein heterogeneity and apolipoprotein B metabolism. Arterioscler Thromb Vasc Biol 1997;(In press).

7. De Graaf J, Hak-Lemmers HLM, Hectors MPC, Demacker PNM, Hendriks JCM, Stalenhoef AFH. Enhanced susceptibility to in vitro oxidation of the dense low density lipoprotein subfraction in healthy subjects. Arteriosclerosis 1991;11:298—306.

8. Tan CE, Forster L, Caslake MJ, Bedford D, Watson TDG, McConnell M, Packard CJ, Shepherd J. Relations between plasma lipids and postheparin plasma lipases and VLDL and LDL subfractions in normolipemic men and women. Arterioscler Thromb Vasc Biol 1995;15: 1839—1848.

9. Lewis GF. Fatty acid regulation of very low density lipoprotein production. Curr Opin Lipid 1997;8:146—153.

10. Gordon DA, Jamil H, Gregg RE, Olofsson S-O, Boren J. Inhibition of the microsomal triglyceride transfer protein blocks, the first step of apolipoprotein β lipoprotein assembly but not the addition of bulk core lipids in the second step. J Biol Chem 1996;271:33047—33053.

11. Wu X, Shang A, Jiang H, Ginsberg HN. Low rates of apoB secretion from HepG2 cells result from reduced delivery of newly synthesized triglyceride to a 'secretion-coupled' pool. J Lipid Res 1996;37:1198—1206.

12. Gaw A, Packard CJ, Lindsay GN, Griffin BA, Caslake MJ, Lorimer AR, Shepherd J. Overproduction of small very low density lipoproteins (Sf 20—60) in moderate hypercholesterolemia: relationship between apolipoprotein B kinetics and plasma lipoproteins. J Lipid Res 1995;36: 158—171.

13. Demant T, Packard CJ, Demmelmair H, Stewart P, Bedynek A, Bedford D, Seidel D, Shepherd J. Sensitive methods to study human apolipoprotein B metabolism using stable isotope labelled amino acids. Am J Physiol 1996;270:E1022—E1036.

14. Malmström R, Packard CJ, Watson TDG, Rannikko S, Caslake M, Bedford D, Stewart P, Yki-Jarvinen H, Shepherd J, Taskinen M-R. Metabolic basis of hypotriglyceridemic effect of insulin in normal men. Arterioscler Thromb Vasc Biol 1997;17:1454—1464.

15. Malmström R, Packard CJ, Caslake M, Bedford D, Stewart P, Yki-Jarvinen H, Shepherd J, Taskinen M-R. Defective regulation of triglyceride metabolism by insulin in the liver in NIDDM. Diabetologia 1997;40:454—462.

16. Lewis GF, Uffelman KD, Szeto LW, Weller B, Steiner G. Interaction between free fatty acids and insulin in the acute control of very low density lipoprotein production in humans. J Clin Invest 1995;95:158—166.

17. Walsh BW, Schiff I, Rosner B, Greenberg L, Ravnikar V, Sacks FM. Effects of postmenopausal estrogen replacement on the concentrations and metabolism of plasma lipoproteins. N Engl J Med 1991;325:1196—1204.

18. Huff MW, Burnett JR. 3-hydroxy-3-methylglutaryl coenzyme A reductase inhibitors and apolipoprotein B secretion. Curr Opin Lipid 1997;8:138—145.

19. Shepherd J, Cobbe SM, Ford I, Isles CG, Lorimer AR, Macfarlane PW, McKillop JH, Packard CJ. Prevention of coronary heart disease with pravastatin in men with hypercholesterolemia. N Engl J Med 1995;333:1301—1307.

20. Jamil H, Gordon DA, Eustice DC, Brooks CM, Dickson JK Jr, Chen Y, Ricci B, Chu C, Harrity TW, Ciosek CP Jr et al. An inhibitor of the microsomal triglyceride transfer protein inhibits apoB secretion from HepG2 cells. Proc Natl Acad Sci USA 1996;93:11991—11995.

Effect of triglyceride-rich lipoproteins on cholesterol transport and atherosclerosis

Josef R. Patsch
University of Innsbruck, Department of Internal Medicine, Innsbruck, Austria

Abstract. The role of triglycerides (TG) in the process of atherosclerosis has been a matter of dispute. This uncertainty originates in most part in the fact that in multivariable epidemiological studies TG are often eliminated as independent risk factor by other lipoproteins, particularly HDL. The biology of the epidemiologically strong risk factors HDL and LDL is, however, controlled strongly by TG.

In this report, clinical examples demonstrating the effect of TG on LDL and HDL are presented. The crucial role of cholesterol ester transfer protein (CETP) in this process is emphasized also by the description of a novel mutation in the CETP gene. As our understanding of the mechanisms by which TG influence cholesterol transport in plasma increases, the important role of TG in the process of atherosclerosis should also be increasingly appreciated.

Keywords: cholesterol ester transfer protein, lipoprotein lipase, triglyceride intolerance, triglyceride supertolerance.

Triglycerides (TG) are transported in blood mainly by chylomicrons and very low density lipoproteins (VLDL), referred to collectively as TG-rich lipoproteins. Cholesterol is mainly transported by low-density lipoproteins (LDL) and high-density lipoproteins (HDL). Increased plasma levels of LDL have clearly been identified as a causal risk factor for atherosclerosis as evidenced by animal studies, epidemiologic observations and prospective trials using medications to lower LDL levels in plasma. As opposed to LDL, plasma concentrations of HDL have been demonstrated to display a continuous negative relationship with atherosclerosis [1].

While the cholesterol-carrying lipoproteins, i.e., LDL and HDL, have been widely accepted to hold strong — albeit opposite — associations with atherosclerosis, the levels of TG-rich lipoproteins are not generally accepted as such risk factors [2]. In recent years, a lipoprotein constellation characterized by the predominance of small dense LDL and the smaller denser subfraction of HDL, i.e., HDL_3, and increased levels of VLDL and IDL has been recognized as a very frequently encountered high-risk lipoprotein phenotype [3].

More recently, TG levels measured after the ingestion of a standardized fatty

---

Address for correspondence: Univ Prof Dr Josef R. Patsch, University of Innsbruck, Department of Internal Medicine, Anichstraße 35, 6020 Innsbruck, Austria. Tel.: +43-512-504-3250. Fax: +43-512-504-3317.

meal have also been shown to hold a risk factor role; when measured in the most appropriate situation, i.e., in the postprandial rather than the postabsorptive state, TGs are a risk factor independent of other lipoproteins, particularly HDL [4]. Other studies have also demonstrated that the magnitude of postprandial lipemia constitutes a risk factor for atherosclerosis [5].

The preponderance of small dense LDL in the entire LDL particle spectrum are considered widely as an independent risk factor for atherosclerosis, and are virtually always the result of high triglyceride levels in plasma [6]. Also, HDL cholesterol shows a strong inverse association with triglyceride levels in plasma, not only in the fasting state [7], but particularly in the postprandial state [8]. All these observations strongly suggest that the above-mentioned lipoprotein characteristics, identified more recently as being atherogenic, are the consequence of impaired TG metabolism due either to overproduction or impaired catabolism of TG-rich lipoproteins or both [9].

Lipoprotein lipase (LPL) is the key enzyme involved in the first catabolic step of TG-rich lipoproteins in plasma. Numerous mutations at the LPL gene locus have been described which impair the function of the enzyme at the levels of synthesis, endothelial attachment or catalytic competence [9]. An example for a point mutation is the single-base transition from guanine to adenine at cDNA position 818 in codon188 which substitutes glutamic acid for glycine and results in the synthesis and secretion of a catalytically inactive enzyme [10]. Inheritance of two defective alleles of the LPL gene causes the inability to catabolize TG-rich lipoproteins, leading to the chylomicronemia syndrome characterized by vast TG elevation, fasting hyperchylomicronemia, lipid deposition in dermal, hepatic and splenic macrophages and bouts of pancreatitis [11]. Carriage of only one defective LPL allele, on the contrary, is not heralded by gross biochemical or clinical abnormalities such as fasting chylomicronemia or abdominal pain. Rather, heterozygous carriers have about half-normal LPL activities which may suffice to keep fasting plasma TG concentrations within normal limits. However, when stress is placed on the plasma lipid transport system, for instance, by obesity, insulin resistance or the use of lipid-raising agents, moderate fasting hypertriglyceridemia may ensue [12].

In one study, even in the absence of such secondary factors, it was demonstrated that a trivial challenge like postprandial lipemia can entirely uncover heterozygous carriage of a defective LPL allele [13]. In two Austrian families, the gene defect was clearly manifested in the postprandial state with an increased magnitude of postprandial lipemia. It was proposed to call this metabolic handicap "impaired TG-tolerance" in order to distinguish it from fasting hypertriglyceridemia and to emphasize that a tolerance test is required for diagnosis. The carriers of the defective allele, uncovered only by augmented postprandial lipemia, showed also typical marks of all lipoprotein classes in fasting plasma; pronounced postprandial lipemia was associated with TG-enriched HDL, low HDL_2 cholesterol, cholesterol-enriched VLDL and intermediate density lipoproteins (IDL), high IDL levels, and small dense LDL. All these stigmata are typical for the atherogenic lipoprotein constellation referred to above.

Because they are all components of a well-defined impairment of TG metabolism, Miesenboeck et al. proposed to call this constellation "the syndrome of TG intolerance" [13]. "TG-intolerance" and the described "syndrome of TG-intolerance" caused by a mutation in the LPL gene clearly demonstrate the importance of TG-rich lipoproteins on cholesterol transport. The lipoprotein distribution characterized by high IDL levels, small dense LDL and low HDL cholesterol can be expected to put heterozygous carriers at an increased risk for atherosclerosis. Future clinical studies, however, are necessary to validate this notion. TG-intolerance and its associated syndrome can probably be caused by several molecular defects other than that in the LPL gene.

If TG-intolerance causes the preponderance of small dense LDL and HDL_3 with low HDL cholesterol, one would expect that a situation of "TG-supertolerance" where TG-rich lipoproteins in plasma are handled very effectively, would cause the preponderance of large buoyant LDL and of large HDL_2 and high HDL cholesterol. Such a situation was indeed described [14,15]. Eleven post-type I diabetic pancreas-kidney transplant recipients (PKT-R) were studied and compared with 11 nondiabetic kidney transplant recipients (KT-R) as controls for the effects of immunosuppressive medication and with 11 healthy control subjects, all matched by age, sex and body mass index. HDL cholesterol was highest in the PKT-R, postprandial lipemia was lowest and LPL activity was highest (average 32 and 154%, respectively, of the mean of the controls). Also, HDL_2 levels were highest and large buoyant LDL were predominant in PKT-R. This distribution of cholesterol-rich lipoproteins can be explained readily by the ability to clear chylomicron-TG very effectively. The low postprandial lipemia found in PKT-R was explained by the high LPL activity in PKT-R, which in turn could be explained by the high insulin level (in the absence of insulin resistance) due to the pancreas transplantation procedure used with systemic venous drainage of the graft. Thus, "TG-supertolerance" as evidenced by very low postprandial lipemia was accompanied by the expected lipoprotein stigmata constituting a phenotype of "TG-supertolerance".

A paradoxical situation where TG-tolerance is not associated with the expected syndrome has also been observed recently (Ritsch et al., Arterioscl Thromb Vasc Biol 1997;(In press)). A woman presented with extremely high HDL cholesterol and, upon lipoprotein analysis exhibited extremely high levels of HDL_2 and even larger HDL populations. From these vastly elevated HDL_2 levels one would expect TG tolerance to be excellent. However, the patient did not exhibit the expected very low postprandial lipemia but, instead, a very pronounced one. This mismatch between the magnitude of postprandial lipemia and HDL cholesterol was explained by a deficiency of cholesteryl ester transfer protein (CETP). CETP activity was less than 5% and CETP mass was less than 2% of that of a normolipidemic plasma pool. The CETP-cDNA of the patient exhibited a mutation (T → G) turning codon 57 (TAT) of exon 2 into a stop codon (TAG) and abolishing an Xcml restriction site. Digestion of directly amplified CETP cDNA from the patient with Xcml indicated the exclusive presence of CETP cDNA containing the mutation. Analysis of the corresponding region of the CETP gene indicated the patient to be heterozygous for the nonsense mutation at codon 57, a finding which can only be explained by the presence of a null allele in addition to the allele with the nonsense mutation. The combination of TG intolerance of uncertain cause together with CETP-deficiency due to a novel mutation produced the paradoxical constellation — high levels of HDL cholesterol (172 mg/dl) associated with a high postprandial lipemia of 1,460 mg triglycerides/dl.8 h — and provided further insight into the role of CETP as mediator between the pools of TG and cholesteryl esters in plasma. This study demonstrated that the effect of TG-rich lipoproteins on cholesterol-carrying lipoproteins is mediated by CETP.

The levels of CETP in plasma vary highly among individuals and are affected by diet, exercise and hormones such as insulin and estrogen [16]. However, in normolipidemic plasma, the transfer of cholesteryl esters from HDL and LDL into TG-rich lipoproteins appears not to be so much a function of CETP levels, but rather of TG levels. Up to a TG concentration of roughly 270 mg/dl the cholesteryl ester enrichment of TG-rich lipoproteins/per unit of time is a linear function of its own concentration and is independent of the concentration of the cholesteryl ester donor particles (LDL and HDL) and of CETP activity [17]. Only at high TG levels, CETP activity becomes rate-limiting, and cholesteryl ester transfer to TG-rich lipoproteins per unit of time reaches a plateau with respect to TG-concentration [17]. This observation is in keeping with a report where high-normal CETP levels were associated with low HDL cholesterol only in hypertriglyceridemic, but not in normotriglyceridemic subjects [18]. Therefore, in mild to moderate fasting and postprandial hypertriglyceridemia, TG concentration appears to be the determining factor for the loss of cholesterol from HDL and LDL to TG-rich lipoprotein [19].

The discussed data from our laboratory, together with those of many other investigators, strongly suggest that TGs hold an important role for cholesterol transport in plasma and for atherosclerosis. The mechanisms by which TG influence cholesterol transport are becoming increasingly understood which should allow prudent strategies to counteract the detrimental effects of impaired TG metabolism in the process of atherosclerosis.

Acknowledgements

The work presented was supported in part by S 07106-MED and by P 11693 MED of the Austrian Fond zur Förderung der Wissenschaftlichen Forschung.

References

1. Castelli WP, Doyle JT, Gordon T, Hames CG, Hjortland MC, Hulley SB, Kagan A, Zukel WJ. HDL-cholesterol and other lipids in coronary heart disease. The cooperative lipoprotein pheno-

typing study. Circulation 1997;55:767—772.
2. Austin ME. Plasma triglyceride and coronary heart disease. Arterioscler Thromb 1991;11: 2—14.
3. Austin MA, King MC, Vranizan KM, Krauss RM. Atherogenic lipoprotein phenotype: a proposed genetic marker for coronary heart disease risk. Circulation 1990;82:495—506.
4. Patsch JR, Miesenboeck G, Hopferwieser T, Muehlberger V, Knapp E, Dunn JK, Gotto AM, Patsch W. Relation of tryglyceride metabolism and coronary artery disease, studies in the postprandial state. Arterioscler Thromb 1992;12:1336—1345.
5. Groot PHE, van Stiphout WAHJ, Krauss XH, Jansen H, van Tol A, van Ramhorst E, Chin-On S, Cresswell SR, Havekes L. Postprandial lipoprotein metabolism in normolipidemic men with and without coronary artery disease. Arterioscler Thromb 1991;11:653—552.
6. McKeone BJ, Patsch JR, Pownall HJ. Plasma trigliycerides determine low density lipoprotein composition, physical properties, and cell-specific binding in cultured cells. J Clin Invest 1993;91:1926—1933.
7. Nikkilä EA, Tskinen M-R, Sane T. Plasma high-density lipoprotein concentration and subfraction distribution in relation to triglyceride metabolism. Am Heart J 1987;113:543—548.
8. Patsch JR, Karlin JB, Scott LW, Smith LC, Gotto AM Jr. Inverse relationship between blood levels of high density lipoprotein$_2$ and magnitude of postprandial lipemia. Proc Natl Acad Sci USA 1983;80:1449—1453.
9. Lalouel J-M, Wilson DE, Iverius PH. Lipoprotein lipase and hepatic triglyceride lipase: molecular and genetic aspects. Curr Opin Lipid 1992;3:86—95.
10. Paulweber B, Wiebusch H, Miesenboeck G, Funke H, Assmann G, Hoelzl B, Sippl MJ, Friedl W, Patsch JR, Sandhofer F. Molecular basis of lipoprotein lipase deficency in two Austrian families with type I hyperlipoproteinemia. Atherosclerosis 1991;86:239—250.
11. Brunzell JD. Familial lipoprotein lipase deficency and other causes of the chylomicronemia syndrome. In: Scriver C, Beaudet A, Sly W, Valle D (eds) The Metabolic Basis of Inherited Disease. New York: McGraw-Hill Book Co., 1989;1165—1180.
12. Sprecher DL, Knauer SL, Black DM, Kaplan LA, Akeson AA, Dusing M, Latter D, Stein EA, Rymaszewski M, Wiginton DA. Chylomicron — retinyl palamitate clearance in type I hyperlipidemic families. J Clin Invest 1991;88:985—994.
13. Miesenboeck G, Hoelzl B, Foeger B, Brandstaetter E, Paulweber B, Sandhofer F, Patsch JR. Heterozygous lipoprotein lipase deficiency due to a missense mutation as the cause of impaired triglyceride tolerance with multiple lipoprotein abnormalities. J Clin Invest 1993;91:448—455.
14. Foeger B, Koenigsrainer A, Palos G, Brandstaetter E, Ritsch A, Koenig P, Miesenboeck G, Lechleitner M, Margreiter R, Patsch JR. Effect of pancreas transplantation on lipoprotein lipase, postprandial lipemia, and HDL cholesterol. Transplantation 1994;58:899—904.
15. Foeger B, Koenigsrainer A, Palos G, Ritsch A, Tröbinger G, Menzel HJ, Lechleitner M, Doblinger A, Koenig P, Utermann G, Margreiter R, Patsch JR. Effects of pancreas transplantation on distribution and composition of plasma lipoproteins. Metabolism 1996;45:856—861.
16. Tall AR. Plasma lipid transfer proteins. J Lipid Res 1986;27:361—367.
17. Mann CJ, Yen FT, Grant AM, Bihain BE. Mechanism of plasma cholesterol ester transfer in hypergtriglyceridemia. J Clin Invest 1991;88:2059—2066.
18. Foeger B, Ritsch A, Doblinger A, Wessels H, Patsch JR. Relationship of plasma cholesterol ester transfer protein to HDL cholesterol, studies in normotriglyceridemia and moderate hypertriglyceridemia. Arterioscler Thromb Vasc Biol 1996;16:1430—1436.
19. Miesenboeck G, Patsch JR. Postprandial hyperlipidemia: the search for the atherogenic lipoprotein. Curr Opin Lipid 1992;3:196—201.

Atherosclerosis XI.
B. Jacotot, D. Mathé and J.-C. Fruchart, editors.

Genetics of elevated apolipoprotein-B and dense LDL in familial combined hyperlipidemia

S.J.H. Bredie[1], L.A. Kiemeney[2], A.F.J. de Haan[3], P.N.M. Demacker[1] and A.F.H. Stalenhoef[1]

Departments of [1]Internal Medicine, [2]Epidemiology and [3]Medical Statistics, University Hospital Nijmegen, The Netherlands

Abstract. *Background.* Familial combined hyperlipidemia (FCH) is characterized by elevations of plasma cholesterol and/or triglycerides in first-degree relatives and an elevation of apolipoprotein-B (apoB). A predominance of small dense atherogenic low-density lipoprotein (LDL) particles is frequently observed. Previously, we have demonstrated a major recessive locus control of dense LDL inheritance and a codominant mechanism involved in the aggregation of elevated apoB levels in 40 FCH families. To establish whether distinct genetic mechanisms express both traits, we now evaluated the inheritance of small dense LDL after correction for the predicted genetic influence of a putative apoB locus.

Methods and Results. By means of a segregation analysis of apoB, individual apoB genotypes could be assigned to 85% of all individuals. LDL subfraction profiles expressed by a continuous variable K differed significantly between apoB genotypes, supporting the metabolic relation between apoB and LDL subfraction profile. Subsequently, LDL subfraction profiles were adjusted for predicted apoB influence by subtracting the apoB genotype specific mean K value from the individual K values. These apoB genotype specific mean K values were obtained from those individuals with their apoB genotype probability $\geq 70\%$. Segregation analysis of residual LDL subfraction profiles provided substantial evidence for a major locus inheritance pattern.

Conclusion. Two distinct genetic mechanisms influence the appearance of elevated plasma apoB and the predominance of dense LDL in these FCH families.

Keywords: atherosclerosis, complex segregation analysis, LDL subfractions.

Introduction

Familial combined hyperlipidemia (FCH) is characterized by elevations of the total plasma cholesterol concentration and/or the plasma triglyceride concentration in first-degree relatives [1,2]. Other characteristics of the disorder are an elevated plasma apolipoprotein-B100 (apoB) concentration and a preponderance of small dense low-density lipoprotein (LDL) particles [2,3]. Originally, FCH was thought to be inherited as a homogeneous single gene disorder with a major effect on triglyceride levels and a secondary effect on plasma cholesterol levels [1]. Although evidence has been provided recently for such a major locus effect

---

Address for correspondence: Prof Dr A.F.H. Stalenhoef MD, Department of Medicine, Division of General Internal Medicine, University Hospital Nijmegen, P.O. Box 9101, 6500 HB Nijmegen, The Netherlands. Tel.: +31-24-3614782. Fax: +31-24-3541734.

802

on triglyceride levels, it was considered that a number of different loci may affect the expression of the FCH phenotype and that the major genes involved still have to be identified [4]. Using segregation analysis, the variation in age- and sex-adjusted apoB levels has been ascribed to a yet unmapped codominant mendelian locus [5,6]. This locus was later found to be predictive of FCH [7,8]. It is noteworthy that elevated plasma apoB levels, corresponding with elevated VLDL and/or LDL levels in FCH, have been metabolically associated with the predominance of small dense LDL [9−11].

Also, the distribution of small dense LDL subfraction profiles appears to have a genetic basis in FCH [3,12]. Because the mechanisms reported for the inheritance of plasma apoB levels were different from those reported for the inheritance of LDL subfraction profiles in FCH, one may wonder whether the presumed inheritance of LDL subfractions is actually caused by the segregation of a trait responsible for elevated plasma apoB concentrations. In order to investigate whether distinct genetic mechanisms underlie the familial aggregation of elevated plasma apoB levels and the predominance of dense LDL subfraction profiles observed in FCH, we conducted a segregation analysis of LDL subfraction profiles adjusted for the inferred genotypic influence of a putative apoB locus.

Materials and Methods

Study population

The FCH pedigrees considered here have been studied for inheritance of LDL subfraction profiles [13] and plasma apoB levels [14]. The families were ascertained through probands exhibiting a combined hyperlipidemia with both plasma cholesterol and triglyceride concentrations above the 90th percentile, adjusted for age and gender.

Low-density lipoprotein subfractionation

LDL subfractions were detected by single spin density gradient ultracentrifugation, according to a method described in detail elsewhere [15]. Up to five LDL subfractions could be distinguished concentrated in the following density ranges: LDL1 (1.030−1.033 g/ml), LDL2 (1.033−1.040 g/ml), LDL3 (1.040−1.045 g/ml), LDL4 (1.045−1.049 g/ml), and LDL5 (1.049−1.054 g/ml). The mean peak heights (h1−h5) of the LDL subfractions (LDL1−LDL5) on densitometric scans were used to calculate the variable K as a continuous variable, that best describes each individual LDL subfraction pattern [16]. A negative value ($-1 < K < 0$) reflects a dense subfraction profile, whereas a complete buoyant profile reveals a positive K value ($0 \leqslant K < 1$) [16].

Segregation analyses

Previous segregation analyses on this data set demonstrated that both the distribution of dense LDL subfraction profiles [12] and the aggregation of elevated plasma apoB levels [17] appeared to have a genetic basis in these FCH families. The segregation of dense LDL subfraction profiles was most consistent with an autosomal recessive locus with a population frequency of 0.42 [12]. In a separate segregation analysis of plasma apoB, the apoB concentrations were adjusted by linear regression for the influence of age, gender, BMI, smoking habits, and alcohol intake prior to the segregation analysis. Subsequently, a codominant model of inheritance plus family correlations and spouse correlation best explained the segregation of adjusted plasma apoB levels [17].

In the present analysis, each individual was classified into their most probable genotype at the apoB locus (i.e., AA, AB, or BB) by segregation analysis of plasma apoB levels. The mean K value of those individuals with one of the apoB genotype probabilities $\geqslant 70\%$ were used to condition the K values for the predicted influence of apoB genotypes. By this arbitrary criterium [18], 53 individuals were assigned to represent apoB genotype AA, 144 to apoB genotype AB and 95 to apoB genotype BB (n = 292 assigned, representing 47% of all subjects), with mean adjusted K values of 0.41, -0.46 and -1.69, respectively. Subsequently, the K values of all 623 subjects were conditioned by subtracting these apoB genotype specific mean K values of the individual K values. For subjects with prob(AA) = prob(AB) $(0.41-0.46)/2$ was subtracted from their K value, and for those with prob(AB) = prob(BB) $(-0.46-1.69)/2$ was subtracted. For those with missing plasma apoB values, $(0.41-0.46-1.69)/3$ was subtracted from the K values. Finally, the residual K values were used in the present segregation analysis.

Results

Sample

566 family members (i.e., 80 probands (40 + 40 additional hyperlipidemic relatives to correct for ascertainment bias) and 486 relatives) and 121 spouses from 40 FCH kindreds (consisting of two to four generations with pedigree size ranges from seven to 104 family members, including spouses) participated. The present segregation analysis involved data of 623 subjects (299 men and 324 women). The mean lipid, (apo)lipoprotein levels and K values of the 80 probands, the FCH relatives and the spouses, adjusted for age, gender, BMI, and smoking habits are presented in Table 1. Due to the inclusion criteria, probands exhibited higher plasma lipid and lipoprotein levels than relatives and spouses. Also, the plasma apoB concentration was higher and the K value was more negative in the probands compared with relatives and spouses. FCH relatives differed significantly from spouses on all parameters except for the LDL cholesterol concentration.

804

Table 1. Mean (±SD) adjusted[a] lipid and (apo)lipoprotein concentrations and K values in probands, FCH relatives and spouses of 40 FCH families.

	Probands	FCH relatives	Spouses
Number	80	480	102
Age (years)	54.6 ± 11.4	38.9 ± 16.8	50.0 ± 11.9[d]
BMI (kg/m^2)	26.7 ± 3.8	24.2 ± 3.7	25.5 ± 3.5[d]
Total plasma cholesterol[b]	6.43 ± 1.40	5.84 ± 1.07	5.58 ± 1.13[d]
Triglycerides[b]	2.58 ± 2.54	1.86 ± 1.47	1.18 ± 0.80[d]
VLDL cholesterol[b]	1.16 ± 1.32	0.77 ± 0.67	0.45 ± 0.41[d]
VLDL triglycerides[b]	1.85 ± 2.19	1.23 ± 1.21	0.67 ± 0.67[d]
HDL cholesterol[b]	1.12 ± 0.27	1.18 ± 0.29	1.31 ± 0.33[d]
LDL cholesterol[b]	4.16 ± 1.15	3.85 ± 0.98	3.91 ± 0.99
Apolipoprotein-B[c]	157.3 ± 42.9	133.4 ± 29.5	117.4 ± 27.1[d]
K value	− 0.32 ± 0.29	− 0.24 ± 0.26	− 0.09 ± 0.23[d]

[a]Values, except for age and BMI, were adjusted for the influence of age, gender, body mass index and smoking habits; [b]in mmol/l; [c]in mg/dl; [d]significant difference between FCH relatives and spouses.

ApoB genotype assignment and effects on lipids, (apo)lipoproteins and K values

Of all 662 individuals (original 687 individuals minus 25 with missing data for apoB standardization) used in the segregation analysis of plasma apoB, one putative apoB genotype was more likely than the other two in 524 subjects (79%), whereas in 37 subjects (6%) two genotypes were equally likely. 101 subjects (15%) could not be classified. In FCH probands and FCH relatives the "high" apoB level genotype BB and the "intermediate" apoB level genotype AB were more frequently assigned compared with spouses, whereas the "low" apoB level genotype AA was more frequently assigned to spouses. Table 2 presents the lipids,

Table 2. Mean (±SD) lipids, (apo)lipoproteins and K value by apoB level genotypes (i.e., AA, AB, or BB) as designated by segregation analysis.

	ApoB AA genotype	ApoB AB genotype	ApoB BB genotype
Number	130	276	118
Age (years)	44.6 ± 16.0	40.6 ± 17.4	45.2 ± 15.3[c]
BMI (kg/m^2)	24.9 ± 4.3	24.3 ± 3.7	24.8 ± 3.0
Total plasma cholesterol[a]	5.04 ± 1.00	5.67 ± 1.14	7.17 ± 1.21[d]
Triglycerides[a]	1.08 ± 0.51	1.51 ± 1.29	2.95 ± 2.05[d]
VLDL cholesterol[a]	0.35 ± 0.21	0.57 ± 0.54	1.38 ± 1.20[d]
VLDL triglycerides[a]	0.59 ± 0.40	0.96 ± 1.16	2.02 ± 1.71[d]
HDL cholesterol[a]	1.33 ± 0.35	1.21 ± 0.36	1.05 ± 0.28[d]
LDL cholesterol[a]	3.36 ± 0.95	3.90 ± 1.06	4.73 ± 1.16[d]
Apolipoprotein-B[b]	106.1 ± 24.5	127.1 ± 30.0	180.8 ± 34.7[d]
K value	− 0.05 ± 0.21	− 0.20 ± 0.29	− 0.46 ± 0.24[d]

[a]In mmol/l; [b]in mg/dl; [c]significantly different from apoB AB genotype; [d]significantly different from apoB AA and AB genotype.

(apo)lipoproteins and K value related to each apoB genotype. Age and BMI did not show significant differences between genotypes. Compared with the apoB AA genotype, the apoB BB genotype corresponded with the highest plasma cholesterol, triglyceride, VLDL cholesterol, VLDL triglyceride and LDL cholesterol levels, and the lowest HDL cholesterol level. Interestingly, the apoB BB genotype was also significantly associated with the lowest K value, representing more dense LDL subfraction profiles. The apoB AB genotype represented values for the parameters in between apoB AA and BB genotypes. Thus, the apoB BB genotype corresponded with a FCH lipid phenotype with elevated plasma lipids and lipoproteins, a decreased HDL cholesterol and a dense LDL subfraction profile. In the entire FCH population without spouses, the variability in crude plasma apoB concentration could account for 42% of the variability in LDL subfraction profiles, revealing a strong correlation between crude values for both variables (Spearman's correlation r = − 0.65). After adjustment for "environmental" influences of both apoB concentrations and K values, this correlation was still significant (r = − 0.47). However, after adjustment of standardized K values for the predicted influence of apoB genotype, the correlation was completely disappeared (Spearman's correlation r = − 0.08). This implicates that LDL subfraction profiles were adequately corrected for inferred genetical influence of plasma apoB concentration.

Segregation of LDL subfraction profiles corrected for apoB genotype

Segregation analysis was carried out using the standardized variable K [12] adjusted for the genetic influence of apoB genotype. Parameter estimates for 13 different models of inheritance were obtained (data not shown). In a sporadic or unimodal model, the spouse, parent-offspring, and sibling correlations were examined to determine multifactorial or polygenic influences (models 1 to 4). The spouse correlation was found to be insignificant and was therefore fixed at 0 in all subsequent models. The parent-offspring and sibling correlations were found to be equal. Therefore, all subsequent models assumed a single correlation among first-degree relatives. The sporadic models (models 1 to 4) and the nongenetic transmission models (models 11 and 12) fitted the data significantly worse than the unrestricted general model 13. This general model, with all variables unrestricted, provided evidence for major locus inheritance of parameter K, because transmission parameters were roughly in accordance with values expected under Mendelian transmission. In order to examine the mode of inheritance, dominant models (models 5 and 6), recessive models (models 7 and 8), and codominant models (models 9 and 10) were fitted by fixing the transmission parameters at their Mendelian expectations. None of the Mendelian models could be rejected. Of the Mendelian models, those including the residual correlations provided the best fit of the data. The residual correlation was used to estimate the polygenic component and was found to be 13% in the dominant model, 15% in the recessive model and 16% in the codominant model. Based on these results the Mendelian models (model 6, 8 and 10) provided the most parsimonious fit of the data, but discrimination between these models appeared to be impossible.

Discussion

Based on data of these FCH families, both the aggregation of elevated apoB levels and the distribution of dense LDL subfraction profiles were shown to have a genetic basis in this lipid disorder. Because inheritance of the traits was investigated for each trait separately, the observed segregation of the individual traits may also have been caused by one genotype controlling both phenotypes. However, the segregation of dense LDL subfraction profiles corrected for putative apoB genotypes assigned by segregation analysis, still provided evidence for the presence of a Mendelian mechanism which exclusively controls the distribution of dense LDL subfractions profiles. Thus, it is likely that the presence of elevated plasma apoB levels and the predominance of small dense LDL are controlled by distinct genetic mechanisms in FCH.

Recently, we have demonstrated that a single major recessive locus controls the predominance of dense LDL subfraction profiles in these FCH families [12]. This was consistent with the findings of Austin et al. [3]. In contrast to an approach using a dichotomous classification of LDL subfraction pattern, or detection of the LDL peak particle diameter as performed by others [3], the great interindividual variation in the LDL subfraction profiles would best be described by the continuous variable K. This K value is characterized by the relative contribution of all detected LDL subfractions to the total LDL subfraction profile [12,16]. Compared with the general population, our analysis revealed a twice as high gene frequency in FCH families [12,16]. Other reports support that also the physical and chemical properties of LDL particles in subjects with FCH differ from those of normolipidemic controls [19]. Many of these properties appeared to be independent of plasma triglyceride concentrations [20], supporting the specificity of dense LDL for this common lipid disorder.

The observed codominant Mendelian model of inheritance explaining the familial cluster of elevated plasma apoB levels in these FCH families [17] was reported previously in two other studies on FCH families [7,8]. Also in families of patients with cardiovascular disease, which did not completely meet the FCH criteria, a codominant major locus effect was observed [5,21]. Therefore, the genetic model for elevated plasma apoB level aggregation could explain both the genetic influence on plasma lipids and the increased incidence of cardiovascular disease in FCH families. So far, linkage analyses were not able to map a gene responsible for elevated apoB levels [22–24], although some markers showed some association [25]. Interestingly, also linkage between markers of the apoB gene and the LDL subclass phenotype B could be excluded [13].

Final proof of the major genes involved must come from the identification of susceptibility loci. Since the apoB locus itself could be excluded, other candidate genes involved in apoB overproduction have to be investigated. Possibly, defects preceding apoB secretion which may result in increased substrate delivery to hepatic apoB synthesizing cells [14], or defects in regulatory components of apoB synthesis such as the microsomal triglyceride transfer protein [26] can be considered. As far as plasma dense LDL is concerned, a locus near the LDL receptor on chromosome 19 has been linked to a predominance of these particles in plasma of normolipidemic subjects [27]. This has been confirmed by a recent study which indicated a multilocus determination of dense LDL, comprising the LDL receptor locus as well, but also the apoAI-CIII-AIV gene cluster, the cholesteryl ester transfer protein locus, and the manganese superoxide dismutase locus [28]. The authors suggested that different genetically determined metabolic mechanisms may give rise to dense LDL particles, without finding evidence for genetic interaction with apoB production. Further studies have to establish these relations in hyperlipidemic families to better understand the atherogenic risk.

References

1. Goldstein JL, Schrott HG, Hazzard WR, Bierman EL, Motulsky AG. Hyperlipidemia in coronary heart disease. II. Genetic analysis of lipid levels in 176 families and delineation of a new inherited disorder, combined hyperlipidemia. J Clin Invest 1973;52:1544–1568.
2. Grundy SM, Chait A, Brunzell JD. Familial combined hyperlipidemia workshop. Arteriosclerosis 1987;7(2):203–207.
3. Austin MA, Brunzell JD, Fitch WL, Krauss RM. Inheritance of low density lipoprotein subclass patterns in familial combined hyperlipidemia. Arteriosclerosis 1990;10:520–530.
4. Cullen P, Farren B, Scott J, Farrall M. Complex segregation analysis provides evidence for a major gene acting on serum triglyceride levels in 55 British families with familial combined hyperlipidemia. Arterioscler Thromb 1994;14:1233–1249.
5. Hasstedt SJ, Wu L, Williams RR. Major locus inheritance of apolipoprotein B in Utah pedigrees. Genet Epidemiol 1987;4:67–76.
6. Pairitz G, Davignon J, Mailloux H, Sing CF. Sources of interindividual variation in the quantitative levels of apolipoprotein B in pedigrees ascertained through a lipid clinic. Am J Hum Genet 1988;43:311–321.
7. Jarvik GP, Beaty TH, Gallagher PR, Coates PM, Cortner JA. Genotype at a major locus with large effects on apolipoprotein B levels predicts familial combined hyperlipidemia. Genet Epidemiol 1993;10:257–270.
8. Jarvik GP, Brunzell JD, Austin MA, Krauss RM, Motulsky AG, Wijsman E. Genetic predictors of FCHL in four large pedigrees. Influence of ApoB level major locus predicted genotype and LDL subclass phenotype. Arterioscler Thromb 1994;14:1687–1694.
9. Deckelbaum RJ, Granot E, Oschry Y, Rose L, Eisenberg S. Plasma triglyceride determines structure-composition in low and high density lipoproteins. Arteriosclerosis 1984;4:225–231.
10. de Graaf J, Hendriks JCM, Demacker PNM, Stalenhoef AFH. Identification of multiple dense LDL subfractions with enhanced susceptibility to in vitro oxidation among hypertriglyceridemic subjects. Normalization after clofibrate treatment. Arterioscler Thromb 1993;13:712–719.
11. Krauss RM. Heterogeneity of plasma low-density lipoproteins and atherosclerosis risk. Curr Opin Lipid 1994;5:339–349.
12. Bredie SJH, Kiemeney LA, De Haan AFJ, Demacker PNM, Stalenhoef AFH. Inherited susceptibility determines the distribution of dense low density lipoprotein subfraction profiles in familial combined hyperlipidemia. Am J Hum Genet 1996;58:812–822.
13. Austin MA, Wijsman E, Guo SW, Krauss RM, Brunzell JD, Deeb S. Lack of evidence for link-

age between low-density lipoprotein subclass phenotypes and the apolipoprotein B locus in familial combined hyperlipidemia. Genet Epidemiol 1991;8:287—297.

14. Sniderman AD, Cianflone KM. Substrate delivery as a determinant of hepatic apoB secretion. Arterioscler Thromb 1993;13:629—636.

15. Swinkels DW, Demacker PNM, Hendriks JCM, van 't Laar A. Low density lipoprotein subfractions and relationship to other risk factors for coronary artery disease in healthy individuals. Arteriosclerosis 1989;9:604—613.

16. de Graaf J, Swinkels DW, De Haan AFJ, Demacker PNM, Stalenhoef AFH. Both inherited susceptibility and environmental exposure determine the low density lipoprotein subfraction pattern distribution in healthy Dutch families. Am J Hum Genet 1992;51:1295—1310.

17. Bredie SJH, van Drongelen J, Kiemeney LA, Demacker PNM, Beaty TH, Stalenhoef AFH. Segregation analysis of plasma apolipoprotein-B levels in familial combined hyperlipidemia. Arterioscler Thromb Vasc Biol 1997;17:834—840.

18. Beaty TH, Prenger VL, Virgil DG, Lewis B, Kwiterovich PO, Bachorik PS. A genetic model for control of hypertriglyceridemia and apolipoprotein B levels in the Johns Hopkins colony of St. Thomas Hospital rabbits. Genetics 1992;132:1095—1104.

19. Hokanson JE, Krauss RM, Albers JJ, Austin MA, Brunzell JD. LDL physical and chemical properties in familial combined hyperlipidemia. Arterioscler Thromb Vasc Biol 1995;15: 452—459.

20. Hokanson JE, Austin MA, Zambon A, Brunzell JD. Plasma triglyceride and LDL heterogeneity in familial combined hyperlipidemia. Arterioscler Thromb 1993;13:427—434.

21. Amos CI, Elston RC, Srinivasan SR, Wilson AF, Cresanta JL, Ward LJ, Berenson GS. Linkage and segregation analyses of apolipoproteins A1 and B, and lipoprotein cholesterol levels in a large pedigree with excess coronary heart disease: the Bogalusa Heart Study. Genet Epidemiol 1987;4:115—128.

22. Deeb SS, Failor RA, Brown BG, Brunzell JD, Albers JJ, Motulsky AG, Wijsman E. Association of apolipoprotein B gene variants with plasma apoB and low density lipoprotein (LDL) cholesterol levels. Hum Genet 1992;88:463—470.

23. Helio T, Palotie A, Totterman KJ, Ott J, Kauppinen-Makelin R, Tikkanen MJ. Lack of association between the apolipoprotein B gene 3′ hypervariable region alleles and coronary artery disease in Finnish patients with angiographically documented coronary artery disease. J Int Med 1992;231:49—57.

24. Coresh J, Beaty TH, Kwiterovich POJ, Antonarakis SE. Pedigree and sib-pair linkage analysis suggest the apolipoprotein B gene is not the major gene influencing plasma apolipoprotein B levels. Am J Hum Genet 1992;50:1038—1045.

25. Laing AE, Amos CI, DeMeester C, Diep A, Xia YR, Elston RC, Srinivasan SR, Berenson GS, Lusis AJ. Linkage between the APOB gene and serum ApoB levels in a large pedigree from the Bogalusa Heart Study. Genet Epidemiol 1994;11:29—40.

26. Scott J, Navaratnam N, Bhattacharya S, Morrison JR. The apolipoprotein B messenger RNA editing enzyme. Curr Opin Lipid 1994;5:87—93.

27. Nishina PM, Johnson JP, Naggert JK, Krauss RM. Linkage of atherogenic lipoprotein phenotype to the low density lipoprotein receptor locus on the short arm of chromosome 19. Proc Natl Acad Sci USA 1992;89:708—712.

28. Rotter JI, Bu X, Cantor RM, Warden CH, Brown J, Gray RJ, Blanche PJ, Krauss RM, Lusis AJ. Multilocus genetic determinants of LDL particle size in coronary artery disease families. Am J Hum Genet 1996;58:585—594.

Hormonal replacement therapy of menopause and atherosclerosis

Atherosclerosis XI.
B. Jacotot, D. Mathé and J.-C. Fruchart, editors.

Estrogen replacement therapy and atherosclerosis

Elizabeth Barrett-Connor
Department of Family and Preventive Medicine, La Jolla, California, USA

Abstract. Multiple observational studies suggest that postmenopausal estrogen use affords a 30% reduction in risk of coronary heart disease (CHD) and has no consistent effect or the risk of stroke. Although the CHD association study results are strong and consistent, and there are several plausible mechanisms whereby estrogen might prevent CHD, many of the known biases would tend to exaggerate estrogen's benefit and no large randomized controlled trials have been completed. Because estrogen therapy clearly carries some increased risks, until randomized trials confirm and quantitate the benefit of estrogen therapy for prevention of CHD, it should not be recommended for this purpose.

Keywords: bias, coronary heart disease, estrogen replacement therapy, prevention, stroke.

Coronary heart disease

Coronary heart disease (CHD) is the most common and most deadly disease of postmenopausal women in nearly all of the industrialized world. Consequently, any significant reduction in CHD risk due to hormone therapy would overwhelm any postulated adverse effect. On this basis, estrogen replacement might be indicated for all postmenopausal women [1,2].

Nearly all observational studies have shown a lower risk of CHD in women using postmenopausal estrogen compared to nonusers — supporting the thesis that estrogen is cardioprotective. Three meta-analyses in the early 1990s reported a 35–50% lower risk of CHD in estrogen users compared to nonusers [1,3,4]. These estimates are based largely on studies conducted in the USA at a time when most women were using unopposed conjugated equine estrogen (CEE) (i.e., estrogen taken without a progestogen). A new meta-analysis [5] of seven studies that assessed the effect of treatment with estrogen plus a progestin found the summary relative risk for CHD to be 0.66 (0.53–0.84), similar to the estimate for unopposed estrogen.

Only one small randomized clinical trial has specifically examined the estrogen-CHD association. Recently, Hemminki and McPherson [6] identified 22 published randomized trials of estrogen therapy of more than 3 months but usually less than 3 years duration, with a total of 1,818 women assigned to hormones and 1,041 assigned to placebo, vitamin supplements, or no treatment. Cardiovascular outcomes were incidental to the purpose of the trial (recorded only as reasons for dropouts or adverse events). The summary calculated odds of cardiovascular events in women taking hormones vs. those not taking hormones was 1.39 (95% confidence interval 0.48–3.95). There is a low probability of finding this odds ratio if estrogen actually reduces the risk of cardiovascular disease by 30%.

Is it plausible that estrogen reduces CHD risk?

Oral estrogen lowers LDL cholesterol and elevates HDL cholesterol; transdermal estrogen appears to have a much smaller effect on HDL, suggesting that estrogen's HDL-lowering is mediated by a "first pass" effect through the liver [7]. In the 3-year postmenopausal estrogen/progestin interventions (PEPI) trial [8], all active treatments significantly reduced LDL cholesterol and increased HDL cholesterol compared to placebo, but estrogen (CEE) alone or with micronized progesterone (MP) raised HDL more than CEE plus either cyclic or continuous medroxyprogesterone acetate (MPA). All active treatment regimens also raised triglycerides and prevented the rise in fibrinogen observed in women assigned to placebo [8]. Hormone therapy did not, however, significantly improve several other risk factors reported in cross-sectional studies to be better in women using estrogen therapy, including no significant effect on weight, waist-hip ratio, blood pressure, fasting glucose or insulin.

Bush et al. [9] and Gruchow et al. [10] used statistical modeling to show that 25—50% of the apparent cardioprotection due to estrogen was mediated by favorable changes in HDL-cholesterol. The fact that the LDL and HDL changes are not large enough to explain all of estrogen's apparent CHD benefit suggests that estrogen has other cardioprotective effects. Several other reported estrogen effects would be expected to reduce CHD risk, including antioxidant inhibition of oxidative modification of LDL cholesterol [11], a calcium antagonist effect [12], and endothelial maintenance against apoptosis [13]. The favorable effects on vascular stiffness and endothelin-dependent and -independent vasodilation [14—16] have attracted the most attention.

The addition of MPA appears to block the coronary vascular effects of estrogen in laboratory models and in nonhuman primates. In cynomolgus monkey's MPA halves the effect of estrogen on coronary artery dilation [17] and essentially ablates estrogen's protective effects on coronary artery atherosclerosis [18]. This is in contrast to the cardioprotective effect observed in monkeys when progesterone is added to the estradiol [19].

Bias and the estrogen-CHD association

Selection bias

Studies of estrogen and CHD are almost entirely observational studies, not clinical trials, and therefore subject to bias. Women prescribed estrogen tend to be more affluent and more educated than untreated women. Education and social class are strongly, independently, and inversely associated with the risk of coronary heart disease [20]. Some of estrogen's putative benefits might reflect "a healthy woman effect". In cross-sectional studies, women taking estrogen have more favorable lifestyles, better levels of several heart disease risk factors, and less diabetes and heart disease than untreated women. Mathews and colleagues [21] found that women who elected to take estrogen after the menopause had more favorable levels of HDL cholesterol, fasting insulin, and blood pressure, and reported more physical activity, alcohol intake, and education than untreated women before the menopause, compared to women who chose not to take estrogen.

Compliance bias

Only 10 to 20% of women prescribed postmenopausal estrogen continue to take it [22]. Compliance reduces the risk of CHD events in randomized double-blind clinical trials, even if the medication is placebo. Thus, women in a β-blocker trial who were compliant with placebo had a 60% decreased risk of mortality compared to women who were noncompliant with placebo [23], similar to the risk reduction attributed to estrogen in some observational studies.

Stroke

In contrast to the remarkably consistent reduced risk of CHD in observational studies, only one of five case-control studies and half of 10 prospective studies with an internal comparison group found significant protection against stroke ([24], Barrett-Connor, unpublished). Most women in these studies were less then 60 years of age, younger than the age when most strokes occur. The studies usually also failed to differentiate hemorrhagic from thromboembolic strokes, which may be related to hormone treatment differently.

Estrogen use and total mortality

Several observational studies have reported a decreased risk of death from nearly all diseases in estrogen users compared to nonusers [9,25–29]. Recently, the 18-year follow-up of a large number of postmenopausal nurses showed that past use of estrogen had no effect on the risk of dying, but current use decreased overall risk by about 25% [30]. Some consider this universal benefit to be too good to be true — additional evidence for a healthy woman effect [31].

Clinical trials

Randomized trials will be necessary to determine how much of the CHD risk reduction in observational studies can be explained by self-selection, confounding and compliance. Two large trials are now underway in the USA. The heart and estrogen-progestin replacement study (HERS) is a secondary prevention trial among 2,763 postmenopausal women with known heart disease who were randomly assigned to daily CEE plus MPA therapy or placebo for 5 years. The primary outcome is new CHD events. This study is scheduled for closure in early 1998, with findings expected later the same year. If the HERS results are positive then the etiologic hypothesis that estrogen is cardioprotective will have been confirmed, but the risk benefit ratio for the treatment of healthy women will remain unknown.

Large clinical trials of women unselected for heart disease will be needed to assess the risk benefit ratio for "universal" estrogen therapy. One such study is the women's health initiative (WHI), a primary prevention trial among 27,500 postmenopausal women. In this trial, women with a uterus are being randomized to daily CEE plus MPA or placebo, and those without a uterus are being randomized to CEE or placebo. Unless the findings require early closure, WHI women will be followed up for about 10 years for CHD events, osteoporotic fractures and cancer. The WHI trial is still enrolling and results are not expected until about 2005. Another large trial (the MRC trial) is beginning in the UK and other European countries [32].

Interim recommendations

The real controversy over hormone replacement therapy is whether all women are likely to benefit. The answer to this question is totally dependent on the effect of hormone therapy on CHD risk. If CHD risk is reduced by at least 30%, as suggested in observational studies, then the benefit would exceed all known and suspected risks [1,2]. However, estrogen therapy clearly increases the risk for endometrial hyperplasia and cancer, hysterectomy, venous thromboembolic events, and gallbladder disease, and long-term therapy almost certainly also increases the risk of breast cancer. (The evidence for other putative benefits, such as the prevention of colon cancer and dementia, is too weak for clinical decision-making.) Therefore, until findings from randomized trials show at least a 25% reduction in CHD risk, it should not be routinely recommended for this purpose. In the meantime, healthy women can reduce their risk of CHD by not smoking, eating a healthy diet, and exercising regularly.

For the women who already have heart disease, estrogen is a plausible but as yet unproven option. Fortunately, recent large clinical trials have shown a 25−35% reduction in cardiovascular events in women who were treated with an acetyl co-A reductase inhibitor [33,34], providing an alternative to estrogen. Statin treatment reduces LDL cholesterol more than daily oral conjugated equine estrogen [35,36]. Sometime soon, new designer estrogens may make it possible to prevent heart disease and preserve bone without cancer risk.

References

1. Grady D, Rubin SM, Petitti DB, Fox CS, Black D, Ettinger B, Ernster VL, Cummings SR. Hor-

mone therapy to prevent disease and prolong life in postmenopausal women. Ann Int Med 1992;117:1016—1037.

2. Col NF, Eckman MH, Karas RH, Pauker SG, Goldberg RJ, Ross EM, Orr RK, Wong JB. Patient-specific decisions about hormone replacement therapy in postmenopausal women. JAMA 1997;277:1140—1147.

3. Bush TL. The epidemiology of cardiovascular disease in postmenopausal women. Ann NY Acad Sci 1990;592:263—271.

4. Stampfer MJ, Colditz GA. Estrogen replacement therapy and coronary heart disease: A quantitative assessment of the epidemiologic evidence. Prev Med 1991;20:47—63.

5. Barrett-Connor E, Grady D. Hormone replacement therapy, heart disease, other other considerations. Ann Rev Pub Health (In press).

6. Hemminki E, McPherson K. Impact of postmenopausal hormone therapy on cardiovascular events and cancer: pooled data from clinical trials. BMJ 1997;315:149—153.

7. Walsh BW, Schiff I, Rosner B, Greenberg L, Ravnikar V, Sacks FM. Effects of postmenopausal estrogen replacement on the concentrations and metabolism of plasma lipoproteins. N Engl J Med 1991;325:1196—1204.

8. Writing Group for the PEPI Trial. Effects of estrogen or estrogen/progestin regimens on heart disease risk factors in postmenopausal women. JAMA 1995;273:199—208.

9. Bush TL, Barrett-Connor E, Cowan LD, Criqui MH, Wallace RB, Suchindran CM, Tyroler HA, Rifkind BM. Cardiovascular mortality and noncontraceptive use of estrogen in women: results from the Lipid Research Clinics Program follow-up study. Circulation 1987;75:1102—1109.

10. Gruchow HW, Anderson AJ, Barboriak JJ, Sobocinski KA. Postmenopausal use of estrogen and occlusion of coronary arteries. Am Heart J 1988;115:954—963.

11. Rifici VA, Khachadurian AK. The inhibition of low-density lipoprotein oxidation by 17-beta estradiol. Metabolism 1992;41:1110—1114.

12. Collins P, Rosano GM, Jiang C, Lindsay D, Sarrel PM, Poole-Wilson PA. Cardiovascular protection by oestrogen — a calcium antagonist effect? Lancet 1993;341:1264—1265.

13. Spyridopoulos I, Sullivan AB, Kearney M, Isner JM, Losordo DW. Estrogen-receptor-mediated inhibition of human endothelial cell apoptosis. Estradiol as a survival factor. Circulation 1997; 95:1505—1514.

14. Gilligan DM, Badar DM, Panza JA, Quyyumi AA, Cannon RO III. Acute vascular effects of estrogen in postmenopausal women. Circulation 1994;90:786—791.

15. Reis SE, Gloth ST, Blumenthal RS, Resar JR, Zacur HA, Gerstenblith G, Brinker JA. Ethinyl estradiol acutely attenuates abnormal coronary vasomotor responses to acetylcholine in postmenopausal women. Circulation 1994;89:52—60.

16. Collins P, Rosano GM, Sarrel PM, Ulrich L, Adamopoulos S, Beale CM, McNeill JG, Poole-Wilson PA. 17 beta-Estradiol attenuates acetylcholine-induced coronary arterial constriction in women but not men with coronary heart disease. Circulation 1995;92:24—30.

17. Williams JK, Anthony MS, Hooré EK, Herrington DM, Morgan TM, Register TC, Clarkson TB. Regression of atherosclerosis in female monkeys. Arterioscler Thromb Vasc Biol 1995;15: 827—836.

18. Adams MR, Register TC, Golden DL, Wagner JD, Williams JK. Medroxyprogesterone acetate antagonizes inhibitor effects of conjugated equine estrogens on coronary artery atherosclerosis. Arterioscler Thromb Vasc Biol 1997;17:217—221.

19. Adams MR, Kaplan JR, Manuck SB, Koritnik DR, Parks JS, Wolfe MS, Clarkson TB. Inhibition of coronary artery atherosclerosis by 17-beta estradiol in ovariectomized monkeys. Lack of an effect of added progesterone. Arteriosclerosis 1990;10:1051—1057.

20. Irbarren C, Luepker RV, McGovern PG, Arnett DK, Blackburn H. Twelve-year trends in cardiovascular disease risk factors in the Minnesota heart survey: are socioeconomic differences widening? Arch Int Med 1997;157:873—881.

21. Matthews KA, Kuller LH, Wing RR, Meilahn EN, Plantinga P. Prior to use of estrogen replacement therapy, are users healthier than nonusers? Am J Epidemiol 1996;143:971—978.

22. Hemminki E, Brambilla DJ, McKinlay SM, Posner JG. Use of estrogens among middle-aged Massachusetts women. Ann Pharmacother (DICP) 1991;25:418–423.

23. Gallagher EJ, Viscoli CM, Horwitz RI. The relationship of treatment adherence to the risk of death after myocardial infarction in women. JAMA 1993;270:742–744.

24. Paganini-Hill A. Estrogen replacement therapy and stroke. Prog Cardiovas Dis 1995;38: 223–242.

25. Rosenberg L, Armstrong B, Jick H. Myocardial infarction and estrogen therapy in postmenopausal women. N Engl J Med 1976;294:1256–1259.

26. Ettinger B, Friedman GD, Bush T, Quesenberry CP Jr. Reduced mortality associated with long-term postmenopausal estrogen therapy. Obstet Gynecol 1996;87:6–12.

27. Heckbert SR, Weiss NS, Koepsell TD, Lemaitre RN, Smith NL, Siscovick DS, Lin D, Psaty BM. Duration of estrogen replacement therapy in relation to the risk of incident myocardial infarction in postmenopausal women. Arch Int Med 1997;157:1330–1336.

28. Henderson BE, Paganini-Hill A, Ross RK. Decreased mortality in users of estrogen replacement therapy. Arch Int Med 1991;151:75–78.

29. Folsom AR, Mink PJ, Sellers TA, Hong C-P, Zheng W, Potter JD. Hormonal replacement therapy and morbidity and mortality in a prospective study of postmenopausal women. Am J Pub Health 1995;85:1128–1132.

30. Grodstein F, Stampfer MJ, Colditz GA, Willett WC, Manson JE, Joffe M, Rosner, B, Fuchs C, Hankinson SE, Hunter DJ, Hennekens CH, Speizer FE. Postmenopausal hormone therapy and mortality. N Engl J Med 1997;336:1769–1775.

31. Vandenbroucke JP. Postmenopausal oestrogen and cardioprotection. Lancet 1991;337:833–834.

32. Vickers MR, Meade TW, Wilkes HC. Hormone replacement therapy and cardiovascular disease: the case for a randomized controlled trial. Ciba Found Symp 1995;191:150–160.

33. Baseline serum cholesterol and treatment effect in the Scandinavian Simvastatin Survival Study (4S). Lancet 1995;345:1274–1275.

34. Sacks FM, Pfeffer MA, Moye LA, Rouleau JL, Rutherford JD, Cole TG, Brown L, Warnica JW, Arnold JM, Wun CC, Davis BR, Braunwald E for the Cholesterol and Recurrent Events Trial Investigators. The effect of pravastatin on coronary events after myocardial infarction in patients with average cholesterol levels. N Engl J Med 1996;335:1001–1009.

35. Davidson MH, Testolin LM, Maki KC, von Duvillard S, Drennan KB. A comparison of estrogen replacement, pravastatin, and combined treatment for the management of hypercholesterolemia in postmenopausal women. Arch Int Med 1997;157:1186–1192.

36. Darling GM, Johns JA, McCloud PI, Davis SR. Estrogen and progestin compared with simvastatin for hypercholesterolemia in ostmenopausal women. N Engl J Med 1997;337:595–601.

Effects of estrogen on the endothelium in postmenopausal women: implications for atherosclerosis

Richard O. Cannon III
Cardiology Branch, NHLBI, National Institutes of Health, Bethesda, Maryland, USA

Keywords: coronary artery disease, fibrinolysis, hormones, nitric oxide.

The beneficial effects of estrogen therapy in postmenopausal women may in part result from increases in high density lipoprotein cholesterol and reduction in low-density lipoprotein cholesterol levels to a more favorable ratio, regarding atherogenesis [1,2], although epidemiological studies question whether alteration in lipid profile alone can account for all of the apparent cardiovascular benefit of estrogen therapy [3]. Animal studies have indicated that estrogen may have vascular effects independent of changes in lipoprotein profile. Thus, intravenous administration of 17 β-estradiol to ovariectomized primates fed an atherogenic diet was found to reverse acutely the epicardial coronary artery response to acetylcholine from constriction to dilation without any effect on nitroglycerin-mediated vasodilation, suggesting estrogen-mediated improvement in endothelial function [4]. This finding was consistent with the demonstration of estrogen-enhanced endothelium-dependent relaxation of rabbit femoral and swine coronary artery rings to acetylcholine [5,6].

We found that 17 β-estradiol infused into the left coronary arteries of 20 postmenopausal women, achieving physiological concentrations in the coronary sinus drainage, augmented acetylcholine-stimulated increases in coronary flow [7]. The enhancement of acetylcholine-mediated vasodilation of the epicardial coronary arteries was minimal, suggesting that most of the vasodilator effect of estradiol was at the microvascular level. This effect of estradiol on acetylcholine-mediated vasodilation was most prominent in women with the most impaired dilator responses to acetylcholine at both the epicardial and microvascular of the coronary circulation. No enhancement of nitroprusside-stimulated flow was noted after estradiol administration, indicative of selective potentiation of endothelium-dependent vasodilation by estradiol at physiological concentrations. Other groups have also reported improvement in endothelium-dependent coronary vasodilator responsiveness following infusions of estrogen into postmeno-

Address for correspondence: Richard O. Cannon III MD, National Institutes of Health, Building 10, Room 7B15, 10 Center Drive MSC-1650, Bethesda, MD 20892-1650, USA. Tel.: +1-301-496-9895. Fax: +1-301-402-0888. E-mail: cannonr@gwgate.nhlbi.nih.gov

pausal women [8,9]. Consistent with the findings of these acute infusion studies is the report of Herrington et al., in which four postmenopausal women chronically taking conjugated equine estrogens at conventional dosages had epicardial coronary dilator responses to intracoronary acetylcholine as opposed to constrictor responses to the same concentrations of acetylcholine noted in six untreated postmenopausal women, with similar dilator responses to nitroglycerin in the two groups [10].

We also found that 17 β-estradiol infused into the brachial arteries of 40 postmenopausal women achieving physiological concentrations in the brachial vein enhanced acetylcholine-stimulated forearm blood flow [11]. The 20 women in this study with risk factors for atherosclerosis also had slight potentiation of endothelium-independent (nitroprusside) blood flow during estradiol infusion. In contrast, the 20 women without risk factors, who had a greater baseline forearm blood flow responses to acetylcholine and to nitroprusside compared with the 20 women with risk factors, showed selective enhancement in endothelium-dependent vasodilation during estradiol infusion. Lieberman et al. reported that oral estradiol administration to 13 postmenopausal women for 9 weeks enhanced flow-mediated brachial artery dilator responses to postischemic hyperemia, without potentiation of the vasodilator response to nitroglycerin [12]. However, the use of an oral estrogen preparation probably caused reduction in low-density lipoprotein and elevation in high-density lipoprotein cholesterol levels (not reported in the article), changes that could have improved endothelial function independent of a direct effect of estrogen on brachial artery vasomotor tone.

The endothelium may also be the source of plasminogen activator inhibitor type 1 (PAI-1), an essential antagonist of fibrinolysis in humans by rapidly and specifically inhibiting both tissue plasminogen activator and urokinase plasminogen activator [13]. PAI-1 has been shown by immunohistochemical analysis and in situ hybridization to be present in endothelial and smooth muscle cells of histologically normal arteries; increased quantities are present in all cellular components of atheromatous arteries [14]. Of potential pathophysiological relevance to women, higher levels of PAI-1 were noted in postmenopausal women than in premenopausal women in the Framingham Offspring Study [15]; this increased level may in part account for the increasing risk of atherosclerosis and its clinical consequences after menopause. In a randomized, crossover study, we investigated the effects of oral conjugated equine estrogens 0.625 mg/day in 30 postmenopausal women and transdermal estradiol 0.1 mg/day in 20 postmenopausal women, either alone or in combination with medroxyprogesterone acetate 2.5 mg daily for 1 month, on plasma PAI-1 antigen levels [16]. Degradation products of cross-linked fibrin (D-dimer) were measured in serum as an index of fibrinolysis. PAI-1 levels were inversely associated with D-dimer levels at baseline (r = -0.540, p = 0.002). Oral estrogen, both alone and in combination with medroxyprogesterone acetate, reduced PAI-1 levels from 32 ± 34 to 14 ± 10 mg/ml (mean ± SD, p > 0.001) and from 31 ± 29 to 15 ± 11 mg/ml (p = 0.003), respectively; there was a significant inverse correlation between pretreatment PAI-1 levels and the degree of reduction in these levels during therapy. The degree of reduction in PAI-1 levels was associated with proportionate increases in D-dimer levels both when oral estrogen was given alone (r = -0.631, p < 0.001) and when combined hormone therapy was given (r = -0.507, p = 0.004). However, transdermal application of estradiol caused no changes in PAI-1 levels, suggesting that the reduction in PAI-1 by oral estrogen therapy may be accomplished more by decreasing the synthesis or increasing the clearance of PAI-1 by the liver rather than decreasing synthesis by the endothelium.

The mechanism of endothelial effects of estradiol in animal and human studies is unknown. Potentiation of acetylcholine-stimulated flow by estrogen could result from vascular smooth muscle relaxation due to enhanced endothelial production or release of relaxing factors such as nitric oxide [17–21] and prostacyclin [22], or inhibition of the release or activity of vasoconstrictor substances such as endothelin [23] and angiotensin II [24]. Because nitric oxide also has other potential antiatherogenic properties that could account for the cardioprotective effects of estrogen [25], as suggested by observational angiographic studies [26] and epidemiological surveys [27], we undertook a study to determine whether the alteration of coronary vascular reactivity observed following administration of estrogen to postmenopausal women is mediated by enhanced bioavailability of nitric oxide [28]. We measured coronary epicardial and microvascular responses to intracoronary acetylcholine (range 3–300 μg/min for 2 min), before and after intracoronary estradiol 75 ng/min for 15 min in 20 postmenopausal women, 16 of whom had angiographic evidence of atherosclerosis or risk factors for atherosclerosis. This testing was repeated following inhibition of nitric oxide synthesis with intracoronary N^G-monomethyl-L-arginine (L-NMMA) 64 μmol/min for 5 min. Estradiol increased acetylcholine-stimulated coronary flow from 54 ± 42% above baseline values prior to estradiol infusion to 100 ± 63% above baseline values (p = 0.007) at a coronary sinus estradiol concentration of 470 ± 192 pg/ml (Fig. 1). Estradiol also tended to lessen the severity of acetylcholine-induced decreases in epicardial coronary artery diameter from 8 ± 11 to 3 ± 11% below baseline values (p = 0.123). However, during L-NMMA infusion, estradiol no longer potentiated the effects of acetylcholine on coronary flow or coronary diameter. Thus, the effects of estradiol at physiological concentrations on endothelium-dependent coronary vasodilator responsiveness at both the epicardial and microvascular levels of the coronary circulation in postmenopausal women are mediated by enhanced bioavailability of nitric oxide.

Estradiol may enhance the synthesis and release of nitric oxide, as suggested by animal tissue and cell culture studies [17–20]. Such an effect could not have been mediated by genomic effects of the hormone in our acute infusion studies, although enhanced synthesis of nitric oxide synthase may be responsible for improvement in endothelium-dependent vasodilation with chronic estrogen therapy. In this regard, estrogen receptors have been demonstrated in bovine aortic and human coronary endothelial cells [29,30], and estrogen response elements have been identified in the promotor region of the gene coding for endothelial

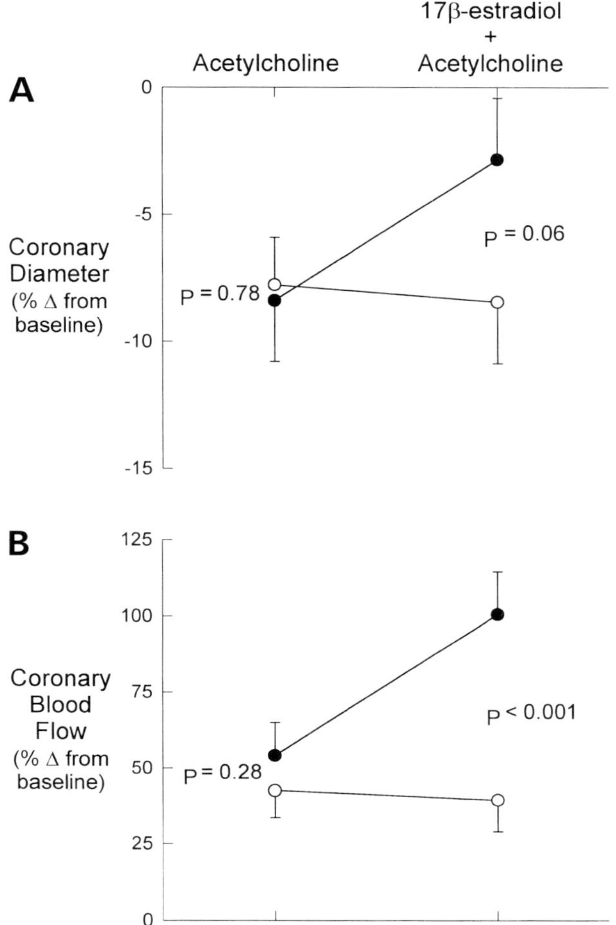

Fig. 1. Epicardial coronary diameter (**A**) and coronary blood flow (**B**) responses to acetylcholine are shown as relative changes from respective preacetylcholine baseline values in 20 postmenopausal women. The dose of acetylcholine represented on these graphs (mode 100 μg/min) produced the coronary flow response that was maximally enhanced during coadministration of 17 β-estradiol. The effects of 17 β-estradiol (75 ng/min) on acetylcholine-stimulated changes in epicardial diameter and coronary flow are shown before (●) and during (○) concomitant infusion of N^G-monomethyl-L-arginine (64 μmol/min), an inhibitor of nitric oxide synthesis. Data are expressed as mean ± SEM. Adapted from [28].

nitric oxide synthase [31]. However, steroid hormones may rapidly initiate intracellular events in the absence of genomic effects, possibly by activation of receptors on the cell membrane [32—34]. Increased intracellular calcium, as has been shown in chicken and pig ovarian granulosa cells following acute estrogen exposure [34], could activate nitric oxide synthase in endothelial cells, with enhanced synthesis and release of nitric oxide. Alternatively, antioxidant effects of estradiol could protect nitric oxide from degradation by superoxide anions and other free radical molecules, resulting in increased bioactivity of nitric oxide [6,21,35].

Increased nitric oxide bioactivity as a result of estrogen administration may not only promote smooth muscle relaxation via increased cyclic GMP, but also benefit other important homeostatic properties of the endothelium, such as inhibition of the activation of proinflammatory genes. In this regard, nitric oxide has been found to inhibit the activation of an important proinflammatory transcription factor, nuclear factor (NF)κB [36—38]. In the presence of reduced cytosolic nitric oxide or increased cytosolic oxidant stress, NFκB is activated by the dissociation from its inhibitor subunit IκB. The heterodimer then translocates to the nucleus where it combines with the promotor regions of several proinflammatory genes, with synthesis of gene products including cytokines, chemokines, and cell adhesion molecules. Inflammatory cells, once activated and attracted into the vessel wall by these gene products, have a variety of proatherogenic effects, including the release of reactive oxygen species, growth factors, prothrombotic factors, and in the case of monocytes, transformation into foam cells upon unregulated uptake of oxidized LDL [39,40]. Accordingly, estrogen-mediated nitric oxide release from the vasculature may account in large part for the cardioprotective effect of estrogen as suggested by experimental and observational studies, the proof of which awaits the completion of randomized clinical trials.

References

1. Walsh BW, Schiff I, Rosner B, Greenberg L, Ravnikar V, Sacks FM. Effects of postmenopausal estrogen replacement on the concentration and metabolism of plasma lipoproteins. N Engl J Med 1991;325:1196—1204.
2. The Writing Group for the PEPI Trial. Effects of estrogen or estrogen/progestin regimens on heart disease risk factors in postmenopausal women: The Postmenopausal Estrogen/Progestin Interventions (PEPI) Trial. JAMA 1995;273:199—208.
3. Bush TL, Barrett-Conner E, Cowan LD, Criqui MH, Wallace RB, Suchindran CM, Tyroler HA, Rifkind BM. Cardiovascular mortality and noncontraceptive use of estrogen in women: results from the Lipid Research Clinics Program Follow-up Study. Circulation 1987;75:1102—1109.
4. Williams JK, Adams MR, Herrington DM, Clarkson TB. Short-term administration of estrogen and vascular responses of coronary arteries. J Am Coll Cardiol 1992;20:452—457.
5. Miller VM. Modulation of endothelium-dependent and vascular smooth muscle responses by oestrogens. Phlebiology 1988;224:19—22.
6. Keaney JF, Shwaery GT, Xu A, Nicolosi RJ, Loscalzo J, Foxall TL, Vita JA. 17β-Estradiol preserves endothelial vasodilator function and limits low-density lipoprotein oxidation in hypercholesterolemic swine. Circulation 1994;89:2251—2259.
7. Gilligan DM, Quyyumi AA, Cannon RO III. Effects of physiological levels of estrogen on coronary vasomotor function in postmenopausal women. Circulation 1994;89:2545—2551.
8. Reis SE, Gloth ST, Blumenthal RS, Resar JR, Zacur HA, Gerstenblith G, Brinker JA. L Ethinyl estradiol acutely attenuates coronary vasomotor responses to acetylcholine in postmenopausal women. Circulation 1994;89:52—60.
9. Collins P, Rosano GM, Sarrel PM, Ulrich L, Adamopoulos S, Beale CM, McNeill JG, Poole-Wilson PA. 17β-estradiol attenuates acetylcholine-induced coronary arterial constriction in women but not men with coronary heart disease. Circulation 1995;92:24—30.
10. Herrington DM, Braden GA, Williams JK, Morgan TM. Endothelium-dependent coronary

822

vasomotor responsiveness in postmenopausal women with and without estrogen replacement therapy. Am J Cardiol 1994;73:951–952.
11. Gilligan DM, Badar DM, Panza JA, Quyyumi AA, Cannon RO III. Acute vascular effects of estrogen in postmenopausal women. Circulation 1994;90;786–791.
12. Lieberman EH, Gebhard MD, Uehata A, Walsh BW, Selwyn AP, Ganz P, Yeung AC, Creager MA. Estrogen improves endothelium-dependent, flow-mediated vasodilation in postmenopausal women. Ann Int Med 1993;121:936–941.
13. Sprengers ED, Kluft C. Plasminogen activator inhibitors. Blood 1987;69:381–387.
14. Lupu F, Bergonzelli GE, Heim DA, Cousin E, Genton CY, Bachmann F, Kruithof EKO. Localization and production of plasminogen activator inhibitor-1 in human healthy and atherosclerotic arteries. Arterioscler Thromb 1993;13:1090–1100.
15. Gebara OCE, Mittleman MA, Sutherland P, Lipinska I, Matheney T, Xu P, Welty FK, Wilson PWF, Muller JE, Tofler GT. Association between increased estrogen status and increased fibrinolytic potential in the Framingham Offspring Study. Circulation 1995;91:1952–1958.
16. Koh KK, Mincemoyer R, Bui MN, Csako G, Pucino F, Guetta V, Waclawiw M, Cannon RO III. Effects of hormone-replacement therapy on fibrinolysis in postmenopausal women. N Engl J Med 1997;336:683–690.
17. Hayashi T, Fukuto JM, Ignarro LJ, Chaudhuri G. Basal release of nitric oxide from aortic rings is greater in female rabbits than male rabbits: Implications for atherosclerosis. Proc Natl Acad Sci USA 1992;89:11259–11263.
18. Weiner CP, Lizasoain I, Baylis SA, Knowles RG, Charles IG, Moncada S. Induction of calcium-dependent nitric oxide synthases by sex hormones. Proc Natl Acad Sci USA 1994;91:5212–5216.
19. Hishikawa K, Nakaki T, Marumo T, Suzuki H, Kato R, Saruta T. Up-regulation of nitric oxide synthase by estradiol in human aortic endothelial cells. FEBS Lett 1995;360:291–293.
20. Hayashi T, Yamada K, Esaki T, Kuzuya M, Satake S, Ishikawa T, Hidaka H, Iguchi A. Estrogen increases endothelial nitric oxide by a receptor-mediated system. Biochem Biophys Res Commun 1995;214:847–855.
21. Arnal JF, Clamens S, Pechet C, Negre-Salvayre A, Allera C, Girolami J-P, Salvayre R, Bayard F. Ethinylestradiol does not enhance the expression of nitric oxide synthase in bovine endothelial cells but increases the release of bioactive nitric oxide by inhibiting superoxide anion production. Proc Natl Acad Sci USA 1996;93:4108–4113.
22. Chang WC, Nakao J, Orimo H, Murota SI. Stimulation of prostacyclin biosynthetic activity by estradiol in rat aortic smooth muscle cells in culture. Biochim Biophys Acta 1980;619:107–118.
23. Polderman KH, Stehouwer CD, van Kamp GI, Dekker GA, Verheugt FW, Gooren LJ. Influence of sex hormones on plasma endothelin levels. Ann Int Med 1993;118:429–432.
24. Proudler AJ, Ahmed AI, Crook D, Fogelman I, Rymer JM, Stevenson JC. Hormone replacement therapy and serum angiotensin-converting enzyme activity in postmenopausal women. Lancet 1995;346:89–90.
25. Cooke JP, Tsao PS. Cytoprotective effects of nitrix oxide. Circulation 1993;88:2451–2454.
26. Sullivan JM, Vander Zwaag R, Lemp GF, Hughes JP, Maddock V, Kroetz FW, Ramanathan KB, Mirvis DM. Postmenopausal estrogen use and coronary atherosclerosis. Ann Int Med 1988;108:358–363.
27. Stampfer MJ, Colditz GA, Willett WC, Manson JE, Rosner B, Speizer EF, Hennekens CH. Postmenopausal estrogen therapy and cardiovascular disease. Ten-year follow-up from the Nurses' Health Study. N Engl J Med 1991;325:756–762.
28. Guetta V, Quyyumi AA, Prasad A, Panza JA, Waclawiw M, Cannon RO III. The role of nitric oxide in the coronary vascular effects of estrogen in postmenopausal women. Circulation 1997;96:November 4 issue.
29. Venkov CD, Rankin AB, Vaughan DE. Identification of authentic estrogen receptor in cultured endothelial cells. A potential mechanism for steroid hormone regulation of endothelial function. Circulation 1996;94:727–733.

30. Kim-Schulze S, McGowan KA, Hubchak SC, Cid MC, Martin MB, Kleinman HK, Greene GL, Schnaper HW. Expression of an estrogen receptor by human coronary artery and umbilical vein endothelial cells. Circulation 1996;94:1402—1407.

31. Venema RC, Nishida K, Alexander RW, Harrison DG, Murphy TJ. Organization of the bovine gene encoding the endothelial nitric oxide synthase. Biochim Biophys Acta 1993;1218: 413—420.

32. Pappas TC, Gametchu B, Yannariello-Brown J, Collins TJ, Watson CS. Membrane estrogen receptors in GH3/B6 cells are associated with rapid estrogen-induced release of prolactin. Endocrine J 1994;2:813—822.

33. Farhat MY, Abi-Younes S, Dingaan B, Vargas R, Ramwell PW. Estradiol increases cyclic adenosine monophosphate in rat pulmonary vascular smooth muscle cells by a nongenomic mechanism. J Pharmacol Exp Ther 1996;276:652—657.

34. Morley P, Whitefield JF, Vanderhyden BC, Tsang BK, Schwartz J-L. A new, nongenomic estrogen action: the rapid release of intracellular calcium. Endocrinology 1992;131:1305—1312.

35. Sack MN, Rader DJ, Cannon RO III. Oestrogen and inhibition of oxidation of low-density lipoproteins in postmenopausal women. Lancet 1994;343:269—270.

36. De Caterina R, Libby P, Peng HB, Thannickal VJ, Rajarashisth TB, Gimbrone MA, Shin WS, Liao JK. Nitric oxide decreases cytokine-induced activation. Nitric oxide selectively reduces endothelial expression of adhesion molecules and proinflammatory cytokines. J Clin Invest 1995;96:60—68.

37. Peng HB, Rajavashisth TB, Libby P, Liao JK. Nitric oxide inhibits macrophage-colony stimulating factor gene transcription in vascular endothelial cells. J Biol Chem 1995;270:17050—17055.

38. Zeiher AM, Fisslthaler B, Schray-Utz B, Busse R. Nitric oxide modulates the expression of monocyte chemoattractant protein-1 in cultured human endothelial cells. Circ Res 1995; 76:980—986.

39. Ross R. The pathogenesis of atherosclerosis: a perspective for the 1990s. Nature 1993;362: 801—809.

40. Berliner JA, Nabyab M, Fogelman AM, Frank JS, Demer LL, Edwards PA, Watson AD, Lusis AJ. Atherosclerosis: basic mechanisms. Oxidation, inflammation, and genetics. Circulation 1995;91:2488—2496.

The influence of hormone replacement therapy usage following successful coronary balloon angioplasty

Guy Lloyd, Nikhil Patel, Kim Tan, Alethea Cooper, Elaine McGing, Sheila Karani and Graham Jackson
The Cardiothoracic Centre, Guy's and St Thomas' Hospitals NHS Trust, St Thomas' Hospital, London, UK

Introduction

Patients undergoing percutaneous coronary angioplasty (PTCA) represent an important patient group for whom hormone replacement therapy (HRT) offers potential benefits. The lipid modulating effects offer potential as secondary prevention from subsequent death and myocardial infarction [1,2]. Other than the risk of subsequent coronary events, patients undergoing PTCA have the additional problem of restenosis that has remained the feature limiting the efficacy of the procedure. Here again the effects of oestrogen alone or in combination with a progestin offer potential advantages with modulation of smooth muscle cell proliferation [3], increased vessel remodeling as a result of vasodilatory [4] effects and reductions in circulating markers of restenosis risk such as fibrinogen [5] and lipoprotein(a) [6]. We hypothesised that use of HRT at PTCA would alter the risk of restenosis or subsequent coronary events. A prospectively collected angioplasty database was therefore examined for differences in outcome between users and nonusers of HRT.

Methods

The Guy's hospital PTCA database is prospectively collected in all patients undergoing PTCA at this institution. For the purposes of this evaluation only the years 1990–95 were evaluated as this represented a period when the introduction of intracoronary stenting became routine and the correct indications for PTCA were well-established. Only patients undergoing first angioplasty were evaluated as restenotic coronary vessels and stents may behave differently.

History of HRT usage was retrospectively ascertained by careful review of hospital case notes, written communication with general practitioners and telephone interviews with patients. Patients were divided into users at PTCA and "ever users".

Univariate comparisons in baseline features were compared using unpaired t tests, χ^2 or Fischer's exact testing where appropriate. Survival functions were

---

Address for correspondence: Guy Lloyd, The Cardiothoracic Centre, Guy's and St Thomas' Hospitals NHS Trust, St Thomas' Hospital, London SE1 7EH, UK.

compared using Kaplan-Meier analysis with adjustment for age performed using Cox's proportional hazard model. Univariate and multivariate hazard ratios were calculated from the Cox's regression.

Results

Population

372 women first underwent PTCA successfully. Full follow-up and ever-used HRT history was available in 303 (81%) with history of use at time of PTCA in 299 (80%). Forty-one patients were HRT users at PTCA with 81 patients "ever users". Of the 41 users at PTCA, 20 (49%) were taking unopposed oestrogen, 12 (29%) cyclical oestrogen/progestin, one (2.5%) continuous combined, four (10%) tibolone and four were taking other hormonally active drugs (e.g., progestin alone or tamoxifen).

Baseline characteristics are presented in Table 1. The only statistically significant difference was the younger age of the HRT users: 57.7 (0.86) vs. 63.0 years (0.62), $p < 0.001$. A trend towards lower cholesterol and less poor left ventricular function were also observed among HRT users. The incidence of hypertension, diabetes and current smoking was not different among users and nonusers.

Repeat angiography

A greater proportion of HRT users underwent repeat coronary angiography (20 (48%) vs. 74 (29%), p = 0.01). Among these patients the incidence of angiographic restenosis (defined as $> 50\%$ stenosis at the target lesion) was lower among the HRT users (20 vs. 50%, p = 0.09). HRT users were more likely to display an incomplete revascularisation at angiography.

Follow-up events

The median follow-up was 23 months (16—39 months) among the HRT users

Table 1. Demographic details of HRT users and nonusers at PTCA.

	Hormone users (n = 41)	Nonhormone users (n = 258)	Significance p value
Age	57.7 (0.86)	63 (0.62)	< 0.001
EF < 40%	0 (0%)	19 (8.9%)	< 0.07
Diabetes	4 (9.8%)	29 (11%)	< 0.54
Hypertension	18 (62.1%)	101 (57.1%)	< 0.61
Current smoker	8 (20%)	46 (19%)	< 0.98
Total cholesterol (mmol/l)	5.86 (0.19)	6.47 (0.25)	< 0.35
Triglycerides (mmol/l)	2.15 (0.22)	2.28 (0.19)	< 0.78

and 22 months (15—38 months) among nonusers. Comparing HRT users with nonusers; death occurred in none vs. four (1.6%), coronary artery bypass grafting (CABG) in three (7.3%) vs. 11 (4.3%), MI in none vs. eight (3.1%) and repeat PTCA in 12 (29 vs. 34 (13%), p = 0.008), respectively. The composite endpoints death/MI, repeat revascularisation and combined adverse clinical endpoints were then examined. Repeat revascularisation occurred more commonly among HRT users (logrank p = 0.049). The hazard ratio was 1.30 (0.94—1.79) after adjustment for age (Fig. 1). This increased risk was reflected in the occurrence of all major adverse cardiac end points (logrank p = 0.17) age-adjusted hazard ratio 1.20 (0.87—1.65). Death/MI occurred less frequently among HRT users but this did not reach statistical significance (p = 0.18) although the hazard ratio was very low for HRT usage (0.012). In order to further explore this finding the occurrence of death/MI was then examined in the 81 ever users and again a similar trend was observed (age-adjusted hazard ratio 0.59 (0.2—1.74, p = 0.12) (Fig. 2).

Discussion

Given the potential benefits of HRT inpatients with or at risk from coronary artery disease, it is disappointing that only 15% of this unselected population were on therapy at the time of angioplasty. This may reflect outdated attitudes that HRT is contraindicated in women with heart disease and other conditions such as diabetes and hypertension.

Two papers that have examined the relationship between HRT usage and PTCA have both demonstrated favourable results. O'Brian et al., in retrospective analysis of the CAVEAT I trial (PTCA vs. directional atherectomy) demonstrated

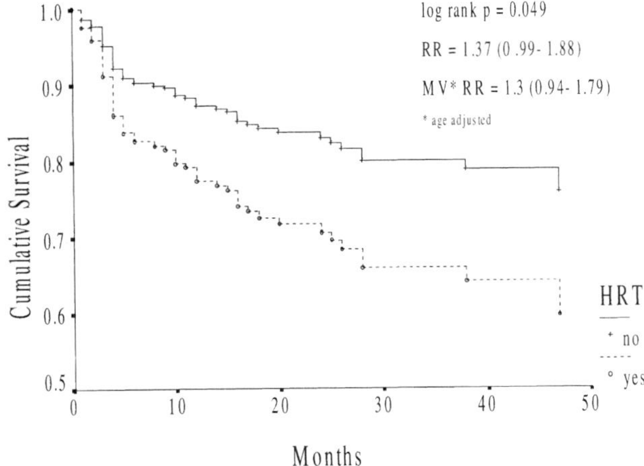

Fig. 1. Freedom from subsequent revascularisation (CABG/MI) procedures in HRT users and non-users at PTCA.

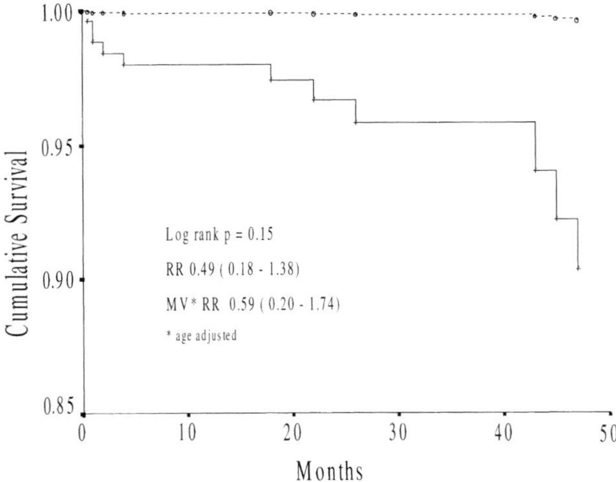

Fig. 2. Freedom from death/MI among "ever" and "never" HRT users.

a lesser degree of luminal renarrowing and a greater minimum vessel lumen diameter at follow-up angiography among HRT users [7]. It is worth noting that this effect was confined to those patients undergoing directional atherectomy. The authors propose that the mechanism of restenosis may be different following the two techniques accounting for this differential HRT effect. Certainly HRT usage has potential to influence the restenotic process at a number of levels. The observed reduction in smooth muscle proliferation along with favorable effects on vessel remodeling and reduction of procoagulent/antifibrinolytic factors all provide mechanisms by which restenosis might be reduced. This data did demonstrate a trend towards reduced restenosis rates among the HRT users undergoing repeat angiography, but this finding must be treated with extreme caution in view of the disparate rates of repeat angiography in the two groups. Many early studies have given encouraging results for drug therapy to tackle restenosis only to be disproved by definitive works with full angiographic follow-up.

HRT users in this cohort underwent more subsequent revascularisation procedures. The reason for this is unclear although at follow-up angiography more HRT users had evidence of incomplete revascularisation. Older women were less likely to undergo repeat revascularisation and this in part explained the disparity between the two groups. HRT users may differ in other ways not investigated, in particular users may be more motivated to seek further health care and compete symptom control.

The primary preventative benefits of HRT have been established in the overwhelming majority of observational cohorts. The study by O'Keefe et al demonstrated a reduction in fatal myocardial infarction among HRT users undergoing successful PTCA [8]. Our data demonstrates a similar trend with an age-adjusted relative risk for "ever use" of 0.6. This did not reach statistical significance which is not surprising because of the low number of events, nevertheless it concords well with other estimates of the benefit from HRT use in the literature.

This study and the work of others suggests that a randomised placebo-controlled study is warranted looking at the effect of HRT on restenosis and mortality following coronary angioplasty.

References

1. Grodstein F, Stampfer MJ, Manson JE et al. Postmenopausal estrogens and progestin use and the risk of cardiovascular disease. N Engl J Med 1996;335:453—461.
2. Bush T, Barrett-Connor E, Cowan L et al. Cardiovascular mortality and noncontraceptive use of estrogen in women: results from the lipid research clinics follow-up study. Circulation 1987;75:1102—1109.
3. Vargas R, Wroblewska B, Rego A, Hatch J, Ramwell P. Oestrodiol inhibits smoth muscle cell proliferation of pig coronary artery. Br J Pharmacol 1993;109:612—617.
4. Collins P, Rosano GM, Sarrel PM, Ulrich L, McNeill J, Poole-Wilson P. 17-beta estrodiol attenuates acetylcholine-induced arterial constriction in women but not men with coronary heart disease. Circulation 1995;92(1):24—28.
5. Montalescot G, Ankra A, Vicaut E, Drobinski G, Grosogeat Y, Thomas D. Fibrinogen after coronary angioplasty as a risk factor for restenosis. Circulation 1995;92(1):31—38.
6. Hearn J, Donohue B, Sgoutas D. Usefullness of serum Lipoprotein (a) as a predictor of restenosis after percutaneous transluminal coronary angioplasty. Am J Cardiol 1992;69:736—739.
7. O'Brien JE, Peterson ED, Keeler GP et al. Relation between estrogen replacement therapy and restenosis after percutaneous coronary interventions. J Am Coll Cardiol 1996;28:1111—1118.
8. O'Keefe JH, Kim SC, Hall RR, Cochran V, Lawhorn SL, McCallister BD. Estrogen replacement therapy after coronary angioplasty in women. J Am Coll Cardiol 1997;29:1—5.

The effect of hormone replacement therapy and route of administration on selected cardiovascular risk factors in postmenopausal women

M. Seed[1], L. Jones[1], M. McLaren[2], G. Kirk[2] and R. Sands[1]

[1] National Heart and Lung Institute, Imperial College School of Medicine, Charing Cross Hospital, London; and [2] Ninewells Hospital & Medical School, University of Dundee, Dundee, UK

Compared to men, premenopausal women have a low risk of coronary heart disease (CHD). This gender gap is reduced after the menopause or oophorectomy, suggesting that gonadal steroids offer protection against CHD [1]. Consistent with this are a number of observational studies suggesting that postmenopausal hormone replacement therapy (HRT) lowers CHD risk [2].

The problem of CHD in women has been understudied. Only in the last 3 years have we seen confirmation from clinical trials (4S, CARE, CCAIT) that the major reduction in cardiovascular risk which can be achieved with lipid lowering therapy in men is also applicable to women, and even in these studies the numbers were too small to demonstrate reduction in mortality as well as in cardiovascular events [3,4]. Furthermore, although gonadal steroids have known effects on a number of CV risk factors (most notably impaired glucose tolerance, hyperlipidaemia, and raised plasma fibrinogen levels) data from randomised controlled trials of the use of HRT to reduce CV risk is not available.

A major problem in studying this topic is that regimes of HRT are selected not for their possible effects on CV risk factors but for convenience of use, relief of menopausal symptoms, prevention of osteoporosis, and avoidance of initiating uterine pathology. This has led to a bewildering variety of regimes and preparations, including single and combined hormone regimes administered by oral, transdermal, intrauterine or implanted routes. As a result, the possible role of HRT in reducing CV risk in postmenopausal women needs to be assessed for several types of regime. This article briefly surveys possible mechanisms of CV risk reduction by gonadal hormones, and reports preliminary results of a study designed to compare different routes and regimes of administration on these risk factors.

Lipoprotein metabolism

Women have lower cholesterol, triglyceride and LDL, and higher HDL levels

---

Address for correspondence: M. Seed, National Heart and Lung Institute, Imperial College School of Medicine, Charing Cross Hospital, London W6 8RF, UK.

until their mid-50s [5]. Oral oestrogen replacement therapy reduces postmenopausal rise in cholesterol and LDL, and overcomes change in HDL [6]. In hyperlipidaemia, the first study of the effect of oral oestrogen showed that the reduction in LDL was greatest in those women with highest LDL levels [7]. HDL concentration was later shown to be inversely related to hormone-sensitive hepatic lipase, the activity of which is reduced by oral oestrogen and increased by androgenic progestogens [8]. A comparison of the effects of HRT and statins in hyperlipidaemic women has shown that such treatments can be combined and are cost-effective [9]. Recently, a comparison of simvastatin and continuous combined oral HRT (oestrogen and medroxyprogesterone acetate MPA) has shown significant reductions in LDL with HRT, though less than with the statin, and with minimal changes in HDL, reflecting the effect of continuous MPA in the hormone-treated group [10]. A number of other studies have shown parenteral to have less effect than oral preparations on lipoprotein metabolism [11].

Carbohydrate metabolism

This is particularly important in women given the greatly increased CHD risk incurred by female diabetics. Oestrogen replacement increases hepatic uptake of insulin and insulin sensitivity. In a community-based study both fasting glucose and insulin levels were lower in women on conjugated equine oestrogen (CEE) but not in those also taking MPA [12]. A study of oral oestrogen replacement in women with non-insulin-dependent diabetes has shown reduced fasting glucose, glycosylated haemoglobin and C-peptide in women, without alteration in fasting insulin [13].

Arterial wall factors

Long-term studies on the effects of gonadal steroids on cynomolgus monkeys has been pivotal in our understanding as arterial wall metabolism and pathology has been accessible. Oestrogen reduces LDL uptake into arterial wall [14].

Doppler ultrasound has shown increased carotid arterial wall compliance with HRT, and animal experiments suggest this is partially due to calcium channel blockade [15].

A number of studies have shown that endothelial function is oestrogen-sensitive; this is particularly important in atherosclerotic vessels [16].

Haemostatic function

The effect of HRT on this important aspect of arterial risk has proved difficult to investigate given the interactions between the many variables and the wide range of normal concentrations. Furthermore the route of administration of HRT appears important. Data from six studies published in the last 2 years can be summarised as follows [17—22]:

- plasminogen activator inhibitor is lowered by oral but not transdermal oestrogen;
- fibrinogen and factor VII are lowered by both oral and transdermal oestrogen;
- factor VII is further lowered by the addition of progestogen;
- antithrombin III is increased by oral HRT; and
- tissue plasminogen activator was reduced, unchanged, or increased in different studies.

The balance of these effects at the low oestrogen dosages used in HRT is towards increased fibrinolysis rather than coagulation. This is in contrast to the prothrombotic effects seen with high-dose oestrogen (e.g., in the oral contraceptive).

The majority of the observational epidemiological studies have been on women taking unopposed oestrogen and the finding of reduced cardiovascular events in such women has been criticised on two counts: 1) that women on HRT are a self-selected healthier population [23], and 2) that added progestogen may be deleterious. However, two recent studies suggest that the use of progestogen together with oestrogen replacement does not impinge on the improvement in cardiovascular events or mortality [24,25]. The majority of women on HRT have not undergone hysterectomy and require the addition of progestogen to protect the endometrium, either cyclically to achieve a regular bleed, or continuously.

The current study is ongoing, and examines the effect both of route of administration and addition of progestogen either cyclically or continuously on selected CV risk factors.

Subjects

Women aged 50—65 years from primary care practices were invited to attend a cardiovascular risk factor lipid clinic at the Charing Cross Hospital. 3,000 women received an invitation; 400 responded, 300 attended the clinic, 100 were recruited as controls and 80 for active therapy. Fifty-three completed the 6-month study on HRT. The study is ongoing.

Nondiabetic, endocrinologically menopausal women aged 50—65 years, without HRT for at least 6 months, were randomised to three HRT regimes or acted as controls. The regimes are: oral cyclical, oral continuous, and transdermal cyclical. Each regime lasts 6 months; for the first 3, oestradiol alone is given by each route; for the second 3 months, norethisterone is added as the progestogen. A further group who had undergone hysterectomy are treated with implants, first oestradiol alone, then oestradiol and testosterone.

Results

Parameters of interest were measured at entry, and at 3 and 6 months. Results to date are summarised in Table 1.

834

Table 1.

Months	Oral (n = 38)			Transdermal (n = 15)			Implant (n = 34)		
	0	3	6	0	3	6	0	3	6
Age	59			58			52		
BMI	26.1	25.4	25.9	25.4	25.2	25.6	25.6	25.8	26.4[c,e]
Oestradiol (pmol/l)	< 50	325[b]	325[b]	< 50	120	185	< 50	343[c]	475[b]
Cholesterol (mmol/l)	6.4	6.0[a]	5.9[a]	6.8	6.3	6.1	6.7	6.2[c]	5.0[c,d]
Triglycerides (mmol/l)	1.1	1.3[a]	1.0[a,d]	1.2	0.9	1.1	1.1	1.0	1.1
HDL (mmol/l)	1.7	1.9[b]	1.6[e]	1.7	1.7	1.6	1.7	1.6	1.6[a]
LDL (mmol/l)	4.2	3.5[c]	3.8[e]	3.8	3.8	3.7	4.4	4.0[b]	3.9[c]
ApoB (g/l)	1.2	1.0[c]	1.0[b]	1.3	1.2	1.1	1.4	1.3[b]	1.2[c,f]
ApoA1 (g/l)	1.6	1.9[a]	1.7[d]	1.6	1.7	1.6	1.6	1.5	1.5
Lp(a) (mg/dl)	12	4[a]	8	6	9	8	8.9	10.1	10.0
Factor VIIc	→	↓[a]	↓[c]	→	→	→			
E-selectin	→	↓[a]	↓[c]	→	→	→			
NO	→	→	↓[a]	→	→	→			

Mean values: cholesterol, HDL, LDL, apoB, apoA1, oestradiol, BMI and age. Median values: triglycerides and Lp(a). Significance values vs. baseline: [a]$p < 0.05$, [b]$p < 0.01$, [c]$p < 0.001$. 6 vs. 3 month value: [d]$p < 0.05$, [e]$p < 0.01$, [f]$p < 0.001$. Control patients (n = 52) showed no change in any parameter. Treatment groups: no change in BP, glucose, insulin and fibrinogen.

Comment

We found no significant change in lipoproteins or haemostatic function in patients on transdermal therapy, possibly due to low numbers. The group on implant (also a parenteral route), showed significant reductions in cholesterol, LDL and apoB, without increase in triglyceride or HDL. The groups on oral therapy showed clear differentiation between the 3 months on oestrogen (E) only and on oestrogen and progestogen (E+P), with increased triglyceride and HDL with E but not with E+P. Cholesterol, LDL and apoB were reduced throughout. The degree of reduction in LDL correlated with initial LDL level and treatment level of oestradiol. The reduction in the vascular endothelial adhesion molecule E-selectin throughout suggests the effect of E on the endothelium is not reduced by the added P. Contrary to experience in the USA, our study does not show that women willing to take hormone replacement therapy are healthier in terms of cardiovascular risk factors than those who do not wish to take it [24].

In conclusion, we have demonstrated changes in lipoproteins in response to oral oestrogen replacement with and without progestogen which would be expected to reduce risk. In terms of lipid lowering, hormone replacement therapy is cost-effective as compared with use of HMG CoA reductase inhibitors and has other useful effects reducing public health costs. However, the recruitment for our study and the uptake of women wishing to start hormone replacement therapy and remain on it illustrate the problems of doing a trial, i.e., getting women to take a hormone without a specific clinical indication and with possible side effects. This may be a problem of motivation in well women as opposed to those with significant risk factors for CHD in whom compliance is improved. In our study, as in others, there is a difficulty in maintaining long-term use of HRT which is needed to accrue cardiovascular risk benefit.

References

1. Bush TL, Barrett-Connor E, Cowan LD, Criqui MH, Wallace RB, Suchindran CM, Tyroler HA, Rifkind BM. Cardiovascular mortality and noncontraceptive use of estrogen in women: results from the Lipid Research Clinics Program Follow-up Study. Circulation 1987;75:1102–1109.
2. Grodstein F, Stampfer M. The epidemiology of coronary heart disease and estrogen replacement in postmenopausal women. Prog Cardiovasc Dis 1995;38:199–210.
3. Randomised trial of cholesterol lowering in 4444 patients with coronary heart disease: the Scandinavian Simvastatin Survival Study (4S). Lancet 1994;344 (8934):1383–1389.
4. Sacks FM, Pfeffer MA, Moye LA, Rouleau JL, Rutherford JD, Cole TG, Brown L, Warnica JW, Arnold JM, Wun CC, Davis BR, Braunwald E. The effect of pravastatin on coronary events after myocardial infarction in patients with average cholesterol levels. Cholesterol and Recurrent Events Trial Investigators. N Engl J Med 1996;335 (14):1001–1009.
5. Heiss G, Tamir I, Davis CE, Tyroler HA, Rifkind BM, Schonfeld G, Jacobs D, Frantz ID Jr. Lipoprotein-cholesterol distributions in selected North American populations: the lipid research clinics program prevalence study. Circulation 1980;61:302–315.
6. Walsh BW, Schiff I, Rosner B, Greenberg L, Ravniker V, Sacks FM. Effects of postmenopausal oestrogen replacement on the concentrations and metabolism of plasma lipoproteins. N Engl J Med 1991;325:1196–1204.
7. Tikkanen MJ, Nikkila EA, Vartiainen E. Natural oestrogen as an effective treatment for type-II hyperlipoproteinaemia in postmenopausal women. Lancet 1978;2:490–491.
8. Tikkanen MJ, Nikkila EA, Kuusi T, Sipinen SU. High density lipoprotein-2 and hepatic lipase: reciprocal changes produced by estrogen and norgestrel. J Clin Endocrinol Metab 1982;54:1113–1117.
9. Seed M, Doherty E. A better strategy than statins in the treatment of postmenopausal hyperlipidaemia? 66th Congress EAS 1996;50.
10. Darling GM, Johns JA, McCloud PI, Davis SR. Estrogen and progestin compared with simvastatin for hypercholesterolemia in postmenopausal women. N Engl J Med 1997;337:595–601.
11. Crook D, Seed M. Endocrine control of plasma lipoprotein metabolism effects of gonadal steroids. (Review) Baillere's Clin Endocrinol Metab 1990;4:851–875.
12. Barrett-Conner E, Laakso M. Ischemic heart disease risk in postmenopausal women. Effects of estrogen use on glucose and insulin levels. Arteriosclerosis 1990;10:531–534.
13. Andersson B, Mattsson LA, Hahn L, Marin P, Lapidus L, Holm G, Bengtsson BA, Bjorntorp P. Estrogen replacement therapy decreases hyperandrogenicity and improves glucose homeostasis and plasma lipids in postmenopausal women with noninsilin-dependent diabetes mellitus. J Clin Endocrinol Metab 1997;82:638–643.
14. Wagner JD, Clarkson TB, St. Clair RW, Schwenke DC, Shively CA, Adams MR. Estrogen and progesterone replacement therapy reduces low density lipoprotein accumulation in the coronary arteries of surgically postmenopausal cynomolgus monkeys. J Clin Invest 1991;88:1995–2002.
15. Gangar KF, Reid BA, Crook D, Hillard TC, Whitehead MI. Oestrogens and atherosclerotic vascular disease — local vascular factors. Baillere's Clin Endocrinol Metab 1993;7:47–59.
16. Collins P, Rosano GM, Sarrell PM, Ulrich L, Adamopoulos S, Beale CM, McNeill JG, Poole-

Wilson PA. 17 beta-Estradiol attenuates acetylcholine-induced coronary arterial constriction in women but not men with coronary heart disease. Circulation 1995;192:24—30.

17. Shahar E, Folsom AR, Salomaa VV, Stinson VL, McGovern PG, Shimakawa T, Chambless LE, Wu KK. Relation of hormone-replacement therapy to measures of plasma fibrinolytic activity. Atherosclerosis Risk in Communities (ARIC) Study Investigators. Circulation 1996;93: 1970—1975.

18. Gilabert J, Estelles A, Cano A, Espana F, Barrachina R, Grancha S, Aznar J, Tortajada M. The effect of estrogen replacement therapy with or without progestogen on the fibrinolytic system and coagulation inhibitors in postmenopausal status. Am J Obstet Gynecol 1995;173: 1849—1854.

19. Koh KK, Mincemoyer R, Bui MN, Csako G, Pucino F, Guetta V, Waclawiw M, Cannon RO. Effects of hormone-replacement therapy on fibrinolysis in postmenopausal women. N Engl J Med 1997;336:683—690.

20. Lindoff C, Peterson F, Lecander I, Martinsson G, Astedt B. Transdermal estrogen replacement therapy: beneficial effects on hemostatic risk factors for cardiovascular disease. Maturitas 1996;24:43—50.

21. Scarabin PY, Vissac AM, Kirzin JM, Bourgeat P, Amiral J, Agher R, Guize L. Population correlates of coagulation factor VII. Importance of age, sex, and menopausal status as determinants of activated factor VII. Arterioscler Thromb Vasc Biol 1996;16:1170—1176.

22. Meade TW. Hormone replacement therapy and haemostatic function. Thromb Haemost 1997; 78:765—769.

23. Mathews KA, Kullar LH, Wing RR. Prior to oestrogen replacement therapy, are users healthier than non-users. Am J Epidemiol 1996;143:971—978.

24. Grodstein F, Stampfer MJ, Manson JE, Colditz GA, Willett WC, Rosner B, Speizer FE, Hennekens CH. Postmenopausal estrogen and progestin use and the risk of cardiovascular disease. N Engl J Med 1996;335:453—461.

25. Falkeborn M, Persson I, Adami HO, Bergstom R, Eaker E, Lithell H, Mohsen R, Naessen T. The risk of acute myocardial infarction after oestrogen and oestrogen-progestogen replacement. Br J Obstet Gynacol 1992;99:821—828.

Hormonal agents used in lowering lipoprotein(a)

Roberta Baetta[1], Fiorenza Bruschi[2], Michele Meschia[2], Piergiorgio Crosignani[2], Rodolfo Paoletti[1] and Maurizio R. Soma[1]

[1]*Institute of Pharmacological Sciences and* [2]*Department of Obstetric and Gynecology, University of Milan, Italy*

Abstract. Lipoprotein(a) (Lp(a)) plasma concentrations in the Caucasian population are classified as a quantitative genetic trait. Although the prevailing view has been that Lp(a) plasma levels are unaffected by age and gender, recent data indicate otherwise. Lp(a) levels change throughout life especially in females after menopause. Lp(a) discriminates CHD cases better in women than in men. In subjects from the ARIC study Lp(a) plasma levels were found to be higher in postmenopausal than in premenopausal women of comparable age while data from the Framingham Offspring Study and our population study refer that Lp(a) values are greater in postmenopause than premenopause, but after controlling for age, this difference disappears. Different sex hormones, namely androgens, estrogen and progestogens, administered alone or in combination lower Lp(a) plasma levels, confirming a direct effect on Lp(a) metabolism. Evidence supports an estrogen influence on Lp(a) synthesis and secretion, as well as catabolism. Regulation of Lp(a) plasma levels by hormone replacement therapy may have clinical relevance since agents able to reduce Lp(a) levels are few or with uncertain effects.

Keywords: estrogen, hormonal replacement therapy, postmenopausal women, progestogen.

Lipoprotein(a) (Lp(a)) is an LDL-like plasma lipoprotein composed of apo B and a large glycoprotein termed apolipoprotein(a) [1−3]. Lp(a) has become a focus of intense research interest because of the epidemiological association of its elevation in plasma with risk for CAD [4] and stroke [5] and because of the striking structural homology between apo(a) and plasminogen. Lp(a) may in fact stand at the crossroads between atherosclerosis and thrombosis.

Aside from the predisposition to CVD, no major physiological function of Lp(a) has been detected thus far. The relative risk of elevated Lp(a) concentrations is significantly increased in patients who also have high levels of LDL cholesterol [2].

The plasma concentration of Lp(a) is mainly determined genetically, however, some common diseases decrease (liver cirrhosis) or increase (renal failure, diabetes) Lp(a) plasma levels [2]. Although the prevailing view has been that Lp(a) plasma levels are unaffected by age and gender, recent data indicate otherwise. Lp(a) levels change throughout life especially in females after menopause [6,7].

Address for correspondence: Maurizio Soma, Institute of Pharmacological Sciences, University of Milan, Via Balzaretti 9, 20133 Milan, Italy. Tel.: +39-2-20488204. Fax: +39-2-29404262.
E-mail: soma@unimi.it

838

Lp(a) discriminates CAD cases better in women than in men [8,9]. We among others reported that different sex hormones, namely androgens, estrogen and progestogen, administered alone or in combination lower Lp(a) plasma levels, confirming a direct effect of sex hormones on Lp(a) metabolism [10–15].

This short review will focus on evidence from prospective and clinical trials of female sex hormones modulation of Lp(a) levels.

Endogenous sex hormones effects on Lp(a) plasma levels

Several publications indicate specific gender differences in Lp(a) plasma concentrations. Lp(a) levels in men and women differ significantly and are influenced by physiological conditions such as pregnancy [16], puberty [17] and menopause [18,19], thus when production of sex hormones are profoundly altered.

Rifai et al. [20] found no gender difference in Lp(a) levels at birth, but a progressive increase in Lp(a) plasma concentration during the first 2 years of life [20]. In the Bogalusa study Lp(a) levels were higher in young females than in young males, in both Blacks and Whites [17]. Lp(a) levels appeared to decrease from age 8–11 years, and rise again between the ages of 11 and 17; however, this trend is significant only in older white females. The gender difference is more evident in adulthood. The first described difference between adult males and females at comparable ages comes from a prospective epidemiological study of company employees in Westfalia [18] in which there was a pronounced positive correlation of age with Lp(a) levels in women, but not in men. These data suggest that endogenous androgens lower Lp(a) concentrations and that endogenous estrogens may theoretically cause a rise in levels, yet several cross-sectional and longitudinal studies have demonstrated that naturally occurring and synthetic estrogens have significant and consistent effect in lowering plasma concentrations of Lp(a). In the same Westfalia study, for example, this rise in Lp(a) was particularly evident in women 40–50 years old, thus at approximately the time of menopause, therefore at estrogen production cessation. In the PROCAM study Lp(a) levels in females continue to rise with age, particularly in the perimenopausal years, while in males they plateau at about 25 years of age [19].

In individuals from the ARIC study [6] Lp(a) plasma levels are found to be higher in postmenopausal than in premenopausal women of comparable age while data from the Framingham Offspring Study [7] refer that Lp(a) values are greater in postmenopause than premenopause, but after controlling for age, this difference disappears.

Based on these conflicting results we investigated the effect of surgical and iatrogen menopause on Lp(a) [12,14]. Surgical menopause causes a sharp rise in plasma Lp(a) concentrations (up to 90 days). Lp(a) levels tend to return to basal value following estrogen treatment (Fig. 1). Menopause induced pharmacologically by LH-RH inhibitors (leuprolide) also increases significantly Lp(a) levels (Fig. 2). These results prove that changes in Lp(a) levels are strictly dependent on the hypoestrogenic state induced by either oophorectomy or drugs and indi-

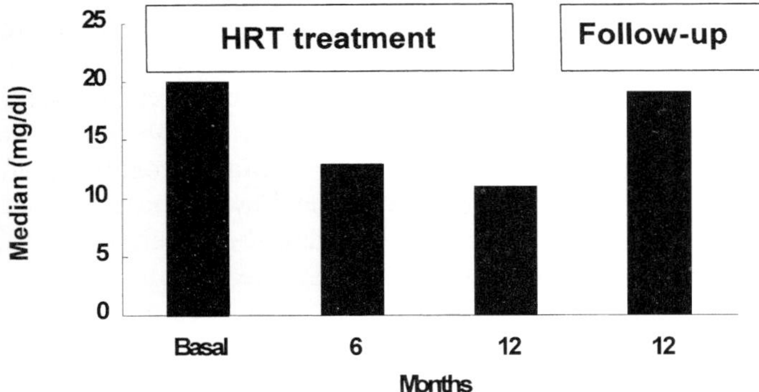

HRT: 1,25 mg CEE + 10 mg cyclic MPA 12 days/months

Fig. 1. Effect of combined HRT on Lp(a).

cate that the higher Lp(a) plasma levels observed in postmenopausal women can be attributed to menopause rather than aging.

Exogenous sex hormones effects on Lp(a) plasma levels

Several groups have reported the influence of sex hormones on Lp(a) plasma levels. In males affected by prostatic cancer estrogen therapy lowers Lp(a) levels by 50%, while orchidectomy treatment slightly increases the plasma concentration of the lipoprotein. Albers et al. [21] reported that stanozolol drastically lowers Lp(a) levels in postmenopausal women. Lp(a) returns to pretreatment levels within 6 weeks after therapy cessation. Crook et al. [22] and we [14] showed similar results with other anabolic steroids such as danazol and gestrinone. A signifi-

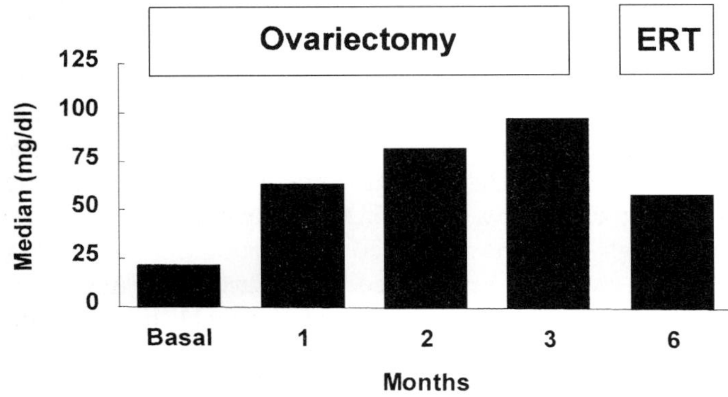

ERT: 0,625 CEE

Fig. 2. Effect of surgical menopause and ERT on Lp(a).

840

cant reduction of Lp(a) was observed in women taking the relatively androgenic progestogen norethisterone [23].

Research on various regimens of postmenopausal hormone replacement, including unopposed estrogen and estrogen plus progesterone, have shown a reduction of 15 to 50% [13,15,24,25]. Also treatments with antiestrogen agents such as tamoxifen decreases plasma levels of Lp(a) in healthy postmenopausal women [26]. Thus overall ERT or HRT treatments confirm the beneficial effect on the basic lipoprotein pattern and demonstrate that these treatments are effective in reducing plasma concentrations of Lp(a) lipoprotein in postmenopausal women.

Conclusions

The mechanisms whereby female sex hormones might affect Lp(a) levels are not well-understood at this time. Estrogen influence hepatic protein and lipid metabolism at multiple regulatory points. Estrogen may influence Lp(a) synthesis and secretion, as well as catabolism.

Recently Zysow et al. [27] investigated the effects of treatment with ethinyl estradiol and progesterone on plasma levels of Lp(a) and liver apo(a) gene expression in ovariectomized female YAC mice transgenic for human apo(a). Estrogen but not progesterone was able to lower plasma Lp(a) by suppressing apo(a) mRNA levels thus suggesting a direct modulation of this hormone on the synthesis of Lp(a) [27]. However, estrogen could also influence Lp(a) by altering the lipoprotein catabolism. Pharmacological doses of estrogen is the most potent way to stimulate hepatic LDL receptor expression in vivo [28]. However, the role of the LDL receptor in the clearance of Lp(a) is still debated and alternative pathways must be considered since in our experience, for example, the Lp(a) decrease is usually more pronounced than that observed for LDL (22 vs. 15% for Lp(a) and LDL, respectively, in [12]) suggesting that different mechanisms are involved in the catabolism of these two plasma lipoproteins. Lp(a) has been reported to form a metastable complex with triglyceride-rich (TG-rich) lipoproteins; this complex could be catabolized through the triglyceride lipoprotein remnant hepatic receptor as supported by previous studies which indicate an inverse relationship between plasma levels of Lp(a) and triglycerides [2]. Oral estrogen consistently increases circulating TG-rich lipoproteins thus potentially increasing Lp(a)-TG-rich lipoprotein complexes. Lp(a) lowering by estrogen could be the results of the catabolism through both the increased number of LDL receptors and the triglyceride lipoprotein remnant hepatic receptor. Furthermore, Harpel and colleagues have recently demonstrated the ability of the VLDL receptor to mediate endocytosis and degradation Lp(a) [29] (Fig. 3).

Because unopposed estrogen replacement therapy increases the risk of endometrial cancer, addition of a progestogen to the therapy is mandatory in nonisterectomized women. The effect of the combined therapy is still controversial since progesterone appears both to counterbalance [25] and act synergistically [11]

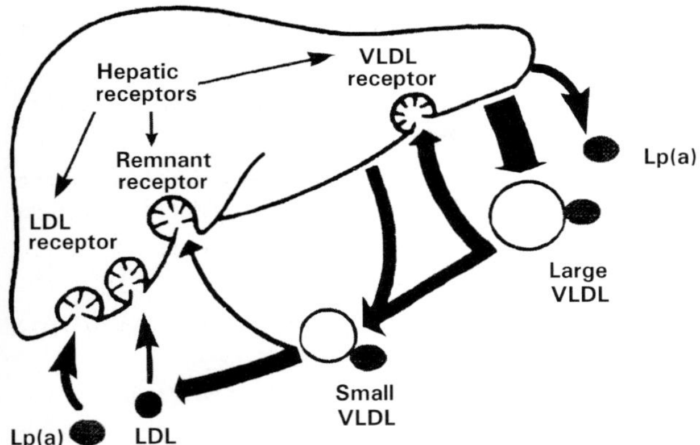

Fig. 3. Lp(a) catabolism: potential mechanisms.

with estrogen to affect lipoprotein(a) plasma levels.

In conclusion, the evidence for a regulatory role of female sex hormones of plasma Lp(a) levels is compelling, even though the effects of sex hormones at the different regulatory points of Lp(a) metabolism remain to be elucidated. Clearly the lack of knowledge about the metabolic regulation of Lp(a) makes impossible any recommendation for clinical practice and hampers the efforts to develop an adequate therapy for lowering serum levels of this lipoprotein. However, regulation of Lp(a) plasma levels by female sex hormones may have clinical relevance since agents able to reduce Lp(a) levels are few or with uncertain effects.

References

1. Scanu AM, Gunther MF. Lipoprotein(a). J Clin Invest 1990;85:1709.
2. Rader DJ, Brewer BH. Lipoprotein(a). Clinical approach to a unique atherogenic lipoprotein. J Am Med Assoc 1992;267:1109.
3. Utermann G. The mysteries of lipoprotein(a). Science 1989;246:904.
4. Rhoads GG, Dahlen G, Berg K, Morton NE, Dannenberg AL. Lp(a) as a risk factor for myocardial infarction. J Am Med Assoc 1986;256:2540.
5. Jurgens G, Koltringer P. Lp(a) in ischemic cerebrovascular disease: a new approach to the assessment of risk for stroke. Neurology 1987;37:513.
6. Nabulsi AA, Folsom AR, White A, Patsch W, Heiss G, Wu KK, Szklo M. Association of hormone-replacement therapy with various cardiovascular risk factors in postmenopausal women. N Engl J Med 1993;328:1069.
7. Jenner JJ, Ordovas JM, Lamon-Fava S, Schaefer MM, Wilson PWF, Castelli WP, Schaefer EJ. Effects of age, sex, and menopausal status on plasma lipoprotein(a) levels. The Framingham offsprings study. Circulation 1993;87:1135.
8. Dahlen GH, Guyton JR, Attar M, Farmer JA, Kautz JA, Gotto AM Jr. Association of levels of lipoprotein Lp(a), plasma lipids, and other lipoproteins with coronary artery disease documented by angiography. Circulation 1986;74:758.

9. Sutton-Tyrrell K, Evans RW, Meilahn E, Alcorn HG. Lipoprotein(a) and peripheral atherosclerosis in older adults. Atherosclerosis 1996;122:11.

10. Soma M, Fumagalli R, Paoletti R, Meschia M, Maini MC, Crosignani P, Ghanem K, Gaubatz J, Morrisett JD. Plasma Lp(a) concentration after oestrogen and progestagen in post-menopausal women. Lancet 1991;337:612.

11. Soma MR, Osnago-Gadda J, Paoletti R, Fumagalli R, Morrisett JD, Meschia M, Crosignani PG. The lowering of lipoprotein(a) induced by estrogen plus progesterone replacement therapy in postmenopausal women. Arch Int Med 1993;153:1462.

12. Bruschi F, Meschia M, Soma M, Perotti D, Paoletti R, Crosignani PG. Lipoprotein(a) and other lipids after oophorectomy and estrogen replacement therapy. Obstet Gynecol 1996;88:950.

13. Soma MR, Meschia M, Bruschi F, Morrisett JD, Paoletti R, Fumagalli R, Crosignani PG. Hormonal agents used in lowering lipoprotein(a). Chem Phys Lipids 1994;67/68:345.

14. The Gestrinone Italian Study Group. Gestrinone versus a gonadotropin releasing hormone agonist for the treatment of the pelvic pain associated with endometriosis: a multicenter, randomized double-blind study. Fertil Steril 1996;66:911.

15. Soma MR, Baetta R, Crosignani PG. The menopause and lipid metabolism: strategies for cardiovascular disease prevention. Curr Opin Lipid 1997;8:229.

16. Zechner R, Desoye G, Schweditsch MO, Pfeiffer KP, Kostner GM. Fluctuations of plasma lipoprotein (a) concentrations during pregnacy and post partum. Metabolism 1986;35:333.

17. Srinivasan SR, Dahlen GH, Jarp RA, Webber LS, Berenson GS. Racial (black-white) differences in serum lipoprotein(a) distribution and its relation to parental myocardial infarction in children. Circulation 1991;84:160.

18. Schriewer H, Assmann G, Sandkamp M, Schulte H. The relationship of lipoprotein(a) (Lp(a)) to risk factors of coronary heart disease: initial results of the prospective epidemiological study on company employees in Westfalia. J Clin Chem Clin Biochem 1984;22:591.

19. Sandkamp M, Assmann G. Lipoprotein(a) in PROCAM participants and young myocardial infarction survivors. In: Scanu AM (ed) Lipoprotein(a): 25 Years of Progress. San Diego: Academic Press, Inc., 1990;205–209.

20. Rifai N, Heiss G, Doetsch K. Lipoprotein(a) at birth, in blacks and whites. Atherosclerosis 1992;92:123.

21. Albers JJ, Taggart HM, Applebaum-Bowden D, Haffner S, Chestnut CH, Hazzard WR. Reduction of lecithin-cholesterol acyltransferase, apolipoprotein D and the Lp(a) lipoprotein with the anabolic steroid stanazolol. Biochim Biophys Acta 1984;795:293.

22. Crook D, Sidhy M, Seed M, O'Donnell M, Stevenson JC. Lipoprotein Lp(a) levels are reduced by danazol, an anabolic steroid. Atherosclerosis 1992;92:41.

23. Farish E, Rolton HA, Barnes JF, Hart DM. Lp(a) concentrations in postmenopausal women taking norethisterone. Br Med J 1991;303:694.

24. Hines C, Chiung T, Chang A, Masarei J, Tomlinson B, Wong E. Effect of oral estradiol on Lp(a) and other lipoproteins in postmenopausal women. Arch Int Med 1996;156:866.

25. Kim CJ, Min YK, Ryu WS, Kwak JW, Ryoo UH. Effect of hormone replacement therapy on lipoprotein(a) and lipid levels in postmenopausal women. Arch Int Med 1996;156:1693.

26. Shewmon DA, Stock JL, Rosen CJ, Heiniluoma KM, Hogue MM, Morrison A, Doyle EM, Ukena T, Weale V, Baker S. Tamoxifen and estrogen lower circulating lipoprotein(a) concentrations in healthy postmenopausal women. Arterioscl Thromb 1994;14:1586.

27. Zysow BR, Kauser K, Lawn RM, Rubanyi GM. Effects of estrus cycle, ovariectomy, and treatment with estrogen, tamoxifen, and progesterone on apolioprotein(a) gene expression in transgenic mice. Arterioscl Thromb Vasc Biol 1997;17:1741.

28. Parini P, Angelin B, Rudling M. Importance of estrogen receptor in hepatic LDL receptor regulation. Arterioscl Thromb Vasc Biol 1997;17:1800.

29. Harpel PC, Argraves KM, Kozarsky KR et al. The human very low density lipoprotein receptor mediates the uptake and degradation of lipoprotein(a). Atherosclerosis 1997;134:15 (Abstract).

HDL reverse cholesterol transport

Structural and functional consequences of nonenzymatic glycation of apolipoprotein A-I and its impact on the reverse cholesterol transport

Carlos Calvo
Department of Clinical Biochemistry and Immunology, University of Concepción, Concepción, Chile

Abstract. Apolipoprotein A-I (apo A-I), the major protein of human high-density lipoproteins (HDL), undergoes a nonenzymatic glycation in diabetic subjects. Nonenzymatic glycation of apoA-I induces a decrease in the stability of the lipid-apolipoprotein interaction and in the apolipoprotein self-association in vitro. Furthermore, glycated apo A-I shows an abnormal association with HDL particles in vivo. These results suggest that the nonenzymatic glycation of apo A-I may affect the structural cohesion of HDL particles. The finding that the preferential site of nonenzymatic glycation of apoA-I is lysine-239, situated on the C-terminal segment, suggests that this modification of lysine in an helical domain locally alters the amphiphilicity of this apolipoprotein.

Nonenzymatic glycation of HDL impairs its recognition by cells and induces a diminished efflux of cholesterol by cell membranes to HDL particles. Moreover, glycated LpA-I particles, isolated from poorly controlled diabetic subjects, were less effective in promoting cholesterol efflux than the nonglycated LpA-I particles.

Finally, glycated apo A-I isolated from diabetic subjects was deficient in its ability to activate lecithin:cholesterol acyltransferase (LCAT). Because LCAT provides a driving force in reverse cholesterol transport by esterifying the cellular cholesterol removed by HDL, this decrease in enzyme reactivity may be associated with a reduction in this process.

Keywords: efflux of cholesterol, glycated apolipoprotein A-I, HDL-structure, LCAT activation.

A significant factor associated with hyperglycaemia in diabetes is the resultant posttraslational nonenzymatic glycation of plasma and cellular proteins. This process which occurs in vivo by direct chemical reaction of glucose with the α- and ε-amino groups of proteins, leads to the loss of charged groups on lysine residues.

It has previously been reported that apo A-I, the major protein constituent of human high-density lipoprotein (HDL), undergoes a nonenzymatic glycation in diabetic subjects [1,2].

This report shows the structural and functional consequences of nonenzymatic glycation of apo A-I and its impact on reverse cholesterol transport process.

Structural consequences

Self-association

In order to study the self-association properties of glycated apo A-I the reversibility of the blue shift of fluorescence in denaturating conditions was measured [3]. The transition of self-associated to monomeric status required less denaturing agent for glycated apo A-I than nonglycated apo A-I. The midpoint for reversing fluorescence shifts were 1.5 and 0.9 M guanidinium chloride (GdmCl), for apo A-I and glycated apo A-I, respectively. These data indicate that the self-association driving force of glycated apo A-I was weaker than that of apo A-I and suggests that the nonenzymatic glycation decreases the stability of the hydrophobicity mediated self-association.

The quenching of tryptophan fluorescence by potassium iodide (KI) was consistent with the concept that the nonenzymatic glycation of apo A-I induces a decrease in the apolipoprotein self-association. The Stern-Volmer constant (Ksv) for apo A-I and glycated apo A-I were 2.0 and 2.6, respectively, demonstrating a better accessibility to water of tryptophan residues in the latter case.

Lipid-binding properties

The affinities of the glycated apo A-I for lipid was measured by monitoring the decrease of the right-angle light scattering of 1-2, di-miristoyl-sn-glycero-3-phosphorylcholine (DMPC) after addition of the apolipoprotein. Although the rates of decrease of DMPC turbidity were not linear, that obtained with nonglycated apo A-I was clearly faster than that observed in the presence of glycated apo A-I.

The effect of the nonenzymatic glycation on the association of apo A-I with HDL in vivo was studied in the rat [4]. The specific tissue distribution volumes obtained after injection of glycated apo A-I was 2- to 3-fold higher in kidney and approximately 30% lower in adrenals and ovaries than that obtained with nonglycated apo A-I. This data indicates that glycated apo A-I behaves differently from the nonglycated apo A-I when injected into rats.

The high uptake of apo A-I by adrenals and ovaries is consistent with previous reports which indicate that HDL are the main suppliers of cholesterol for steroidogenic tissues in the rat. The smaller uptake of glycated apo A-I compared with nonglycated apo A-I in these organs may reflect the diminished association of glycated apo A-I with HDL. These results agree with those of other authors who established that adrenals and ovaries bind to HDL-bound apo A-I [5]. In contrast, the preferential uptake of glycated apo A-I by kidneys cannot be explained by uptake of intact HDL particles, but may rather be attributed to glomerular filtration and tubular reabsorption of apo A-I not associated with HDL. This is consistent with the large amount of free glycated apo A-I detected by gel filtration chromatography in plasma of rats injected with this apolipoprotein. In contrast, plasma of rats injected with nonglycated apo A-I shows that virtually all of the apo A-I was reassociated with HDL and very little free apo A-I was detected.

The mechanism by which the glycation of apo A-I may alter the structural cohesion of HDL particles is not clear. Much evidence has established that lysine appears at the polar nonpolar interface of the amphipathic helical segments of apolipoproteins. Therefore the presence of covalently linked glucose molecules on lysine residues in an amphipathic helical domain of apo A-I could alter the lipid protein interaction.

In a study with synthetic peptides corresponding to the eight tandem repeating 22-mer domains of apo A-I, only the N- and C-terminal peptides (45–65 and 220–241) were effective in clarifying multilamellar vesicles of DMPC. This result suggests that the strong lipid-associating properties of apo A-I are localized to the N- and C-terminal amphipathic domains and that these terminal amphipathic helical domains are involved in the initial binding of apo A-I to the lipid surface to form HDL particles, followed by cooperative binding of the middle six amphipathic helical domains [6].

Extensive glycation may not be required to ensure derivatization of a critical lysine residue. Therefore, if particular lysine residues are preferentially glycated in vivo, then modification of apolipoprotein function could occur with only minor degrees of absolute glycation.

In order to identify the preferential site of nonenzymatic glycation of human apo A-I in vivo we carried out competitive assays with two monoclonal antibodies to human apo A-I, addressed to the N-(CNBr1) and C-(CNBr4) terminal segments, respectively, and other addressed to a conformational epitope. No recognition of the monoclonal antibody addressed to the C-terminal segment was obtained with glycated apo A-I indicating that glycation occurs probably on the C-terminal segment. Moreover, treatment of apo A-I with acetic anhydride only abolished the reactivity of the monoclonal antibody addressed to the C-terminal segment, suggesting that a lysine residue contribute to the epitope recognized by this antibody [7].

Digestion with carboxypeptidase Y showed that glycated and nonglycated apo A-I yield the same four first residues which correspond exactly to the C-terminal sequence of apo A-I (240–243). Moreover, nonglycated apo A-I released 1 mol of lysine per mol of protein. In contrast no liberation of lysine was obtained when the experiment was carried out with glycated apo A-I. Thus, based on these results, we propose that lysine-239 is the preferential site of nonenzymatic glycation of apo A-I. Finally, we hypothesize that this modification in a lysine residue situated in a helical domain of apo A-I alters the amphyphilicity of this apolipoprotein.

Functional consequences

Efflux of cholesterol

The efflux of unesterified cholesterol from cells to acceptor lipoproteins represent the first step in the transport from extrahepatic cells to the liver for excretion, a process termed reverse cholesterol transport.

Previous studies have shown that nonenzymatic glycation of HDL in vitro inhibits high-affinity binding to cultured cells and the candidate of HDL-receptor protein [8]. Based on the HDL-receptor hypothesis of cholesterol efflux the authors proposed that nonenzymatic glycated HDL may have reduced ability to remove excess of cholesterol from extrahepatic cells during reverse cholesterol transport.

Recently it has been demonstrated [9] that glycated-HDL$_3$ has a slightly greater ability than control HDL$_3$ to sequester cholesterol directly from the plasma membrane, as predicted by changes in lipid composition. This process is independent of HDL-receptor binding and should not be influenced by reduced binding of HDL$_3$. In contrast, efflux of intracellular cholesterol from cells, which is HDL-receptor-dependent, was reduced by 25% by nonenzymatic glycation of HDL$_3$ and the efflux of acetylated-LDL-derived ^{3}H-cholesterol from human monocyte-derived macrophage was reduced by 30–40% by nonenzymatic glycation of HDL$_3$. The ability of glycated HDL$_3$ to diminish cholesterol esterification was significantly reduced, indicating reduced net cholesterol efflux. Steady-state efflux of LDL-derived cholesterol was also markedly reduced. These in vitro studies suggest that nonenzymatically glycated HDL$_3$ may have reduced ability to remove cholesterol from extrahepatic cells in vivo.

Because the removal of cholesterol from extrahepatic cells by HDL is believed to be the first step in reverse cholesterol transport, it is possible that nonenzymatic glycation of HDL may be associated with a reduction in this process.

It is now recognized that HDL contains at least two types of apo A-I containing lipoprotein particles that might have different metabolic functions and clinical significance. One species contains as main protein components both apo A-I and apo A-II (Lp A-I:A-II), while in the other apo A-II is absent (Lp A-I) [10,11].

It has been demonstrated that cholesterol efflux from cells is mediated by Lp A-I and not by Lp A-I:A-II and that the lower HDL concentration in coronary artery disease was linked with lower Lp A-I levels, while Lp A-I:A-II was unchanged [12].

When Lp A-I, isolated from poorly controlled insulin-dependent diabetic patients, was compared in its ability to promote cholesterol efflux from cultured adipose cells with the same particles purified from nondiabetic control subjects, no differences were noted between the two types of Lp A-I preparations. In this study the total efflux was only measured without distinguishing between intracellular and plasma membrane origins, and so it is not surprising that Lp A-I particles from diabetic subjects and control subjects were equally effective in producing cholesterol efflux. However, when Lp A-I from poorly controlled diabetic subjects were separated by degree of glycation, the specifically glycated subfractions were about 50% less effective in producing cholesterol efflux than the nonglycated particles [13].

LCAT-activation

The second step in the reverse cholesterol transport process consists of the esterification of cholesterol on the surface of HDL by the enzyme lecithin:cholesterol acyltransferase (LCAT).

The cholesteryl esters formed in the reaction move into the centre of the HDL, leaving the surface of the particle depleted of cholesterol. This creates a concentration gradient which promotes the transfer of cholesterol from cell membranes to HDL.

Apo A-I is the most important LCAT activator. Additionally, apo A-IV, apo C-I and apo E have been shown to activate LCAT in vitro [12].

We tested the ability of glycated apo A-I isolated from diabetic subjects to activate LCAT in vitro. Activation by glycated apo A-I was significantly lower at all concentrations than the activation by nonglycated apo A-I. An increase in Km (5.29 vs. 10.82 μmol/l) and a reduction in both Vmax (4.14 vs. 3.13 nmol/h) and enzyme reactivity, Vmax/Km (0.78 vs. 0.29 nmol $\times$ l/h $\times$ μmol) was observed when glycated apo A-I was used as activator [14]. This decrease in LCAT reactivity suggests that the efficiency of the enzyme towards the substrate was reduced and that this abnormal activation may be associated with a reduction in the reverse cholesterol transport process.

Assays with a panel of monoclonal antibodies addressed to locate specific areas of apo A-I required for LCAT activation show an inhibitory effect with those whose epitopes covered the areas of apo A-I encompassing amino acids 96—174 [15]. This finding suggests that several areas spanning the middle region of apo A-I may act in unison to stimulate LCAT activity, possibly by cooperative interaction with the enzyme.

Since glycation does not involve lysine residues located in the LCAT-activating domain in apo A-I, differences observed in LCAT activities could be related to progressive changes in apo A-I conformation due to nonenzymatic glycation.

In summary, although it is difficult to extrapolate from in vitro studies to in vivo systems, findings in all these studies suggest that glycated apo A-I may be structurally and functionally abnormal.

Acknowledgements

This study was supported in part by grant 90-0274 from FONDECYT and grant 20.72.04 from the University of Concepción, Chile. This work was also supported by a grant from INSERM U-197, France.

References

1. Calvo C, Ponsin G, Berthezene F. Characterization of the non-enzymatic glycation of high density lipoprotein in diabetic patients. Diabet Metab 1988;14:264—269.
2. Curtis LK, Witztum JL. Plasma apolipoprotein A-I, A-II, B, C-I and E are glycosilated in hyperglycemic diabetic subjects. Diabetes 1985;34:452—461.
3. Calvo C, Talussot C, Ponsin G, Berthezene F. Non-enzymatic glycation of apolipoprotein A-I. Effects on its self-association and lipid binding properties. Biochem Biophys Res Commun 1988;153:1060—1067.
4. Calvo C, Verdugo C. Association in vivo of glycated apolipoprotein A-I with high density lipo-

proteins. Eur J Clin Chem Clin Biochem 1992;30:3—5.

5. Ponsin G, Sparrow JT, Gotto AM, Pownal H. In vivo interaction of synthetic acylated apopeptides with high density lipoprotein in rat. J Clin Invest 1986;77:559—567.

6. Palgunachari MN, Mishra VK, Lund-Katz S, Phillips MC, Adeyeye SO, Alluri S, Anantharamaiah GM, Segrest JP. Only the two end helixes of eight tandem amphipathic helical domain of human apo A-I have significant lipid affinity. Arterioscler Thromb Vasc Biol 1996;16: 328—338.

7. Calvo C, Ulloa N, Campos M, Verdugo C, Ayrault-Jarrier M. The preferential site of non-enzymatic glycation of human apolipoprotein A-I in vivo. Clin Chim Acta 1993;217:193—198.

8. Duell PB, Oram JF, Bierman EL. Nonenzymatic glycosylation of HDL resulting in inhibition of high-affinity binding to cultured human fibroblasts. Diabetes 1990;39:1257—1263.

9. Duell PB, Oram JRF, Bierman EL. Nonenzymatic glycosylation of HDL and impaired HDL-receptor-mediated cholesterol efflux. Diabetes 1991;40:377—384.

10. Cheung MC, Albers JJ. Characterization of lipoprotein particles isolated by immunoaffinity chromatography: particles containing AI and AII particles and particles containing AI but no AII. J Biol Chem 1984;256:12201—12209.

11. Calvo C, Bustos P, Sepúlveda J, Ulloa N, Sepúlveda V. Development of monoclonal antibodies for the selective isolation of human plasma apolipoprotein A-containing particles. Hybridoma 1995;14:603—608.

12. Tailleux A, Fruchart JC. HDL heterogeneity and atherosclerosis. Crit Rev Clin Lab Sci 1996;33: 163—201.

13. Fievet C, Theret N, Shojaee N, Duchateau P, Castro G, Ailhaud G, Drouin P, Fruchart JC. Apolipoprotein A-I-containing particles and reverse cholesterol transport in IDDM. Diabetes 1992;41:81—85.

14. Calvo C, Ulloa N, Del Pozo R, Verdugo C. Decreased activation of lecithin:cholesterol acyltransferase by glycated apolipoprotein A-I. Eur J Clin Chem Clin Biochem 1993;31:217—220.

15. Uboldi P, Spoladore M, Fantappie S, Marcovina S, Catapano AL. Localization of apolipoprotein A-I epitopes involved in the activation of lecithin:cholesterol acyltransferase. J Lipid Res 1996;37:2557—2568.

Caveolin-dependent free cholesterol efflux

Christopher J. Fielding[1], Phoebe E. Fielding[2] and Anita Bist[1]
Cardiovascular Research Institute and Departments of [1]Physiology and [2]Medicine, University of California Medical Center, San Francisco, California, USA

Introduction

It has recently become clear that multiple mechanisms contribute to cellular cholesterol homeostasis. In addition to the well-known pathways involving low-density lipoprotein (LDL) receptor-mediated endocytosis and cholesterogenesis [1] additional contributors more recently described include the selective uptake of cholesteryl esters from HDL via SR-B1 receptors [2] and of free cholesterol (FC) from LDL [3].

Most peripheral tissues in vivo synthesize no bile acids, steroid hormones of plasma lipoproteins. The mitotic rate is very low. Similar conditions can be reproduced in confluent monolayers of many peripheral cells, including fibroblasts, vascular smooth muscle cells and endothelial cells. These cells have little demand for new cholesterol. Nevertheless when labeled to equilibrium with isotopically labeled FC, these cells demonstrate a rapid rate of FC efflux. Total FC mass remains unchanged [3]. It follows there must be an equivalent and opposite influx of unlabeled cholesterol from plasma lipoproteins into the cell. Most vascular cells express only very low levels of cell surface LDL and SR-B1 receptors. Cholesterol influx via these pathways can be calculated to contribute only a few percent of the required rate of total influx. Until recently it was often assumed that the residuum reflected a passive, probably diffusional exchange of plasma membrane FC between the cell surface and plasma lipoproteins. New data of several kinds now makes this explanation unlikely, at least as a major contributor to FC homeostasis. Very little plasma membrane FC was found to be directly accessible to the extracellular medium. Most FC entering the cell delivered from LDL. Following intracellular transport that included several different membrane compartments; FC that returned to the cell surface was transferred mostly to HDL, particularly its small, lipid-poor pre-β-migrating fraction [3]. In quiescent peripheral cells, the majority of FC entering the cell may originate from LDL-FC.

Address for correspondence: Christopher J. Fielding, Cardiovascular Research Institute and Departments of Physiology, University of California Medical Center, San Francisco, CA 94143, USA.

The LDL-FC recycling pathway

Selective LDL-FC internalization was independent of the presence of LDL receptors. Its rate was similar in LDL-receptor-deficient and normal cells. Several pieces of evidence suggest that LDL-derived FC enters the cell as part of the endocytic mechanism involving clathrin-coated pits. Hyperosmotic and K^+-free media, which selectively inhibit this pathway, proportionately reduced the uptake into human skin fibroblasts of ^{3}H-FC from LDL and ^{125}I-transferrin, a ligand internalized exclusively via clathrin-coated pits in these cells. FC and transferrin subsequently colocalized with clathrin in dense vesicles following density-gradient fraction of cell homogenates fractionated at ice temperature. Subsequently the label was identified in a lighter vesicle fraction comigrating with protein markers of the *trans*-Golgi network. Finally, after 3—5 min, label was recovered in a plasma membrane fraction enriched with caveolin, the structural protein of caveolae [4]. These data provide support for the hypothesis that LDL-derived FC, like newly synthesized FC, and FC from cholesteryl esters internalized by the LDL receptor pathway, is transported intracellularly. LDL-derived C would be available, along with FC from other sources, in regulating cholesterogenesis and potentially, FC efflux.

FC and caveolae

Caveolin is a major structural protein of caveolae, which are clathrin-free invaginations, 60—80 nm in diameter, at the surface of many cells [5]. Caveolae and caveolin are particularly enriched in quiescent peripheral cells. Caveolae were downregulated in cells FC-depleted with lipoprotein-deficient plasma [6]. Cells actively involved in FC catabolism, such as hepatocytes, adrenal and gonadal cells, have few caveolae and relatively high levels of LDL-receptors and/or SR-B1 receptors. Oncogenic transformation of fibroblasts led to a reduction in the expression of caveolae and an upregulation of LDL receptors [7]. Caveolae are FC-rich, relative to the rest of the plasma membrane, but only FC associated with caveolae was accessible to cholesterol oxidase in unfixed fibroblast monolayers [8]. This probably indicates that in caveolae, FC is located within, or accessible to, the exofacial leaflet of the plasma membrane bilayer. Caveolin may be present in caveolae in the form of a looped polypeptide whose N- and C-termini extend into the cytoplasm, and whose central, hydrophobic domain extends between the exofacial and cytofacial leaflets of the bilayer [9]. These data suggested that the expression of caveolin and caveolae might be linked to cell FC homeostasis. Caveolin-1 was the first member identified in the caveolin family, and is a major protein component of cell surface caveolae in peripheral cells. Caveolin-1 was chosen as a possible target for regulatory control by FC.

Regulation of the expression of caveolin

A full-length caveolin cDNA was cloned from a human lung library. Its sequence was consistent with previously published data with the exception of three single-base modifications [10]. Following end-labeling, the cDNA was used as a probe of the relative concentration of caveolin mRNA in cells exposed to different concentrations of LDL, isolated or in native plasma. Studies were also carried out using plasma from which LDL had been removed by affinity chromatography on heparin-agarose. Following electrophoresis on 1% agarose/formaldehyde gels, RNA was transferred to nylon membranes, and hybridized with ^{32}P-caveolin cDNA. Annexin-2 and GAPD probes were used as internal controls.

Fibroblast monolayers were transferred from 10% plasma-DME medium to medium containing 80% plasma, LDL at 80% plasma concentration, or 80% plasma from which LDL had been removed. Over 3 h at 37°C, there was a 4- to 6-fold increase in caveolin mRNA levels, without change in the concentration of internal "housekeeping" control mRNAs, with plasma or purified LDL. No change, or a decrease in caveolin mRNA levels, was observed with plasma-LDL. FC efflux was measured in fibroblast monolayers pre-equilibrated with 1,2-^{3}H-FC, treated under identical conditions. FC efflux increased in proportion to the expression of caveolin mRNA. Incubation of cells with 10 or 80% lipoprotein-deficient plasma decreased caveolin mRNA levels 4- to 5-fold below baseline (10% plasma) values. When fibroblast monolayers were transfected with caveolin antisense-DNA, an equivalent decrease in FC efflux was observed (-42 vs. -47%). Finally, when fibroblasts were treated with several oxysterol inhibitors of intracellular FC transport there was an equivalent decrease in caveolin mRNA levels and FC efflux. Together these data suggested a relationship between the expression of caveolin mRNA and cellular FC homeostasis, mediated at the level of FC efflux.

Regulation of caveolin gene transcription

About 1 kB of 5′-flanking sequence of caveolin genomic cDNA was cloned and sequenced, together with exon 1, intron 1, exon 2 and part of intron 2 [11]. Rapid amplification of DNA ends was used to identify alternative transcriptional start sites at -62 and -106 bp, relative to the ATG translational start site (+1 bp). The promoter sequence also included a consensus Sp1 site at -148 bp, and three other G/C-rich boxes showing sequence homology with sterol regulatory elements (SREs) in the HMGCoa reductase and LDL receptor protein gene promoters. Transcriptional regulation requires the interaction of these sequences with an SRE-binding protein (SREBP). The caveolin SRE-like sequences were located at -287, -396 and -646 bp in the promoter sequence of this gene.

Three DNA promoter fragments were prepared by deletional mutagenesis, in each of which one of these sequences had been excised. These were ligated to the pGL3 luciferase gene expression vector. Wild-type promoter was ligated into pGL3 in the forward and reverse directions. Each construct was then transiently expressed in fibroblast monolayers incubated in 10 or 80% plasma medium. Cotransfection with pSV-β-galactosidase expression vector was carried out to provide an internal control.

Cells transfected with caveolin wild-type promoter stimulated luciferase expression by 5- to 6-fold. (Promoter with the wild-type promoter in the reverse orientation was without activity.) Caveolin promoter from which either the -646 or -395 bp G/C-rich site had been removed showed little or no increase in expression in 7% (vs. 80%) plasma, while the mutant promoter in which the -287 bp G/C-rich box had been excised was fully active. These data indicated that two (of three) SRE-like G/C-rich sites were required for FC to stimulate caveolin transcription.

Gel-shift analysis was carried out to obtain further information on transcription factors binding to these "essential" promoter sites. DNA fragments including either SRE-like sequence were end-labeled with ^{32}P. The labeled oligonucleotide was then incubated with the total protein of purified fibroblast nuclei. Incubations were carried out in the presence or absence of antibodies to SREBP-1 or Sp-1, a transcription factor also reactive with G/C rich promoter sequences. Successful binding of antibody to transcription protein would be indicated by a "supershift" after electrophoresis, in which labeled DNA was further separated from the corresponding labeled protein-DNA complex formed in the absence of antibody. A supershift was obtained with anti-SREBP-1 with the -395 bp G/C-rich labeled oligonucleotide. No supershift shift was obtained with anti-Sp-1. No supershift was obtained with either antibody with the -646 bp oligonucleotide. These data suggest that the effect of FC on caveolin was mediated in part by transcription factor SREBP-1, binding at -395 bp. It was also mediated by the reaction of a transcription factor, as yet unidentified, binding at -646 bp.

Overall, the study suggests that transcription of the caveolin gene, like the genes for LDL receptor protein, HMGCoA reductase, and several other genes of cholesterogenesis, is mediated by SREBPs [12–15]. Caveolin appears to play an important role in the regulation of cell cholesterol content, presumably by regulating FC efflux. The role of SREBP-1 as a key regulator not only of FC synthesis and influx, but now also of FC efflux, is suggested.

Acknowledgements

This research was supported by the National Institutes of Health via HL 14237 and HL 57976.

References

1. Brown MS, Goldstein JL. A receptor-mediated pathway for cholesterol homeostasis. Science 1985;232:34–47.
2. Acton S, Rigotti A, Landschulz KT, Xu S, Hobbs HH, Krieger MM. Identification of scavenger

receptor SR-B1 as a high density lipoprotein receptor. Science 1996;271:518—520.

3. Fielding CJ, Fielding PE. Role of an N-ethylmaleimide-sensitive factor in the selective cellular uptake of low density lipoprotein free cholesterol. Biochemistry 1995;34:14237—14244.

4. Fielding PE, Fielding CJ. Intracellular transport of low density lipoprotein-derived free cholesterol begins at clathrin-coated pits and terminates at cell surface caveolae. Biochemistrty 1996; 35:14932—14938.

5. Dupree P, Parton RG, Raposo G, Kurzchalia TV, Simons K. Caveolae and sorting in the trans-Golgi network. EMBO J 1993;12:1597—1604.

6. Chang WJ, Rothberg KG, Kamen BA, Anderson RGW. Lowering the cholesterol content of MA104 cells inhibits receptor-mediated transport of folate. J Cell Biol 1992;118:63—69.

7. Koleske A, Baltimore D, Lisanti MP. Reduction of caveolae and caveolin in oncogenically transformed cells. Proc Natl Acad Sci USA 1995;92:1381—1385.

8. Smart EJ, Ying YS, Conrad PA, Anderson RGW. Caveolin moves from caveolae to the Golgi apparatus in response to cholesterol oxidation. J Cell Biol 1994;127:1185—1197.

9. Parton RA, Simons K. Digging into caveolae. Science 1995;269:1398—1399.

10. Fielding CJ, Bist A, Fielding PE. Caveolin mRNA levels are upregulated by free cholesterol and downregulated by oxysterols in fibroblast monolayers. Proc Natl Acad Sci USA 1997;94: 3753—3758.

11. Bist A, Fielding PE, Fielding CJ. Two sterol regulatory element-like sequences mediate up-regulation of caveolin gene transcription in response to low density lipoprotein free cholesterol. Proc Natl Acad Sci USA 1997;94:10693—10698.

12. Yokoyama C, Wang X, Briggs MR, Admon A, Wu J, Hua X, Goldstein JL, Brown MS. SREBP-1, a basic-helix-loop-helix-leucine zipper protein than controls transcription of the low density lipoprotein receptor gene. Cell 1993;75:187—197.

13. Vallett SM, Sanchez HB, Rosenfeld JM, Osborne TF. A direct role for sterol regulatory element binding protein in activation of 3-hydroxy-3-methylglutaryl coenzyme A reductase gene. J Biol Chem 1996;271:12247—12253.

14. Ericsson J, Jackson SM, Lee BC, Edwards PA. Sterol regulatory element binding protein binds to a cis element in the promoter of the farnesyl diphosphate synthase gene. Proc Natl Acad Sci USA 1996;93:945—950.

15. Guan G, Jiang G, Koch RL, Schechter I. Molecular cloning and functional analysis of the human squalene synthase gene. J Biol Chem 1995;270:21958—21965.

Is plasma HDL concentration rate-limiting for reverse cholesterol transport?

Norman E. Miller
Department of Cardiovascular Biochemistry, St Bartholomew's and the Royal London School of Medicine and Dentistry, London, UK

Abstract. Plasma high-density lipoprotein (HDL) concentration is a major risk factor for atherosclerosis in humans, and there is strong experimental evidence that HDLs and apolipoprotein (apo) A-I retard atherogenesis in animals. Although it is well-established that HDLs play a central role in reverse cholesterol transport, it is not yet clear that this explains their antiatherogenic activity. Although plasma HDL concentration can be rate-limiting for cholesterol efflux from cultured cells, more work is needed to determine whether or not this is also true in vivo.

Keywords: apolipoprotein A-I, atherosclerosis, lipids, phospholipid.

Plasma high-density lipoprotein (HDL) concentration is a major risk factor for atherosclerosis in humans. Studies in transgenic animals [1,2] and in animals infused with HDLs [3] have provided unequivocal evidence that HDLs are directly antiatherogenic. It is now also well-established that the HDLs play a central role in the transport of cholesterol from peripheral tissues to the liver (reverse cholesterol transport, RCT). However, other mechanisms unrelated to the function of HDLs in RCT might be responsible for their antiatherogenicity [4,5]. Theoretically, variations in plasma HDL cholesterol could reflect changes not only in RCT, but also in the transfer of cholesterol from triglyceride-rich lipoproteins to HDLs, transfer of cholesteryl esters (CEs) in the reverse direction, reduced catabolism of HDL particles and/or reduced transfer of CEs from HDLs to the liver [6]. Thus, although HDL concentration can be rate-limiting for cholesterol efflux from cultured cells [7,8], it is not certain that this is also true in vivo, when RCT is a more complex dynamic process with extravascular, intravascular and intrahepatic components [9]. The rate-limiting step for RCT in vivo is not known, and in particular the extent to which plasma HDL concentration influences the efficiency of the process is unclear. Studies in cholesteryl ester transfer protein transgenic mice have shown that, in that species at least, variations in plasma HDL cholesterol do not necessarily reflect concordant changes in cholesterol flux from tissues [10]. The problem is compounded by the fact that there is no accepted method for quantifying cholesterol transport from tis-

---

Address for correspondence: Prof Norman E. Miller, Department of Cardiovascular Biochemistry, St Bartholomew's and the Royal London School of Medicine and Dentistry, Charterhouse Square, London EC1M 6BQ, UK.

sues in vivo. One approach might be to acutely load peripheral tissues with cholesterol, and then to quantify the rate of release of cholesterol into plasma. Two potential models are available [11,12], but neither has yet been applied to study RCT in relation to genetic, physiologic or pharmacologic changes in HDL concentration. Complex multicompartmental models of plasma cholesterol specific radioactivity: time curves may be informative, but involve many assumptions of uncertain validity [13]. Preliminary work on long-term peripheral lymph collections in humans offers promise for quantifying changes in RCT, particularly when combined with labelling of peripheral tissues with radioactive cholesterol [14]. However, the only information in humans of direct relevance to date has been provided by studies of the effects of intravenous infusion of apo A-I or reconstituted HDLs. When Nanjee et al. infused lipid-free apo A-I (Swiss Red Cross, Bern, Switzerland) into healthy men, no increase in plasma HDL cholesterol concentration was recorded [15]. However, no conclusions regarding the effects of lipid-free apo A-I on RCT could be drawn, as the infusions produced major increases in plasma triglycerides, apparently due to combined inhibition of hepatic lipase and lipoprotein lipase activities. Subsequent studies by the same group showed that intravenous infusion of apo A-I/phosphatidylcholine discs (Swiss Red Cross, Bern, Switzerland) resembling nascent HDLs, increased plasma HDL cholesterol concentration before any significant effect on plasma triglycerides [16]. Increases were also observed in non-HDL CEs. These changes in lipids were associated with increases in plasma pre-β HDLs, the putative primary acceptor of cell-derived cholesterol [7]. Studies in vitro, using incubations of whole blood or plasma, showed that the new HDL cholesterol could not have been derived from circulating erythrocytes. Thus, these results provided the first evidence in vivo that plasma HDL concentration might be rate-limiting for RCT. In a third study by the same group intravenous infusion of recombinant pro-apo A-I/phosphatidylcholine discs (UCB Pharma, Brussels) produced similar changes in plasma, and also increased the cholesterol concentration, pre-β HDL concentration and cholesterol specific radioactivity in peripheral lymph [14].

In summary, the extent to which plasma HDL concentration determines the efficiency of RCT in vivo is unresolved, and more work is needed both in humans and in animals. However, recent studies in humans have supported the notion that at least under some circumstances the circulating concentration of apo A-I containing lipoproteins, and in particular the pre-β HDL subclass, may have a significant impact on the efficiency with which cholesterol is cleared from tissues.

References

1. Rubin EM, Krauss RM, Spangler EA, Verstuyft JG, Clift SM. Inhibition of early atherogenesis in transgenic mice by human apolipoprotein AI. Nature 1991;353:265–267.
2. Paszty C, Maeda N, Verstuyft J, Rubin EM. Apolipoprotein AI transgene corrects apolipoprotein E deficiency-induced atherosclerosis in mice. J Clin Invest 1994;94:899–903.

3. Badimon JJ, Badimon L, Fuster V. Regression of atherosclerotic lesions by high density lipoprotein plasma fraction in the cholesterol-fed rabbit. J Clin Invest 1990;85:1234—1241.
4. Cockerill GW, Rye K-A, Gamble JR, Vadas MA, Barta PJ. High density lipoproteins inhibit cytokine-induced expression of endothelial cell adhesion molecules. Arterioscler Thromb Vasc Biol 1995;15:1987—1994.
5. Watson AD, Berliner JA, Hama SY, La Du BN, Full KF, Fogelman AM, Navab M. Protective effect of high density lipoprotein associated paraoxonase. J Clin Invest 1995;96:2882—2891.
6. Miller NE. Reverse cholesterol transport. In: Born GVR, Schwartz CJ (eds) New Horizons in Coronary Heart Disease. London: Science Press, 1993;8.1—8.9.
7. Kawano M, Miida T, Fielding CJ, Fielding PE. Quantitation of pre-beta-HDL-dependent and nonspecific components of the total efflux of cellular cholesterol and phospholipid. Biochemistry 1993;32:5025—5028.
8. De la Llera Moya, Atger V, Pool JL, Fournier N, Moatti N, Giral P, Friday K, Rothblat G. A cell culture system for screening human serum for ability to promote cellular cholesterol efflux. Arterioscler Thromb 1994;14:1056—1065.
9. Miller NE. Disorders of HDL metabolism: clues to the pathophysiology of reverse cholesterol transport. In: Carson LA (ed) Disorders of HDL. London: Smith-Gordon & Co., Ltd., 1990; 1—6.
10. Osono Y, Woollett LA, Marotti KR, Melchior GW, Dietschy JM. Centripetal cholesterol flux from extrahepatic organs to the liver is independent of the concentration of high density lipoprotein cholesterol in plasma. Proc Natl Acad Sci USA 1996;93;4114—4119.
11. Miller NE, La Ville A, Crook D. Direct evidence that reverse cholesterol transport is mediated by high density lipoprotein in rabbit. Nature 1985;314:109—111.
12. Stein O, Dabach Y, Hollander G, Ben-Naim M, Halperin G, Okon E, Stein Y. Cholesterol efflux in vivo from a depot of cationized LDL injected into a thigh muscle of small rodents. Atherosclerosis 1997;133:15—22.
13. Schwartz CC, Berman M, Vlahcevic ZR, Halloran LG, Gregory DH, Swell L. Multi-compartmental analysis of cholesterol metabolism in men. J Clin Invest 1978;61:408—423.
14. Nanjee MN, Cook CJ, Olszewski WL, Miller NE. Regulation of pre-beta high density lipoproteins in human tissue fluids in vivo. Circulation (In press) (Abstract).
15. Nanjee MN, Crouse JR, King JM, Hovorka R, Rees SE, Carson ER, Morgenthaler JJ, Lerch P, Miller NE. Effects of intravenous infusion of lipid-free apolipoprotein A-I in humans. Arterioscler Thromb Vasc Biol 1996;16:1203—1214.
16. Nanjee MN, Miller NE. Effects of intravenous apolipoprotein A-I/phosphatidylcholine discs in humans. Circulation 1996;94(Suppl 1):1—463 (Abstract).

High-density lipoproteins and cellular cholesterol efflux

Michael C. Phillips, Kristin Gillotte, Sissel Lund-Katz, William Johnson and George Rothblat
Department of Biochemistry, Allegheny University of the Health Sciences, MCP/Hahnemann School of Medicine, Philadelphia, Pennsylvania, USA

Abstract. High-density lipoprotein (HDL) particles and their principal protein component, apolipoprotein (apo) A-I, can mediate efflux of cellular cholesterol. There is a bidirectional flux of unesterified cholesterol molecules between the plasma membrane of cells and HDL particles in the extracellular medium. Net efflux of cholesterol mass from the cells involves passive diffusion of cholesterol molecules through the aqueous phase and down their concentration gradient between the membrane and HDL; the concentration gradient is maintained by lecithin-cholesterol acyltransferase (LCAT)-mediated esterification of cholesterol molecules in the HDL particles. Fully lipidated apo A-I in HDL particles is important in promoting this "aqueous diffusion" mechanism because: 1) it has solubilized phospholipid into small HDL-sized particles that are efficient at absorbing cholesterol molecules diffusing away from the cell surface; and 2) it can act as a cofactor for LCAT. In contrast, incompletely lipidated apo A-I molecules are able to acquire more lipid by solubilizing phospholipid and cholesterol directly from the plasma membrane of cells. This "membrane-microsolubilization" process is enhanced by enrichment of cells with cholesterol and is the mechanism by which pre-β HDL particles in the extracellular medium remove cholesterol and phospholipid from cells.

Introduction

The efflux of cholesterol from the plasma membranes of peripheral cells to high-density lipoprotein (HDL) is the first step in reverse cholesterol transport (for a review, see [1]). Promotion of this step is antiatherogenic because of the reduced possibility of overaccumulation of cholesterol in peripheral cells such as those in the walls of blood vessels. Apo A-I is the primary protein of HDL and, as expected from the above observations, is antiatherogenic. This effect has been demonstrated by the observation that transgenic mice expressing very high levels of human apo A-I have fewer atherosclerotic lesions than control mice [2]. More than 90% of HDL particles in human plasma contain apo A-I and the apo A-I molecules can recycle between lipid-associated and lipid-free (poor) pools as HDL particles are remodelled and change size [3]. The mechanisms by which these two pools of apo A-I remove cholesterol from cells are different. Fully lipidated apo A-I in HDL particles removes cell cholesterol by an "aqueous diffusion" mechanism whereas lipid-free (poor) apo A-I removes cell cholesterol by a "membrane microsolubilization" process. Interaction of HDL with the scavenger

---

Address for correspondence: Michael C. Phillips, Department of Biochemistry, Allegheny University of the Health Sciences, MCP/Hahnemann School of Medicine, 2900 Queen Lane, Philadelphia, PA 19129 USA.

receptor (SR)-B1 can promote cell cholesterol efflux [4]. In this article, we summarize the mechanisms of the aqueous diffusion and membrane microsolubilization processes, with emphasis on the roles of apo A-I.

Fully lipidated apo A-I as an acceptor of cell cholesterol

The fully lipidated apo A-I molecules in either discoidal or spherical HDL particles associate with phospholipid (PL) via their amphipathic α-helices [5]. Mature HDL_2 and HDL_3 particles participate in a bidirectional flux of free cholesterol (FC) molecules between the lipoprotein and cells with the direction of net transfer of cholesterol mass being determined by the gradient in cholesterol concentration [1,6]. This exchange or transfer of FC occurs by a so-called aqueous diffusion mechanism in which cholesterol molecules desorb from the donor lipid-water interface and diffuse through the intervening aqueous layer until they collide with and are absorbed by an acceptor particle. The rate of cholesterol exchange or transfer is first order with respect to the concentration of FC in the donor particle and is strongly temperature-dependent. The rate constant for cholesterol transfer is about an order of magnitude greater than that for PL transfer [6].

More rapid FC efflux occurs when the PL acceptor in the extracellular medium is dispersed as small particles [6]. Thus, the same concentration of PL present as a discoidal HDL particle causes faster efflux than when it is present as small unilamellar vesicles [7]. The amphipathic α-helical segments in the apo A-I molecule [5] can interact with PL molecules to create small HDL particles that are efficient at absorbing cholesterol molecules as they diffuse away from the cell surface. The general amphipathic nature of the α-helices rather than the specific amino acid sequences are important in the FC efflux process. Thus, reconstituted discoidal HDL particles containing synthetic α-helical peptides with no sequence homology to apo A-I can sustain cell cholesterol efflux [8]. Consistent with this, engineered apo A-I molecules containing deletions of helical segments in the N-terminal, central and C-terminal domains all form discoidal HDL particles with similar abilities to mediate cell FC efflux [9]. It follows that a key structural feature of apo A-I required for promoting FC efflux by the aqueous diffusion mechanism is the presence of amphipathic helical segments that stabilize small HDL-sized particles. Another important feature of the apo A-I molecule is its ability to activate LCAT [10].

Incompletely lipidated apo A-I as an acceptor of cell cholesterol

Approximately 5% of the apo A-I in human plasma exists in a lipid-free (poor) pool [11,12] which exhibits pre-β mobility on agarose gel electrophoresis. This pool of incompletely lipidated apo A-I is created by remodelling of HDL particles, in particular by the reduction in particle size due to the actions of cholesteryl ester transfer protein and hepatic lipase [3]. Some of this apo A-I is thought to reassociate with HDL particles as they increase in size due to the activity of LCAT. The lipid-free apo A-I in the pre-β HDL pool can also diffuse from the plasma compartment into the interstitial space where it can promote efflux of cholesterol from peripheral cells [3,11]. In agreement with these ideas, the pre-β pool of apo A-I is preferred over fully lipidated apo A-I in spherical HDL particles as the acceptor of cell cholesterol when fibroblasts are incubated with plasma for 1 min [11]. It is now well-established that lipid-free apo A-I can remove FC and PL from cells (for a review, see [13]).

Enrichment of cells with cholesterol can stimulate apo A-I-mediated release of PL and FC. To test the hypothesis that cellular PL may contribute to HDL structure and the removal of sterol from cells, the efflux of [^{3}H]FC and [^{32}P]PL from control and cholesterol-enriched fibroblasts to apolipoproteins has been examined [14]. Strikingly, enrichment of cells with FC enhances the efflux of both PL and FC to human apo A-I over a 24-h period. Doubling the cell cholesterol content increases the fractional efflux of both lipids by 5- to 7-fold. Several classes of PL are released but PC accounts for 70% of the total PL released from cholesterol-enriched fibroblasts. The reasons for this stimulation remain to be established. A possible explanation is that the plasma membrane content of cholesterol-rich domains such as caveolae is increased [15]; the poorly lipidated apo A-I (pre-β HDL) may preferentially access this pool in the plasma membrane [16]. The molecular mechanism by which apo A-I causes efflux of cell PL and FC probably involves interaction with plasma membrane domains [11,17] but the nature of the binding site is not known. Apolipoprotein/membrane PL and apolipoprotein/membrane protein interactions are possible. There are indications that membrane proteins are involved in lipid efflux to apo A-I. Thus, some macrophage cell lines express a cAMP-inducible receptor which binds apo E or apo A-I and mediates release of cellular FC and PL [18].

Apolipoproteins A-I, A-II, A-IV, C and E all mediate release of cell FC and PL from cholesterol-enriched fibroblasts [14]. Synthetic peptides containing amphipathic α-helical segments that mimic those present in human apo A-I have been used to examine the structural features of the apolipoproteins that stimulate lipid efflux [19]. Peptides containing only 1 or 2 amphipathic helical segments stimulate as much FC efflux from both mouse macrophages and L-cells as apo A-I. Acceptor efficiency is dependent on the number of amphipathic helices per molecule and increasing the lipid affinity of the peptides decreases the concentration required to achieve half-maximal efflux of both FC and PL. The fact that various exchangeable apolipoproteins, as well as synthetic peptides, can remove cell PL and FC indicates that the structural requirements for the apoprotein are not highly specific. It seems that the characteristic distribution of amphipathic α-helices with appropriate properties confers functionality to the apo A-I molecule.

Summary and Conclusions

The pathway by which apo A-I mediates efflux of cellular cholesterol depends upon its degree of lipidation. HDL particles that contain fully lipidated apo A-I molecules participate in the aqueous diffusion process. Incompletely lipidated apo A-I molecules in the lipid-free (poor) pre-β HDL pool remove FC and PL from the plasma membrane of cells by a membrane microsolubilization process. It is likely that the relative contributions of these two pathways to cellular cholesterol efflux in vivo vary depending upon the local environment. High LCAT activity tends to reduce the size of the lipid-free pool of apo A-I in plasma, and presumably in interstitial fluid, thereby reducing the relative contribution of membrane microsolubilization.

Acknowledgements

The research from this laboratory described here was supported by NIH grants HL07443 and HL22633.

References

1. Johnson WJ, Mahlberg FH, Rothblat GH, Phillips MC. Cholesterol transport between cells and high density lipoproteins. Biochim Biophys Acta 1991;1085:273−298.
2. Schultz JR, Rubin EM. The properties of HDL in genetically engineered mice. Curr Opin Lipid 1994;5:126−137.
3. Barter PJ, Rye K-A. Molecular mechanisms of reverse cholesterol transport. Curr Opin Lipid 1996;7:82−87.
4. Ji Y, Jian B, Wang N, Sun Y, de la Llera Moya M, Phillips MC, Rothblat GH, Swaney JB, Tall AR. Scavenger receptor BI promotes high density lipoprotein-mediated cellular cholesterol efflux. J Biol Chem 1997;272:20982−20985.
5. Brouillette CG, Anantharamaiah GM. Structural models of human apolipoprotein A-I. Biochim Biophys Acta 1995;1256:103−129.
6. Phillips MC, Johnson WJ, Rothblat GH. Mechanisms and consequences of cellular cholesterol exchange and transfer. Biochim Biophys Acta 1987;906:223−276.
7. Davidson WS, Rodrigueza WV, Lund-Katz S, Johnson WJ, Rothblat GH, Phillips MC. Effects of acceptor particle size on the efflux of cellular free cholesterol. J Biol Chem 1995;270: 17106−17113.
8. Davidson WS, Lund-Katz S, Johnson WJ, Anantharamaiah GM, Palgunachari N, Segrest JP, Rothblat GH, Phillips MC. The influence of apolipoprotein structure on the efflux of cellular free cholesterol to high density lipoprotein. J Biol Chem 1994;269:22975−22982.
9. Gillotte KL, Davidson WS, Lund-Katz S, Rothblat GH, Phillips MC. Apolipoprotein A-I structural modification and functionality of reconstituted high density lipoprotein particles in cellular cholesterol efflux. J Biol Chem 1996;271:23792−23798.
10. Jonas A. Lecithin-cholesterol acyltransferase. In: Gotto AM Jr (ed) Plasma Lipoproteins. Amsterdam: Elsevier, 1987;299−333.
11. Fielding CJ, Fielding PE. Molecular physiology of reverse cholesterol transport. J Lipid Res 1995;36:211−228.
12. Asztalos BF, Roheim PS. Presence and formation of 'free apolipoprotein A-I-like' particles in human plasma. Arterioscler Thromb Vasc Biol 1995;15:1419−1423.
13. Oram JF, Yokoyama S. Apolipoprotein-mediated removal of cellular cholesterol and phospholipids. J Lipid Res 1996;37:2473−2491.
14. Bielicki JK, Johnson WJ, Weinberg RB, Glick JM, Rothblat GH. Efflux of lipid from fibroblasts to apolipoproteins: dependence on elevated levels of cellular unesterified cholesterol. J Lipid

Res 1992;33:1699—1710.

15. Fielding CJ, Bist A, Fielding PE. Caveolin mRNA levels are up-regulated by free cholesterol and down-regulated by oxysterols in fibroblast monolayers. Proc Natl Acad Sci USA 1997;94: 3753—3758.

16. Fielding PE, Fielding CJ. Plasma membrane caveolae mediate the efflux of cellular free cholesterol. Biochemistry 1995;34:14288—14292.

17. Rothblat GH, Mahlberg FH, Johnson WJ, Phillips MC. Apolipoprotein, membrane cholesterol domains, and the regulation of cholesterol efflux. J Lipid Res 1992;33:1091—1098.

18. Smith JD, Masaaki M, Ginsberg M, Grigaux C, Shmookler E, Plump AS. Cyclic AMP induces apolipoprotein E binding activity and promotes cholesterol efflux from a macrophage cell line to apolipoprotein acceptors. J Biol Chem 1996;271:30647—30655.

19. Yancey PG, Bielicki JK, Johnson WJ, Lund-Katz S, Palgunachari MN, Anantharamaiah GM, Segrest JP, Phillips MC, Rothblat GH. The efflux of cellular cholesterol and phospholipid to lipid-free apolipoproteins and class A amphipathic peptides. Biochemistry 1995;34:7955—7965.

Genetic determinants of HDL and their relationships to atherosclerosis

Alan R. Tall, Can Bruce, Dan Sharp, Yong Ji, Yu Sun and Nan Wang
Division of Molecular Medicine, Department of Medicine, Columbia University, New York, New York, USA

Abstract. We have investigated the role of cholesteryl ester transfer protein (CETP) and scavenger receptor B1 (HDL receptor, SRB) in high-density lipoprotein (HDL) metabolism and atherogenesis. Studies in Japanese-American subjects indicate that heterozygous CETP deficiency (D442G mutation) is associated with moderately increased HDL levels but increased CHD risk; however, when CETP deficiency is associated with high HDL levels (HDL chol > 60 mg/dl), CHD prevalence is low. Recently, we have investigated the impact of the ileu405:val CETP polymorphism, found in many ethnic groups. Subjects with the VV polymorphism were found to have higher HDL chol and lower plasma CETP levels; this effect was primarily observed in subjects with plasma TG > 160 mg/dl. Hypertriglyceridemic VV subjects had increased CHD risk compared to normotriglyceridemic VV or II subjects (p < 0.05). CETP distribution was bimodal in VV subjects but unimodal in II subjects, suggesting that a functionally significant CETP gene mutation has arisen on a subset of chromosomes containing V alleles. SRB transgenic mice (liver-specific promoter) had profound reductions in HDL cholesterol and apoA-I levels, confirming that SRB1 is a functional HDL receptor. CHO cells transfected with SRB1 showed increased selective uptake of HDL CE, C and phospholipid and were also found to have a 2- to 4-fold increase in the initial rate of HDL-mediated free cholesterol efflux. In situ hybridization showed that SRB1 mRNA was expressed by macrophage-like cells in atheroma of apoE0 mice. Thus, SRB1 may also be involved in HDL-mediated cholesterol efflux from cells in the arterial wall, as well as in the uptake of HDL C and CE by the liver.

Keywords: atherosclerosis, cholesteryl ester transfer protein, high-density lipoproteins, scavenger receptor B1.

Plasma high-density lipoproteins (HDL) show a general inverse relationship with atherosclerosis. A major hypothesis to explain the antiatherogenic properties of HDL is related to the role of HDL in reverse cholesterol transport (RCT). The process of RCT involves the removal of cholesterol from cells in the arterial wall with subsequent transport to the liver by plasma lipoproteins; cholesterol taken up from plasma lipoproteins in the liver may then be excreted into bile. Cholesterol transported to the liver by HDL may be taken up directly by hepatocytes as free cholesterol (FC) or cholesteryl ester (CE). Recent evidence indicates that the transfer of FC or CE from HDL to the liver may be facilitated by an HDL receptor, scavenger receptor B1. Alternatively, CE may be transferred from

Address for correspondence: Alan R. Tall MD, College of Physicians and Surgeons of Columbia University, 622 West 168th Street, New York, NY 10032, USA. Tel.: +1-212-305-9418. Fax: +1-212-305-5052. E-mail: art1@columbia.edu.

HDL to triglyceride-rich lipoproteins (TRL) by cholesteryl ester transfer protein (CETP), with subsequent metabolism and hepatic uptake of TRL. This review will focus on recent research on the role of CETP and SRB1 in HDL metabolism and atherogenesis.

Human genetic deficiency of CETP results in increased HDL levels, reflecting the role of CETP in the catabolism of HDL CE [1,2]. Two common genetic deficiency states have been described in the Japanese, an intron 14 splicing defect which in the homozygous state results in complete absence of CETP and marked 3- to 4-fold elevations of HDL cholesterol, and a missense mutation (aspartate 442:glycine) causing partial CETP deficiency and more moderate increases in HDL cholesterol [3—5]. The corresponding heterozygous deficiency states are exceedingly common, representing about 2 and 5%, respectively, of the general Japanese population [3]. The heterozygous deficiency states result in 30—40% reductions in plasma CETP levels and in population-based samples only small increases in mean HDL cholesterol, 10—15% for the missense mutation and about 30% for the intron 14 defect [3,4]. In elderly men of the Honolulu Heart Program study, heterozygous CETP deficiency (principally the missense mutation) is associated with a significant excess of coronary heart disease (CHD) [4]. The relative risk of CHD is about 1.3 for men with the mutation, and increases to about 1.7 after adjustment for other risk factors and HDL levels. Although a survival artifact cannot be excluded, these findings are consistent with the idea that the overall role of CETP is to promote reverse cholesterol transport, resulting in an antiatherogenic effect. However, it should be noted that subjects with genetic CETP deficiency with HDL cholesterol > 60 mg/dl have a very low prevalence of CHD, similar to that of subjects with high HDL who do not have CETP deficiency [5]. Thus, a qualitative defect in RCT resulting from partial CETP deficiency may be overcome when HDL concentration rises above a threshold level.

Recently, we have explored the relationship of a common CETP gene polymorphism (isoleucine 405:valine) to HDL levels and CHD (C. Bruce, D. Sharp, A.R. Tall, unpublished). In 576 Japanese-American men from the Honolulu Heart Program, this conservative substitution was associated with significantly altered plasma CETP concentrations (1.95, 1.91 and 1.77 µg/ml for the II, IV and VV genotypes, respectively) and HDL cholesterol concentrations (51.1, 51.3 and 55.4 mg/dl, respectively, p < .04). However, the increase in HDL cholesterol was only significant in VV men with plasma triglyceride > 165 mg/dl. Although CHD prevalence was not significantly different among the three genotypes in this population, in the subgroup with high plasma TG, CHD prevalence was significantly higher in VV than II subjects (38 vs. 18%, p < 0.05). Like the intronic Taq 1B polymorphism of the CETP gene, the I405V polymorphism seems to be consistently associated with increased HDL levels, even though it is unlikely that the conservative substitution is the direct cause of reduced plasma CETP levels. Consistent with this idea we found that the specific activity of plasma CETP was identical in fresh plasma from normolipidemic VV, IV and II subjects. Moreover, the distribution of plasma CETP levels in VV subjects of the Honolulu Heart Program was found to be bimodal, while for II subjects the distribution was unimodal. The data suggests that the V polymorphism is in linkage disequilibrium with a widespread, functionally significant mutation which reduces expression of the CETP gene. The impact of this putative mutation on HDL levels and CHD may be modulated by the coexistence of hypertriglyceridemia. These findings are consistent with in vitro and transgenic mouse studies indicating that the effects of CETP on HDL and atherosclerosis are modified by hypertriglyceridemia [6,7].

The original studies of Glass, Pittman and colleagues [8,9] defined a process for catabolism of HDL cholesteryl esters (CE) where CE would be taken up by tissues without catabolism of HDL protein. The selective uptake of CE was prominent in steroidogenic tissues and liver. Recently, Acton et al. [10] showed that scavenger receptor B1 could mediate selective uptake of HDL CE in cultured cells. Moreover, SRB1 was found to be highly expressed in steroidogenic tissues and moderately expressed in liver. SRB1 was found to be upregulated in the adrenal gland in apoA-I knockout mice, which have depleted adrenal cholesterol stores, and also upregulated by stress or ACTH in the adrenal [11], consistent with a role of SRB1 in taking up HDL cholesterol for corticosteroid synthesis. Overexpression of SRB1 in the liver using adenovirus resulted in marked decreases in HDL cholesterol, and increases in biliary cholesterol output, consistent with a role of SRB1 in the catabolism of HDL cholesterol and transport into bile [12]. We have also overexpressed SRB1 in the liver by a transgenesis approach, resulting in marked decreases in HDL cholesterol, apoA-I and apoA-II (N. Wang, A.R. Tall, unpublished). In contrast to the results with adenovirus overexpression, where 7 or 10 days after injection of the virus plasma cholesterol was increased due to increased VLDL and LDL cholesterol, plasma cholesterol was profoundly reduced with chronic overexpression in the transgenic model.

We have also evaluated a possible role of SRB1 in the efflux of cholesterol from cells [13]. CHO cells transfected with the SRB1 cDNA showed a 2- to 3-fold increase in the HDL-mediated efflux of cellular cholesterol. The increased efflux was time-dependent and proportional to the concentration of HDL in media. When discoidal phospholipid/apoA-I complexes were provided, stimulation of net cholesterol efflux could be demonstrated. SRB1 stimulation of efflux was limited to free cholesterol, even in cells where radiolabel was present in CE. In contrast, SRB1-transfected cells showed increased uptake of both free and esterified cholesterol from HDL. In a variety of different cell types, including cultured macrophages, the rate constant for cholesterol efflux per µg HDL in media was closely correlated with the log of cellular SRB1 levels. This suggests a physiological role for SRB1 in mediating cellular cholesterol efflux in a variety of cell types, even those expressing low levels of SRB1. Moreover, SRB1 was readily detectable on an mRNA level by in situ hybridization of atheromatous aorta from apoE KO mice. The signal appeared to colocalize with macrophages. Thus, SRB1 may be involved in the initial steps of cholesterol efflux in the arterial wall, as well as the final stages of reverse cholesterol transport in the liver.

The recent findings on CETP and SRB1 illustrate a metabolic paradox, i.e., that the stimulation of reverse cholesterol transport by overexpression of either molecule is associated with a decrease in HDL levels. In the case of CETP, the net effects on atherogenesis appear to be modulated by plasma triglyceride and HDL levels. For SRB1, it seems likely that relationships to atherogenesis will also be complex. A challenge for the future will be to successfully target CETP or SRB1 molecules to influence atherogenesis in a beneficial way.

References

1. Brown ML, Inazu A, Hesler CB, Agellon LB, Mann C, Whitlock ME, Marcel YL, Milne RW, Koizumi J, Mabuchi H et al. Molecular basis of lipid transfer protein deficiency in a family with increased transfer protein deficiency in a family with increased high density lipoproteins. Nature 1989;342:448—451.
2. Inazu A, Brown ML, Hesler CB, Agellon LB, Koizumi J, Takata K, Maruhama Y, Mabuchi H, Tall AR. Increased high density lipoprotein casued by a common cholesteryl ester transfer protein gene mutation. N Engl J Med 1990;323:1234—1238.
3. Inazu A, Jiang X-C, Haraki T, Kamon N, Koizumi J, Mabuchi H, Takeda R, Takata K, Moriyama Y, Doi M et al. Genetic cholesteryl ester transfer protein deficiency caused by two prevalent mutations as a major determinant of increased levels of high density lipoprotein cholesterol. J Clin Invest 1994;94:1872—1882.
4. Takahashi K, Jiang X-C, Sakai N, Yamashita S, Hirano K, Bujo H, Yamazaki H, Kusunoki J, Miura T, Kussie P et al. A missense mutation in the cholesteryl ester transfer protein gene with possible dominant effects on plasma high density lipoprotein. J Clin Invest 1993;92:2060—2064.
5. Zhong S, Sharp DS, Grove JS, Bruce C, Katsuhiko Y, Curb JD, Tall AR. Increased coronary heart disease in Japanese-American men with mutations in the cholesteryl ester transfer protein gene despite increased HDL levels. J Clin Invest 1996;97:2917—2923.
6. Hayek T, Azrolan N, Verdery RB, Walsh A, Chajek-Shaul T, Agellon LB, Tall AR, Breslow JL. Hypertriglyceridemia and cholesteryl ester transfer protein interact to dramatically alter high density lipoprotein levels, particles sizes, and metabolism. J Clin Invest 1993;92:1143—1152.
7. Masucci-Magoulas L, Goldberg IJ, Bisgaier CL, Serajudin H, Francone OL, Breslow JL, Tall AR. A mouse model with features of familial combined hyperlipidemia. Science 1997;275: 391—394.
8. Glass C, Pittman RC, Civen M, Steinberg D. Uptake of high-density lipoprotein-associated apoprotein A-I and cholesterol esters by 16 tissues of the rat *in vivo* and by adrenal cells and hepatocytes *in vitro*. J Biol Chem 1985;260:744—750.
9. Glass C, Pittman RC, Weinstein DB, Steinberg D. Dissociation of tissue uptake of cholesterol ester from that of apoprotein A-I of rat plasma high density lipoprotein: selective delivery of cholesterol ester to liver, adrenal, and gonad. Proc Natl Acad Sci USA 1983;80:5435—5439.
10. Acton S, Rigotti A, Landschulz KT, Xu S, Hobbs HH, Krieger M. Identification of scavenger receptor SR-BI as a high density lipoprotein receptor. Science 1996;271:518—520.
11. Wang N, Weng W, Breslow JL, Tall AR. Scavenger receptor B1 (SR-B1) is up regulated in apolipoprotein A-I and hepatic lipase as a response to depletion of cholesterol stores. J Biol Chem 1996;271:21001—21004.
12. Kozarsky KF, Donahee MH, Rigotti A, Iqbal SN, Edelman ER, Krieger M. Overexpression of the HDL receptor SR-B1 alters plasma HDL and bile cholesterol levels. Nature 1997;387: 414—417.
13. Ji Y, Jian B, Wang N, Sun Y, Moya L, Phillips MC, Rothblat GH, Swaney JB, Tall AR. Scavenger receptor B1 promotes high density lipoprotein-mediated cellular cholesterol efflux. J Biol Chem 1997;272:20982—20985.

Lipoprotein cell interactions

Cellular catabolism of triglyceride-rich lipoproteins

Jörg Heeren and Ulrike Beisiegel
Medical Clinic, University Hospital, Hamburg, Germany

Abstract. The intravascular metabolism of lipoproteins has been quite extensively studied, however, the intracellular destiny of lipoproteins other than low-density lipoproteins (LDLs) has not yet been further elucidated. We studied the intracellular fate of triglyceride-rich lipoproteins (TRL) associated with lipoprotein lipase (LpL) in human hepatoma cells and fibroblasts. By pulse chase experiments, it was demonstrated that apolipoprotein E (apoE), other surface apolipoproteins and LpL escape lysosomal hydrolysis and are released intact into the medium, whereas apolipoprotein B (apoB) and other high molecular weight proteins are degraded. Kinetic studies revealed that recycling apolipoproteins are retained inside the cell much longer than transferrin (Tf), a well-established marker for the recycling pathway, is. The intracellular pathway of TRL was further investigated using indirect immunofluorescence for apoE, LpL and lipids. In contrast to fluorescence-labeled lipids, which are delivered to lysosomal compartments, apoE and LpL follow a distinct route to a sorting compartment, clearly distinguishable from the well-established perinuclear Tf recycling compartment. The surface apoproteins remain therefore accessible for slow recycling back to the plasma membrane, and possible reintegration into lipoproteins.

Keywords: apoE, degradation pathway, lipoprotein lipase, recycling, retroendocytosis.

Introduction

The transport of triglycerides through the circulation to the peripheral tissues and to the liver involves two distinct classes of TRL: chylomicrons (CM) and very low density lipoproteins (VLDL). Both are composed of several apolipoproteins which serve as solvents for the hydrophobic lipid moiety, as cofactors for enzymatic activity and as ligands for cellular receptors [1].

The exogenous pathway originates in the intestine, where CM are synthesized and subsequently transported via lymph into the bloodstream. The structural protein apoB$_{48}$ is characteristic for intestinally derived lipoproteins and does not possess binding properties for lipoprotein receptors. The action of LpL converts CM at the endothelial surface to remnant lipoproteins [2], which are further hydrolyzed by hepatic lipase (HL) in the liver. These chylomicron remnants are rapidly cleared from the circulation by hepatocytes, foremost a consequence of high-affinity binding of apoE to the LDL receptor and LRP [3,4]. Additionally particle-associated LpL and HL can facilitate their clearance via the LDL receptor related protein (LRP) [5—8].

Address for correspondence: Prof Dr Ulrike Beisiegel, Medical Clinic, University Hospital Eppendorf, Martinistrasse 52, 20249 Hamburg, Germany. Tel.: +49-40-47173917. Fax: +49-40-47174592.
E-mail: beisiegel@uke.uni-hamburg.de

The endogenous pathway starts in the liver with the secretion of VLDL from the hepatocytes. In plasma VLDL are remodeled to relatively cholesterol-enriched IDL and subsequently to triglyceride poor LDL by LpL and HL. In contrast to LDL, VLDL and IDL contain apoE which contributes to its receptor recognition [9]. In humans all liver-derived VLDL and LDL are characterized by the presence of apoB$_{100}$, which is recognized by the LDL receptor.

LDL taken up by the LDL receptor enter the cell via clathrin-coated pits. After endosomal acidification LDL dissociate from their receptors and remain within the lumen of the sorting endosome. Subsequently LDL are degraded in lysosomes and thereby deliver their cholesterol to the cell [10], while the receptors recycle back to the cell surface. In contrast to this classical degradation pathway, slow transport and degradation of VLDL were observed in the hepatoma cell line HepG2 [11]. Rabbit β-VLDL used as a model particle for TRL appeared in a set of widely distributed vesicles and had a delayed protein degradation rate in comparison to LDL in mouse peritoneal macrophages [12,13]. However, fluorescent-labeled lipid analogues incorporated into β-VLDL are finally delivered to perinuclear-located lysosomal compartments [14].

Results

Lipoprotein uptake and degradation

Studies on the metabolism of lipoproteins in cultured cells can provide useful information regarding their intracellular trafficking. TRL (isolated from patients with type-I hyperlipidemia due to LpL or apoC-II deficiency), and LDL were labeled by ^{125}I-iodine for quantitative analysis of the intracellular pathway. TRL of type-I patients have apoB$_{100}$ in addition to apoB$_{48}$, which indicated that TRL contain both CM and VLDL. The major apolipoproteins of TRL were apoE and apoC. In contrast LDL contained solely apoB$_{100}$ as structural protein, which is also responsible for the binding to the LDL receptor.

To compare intracellular degradation of TRL and LDL, Hep3b cells were incubated with either ^{125}I-LDL or ^{125}I-TRL in the presence or absence of additional bovine LpL for 6 h at 37°C. Degradation assays were performed to measure ^{125}I-tyrosine in the medium. The majority of apoB$_{100}$ was found to be degraded after 6 h. In the case of the TRL apolipoproteins only a few degradation products were detected within the same time. The addition of LpL decreased the amount of degradation. By indirect immunofluorescence we found that the reduced proteolytic degradation of the apolipoproteins of TRL in comparison to apoB$_{100}$ from LDL might be due to a different endocytic pathway. In contrast to the perinuclear distribution of LDL characteristic for lysosomal targeting, we observe a diffuse pattern throughout the cytoplasm for TRL associated apoE. After internalization, lysosome-directed ligands such as LDL remain within the sorting endosomes [15], which mature to late endosomes and finally fuse with lysosomes [16].

To follow the intracellular metabolism of the lipids from LDL and TRL the nontransferable fluorescent lipid analogue DiI was incorporated into these lipoproteins. With DiI as a direct incorporated label of either LDL or TRL lipids we visualized this classic pathway in accordance to described data [12]. DiI-labeled LDL and TRL colocalize after a 20-min uptake with the typical perinuclear staining pattern of lysosome-associated membrane protein 1 as a marker for lysosomal compartments. Since, however, apoE remains in peripheral vesicles for at least 1 h, an unexplained mechanism of particle disintegration must occur for TRL in sorting endosomes.

Recycling of apolipoproteins

To examine the possibility that apolipoproteins might be recycled, we performed pulse chase experiments. The degree of retention, degradation and recycling kinetics of apolipoproteins from TRL was compared with previously described data for transferrin [17] and LDL [18]. Transferrin was released intact with a half-life of ~ 30 min (Fig. 1A) and no degradation products in the supernatant of the TCA precipitable material were found. ^{125}I-LDL degradation products appeared in the medium after ~ 60 min, while very few LDL particles were resecreted intact (Fig. 1B). After an initial fast release most of the radioactivity of endocytosed TRL was retained longer inside the cell than ^{125}I-Tf, suggesting that constituents of TRL might be trapped in the endosomal system. Their apolipoproteins, however, escaped proteolytic degradation and can be resecreted into the medium (Fig. 1C). In previous studies we demonstrated that TRL core apolipoproteins are degraded while the surface apolipoproteins, predominantly apoE and apoC are resecreted [19]. In order to analyze this in more detail, we produced apoE-containing proteoliposomes. Figure 1D shows that apoE from these liposomes is also released intact with a half-life of 90 min. The recycled apolipoproteins attach mainly to high-density acceptor lipoproteins in the chase medium.

To confirm these data with different techniques, immunofluorescence experiments were performed. Human fibroblasts were incubated with TRL and additional LpL for 20 min at 37°C. ApoE and LpL were colocalized at 20 min, and even after 60-min chase time, as demonstrated by confocal laser scanning microscopy. The distribution pattern of vesicles throughout the cytoplasm did not change over the period of chase time, but the amount of apoE- and LpL-containing vesicles decreased, as expected, with increasing resecretion. ApoE retention and recycling might be either determined by an LRP-mediated process, or dependent on the cross-linking of different lipoprotein receptors, thus preventing the uncoupling of ligand and receptors.

Intracellular fate of apoE and Tf

With morphological methods we compared the recycling of apoE, the well-estab-

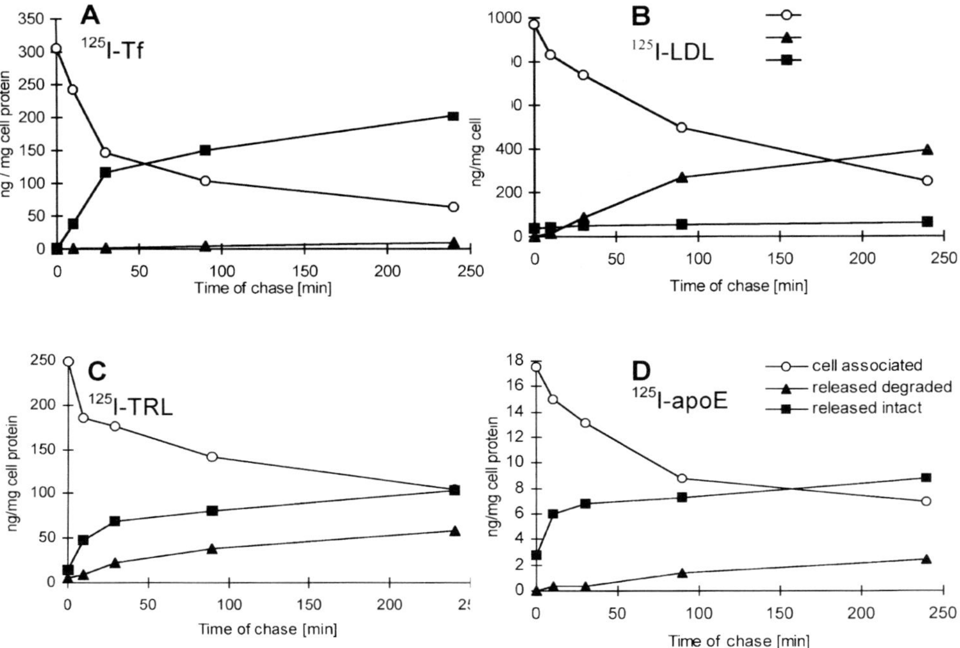

Fig. 1. To compare recycling kinetics of different ligands human hepatoma cells were incubated either with ^{125}I-Tf (**A**), ^{125}I-LDL (**B**), ^{125}I-TRL plus LpL (**C**) or ^{125}I-apoE proteoliposomes (**D**) for 60 min at 37°C. Surface-bound ligands were removed by heparin or by a mild acid wash (^{125}I-Tf), respectively. The cells were incubated with fresh preheated medium at 37°C for various chase times. The supernatant of each sample was separated in TCA precipitable proteins (released intact, squares) and ^{125}I-tyrosine (degradation products, triangles). The cells were solubilized with 0.1 N NaOH, and defined as cell associated fraction (open circles). The data presented are from one representative experiment out of four and the mean of duplicates is shown.

lished recycling pathway described for transferrin. As shown in Fig. 2B apoE-containing endosomes are widely dispersed throughout the cytoplasm, while transferrin (Fig. 2A) is found in the well-described perinuclear recycling compartment. The morphology of the perinuclear recycling compartment, which is not connected to the sorting endosomes, resembles the well characterized recycling compartment demonstrated in CHO cells [20]. Furthermore, recycling times for transferrin to the plasma membrane (~15 min) are also comparable to kinetics observed earlier [21]. In summary, recycling of apoE in human fibroblasts is clearly distinguishable from the transferrin pathway both in kinetic experiments (Fig. 1) and immuncytological pictures (Fig. 2).

Conclusion

Here we report on the recycling of TRL surface apolipoproteins via a peripheral sorting compartment in human hepatoma cells and in human fibroblasts. After

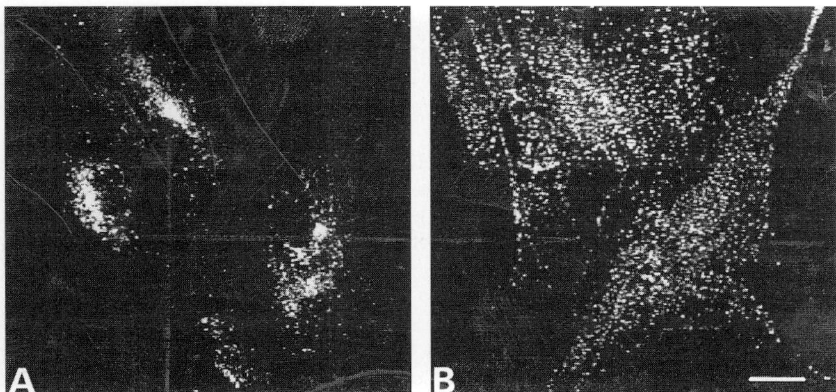

Fig. 2. Human skin fibroblasts were incubated either with 15 µg/ml Tf (**A**) or 5 µg/ml TRL plus 1 µg/ml LpL (**B**) for 20 min at 37°C. Cell surface bound material was released by heparin treatment or in case of Tf by a mild acid wash. After 10 min chase time with fresh preheated medium cells were rinsed in PBS, fixed and processed for indirect immunofluorescence with polyclonal antibody to Tf (**A**) or to apoE (**B**), followed by Cy3-goat antirabbit. Bar, 10 µm.

receptor-mediated endocytosis, TRL disintegrate and apolipoproteins apoE and apo C, as well as particle-associated LpL, remain within these compartments, while lipids and core apolipoproteins are directed to late endosomal compartments and lysosomes. In summary, we propose a mechanism of selective apolipoprotein recycling, which involves a class of sorting vesicle, in which disintegration of TRL components occurs thus explaining the differential fates of lipids vs. apolipoproteins and associated lipases. Considering that lipids satisfy the nutritional needs of the cell while apoE might be reused for lipoprotein formation or may be involved in regulating cholesterol efflux from cells, the TRL disintegration might be of physiological relevance.

Acknowledgements

We would like to thank Dr Senen Vilaro (University of Barcelona, Spain) for the help in establishing the immunocytochemistry in our laboratory. This work was supported by a grant of the Deutsche Forschungsgemeinschaft (Klinische Forschergruppe Gr 258/10-1).

References

1. Mahley RW, Hussain MM. Chylomicron and chylomicron remnant catabolism. Curr Opin Lipid 1991;2:170–176.
2. Olivecrona T, Bengtsson-Olivecrona G. Lipoprotein lipase and hepatic lipase. Curr Opin Lipid 1993;4:187–196.
3. Beisiegel U. Receptors for triglyceride-rich lipoproteins and their role in lipoprotein metabolism. Curr Opin Lipid 1995;6;117–122.

4. Willnow TE, Sheng Z, Ishibashi S, Herz J. Inhibition of hepatic chylomicron remnant uptake by gene transfer of a receptor antagonist. Science 1994;264:1471—1474.

5. Beisiegel U, Weber W, Bengtsson-Olivecrona G. Lipoprotein lipase enhances the binding of chylomicrons to low density lipoprotein receptor-related protein. Proc Natl Acad Sci USA 1991; 88:8342—8346.

6. Krapp A, Ahle S, Kersting S, Hua Y, Kneser K, Nielsen M, Gliemann J, Beisiegel U. Hepatic lipase mediates the uptake of chylomicrons and beta-VLDL into cells via the LDL receptor-related protein (LRP). J Lipid Res 1996;37:926—936.

7. Ji ZS, Lauer SJ, Fazio S, Bensadoun A, Taylor JM, Mahley RW. Enhanced binding and uptake of remnant lipoproteins by hepatic lipase-secreting hepatoma cells in culture. J Biol Chem 1994; 269:13429—13436.

8. Beisiegel U, Krapp A, Weber W, Olivecrona G. The role of alpha 2M receptor/LRP in chylomicron remnant metabolism. Ann NY Acad Sci 1994;737:53—69.

9. Havel RJ. The formation of LDL: mechanisms and regulation. J Lipid Res 1984;25:1570—1576.

10. Brown MS, Anderson RG, Goldstein JL. Recycling receptors: the round-trip itinerary of migrant membrane proteins. Cell 1983;32:663—667.

11. Lombardi P, Mulder M, van der Boom H, Frants RR, Havekes LM. Inefficient degradation of triglyceride-rich lipoprotein by HepG2 cells is due to a retarded transport to the lysosomal compartment. J Biol Chem 1993;268:26113—26119.

12. Tabas I, Lim S, Xu XX, Maxfield FR. Endocytosed beta-VLDL and LDL are delivered to different intracellular vesicles in mouse peritoneal macrophages. J Cell Biol 1990;111:929—940.

13. Tabas I, Myers JN, Innerarity TL, Xu XX, Arnold K, Boyles J, Maxfield FR. The influence of particle size and multiple apoprotein E-receptor interactions on the endocytic targeting of beta-VLDL in mouse peritoneal macrophages. J Cell Biol 1991;115:1547—1560.

14. Myers JN, Tabas I, Jones NL, Maxfield FR. Beta-very low density lipoprotein is sequestered in surface-connected tubules in mouse peritoneal macrophages. J Cell Biol 1993;123:Pt-402.

15. Goldstein JL, Brown MS. Binding and degradation of low density lipoproteins by cultured human fibroblasts. Comparison of cells from a normal subject and from a patient with homozygous familial hypercholesterolemia. J Biol Chem 1974;249:5153—5162.

16. Stoorvogel W, Strous GJ, Geuze HJ, Oorschot V, Schwartz AL. Late endosomes derive from early endosomes by maturation. Cell 1991;65:417—427.

17. Ciechanover A, Schwartz AL, Dautry-Varsat A, Lodish HF. Kinetics of internalization and recycling of transferrin and the transferrin receptor in a human hepatoma cell line. Effect of lysosomotropic agents. J Biol Chem 1983;258:9681—9689.

18. Goldstein JL, Brown MS. The low-density lipoprotein pathway and its relation to atherosclerosis. Ann Rev Biochem 1977;46:897—930.

19. Beisiegel U, Weber W, Heeren J, Hilpert J. Intracellular consequences of chylomicron uptake. Circulation 1995;92:691.

20. Yamashiro DJ, Tycko B, Fluss SR, Maxfield FR, Willingham MC, Hanover JA, Dickson RB, Pastan I. Segregation of transferrin to a mildly acidic (pH 6.5) para-Golgi compartment in the recycling pathway. Cell 1984;81:175—179.

21. Mayor S, Presley JF, Maxfield FR. Sorting of membrane components from endosomes and subsequent recycling to the cell surface occurs by a bulk flow process. J Cell Biol 1993;121: 1257—1269.

The effect of leukaemia inhibitory factor on experimental atherosclerosis*

Julie H. Campbell, Corey S. Moran and Gordon R. Campbell
Centre for Research in Vascular Biology, Department of Anatomical Sciences, The University of Queensland, Brisbane, Queensland, Australia

Abstract. Human leukaemia inhibitory factor (hHIF) is a polyfunctional cytokine, related to oncostatin M and interleukin-6, whose effects include stimulation of monocyte/macrophage differentiation and inhibition of lipoprotein lipase activity. In order to determine whether it influences atherosclerosis or vascular repair processes, hLIF at 30 µg/kg/day was administered for 28 days to rabbits on either a normal or 1% cholesterol diet via an osmotic minipump in the peritoneal cavity. At the same time, the right carotid artery was either balloon catheter de-endothelialized or ensheathed in a silicon periadventitial cuff. In cholesterol-fed rabbits, LIF reduced plasma cholesterol levels from 10.7 ± 0.1 to 8.0 ± 0.6 mmol/l ($p < 0.05$). Aortic arch cholesterol was reduced from 1.4 ± 0.3 to 0.6 ± 0.1 mg/g tissue and thoracic fatty streak formation was almost entirely inhibited. LIF (100 ng/ml) failed to prevent lipid uptake by either cultured SMC or macrophages when exposed to β-VLDL, but induced a 3-fold increase in lipid accumulation in human hepatoma cells (HepG2) via upregulation of LDL-receptors. Neointima formation induced by the cuff or balloon injury was significantly inhibited by LIF (19.3 ± 5.3 vs. $2.1 \pm 5.4\%$ and 85.3 ± 5.5 vs. $30.0 \pm 4.6\%$ wall area, respectively). In the presence of the nitric oxide (NO) substrate L-arginine, LIF (5 ng/ml) induced maximal SMC nitric oxide synthase (NOS) activity and significantly inhibited SMC DNA synthesis in vitro. In vivo neointimal thickening was augmented by treatment with L-NAME (a NOS-inhibitor), but the potent inhibitory effect of hLIF on neointimal formation was not prevented by simultaneous administration of L-NAME. Significantly L-NAME only partially ameliorated the potent induction of NOS activity by hLIF in both cuffed arteries and in SMC culture. This suggests there may be "superinduction" of NO formation by hLIF in the vessel wall that overrides the effect of the NOS inhibitor. We suggest that hLIF may be useful to inhibit restenosis following angioplasty particularly in hypercholesterolaemic patients.

Keywords: cytokine, lipoprotein, myointimal thickening, nitric oxide, vascular smooth muscle.

Introduction

The cytokine LIF is a secreted glycoprotein related to oncostatin M, interleukin-6 and ciliary neurotrophic factor. It was originally purified, characterized and cloned by virtue of its ability to induce the terminal differentiation and suppression of clonogenicity of myeloid leukaemic cells [1,2]; however, it is now clear

Address for correspondence: Prof Julie H. Campbell, Centre for Research in Vascular Biology, Department of Anatomical Sciences, The University of Queensland, Brisbane, Queensland 4072, Australia. Tel.: +61-7-33654658. Fax: +61-7-33651299. E-mail: julie.campbell@mailbox.uq.edu.au
*The work in this manuscript has been published in Arterioscler Thromb 1994;14:1356—1363 and Arterioscler Thromb Vasc Biol 1997;17(7):1267—1273, and is in press in J Vasc Res 1997. The current manuscript is a consolidation of these results into one document.

that LIF possesses a diverse range of biological activities in a variety of tissue systems. Recombinant human LIF, now known as AM424, directs neurotransmitter choice and neuron survival [3] and is in clinical development for neurological indications. LIF is essential for embryo implantation [4], and acts directly or synergistically to stimulate osteoblast/osteoclast activity, release of acute-phase proteins by hepatocytes, differentiation of megakaryocytes into platelets and proliferation of skeletal myoblasts and some haemopoietic cells [5].

Since LIF also inhibits adipocyte lipoprotein lipase activity [6] and induces cytokine expression in human blood monocytes [7], we questioned whether it could influence experimental atherosclerosis or vascular injury/repair processes.

Materials and Methods

Recombinant human (h)LIF was a gift from Dr Nic Gough of the Australian Medical Research and Development Corporation (AMRAD) Victoria, Australia. The recombinant hLIF was produced using the pGEX bacterial (*(Escherichia coli)* expression system [8] and purified to homogeneity as described by Gearing et al. [9].

Human LIF at 30 μg/kg/day was administered for 28 days to rabbits on either a normal or 1% cholesterol-enriched diet via an osmotic minipump in the peritoneal cavity [10]. At the same time, the right carotid artery was either balloon catheter de-endothelialized [11] or ensheathed in a silicon periadventitial cuff [10], both of which result in the formation of a neointimal thickening after 28 days. The protocols adopted are summarized in Fig. 1. There were eight rabbits per experimental group.

Plasma cholesterol levels were determined by an automated version of an enzymatic colorimetric method (CHOD-PAP) on the COBAS Bioanalyzer (Roche) and a commercially available kit (Monotest Cholesterol, Boehringer Mannheim). Fatty streaks on the luminal surface were stained en face with Oil-Red-O [10]. The cuffed or balloon de-endothelialized regions of the right carotid artery, and the same regions of the unmanipulated left carotid artery, were cut into 12 ring segments and every second ring fixed in 10% neutral buffered formaldehyde, sectioned at 6 μm and stained with toluidine blue. The size of the intima as a percentage of the total vessel wall area was determined by morphometric analysis using a digitizing tablet interfaced to an IBM-AT-compatible PC and MEASURE software (Capricorn Scientific) of four random sections per ring, six rings per vessel and eight vessels per experimental group (i.e., 192 sections per group).

Aortic smooth muscle cells were obtained from thoracic and abdominal aortas of 9- to 12-week-old New Zealand White rabbits via enzymatic dispersion as previously described [12]. Macrophages were the J774A.1 cell line derived from the BALB/c mouse strain. The human hepatoma cell line HepG2 was obtained from the American Type Culture Collection. Nitric oxide (NO) production was measured using a modification of the method of Busse and Mülsch [13].

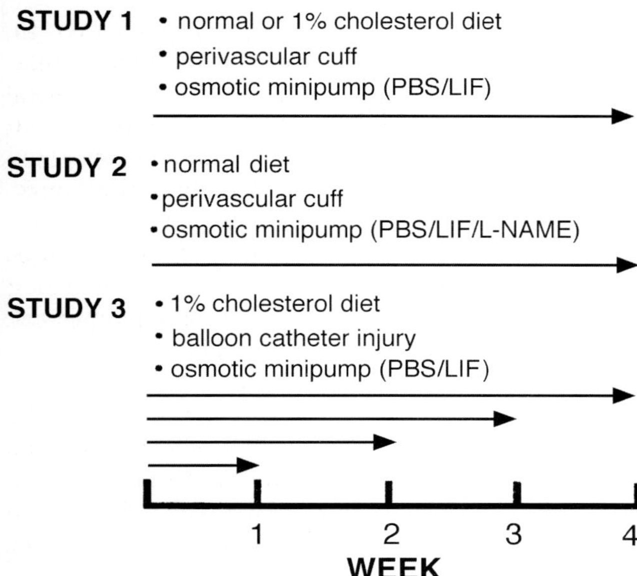

Fig. 1.

Results

In the rabbit, hLIF induced a 2- to 3-fold increase in plasma platelet number under both normo- and hyperlipidaemic conditions compared with appropriate controls. There was also an accelerated erythrocyte sedimentation rate (ESR). Human LIF initially inhibited the normal increase in body weight, however, after 2 weeks of hLIF treatment, animals proceeded to gain weight to be within the control weight ranges after a further 2 weeks [10].

Plasma cholesterol levels were significantly lowered with hLIF treatment compared to control cholesterol-fed rabbits over the full 28 days of treatment (8.0 ± 0.6 compared with 10.7 ± 0.1 mmol/l, $p < 0.05$) but were still significantly greater than that of normal diet animals (0.98 ± 0.1 mmol/l) [10]. This decrease in plasma cholesterol was associated mainly with a decrease in LDL-cholesterol ($p = 0.01$); other lipoprotein species were reduced, but not significantly. There was no difference in cholesterol levels or lipoprotein species of normolipidaemic rabbits with or without hLIF ($p < 0.05$).

The administration of hLIF to rabbits on a cholesterol-enriched diet significantly inhibited cholesterol accumulation in the aortic arch, reducing levels by 60% from 1.4 ± 0.3 to 0.6 ± 0.1 mg/g tissue. Similarly, fatty lesions which covered approximately 82% of the thoracic aorta of rabbits following cholesterol feeding were significantly reduced to cover only 12% of the luminal surface with hLIF treatment [10].

In carotid arteries of both normal and cholesterol-fed rabbits encapsulated with a silastic cuff, a concentric thickening of neointima developed over 28 days. In both cases with hLIF treatment there was a 90% decrease in neointimal formation (e.g., in cholesterol-fed rabbits from 19.3 ± 5.3 vs. 2.1 ± 5.4% wall area). Similarly, hLIF resulted in a 65% decrease in neointimal thickening development in rabbit carotid arteries subjected to balloon catheter de-endothelialization injury from 85.3 ± 5.5 vs. 30.0 ± 4.6% wall area. This was in spite of the degree of endothelial cell regrowth (as observed by Evan's blue staining) being significantly less in the rabbits receiving hLIF compared to non-hLIF-treated rabbits (5.4 ± 2.9 mm vs. 16.0 ± 3.6 mm; p < 0.05) [14].

In order to examine the mechanism by which LIF exerts these antiatherogenic effects, the influence of hLIF on lipoprotein uptake by SMC, macrophages, and hepatocytes was examined in cell culture. hLIF at concentrations 50−500 ng/ml had little effect on the uptake of βVLDL by either SMC or macrophages compared to cells exposed to βVLDL alone. In contrast, LIF (100 ng/ml) in the presence of LDL (20 μg/ml) significantly increased cholesterol accumulation in HepG2 liver cells 3-fold from 163 ± 8 to 505 ± 9 ng/mg protein. This was as a result of an increase in LDL-receptor expression by approximately 35% compared to that by control cells exposed to LDL only [15].

Thus hLIF has no effect on SMC and macrophage accumulation of lipid, but it stimulates both LDL receptor expression and cholesterol accumulation by liver cells, indicating that one mechanism by which hLIF reduces plasma cholesterol is through increased cholesterol clearance in the liver.

In order to examine the mechanism by which hLIF inhibits the development of a myointimal thickening following cuff- or balloon catheter-induced injury, its effect on SMC phenotype and proliferation in culture was examined. After 5 days in primary culture, SMC incubated in hLIF (at a concentration of 200 ng/ml) had a volume fraction of myofilaments ($V_v$myo) significantly higher than that for cells incubated in medium alone. A bell-shaped dose-response curve was observed, with higher and lower doses of hLIF being less effective.

In the presence of either 0.5 or 5% foetal calf serum, hLIF at all concentrations tested had no effect on SMC number when compared with controls, indicating that hLIF does not exert a direct influence on SMC growth. However, when SMCs were grown in the presence of hLIF plus the NO precursor L-arginine (10 μg/ml) DNA synthesis was significantly reduced compared to levels observed in control cells with L-arginine only [14].

The effect of hLIF on SMC nitric oxide synthase (NOS) induction by rabbit aortic SMC in culture was then examined. The production of NO ([^{3}H]-L-citrulline) following a 24-h preincubation with hLIF [^{3}H]-L-arginine was concentration-dependent with NOS activity evident at 50 pg/ml hLIF and maximal stimulation of a massive 450-fold above that of control at 5 ng/ml. In the presence of 5 ng/ml hLIF, a rapid increase in [^{3}H]-L-citrulline formation occurred after 4 h reaching a maximum at 12 h, after which production plateaued. The superinduction of NO synthesis by SMC through stimulation with 5 ng/ml hLIF in vitro for 24 h was reduced by approximately 86% in the presence of 30 ng/ml of the

NOS inhibitor L-NAME, but was still significantly elevated when compared with control cells. That is, 30 ng/ml L-NAME could not completely override the stimulatory effect of 5 ng/ml hLIF on NOS activity with there still being a massive 63-fold increase in NO production [14].

It was then determined whether L-NAME (12 mg/kg/day) administered to rabbits via an osmotic minipump in the peritoneal cavity could prevent the inhibition of a cuff-induced neointima in the presence of hLIF. In normolipidaemic animals, the effect of the cuff on the vessel wall was augmented in the presence of L-NAME, resulting in a significantly larger neointima 27.0 ± 2.0% compared with 19.3 ± 5.4% of the total vessel wall cross-sectional area; p = 0.01). The NO precursor L-arginine decreased neointimal formation (11.3 ± 2.0%), however, this reduction, while significant when compared to the controls, was considerably less than that in hLIF-treated rabbits where there was almost complete inhibition of neointimal formation with only the occasional appearance of SMC one to two layers thick comprising 2.1 ± 5.4% of the total cross-sectional area. This inhibition was accompanied by a significant increase in arterial NOS activity which was 2.7-fold higher than in the cuffed artery with no hLIF. In the animals receiving the dual L-NAME/L-arginine regime, L-NAME counteracted the inhibitory effect of L-arginine, increasing the area of intimal thickening (16.4 ± 1.5). In contrast, L-NAME did not remove the potent inhibitory effect of 30 μg/kg/day hLIF on cuff-induced myointimal thickening (3.2 ± 2.5%; p < 0.001). L-NAME significantly reduced NOS activity in the hLIF-treated cuffed vessels (p = 0.01), but this was still 1.9-fold higher than the cuffed controls [14].

Discussion

This study showed that hLIF-lowered serum cholesterol levels in the cholesterol-fed rabbit by about 30%, which was associated with a decreased LDL level. hLIF inhibited fatty streak formation (by about 80%) on the luminal surface of thoracic aorta of cholesterol-fed rabbits and decreased cholesterol content of the aortic arch by 60% but had no direct inhibitory effect on lipoprotein (βVLDL) uptake by either SMC or macrophages in vitro. LIF is a known lipoprotein lipase-inhibitor and a potent inhibitor of proteoglycan synthesis. By inhibiting the activity of lipoprotein lipase (and thus generation of LDL) and/or interfering with the biological properties of extracellular matrix, hLIF may be acting to prevent the entrapment of lipoprotein in the vessel wall, thus preventing its modification and ingestion by SMC and macrophages. However, in a non-dose-dependent manner, hLIF also increased both LDL-receptor expression and LDL uptake in vitro by the human hepatoma cell line HepG2 indicating that the reduced serum cholesterol levels in the presence of hLIF may be due to up-regulation of hepatic LDL-receptors.

Human LIF also increased NOS activity and thus the production of NO following cuff or balloon-induced injury and potently inhibited neointimal formation in these vessels. Nitric oxide is also known to have other antiatherogenic properties such as inhibition of expression of endothelial adhesion molecules and of various chemokines and cytokines which are mediated in a coordinated fashion through reduction in the transcription factor NF-κB [16]. At 100 ng/ml in culture hLIF prevented SMC phenotypic change to the "synthetic" state in which mature cells become responsive to mitogens. It inhibited DNA synthesis by SMC in the presence (but not absence) of the NO precursor L-arginine, and superinduced NO synthesis in SMC in vitro which was only partially inhibited by L-NAME. Likewise, the inhibitory effect of neointimal formation in vivo was not counteracted by L-NAME at 12 mg/kg/day, leaving open the possibilities that either the concentration of L-NAME was insufficient to block the superinduction of NO, or that an additional unknown mechanism is operating.

Thus hLIF inhibits SMC phenotypic change and stimulates SMC nitric oxide production which in turn decreases SMC proliferation and neointimal formation. Human LIF also decreases plasma cholesterol levels and aortic tissue accumulation of lipid and fatty streak formation. This suggests that hLIF is of potential use in the inhibition of progression of primary atherosclerosis, where high plasma cholesterol and vessel wall deposition of lipid feature, and may prevent hyperplastic restenosis following surgical intervention to remove occluding lesions as in angioplasty or endarterectomy.

Acknowledgements

The work in this manuscript was supported by research grants from AMRAD (Australia) and Glaxo-Wellcome (UK). Julie H. Campbell was supported by the National Health and Medical Research Council of Australia, and Corey S. Moran by an Australian Postgraduate Award (Industry) from AMRAD (Australia).

References

1. Tomida M, Yamamoto-Yamaguchi Y, Hozumi M. Purification of a factor inducing differentiation of mouse myeloid leukemic M1 cells from conditioned medium of mouse fibroblast 1929 cells. J Biol Chem 1984;259:10978−10986.
2. Gearing DP, Gough NG, King JA, Hilton DJ, Nicola NA, Simpson RJ, Nice EC, Kelso A, Metcalf D. Molecular cloning and expression of cDNA encoding a murine myeloid leukemia inhibitory factor (LIF). EMBO J 1987;6:3995−4010.
3. Yamamori T, Fukuda K, Abersold R, Korsching S, Fann M-J, Patterson PH. The cholinergic neuronal differentiation factor is a hemopoietic regulator. Science 1989;246:1412−1416.
4. Cullinan EB, Abbondanzo SJ, Anderson PS, Pollard JW, Lessey BA, Stewart CL. Leukemia inhibitory factor (LIF) and LIF receptor expression in human endometrium suggests a potential autocrine/paracrine function in regulating embryo implantation. Proc Natl Acad Sci USA 1996;93:3115−3120.
5. Hilton DJ, Gough NM. Leukemia inhibitory factor: a biological perspective. J Cell Biochem 1991;46:21−27.
6. Mori M, Yamaguchi K, Abe K. Purification of a lipoprotein lipase-inhibiting protein produced by a melanoma cell line associated with cancer cachexia. Biochem Biophys Res Commun 1989;160:1085−1092.

7. Villiger PM, Geng Y, Lotz M. Induction of cytokine expression by leukemia inhibitory factor. J Clin Invest 1993;91:1575–1581.

8. Smith DB, Johnson KS. Single-step purification of polypeptides expressed in *E. coli* as fusions with glutathione S-transferase. Gene 1988;67:31–42.

9. Gearing DP, Nicola NA, Metcalf D, Foote S, Wilson TA, Gough NM, Williams RL. Production of leukemia inhibitory factor (LIF) in *Escherichia coli* by a novel procedure and its use in maintaining embryonic stem (ES) cells in culture. Biotechnology 1989;7:1157–1166.

10. Moran CS, Campbell JH, Simmons DL, Campbell GR. Leukaemia inhibitory factor and atherosclerosis. Arterioscler Thromb 1994;14:1356–1363.

11. Manderson JA, Mosse PRL, Safstrom JA, Young SB, Campbell GR. Balloon catheter injury to the rabbit carotid artery. I. Changes in smooth muscle phenotype. Arteriosclerosis 1989;9:289–298.

12. Campbell JH, Kocher O, Skalli O, Gabbiani G, Campbell GR. Cytodifferentiation and expression of alpha smooth muscle actin mRNA and protein during culture of aortic SMC. Correlation with cell density and proliferative state. Arteriosclerosis 1989;9:633–643.

13. Busse R, Mülsch A. Induction of nitric oxide synthase by cytokines in vascular smooth muscle cells. FEBS Lett 1990;275:87–90.

14. Moran CS, Campbell JH, Campbell GR. Induction of smooth muscle cell nitric oxide synthase by human leukaemia inhibitory factor: effects in vitro and in vivo. J Vasc Res 1997;(In press).

15. Moran CS, Campbell JH, Campbell GR. Human leukaemia inhibitory factor upregulates LDL receptors on liver cells and decreases serum cholesterol in the cholesterol-fed rabbit. Arterioscler Thromb Vasc Biol 1997;17:1267–1273.

16. De Caterina R, Libby P, Peng HB, Thannickal VJ, Rajavashisth TB, Gimbrone MA Jr, Shin WS, Liao JR. Nitric oxide decreases cytokine-induced endothelial activation. Nitric oxide selectively reduces endothelial expression of adhesion molecules and proinflammatory molecules. J Clin Invest 1995;96:60–68.

Lipoprotein association with cells and matrix: modulation by lipase and proteoglycans

Ira J. Goldberg[1], Sivaram Pillarisetti[1], Joseph C. Obunike[1], William S. Blaner[1], William D. Wagner[2] and John C. Rutledge[3]

[1]Columbia University College of Physicians and Surgeons, New York, New York; [2]Bowman Gray School of Medicine, Winston-Salem, North Carolina; and [3]University of California, Davis, California, USA

Abstract. How LDL associates with matrix proteins is unknown. The speculations about this atherosclerosis initiating process are that the LDL is retained because either the LDL is altered in the subendothelial space, or the native LDL binds to specific matrix proteins, some of which may be more abundant in advanced lesions. One class of potential LDL-binding proteins is proteoglycans (PGs). LDL, however, binds poorly to most vessel wall PGs in physiologic ionic strength buffers. We have obtained data both in vitro and in perfused blood vessels that LDL retention by matrix is increased by an intermediary molecule, lipoprotein lipase (LpL). This occurs because of a dual interaction of LpL with PGs and the amino-terminal region of apoB. In addition, lipoproteins may interact with other matrix components, e.g., Lp(a) binds to fibronectin and other matrix molecules.

Associations of molecules with the subendothelial matrix are altered when oxidized LDL or lysolecithin stimulates endothelial cells. We have shown that stimulated endothelial cells produce a heparanase that reduces the heparan sulfate (HS) PG content of the matrix, thereby increasing its ability to retain monocytes and some lipoproteins. Since vessel wall HSPG are reduced with aging and atherosclerosis, these matrix alterations may be primary abnormalities that predispose to atherosclerosis.

Keywords: apolipoprotein B, atherosclerosis, heparin, lipolysis, low density lipoprotein, triglyceride.

Introduction

Aside from its actions as a triglyceride and phospholipid hydrolase, LpL has been shown in vitro to function as a "bridging" molecule between lipoproteins and proteoglycans (PGs) on cell surfaces and within the matrix. Moreover, by virtue of its dimeric configuration, it can bind to PGs on two different cell types, thus increasing, for example, the association of monocytes with endothelial cells [1]. These actions of LpL do not require it to be enzymatically active, but require an appropriate three-dimensional structure. This article will review LpL-mediated processes that increase the association of lipoproteins with cells and increase the uptake of lipids by tissues. It will focus on progress made in understanding the biochemistry of LpL-mediated interactions with lipoproteins and PGs. In addition, newly discovered information about how lipolysis and lipolysis products

Address for correspondence: Ira J. Goldberg MD, Department of Medicine, Columbia University College of Physicians and Surgeons, 630 West 168th Street, New York, NY 10032, USA. Tel.: +1-212-305-5961. Fax: +1-212-305-5384. E-mail: IJG3@columbia.edu

such as lysolecithin alter endothelial cell biology and create atherogenic stimuli will be reviewed.

Lipoprotein uptake and retention via LpL: in vitro observations

LpL interaction with lipoproteins is required for the delivery of fatty acids to the peripheral tissues and conversion of triglyceride-rich particles into lipoproteins that predominantly contain core cholesteryl ester. Although students of this field had long postulated that LpL had additional functions, this hypothesis became much less speculative after Beisiegel and her colleagues [2] demonstrated that LpL could interact with the LDL receptor related protein (LRP). Thus, a plausible in vivo function for LpL as a receptor ligand was reconsidered.

The earliest models of LpL-mediated hydrolysis of triglyceride-rich lipoproteins showed LpL bridging the space between its substrate triglyceride-rich lipoproteins and the endothelial cell surface. Bridging, however, was not thought to occur with nonsubstrate lipoproteins. Saxena et al. [3], while studying the effects of LpL on the transport of lipoproteins across monolayers, observed that LpL markedly increased the amount of LDL that was retained within the subendothelial space. LpL anchors lipoproteins and modified lipoproteins to subendothelial cell matrix and enhances the cellular uptake of the lipoproteins (reviewed in [4]). The LpL-mediated pathway appears to be most important in cells containing fewer classical lipoprotein receptors; in the presence of a large number of cell surface receptors and adequate ligands it may be relatively less important. LpL-mediated uptake of LDL is proportionately greater in LDL receptor deficient cells than in normal fibroblasts, whereas uptake of acetyl LDL by scavenger receptor-rich macrophages is minimally increased by LpL [5].

How does LpL increase lipoprotein uptake by cells? Three postulated mechanisms are reviewed in Fig. 1. While some lipoprotein uptake appears to be via direct interaction of LpL with cell surface lipoprotein receptors or by increasing the probability of a lipoprotein interacting with receptors, additional uptake is independent of these receptors. Because the turnover of cell surface PGs is fairly rapid [5], one route of LpL-mediated lipoprotein uptake appears to be via the recycling of cell surface PGs to which the lipoproteins are associated.

Biochemistry of the LpL-LDL-proteoglycan interaction

Several interactions are required for LpL to form an anchor between lipoproteins and PGs. LpL binds to heparan sulfate HSPGs and we [6] and others [7] have isolated a 10 unit oligosaccharide that contains high-affinity LpL-binding sequences. LpL also binds to other highly sulfated PGs that are made by differentiated macrophages [8] and perhaps other cells.

A second interaction is that between LpL and the lipoprotein. LpL has a lipid-binding lid structure that confers specificity for substrate lipoproteins. Presumably, this is the reason that LpL is the primary enzyme hydrolyzing large triglyc-

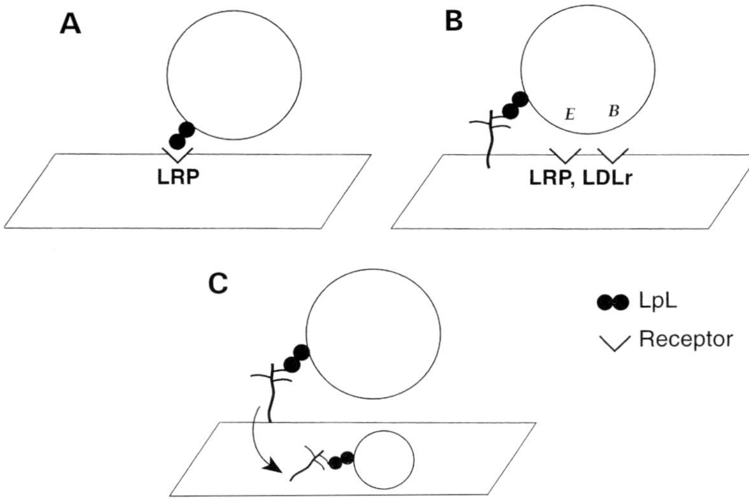

Fig. 1. LpL-mediated cellular uptake of lipoproteins. There are at least three postulated pathways by which LpL can modulate the uptake of lipoproteins by cells. **A**: LpL is the ligand for cell surface receptors, especially those of the LDL receptor related protein class. **B**: By increasing the association of lipoproteins with the surface of cells, the effective concentration of the lipoproteins is increased. This, in turn, increases conventional lipoprotein-receptor uptake. **C**: Lipoprotein-LpL complexes attached to cell surface proteoglycans are internalized as a complex, perhaps in conjunction with the recycling of the cell membrane. This is a higher capacity but kinetically slower process than that of classical receptor mediated endocytosis.

eride-rich lipoproteins. As those particles become smaller, they become more suited to hydrolysis by hepatic lipase. In part, this improves their interaction with the hepatic lipase lid. It appears, however, that a second interaction with lipoproteins also exists; one that does not position the LpL to perform lipolysis but allows the LpL to bind to nonsubstrate lipoproteins like LDL. A series of studies using fragments of apolipoprotein B and monoclonal antibodies showed that LpL-LDL interactions are mediated by the NH_2-terminal region of apoB (NTAB) [9]. Antibodies against this region of apoB will decrease LpL-LDL complex formation and block LpL-mediated retention of LDL in perfused blood vessels [10]. In contrast, antibodies to NTAB do not inhibit LpL-mediated hydrolysis of VLDL in solution assays. Thus, a distinct biochemical interaction is involved in the LpL-LDL bridging process that is independent of the LpL interactions required for hydrolysis of triglyceride-rich lipoproteins.

Other postulated interactions involving NTAB

NTAB is a large, greater than 80 kb, region of apoB that contains seven pairs of disulfide bonds. This region of apoB is thought to extend away from the lipid core of LDL. This portion of the protein has no well-established function. Several groups [11,12] have provided data suggesting that NTAB is required for apoB

890

synthesis. One hypothesis is that NTAB inserts into the ER membrane and then allows the more hydrophobic regions of apoB to traverse into the ER lumen. Because this region extends away from the more hydrophobic portions of apoB it could also provide for protein-protein interactions. Evidence exists for NTAB interaction with the scavenger receptor [13], the macrophage triglyceride-rich lipoprotein receptor [14], and LpL.

NTAB has several clusters of basic amino acids and small peptides of this region will associate with heparin; some peptides from near the LDL receptor binding portion of apoB have a greater affinity for heparin [15]. Nonetheless, if lipoprotein retention by subendothelial cell PGs is one of the processes that initiates atherogenesis, it is likely to be a process that can utilize both apoB100- and apoB48-containing lipoproteins. We have recently obtained data showing that LDL interaction with heparin and subendothelial matrix is mediated, at least in part, by NTAB [16]. These data include the following:
1) NTAB, produced by expressing apoB17 in cultured cells, will associate with heparin affinity columns better than LDL.
2) Medium containing apoB17 will decrease LDL association with subendothelial matrix and purified PGs.
3) Monoclonal antibodies to NTAB will decrease LDL association with heparin and with matrix.
4) Antibodies to the amino terminal region of apoB decrease LpL-mediated LDL retention in perfused blood vessels [10]. We therefore hypothesize that this is the atherogenic region of apoB since it promotes retention of apoB containing lipoproteins by matrix molecules.

Nonenzymatic actions of LpL: do they operate in vivo?

Although there is in vitro evidence for a nonenzymatic role of LpL in lipoprotein metabolism, proof that this occurs in vivo is required. Methods to study LpL nonenzymatic functions in animals have recently been developed. Using adenoviruses, Dugi et al. [17] have recently reported that adenovirus expression of very high concentrations of enzymatically inactive hepatic lipase led to lipoprotein uptake by the liver. Another way to test whether LpL removes lipoproteins via a nonenzymatic pathway is to assess the effect of adding this enzyme to mice that have increased concentrations of cholesterol-rich lipoproteins that are not substrates for LpL actions. When a LpL transgene was crossed onto the LDL knockout mice, there was a marked decrease in circulating LDL [18]. Similarly, muscle LpL overexpression in apoE knockout mice reduced the levels of circulating cholesterol-rich remnant lipoproteins (Weinstock and Breslow, personal communication). Although these experiments are not conclusive because LpL enzymatic actions could have altered lipoprotein metabolism, they do support the hypothesis that LpL has actions other than triglyceride hydrolysis.

Other markers that can be used to assess the role of LpL in lipoprotein uptake by tissues are fat-soluble vitamins. Studies by Traber et al. [19] and Blaner et al.

[20] showed that LpL increased vitamin E and A uptake by cultured cells. The following questions remained to be answered. Does LpL affect vitamin uptake in vivo? Does LpL expression alter tissue stores of vitamins A or E? Does uptake of vitamins A and E require enzymatic LpL actions? Data showing that LpL overexpression increased the vitamin E content of skeletal muscle was recently published [21]. To determine whether tissue LpL affected vitamin A uptake from the circulation, wild-type and mice expressing human LpL in muscle on the wild-type and LpL knockout backgrounds were studied. Rat chylomicrons were labeled with (^{3}H)retinyl ester. The plasma clearance and tissue uptake and content of this vitamin were assessed. Tissue uptake of vitamin A correlated with the LpL activity of the muscle. Surprisingly, although overexpression of LpL in muscle increased (^{3}H)-vitamin A uptake, it did not affect overall muscle vitamin A levels. Therefore, vitamin A stores did not correlate with uptake of chylomicron retinyl ester. This suggests that tissue content of retinoid is dependent on other pathways of vitamin uptake or on the capacity of the tissues to store this fat-soluble vitamin.

Retinyl ester has been used as a marker for the core lipids of chylomicrons. Therefore its uptake by tissues requires one of the following: 1) hydrolysis of the vitamin, as we observed in in vitro studies [20], 2) uptake of retinyl ester as a component of the surface lipid that is shed from the chylomicron during lipolysis, or 3) uptake of the entire chylomicron or chylomicron remnant. A preliminary study was performed to assess tissue uptake of retinyl ester and the nonhydrolyzable analogue retinyl ether in rats during the fed and fasting state (LpL activity in the muscle is greater with fasting). Uptake of both labels was greater in the muscle, but uptake of ester exceeded that of ether. This suggests that hydrolysis of the ester was, to some degree, involved in the vitamin A uptake. The final proof that nonenzymatic LpL actions operate in vivo will, however, require studies using lipoproteins that are nonhydrolyzable and/or transgenic mice containing enzymatically inactive LpL (Fig. 2).

Lipoprotein interactions with matrix

A key step in the atherosclerotic process is the interaction and then retention of lipoproteins within the arterial wall. LDL is found within PG-rich regions of atherosclerotic plaques. Ways to increase lipoprotein matrix interaction include increasing LDL transit into the vessel wall, increasing the amount or affinity of matrix molecules for LDL, modifying the lipoproteins to increase their matrix-binding characteristics, and including anchoring molecules that promote lipoprotein-matrix interaction. LpL, a product of arterial wall macrophages and a component of atherosclerotic lesions, increases LDL retention in subendothelial matrix [3] and in perfused blood vessels [10] via this latter mechanism. In addition, since hydrolysis of hypertriglyceridemic human plasma within the lumen of a perfused artery increased vessel wall permeability [10], LpL may also promote lipoprotein transit into the artery wall. This could be a mechanism for the

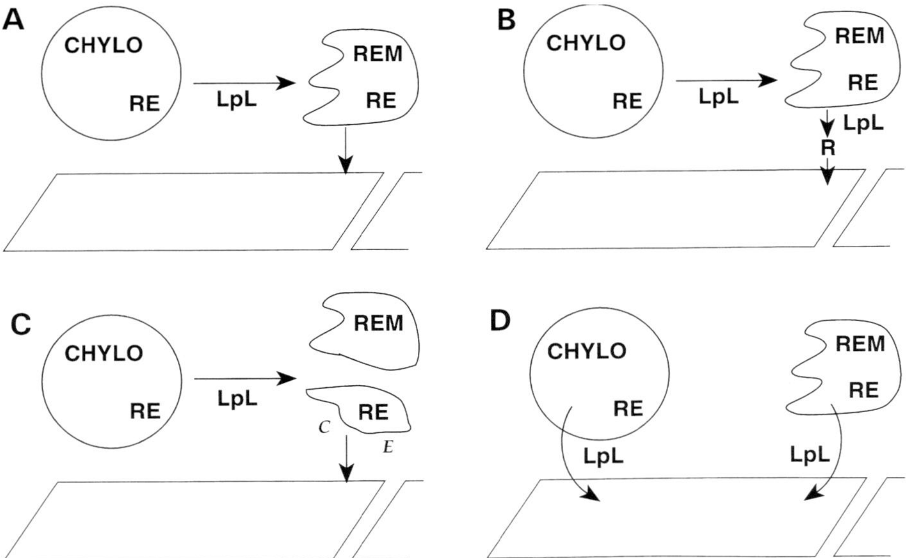

Fig. 2. Mechanisms for LpL-mediated uptake of retinyl ester (RE). **A**: LpL hydrolyzes chylomicrons (denoted CHYLO) and the remnants (denoted REM) containing RE are internalized via receptor-mediated processes. **B**: LpL hydrolyzes chylomicron triglyceride and then hydrolyzes the RE to free retinol (R) that can diffuse across cell membranes. **C**: Lipolysis releases surface lipid from the chylomicrons that in addition to phospholipids and some apolipoproteins (E and Cs) also contains some core lipid, including RE. The lipolysis products, e.g., lysophospholipids, could disrupt the endothelial barrier function. Liberated surface lipid is internalized either via apoE and/or LpL interaction with lipoprotein receptors or receptors for negatively charge lipids. **D**: LpL increases uptake of chylomicrons and remnants by promoting their interaction with the cell surface (see Fig. 1). Three of these processes, A—C, require LpL enzymatic activity; D does not.

atherogenicity of postprandial lipoproteins.

Although LDL retention is thought to occur via interaction with chondroitin and dermatan sulfate PGs, Lp(a) associates with matrix adhesion molecules. The most prominent of these is fibronectin. While LpL anchoring of LDL to matrix occurs via its interaction with HSPG, we have obtained evidence that HSPGs inhibit Lp(a) retention. Removal of HSPG by heparinase-treatment increased Lp(a) binding by 2- to 10-fold [22]. Antibodies to fibronectin inhibited much of this increase. Inclusion of lysolecithin in the medium of cultured endothelial cells resulted in less HSPG in the subendothelial matrix [23]. Oxidized-LDL, a lipoprotein high in lysolecithin content, also decreased the content of HSPG in the subendothelial matrix [22]. These decreases in matrix HSPG were associated with the production of a heparanase that was secreted preferentially from the basolateral side of the cultured endothelial cells [24]. Although increases in matrix chondroitin and dermatan sulfate accompany atherosclerosis and are thought to accelerate lipoprotein retention, less HS is often found in lesions and may be pathogenic.

Summary

In general, greater activity of LpL leads to a less atherogenic lipoprotein profile because it increases the removal rate of postprandial lipoproteins, reduces fasting triglyceride and raises HDL. Another consequence of reduced LpL activity in peripheral tissues, i.e., muscle and adipose, is an increase in circulating triglyceride containing lipoproteins that can, theoretically, be lipolyzed by the small amount of LpL on the surface of medium and large blood vessels. Some of this LpL is synthesized by macrophage foam cells and is the reason that atherosclerotic vessels have an increase in vessel wall LpL.

Many potential physiologic and pathophysiologic effects of LpL and lipolysis have been demonstrated using cell culture techniques. More recently, experiments in perfused vessels and genetically modified mice have corroborated many of the findings. These include showing that LpL: 1) retains LDL within the artery wall, 2) decreases plasma levels of LDL, and 3) increases uptake of fat-soluble vitamins. It is, however, likely that not all tissue culture observations will prove to be of physiological importance. A goal for the near future is to establish the importance of nonenzymatic LpL processes in vivo.

References

1. Obunike JC, Paka S, Sivaram P, Goldberg IJ. Lipoprotein lipase can function as a monocyte adhesion protein. Arterioscler Thromb Vasc Biol 1997;17:1414–1420.
2. Beisiegel U, Weber W, Bengtsson-Olivecrona G. Lipoprotein lipase enhances the binding of chylomicrons to low density lipoprotein receptor-related protein. Proc Natl Acad Sci USA 1991;88:8342–8346.
3. Saxena U, Klein MG, Vanni TM, Goldberg IJ. Lipoprotein lipase increases low density lipoprotein (LDL) retention by subendothelial cell matrix. J Clin Invest 1992;89:373–380.
4. Goldberg IJ. Lipoprotein lipase and lipolysis: central roles in lipoprotein metabolism and atherosclerosis. J Lipid Res 1996;37:693–707.
5. Obunike JC, Edwards IJ, Rumsey SC, Curtiss LK, Wagner WD, Deckelbaum RJ, Goldberg IJ. Cellular differences in lipoprotein lipase mediated uptake of low density lipoproteins. J Biol Chem 1994;269:13129–13135.
6. Parthasarathy N, Goldberg IJ, Sivaram P, Mulloy B, Flory DM, Wagner WD. Oligosaccharide sequences of endothelial cell surface heparan sulfate proteoglycan with affinity for lipoprotein lipase. J Biol Chem 1994;269:22391–22396.
7. Larnkjaer A, Nykjaer A, Olivecrona G, Thogersen H, Ostergaard P. Structure of heparin fragments with high affinity for lipoprotein lipase and inhibition of lipoprotein lipase binding to alpha2-macrophglobulin-receptor/low density lipoprotein receptor-related protein by heparin fragments. Biochem J 1995;307:205–214.
8. Edwards IJ, Xu H, Goldberg IJ, Wagner WD. Cell surface proteoglycans which bind lipoprotein lipase are upregulated in differentiated macrophages. Arterioscler Thromb Vasc Biol 1995;15:400–409.
9. Choi SY, Sivaram P, Walker DE, Curtiss LK, Gretch D, Sturley S, Attie A, Deckelbaum RJ, Goldberg IJ. Lipoprotein lipase association with lipoproteins involves protein-protein interaction with apolipoprotein B. J Biol Chem 1995;270:8081–8086.
10. Rutledge JC, Woo MW, Rezai AA, Curtiss LK, Goldberg IJ. Lipoprotein lipase increases lipoprotein binding to the artery wall and increases endothelial layer permeability by formation of

lipolysis products. Circ Res 1997;80:819—828.

11. Gretch DG, Sturley SL, Wang L, Lipton BA, Dunning A, Grunwald KA, Wetterau JR, Yao Z, Talmud P, Attie AD. The amino terminus of apolipoprotein B is necessary but not sufficient for microsomal triglyceride transfer protein responsiveness. J Biol Chem 1996;271:8682—8691.

12. Ingram MF, Shelness GS. Folding of the amino-terminal domain of apolipoprotein B initiates microsomal triglyceride transfer protein-dependent lipid transfer to nascent very low density lipoprotein. J Biol Chem 1997;272:10279—10286.

13. Kreuzer J, White AL, Knott TJ, Jien ML, Mehrabian M, Scott J, Young SG, Haberland ME. Amino terminus of apolipoprotein B suffices to produce recognition of malondialdehyde-modified low density lipoprotein by the scavenger receptor of human monocyte-macrophages. J Lipid Res 1997;38:324—342.

14. Gianturco SH, Ramprasad MP, Lin A-Y, Song R, Bradley WA. Cellular binding site and membrane binding proteins for triglyceride-rich lipoproteins in human monocyte-macrophages and THP-1 monocytic cells. J Lipid Res 1994;35:1674—1687.

15. Camejo G, Olofsson SO, Lopez F, Carlsson P, Bondjers G. Identification of apo B-100 segments mediating the interaction of low density lipoproteins with arterial proteoglycans. Arteriosclerosis 1988;8:368—377.

16. Goldberg IJ, Paka L, Pang L, Obunike JC, Pillarisetti S. Evidence that the amino-terminal region of apolipoprotein B is the atherogenic portion of low density lipoprotein. Circulation (In press) (Abstract).

17. Dugi KA, Knapper CL, Applebaum-Bowden D, Bensadoun A, Meyn SM, Le TT, Maeda N, Brewer HB Jr, Santamarina-Fojo S. In vivo evidence for a nonlipolytic role of hepatic lipase in the metabolism of high density lipoproteins. Circulation 1996;94:I—398.

18. Shimada M, Ishibashi S, Inaba T, Yagayu H, Harada K, Oshuga J, Yazaki Y, Yamada N. Overexpression of lipoprotein lipase reduced atherosclerotic lesions in low density lipoprotein receptor deficient mice. Proc Natl Acad Sci USA 1996;93:7242—7246.

19. Traber M, Olivecrona T, Kayden H. Bovine milk lipoprotein lipase transfers tocopheral to human fibroblasts during triglyceride hydrolysis in vitro. J Clin Invest 1985;75:1729—1734.

20. Blaner WS, Obunike JC, Kurlandsky SB, Al-Haideri M, Piantedosi R, Deckelbaum RJ, Goldberg IJ. Lipoprotein lipase hydrolysis of retinyl ester: possible implications for retinoid uptake by cells. J Biol Chem 1994;269:16559—16565.

21. Sattler W, Levak-Frank S, Radner H, Kostner GM, Zechner R. Muscle-specific overexpression of lipoprotein lipase in transgenic mice results in increased alpha-tocopherol levels in skeletal muscle. Biochem J 1996;318:15—19.

22. Pillarisetti S, Paka S, Obunike JC, Berglund L, Goldberg IJ. Subendothelial retention of lipoprotein (a): evidence that reduced heparan sulfate promotes lipoprotein binding to subendothelial matrix. J Clin Invest 1997;100:867—874.

23. Sivaram P, Obunike JC, Goldberg IJ. Lysolecithin induced alteration of subendothelial heparan sulfate proteoglycans increases monocyte binding to matrix. J Biol Chem 1995;270:29760—29765.

24. Pillarisetti S, Paka S, Sasaki A, Vanni-Reyes T, Yin B, Parthasarathy N, Wagner WD, Goldberg IJ. Endothelial cell heparanase modulation of lipoprotein lipase activity: evidence that heparan sulfate oligosaccharide is an extracellular chaperone. J Biol Chem 1997;272:15753—15759.

Arterial-wall sphingomyelinase and atherogenesis

Ira Tabas[1], Scott L. Schissel[1], Kevin Jon Williams[2], Edward H. Schuchman[3], Joseph H. Rapp[4] and Judith Tweedie-Hardman[4]

[1]*Departments of Anatomy and Cell Biology and Medicine, Columbia University, New York, New York;* [2]*Dorrance H. Hamilton Research Laboratories, Division of Endocrinology, Diabetes and Metabolic Diseases, Thomas Jefferson University, Philadelphia, Pennsylvania;* [3]*Department of Human Genetics, Mount Sinai School of Medicine, New York, New York; and* [4]*Department of Surgery, University of California-San Francisco and the San Francisco Veterans Affairs Medical Center, San Francisco, California, USA*

Abstract. *Background.* The subendothelial retention and aggregation of atherogenic lipoproteins are key events in atherogenesis. Lipoprotein aggregation leads to massive macrophage foam cell formation and further promotes lipoprotein retention. We have probed one potential mechanism of lesional lipoprotein aggregation, namely hydrolysis of lesional lipoproteins by the enzyme sphingomyelinase (SMase).

Methods. Plasma and lesional lipoproteins were analyzed directly for ceramide content or incubated in vitro with bacterial SMase, rabbit aortic strips or SMase isolated from the conditioned medium of cultured cells, and then assayed for ceramide and lipoprotein aggregation.

Results. Treatment of LDL with a bacterial SMase led to the formation of LDL aggregates that appeared similar to those that form in lesions (that greatly enhance lipoprotein retention to matrix and that are able to induce massive macrophage foam cell formation). The mechanism involves the generation of lipoprotein-ceramide. Most importantly, aggregated LDL isolated from human lesions (but not unaggregated lesional LDL or plasma LDL) was enriched in ceramide, indicating action by an arterial-wall SMase. Furthermore, when (^{3}H)SM-labeled LDL was incubated with strips of rabbit aorta ex vivo, (^{3}H)ceramide was increased in the retained (but not the unretained) LDL. As a potential source of extracellular SMase in lesions, cultured macrophages and endothelial cells were found to secrete a SMase activity (S-SMase) that can hydrolyze and aggregate atherogenic lipoproteins.

Conclusions. Lipoproteins in lesions are hydrolyzed by an arterial-wall SMase, a process that might promote lipoprotein aggregation, enhanced lipoprotein retention and macrophage foam cell formation. A leading candidate for this arterial-wall SMase is S-SMase, which secreted by macrophages and endothelial cells can hydrolyze and aggregate atherogenic lipoproteins.

Keywords: ceramide, endothelial cells, foam cells, LDL, lipoprotein aggregation, macrophages.

Introduction

The subendothelial retention and aggregation of atherogenic lipoproteins, including LDL [1,2] lipoprotein(a) (Lp(a)) [3,4] and triglyceride-rich lipoproteins [5] are important early events in atherosclerosis [6]. In particular, a number of laboratories have demonstrated by both biochemical and morphological

---

Address for correspondence: Dr Ira Tabas, Department of Medicine, Columbia University, 630 West 168th Street, New York, NY 10032, USA.

896

approaches that lipoproteins retained in the subendothelial matrix are often extensively aggregated [2,7–9]. Lipoprotein aggregation which occurs in both prelesional and macrophage-rich lesional sites [2,8], is likely to play an important role during atherogenesis. Aggregation greatly increases the quantity of lipoprotein retained (below and [10]) and thus would be expected to amplify the atherogenic arterial-wall responses to retained lipoproteins [6]. Moreover, aggregated LDL (but not unaggregated LDL) leads to massive cholesteryl ester accumulation in macrophages [11–14] and appears to be more potent than even oxidized LDL in inducing foam-cell formation (e.g., see [15]).

Lipoprotein self-aggregation can be induced in vitro by vortexing [12], extensive phospholipase C hydrolysis [13], extensive oxidation [16], and (in work from our laboratories) by limited hydrolysis with sphingomyelinase (SMase) (below and [14]). Vortexing and extensive hydrolysis by phospholipase C are unlikely to be physiologically important. LDL oxidation does occur in arteries [17], but subendothelial LDL aggregates have been shown to be present in normal rabbit aorta as early as 2 h after an intravenous bolus injection of LDL [2], which is almost certainly too soon for extensive LDL oxidation to occur in these normal vessels. Recently, we have obtained evidence (including human data) to indicate that LDL-SM hydrolysis may be physiologically important in both prelesional and lesional sites. The focus of this chapter is to present evidence supporting a role for arterial-wall SMase in lipoprotein retention and aggregation and atherogenesis.

Materials and Methods

SMase from *B. cereus*, sphingomyelin and ceramide were purchased from Sigma, and (N-palmitoyl-9-10-^{3}H)sphingomyelin was synthesized as described [14]. Lipoprotein lipase was purified from bovine milk [10] and plasma lipoproteins were isolated by preparative ultracentrifugation [18]. Acid SMase knockout mice were developed as described [19], and fibroblasts were obtained from patients with types A and B Niemann-Pick disease [20]. The following procedures and assays are described in the indicated citations: treatment of lipoproteins with bacterial SMase and aggregation assay [14]; incubation of lipoproteins with cultured macrophages and cholesteryl ester assay [14]; incubation of lipoproteins with smooth muscle cells and lipoprotein retention assays [10]; isolation and characterization of lesional LDL and ceramide assay [21]; ex vivo rabbit aortic strip SMase assay [21]; and harvesting of conditioned media (CM) and assay of mammalian SMase activity in cell lysates and CM [20].

Results and Discussion

Initial studies from our laboratory indicated that partial hydrolysis of human plasma LDL with bacterial SMase led to the formation of LDL aggregates that appeared similar to those have been shown to form in the arterial wall in vivo [14]. When these aggregates were added to cultured macrophages, cholesteryl ester accumulation was stimulated 3- to 5-fold compared with the addition of untreated LDL [14]. To explore the potential role of SMase-induced aggregation in a more physiological experimental system, we showed that bacterial SMase plus lipoprotein lipase (LpL) (which can act as "bridge" between lipoproteins and extracellular matrix [22]) led to 50- to 100-fold increases in LDL and lipoprotein(a) (Lp(a)) retention onto SMC-surface chondroitin sulfate proteoglycans (CSPGs); this effect was 10-fold greater than that seen with SMase or LpL alone [10]. Macrophages added to these cell-surface-bound lipoprotein aggregates were converted into foam cells within 24 h [10]. Interestingly, we have also found that apolipoprotein AI potently inhibits SMase-induced LDL aggregation (unpublished data). Thus, one of the mechanisms involved in the known anti-atherogenic properties of apo AI [23—25] may be its ability to inhibit or alter lipoprotein aggregation.

Studies on how SMase causes LDL aggregation led to two important findings. First, we showed that the role of SMase in LDL aggregation is enzymatic, not structural [21]. Thus, although our initial experiments used bacterial SMase, similar results can be expected for mammalian SMases. Second, we showed that SMase-induced LDL aggregation was due to an increase in LDL ceramide content, not due to low LDL SM content or to the generation of choline phosphate [21]. In fact, SM enrichment of particles was shown to enhance subsequent SMase-induced aggregation [21]. This was an important finding, since aggregation that depends on a low LDL SM content could not be physiologically significant: lesional LDL is enriched in SM [26,27].

The above findings led us to examine a previously unreported parameter of retained lesional LDL, namely its ceramide content. Thus, LDL was extracted from human lesions in the presence of EDTA (an inhibitor of many SMases) and purified by density gradient ultracentrifugation (d, 1.019—1.063 g/dl) as previously described [5]. Note that despite the fact that the LDL originated from advanced lesions, the apo B-100 of the LDL was intact [5]. As our model predicts, we found that the lesional LDL was 10- to 30-fold enriched in ceramide compared with same-donor plasma LDL [21]. When the atherectomy specimen was extracted in buffers that contained (^{3}H)SM-LDL, the labeled LDL was not hydrolyzed, indicating no artifactual SM hydrolysis during the extraction procedure [21]. No diacylglycerol was detected in human lesional LDL, indicating an absence of phospholipase C activity [21]. Similar data were obtained with lipoproteins extracted from early animal and human lesions [21]. Most importantly, when the lesional LDL was fractionated by low-speed centrifugation and gel filtration into aggregated ($\sim$80%) and unaggregated ($\sim$20%) forms, only the aggregated lesional LDL demonstrated increased ceramide content [21]. In a follow-up experiment, we incubated (^{3}H)SM-labeled LDL with strips of rabbit aorta ex vivo and directly demonstrated the presence of a nonlysosomal, cation-dependent SMase that can act directly on retained LDL [21].

To further characterize SMase activities that might be present in macrophage-rich atherosclerotic lesions, we examined homogenates and conditioned medium

(CM) of macrophages for SMase activity. Using (^{3}H)SM-containing detergent micelles as our assay substrate, we found that cellular homogenates of cultured J774 and mouse peritoneal macrophages contained primarily the cation-independent pH-5.0 activity, presumably lysosomal SMase (L-SMase). Conditioned medium, however, revealed the presence of a pH 5.0 SMase activity (secretory, or S−, SMase) that was inhibited by EDTA, unlike L-SMase; remarkably, optimal activity of this macrophage-secreted SMase required zinc. We also found that human monocyte-derived macrophages secrete S-SMase activity and that this activity is upregulated by monocyte-to-macrophage differentiation [20]. Furthermore, human endothelial cells are an abundant source of S-SMase (manuscript in preparation), a finding that could possibly explain LDL aggregation in prelesional (i.e., macrophage-poor) sites [2]. Moreover, certain cytokines known to be in atherosclerotic lesions (such as interferon-γ and interleukin-1β) stimulate secretion of S-SMase from endothelial cells (manuscript in preparation).

The cellular origin of S-SMase represents a fascinating cell biological phenomenon. In brief, we have proven that S-SMase arises from the same gene as L-SMase, namely the acid SMase (ASM) gene [20]. Our current working hypothesis on how the L- and S-SMase arise is as follows (manuscript submitted for publication): L-SMase comes from a portion of the newly translated product of the acid SMase gene that is mannose-phosphorylated and targeted to late endosomes, then lysosomes according to the well-described mannose-phosphate receptor (MPR)-mediated lysosomal targeting pathway. In this pathway, L-SMase acquires Zn^{2+} from cellular pools and binds it very avidly; thus, Zn^{2+} is not required at the time of assay of L-SMase, and EDTA (a relatively weak Zn^{2+}-chelator) does not inhibit its activity. S-SMase arises from another substantial portion of the gene product that escapes mannose-phosphorylation and thus is secreted instead of being targeted to lysosomes. In the secretory pathway, S-SMase is sequestered from cellular pools of Zn^{2+} and thus the metal is required at the time of assay.

The finding that S-SMase is secreted by macrophages and endothelial cells clearly establish S-SMase as a leading candidate for the arterial-wall SMase that we have shown acts on lesional LDL. In fact, we have recently obtained immunohistochemical data showing that S-SMase is present both in prelesional sites and in atherosclerotic lesions of mice and rabbits (manuscript in preparation). Nonetheless, the properties of S-SMase raise two important issues regarding its potential role in hydrolyzing lesional lipoproteins. First, given its requirement for Zn^{2+} is the enzyme likely to be active in lesions? The zinc requirement of S-SMase is similar to that of zinc-metalloenzymes [20,28] and zinc-metalloenzymes have been shown to be active in atherosclerotic lesions [29]. Thus, lesional zinc levels should be high enough to activate S-SMase.

Second, and more importantly, the enzyme has an acidic pH optimum when assayed using SM in detergent micelles [20,28]. Although advanced lesions may have pockets of acidity [30], a role for S-SMase in prelesional susceptible areas or in early lesions would require its ability to hydrolyze lipoprotein-SM at neutral pH. Interestingly, studies by Callahan et al. [31] demonstrate that only the affinity of L-SMase for SM-micelles (i.e., K_m) is highly sensitive to changes in pH, whereas the maximal velocity (V_{max}) for SM hydrolysis is pH independent. Since the kinetic properties of S-SMase and L-SMase should be similar [20], we reasoned that LDL-SM would be hydrolyzed at neutral pH if it could access the active site of S-SMase. Moreover, several physiologically relevant modifications of LDL (including oxidation, hydrolysis with phospholipase A_2 and sphingomyelin enrichment) alter the structure of the lipoprotein surface, perhaps allowing S-SMase to bind LDL-SM at neutral pH. These ideas prompted us to test whether modified forms of LDL are better substrates than native LDL for S-SMase at neutral pH (manuscript submitted for publication). Initially, we found that S-SMase could hydrolyze and aggregate native plasma LDL, but only at acid pH. Oxidized LDL, however, was an excellent substrate for S-SMase at neutral pH. In addition, lipoproteins from two atherogenic mouse models, apo E0 mice and LDLR0 x apolipoprotein CIII transgenic mice, were hydrolyzed and aggregated by S-SMase at neutral pH. Most importantly, LDL from human atherosclerotic lesions was also an excellent substrate for S-SMase at neutral pH.

In conclusion, aggregation of lesional lipoproteins is a prominent and likely important event during both early and advanced atherogenesis. We have explored a hypothesis in which an arterial wall SMase activity, by hydrolyzing the SM of retained lipoproteins, is at least one cause of lesional lipoprotein aggregation. Aggregated lesional lipoproteins are acted upon by an arterial-wall SMase and both macrophages and endothelial cells secrete a SMase that is a leading candidate for this arterial-wall enzyme. Current studies are directed towards elucidating factors that influence lipoprotein susceptibility to S-SMase, determining the regulation of S-SMase secretion and developing induced mutant mouse models to test the role of S-SMase in atherogenesis in vivo.

Acknowledgements

The work cited in this chapter was supported by National Institutes of Health (NIH) Grants HL-39703 and 21006 (IT), HD-28607 (EHS), HL-38956 (KJW), and HL-56984 (IT and KJW); a NIH Medical Scientist Training Grant award (SLS); Established Investigator Awards from the American Heart Association and Boehringer-Ingelheim (IT) and Genentech (KJW); a grant-in-aid from the American Heart Association, Southeastern Pennsylvania Affiliate (KJW); a March of Dimes Birth Defects Foundation Basic Research Grant 1-1224 (EHS); a cardiovascular research grant from the W.W. Smith Charitable Trust (KJW); and a Veterans Affairs Research Service award (JHR). We would like to acknowledge our other coauthors on these studies, including Dr Xiang-Xi (Michael) Xu, Dr Yueqing Li, Robert W. Brocia, Shu Wen Xu, Dr Theresa L. Swenson, George Graham, Dr Xian-cheng Jiang, Dr Tae-sook Jeong, Dr Eva Hurt Camejo, Dr Jamila Najib and Dr Michael Yellin.

References

1. Schwenke DC, Carew TE. Initiation of atherosclerotic lesions in cholesterol-fed rabbits: I. Focal increases in arterial LDL concentrations precede development of fatty streak lesions. Arteriosclerosis 1989;9:895—907.
2. Nievelstein PFEM, Fogelman AM, Mottino G, Frank JS. Lipid accumulation in rabbit aortic intima 2 h after bolus infusion of low-density lipoprotein. Arterioscl Thromb 1991;11: 1795—1805.
3. Kreuzer J, Lloyd MB, Bok D et al. Lipoprotein(a) displays increased accumulation compared with low-density lipoprotein in the murine arterial wall. Chem Phys Lipids 1994;67/68: 175—190.
4. Nielsen LB, Stender S, Jauhiainen M, Nordestgaard BG. Preferential influx and decreased fractional loss of lipoprotein(a) in atherosclerotic compared with nonlesioned rabbit aorta. J Clin Invest 1996;98:563—571.
5. Rapp JH, Lespine A, Hamilton RL et al. Triglyceride-rich lipoproteins isolated by selected-affinity antiapolipoprotein B immunosorption from human atherosclerotic plaque. Arterioscl Thromb 1994;14:1767—1774.
6. Williams KJ, Tabas I. The response-to-retention hypothesis of early atherogenesis. Arterioscl Thromb 1995;15:551—561.
7. Steinberg D, Parthasarathy S, Carew TE, Khoo JC, Witztum JL. Beyond cholesterol: modifications of low-density lipoprotein that increase its atherogenicity. N Engl J Med 1989;320: 915—924.
8. Hoff HF, Morton RE. Lipoproteins containing apo B extracted from human aortas: structure and function. Ann NY Acad Sci 1985;454:183—194.
9. Guyton JR, Klemp KF. Development of the lipid-rich core in human atherosclerosis. Arterioscl Thromb Vasc Biol 1996;16:4—11.
10. Tabas I, Li Y, Brocia RW, Wu SW, Swenson TL, Williams KJ. Lipoprotein lipase and sphingomyelinase synergistically enhance the association of atherogenic lipoproteins with smooth muscle cells and extracellular matrix. A possible mechanism for low-density lipoprotein and lipoprotein(a) retention and macrophage foam cell formation. J Biol Chem 1993;268:20419—20432.
11. Hoff HF, O'Neill J, Pepin JM, Cole TB. Macrophage uptake of cholesterol-containing particles derived from LDL and isolated from atherosclerotic lesions. Eur Heart J 1990;11:105—115.
12. Khoo JC, Miller E, McLoughlin P, Steinberg D. Enhanced macrophage uptake of low-density lipoprotein after self-aggregation. Arteriosclerosis 1988;8:348—358.
13. Suits AG, Chait A, Aviram M, Heinecke JW. Phagocytosis of aggregated lipoprotein by macrophages: low-density lipoprotein receptor-dependent foam-cell formation. Proc Natl Acad Sci USA 1989;86:2713—2717.
14. Xu X, Tabas I. Sphingomyelinase enhances low-density lipoprotein uptake and ability to induce cholesteryl ester accumulation in macrophages. J Biol Chem 1991;266:24849—24858.
15. Hoppe G, O'Neill J, Hoff HF. Inactivation of lysosomal proteases by oxidized low-density lipoprotein is partially responsible for its poor degradation by mouse peritoneal macrophages. J Clin Invest 1994;94:1506—1512.
16. Hoff HF, Whitaker TE, O'Neill J. Oxidation of low-density lipoprotein leads to particle aggregation and altered macrophage recognition. J Biol Chem 1992;267:602—609.
17. Witztum JL, Steinberg D. Role of oxidzed low-density lipoprotein in atherogenesis. J Clin Invest 1991;88:1785—1792.
18. Havel RJ, Eder H, Bragdon J. The distribution and chemical composition of ultracentrifugally reported lipoproteins in human serum. J Clin Invest 1955;34:1345—1353.
19. Horinouchi K, Erlich S, Perl D et al. Acid sphingomyelinase deficient mice: a model of types A and B Niemann-Pick disease. Nature Genet 1995;10:288—293.
20. Schissel SL, Schuchman EH, Williams KJ, Tabas I. Zn^{2+}-stimulated sphingomyelinase is secreted by many cell types and is a product of the acid sphingomyelinase gene. J Biol Chem

1996;271:18431–18436.

21. Schissel SL, Tweedie-Hardman J, Rapp JH, Graham G, Williams KJ, Tabas I. Rabbit aorta and human atherosclerotic lesions hydolyze the sphingomyelin of retained low-density lipoprotein. Proposed role for arterial-wall sphingomyelinase in subendothelial retention and aggregation of atherogenic lipoproteins. J Clin Invest 1996;98:1455–1464.

22. Williams KJ, Fless GM, Petrie KA, Snyder ML, Brocia RW, Swenson TL. Mechanisms by which lipoprotein lipase alters cellular metabolism of lipoprotein(a), low-density lipoprotein, and nascent lipoproteins. Roles for low-density lipoprotein receptors and heparan sulfate proteoglycans. J Biol Chem 1992;267:13284–13292.

23. Rubin EM, Krauss RM, Spangler EA, Verstuyft JG, Clift SM. Inhibition of early atherogenesis in transgenic mice by human apolipoprotein AI. Nature 1991;353:265–267.

24. Pászty C, Maeda N, Verstuyft J, Rubin EM. Apolipoprotein AI transgene corrects apolipoprotein E deficiency-induced atherosclerosis in mice. J Clin Invest 1994;94:899–903.

25. Plump AS, Scott CJ, Breslow JL. Human apolipoprotein A-I gene expression raises HDL and suppresses atherosclerosis in the apo E-deficient mouse. Proc Natl Acad Sci USA 1994;91: 9607–9611.

26. Hoff HF. LDL in the arterial wall: localization, quantitation, and characterization. In: Lewis LA (ed) Handbook of Electrophoresis, vol III. Lipoprotein Methodology and Human Studies. Boca Raton, FL: CRC Press, 1983;133–165.

27. Ylä-Herttuala S, Palinski W, Rosenfeld ME et al. Evidence for the presence of oxidatively modified low-density lipoprotein in atherosclerotic lesions of rabbit and man. J Clin Invest 1989;84: 1086–1095.

28. Spence MW, Byers DM, Palmer FB, Cook HW. A new Zn^{2+}-stimulated sphingomyelinase in fetal bovine serum. J Biol Chem 1989;264:5358–5363.

29. Galis ZS, Sukhova GK, Lark MW, Libby P. Increased expression of matrix metalloproteinases and matrix degrading activity in vulnerable regions of human atherosclerotic plaques. J Clin Invest 1994;94:2493–2503.

30. Smith EB. Metabolic activities in the arterial wall. Adv Exp Med Biol 1979;115:245–297.

31. Callahan JW, Jones CS, Davidson DJ, Shankaran P. The active site of lysosomal sphingomyelinase: evidence for the involvement of hydrophobic and ionic groups. J Neurosci Res 1983;10: 151–163.

Lipid oxidation products as regulators of macrophage function in atherosclerosis

Olov Wiklund, Lillemor Mattsson-Hultén, Bertil Ohlsson, Yani Liu-Wu, Eva Hurt-Camejo and Göran Bondjers
Wallenberg Laboratory, Sahlgrenska University Hospital, Göteborg, Sweden

Abstract. *Background.* It is still not known which of the potential capacities of macrophages are expressed in the atherosclerotic lesions, and how these are regulated. Oxysterols are present in oxLDL and accumulated in macrophage-derived foam cells. In the present study, we analyse the role of oxysterols as regulators of macrophage functions.

Methods. Cells were isolated from tissue by an immunomagnetic method. Monocyte-derived macrophages were studied in culture. Protein secretion and mRNA expression was studied after exposure to oxLDL or oxysterols in vitro. Binding of proteins to DNA was studied by electrophoretic mobility shift assay.

Results. In tissue-derived cells there was a low expression of lipoprotein lipase but a high level of IL-8. Exposure to oxysterols did downregulate the expression of lipoprotein lipase and increase the synthesis of IL-8. After exposure to oxidised low-density lipoprotein (oxLDL) or oxysterols, macrophages showed a reduced response to stimulation by endotoxin. This was paralleled by a reduced binding of NF-κB to DNA. Furthermore, our data suggest that oxysterols induce a repressing transcription factor.

Conclusions. OxLDL and oxysterols may regulate the function of macrophages. Our data also suggest that the macrophage population in the lesion is heterogenous with a wide variety of potential responsiveness to different stimuli.

Keywords: cytokines, lipoprotein lipase, oxidized LDL, oxysterols.

Introduction

Macrophages constitute one of the major cell populations of the atherosclerotic lesions. Macrophage-derived foam cells are the dominating cells of the early fatty streaks, while in the fibrous plaque and the complicated lesions these cells are found together with smooth muscle cells and lymphocytes. Although the presence of macrophages has been documented in a series of studies, their actual role during the development of the atherosclerotic lesion still is largely unknown. The macrophages are cells with a very varied potential capacities expressed under different conditions. Several of the potential roles of the macrophages may have a crucial role during the development of atherosclerosis, and also during the transition of the stable fibrous plaque into a rupture prone or thrombo-

Address for correspondence: Olov Wiklund MD, PhD, Wallenberg Laboratory, Sahlgrenska Sjukhuset, 413 45 Göteborg, Sweden. Tel.: +46-31-412242. Fax: +46-31-823762.
E-mail: wiklund@wlab.wall.gu.se

gentic inflammatory active lesion. Thus, the macrophages are not only active phagocytic cells but also show a wide spectrum of secretory activities with a potential to secrete a variety of cytokines and growth factors as well as proteolytic enzymes and lipases [1]. Several of the secretory products of macrophages have also been shown in atherosclerotic lesion. For example, the presence of inflammatory cytokines as IL-1β and TNF-α has been shown using immune histochemistry or in situ hybridisation. In other studies the presence of lipoprotein lipase or metalloproteinases has been shown.

Although the role of macrophages in atherogenesis has been emphasized by several investigators for many years, the actual activity of these cells in the lesion is still controversial, and the regulation or mechanisms of activation of macrophages in atherosclerosis still has to be studied. In the present study, we have focused on some aspects of the regulation of macrophages with emphasis on the role of oxidized low-density lipoprotein (LDL) and lipid oxidation products.

During oxidation of LDL a series of different lipid oxidation products are generated. Among these are the oxidation products of cholesterol, the oxysterols. As shown by Dzeletovic et al. [2] these oxysterols are also generated during different oxidation procedures. We have studied the composition of oxysterols in foam cells isolated from human atherosclerotic lesions, and shown that the pattern of oxysterols is very similar to that found in in vitro oxidized LDL [3]. However, in foam cells we also find high concentrations of the enzymatically derived 27-hydroxy cholesterol, which is lacking in in vitro oxidized LDL. Oxysterols are potentially biologically active components which might be of importance for the regulation of cellular functions in the atherosclerotic lesions. Therefore, we have focused interest on the role of oxysterols as regulators of macrophage functions.

Methods

Cells

Cells were isolated from human atherosclerotic tissue obtained preoperatively. Macrophage-derived foam cells were isolated after digestion of the tissue with collagenase. Specific cells were extracted from the cell suspension using specific antibodies (antiCD14) and magnetic microspheres [4].

Monocyte-derived macrophages were obtained from buffy coats. Macrophages were isolated after adhesion to plastic dishes as described [5]. The cells were then allowed to differentiate to macrophages in culture for up to 7 days.

Biochemical analyses

Lipoprotein lipase activity was analysed as heparin releasable activity according to Nilsson-Ehle [6]. mRNA was quantified by a RT-PCR method, using an internal standard essentially as described by Wang et al. [7]. The concentrations of IL-8 were determined with commercially available ELISA kit (R&D Systems).

The binding of transcription factors to DNA was analysed with electrophoretic mobility shift assay as described [8].

Results

Oxysterols as regulators of lipoprotein lipase

Expression of lipoprotein lipase (LPL) is an early differentiation marker for macrophages. Whether macrophage-derived foam cells in atherosclerotic lesions express lipoprotein lipase (LPL) has been controversial [9,10]. In cells isolated from human atherosclerotic lesions we found very low levels of LPL activity, as well as low levels of mRNA for LPL [11]. In contrast, monocyte-derived macrophages did express LPL activity and LPL mRNA. Furthermore, the tissue-derived cells could not be stimulated by PMA (Fig. 1).

In order to explore if oxysterols regulate the expression of lipoprotein lipase, we exposed monocyte derive macrophages to oxysterols. We could then show that oxysterols downregulate the expression of LPL. This was true for several oxysterols but most prominently for 7-hydroxy cholesterol and 25-hydroxy cholesterol [3]. We suggest, therefore, that the accumulation of oxysterols in macrophages modulate the expression of LPL in atherosclerosis.

Oxysterols as regulators of IL-8

It has been shown in earlier studies [12] that oxLDL may induce IL-8 production in macrophages. IL-8 is an important chemkine and may contribute to the propagation of an inflammatory reaction in the arterial intima. In studies of the presence of IL-8 in cells derived from arterial tissue, we could show that these

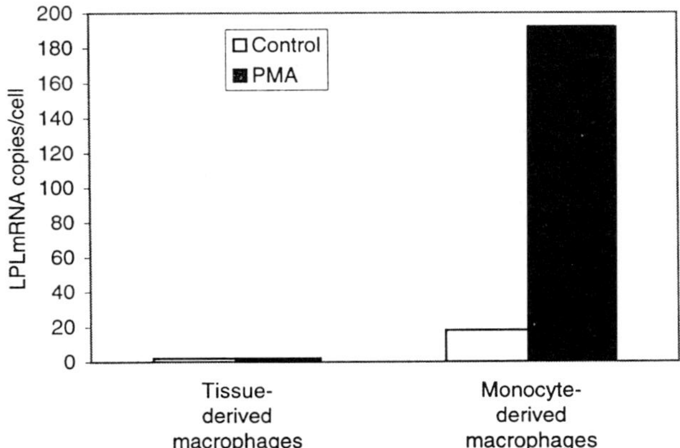

Fig. 1. Expression of lipoprotein lipase (LPL) mRNA in macrophages derived from human atherosclerotic tissue and in human monocyte derived macrophages. mRNA was analysed by RT-PCR in freshly isolated cells and in cells after stimulation with PMA (10 nM) for 24 h.

cells express very high levels of IL-8, while monocytes and monocyte-derived macrophages express low levels [13]. In line with our earlier observations of oxysterols in macrophages, we then explored the possibility that oxysterols induce IL-8 production in macrophages. All oxysterols (but most significantly 25-hydroxycholesterol) could induce IL-8 production. This response was dose- and time-dependent.

OxLDL and oxysterols reduce the response to endotoxin

Bacterial endotoxins (LPS) is a potent activator of macrophages. In order to study how oxLDL or oxysterols affect the capacity of macrophages to respond to activation, we used LPS-stimulation as a model for inflammatory activation of macrophages. Monocyte-derived macrophages were exposed to oxysterols or oxLDL for 24 h followed by stimulation with LPS for 1 h. We then found that pre-incubation with oxLDL or with 25-hydroxycholesterol dramatically reduced the response to LPS stimulation. This response was measured as synthesis of TNF-α or IL-1β [14].

The possibility that this response was mediated by a reduced binding of the proinflammatory transcription factor NF-κB was explored using electrophoretic mobility shift assay (EMSA). In these studies we used a DNA construct corresponding to a NF-κB binding site in the TNF-α promoter. It was then observed that oxLDL reduced the LPS-induced binding of NF-κB to DNA. These data strongly supported that the reduced LPS response was mediated by a reduced activation of NF-κB (Fig. 2).

Regarding the response to oxysterols our observations were contradictory. Although 25-hydroxycholesterol quite dramatically reduced the response to LPS no reduction in the binding of NF-κB to the TNF-α promoter was seen. This was taken as evidence for the presence of other mechanisms, possibly the induction of an inhibitory transcription factor. We have then been able to show that 25-hydroxycholesterol induces the binding of a protein to a site close to the TATA box of the TNF-α promoter. This transcription factor probably belongs to the SP family. The present working hypothesis is that the oxysterol induces an inhibitory transcription factor. The hypothesis is supported by the fact that the production of IL-1β (that lacks the SP binding site in its promoter) is not inhibited by 25 hydroxycholesterol.

Conclusions

The data presented show that oxysterols may mediate a differentiated modulation of the macrophage function in atherosclerosis. In monocytes and early macrophages, oxysterols may promote inflammation by the induction of IL-8 synthesis. On the other hand, in mature macrophages or cells after prolonged exposure to oxLDL or oxysterols the responsiveness seems to be reduced. This was found both for the secretion of lipoprotein lipase and for the responsiveness to LPS.

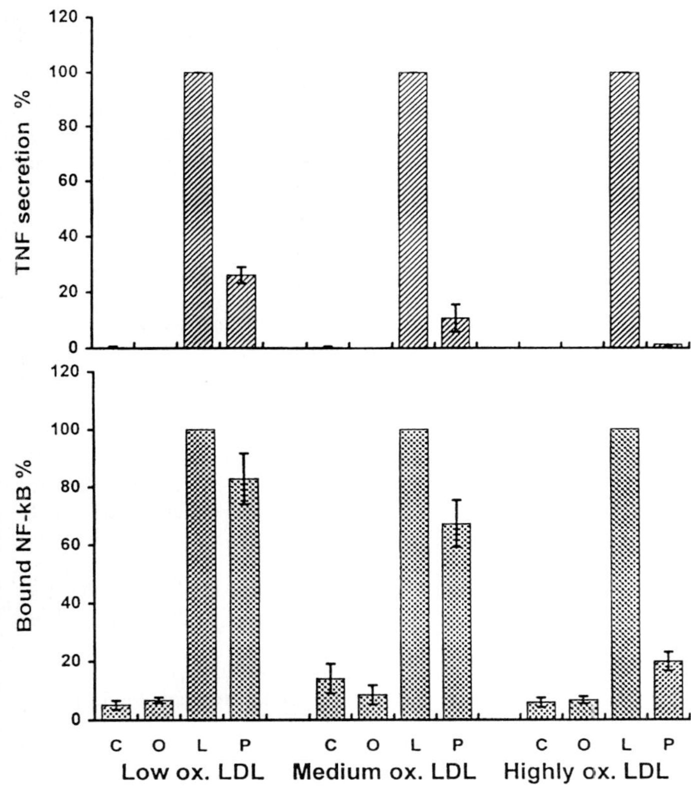

Fig. 2. Effect of oxidized LDL on the response of macrophages from LPS treatment. The response was measured as TNF-α secretion and as the binding of NF-κB to the TNF-α promoter. The TNF-α secretion was measured in the cell-culture medium and nuclear protein extracts were analysed for binding to DNA by EMSA. The TNF-α secretion and nuclear protein extracts were compared from untreated macrophages (C), macrophages treated with oxLDL (50 µg/ml) for 24 h (O), cells stimulated with LPS (1 µg/ml) for 3 h and cells pretreated with oxidized LDL (50 µg/ml) for 24 h before exposure to LPS (1 µg/ml) for 3 h (P). Data are expressed as percent of the levels in cells treated only with LPS (100%).

Since foam cells have been shown to accumulate oxysterols, the oxysterols may play a key role for the capacities of these cells that are expressed. Our data would suggest that mature foam cells have a limited capacity to respond to activation. Our data also suggest that the macrophage population of the atherosclerotic lesion is very heterogenous with a wide variety of potential responsiveness to different stimuli.

References

1. Adams DO, Hamilton TA. The cell biology of macrophage activation. Ann Rev Immunol 1984; 2:283–318.

2. Dzeletovic S, Babiker A, Lund E, Diczfalusy U. Time course of oxysterol formation during in vitro oxidation of low-density lipoprotein. Chem Phys Lipids 1995;78:119—128.
3. Mattsson-Hultén L, Johansson H, Diczfalusy U, Björkhem I, Ottosson M, Liu Y, Bondjers G, Wiklund O. Oxysterols present in atherosclerotic tissue decrease the expression of lipoprotein lipase mRNA in human monocyte-derived macrophages. J Clin Invest 1997;97:461—468.
4. Mattsson L, Bondjers G, Wiklund O. Isolation of cell populations from arterial tissue, using monoclonal antibodies and magnetic microspheres. Atherosclerosis 1991;89:25—34.
5. Böyum A. Isolation of lymphocytes, granulocytes and macrophages. Scand J Immunol 1976; 5:9.
6. Nilsson-Ehle P, Törnqvist H, Belfrage P. Rapid determination of lipoprotein lipase activity in human adipose tissue. Clin Chim Acta 1972;42:383—390.
7. Wang AM, Doyle MV, Mark DF. Quantification of mRNA by the polymerase chain reaction. Proc Natl Acad Sci USA 1989;86:9717—9721.
8. Garner MM, Revzin A. A gel electrophoresis method for quantifying the binding of proteins to specific DNA regions: application to components of the *Escherichia coli* lactose operon regulatory system. Nucl Acid Res 1981;9:3047—3060.
9. Jonasson L, Bondjers G, Hansson GK. Lipoprotein lipase in atherosclerosis: its presence in smooth muscle cells and absence from macrophages. J Lipid Res 1987;28:437—445.
10. O'Brien KD, Gordon D, Deeb S, Ferguson M, Chait A. Lipoprotein lipase is synthesized by macrophage-derived foam cells in human coronary atherosclerotic plaques. J Clin Invest 1992; 89:1544—1550.
11. Mattsson L, Johansson H, Ottosson M, Bondjers G, Wiklund O. Expression of mRNA for lipoprotein lipase and enzyme secretion in macrophages isolated from human atherosclerotic tissue. J Clin Invest 1993;92:1759—1765.
12. Terkeltaub R, Banka CL, Solan J, Santoro D, Brand K, Curtiss LK. Oxidized LDL induces monocytic cell expression of interleukin-8, a chemokine with T-lymphocyte chemotactic activity. Arterioscl Thromb 1993;14:47—53.
13. Liu Y, Mattsson L, Wiklund O. Macrophages isolated from human aterhosclerotic plaques produce IL-8, and oxysterols may have a regulatory function for IL-8 production. Arterioscl Thromb 1997;17:317—323.
14. Ohlsson BG, Englund M, Karlsson A-L, Knutsen E, Erixon C, Skribeck H, Liu Y, Bondjers G, Wiklund O. Oxidized low-density lipoprotein inhibits lipopolysaccharide-induced binding of nuclear factor-κB to DNA and the subsequent expression of the TNF-α and IL-1β in macrophages. J Clin Invest 1996;98:1—12.

Health economy and hypolipidemic drugs

Atherosclerosis XI.
B. Jacotot, D. Mathé and J.-C. Fruchart, editors.

Rationale and effectiveness of lipid therapy

Eberhard Windler, Birgit-Christiane Zyriax and Heiner Greten
Medizinische Kernklinik und Poliklinik, Universitäts-Krankenhaus Eppendorf, Hamburg, Germany

Abstract. Coronary artery disease still has a grave prognosis. More than half of the patients die within 24 h, mostly before reaching a hospital. A minority survive the 1st year even with the conditions of advanced medical care in Western industrial countries. Only more intense methods of prevention will lead to a fundamental change in the fate of coronary patients.

Primary prevention, in its narrowest sense, refers to avoiding the development of initial lesions early in life. Therefore, it can only be the result of an education directed towards a healthy lifestyle and is the responsibility of educational institutions.

In our population, the majority of the middle-aged are likely to have developed arteriosclerosis. Thus, the use of the term "primary prevention" no longer refers to avoiding arteriosclerosis, but rather to avoiding the complications of coronary artery disease in still asymptomatic patients. The outstanding effects of lipid therapy in patients at risk will result primarily from delaying progression, thereby circumventing the evolution of stable (and particularly unstable) plaques.

However, lipid therapy is most effective in patients with proven coronary artery disease. Reduction of LDL-cholesterol and an increase of HDL-cholesterol results in a 30–40% lower rate of major coronary events, and a decrease of the total mortality in the same order of magnitude. Evidently, the majority of coronary events can be prevented by idealizing the lipid parameters, i.e., lowering the LDL-cholesterol below 100 mg/dl or reducing the ratio of LDL- and HDL-cholesterol to less than 2.

The chronic coronary syndrome is still the domain of interventional cardiology. Lipid therapy will lead only gradually to a reduction of significant coronary stenoses. Recently, there has been evidence accumulating that the correction of the lipid metabolism has the potential of improving endothelial dysfunction and reducing silent ischemia and angina within weeks. This promises an additional conservative approach to one of the manifestations of coronary artery disease.

Thus, lipid therapy is an effective measure to stop the development of coronary atherosclerosis, avoid its often lethal complications and ameliorate the clinical sequelae of late-stage coronary artery disease. Costs and long-term safety seem to be the major limitations for a broad application of lipid-lowering drugs in the prevention and treatment of coronary artery disease.

Do we need new strategies to fight coronary artery disease?

In general, patients and doctors overestimate the prognosis of coronary artery disease because both emergency care and established medical and invasive treatment have decreased the mortality of hospitalized patients to 10–15% within 1 year. However, the prehospital mortality is exceedingly high. About one-third of the patients die before reaching a hospital, and another 20% die within the first 24 h from onset of symptoms. Mortality rates have been reported to be similarly

Address for correspondence: Eberhard Windler MD, Prof, Medizinische Kernklinik und Poliklinik, Universitäts-Krankenhaus Eppendorf, Martinistraße 52, D-20246 Hamburg, Germany. Tel.: +49-40-47173947. Fax: +49-40-47175059.

high in all the Western industrial countries by the MONICA project [1,2]. It is this fact that calls for more effective regimes in the prevention and treatment of coronary artery disease. Lipid therapy has evolved as a new promise for patients at risk.

What is the clinical impact of primary prevention?

The term "primary prevention" in its narrow sense refers to measures to avoid initial atherosclerotic lesions. However, fatty streaks already develop from childhood onwards [3–6]. Thus, early lifestyle modification through health education is the only realistic way to circumvent the progression to advanced lesions.

In the adult population of Western industrial countries, however, arteriosclerosis is so prevalent that primary prevention implies the treatment of risk factors to avoid complications of already developed atherosclerotic lesions. After several randomized trials in asymptomatic patients, the "West of Scotland Coronary Prevention Study" (WOSCOP) [7] has recently examined the potential benefit of a lipid-lowering therapy in asymptomatic middle-aged men with hypercholesterolemia, but no history of myocardial infarction. Prevalence of other risk factors such as smoking or hypertension was high. Lipid therapy unequivocally reduced the morbidity and mortality of myocardial infarction and the total mortality. The rate of strokes was decreased and a high percentage of PTCAs and bypass operations were avoided. These results demonstrate the benefit of a lipid-lowering therapy in the prevention of complications of arteriosclerosis in the population.

Numerous coronary prevention studies show on average that for each 10% decrease in cholesterol the rate of myocardial infarction drops by 25%. This effect is reached within 3 years and can last for decades. In agreement with many international guidelines, an LDL-cholesterol below 160 mg/dl and an HDL-cholesterol above 40 mg/dl is desirable in low-risk patients, corresponding to an LDL/HDL ratio below 4 [8,9]. As the coronary risk increases with the number of risk factors exponentially [10], an LDL-cholesterol below 130 mg/dl is requested to achieve a reasonable low risk in the presence of at least one risk factor (e.g., hypertension, smoking, diabetes or Lp(a) or an HDL below 40 mg/dl) [11]. This corresponds to an LDL/HDL ratio below 3. Primary prevention can be achieved through lifestyle modifications, but in many cases medical treatment will be required to achieve these goals, making cost-effectiveness a question of prime importance. Screening programs for patients at risk will be the basis for a cost-effective practice of the prevention of coronary artery disease.

Can lipid therapy prevent the acute coronary syndrome?

In patients with established coronary artery disease, the effect of coronary interventions like angioplasty on the long-term prevention of acute coronary events is commonly overestimated. Revascularization may add to the prognostic value of measures proven to reduce coronary events like aspirin, β-blockers and (in certain settings) ACE-inhibitors [12]. However, lipid therapy is still underestimated in its effect although it has to be part of such a regime, since it appears to act directly on the cause of coronary events in the arterial wall.

In advanced stages of coronary artery disease cholesterol seems to destabilize the arteriosclerotic plaques and promote plaque rupture [13]. An evolving thrombus may cause unstable angina and myocardial infarction [14]. Such plaque ruptures or erosions have to be prevented. Since the majority of these events occur independently of coronary stenoses, localized interventions are not likely to affect the great number of myocardial infarctions [15—17]. Moreover, high degree coronary stenoses may even progress to coronary occlusion, yet not necessarily to an infarct due to the development of collaterals preventing ischemia [18]. Thus, lipid therapy may be more effective in the prevention of the acute coronary syndrome than the conventional cardiologic procedures routinely applied because of its systemic and causative effect [19,20].

Proof of this concept was furnished by the "Scandinavian Simvastatin Survival Study" (4S study) [21]. A reduction of the LDL-cholesterol and an increase of the HDL-cholesterol resulted in a 30—40% lower rate of major coronary events and a decrease of the total mortality in the same order of magnitude. For two reasons the results that can be achieved by lipid therapy are underestimated in trials like the 4S study. The effect increases with time, and lipids are not lowered to target values. Optimal results require that the LDL-cholesterol is lowered to below 100 mg/dl.

Which coronary patient will profit from lipid therapy?

The effect depends upon both a reduction of the LDL-cholesterol and an elevation of the HDL-cholesterol [22]. HMG-CoA-reductase inhibitors act optimally due to their dual effect on the LDL-cholesterol and HDL-cholesterol. The "Bezafibrate Coronary Atherosclerosis Infarction Prevention Trial" (BECAIT) used a fibrate and underlined the value of an elevation of the HDL-cholesterol [23]. In agreement with the documented risk of hypertriglyceridemia, the correction of the prevalent lipid profile of high triglycerides and low HDL-cholesterol is an effective part of lipid therapy [24]. For optimal results of the treatment of coronary heart disease the ratio of LDL- and HDL-cholesterol should be reduced to less than 2. Evidently, the majority of coronary events can be prevented by idealizing the lipid parameters [22]. Thus, lipid therapy is one of the most effective measures to treat coronary artery disease.

Lipid therapy in the treatment of coronary artery disease has a broad application. Its efficacy is independent of a wide range of baseline cholesterol values. Susceptible patients appear to develop coronary artery disease despite only marginally elevated cholesterol concentrations. But likewise they profit from a reduction of the individually too high, though comparatively moderate cholesterol value. This has been examined in the "Cholesterol and Recurrent Event Study" (CARE) which showed that even reduction of baseline LDL-cholesterol values of 130 mg/dl effectively lowered the rate of coronary events including death [25].

The effectiveness of lipid therapy proved to be independent of the risk factors that led to atherosclerosis. Smokers and patients with hypertension or diabetes mellitus profited alike [26]. Plaque stabilization seems to be a universal mechanism, independent of the individual's genesis of coronary artery disease. In these high-risk populations the effect was especially pronounced. In agreement with these findings, there is no evidence for a difference between gender. Thus, because of its effectiveness, costs can only be a second-line argument for the application of lipid therapy in coronary patients.

Is lipid therapy useful in the chronic coronary syndrome?

The chronic coronary syndrome is characterized by ischemia that may cause stable angina and myocardial dysfunction due to high-percentage stenoses, commonly $> 75\%$. Neither the detection of ischemia (e.g., by stress-ECG) or stenoses (e.g., by angiography), however, are sensitive predictors for myocardial infarction since they are the result of unpredictable plaque ruptures [14]. Thus, in the chronic coronary syndrome one therapeutic goal is relieving chest pain and improving myocardial function. This may be achieved by revascularization procedures although their prognostic value is only documented for specific indications and for a limited time [12,19]. Chest pain on its own may also be treated by the established anti-ischemic drugs, some of which even provide a prognostic advantage [27].

Lipid therapy for the treatment of the chronic coronary syndrome has been evaluated in about 30 angiographically controlled trials using hypolipidemic drugs or lifestyle changes (including diet) [28–31]. The effect on coronary stenoses ranged from reduced progression to regression. The major outcome appears to be that with adequate lipid changes coronary artery disease can be stopped, which is a major aim not achieved by other measures. This alone may be reason enough to apply lipid therapy to every coronary patient.

In these trials reduction of coronary stenoses was limited to a few percent per year. This may still lead to a measurable improvement of the blood flow, since it is only significantly impaired with a very high degree of coronary stenosis [32]. But, this can only be a byproduct of lipid therapy in the light of the drastic improvements by interventional procedures. However, these procedures call for long-term adjunctive treatment to preserve the acutely achieved result. This is often neglected in view of the remarkable success of the local therapy. Progression of the disease has to be stopped, and after bypass surgery the development of lesions in the new vessels has to be avoided. However, this is commonly omitted as recently demonstrated in the "Munich Coronary Bypass Intervention Trial" (MCBIT) (J. Thiery, D. Seidel, B. Meisser and B. Reichart, personal communication, 1997), although the efficacy of lipid therapy has been repeatedly documented [33]. Thus, lipid therapy is a necessary adjunct to interventional cardiology.

Is lipid therapy effective in symptomatic patients?

Despite the protracted effect on coronary stenoses, lipid therapy may have a major impact on the symptomatic improvement of coronary patients. An early dysfunction in atherosclerotic blood vessels is an impaired endothelium-dependent vasomotor function reflected in a pathologic tendency towards vasoconstriction. Repeatedly, it has been shown that the degree of this dysfunction is vastly dependent on the plasma concentration of LDL-cholesterol, and reciprocally of HDL-cholesterol [34]. Lipid therapy ameliorates this reaction. This mechanism may be the basis for the clinical experience that in patients with coronary artery disease compromised myocardial perfusion improves (without exception), with drastically lowered LDL-cholesterol as determined by positron emission tomography [35]. This effect can be detected within weeks and is much faster than any regression of plaques.

In agreement with these results in the "Lifestyle Heart Trial" it has been observed that the rate of angina pectoris was diminished by 90% within 1 year in the treated group, as compared to the controls [28]. Likewise, in the 4S study, angina was reduced in parallel to the reduction of coronary events (T. Pedersen, Oslo, personal communication). Recently, the effect of lipid therapy on vasomotor function has been subjected to randomized trials. Within weeks the number of episodes of ischemia were substantially lowered with no detectable ischemia in the majority of subjects [36]. With these results, a new perspective for the application of lipid therapy in the treatment of the chronic coronary syndrome appears to open up. Since it is a byproduct of the lipid therapy in coronary patients, costs are no limitation. On the contrary, since other measures may be saved, this symptomatic effect will perhaps add to the cost-effectiveness of lipid therapy.

Should lipid therapy be part of the standard treatment of coronary artery disease?

Lipid therapy is effective in the prevention of arteriosclerosis and the treatment of the sequelae of coronary artery disease, not only symptomatic, but also by improving the prognosis. Despite its overwhelming effectiveness, lipid therapy has only limited use in the treatment of coronary patients. This may be based on the arbitrary semantic differentiation between treatment which is accepted as being indispensable and lipid therapy as part of preventive measures which are often rated as not obligatory. Doubts about its cost-effectiveness appear to be the major obstacle brought forward by clinicians as an argument to neglect this promising therapeutic option.

References

1. Löwel H, Dobson A, Keil U, Herman B, Hobbs MST, Stewart A, Arstila M, Miettinen H, Mustaniemi H, Tuomilehto J. Coronary heart disease case fatality in four countries — a community

study. Circulation 1993;88:2524–2531.

2. WHO Monica Project. Myocardial infarction and coronary deaths in the World Health Organization MONICA project. Registration procedures, event rates, and case-fatality rates in 38 populations from 21 countries in four continents. Circulation 1994;90:583–612.

3. Faggiotto A, Ross R, Harker L. Studies of hypercholesterolemia in the nonhuman primate. I. Changes that lead to fatty streak formation. Arteriosclerosis 1984;4:323–340.

4. Faggiotto A, Ross R. Studies of hypercholesterolemia in the nonhuman primate. II. Fatty streak conversion to fibrous plaque. Arteriosclerosis 1984;4:341–356.

5. Steinberg D. Modified forms of low-density lipoprotein and atherosclerosis. J Int Med 1993;233:227–232.

6. Stary HC. The sequence of cell and matrix changes in atherosclerotic lesions of coronary arteries in the first forty years of life. Eur Heart J 1990;11(Suppl E):3–19.

7. Shepherd J, Cobbe SM, Ford I, Isles CH, Lorimer AR, MacFarlane PW, McKillop JH, Packard CJ, for the West of Scotland Coronary Prevention Study Group. Prevention of coronary heart disease with pravastatin in men with hypercholesterolemia. N Engl J Med 1995;333:1301–1307.

8. Pyörälä K, DeBacker G, Graham I, Poole-Wilson P, Wood D on behalf of the Task Force. Prevention of coronary heart disease in clinical practice: recommendations of the Task Force of the European Society of Cardiology, European Atherosclerosis Society and European Society of Hypertension. Atherosclerosis 1994;110:121–161.

9. National Cholesterol Education Program. Second report of the expert panel on detection, evaluation, and treatment of high blood cholesterol in adults. Circulation 1994;89:1333–1445.

10. Kannel WB. High-density lipoproteins: epidemiologic profile and risks of coronary artery disease. Am J Cardiol 1983;52:9b–12b.

11. Cremer P, Nagel D, Labrot B, Muche R, Elster H, Mann H, Seidel D. Göttinger Risiko-, Inzidenz- und Prävalenzstudie (GRIPS). Heidelberg: Springer Verlag, 1991.

12. Yusuf S, Zucker D, Peduzzi P, Fischer LD, Takaro T, Kennedy JW, Davis K, Killip T, Passamani E, Norris R, Morris C, Mathur V, Varnanskas E, Chalmas TC. Effect of coronary artery bypass graft surgery on survival: overview of 10-year results from randomised trials by the Coronary Artery Bypass Graft Surgery Trialists Collaboration. Lancet 1994;344:563–570.

13. Davies MJ. Pathology of atherosclerosis, plaque disruption, and thrombus formation. Curr Opin Cardiol 1989;4:464–467.

14. Fuster V, Badimon L, Badimon JJ, Chesebro JH. The pathogenesis of coronary artery disease and the acute coronary syndromes. N Engl J Med 1992;326:310–318.

15. Giroud D, Li JM, Urban P, Meier B, Rutishauser W. Relation of the site of acute myocardial infarction to the most severe coronary arterial stenosis at prior angiography. Am J Cardiol 1992;69:729–732.

16. Pétursson MK, Jónmundsson EH, Brekkan A, Hardarson T. Angiographic predictors of new coronary occlusions. Am Heart J 1995;129:515–520.

17. Shahar E, Lewis M, Keil U, McGovern PG, Löwel H, Luepker RV. Hospital care and survival of acute myocardial infarction patients in Minnesota and southern Germany: a comparative study. Pathophysiol Nat Hist 1996;7:467–473.

18. Yellon DM, Baxter GF, Marber MS. Angina reassessed: pain or protection. Lancet 1996;347:1059–1062.

19. RITA-2 trial participants. Coronary angioplasty versus medical therapy for angina: the second Randomised Intervention Treatment of Angina (RITA-2) trial. Lancet 1997;350:461–468.

20. Levine GN, Keaney JF, Vita JA. Cholesterol reduction in cardiovascular disease: clinical benefits and possible mechanisms. N Engl J Med 1995;332:512–521.

21. Scandinavian Simvastatin Survival Study Group. Randomised trial of cholesterol lowering in 4444 patients with coronary heart disease: the Scandinavian Simvastatin Survival Study (4S). Lancet 1994;344:1383–1389.

22. Pedersen TR, Olsson AG, Færgeman O, Berg K, Miettinen T, Wedel H for the 4S Group. Sim-

vastatin-induced reduction in risk of major coronary events is related to both reduction in LDL-cholesterol and increase in HDL-cholesterol. Circulation 1995;92:I—198.

23. Ericsson C-G, Hamsten A, Nilsson J, Grip L, Svane B, de Faire U. An angiographic evaluation of the effects of bezafibrate on the progression of coronary artery disease in young male postinfarction patients. The bezafibrate coronary atherosclerosis intervention trial (BECAIT). Lancet 1996;347:849—853.

24. Assmann G. Lipid Metabolism Disorders and Coronary Heart Disease. München: MMV Medizin Verlag, 1993.

25. Sacks FM, Rouleau J-L, Moye LA, Pfeffer MA, Warnica JW, Arnold MO, Nash DT, Brown LE, Sestier F, Rutherford J, Davis BR, Hawkins CM, Braunwald E for the CARE Investigators. Baseline characteristics in the Cholesterol and Recurrent Events (CARE) Trial of secondary prevention in patients with average serum cholesterol levels. Am J Cardiol 1995;75:621—623.

26. Kjekshus J, Pedersen TR, Pyörälä K, for the 4S Group. Impact of hypertension, diabetes and smoking on the effect of simvastatin on coronary events in coronary heart disease patients. Circulation 1995;92:I—18.

27. Parisi AF, Folland ED, Hartigan P. Veterans Affairs ACME Investigators: a comparison of angioplasty with medical therapy in the treatment of single-vessel coronary artery disease. N Engl J Med 1992;326:10—16.

28. Ornish D, Brown SE, Scheerwitz LW, Billings JH, Armstrong WT, Ports TA, McLanahan SM, Kirkeeide RL, Brand RJ, Gould KL. Can lifestyle changes reverse coronary heart disease? — the lifestyle heart trial. Lancet 1990;336:129—133.

29. Kane JP, Malloy MJ, Ports TA, Phillips NR, Diehl JC, Havel RJ. Regression of coronary atherosclerosis during treatment of familial hypercholesterolemia with combined drug regimens. JAMA 1990;264:3007—3012.

30. Brown BG, Zhao X-Q, Albers JJ. Plaque regression and clinical events in coronary disease. Prim Cardiol 1992;18:6—54.

31. MAAS investigators. Effect to simvastatin on coronary atheroma: the Multicentre Anti-Atheroma Study (MAAS). Lancet 1994;344:633—638.

32. Cashinhemphill L, Mack WJ, Pogoda JM, Sanmarco ME, Azen SP, Blankenhorn DH. Beneficial effects of colestipol-niacin on coronary atherosclerosis — a 4-year follow-up. JAMA 1990; 264:3013—3017.

33. The Postcoronary Artery Bypass Graft Trial Investigators. The effect of aggressive lowering of low-density lipoprotein cholesterol levels and low-dose anticoagulation on obstructive changes in saphenous-vein coronary-artery bypass grafts. N Engl J Med 1997;336:153—162.

34. Zeiher AM, Schaechlinger V, Hohnloser SH, Saurbier B, Just H. Coronary atherosclerotic wall thickening and vascular reactivity in humans. Elevated high-density lipoprotein levels ameliorate abnormal vasoconstriction in early atherosclerosis. Circulation 1994;89:2525—2532.

35. Gould KL, Martucci JP, Goldberg DI, Hess MJ, Edens RP, Latifi R, Dudrick SJ. Short-term cholesterol lowering decreases size and severity of perfusion abnormalities by positron emission tomography after dipyridamole in patients with coronary artery disease. A potential noninvasive marker of healing coronary endothelium. Circulation 1994;89:1530—1538.

36. Andrews THC, Raby K, Barry J, Naimi CL, Allred E, Ganz P, Selwyn AP. Effect of cholesterol reduction on myocardial ischemia in patients with coronary disease. Circulation 1997;95: 324—328.

The economic implications of lipid-lowering therapy: vice or virtue

T.D. Szucs

Centre of Pharmacoeconomics, School of Pharmacy, University of Milan, Milan, Italy

Upwardly spiralling medical costs across Europe as well as the unique burden associated with managing diseases have sensitised health care decision makers in both the private and the public sector to the problems of scarce resources and competing interventions. Providers, insurers, employers and other decision makers are finding it more and more difficult to allocate resources efficiently, due to the lack of sufficient economic data. Economic assessment in health care has developed in response to the needs of those making decisions, to understand the consequences of technological change in health care. They are no longer content, as they may have been in the past, to have a simple faith in the benefits and costs of health care interventions. Now, they are increasingly insisting on hard data. In any case, previous decisions about the use of health care technologies were based almost entirely on the clinical safety, efficacy and quality of the therapeutics used.

In the light of these changes, public health policy in the field of coronary artery disease will depend highly on the economic impact of this disease and will require subsequent and appropriate research activities. An important aspect in evaluating the economic impact of treatment is to consider the individual perspective taken. This would mean addressing the specific needs and views of the individual to whom the results of the economic study are addressed.

The burden of CHD

We have estimated that the burden of CHD as a percentage of total health care expenditure is approximately 2.6% in Germany, 7.9% in the USA and 1% in the UK. The largest share of direct costs are due to hospitalisation, whereas productivity losses are the main component of indirect costs.

The rationale for pharmacoeconomic research

In the past few years the discipline of health economics has experienced an extra-

---

Address for correspondence: Prof Dr Thomas D. Szucs, Centre of Pharmacoeconomics, School of Pharmacy, University of Milan, Via Balzaretti 9, I-20031 Milan, Italy.

ordinary boom within the health care sector. Researchers from a wide range of disciplines have developed new techniques to evaluate the impact of clinical care and medical technology. Clinicians, pharmacists, economists, epidemiologists and operations researchers have contributed to the new field of clinical economics to study how different approaches to patient care influence the resources consumed in clinical medicine. In front of the basic economic notion that resources are limited and desires as well as needs are infinite, health economists try to find solutions on how these resources are allocated appropriately to maximise the production of health. The common denominator is to the search for increased efficiency and effectiveness (Table 1) of health care services and products.

Forms of economic evaluation

The most common methods employed by health economists are classical research designs such as cost-of-illness, cost-benefit, cost-effectiveness, cost-utility, and cost-minimisation analyses [1—3].

Cost-of-illness studies

In the economic literature one will also find references to cost of illness. Definitions vary, but generally "cost of illness" refers to all the costs as they are borne by society. The cost of illness to society is reflected by such factors as loss of productivity in the work force and loss of income by the patient, which results in the loss of tax revenues and inability to purchase the goods and services that drive the economy. The important point is that everyone in society bears the cost health care: providers, patients, third-party payers, and business and industry.

Cost-minimisation analyses (CMA)

Cost-minimisation analysis is concerned with comparing the costs of different

Table 1.

Effectiveness

The extent to which a specific intervention, when deployed in the field, does what it is intended to do.

Efficacy

The extent to which a specific intervention produces a beneficial result under ideal conditions.

Efficiency

The extent to which the resources used to provide a specific intervention of known efficacy and effectiveness are minimised.

treatment modes which produce the same result. For example, this form of analysis could be used to compare the cost of two programs which involve minor surgery for adults. Both have the same outcome in terms of the surgical procedure, but the first program might require the patient to stay overnight at the hospital, and the second might be done through day surgery without requiring hospitalisation. Given these two alternatives the search would be for the least costly treatment.

As far as pharmaceuticals are concerned, this type of study is used most frequently when a new drug is introduced into a therapeutic class which includes close competitors and no measurable therapeutic effect between them has been documented. When the cost of two interventions is being compared, cost-minimisation analysis often assumes they lead to the identical health outcome. Studies of this nature should report evidence to support the contention that outcome differences are nonexistent or trivial in nature. In most cases, however, the issues are more than one of solely cost. It is rarely the case where two therapies having the same indication produce identical health outcomes in every respect.

Cost-benefit analyses (CBA)

As applied to healthcare, cost-benefit analysis (CBA) measures all costs and benefits of competing therapies in terms of monetary units. Generally, a ratio of the discounted value of benefits to costs (the present value of both) is calculated for each competing therapy. The ratios for each of the competing therapies and for competing programs (e.g., intensive care unit vs. new diagnostic equipment) can be readily compared. CBA has the shortcoming of requiring the assignment of a dollar value to life and to health improvements including quality of life variables. This presents equal benefit issues as well as substantial measurement problems. CBA, for these reasons, has not been widely used in recent years for evaluating drug therapies.

Cost-effectiveness analyses (CEA)

Cost-effectiveness studies do not measure changes in the cost of all relevant treatment alternatives, but measure the differences in outcomes in some natural unit such as actual lives saved, years of lives saved or children immunised. CEA can also be applied equally to cases where the outcome is in terms of quality of life. Cost-effectiveness analysis is useful in comparing alternative therapies which have the same outcome units (e.g., years of life expectancy, or of lives saved) but the treatments do not have the same effectiveness (i.e., one drug may lead to greater life expectancy). The measure compared is the cost of therapy divided by the units of effectiveness and, hence a lower number signifies a more cost-effective outcome.

922

Cost-utility analyses (CUA)

Cost-utility analysis compares the added costs of therapy with the number of quality-adjusted life years gained. The quality adjustment weight is a utility value which can be measured as part of clinical trials or independently. The advantage of cost-utility analysis is that therapies which produce different or multiple results can be compared. As explained in the previous section, the QALY, which has been the standard measure of benefit thus far, is arrived at in each case by adjusting the length of time affected through the health outcome by the utility value (on a scale of 0 to 1) of the resulting health status. Many analysts are more comfortable with this measure of the consequence of medical care than with the use of money as the measure of benefits [4].

Cost-utility analysis is an improvement on cost effectiveness analysis because it can measure the effects of multiple outcomes (such as the impact of medicines on both morbidity and mortality or the impact on both pain and physical functional status).

Pharmacoeconomic evaluation of statins in primary and secondary coronary prevention

The clinical usefulness and benefit of statins in secondary and primary cardiovascular prevention has been clearly established in well-controlled, large outcome studies. The remaining issue, however, is whether health care decision makers are willing or able to pay for these medicines. A means of facilitating the decision-making process is to consider pharmacoeconomic analyses of statin therapy. These types of analyses have become extremely important in substantiating the true economic value of drug therapies, making them comparable to other commonly accepted medical interventions. Several economic studies have already been performed on the basis of the 4S, PLAC I and II, CARE and WOSCOPS studies, employing various methodologies [5—8] (Figs. 1 and 2). These studies have clearly demonstrated that statin therapy in primary and secondary prevention is cost-effective in comparison to other health care interventions. The cost effectiveness is, however, strongly related to the constellation of risk factors and the extent of cardiovascular risk reduction through the intervention.

Putting economic study results into policy decisions

The degree of impact on a study will be greater if the relevant decision makers are involved in the conducting and/or the commissioning of the study. Thus, researchers must "sell" their research before it is started. Also, an economic study will only be one of various pieces of information available to decision makers so that researchers must aim to convince decision makers of the relevance of their work. Another important aspect is that the greater the number of relevant decision makers who are aware of the study the greater the possibility of impact

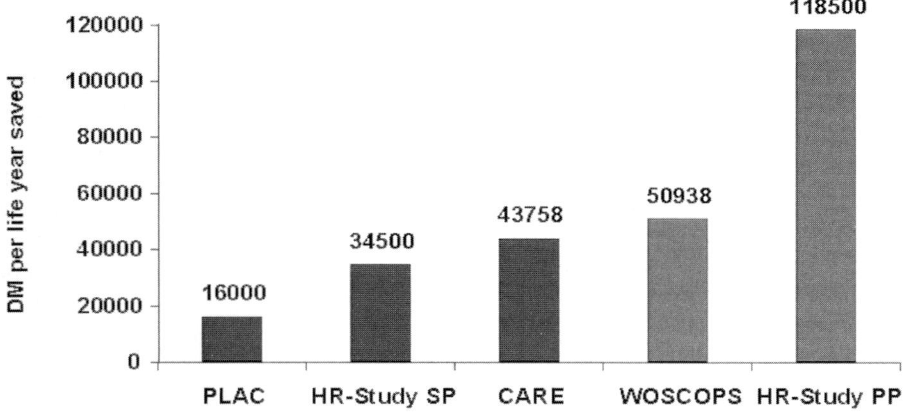

Fig. 1.

might be. This will require that researchers disseminate their work appropriately convincing decision makers of the necessity to make decisions on the basis of efficiency. Preferably, the results of an economic study must be available prior to the health policy decision to be taken and must meet the criteria of high methodological standards.

Despite certain methodological challenges, economic analyses will be critical to rational allocation of resources by manufacturers, providers and payers. These analyses can help payers and providers make coverage and utilisation decisions,

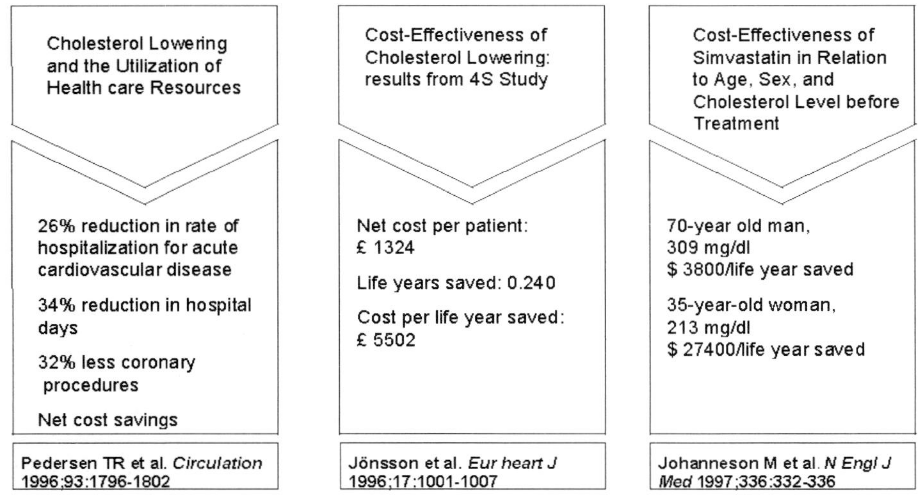

Cholesterol Lowering and the Utilization of Health care Resources	Cost-Effectiveness of Cholesterol Lowering: results from 4S Study	Cost-Effectiveness of Simvastatin in Relation to Age, Sex, and Cholesterol Level before Treatment
26% reduction in rate of hospitalization for acute cardiovascular disease 34% reduction in hospital days 32% less coronary procedures Net cost savings	Net cost per patient: £ 1324 Life years saved: 0.240 Cost per life year saved: £ 5502	70-year old man, 309 mg/dl $ 3800/life year saved 35-year-old woman, 213 mg/dl $ 27400/life year saved
Pedersen TR et al. *Circulation* 1996;93:1796-1802	Jönsson et al. *Eur heart J* 1996;17:1001-1007	Johanneson M et al. *N Engl J Med* 1997;336:332-336

Fig. 2. Economic benefit of simvastatin in secondary CHD prevention.

and help manufacturers document the value of the products they are marketing. Rational use of new and established technology is going to require increased technology assessment, better assessment of patient preferences, and more rigorous economic evaluation. The benefit of such assessments, however, will be worth their cost.

The challenge for conducting more economic research is not only pressing but also rewarding. It can be expected that this type of information will become an important cornerstone in health care policy formulation, as a basis for better health care decision making. This will be especially true for such indications where an imminent public health impact can be expected. There is no doubt that this holds true for coronary heart disease.

References

1. Luce BR, Elixhauser A. Standards for the Socioeconomic Evaluation of Health Care Services. Berlin (Springer), 1990.
2. Drummond MF, Stoddard GL, Torrance GW. Methods for the Economic Evaluation of Health Care Programmes. Oxford: Oxford Medical Publishers, 1987.
3. Szucs TD, Schramm W. Die sozioökonomische Evaluation. Einführing in die Methodologie. Hämostaseologie 1994;14:84—89.
4. Drummond M. Cost-effectiveness league tables: more harm than good. Soc Sci Med 1993;37: 33—40.
5. Berger K, Klose G, Szucs TD. Die Wirtschaftlichkeit von Arzneimiteltherapien. Eine sozioökonomische Analyse der HMG-CoA-Reduktase-Hemmung bei KHK-Patienten am Beispiel von Pravastatin. Med Klin 1997;(In press).
6. Pedersen TR et al. Cholesterol lowering and the use of healthcare resources. Circulation 1996; 93(11):1—7.
7. Jönsson B et al. Cost-effectiveness of cholesterol. Eur Heart J 1996;17:1001—1007.
8. Johannesson M et al. Cost effectiveness of simvastatin to lower cholesterol levels in patients with coronary heart disease. N Engl J Med 1997;336:332—336.

The cost-effectiveness of simvastatin treatment to lower cholesterol in patients with coronary heart disease

Flemming Ørnskov
Merck & Co. Inc., West Point, Pennsylvania, USA

Coronary artery disease is a leading health problem in the USA and most developed nations. Due to economic development and availability of drug therapy and health care technology, more and more people in developing countries also suffer from coronary heart disease (CHD). Treatment of cardiovascular diseases consumes around 10–15% of total health care budgets in developed countries. The direct and indirect costs of cardiovascular diseases and stroke in the USA alone were estimated at US$259 billion in 1996 [1]. Much emphasis has been placed on risk factor identification, modification and reduction by lifestyle changes and/or drug and medical interventions. Hyperlipidaemia is one of the risk factors for CHD. Clinical studies have shown that lowering blood-cholesterol levels reduces morbidity and mortality from CHD. In the Scandinavian Simvastatin Survival Study (4S), simvastatin therapy decreased total mortality by 30%, coronary mortality by 42%, and reduced the incidence of costly CHD events over a 5.4-year period [2].

Cost-effectiveness of simvastatin: results from the 4S study

In the 4S study, 4,444 men and women 35–70 years of age who had CHD, serum total cholesterol levels of 5.5–8.0 mmol/l (212–309 mg/dl) and triglycerides of $\leqslant 2.5$ mmol/l (221 mg/dl) while on a lipid-lowering diet were randomized to treatment with placebo (n = 2,223) or simvastatin 20–40 mg (n = 2,221) daily. Dosage was adjusted at week 12 and month 6 if the treatment goal of total cholesterol between 3.0 and 5.2 mmol/l (116 and 200 mg/dl) was not achieved. The objective of the study was to investigate whether simvastatin therapy was effective in treatment of patients with postmyocardial infarction and/or angina. The median length of follow-up was 5.4 years (range 4.9–6.3 years).

Upon entry into the study the mean blood cholesterol was 6.8 mmol/l (263 mg/dl), the mean LDL cholesterol was 4.9 mmol/l (189 mg/dl), the mean HDL cholesterol 1.2 mmol/l (46 mg/dl) and the mean triglycerides 1.5 mmol/l (133 mg/dl). The mean age was 59 years and 19% of enrollers were women. Elevated total cholesterol, but not elevated LDL cholesterol, was part of the entry criteria [2]. At the end of the study period, the mean blood cholesterol changes from baseline

The work presented in this paper was originally done at the Stockholm School of Economics, Centre of Health Economics by Professor Bengt Jönsson and his group in collaboration with the 4S study steering committee.

926

Table 1. 4S: surrogate outcomes.

	Treated group	Control group	Change
Total cholesterol (%)	− 25	+1	− 26
LDL cholesterol (%)	− 35	+1	− 36
HDL cholesterol (%)	+8	+1	+7
Triglycerides (%)	− 10	+7	− 17

were as shown in Table 1.

In addition (as shown in the figures), simvastatin therapy reduced the risk of total mortality by 30%, CVD death by 35%, coronary deaths by 42%, fetal and nonfetal coronary events by 34%, fetal and nonfetal strokes by 28% and hospitalizations days by 34% [2,3]. All results are statistically significant. There was no significant difference in non-CVD deaths or overall cancer incidence between the two groups.

Two studies have been conducted to evaluate the cost-effectiveness of simvastatin therapy in secondary prevention based on the 4S results [4,5]. Presented below are the results from the 4S study and the cost-effectiveness analysis by Jönsson et al. [4]. In the cost-effectiveness analysis by Jönsson et al. [4] the cost-effectiveness ratio is defined as a net cost per life year saved (LYS) (drug costs minus savings from reduced events) below a defined threshold value. The question to evaluate is what are the extra benefits and costs of adding simvastatin to the treatment of patients post-MI and with angina using a societal perspective.

The benefits were assessed in terms of the following effectiveness measures: number of additional survivors at the end of the trial; and number of life years gained per patient treated in the trial. The costs included in the analysis included:
1) cost of simvastatin;
2) cost of cardiovascular hospitalizations;
3) cost for treatment of side effects; and
4) cost for physician visits.

The following costs were not included in the analysis:
1) cost for screening;
2) cost for monitoring cholesterol levels;
3) indirect costs (i.e., productivity and wage loss due to CHD); and
4) cost in added years of life.

The cost-effectiveness analysis hence expresses net costs as costs of simvastatin minus costs due to CVD hospitalization avoided during the study period (median 5.4 years). Effectiveness is calculated as the number of life years gained. This gives the output: cost (in Swedish kronor) per life year saved (SEK/LYS).

The costs per life year saved (SEK/LYS) calculations were performed based on the following data input. Utilization of health care resources prospectively collected in the trial. These included hospitalizations, diagnostic procedures and medical usage. Hospitalizations were classified by diagnosis-related groups (DRG) codes. Swedish costs were applied for each DRG code. The number of

Table 2. Simvastatin dose and cost/day.

Simvastatin dose	Percentage of follow-up time	Daily drug cost
No drug	6.7%	N/A
10 mg/day	0.1%	7.46 SEK
20 mg/day	61.6%	12.20 SEK
40 mg/day	31.6%	14.91 SEK
Undiscounted average	100.0%	12.23 SEK (£1.19)

life years saved were estimated by two methods:
1) Kaplan-Meier analysis within trial plus age specific life expectancy post-MI.
2) Proportional hazards projection of survival curves.
Both costs and benefits were discounted with 5%.

The 4S study allowed simvastatin dosage titration. Of the 2,221 patients randomized to simvastatin 20 mg/day, 63% stayed at this dosage and 37% titrated within the first 6 months to 40 mg/day. The treatment costs were, therefore, calculated as illustrated in Table 2.

The intervention cost was 21,210 SEK (£2,059) in 1995 Kronor, which is the cost of simvastatin during 5 years, discounted at 5%.

The rate of adverse events in the simvastatin and placebo groups were similar [2], so for the purposes of a cost-effectiveness analysis the costs of treating adverse events did not need to be included. Also, the use of other (primarily cardiovascular) medications was similar in both the simvastatin and placebo groups, so this was not included into the cost-effectiveness analysis (Table 3).

Within the 5.4-year period, in the placebo group (n = 2,223), 937 patients had 1,905 hospitalizations for acute cardiovascular events or coronary revascularization procedures, whereas in the simvastatin group (n = 2,221), 720 had 1,403 such hospitalizations [2,4] (Table 4).

The reductions in hospitalization were consistent in all participating countries in the 4S trial (Table 5).

Simvastatin significantly reduced hospital length of stay (7.1 days for simvastatin group vs. 7.9 days for placebo). In terms of costs, treatment with simvastatin reduced hospitalization costs by 32% (Fig. 1).

In the USA, the resulting reduction in hospitalization costs alone would reduce

Table 3. Average daily medication usage.

	Placebo	Simvastatin
Type of medication	Average (standard)	Average (standard)
Antianginal	1.58 (1.18)	1.54 (1.14)
Other cardiovascular	0.77 (0.74)	0.71 (0.70)
Total cardiovascular	2.35 (1.50)	2.25 (1.47)
Noncardiovascular	0.59 (0.88)	0.59 (0.88)
Total medications	2.94 (1.93)	2.85 (1.89)

928

Table 4. 4S outcome measures.

Outcomes	Placebo (n = 2223	4S (n = 2221)	Percentage reduction	p value
Number of cardiovascular disease Hospitalizations	1905	1403	26%	p < 0.001
AMI	395	630		
Prolonged chest pain	401	312		
LV failure	45	23		
Arrhythmia	150	93		
Stroke	80	61		
TIA	30	19		
CABG/PTCA	278	411		
Other cardiac	215	165		
Total days in hospital	15089	9951	34%	p < 0.0001
Revascularization procedures	413	279	32%	p < 0.0001

the effective cost of simvastatin by 88% to US$0.28 per day [6]. Savings in costs for CHD hospitalization amounted to (discounted at 5%) 7,560 SEK.

The per patient gain in life years during 4S was 0.065 years, which discounted at 5% for the cost-effectiveness analysis equals 0.054 years/patient. For the cost-effectiveness analysis, it was assumed that there were no additional mortality benefits after the end of the trial due to treatment with simvastatin. Both the simvastatin and placebo group were assumed to have the same average life expectancy of 10 additional years based on Swedish epidemiological data for 65-year-old post-MI patients. Assuming a constant rate of death, half of the survivors at the end of study would be dead at 10 years, and all patients would be dead by 20 years. This would equal (for cost-effectiveness modeling purposes) a gain in life years per patient of 0.312 (0.186 discounted at 5%) after the end of the study, and through the remaining lifetime of the patient. Adding this up, the combined within and posttrial gain in life years (in the cost-effectiveness analysis expressed as life years saved) would be 0.377 years (0.065 + 0.312), or 0.240 years discounted at 5%, assuming, as stated above, that patients alive at the end of the study have an average life expectancy of 10 additional years (Fig. 2).

Table 5. Hospital reductions by country.

	Denmark	Sweden	Norway	Iceland	Finland	χ^{2} [a]	p value
n (placebo/simvastatin)	355/358	845/836	845/836	511/514	79/78	433/435	
CHD hosp.	−32.0	−28.8	−32.2	−39.1	−38.5	−1.20	NS
CABG/PTCA	−21.1	−33.3	−30.5	−44.0	−35.0	−0.81	NS
All CVD hosp.	−30.7	−24.1	−29.5	−39.7	−20.3	−2.89	NS

[a]Based on a number of hospitalization in each group.

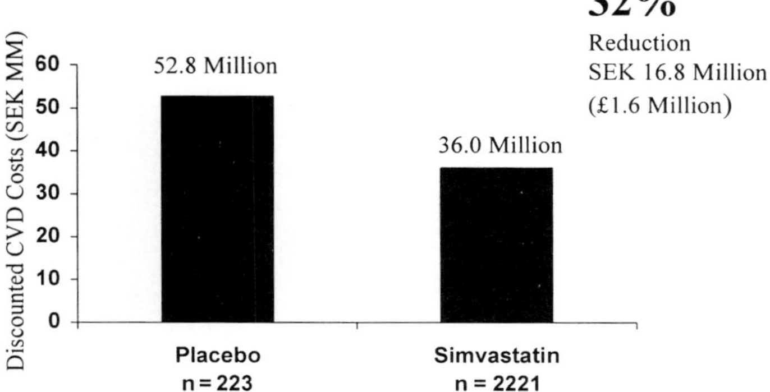

Fig. 1. Hospitalization costs.

The net costs, calculated as the drug costs (21,100 SEK) minus the reductions in hospital costs (7,560 SEK), amounted to 13,540 SEK. By dividing this amount by the discounted number of life years (i.e., 0.240) a cost-effectiveness ratio of 56,400 SEK/life years saved (£5,500/life years saved) is obtained. A key question in cost-effectiveness analysis (modeling) is how robust the ratio is to changes if the underlying assumptions are changed. Sensitivity analysis was performed on the key variables (Table 6).

In general, the cost-effectiveness ratio is fairly robust to changes in assumptions regarding life expectancy at the end of the trial. Using a less conservative approach (than the Kaplan-Meier approach used) in estimating the number of life years saved within and posttrial (namely the Weibull method) would lead to a lower cost-effectiveness ratio, as would not discounting cost and benefits, or only discounting costs. If the costs of screening and monitoring patients were

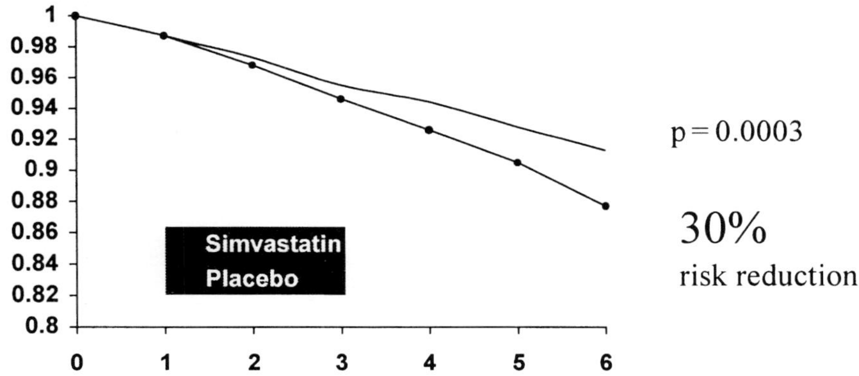

Adapted from the Scandinavian Simvastatin Survial Study Group: *Lancet 344*, 1994

Fig. 2. Survival during 4S trial.

930

Table 6. Sensitivity analysis of cost/LYS.

	Cost per LYS in SEK (£)
Standard analysis	SEK 56,400 (£5254)
Adjusted life expectancy	
8 years	SEK 64,100 (£6254)
12 years	SEK 51,100 (£4985)
Weibull estimate of LYS	SEK 37,600 (£3668)
Costs of initiating and monitoring	
Laboratory tests only	SEK 69,400 (£6771)
Laboratory tests and office visits	SEK 96,100 (£9376)
Discount rate	
Costs 10%, Benefits 10%	SEK 76,040 (£7419)
Costs 0%, Benefits 0%	SEK 39,500 (£3854)
Costs 5%, Benefits 0%	SEK 36,000 (£3512)

included, the cost-effectiveness ratio would increase.

A more crucial question is what a cost-effectiveness ratio actually means. A cost per life year saved can be interpreted as an explicit assessment of willingness to pay for increased survival or an implicit comparison of what is spent on similar programs. However, there is no clear definition of what constitutes a cost-effective treatment or intervention. However, a number of rough guidelines in interpreting cost-effectiveness ratios have been identified (Fig. 3).

In conclusion, the health economics analysis based on data prospectively collected from hospital admissions in the 4S demonstrated that simvastatin was cost-effective in the treatment of hyperlipidaemia in patients with CHD [2]. The cost-effectiveness ratio was also converted to 11 countries [2] (Table 7).

Another study [4] found in a cost-effectiveness analysis limited to direct costs

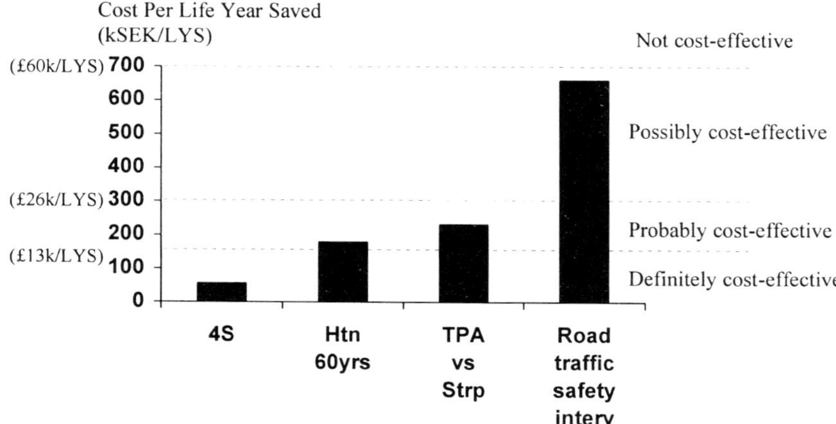

Fig. 3. Interpreting cost-effectiveness ratios.

Table 7. Local costs applied to 4S data.

Country	Cost/LYS (NCU)	Cost/LYS (£UK)
Sweden	56,400 SEK	£5500
Norway	62,300 NOK	£6400
Belgium	235,500 BEF	£5200
France	31,600 FFr	£4100
Germany	17,200 DM	£7200
Italy	15,336,000 Lit	£6200
Portugal	1,933,000 Esc	£8300
Spain	1,160,600 Pta	£6100
UK	—	£7000
Australia	AUS$12,400	£6000
New Zealand	NZ$20,800	£8800

that the cost per life year gained ranged from US$3,800 for 70-year-old men with 309 mg of cholesterol per dl to US$27,400 for 35-year-old women with 213 mg of cholesterol per dl. When indirect costs were included, the results ranged from cost savings in the 35-year-old patients to a cost of US$13,300 per year of life gained in 70-year-old women with 213 mg of cholesterol per dl.

Conclusion

In summary, clinical and economics studies have demonstrated that simvastatin is effective in lowering blood cholesterol and reducing morbidity and mortality from CHD, and is cost-effective for the treatment of hyperlipidaemia in patients with CHD [7]. Treatment with simvastatin reduced hospital utilization for CVD admissions by 26%. Days in hospital were reduced from 15,089 to 9,951 days, a reduction of 34%. CVD hospital costs were reduced with 16.8 million SEK (£1.6 million), equal to 32%. Treatment with simvastatin is cost-effective in CHD patients, with a cost-effectiveness ratio of 56,400 SEK/LYS (£5,500/LYS). Simvastatin produces cost savings among younger patients when indirect costs are included [5].

References

1. 1997 Heart and Stroke Statistical Update, American Heart Association, Dallas, Texas. 1996;28.
2. Scandinavian Simvastatin Survival Study Group. Randomized trial of cholesterol lowering in 4444 patients with coronary heart disease: The Scandinavian Simvastatin Survival Study (4S). Lancet 1994;344:1383—1389.
3. Hebert PR et al. Cholesterol lowering with statin drugs. Risk of stroke, and total mortality. JAMA 1997;278:313—21.
4. Jönsson B, Johannesson M, Kjekshus J et al. Cost-effectiveness of cholesterol lowering. Results from the Scandinavian Simvastatin Survival Study (4S). Eur Heart J 1996;17:1001—1007.
5. Johannesson M, Jönsson B, Kjekshus J et al. Cost effectiveness of simvastatin treatment to lower cholesterol levels in patients with coronary heart disease. N Engl J Med 1997;336:332—336.

6.   Pedersen TR, Kjekshus J, Berg K et al. Cholesterol lowering and the use of healthcare resources. Results from the Scandinavian Simvastatin Survival Study. Circulation 1996;93:1796—1802.
7.   Goa KL, Barradell LB, McTavish D. Simvastatin. A reappraisal of its cost-effectiveness in dyslipidaemia and coronary heart disease. Pharmaco Economics 1997;11:89—110.

Cost-effectiveness of primary prevention of myocardial infarction using statins inermany

Karl W. Lauterbach and Marion Danner
Department of Health Economics, University of Cologne Medical School, Cologne, Germany

Abstract. *Aim.* To determine the cost-effectiveness of primary prevention of myocardial infarction using statins, in Germany.

Methods. We estimated the effectiveness of the treatment of 1,000 patients with pravastatin for 10 years, the associated direct costs and savings in the German population using published data from the West of Scotland Coronary Prevention Study (WOSCOP study) and primary cost data from sickness funds and hospitals in Germany. A cost-effectiveness analysis from the perspective of society was performed determining the cost-effectiveness ratio (CER) measured in US\$/life-year-saved (\$/ LYS) as the outcome; analysis included discounting of all direct costs and benefits, sensitivity analysis and a hypothetical "incremental analysis" using aspirin as a possible alternative treatment (in which the CER was based on the estimated differences in costs and effectiveness between these treatment alternatives).

Data. Effectiveness data: published data of the WOSCOP study for the treatment with pravastatin 40 mg for primary prevention of myocardial infarction; and cost data: data of German hospitals and sickness funds for the utilization of angiography, CABG surgery, PTCA and medical treatment after MI and newly diagnosed CHD; data from sickness funds for the utilization of rehabilitation programs after MI and CHD, and average treatment costs in ambulatory care in year 1 and in years 2−5 after diagnosis.

Results. The CER of treatment vs. no treatment ranged from US\$56,000/LYS (best case) to US\$180,000/LYS (worst case). The incremental analysis with aspirin treatment worsened the best case CER of pravastatin by about 30%, resulting in a CER of US\$78,000/LYS.

Introduction

In Germany, no consensus on the treatment of hypercholesteremia for the primary prevention of cardiovascular disease using drugs has been achieved so far. This also holds for the prescription of statins, despite evidence from the West of Scotland Coronary Prevention (WOSCOP) Study which demonstrated a reduction of cardiovascular mortality in high-risk groups [1]. The main reason for the remaining controversy appears to be economic rather than medical [2]. The cost-effectiveness of primary prevention of myocardial infarctions using statins may be unacceptably high, in contrast to that of secondary prevention where several studies have been published showing good or acceptable cost-effectiveness [3]. Pharaoh and Hollingworth conducted a study exploring the cost effectiveness of primary prevention of myocardial infarction with statins, applying the results of the WOSCOP study to a health-district population in the UK, coming to the conclusion that "lowering serum cholesterol concentration in patients with and without pre-existing coronary heart disease is effective and safe, but treatment for all those in whom treatment is likely to be effective is not sustainable within current NHS resources" [1]. Similar conclusions for primary prevention through lipid-lowering drugs were drawn by Thorvik and Aursnes [4].

The economic controversy about the economic feasibility of primary prevention through lipid-lowering drugs may become more pronounced in Germany in the future because of growing problems in financing health insurance. These problems are mainly due to high unemployment on the one hand, and increasing costs for health care on the other hand. The government has responded to this problem by calling for tight caps on expenditure, naming drug expenditures as an important cause of rising costs. Thus, the cost-effectiveness of the treatment of hypercholesteremia for the primary prevention of coronary heart disease has become an important public health issue in Germany. Mortality of coronary heart disease and rates of myocardial infarction remain high. In men aged 35–64 years, mortality is 160/100,000 [5]. 28% of the population between 35 and 59 years have total cholesterol levels of 250 mg/dl and higher, and 6% have levels higher than 300 mg/dl. However, only 3% of the general population aged 50–69 years and only 8% of all diabetics in this age group take lipid-lowering drugs. In Germany we conducted a cost-effectiveness analysis (similar to that of Pharaoh and Hollingworth in the UK) for the treatment of men aged 45–64 years. A better CER may be expected in Germany since the treatment costs and associated costs for each case of coronary heart disease may be higher in the German population than in the UK (i.e., more invasive procedures and more rehabilitation programs) while little difference in the costs of prevention may be expected.

Methods

We assumed that the results of the WOSCOP study could be generalized to apply to a population in Germany which has a similar risk profile for myocardial infarction to the one treated in the study. We also assumed that the treatment effects would hold for the treatment of 10 years with a linear distribution of their effectiveness. We modelled the treatment of 1,000 men aged 45–64 for 10 years, in a similar manner to the cost-effectiveness study done by Pharoah and Hollingworth, applying the published effectiveness data from the WOSCOP study. Direct costs were taken from German data sources. Costs and medical benefits were discounted at a rate of 5% using 1995 as the reference year. Sensitivity analysis was performed including price reduction of pravastatin, an assumed increase in the effectiveness of pravastatin by 33% achieved by selecting high-risk groups within the study population, the additional consideration of indirect costs, and the consideration of aspirin as a hypothetical treatment alternative which we assumed to be less expensive and less effective.

Data sources

In the WOSCOP study, pravastatin 40 mg was used in 3,302 men who were 45–64 years old at study entry. Pravastatin reduced LDL-cholesterol by 26%, raised HDL-cholesterol by 5%, reduced coronary deaths by 28% (analyzing confirmed cases only), reduced cardiovascular deaths by 32% (p = 0.033), and reduced total mortality by 22% (p = 0.051). At entry into the study 5% of patients had angina, 1% diabetes, 15% hypertension, 44% were smokers, and 8% had ECG abnormalities. For inclusion, total cholesterol levels had to be greater than 232 mg/dl or LDL cholesterol had to be greater than 174 mg/dl. Mean total cholesterol levels of the study population were 272 mg/dl. We used the data on reduced cardiovascular mortality to estimate the effects of the treatment of 1,000 men for 10 years, which would imply 70 LYS without discounting for future health benefits, and 57 LYS if discounted at 5% per year.

In addition to the benefits of reduced cardiovascular mortality which were observed in the study, a reduced cardiovascular morbidity was assumed: using Framingham data it was estimated that for one diagnosed coronary event there are two new cases of coronary disease that need treatment. These cases were considered for estimating direct costs and savings only, but not as a medical outcome influencing quality of life. This may lead to an underestimation of the effectiveness of treatment.

Germany has a high utilization rate of diagnostic and therapeutic procedures for coronary artery disease, in particular angiography, coronary artery bypass grafting (CABG), angioplasty (PTCA) and rehabilitation programs. The costs of

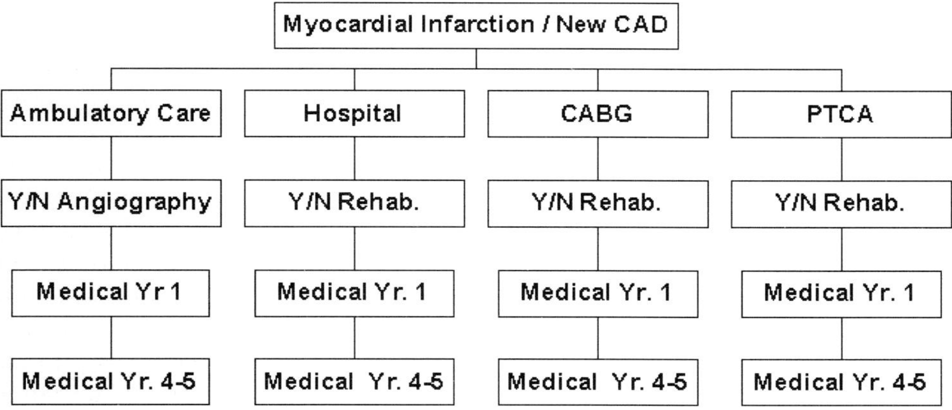

Fig. 1. The likelihood of a new MI or a new case of coronary artery disease that was diagnosed but not an MI (angina or heart failure), was seperately analyzed for leading to ambulatory care only, hospital care only, CABG, or PTCA was estimated from sickness funds data and hospital data. For ambulatory care the likelihood of angiography was determined. For hospital care, CABG, and PTCA the likelihood of taking part in a rehabilitation program was estimated. The average costs were estimated using sickness fund data.

these interventions were estimated using primary data sources. Figure 1 shows the interventions that were considered. The likelihood of having each of the different interventions was estimated seperately for either myocardial infarctions or new cases of CAD without myocardial infarction on the basis of sickness-fund data and primary care hospital data. Costs were estimated from sickness-fund data and cost data which were used to calculate DRGs in Germany. A further assumption was made that these procedures would not significantly reduce cardiovascular mortality as compared to the cardiovascular mortality observed in the WOSCOP study. Otherwise, one may argue that the reduction of cardiovascular mortality observed in the WOSCOP study could not be expected in Germany due to more effective treatment of myocardial infarction or manifest CAD. The hypothesis that a possibly more aggressive treatment of MI and CAD would lead to a significantly lower mortality of CAD in Germany, however, is not supported by MONICA study data which do not show a significant improvement of mortality after MI during the last decade in Germany, despite a sharp increase in the use of more invasive procedures after MI [6].

For the treatment with pravastatin it was assumed that only drug costs, laboratory costs, and costs for a checkup for the effectiveness of treatment 4—6 weeks after treatment initiation are incurred. All costs for treatment with pravastatin and costs savings for reduced cardiovascular morbidity were discounted at the same rate as effectiveness was discounted (5%). The price for pravastatin was estimated from the Red List in Germany.

Results

The cost-effectiveness ratio was US$180,000/LYS if daily dose costs were assumed to be US$3.80 (Red List Price 1995). Since then the price of pravastatin fell. If daily dose costs were estimated at US$2 the cost-effectiveness ratio would improve to US$90,000/LYS.

Sensitivity analysis

Varying the discount rate from 2 to 10% has very little influence on CER because costs and benefits accrue over time in an almost parallel way. We doubled the direct savings by including indirect costs for lost productivity and costs assumed for additional procedures, in particular redo-PTCAs and CABG after PTCA. However, this assumption improves CER by only 10% at costs per daily dose of US$3.8 or by 15% at daily dose costs of US$2 (CER: US$75,000/LYS). If additionally a 33% higher effectiveness of treatment is assumed because only the group with one additional risk factor would be treated a CER of US$56,000/LYS would result. This is the best case scenario (Fig. 2) which appears to approximate realistic conditions.

A further sensitivity analysis was performed with a hypothetical incremental analysis of aspirin as an alternative treatment. Several assumptions were made:

	Costs per daily dose 3.80 US-$	2.00 US-$
No indirect savings, no redos, full group treated	180.000 $/LYS	
Indirect savings, redos, 33% gain in effectiveness		56.000 $/LYS

Fig. 2. Best- and worst-case scenario. Under the assumption of of a 33% higher effectiveness than WOSCOP data in the group of those with one additional risk factor (indirect costs and redo-procedures considered) and a daily dose price of US$2.00 the best case scenario of US$56,000/LYS can be achieved.

Assumption 1: 33% of the effect in the high-risk group (with one additional risk factor) can be achieved with aspirin as an alternative treatment to pravastatin.

Assumption 2: Costs per daily dose of aspirin is US$0.10. This scenario pursues the question whether pravastatin can be expected to be cost-effective given the assumption that the high-risk group could be treated with aspirin alone at lower costs, but also at only one-third of the benefit of pravastatin. The baseline assumption is the best case scenario, having a CER of US$56,000/LYS. Under these assumptions aspirin as a treatment alternative worsens the CER to US$78,000/LYS. This is worse than the CER that could be expected if both pravastatin and aspirin are given, but are no more effective than pravastatin alone (CER US$60,000/LYS). This option should, however, not be considered because it is unlikely and would then be dominated by using pravastatin alone (Fig. 3).

Discussion

The treatment of hypercholesteremia for the primary prevention of CAD in Germany can be cost-effective if one additional risk factor is assumed and costs per daily dose are moderate. This assumed best-case scenario is actually more realistic than the worst-case scenario because it better approximates current drug prices and the current recommendations for the treatment of hypercholesteremia. If aspirin is hypothetically considered as an alternative treatment, these results are not altered in principle under the assumption that aspirin is only one third as effective as pravastatin. This assumption, however, is made quite arbitrarily since there are no head-to-head data for comparison in this high-risk

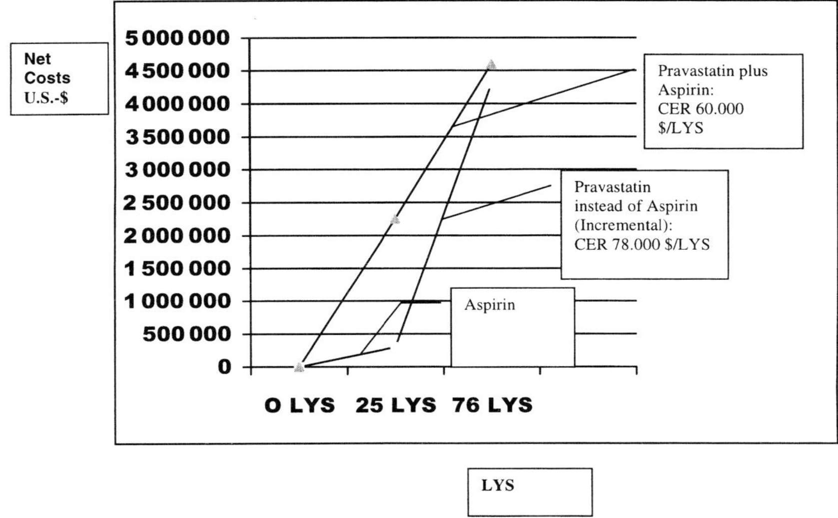

Fig. 3. The cost-effectiveness of pravastatin drops from the best case scenario (US$56,000/LYS) to US$78,000/LYS if one assumes that one-third of the effectiveness of pravastatin could be achieved by aspirin alone.

group available. The incremental comparison performed here is, therefore, only a test for the robustness of the CER obtained in the analysis and does not approximate real comparative data. It is illustrative, however, since aspirin may be the drug with the best CER for the patient group considered and may offer an alternative treatment for many of these patients.

In the study by Pharoa and Hollingworth "the average cost effectiveness of treating men aged 45—64 with no history of coronary heart disease and a cholesterol concentration 6.5 mmol/l for 10 years with a statin was £136,000 per life year saved and the average cost effectiveness for patients with pre-existing coronary heart disease and a cholesterol concentration 5.4 mmol/l was £32,000" [1]. Our results are similar, but also imply that pravastatin for primary prevention can be cost-effective in the patient group with one additional risk factor if indirect costs are included, cardiovascular morbidity is considered and drug costs are moderate.

References

1. Pharoah PD, Hollingworth W. Cost effectiveness of lowering cholesterol concentration with statins in patients with and without pre-existing coronary heart disease: life table method applied to health authority population. Br Med J 1996;312(7044):1443—1448.
2. Diewitz M. Critical and heretical thoughts on the development of cardiology. Limits of mental and social compliance attitude of the population. Versicherungsmedizin 1996;48(2):43—45.
3. Ashraf T, Hay JW et al. Cost-effectiveness of pravastatin in secondary prevention of coronary artery disease. Am J Cardiol 1996;78(4):409—414.

4. Thorvik E, Aursnes I et al. Cost-effectiveness of cholesterol-lowering drugs: a review of the evidence. Wien Klin Wochenschr 1996;108(8):234—243.
5. Barth W, Lowel H et al. Coronary heart disease mortality, morbidity, and case fatality in five east and west German cities 1985—1989. Acute Myocardial Infarction Register Teams of Augsburg, Bremen, Chemnitz, Erfurt and Zwickau. J Clin Epidemiol 1996;49(11):1277—1284.
6. Marques-Vidal P, Ferrieres J et al. Trends in coronary heart disease morbidity and mortality and acute coronary care and case fatality from 1985—1989 in southern Germany and south-western France. Eur Heart J 1997;18(5):816—821.

Cellular and haemodynamic regulation of endothelial function

Hemodynamic forces and vascular cell communication

Peter F. Davies[1], Natacha DePaola[2] and Denise Polacek[1]

[1]*Institute for Medicine and Engineering, University of Pennsylvania, Philadelphia, Pennsylvania;* [2]*Department of Biomedical Engineering, Rensselaer Polytechnic Institute, Troy, New York, USA*

Abstract. The regulation of Connexin43 (Cx43), the predominant gap junctional protein expressed in cultured endothelium, was studied in an in vitro model of steady disturbed flow to investigate the role of gap junction-mediated intercellular communication in relation to hemodynamics. Disturbed flow lesion-prone regions of the arterial circulation were modeled in steady flow by the creation of flow separation (recirculation) zones. Cx43 mRNA levels and Cx43 protein expression were related to spatial variations in fluid forces. Cx43 mRNA expression in regions of steady undisturbed flow were transiently elevated, returning to control no-flow levels after 16 h. However, endothelial Cx43 mRNA expression in areas of flow recirculation (disturbed flow) were significantly increased and remained elevated up to 16 h. These changes in message levels were paralleled by the disassembly of normal gap junctional structures at intercellular junctions in both undisturbed and disturbed flow regions within 5 h. However, by 16 and 24 h there was reassembly of gap junctions in the region of undisturbed flow whereas gap junctions failed to reform in the regions of disturbed flow. The sustained changes of Cx43 transcript and gap junctions correlated with regions of high shear stress gradients within the flow fields. These studies demonstrate that Cx43 gap junction assembly in vascular endothelial cells is dynamically regulated by specific flow parameters in vitro and suggest that spatial and temporal regulation may modulate interendothelial communication resulting from localized areas of altered cell functions.

Keywords: Connexin43, disturbed flow and gene regulation, gap junctional cell communication.

Introduction

The localization of atherosclerotic lesions coincides with disturbed blood flow where endothelial cells exhibit altered morphological and functional characteristics [1,2]. We propose that one manifestation of regional differences is the modulation by hemodynamic forces of interendothelial gap junctional communication. An important intercellular communication pathway between endothelial cells, and possibly between endothelium and underlying smooth muscle, is direct transfer of ions and small molecules through transmembrane gap junctions composed of connexin (Cx) protein subunit assemblies [3]. Endothelial cells express Cx37, 40, and 43, of which Cx43 is most prominently expressed in vitro. Although the influence of flow-related forces upon endothelial signaling, gene expression and function is well-documented [2], few studies have addressed the effects upon this form of intercellular communication. Previous studies have supported the

Address for correspondence: Peter F. Davies PhD, Institute for Medicine and Engineering, University of Pennsylvania, Vagelos Laboratories, 3340 Smith Walk, Philadelphia, PA 19104-3357, USA. Tel.: +1-215-898-4647. Fax: +1-215-573-6815. E-mail: pfd@pobox.upenn.edu

944

hypothesis that local shear stress gradients rather than the magnitude of shear stress alone mechanically regulate endothelial structure and function [4]. We therefore created an in vitro flow model that included distinct regions of precisely defined flow separation and recirculation as well as steady undisturbed flow. Cx43 expression and gap junction distribution were then mapped as a function of the spatial distribution of shear stresses acting on the cells.

Materials and Methods

A disturbed flow apparatus was constructed that consisted of a flow loop connected to a parallel plate chamber in which a 22 × 22 mm glass coverslip with a surface step was placed and upon which a confluent monolayer of bovine aortic endothelial cells was grown (Fig. 1). The step on the coverslip surface created a localized region of flow separation and recirculation (disturbed flow) within the chamber as described previously [5]. In the disturbed flow region, the wall shear stress was nonuniform. Spatial variations in shear stress in regions of flow separation and recirculation were calculated from the numerical solutions of the flow equations. The computational domain was a two-dimensional straight channel with a rectangular step on one of the walls. The aspect ratio of the step was 0.4 and the ratio of the channel gap to the step height was 2.5. The two-dimensional steady Navier-Stokes equations were solved using the computational pro-

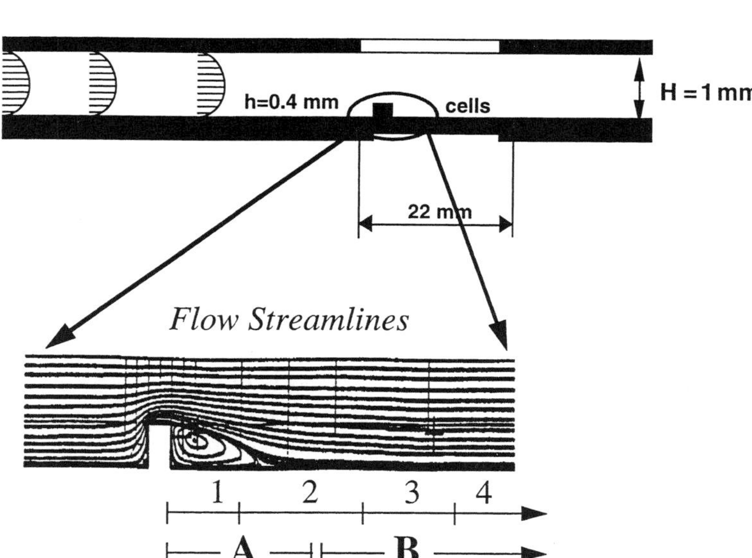

Fig. 1.

gram NEKTON [6]. A total of 22 spectral elements were considered and all calculations were performed using n = 5 for a total of 550 grid points. On the basis of these calculations, the flow and medium viscosity were adjusted to produce regions of flow separation, reattachment and flow recovery over the same endothelial monolayer at physiological levels of shear stress (13.5 dyn/cm^2 in the downstream undisturbed flow region). Confluent endothelial monolayers were exposed to steady disturbed flows for time periods up to 24 h. Low Reynolds numbers were chosen to produce disturbed flow fields in which flow separation and recovery could be observed within a 10-mm region downstream of the surface step. The protocols for cell culture, preparation of Cx43 riboprobes, in situ hybridization, immunocytochemistry, and image analysis were as described previously [7].

Results

Flow streamlines were calculated that demonstrated a recirculation area with a steady two-dimensional vortex immediately downstream of the surface step (region A, Fig. 1). This was a region of flow disturbance in which the shear stress distribution showed an area of reverse flow characterized by a negative shear stress. The absolute value (positive or negative) of the wall shear stress within the recirculation region ranged from zero to 8.5 dyn/cm^2. Shear stress was zero at the downstream boundary of the separated flow (stagnation point), beyond which shear stress became positive and increased in the axial direction, rapidly reaching a value (13.5 dyn/cm^2) corresponding to fully developed downstream flow at a distance 1.3 mm beyond the step point. A schematic is shown in Fig. 1 in which the disturbed flow region is designated region A and the fully developed downstream flow region is B. Within the entire flow field, four distinct areas of shear stress gradients (SSG) were defined. The largest SSG were within the recirculation zone and extending 0.8 mm downstream of flow reattachment (SSGR 1 and 2). These gradients were more than 10-fold greater than further downstream (Table 1). Beyond the downstream boundary of SSG region 2, the shear stress recovered to 80% of that in the fully developed downstream flow region. Consequently, the average SSG in region 3 was significantly lower than that of region 2 and in region 4 the flow was 98% recovered and the SSG was negligible.

Table 1 outlines the levels of Cx43 mRNA expression in endothelial cells in different regions of the flow field after 5 and 16 h. The silver grain distribution corresponding to the location and extent of mRNA expression following in situ hybridization was quantitated in darkfield photomicrographs. The average level of expression in regions A and B were normalized to the expression levels measured in no-flow control monolayers. Within 5 h, there was an averaged 7-fold induction of Cx43 message in region A that was sustained at the same level after 16 h. In contrast, in region B, where fully developed downstream flow was reestablished, there was an approximate 4-fold increase at 5 h which returned to control levels by 16 h.

Table 1. Spatial distribution of endothelial Connexin43 mRNA expression in disturbed laminar flow.

Region		Cx43 mRNA expression[a]	
		5 h	16 h
A		7.2 ± 0.6	8.4 ± 1.9
B		3.7 ± 0.3	1.1 ± 0.1
SSGR[b]	SSG[c]		
1	192	7.1 ± 0.8	6.6 ± 0.2
2	179	7.0 ± 0.6	9.0 ± 1.5
3	16	4.7 ± 0.4	1.5 ± 0.1
4	0	3.71 ± 0.3	1.1 ± 0.1
No flow (control)	0	1.0	1.0

[a]Grains/cell normalized to no-flow control; [b]SSGR: Shear stress gradient region; [c]SSG: Shear stress gradients ($dyn/cm^2.cm$).

Sustained overexpression of Cx43 mRNA was associated with regions corresponding to high shear stress gradients (Table 1). Statistical analysis indicated that message expression in areas of high SSG when compared with areas of low SSG (regions 1 and 2 vs. regions 3 and 4) was significantly different in all cases ($p < 0.05$). We conclude that there was a transient increase in Cx43 mRNA expression induced by a steady laminar flow but a sustained, spatially dependent increase in regions of disturbed flow that correlated with high gradients of shear stress.

Immunocytochemical localization of Cx43 protein showed marked changes in the normal band-type distribution of gap junctional protein localized at the periphery of the cells (not shown). After 1 h of disturbed flow, there was disassembly in the pattern of Cx43 immunoreactivity with partial disaggregation of the normal junctional pattern. These changes occurred in both the disturbed flow region A and the fully developed downstream flow region B, although the changes were more marked in the disturbed flow region. After 5 h, the typical pattern of gap junctional distribution in the disturbed flow region was largely absent, there being small amounts of Cx43 protein aggregates located in the interior of the cell with no localization to the cell perimeter. In the downstream undisturbed flow region (B) at 5 h, there was a mixture of both disaggregation and typical band-like peripheral staining. However, after 16 h the reassembly of gap junction connexin was in evidence in region B, a process which had fully recovered by 24 h. In contrast, the disturbed flow region (A) junctional pattern never recovered to the normal configuration. Measurement of endothelial cell DNA synthesis (BrdU labeling) at 5 h demonstrated a correlation with high shear stress gradient regions. By 24 h in undisturbed flow (low stress gradients; low DNA synthesis, normal Cx43 mRNA expression; reassembled gap junctions) there was partial alignment of the cells with the direction of flow. In contrast, in disturbed flow (high stress gradients; elevated DNA synthesis; sustained elevated Cx43 mRNA; disassembled gap junctions) cells remained unaligned.

Discussion

These studies demonstrate that in regions of undisturbed flow an increase of shear stress resulted in transient changes of Cx43 gene expression and gap junction distribution. The results are consistent with a number of responses of endothelium to sustained changes in the mechanical environment [8,9] that represent adaptive responses. Cx43 mRNA was elevated coincident with disassembly of normal gap junctional distributed at the cell periphery. After 24 h the pattern was reversed. In contrast, in regions of high stress gradients even under steady flow conditions disassembly of gap junctions persisted despite continued elevation of Cx43 mRNA levels. There appears, therefore, to be inhibition of adaptive responses associated with the high shear stress gradients, at least within the time frame of this study; eventual restabilization of Cx43 gene expression and gap junction assembly in disturbed flow cannot be precluded. There was a strong correlation in these studies between stress gradients and gap junction distribution, suggesting that interendothelial gap junctional communication may be significantly inhibited in regions of disturbed flow that exhibit steep shear stress gradients. In vivo, pulsatility and arterial wall compliance add further complexity to the characteristics of the disturbed flow regions. These regional effects upon gene expression and junctional assembly will compromise interendothelial communication in which Cx43 gap junctions are utilized. Hemodynamic effects upon cell communication may be associated with the predilection of the sites to the development of atherosclerosis.

Acknowledgements

Supported by grants from the NHLBI (HL36049) and the Whitaker Foundation.

References

1. Stehbens WE. Haemodynamics and atherosclerosis. Exp Mol Pathol 1974;20:412—425.
2. Davies PF. Flow-mediated endothelial mechanotransduction. Physiol Rev 1995;75:519—560.
3. Beyer EC. Gap junctions. Int Rev Cytol 1993;137C:1—37.
4. Davies PF, Remuzzi A, Gordon EJ, Dewey CF, Gimbrone MA. Turbulent shear stress induces endothelial cell turnover in vitro. Proc Natl Acad Sci USA 1986;83:2114—2117.
5. DePaola N, Gimbrone MA, Davies PF, Dewey CF. Vascular endothelium responds to fluid shear stress gradients. Arterioscl Thromb 1993;13:465—469.
6. Maday Y, Patera AT. Spectral element methods for the Navier-Stokes equations. In: Noor AK, Oden JT (eds) State of the Art Surveys on Computational Mechanics. Am Soc Mech Eng Baltimore USA. 1989;71—143.
7. Polacek D, Bech F, McKinsey JF, Davies PF. Connexin 43 gene expression in the rabbit arterial wall: effects of hypercholesterolemia, balloon injury, and their combination. J Vasc Res 1997;34:19—30.

8. Davies PF, Dewey CF Jr, Bussolari SR, Gordon EJ, Gimbrone MA Jr. Influence of hemodynamic forces on vascular endothelial function. J Clin Invest 1983;73:1121–1129.
9. Resnick N, Gimbrone MA Jr. Hemodynamic forces are complex regulators of endothelial gene expression. FASEB J 1995;9:874–882.

Vascular endothelium, hemodynamic forces and atherogenesis

Michael A. Gimbrone Jr and James N. Topper
Vascular Research Division, Departments of Pathology, Brigham and Women's Hospital, Harvard Medical School, Boston, Massachusetts, USA

Abstract. The localization of atherosclerotic lesions to arterial geometries associated with disturbed flow patterns suggests an important role for local hemodynamic forces in atherogenesis. There is increasing evidence that the vascular endothelium, which is directly exposed to fluid mechanical forces generated by blood flow, can discriminate among these stimuli and transduce them into genetic regulatory events. At the level of individual genes, this regulation is accomplished via the interaction of various transcription factors, such as NF-κB and Egr-1, with "shear-stress response elements" or SSREs, such as the GAGACC motif in the proximal promoter of the human PDGF-B gene, or the Egr-1/Sp1-binding sites in the PDGF-A gene. At the level of multiple genes, distinct patterns of up- and downregulation appear to be elicited by exposure to steady laminar shear stresses vs. comparable levels of nonlaminar (e.g., turbulent) shear stresses or cytokine stimulation (e.g., IL-1β). Certain genes that are upregulated by a steady laminar shear-stress stimulus (such as ecNOS, COX-2 and Mn-SOD) support "vasoprotective" (anti-inflammatory, antithrombotic, antioxidant) functions in the endothelium. The selective and sustained expression of these and related "antiatherogenic genes" in the endothelial lining of lesion-protected areas represent a mechanism whereby hemodynamic forces can influence lesion formation and progression.

Keywords: biomechanical forces, fluid shear stress, gene regulation.

Vascular endothelium and atherogenesis

The involvement of vascular endothelium in disease processes such as atherosclerosis has been recognized since the time of Virchow [1], but a working knowledge of the relevant pathobiology of this tissue has been developed only recently, largely as a result of the application of modern cellular and molecular biological techniques. We now appreciate that this single-cell-thick lining of the circulatory system is in fact a vital organ whose health is essential to normal vascular physiology and whose dysfunction can be a critical factor in the pathogenesis of vascular disease [2]. It has been our laboratory's working concept that the vascular endothelium is a dynamically mutable interface, whose structural and functional properties are responsive to a variety of stimuli, both local and systemic, and further that its phenotypic modulation to a dysfunctional state can constitute a pathogenic risk factor for vascular diseases [3]. In the arterial wall, certain consequences of endothelial dysfunction are directly related to the pathogenesis of

Address for correspondence: Michael A. Gimbrone Jr MD, Vascular Research Division, Brigham and Women's Hospital, 221 Longwood Avenue, LMRC-401, Boston, MA 02115-5817, USA. Tel.: +1-617-732-5901. Fax: +1-617-732-5933. E-mail: gimbrone@bustoff.bwh.harvard.edu

atherosclerosis and its complications [4,5]. These include: altered vascular reactivity and vasospasm; altered intimal permeability to lipoproteins; enhanced mononuclear leukocyte recruitment and intimal accumulation as foam cells; altered vascular cell growth regulation (e.g., decreased endothelial regeneration, increased smooth muscle proliferation); and altered hemostatic/fibrinolytic balances (favoring thrombin generation, platelet and fibrin deposition). Pathophysiologic stimuli of arterial endothelial dysfunction that are especially relevant to atherogenesis include: activation by cytokines and bacterial endotoxin; infection (and possible transformation) by viruses; advanced glycosylation endproducts (AGEs) that are generated in diabetes and with aging; hyperhomocysteinemia; and hypercholesterolemia (per se), as well as oxidized lipoproteins and their components (e.g., lyso-phosphatidylcholine). In addition to these humoral stimuli, it is now clear that biomechanical forces, generated by flowing blood, can also influence structure and function of endothelial cells and even modulate their expression of pathophysiologically relevant genes [6—8].

The possibility that hemodynamic forces can act as pathophysiologic stimuli for endothelial dysfunction provides a conceptual rationale for the long-standing observation that the earliest lesions of atherosclerosis characteristically develop in a nonrandom pattern, the geometry of which correlates with branch points and other regions of altered blood flow [9,10]. In this brief review, we summarize recent studies in our laboratory that are focused on the molecular mechanisms involved in the regulation of endothelial gene expression by biomechanical forces. The results of these studies, as well as the working hypotheses they are generating, promise to provide some basic mechanistic insights into the role of hemodynamics in the pathogenesis of atherosclerosis.

Hemodynamic forces and endothelial function

Because of its anatomical position, the vascular endothelial lining of the cardiovascular system is constantly subjected to a variety of mechanical forces resulting from pulsatile blood flow. These include fluid shear stresses, cyclic strains and hydrostatic pressures. As the cellular layer in direct contact with blood, endothelium bears (in particular) the frictional forces (wall shear stress) derived from the flow of this viscous fluid. A number of in vivo observations suggest that these hemodynamic forces can alter endothelial structure and function (reviewed in [2,6]). These include the demonstration of increased macromolecular permeability, lipoprotein accumulation, endothelial cell damage and repair, leukocyte adhesion molecule expression and mononuclear leukocyte recruitment near branch points and bifurcations (i.e., in areas of complex, nonuniform disturbed laminar flows), as well as the topographical mapping of ellipsoidal endothelial cell (and nuclear) shape and axial alignment (in the flow direction) to laminar flow regions and the disruption of this orderly pattern in regions of disturbed flow. In addition, experimental alterations of vascular architecture, (e.g., surgical coarctation and shunts) result in both acute and chronic vessel wall changes that appear to be (at least in part) endothelium-dependent [11,12], and in the presence of hypercholesterolemia can result in lesions resembling atherosclerosis [13]. Taken together, these in vivo observations are consistent with a direct or indirect effect of one or more hemodynamic stimuli on endothelial function/dysfunction in the context of atherogenesis.

Evidence of the direct action of hemodynamic forces on endothelial structure and function has come from in vitro studies in which cultured monolayers of human and animal endothelial cells have been subjected to defined fluid mechanical forces, under well-controlled experimental conditions. Our laboratory in the Vascular Research Division (Brigham and Women's Hospital, Harvard Medical School), in conjunction with Prof C. Forbes Dewey and his colleagues in the Fluid Mechanics Laboratory (Massachusetts Institute of Technology), was among the first to develop experimental apparatuses that could reproducibly generate defined laminar, turbulent and disturbed laminar flow fields on confluent cultured endothelial monolayers [14—16]. Using a modified cone and plate viscometer, we found that unidirectional steady laminar shear stresses could induce a time- and force-dependent cell shape change and alignment in cultured endothelial monolayers that was gradually reversible upon cessation of flow. These shear-induced changes were accompanied by reorganization of actin-containing stress fibers, as well as other cytoskeletal components, thus mimicking the morphology of aortic endothelium in vivo. Further studies by our group and several others, have also documented a variety of changes in the metabolic and synthetic activities of endothelial cells in response to defined biomechanical forces, including the production of arachidonate metabolites (in particular, prostacyclin), growth factors (e.g., PDGF), coagulation and fibrinolytic components, extracellular matrix components and vasoactive mediators (angiotensin-converting enzyme, EDRF/nitric oxide, ET-1) [2,6—8]. Some of these more acute shear-induced changes appear to involve regulation at the level of rate-limiting enzymes and/or substrate availability (e.g., arachidonic release by calcium-sensitive phospholipases, NO production by nitric oxide synthase). However, especially in the case of delayed responses in which de novo protein synthesis is occurring, upregulation of gene expression appears to be occurring as a direct consequence of exposure to fluid mechanical forces.

Hemodynamic forces modulate endothelial gene expression

In vitro studies have demonstrated that the direct application of physiological levels of laminar shear stress to cultured monolayers of endothelial cells can modulate the expression of a broad spectrum of (patho)physiologically relevant genes, including growth factors such as the A- and B-chains of PDGF and transforming growth factor-β, fibrinolytic factors such as tPA, and adhesion molecules such as ICAM-1 and VCAM-1 [6—8]. The force-dependences and kinetic profiles for these various genes show qualitatively different patterns, suggesting that the molecular mechanisms linking an externally applied force to genetic regulatory events in the nucleus are complex [7,8]. These patterns could reflect a complex interplay of stimuli and responses at several levels, including intracellular second messenger pathways, transcriptional activators and inhibitors, and post-transcriptional effects at the mRNA and/or protein level.

To experimentally dissect the molecular mechanisms involved in the biomechanical regulation of endothelial genes, we have utilized a well-characterized cone-plate flow apparatus [14] to expose confluent monolayers of cultured human umbilical vein (HUVEC) or bovine aortic (BAEC) enothelial cells to a uniform laminar shear stress stimulus of physiological amplitude (e.g., $5-10$ dyne/cm^2), and have analyzed gene expression by various techniques (e.g., Northern blotting, transfection of shear-responsive reporter gene constructs, nuclear run-on assay, differential display of expressed transcripts, etc.). Initially, we studied individual genes (e.g., PDGF-A, PDGF-B, ICAM-1) as molecular model systems, focusing on the analysis of their promoters and interacting transcription factors. More recently, we have begun to analyze the patterns of multiple endothelial genes that respond in a coordinated fashion to different types of biomechanical stimuli.

Our early studies [17] focused on the transcriptional regulation of the human PDGF-B gene, which had been previously shown [6,7] to be "shear-sensitive" at the level of steady-state mRNA. Our nuclear run-on assays confirmed increased transcriptional activity after 1 h of flow exposure, and a reporter gene (consisting of a 1.3 kb fragment of the human PDGF-B promoter coupled to chloramphenicol acyltransferase (CAT)), when transfected into BAEC monolayers that were exposed to laminar shear stress registered several-fold increases in expression compared to "no flow" controls. Through the use of 5′ nested deletional mutations of the PDGF-B promoter, shear-responsiveness was localized to a relatively short region situated near the transcriptional start site (at position -153 to -101). Oligonucleotide probes spanning this region were then used in "gel-shift" assays of nuclear extracts from large samples (10^7 cells) of both static and laminar shear stimulated endothelial monolayers. A specific, shear-inducible DNA-nuclear protein complex was consistently observed, which was localized to a 12 basepair portion within the shear-responsive region. Mutational analysis defined a 6 basepair "core-binding sequence", GAGACC, which was termed the "shear-stress response element" or "SSRE". Nuclear protein-DNA binding events could be demonstrated with probes based on this SSRE as early as 30 min after the onset of flow, and thus were consistent with the kinetics of transcriptional activation of the intact endothelial PDGF-B gene, as seen by nuclear run-on analysis. Hybrid promoters consisting of this core-binding sequence (GAGACC) coupled to a nonshear-sensitive reporter gene construct were activated by shear stress, thus demonstrating that the SSRE motif was sufficient to confer "shear-responsiveness". Interestingly, computer analysis of gene sequence databases revealed that there was conservation of this sequence across species (human, murine and feline) within the PDGF-B promoter [17], suggesting that this mechanism of genetic response to biomechanical stimuli in endothelial cells has been conserved in this gene over many years of evolution.

Recent studies now have defined other positive and negative shear-stress-responsive elements, in addition to the SSRE motif (GAGACC) identified in the PDGF-B promoter, that appear to mediate the biomechanical responsiveness of other pathophysiologically relevant genes in vascular endothelium. These include: a TRE (AP-1 family) site in the human MCP-1 promoter, and Egr-1/SP1 binding sites in the PDGF-A promoter, each of which mediate shear-induced upregulation of these genes [5,18]; in addition, "negative SSRE's" have been mapped in the promoters of other genes, such as VCAM-1 and endothelin-1, which appear to function in their downregulation in response to a shear stress stimulus [5,7,19].

In parallel with these promoter analyses, considerable attention has also been focused on the influence of biomechanical forces on the expression and activation of various known transcription factors. For example, certain "immediate-early response genes", such as c-fos and Egr-1, whose encoded proteins function as transactivating factors, are directly and rapidly induced by shear stress in vascular endothelial cells. Other transcription factors such as the NF-κB system show their typical pattern of activation (cytoplasmic to nuclear translocation) immediately following the onset of a shear stress stimulus [7]. Recent studies in our group have demonstrated that NF-κB components (p50, p65) can interact directly with the SSRE motif in the human PDGF-B promoter, thus providing further insight into the distal mechanisms involved in shear-induced gene expression [20]. Clearly, further studies will be needed to define the complexities of combinatorial transactivation of a given gene in response to the various input stimuli, both humoral and biomechanical, that vascular endothelium encounters in its (patho)physiologic milieu in vivo [8].

Do different biomechanical forces elicit different patterns of endothelial gene expression? Does this correlate with atherogenesis in vivo?

To more systematically approach the question of differential patterns of endothelial gene regulation by biomechanical stimuli, we have undertaken a new experimental strategy, in collaboration with Dr Dean Falb's group at Millennium Pharmaceuticals, Inc. (Cambridge, Massachusetts). We are utilizing an RT-PCR based, high throughput, differential display of transcripts to compare the patterns of genes that are up- (or down-) regulated in human endothelial cells in response to a physiological level of steady laminar shear stress, a comparable level of turbulent (nonlaminar) shear stress, and a soluble cytokine stimulus (IL-1β) at a maximally effective concentration. This approach has revealed distinctive patterns of endothelial gene expression not previously appreciated, including a set of genes that appear to be upregulated in a sustained fashion by steady laminar shear stress, but not by turbulent shear stress. Certain of these differentially regulated transcripts encode known endothelial genes of relevance to atherogenesis, such as ecNOS (the endothelial isoform of nitric oxide synthase), COX-2 (the inducible isoform of cyclooxygenase), and Mn-SOD (manganese-dependent superoxide dismutase). These endothelial genes encode enzymes that exert potent antithrombotic, antiadhesive, antiproliferative, anti-inflammatory, and antioxidant effects both within the endothelial lining and also with interacting cells, such as platelets, leukocytes and vascular smooth muscle. The biological consequences of these steady laminar shear upregulated endothelial genes thus would be predicted to be "vasoprotective" or "antiatherogenic" [21].

Given that uniform laminar shear stresses are characteristically associated with atherosclerotic lesion-protected arterial geometries in vivo, these observations have led us to hypothesize that laminar shear stresses can act to upregulate the expression of a set of "atheroprotective genes" in endothelial cells, which then act locally in the lesion-protected areas to offset the effects of systemic risk factors, such as hypercholesterolemia, hyperhomocysteinemia, diabetes, hypertension, etc. [21]. The coordinated and selective upregulation of atheroprotective genes by laminar shear stress provides a possible mechanistic link between the local hemodynamic milieu, endothelial gene expression, and early events in atherogenesis, and thus a potential explanation for the nonrandom localization of early atherosclerotic lesions. We are currently pursuing the experimental validation of this hypothesis in murine models of atherosclerosis. In addition, we are also characterizing the function and in vivo patterns of expression of several novel human genes that also have been identified and cloned via this approach [22]. Hopefully, the information gleaned from these studies will provide new basic insights into the interrelationship of hemodynamic forces, endothelial gene expression, and the atherogenic process.

Acknowledgements

The original research studies summarized in this review were supported primarily by research grants from the National Heart Lung and Blood Institute (PO1-HL36028; R37-HL51150; P50-HL56985), and a sponsored research agreement with the Brigham and Women's Hospital from Millennium Pharmaceuticals, Inc. (Cambridge, Massachusetts, USA). The authors wish to acknowledge the collaboration of Prof C.F. Dewey and colleagues in the Fluid Mechanics Laboratory at the Massachusetts Institute of Technology; Dr D. Falb and colleagues at the Millennium Pharmaceutical Corporation (Cambridge, Massachusetts); and in particular, our colleagues, N. Resnick, T. Nagel, T. Collins, L. Khachigian, W. Atkinson, K. Anderson and S. Wasserman who directly participated in these and related studies in the Vascular Research Division.

References

1. Virchow R. Der ateromatose Prozess der Arterien. Wien Med Wochenschr 1856;6:825—841.
2. Gimbrone MA Jr, Topper JN. Biology of the vessel wall: endothelium. In: Chien KR et al. (eds) Molecular Basis of Heart Diseases. Philadelphia, PA: W.B. Saunders Inc., 1998;(In press).
3. Gimbrone MA Jr. Vascular endothelium in health and disease. In: Haber E (ed) Molecular Cardiovascular Medicine. New York, NY: Scientific American Medicine, 1995;4:49—61.
4. Gimbrone MA Jr, Cybulsky MI, Kume N, Collins T, Resnick N. Vascular endothelium: an inte-

grator of pathophysiological stimuli in atherogenesis. In: Numano F, Wissler RW (eds) The Third Saratoga International Conference on Atherosclerosis, Ann NY Acad Sci, 1995;748: 122—132.

5. Gimbrone MA Jr, Resnick N, Nagel T, Khachigian L, Collins T, Topper JN. Hemodynamics, endothelial gene expression and atherogenesis. In: Numano F, Ross R (eds) The Fourth Saratoga International Conference on Atherosclerosis, Ann NY Acad Sci, 1997;811:1—11.

6. Davies PF. Flow-mediated endothelial mechanotransduction. Physiol Rev 1995;75:519—560.

7. Resnick N, Gimbrone MA Jr. Hemodynamic forces are complex regulators of endothelial gene expression (Review). FASEB J 1995;9:874—882.

8. Gimbrone MA Jr, Nagel T, Topper JN. Biomechanical activation: an emerging paradigm in endothelial adhesion biology. J Clin Invest 1997;99(8):1809—1813.

9. Cornhill JF, Roach MR. A quantitative study of the localization of atherosclerotic lesions in the rabbit aorta. Atherosclerosis 1976;23:489.

10. Glagov S, Zarins C, Giddens DP, Ku DN. Hemodynamics and atherosclerosis: insights and perspectives gained from studies of human arteries. Arch Pathol Lab Med 1988;112:1018—1031.

11. Langille BL, O'Donnell F. Reductions in arterial diameter produced by chronic decreases in blood flow are endothelium-dependent. Science 1986;231:405—407.

12. Walpola PL, Gottlieb AI, Cybulsky MI, Langille BL. Expression of ICAM-1 and VCAM-1 and monocyte adherence in arteries exposed to altered shear stress. Arterioscl Thromb Vasc Biol 1995;15:2—10.

13. Joris I, Zand T, Majno G. Hydrodynamic injury of the endothelium in acute aortic stenosis. Am J Pathol 1982;106:394—408.

14. Bussolari SR, Dewey CF Jr, Gimbrone MA Jr. Apparatus for subjecting living cells to fluid shear stress. Rev Sci Instrum 1982;53(12):1851—1854.

15. Dewey CF Jr, Bussolari SR, Gimbrone MA Jr, Davies PF. The dynamic response of vascular endothelial cells to fluid shear stress. J Mech Eng 1981;103:177—185.

16. DePaolo N, Gimbrone MA Jr, Davies PF, Dewey CF Jr. Vascular endothelium responds to fluid shear stress gradients. Arterioscl Thromb 1992;12:1254—1257.

17. Resnick N, Collins T, Atkinson W, Bonthron DT, Dewey CF Jr, Gimbrone MA Jr. Platelet-derived growth factor B chain promoter contains a cis-acting fluid shear-stress-responsive element. Proc Natl Acad Sci USA 1993;90:4591—4595.

18. Khachigian LM, Anderson KR, Halnon NJ, Gimbrone MA Jr, Resnick N, Collins T. Egr-1 is activated in endothelial cells exposed to fluid shear stress and interacts with a novel shear-stress response element in the PDGF A-chain promoter. Arterioscl Thromb Vasc Biol 1997;(In press).

19. Malek AM, Izumo S. Molecular aspects of signal transduction of shear stress in the endothelial cell (Editorial Review). J Hypertension 1994;12:989—999.

20. Khachigian LM, Resnick N, Gimbrone MA Jr, Collins T. Nuclear factor-κB interacts functionally with the platelet-derived growth factor B-chain shear-stress response element in vascular endothelial cells exposed to fluid shear stress. J Clin Invest 1995;96:1169—1175.

21. Topper JN, Cai J, Falb D, Gimbrone MA Jr. Identification of vascular endothelial genes differentially responsive to fluid mechanical stimuli: cyclooxygenase-2, manganese superoxide dismutase, and endothelial cell nitric oxide synthase are selectively upregulated by steady laminar shear stress. Proc Natl Acad Sci USA 1996;93:10417—10422.

22. Topper JN, Cai J, Qiu Y, Anderson KR, Xu Y-Y, Deeds JD, Feeley R, Gimeno CJ, Woolf EA, Tayber O, Mays GG, Sampson BA, Schoen FJ, Gimbrone MA Jr, Falb D. Vascular MADs: two novel MAD-related genes selectively inducible by flow in human vascular endothelium. Proc Natl Acad Sci USA 1997;94:9314—9319.

Endothelial VCAM-1 gene regulation by steady and oscillatory shear stress

Signe E. Varner[1], R. Wayne Alexander[2], Russell M. Medford[2] and Robert M. Nerem[1]

[1]*Institute for Bioengineering and Bioscience, Georgia Institute of Technology, Atlanta; and* [2]*Division of Cardiology, Emory University School of Medicine, Atlanta, Georgia, USA*

Abstract. *Background.* Atherosclerotic lesions localize to regions characterized by low and oscillatory fluid shear stresses. The goal of this study was to determine the correlative relationship between fluid shear stress and endothelial vascular cell adhesion molecule-1 (VCAM-1) expression in vitro.

Methods. Human vascular endothelial cells were subjected to both steady and oscillatory fluid flow. The subsequent effects on VCAM-1 gene expression were measured by Northern analysis. The mechanism of VCAM-1 gene modulation was investigated by promoter activation studies and by gel shift.

Results. While steady flow had no effect on constitutive VCAM-1 gene expression, oscillatory flow transiently induced VCAM-1. Steady laminar shear stress and oscillatory shear stress preconditioning suppressed subsequent cytokine (IL-1β) induction of VCAM-1 mRNA by 95 and 40% (compared to static controls), respectively. The steady shear stress suppression was found to be transcriptional and unaccompanied by inhibition of nuclear factor-kappa B (NF-κB) binding activity.

Conclusions. These results clearly demonstrate that the pattern of gene regulation by shear is specific to the dynamic character of the flow field (steady vs. oscillatory). These effects could at least in part explain the predilection of atherosclerotic lesions for areas of the vessel wall experiencing reversing blood flow.

Keywords: emodynamic force, leukocyte adhesion, nuclear factor-kappa B.

Introduction

Atherosclerosis is a chronic inflammatory disease of the vasculature characterized by a focal predisposition for areas of low and oscillatory wall shear stress [1]. These atherogenic prone regions are further characterized by monocyte adhesion and expression of oxidation-reduction (redox) sensitive inflammatory genes such as VCAM-1 [2] as well as regulatory transcriptional factors such as nuclear factor-kappa B (NF-κB) [3] important in mediating vascular inflammatory responses. These characteristics suggest a direct regulatory linkage between fluid shear stress and the ability of vascular endothelial cells to modulate redox-sensitive inflammatory response pathways.

The goal of the present study was to determine whether there might be a corre-

Address for correspondence: Robert M. Nerem, Institute for Bioengineering and Bioscience, Georgia Institute of Technology, 281 Ferst Drive, N.W., Atlanta, GA 30332-0363, USA.

lative relationship between fluid shear stress and endothelial VCAM-1 expression.

Materials and Methods

Cell culture

Cryopreserved primary human umbilical vein endothelial cells (HUVECs) were obtained from Clonetics, Inc. (San Diego, California). HUVECs were cultured in M199 medium supplemented with 20% FBS, 16 U/ml heparin, 50 µg/ml endothelial cell growth supplement, 25 mM Hepes buffer, 2 mM L-glutamine, 100 U/ml penicillin, and 100 µg/ml streptomycin, and grown in tissue culture dishes coated with 0.1% gelatin. The human microvascular endothelial cell (HMEC-1) line [4] was obtained from the Centers for Disease Control (CDC), and was cultured in EBM medium supplemented with 10% FBS and EGM "Singlequots" (Clonetics).

Experimental design

Endothelial cell monolayers grown to confluence on tissue culture plastic slides were placed in parallel plate flow chambers containing 50 ml of recirculating media. The parallel plate flow chamber utilized for generating defined fluid shear stresses has been described [1]. Cells were subjected to either a laminar steady shear stress of 5 dyn/cm^2 or an oscillatory shear stress peaking at ±5 dyn/cm^2 at a frequency of 1 Hz, with there being for all practical purposes no mean shear stress component. Confluent endothelial cell monolayers (removed from flow chambers or parallel controls from static culture) were incubated in fresh media containing 10 U/ml of interleukin 1-beta (IL-1β) for 1 h for gel shift analysis, 4 h for mRNA analysis, or 8 h for promoter analysis.

Northern analysis

Total cellular RNA was isolated and 20 µg size fractionated using 1% agarose-formaldehyde gels. The ^{32}P-labeled DNA probes for hybridization were prepared from human VCAM-1 cDNA, human intercellular adhesion molecule-1 (ICAM-1) cDNA, human E-Selectin cDNA, and a 1.2 kb Pst I fragment of human glyceraldehyde phosphate dehydrogenase (GAPDH) cDNA. Expression levels of cell adhesion molecule mRNA were normalized as a fraction of the GAPDH expression level.

Transient DNA transfection and CAT assay

HMECs were transiently transfected with 40 µg of reporter plasmid by calcium phosphate coprecipitation according to standard protocols. Cells were then subjected to a steady fluid shear stress of 5 dyn/cm^2 for 24 h. Following an 8-h static incubation in 10 U/ml IL-1β, cell extracts were prepared and chloramphenicol acetyltransferase activity assayed by thin layer chromatography. The reporter plasmid p(HIVκβ)$_4$CAT contains four tandem copies of the κB DNA sequences cloned upstream of the human immunodeficiency virus-1 long terminal repeat and fused to the coding region of the bacterial CAT gene [5]. The reporter gene p85VCAMCAT contains coordinates −85 to +12 of the human VCAM-1 promoter, while p288VCAMCAT contains coordinates −288 to +22 [6]. The 77/63VCAMCAT promoter contains coordinates −77 to −48 fused to the SV40 promoter.

Gel shift analysis

Nuclear extracts were prepared as previously described [7] and subjected to binding conditions in the presence of ^{32}P-labeled oligonucleotide wt VCAM synthesized to encompass the two NF-κB sites (underlined) found at coordinates −73 and −58 of the human VCAM-1 promoter: 5′-CTGCCCT<u>GGGTTTCCCC</u>TTGA<u>AGGGATTTCCC</u>TCCGCCTCTGCAACAA. After the binding reaction, the samples were subjected to electrophoresis in a 1 × Tris-glycine buffer using 4% polyacrylamide gels.

Results

The effects of fluid flow on both constitutive and cytokine-inducible VCAM-1 gene expression was determined by Northern analysis. While steady shear stress had no effect on constitutive VCAM-1 gene expression, oscillatory shear stress resulted in a transient increase of VCAM-1 mRNA levels, peaking at 4 h and returning to baseline by 24 h after the onset of flow. Exposure to a steady laminar shear stress of 5 dyn/cm^2 for 24 h was found to have a "protective" effect on endothelial cells, suppressing subsequent inflammatory cytokine (IL-1β) induction of VCAM-1 mRNA by 96% compared to static controls. An oscillatory shear stress shared this suppressive effect, though much less dramatically, suppressing inflammatory VCAM-1 induction by 40%. This shear-induced suppression was selective for VCAM-1, as the cytokine-induction of another cell adhesion molecule, ICAM-1, was not inhibited by shear preconditioning.

The steady shear suppression of inducible VCAM-1 was further investigated in promoter studies and by nuclear protein binding assay. Steady shear preconditioning suppressed the cytokine-induced transactivation of abbreviated VCAM-1 promoter/reporter constructs (p85VCAMCAT and p288VCAMCAT) in HMECs by 80% compared to cells maintained in static culture. As measured by gel shift, the binding activity of NF-κB remained intact in both HUVECs and HMECs subjected to identical conditions. In an assay of functional of NF-κB activity, the inducible transactivation of two NF-κB driven promoters, p(HIVκB)$_4$CAT and p77/63VCAMCAT, remained unaffected by shear preconditioning. These

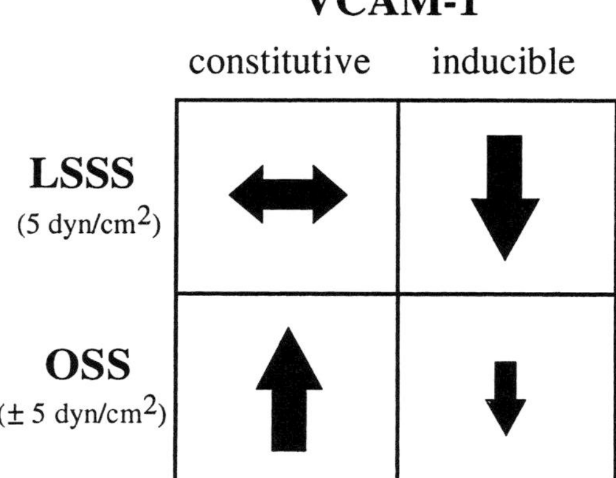

Fig. 1. Effects of laminar steady shear stress (LSSS) and oscillatory shear stress (OSS) on both constitutive and IL-1β inducible VCAM-1 gene expression in HUVCs.

studies clearly demonstrate that shear stress suppresses inducible VCAM-1 through a transcriptional mechanism independent of NF-κB.

Discussion

This work establishes that steady laminar shear selectively suppresses IL-1β-mediated endothelial VCAM-1 expression at the mRNA and transcriptional level. Binding of the transcription factor NF-κB to its tandem consensus binding sites (coordinates -73 and -58) has previously been shown to be necessary for VCAM-1 promoter activation by cytokine [7]. Steady shear stress inhibits the transactivation of the VCAM-1 promoter through a mechanism that does not involve inhibition of the transcription factor NF-κB. These results strongly suggest the activation of a repressor protein by shear which may interact with the VCAM-1 promoter downstream of the NF-κB consensus binding sequences.

It has also been demonstrated that the VCAM-1 gene is exquisitely sensitive to the dynamic composition of the shear stress signal. A reversing shear stress (±5 dyn/cm^2) resulted in a transient induction of VCAM-1 transcript over basal level, and had a milder inhibitory effect on subsequent inflammatory activation by IL-1β compared to steady shear stress (summarized in Fig. 1).

Through these molecular pathways shear stress may mediate, at least in part, the predisposition of focal areas of the vessel wall to inflammatory processes leading to atherosclerotic lesions.

Acknowledgements

This study was supported by grant P01 HL48667 from the National Institutes of Health.

References

1. Levesque MJ, Nerem RM. The elongation and orientation of cultural endothelial cells in response to shear stress. ASME J Biomech Eng 1985;176:341—347.
2. O'Brian KD, McDonald TO, Chait A, Allen MD, Alpers CE. Neovascular expression of E-Selectin, intercellular adhesion molecule-1, and vascular cell adhesion molecule-1 in human atherosclerosis and their relation to intimal leukocyte content. Circulation 1996;93:672—682.
3. Brand K, Page S, Rogler G, Bartsch A, Brandl R, Knuechel R, Page M, Kaltschmidt C, Baeuerle PA, Neumeier D. Activated transcription factor nuclear factor-kappa B is present in the atherosclerotic lesion. J Clin Invest 1996;97:1715—1722.
4. Xu Y, Swerlick RA, Sepp N, Bosse D, Ades EW, Lawley TJ. Characterization of expression and modulation of cell adhesion molecules on an immortalized human dermal microvascular endothelial cell line (HMEC-1). J Invest Dermatol 1994;102:833—837.
5. Kunsch C, Ruben SM, Rosen CA. Selection of optimal kB/Rel DNA binding motifs: interaction of both subunits of NF-kappa B with DNA is required for transcriptional activation. Molec Cell Biol 1992;12:4412—4421.
6. Iademarco MF, McQuillan JJ, Rosen GD, Dean DC. Characterization of the promoter for vascular cell adhesion molecule-1 (VCAM-1). J Biol Chem 1992;267:16323—16329.
7. Neish A, Williams A, Palmer H, Whitley M, Collins T. Functional analysis of the human vascular cell adhesion molecule 1 promoter. J Exp Med 1992;176:1583—1593.

Interaction between red blood cells and endothelium

Jean-Luc Wautier and Marie-Paule Wautier
Laboratoire Biologie Vasculaire et Cellulaire, Hôpital Lariboisière, Paris, France

The interaction between blood cells and the vessel wall has been observed ever since the microscope was invented. Leukocytes and erythrocytes were first recognized and named according to their color, white and red, as they appear in absence of staining. Platelets discovered in late 1840 were in the 1970s the subject of several investigations and a great number of studies were focused on platelet adhesion to the vessel wall and particularly the subendothelium [1]. Major developments of leukocyte endothelium interactions have been possible following identification of the molecular bases of these processes [2]. Since the observation of an abnormal adhesion of erythrocytes with the endothelium in sickle cell anemia, diabetes mellitus and malaria, the molecules involved in the adhesion mechanism have been identified in recent years.

Diabetes mellitus

In diabetic patients, one of the biological consequences of the high plasma glucose concentration is the nonenzymatic glycosylation (glycation) of a variety of intra- and extracellular proteins. Erythrocyte membrane proteins are glycated and the membrane content in glucose is 2-fold higher in diabetic as compared to nondiabetic subjects. Band 3, the major transmembrane protein, is easily accessible to glycation, while another protein, band 4.1, can be glycated. It has been estimated that 20—40% of band 4.1 is glycated, although this modification has no apparent effect on the electrophoretic mobilities of the bands 4.1a and 4.1b. Whether the biological functions of the glycated band 4.1 protein are different from those of nonglycated band 4.1 as yet remains unknown [3].

Diabetic erythrocytes adhere abnormally to cultured human endothelial cells [4]. The increase in adhesion is correlated with the extent of vascular complications as evaluated by the severity of retinopathy, neuropathy, peripheral vascular disease and myocardial ischemia. The abnormal interaction also affects the endothelial cell arachidonic acid pathway, erythrocyte adhesion being correlated with an increased in PGI_2 as assessed by the increase in release of 6-keto-PGF1α from the endothelium. Schmidt et al. [5] have identified two receptors

Address for correspondence: Prof J.-L. Wautier, INTS, 6, rue Alexandre Cabanel, 75739 Paris Cedex 15, France. Tel.: +33-1-44-49-30-35. Fax: +33-1-43-06-04-83.

for the advanced glycosylation end-product (AGE). These receptors are expressed on the macrophage and endothelial cell surfaces. Special structures present on endothelial cells were found to bind advanced glycated end products (AGE). One of the structures was found to be identical to lactoferrin. A 35 KDa molecule binds AGE protein and diabetic RBC(s). This molecule was purified, characterized and cloned, and considered to be a receptor for AGE (RAGE). RAGE belongs to the immunoglobulin superfamily of membrane molecules. Antibodies directed against AGE or RAGE block the interaction between diabetic RBC and endothelium suggesting that RAGE is the receptor for the diabetic RBCs and that AGE present on the cell membranes are the counterpart [6]. A truncated form of the receptor (sRAGE) when preincubated with diabetic RBCs inhibited the adherence to endothelium in culture.

RBCs obtained from diabetic rats when injected in normal syngeneic rats had a reduced life span which was corrected when the animal received anti-RAGE antibodies while antithrombomodulin antibodies which recognize an endothelial cell component were without effect [7].

Diabetic RBCs bearing AGE when bound to endothelial cell RAGE induced an oxidant stress as evidenced by an increase in thiobarbituric reactive substances (TBARS) similarly when injected into rats liver TBARS are enhanced. In addition to the TBARS level, AGE-RAGE interaction induces an activation of the nuclear factor Kappa B (NFκB). The endothelium barrier function was altered by AGE-RBC binding to RAGE. The vascular hyperpermeability observed in diabetic rats can be prevented by blocking RAGE with specific anti-RAGE antibodies. The vascular permeability measured by radiolabelled albumin transfer to the extravascular compartment is augmented when diabetic RBCs are infused in normal rats. This effect was blocked when diabetic RBCs were incubated with sRAGE before infusion in the animal.

To further evaluate whether oxidant stress was involved in the transmission of the intracellular message responsible for the enhanced permeability, we have incubated the endothelial cells with antioxidant (Probucol, vitamin E) or treated the animal with the two drugs. Both drugs reduced in vitro and in vivo the hyperpermeability produced by RBC AGE-RAGE interaction [8].

Several endothelial cell functions are modified by RAGE occupation. Vascular cell adhesion molecule expression is induced after AGE binding to RAGE, as is the case for tissue factor. AGE-RBC binding to endothelial cell potentiates interleukin 6 production. All these alterations may play a determinant role in the genesis of vascular dysfunctions observed in the diabetic vasculopathy [8].

Sickle cell anemia

In sickle cell anemia the erythrocyte population is extremely heterogeneous and characterized by an increase in the proportion of the reticulocytes.

Erythrocytes from patients with sickle cell anemia exhibit an abnormal propensity to adhere to vascular endothelium or monocytes [9]. As red cells from HbSS patients are widely heterogeneous, the abnormalities already considered may be partly responsible for their increased adhesion to endothelium.

Sickle erythrocytes differ in their ability to adhere to large and microvascular vessels. Since HbSS erythrocytes adhere mainly to the postcapillary venules, obliteration starts with adhesion of young sickle cells to postcapillary vessels and occlusion is achieved by recruitment of irreversibly sickled erythrocytes. Flow modifications favor increased adherence and promote local hypoxia and acidosis. These biochemical and hemodynamic changes induce further sickling, adhesion and trapping of dense sickle erythrocytes, thus creating a self-maintained cycle of sickling. Erythrocytes from patients with HbSS adhere to endothelial cells of large vessel and microvascular sites by quantitatively and qualitatively different mechanisms and autologous plasma differently promotes adherence to microvascular and venous endothelial cells. Recently, Swerlick et al. [10] have postulated that the interactions between reticulocytes of patients with sickle cell anemia and endothelium may initiate vascular occlusion. Binding is mediated by the $\alpha_4\beta_1$-integrin complex (VLA4) which is expressed on the membrane of the reticulocytes and by VCAM-1 (vascular cell adhesion molecule-1) on the "activated" endothelial cell surface. This phenomenon could be important in cases of disease with a high reticulocyte count, sickle erythrocytes attached to subendothelial components such as thrombospondin and laminin [11].

Plasma depleted in divalent cations or collagen-binding proteins does not enhance the adherence of erythrocytes as well as a normal plasma, while fibrinogen and fibronectin have been identified as adhesion promoting factors and could constitute the required collagen-binding proteins [12]. Finally, the abnormal interaction with sickle erythrocytes stimulates the production and release of prostacyclin by endothelial cells, as revealed by a significant rise of 6-keto-PGF1α in plasma [13]. The increase in prostacyclin synthesis is correlated to the extent of sickle erythrocyte adhesion.

Plasmodium falciparum malaria

Clinical complications are favored by mechanical intravascular obstruction with erythrocytes containing asexual stages of the parasite and postmortem analyses of patients dying from cerebral malaria have revealed parasitized erythrocytes sequestrated within capillaries and postcapillary venules.

The adhesion of erythrocytes to endothelium is associated with the occurrence of knobs on the cell membrane. As observed by electron microscopy, these knobs appear regular and symmetrical and are thought to be the exclusive site at which the parasitized erythrocytes bind to the endothelium. *P. falciparum* erythrocyte membrane protein 1 (P*f*EMP 1), a family of high molecular weight proteins (220—350 KDa) specifically located at knob sites on the outer membrane surface, presents a wide range of phenotypic antigens and is probably responsible in part for the immune response. P*f*EMP 1, considered as a high-affinity adhesion molecule, is a candidate for a number of ligands such as CD36, ICAM-1 and thrombospondin. Recently, a recognition protein for CD36, termed sequestrin, was identified as a mediator in the adhesion of infected erythrocytes to endothelium. *P. falciparum* induced alterations such as protein dephosphorylation inhibit new parasite invasion, as this process requires high levels of phosphoproteins.

Nash et al. [14] have found that the adhesion, which is initially weak and shear reversible, is subsequently stabilized by cooperative effects of multiple receptor interactions and three endothelial proteins have been identified in vitro as receptors for infected erythrocytes: thrombospondin, CD36 and ICAM-1 [15]. CD36 is a receptor for thrombospondin and collagen type I. Using MAbs which recognize different epitopic sites of ICAM-1, the molecular domain 1 has been identified as the binding site for infected erythrocytes and been shown to be distinct from the LFA-1 sites. Ockenhouse et al. [16] have further demonstrated the importance of domains 1 and 2 in the interaction of ICAM-1 with infected erythrocytes by means of mutant ICAM cDNA transfected COS cells expressing all or part of the peptide chains. Soluble ICAM and synthetic peptides of ICAM bind to infected erythrocytes, results which suggest that such molecules could be employed in the treatment of severe and cerebral malaria.

Among other endothelial cell molecules constituting putative receptors for malaria-infected erythrocytes, the adhesion molecules induced by cytokines can also mediate the cytoadhesion of parasitized cells to endothelium. Adhesion is inhibited by antibodies against VCAM-1 and E-selectin (ELAM-1). E-selectin and VCAM-1 are present on the endothelium of postmortem brain tissue from patients dying of cerebral malaria, while during clinical episodes of malaria, increases in the plasma levels of soluble ICAM-1 and E-selectin are positively correlated with plasma concentrations of soluble IL-2. A recent report indicated that the interaction between *P. falciparum* infested erythrocytes and endothelial cell receptor are also dependent of individual factors [17]. In that study, the parasitized erythrocytes always bind to ICAM and CD36 but to different extents. No, or infrequent, adhesion was observed to VCAM1 or E-selectin [17].

References

1. Wautier JL, Caen JP. Pharmacology of platelet suppressive agents. Sem Thromb Hemostas 1979; 4:293—315.
2. Rainger E, Wautier MP, Nash G, Wautier JL. Prolonged E-selectin induction by monocytes potentiates the adhesion of flowing neutrophils to cultured endothelial cells. Br J Haematol 1996;92:192—199.
3. Chappey O, Wautier MP, Wautier JL. Adhesion of erythrocytes to endothelium in pathological situations: a review article. Nouv Rev Fr Hématol 1994;36:281—288.
4. Wautier JL, Paton C, Wautier MP, Pintigny D, Abadie E, Passa P, Caen J. Increased adhesion of erythrocytes to endothelial cells in diabetes mellitus and its relation to vascular complications. N Engl J Med 1981;305:237—242.
5. Schmidt AM, Hori O, Brett J, Yan SD, Wautier JL, Stern D. Cellular receptors for advanced glycation end products: implications for induction of oxidant stress and cellular dysfunction in the pathogenesis of vascular lesions. Arterioscl Thromb 1994;10:1521—1528.

6. Wautier JL, Wautier MP, Schmidt AM, Zoukourian C, Capron L, Chappey O, du Yan S, Brett G, Guillausseau PJ, Stern D. Advanced glycation end products (AGE) on the surface of diabetic red cells bind to the vessel wall via a specific receptor inducing oxidant stress in the vasculature: a link between surface-associated AGEs and diabetic complications. Proc Natl Acad Sci 1994;91:7742−7746.

7. Wautier JL, Zoukourian C, Chappey O, Wautier MP, Guillausseau PJ, Cao R, Hori O, Stern D, Schmidt AM. Receptor-mediated endothelial cell dysfunction in diabetic vasculopathy. Soluble receptor for advanced glycation end products blocks permeability in diabetic rats. J Clin Invest 1996;1:238−243.

8. Chappey O, Dosquet C, Wautier MP, Wautier JL. Advanced glycation end products, oxidant stress and vascular lesions. Eur J Clin Invest 1997;27:97−108.

9. Hebbel RP, Yamada O, Moldow CP, Jacobs MS, White JG, Eaton JW. Abnormal adherence of sickle erythrocytes to cultured endothelium. Possible mechanism for microvascular occlusion in sickle cell anemia. J Clin Invest 1980;65:154−160.

10. Swerlick KA, Eckman JR, Kumar A, Jeitler M, Wick TM. $\alpha4\beta1$ integrin expression on sickle erythrocytes: vascular wall adhesion molecule 1 dependent binding to endothelium. Blood 1993;82:1891−1899.

11. Hilery C, Du M, Montgomery R, Scott J. Increased adhesion of erythrocytes to components of the extracellular matrix: isolation and characterization of a red blood cell lipid that binds thrombospondin and laminin. Blood 1996;87:4879−4886.

12. Wautier JL, Pintigny D, Wautier MP, Paton RC, Galacteros F, Courillon-Mallet A, Passa P, Caen JP. Fibrinogen, a modulator of erythrocyte adhesion to vascular endothelium. J Lab Clin Med 1983;101:911−918.

13. Wautier JL, Pintigny D, Maclouf J, Wautier MP, Corvazier E, Caen JP. Release of prostacyclin after erythrocyte adhesion to cultured vascular endothelium. J Lab Clin Med 1986;107:210−215.

14. Nash GB, Cook BM, Marsh K, Berendt A, Newbold C, Stuart J. Rheological properties of the adhesive interactions of red blood cells paratized by *Plasmodium Falciparum*. Blood 1992;79:788−807.

15. Berendt AR, Simmons PL, Tansey S. Intracellular adhesion molecule-1 is an endothelial receptor for *Plasmodium falciparum*. Nature 1989;341:57−59.

16. Ockenhouse CF, Tegoshi T, Maeno Y. Human vascular endothelial cell adhesion receptor for Plasmodium Falciparum infected erythrocytes: roles for endothelial leukocyte adhesion molecule -1 and vascular adhesion molecule-1. J Exp Med 1992;176:1183−1189.

17. Udomsangpetch R, Taylor B, Looareesuwan S, White N, Elliott J, Ho M. Receptor specifiy of clinical Plasmodium Falciparum isolates: non adherence to cell-bound E-selectin and vascular cell adhesion molecule-1. Blood 1996;88:2754−2760.

Suppression of gap junctional intercellular communication in HUVEC by neutrophil adhesion

Sei-itsu Murota, Masamichi Nishida and Ikuo Morita
Department of Physiological Chemistry, Tokyo Medical and Dental University, Tokyo, Japan

Abstract. Interaction between leukocytes and endothelium is believed to be important in many pathophysiological states. But little is known about the influence of leukocytes on gap junctional intercellular communication (GJIC) between endothelial cells. The activity of GJIC was measured by the the method of fluorescence recovery after photobleaching using an interactive lase cytometer. For adhesion assay, human umbilical vein endothelial cells (HUVEC) grown to confluency were stimulated for 5 h with LPS and then exposed to a LPS-stimulated neutrophils suspension. After incubation for 1 h, nonadherent neutrophils were removed by washing. Then the GJIC was measured. GJIC of HUVEC which had adherent neutrophils was suppressed. This suppression was abolished by inhibiting neutrophils adhesion to HUVEC with antihuman ICAM-1 antibody. Assay using intercell chambers which prevented the direct contact of neutrophils with HUVEC, showed that no suppression of GJIC was observed. The suppression of HUVEC GJIC by adherent neutrophils was not abolished by protease inhibitors. This suppression was abolished by pretreatment of HUVEC with tyrosine kinase inhibitors. To characterize the nature of this suppression, we examined the GJIC by anti-ICAM-1 antibody cross-linking. Cross-linking of ICAM-1 in HUVEC suppressed the GJIC. These results indicate that: 1) the suppression of GJIC by adherent neutrophils is not affected by proteases, and 2) this suppression is attributed to tyrosine phosphorylation of the gap junction protein, caused by adhesion to HUVEC through integrin and ICAM-1 binding.

Keywords: activated leukocyte, adhesion molecule, cross-linking, endothelial cell, gap junction, ICAM-1, integrin.

Introduction

Parenchymal cells in tissues are known to communicate with each other through gap junctions, which are intercellular membrane channels that permit the diffusion of ions, small molecules and second messengers between adjacent cells. The structural unit of the gap junction is the connexon, a proteinaceous cylinder with a hydrophilic channel. The connexon is composed of six subunits called connexin. Gap junctional intercellular communication is an important mechanism for controlling cellular homeostasis, proliferation and differentiation. Since little is known about the influence of activated leukocytes on gap junctional intercellular communication of vascular endothelial cells, we examined it by using cultured human umbilical vein endothelial cells (HUVEC).

Address for correspondence: Sei-itsu Murota, Department of Physiological Chemistry, Graduate School, Tokyo Medical and Dental University, 1-5-45 Yushima, Bunkyo-ku, Tokyo 113, Japan.

Experimental

Endothelial cell culture HUVEC were obtained from fresh umbilical cords. HUVEC were grown to confluency in a culture medium supplemented with 10% heat inactivated fetal bovine serum, heparin (10 u/ml), endothelial cell growth supplement (30 µg/ml), and HEPES (15 mM) [1].

The activity of gap junctional intercellular communication was assayed according to the fluorescence recovery after photobleaching technique by means of an interactive laser cytometer ACAS 570 [2]. Cultured HUVEC were prelabeled with fluorescent dye CFDA, so that each cell could easily be distinguished from another under a fluorescence microscope. Then the target cells chosen at random were photobleached by laser beam, which caused the cells to lose their fluorescence. The lost fluorescence emission in the bleached cells, however, recovered gradually if the gap junctional intercellular communication was kept intact. Under normoxia condition, 14 min after the bleaching, the fluorescence level recovered completely to the original level as a result of the influx of fluorescent dye from adjacent cells through connexin channels.

Results and Discussion

Fluorescence recovery after photobleaching in HUVEC under the normoxia condition was monitored. In individual cells the lost fluorescence has recovered gradually with time. The data show that if gap junctional intercellular communication is normal, $10 \sim 15$ min is enough for the cells to resume to the original level.

HUVEC were treated with LPS for 5 h to have these endothelial cells express their adhesion molecules including ICAM-1. Similarly LPS-treated leukocytes were placed onto these cells. Then 1 h later nonadherent leukocytes were washed out. Only the leukocytes adhered firmly to endothelial cells with integrin were left on the cell layer. We examined fluorescence recovery after photobleaching in the cells to which some leukocytes were adhered. LPS itself (at least at the dose used of 100 ng/ml) did not affect gap junctional intercellular communication at all. When leukocytes were treated with LPS (100 ng/ml), oxygen burst occurred at the early stage. We waited for 60 min and then the leukocytes were washed with a buffered saline before adding to the endothelial monolayer.

The fluorescence recovery in the cells with leukocyte adhesion was very suppressed; far from the original level even after 14 min. In the cells without leukocyte adhesion, the bleached fluorescence recovered quickly to the original level. In cells with leukocyte adhesion, fluorescence recovery was suppressed, however, this suppression was abolished in the presence of an anti-ICAM-1 antibody, suggesting that integrin and ICAM-1 binding is deeply involved in the reduced gap junctional intercellular communication due to the activated leukocytes.

To confirm the fact that the reduced gap junctional intercellular communication due to the LPS-activated leukocytes was actually mediated by adhesion molecules, we used a special device which had been developed for culturing two different types of cells without them having contact with each other. When leukocytes were placed directly on a monolayer of endothelial cells, a severe suppression of fluorescence recovery was observed. However, when leukocytes were placed on a filter which was set apart from the monolayer of endothelial cells, no suppression was observed. These results strongly suggest that the substance responsible for the reduced gap junctional intercellular communication due to the activated leukocytes cannot be humoral substances released from LPS-stimulated leukocytes, but presumably is adhesion molecules.

The reduced gap junctional intercellular communication due to the activated leukocytes was not abolished by protease inhibitors (i.e., a mixture of aprotinin, leupeptin and pepstatin A) suggesting again that the substance responsible for the reduced gap junctional intercellular communication due to the activated leukocytes is not humoral substances, such as proteases.

The reduced gap junctional intercellular communication due to the activated leukocytes was abolished in the presence of genistein and herbimysin, suggesting that tyrosine kinase is involved in the connexin protein disfunction.

Since we found that integrin and ICAM-1 binding is deeply involved in the reduced gap junctional intercellular communication due to the activated leukocytes, we next stimulated endothelial ICAM-1 directly with anti-ICAM-1 antibody, and at the same time stimulated its secondary antibody to induce ICAM-1 clustering.

Even in the absence of activated leukocytes, if endothelial ICAM-1 was stimulated with cross-linking (that is a mixture of anti-ICAM-1 antibody and its secondary antibody) gap junctional intercellular communication was suppressed significantly, suggesting that ICAM-1 clustering is necessary for the cells to induce the reduced gap junctional intercellular communication in endothelial cells.

Conclusions

1. LPS-activated leukocytes suppressed the gap junctional intercellular communication of cultured HUVEC pretreated with LPS in the subthreshold dose.
2. The reduced gap junctional intercellular communication of the HUVEC due to the activated leukocytes was abolished in the presence of specific antibody against ICAM-1 as well as tyrosine kinase inhibitors, suggesting the involvement of adhesion molecules and tyrosine kinase in this phenomenon.
3. Even in the absence of activated leukocytes, if endothelial ICAM-1 was stimulated with cross-linking (i.e., the mixture of anti-ICAM-1 antibody and its secondary antibody) gap junctional intercellular communication was significantly suppressed, suggesting that ICAM-1 clustering may be necessary for the endothelial cells to induce connexin protein dysfunction, followed by inhibiting gap junctional intercellular communication.

References

1. Jaffe EA, Nachman RL, Becker CG. Culture of human endothelial cells derived from umbilical veins. J Clin Invest 1973;52:2745—2756.
2. Wade MH, Trosko JE, Achindler M. A fluorescence photobleaching assay of gap junction-mediated communication between human cells. Science 1986;232:525—528.

Immune and infectious factors in atherogenesis

Cytomegalovirus and vasculopathy — an overview

Cathrien A. Bruggeman
Department of Medical Microbiology, Cardiovascular Institute Maastricht, Maastricht, The Netherlands

Abstract. Cytomegalovirus (CMV) infections occur mostly without clinical symptoms but severe pathology is induced in the immunocompromised host. After primary infection the virus persists in the host in a latent state. The vessel wall, especially the smooth muscle cell layer is probably a site of latency. There is increasing evidence that CMV is involved in vasculopathology. Several reports indicate that CMV infections are thought to play a role in neointima formation and more recently in restenosis. It is also clear that CMV infections have an influence on the pathogenesis of transplant-associated arteriosclerosis. Using a rat model we studied the infection of vascular cells and the role of the virus on the development of vessel-wall pathology. Using the balloon denudation model it was found that neointimal smooth muscle cells are permissive cells for viral replication. Infections in rats resulted in activation of endothelium leading to enhanced adhesion of leukocytes, while viral infection in the transplanted graft resulted in an accelerated transplant-associated athero-sclerosis.

From these data we conclude that the vessel wall is a preferential site of infection and that infec-tion leads to activation of the vascular system, which in the end might lead to the development of vascular disease.

Keywords: atherosclerosis, cytomegalovirus, endothelium, smooth muscle cells.

Relation between cytomegalovirus infection and atherosclerosis?

Several reports suggest that immunological factors and infectious agents are involved in the development of atherosclerosis.

The role of herpes viruses in vasculopathy had been reported for the first time at the end of the 70s by Fabricant [1]. In these studies, the development of athe-rosclerosis was described in chickens infected with Marek's disease virus (MDV), an avian herpesvirus.

Later, Melnick [2] reported the presence of cytomegalovirus (CMV), a member of the herpesvirus family, in atherosclerotic lesions of humans. They showed that more than 25% of the smooth muscle cell cultures of the arterial samples of patients with atherosclerosis contained CMV.

Epidemiological studies indicate that antibodies against CMV were signifi-cantly higher in patients with coronary atherosclerosis compared to control sub-jects [3].

More recently, Nieto [4] reported the association between intimal thickening

Address for correspondence: Cathrien A. Bruggeman, Department of Medical Microbiology, Univer-sity of Maastricht, c/o University Hospital Maastricht, P.O. Box 5800, 6202 AZ Maastricht, The Neth-erlands. Tel.: +31-43-3876644. Fax: +31-43-3876643.

and CMV antibody titers. In this study, elevated levels of CMV antibody titers in sera collected in 1974 were shown to be associated with increased risk of carotid intimal-medial thickening (IMT) 13–18 years later. These data suggest a correlation between generalized CMV infection and atherogenesis.

No clear answer can be given yet about the possible mechanism. The fact that a high antibody titer is correlated with development of carotid IMT suggests that recurrent infections (probably by reactivation of latent virus) leading to high antibody titers, is a prerequisite for its role in vasculopathy. In general, reactivation of CMV is associated with immune suppression [5], although other factors such as stress factors are also thought to play a role in reactivation of the latent virus.

Interaction of CMV with vascular cells

With the exception of immunosuppressed individuals and newborns, CMV infections occur without clinical symptoms. The virus infects a wide variety of cells (among them monocytes/macrophages, fibroblasts, endothelial cells) in different organs [5].

After primary infection, the virus persists in the host in a so-called latent state. In this state the virus remains in several cells such as monocytes/macrophages (or their progenitor cells), and probably in other cells such as vascular cells (endothelial and smooth muscle cells). Although endothelial cells of the large vessels are in general not infected in the normal (i.e., immunocompetent host), in the severely immune-suppressed host, endothelial cells are often infected [6,7].

Studies in animal models confirm this observation [8,9] suggesting that in the normal situation endothelial cells form an efficient barrier, protecting underlying tissues against infections. In vitro experiments further support these observations and show that infection of endothelial cells is limited [10–12], and is largely dependent on factors such as activation state of the cells and oxidative stress [13,14].

In smooth muscle cells the presence of CMV was first described by Melnick [2]. This study was followed by several studies confirming this observation, all indicating that CMV genome persists in the smooth muscle cell layer [15–17].

In these cells the viral genome but no infectious virus or viral antigens were detectable, suggesting that the smooth muscle cell layer is a site of persistence of latent virus. In contrast, active CMV replication (characterized by presence of intracellular viral antigens) is not very common in the vessel wall, and is probably dependent on the activation and on the cellular differentiation state of the cells [18–20].

Does CMV induce vasculopathy?

The pathogenesis of CMV is not only affected by the cell type infected, but also by the state of the immune response of the host.

Pathology can be induced either by the virus itself (direct effect) or by virus-induced immunomodulation (indirect effect). The latter is thought to be the most important in the case of CMV-induced vasculopathy.

Among the mechanisms involved several are probably known:

1) the first mechanism concerns the activation of endothelium by entry of the virus into the cells leading to membrane perturbation, induction of adhesion molecules, upregulation of membrane antigens and production of cytokines [10,21—25];

2) the second mechanism is the alteration of the lipid metabolism of smooth muscle cells induced by virus infection [1,26];

3) the third mechanism is the interaction between CMV and p53 leading to enhanced proliferation of smooth muscle cells in restenosis after angioplasty [27]; and

4) the fourth mechanism occurs in transplant-associated atherosclerosis and is mediated by interaction of CMV with the immune response leading to enhanced inflammation in the allograft and proliferation of smooth muscle cells resulting in neointimal formation [28,29].

More research is needed in the future on this topic. The use of appropriate animal models and more sensitive techniques for detection of virus and viral products will help to define if CMV is a causal agent or an innocent bystander in the development of vasculopathy.

References

1. Fabricant CG, Fabricant J, Litrenta MM, Minick CR. Virus-induced atherosclerosis. J Exp Med 1978;148:335—340.
2. Melnick JL, Petrie BL, Dreesman GR, Burek J, McCollum CH, DeBakey ME. Cytomegalovirus antigen within human arterial smooth muscle cells. Lancet 1983;2:644—647.
3. Adam E, Melnick JL, Probtsfield JL et al. High levels of cytomegalovirus antibody in patients requiring vascular surgery for atherosclerosis. Lancet 1987;2:291—293.
4. Nieto FJ, Adam E, Sorlie P et al. Cohort study of cytomegalovirus infection as a risk factor for carotid intimal-medial thickening, a measure of subclinical atherosclerosis (see comments). Circulation 1996;94:922—927.
5. Bruggeman CA. Cytomegalovirus and latency: an overview. Virchows Arch B Cell Pathol Incl Mol Pathol 1993;64:325—333.
6. Myerson D, Hackman RC, Nelson JA, Ward DC, McDougall JK. Widespread presence of histologically occult cytomegalovirus. Hum Pathol 1984;15:430—439.
7. Grefte A, van der Giessen M, van Son W, The TH. Circulating cytomegalovirus (CMV)-infected endothelial cells in patients with an active CMV infection. J Infect Dis 1993;167:270—277.
8. Span AH, Frederik PM, Grauls G, van Boven GP, Bruggeman CA. CMV induced vascular injury: an electron-microscopic study in the rat. In Vivo 1993;7:567—573.
9. Span AH, Grauls G, Bosman F, van Boven CP, Bruggeman CA. Cytomegalovirus infection induces vascular injury in the rat. Atherosclerosis 1992;93:41—52.
10. Span AH, van Boven CP, Bruggeman CA. The effect of cytomegalovirus infection on the adherence of polymorphonuclear leucocytes to endothelial cells. Eur J Clin Invest 1989;19:542—548.
11. Slobbe ME, Hendrickx A, Vossen RC, Speel EJ, van Dam-Mieras MC, Bruggeman CA. Cytomegalovirus infection of endothelial cells: restricted viral or limited nuclear transport. Sixth International Cytomegalovirus Workshop Alabama, USA, 1997;(Abstract).
12. Vossen RCRM, Derhaag JG, Slobbe-van Drunen MEP, Duijvestijn AM, van Dam-Mieras

MCE, Bruggeman CA. A dual role for endothelial cells in cytomegalovirus infection? A study of cytomegalovirus infection in a series of rat endothelial cell lines. Virus Res 1996;46:65—74.

13. Vossen RCRM, Persoons MCJ, Slobbe-van Drunen MEP, Bruggeman CA. Intracellular thiol redox status affects cytomegalovirus infection of vascular cells. Virus Res 1997;48:173—183.

14. Scholz M, Cinatl J, Gross V et al. Impact of oxidative stress on human cytomegalovirus replication and on cytokine-mediated stimulation of endothelial cells. Transplantation 1996;61: 1763—1770.

15. Yamashiroya HM, Ghosh L, Yang R, Robertson AL Jr. Herpesviridae in the coronary arteries and aorta of young trauma victims. Am J Pathol 1988;130:71—79.

16. Hendrix MG, Dormans PH, Kitslaar P, Bosman F, Bruggeman CA. The presence of cytomegalovirus nucleic acids in arterial walls of atherosclerotic and nonatherosclerotic patients. Am J Pathol 1989;134:1151—1157.

17. Hendrix MG, Salimans MM, van Boven CP, Bruggeman CA. High prevalence of latently present cytomegalovirus in arterial walls of patients suffering from grade III atherosclerosis. Am J Pathol 1990;136:23—28.

18. Tumilowicz JJ, Gawlik ME, Powell BB, Trentin JJ. Replication of cytomegalovirus in human arterial smooth muscle cells. J Virol 1985;56:839—845.

19. Persoons MCJ, Daemen MJAP, Bruning JH, Bruggeman CA. Active cytomegalovirus of arterial smooth muscle cells in immunocompromides rats. A clue to herpesvirus-associated atherogenesis? Circulation Res 1994;75:214—220.

20. Persoons MCJ, Daemen MJAP, van Kleef EM, Grauls GELM, Wijers E, Bruggeman CA. Does the phenotype of neointimal smooth muscle cells affect their susceptibility to cytomegalovirus (CMV) infection? Cardiovasc Res 1997;(In press).

21. van Geelen AG, Slobbe van Drunen ME, Muller AD, Bruggeman CA, van Dam-Mieras MC. Membrane-related effects in endothelial cells induced by human cytomegalovirus. Arch Virol 1995;140:1601—1612.

22. Span AH, Mullers W, Miltenburg AM, Bruggeman CA. Cytomegalovirus induced PMN adherence in relation to an ELAM-1 antigen present on infected endothelial cell monolayers. Immunology 1991;72:355—360.

23. Ustinov J, Loginov R, Bruggeman C, Suni J, Hayry PJ, Lautenschlager I. CMV-induced class II antigen expression in various rat organs. Transpl Int 1994;7:302—308.

24. Waldman WJ, Adams PW, Orosz CG, Sedmak DD. T lymphocyte activation by cytomegalovirus-infected, allogeneic cultured human endothelial cells. Transplantation 1992;54:887—896.

25. Waldman WJ, Knight DA. Cytokine-mediated induction of endothelial adhesion molecule and histocompatibility leukocyte antigen expression by cytomegalovirus-activated T cells. Am J Pathol 1996;148:105—119.

26. Fabricant CG, Krook L, Gillespie JH. Virus-induced cholesterol crystals. Science 1973;181: 566—567.

27. Speir E, Modali R, Huang ES et al. Potential role of human cytomegalovirus and p53 interaction in coronary restenosis (see comments). Science 1994;265:391—394.

28. Lemstrom KB, Bruning JH, Bruggeman CA, Lautenschlager IT, Hayry PJ. Cytomegalovirus infection enhances smooth muscle cell proliferation and intimal thickening of rat aortic allografts. J Clin Invest 1993;92:549—558.

29. Li F, Grauls G, Yin M, Bruggeman CA. Initial endothelial injury and cytomegalovirus infection accelerate the development of allograft arteriosclerosis. Transplant Proc 1995;27:3552—3554.

Atherosclerosis XI.
B. Jacotot, D. Mathé and J.-C. Fruchart, editors.

Autoimmunity in atherosclerosis

Göran K. Hansson, Sten Stemme, Gabrielle Paulsson, Xinghua Zhou, Martin Bruzelius, Giuseppina Caligiuri, Antonino Nicoletti, Allan Sirsjö, Dirk Wuttge and Zhong-qun Yan
Center for Molecular Medicine, Karolinska Institute, Stockholm, Sweden

Atherosclerosis is accompanied by a local immune response in the plaque. Analysis of human endarterectomy specimens have shown the presence of activated T cells and macrophages, proinflammatory cytokines, immunoglobulins and complement factors [1]. Phenotypic analysis of plaque T cells reveal that they largely are CD4+ cells of the Th1 type, which activate macrophages and induce local inflammation [2].

The pathophysiological consequences of such an inflammation have been unclear and both proatherogenic and antiatherogenic effects have been proposed. Cell-culture studies have shown that the Th1 cytokine, interferon-γ (IFN-γ) activates macrophages and downregulates its scavenger receptors [3]. IFN-γ also induces endothelial expression of adhesion molecules [4] and inhibits the growth, α-actin expression and collagen secretion of vascular smooth muscle cells [5,6]. The activated macrophage secretes interleukin-1 (IL-1) and tumor necrosis factor-α (TNF-α), the latter of which is also produced by Th1 cells. IL-1 and TNF-α are proinflammatory cytokines that activate endothelial cells [7] and induce smooth muscle cells to synthesize nitric oxide (NO) via the cytokine-inducible pathway [8]. Although IFN-γ and the proinflammatory cytokines often act in concert, there are also situations in which they counteract each other. For instance, IFN-γ inhibits while TNF-α and IL-1 induce 92 kDa gelatinase (MMP-9) expression by macrophages [9].

IFN-γ is a potent growth inhibitor for smooth muscle cells and also inhibits their production of collagen. In vivo studies have shown that recombinant IFN-γ and the presence of IFN-γ producing T cells inhibits smooth muscle proliferation after balloon angioplasty [10,11]. As mentioned, this cytokine also acts on endothelial cells to induce adhesion molecules. An important action of this cytokine may be on macrophages, which are induced to synthesize oxygen radicals, proteases, cytokines and coagulation factors [12]. The effects on smooth muscle cells are likely to reduce stenosis, but the mechanical strength of a plaque and the macrophage effects may also increase tissue destruction and enhance thrombus formation. Together, this could increase the risk for plaque rupture. Interestingly, macrophages and activated T cells are particularly frequent at sites of plaque rupture in advanced human atherosclerosis [13].

The effects of Th1, IFN-γ and inflammation on the formation of plaques and in the early phase of atherosclerosis have been controversial. However, recent studies of gene-targeted apoE-knockout mice have revealed that cellular immune responses are vivid in atherosclerotic lesions of such mice [14,15], that macrophages are essential for plaque growth [16], that T and B cells play an important aggravating role [17], and that the Th1 cytokine (IFN-γ) significantly increases atherosclerosis [18]. Lesions at the transition stage between fatty streak and fibrous plaque were less cellular, more fibrous and contained less lipid in compound knockout mice with targeted gene deletions of both apoE and the IFN-γ receptor [18]. This suggests that IFN-γ inhibits collagen formation and, perhaps through secondary mechanisms, also reduces cell proliferation and cholesterol elimination from the plaque. In conclusion, the studies of apoE knockout mice have shown (i) that immune cells are activated in the plaque, (ii) that their elimination by gene targeting reduces lesion development, and (iii) that IFN-γ is an important, aggravating factor for atherosclerosis.

The important roles for T cells and immune mechanisms in atherosclerosis suggest that specific immune responses may be involved in atherosclerosis. Several candidate antigens have been discussed, among them both microorganisms and autoantigens. At present, there are suggestive epidemiological and histological data implying a relationship between atherosclerosis and infections with *Chlamydia pneumoniae* [19,20] and possibly also *Helicobacter pylori*. Experimental and histopathological studies have suggested that viruses of the herpes family (e.g., cytomegalovirus and herpes simplex type I) may play a role [21]. Although we lack mechanistic explanations for all these correlations, it is possible that viral infections aggravate metabolically initiated atherogenesis.

Two autoantigens have been linked to atherosclerosis, oxidized LDL and heat shock protein 60 (hsp60). The latter is expressed during cell injury in endothelial cells and induces strong immune responses during several inflammatory conditions [22]. In rabbits, immunization with hsp65, the mycobacterial equivalent of hsp60, aggravates atherosclerosis [23]. Wick and Xu have, therefore, proposed that an autoimmune response to hsp60 is an initiating event in atherosclerosis.

Oxidized LDL is strongly correlated to atherosclerosis [24]. LDL is protected from oxidation by antioxidants in the blood, but these are apparently sequestered in the extracellular space. LDL oxidation, therefore, takes place in the arterial intima, particularly if macrophages or activated endothelial cells are present [25]. Oxidation generates proinflammatory lipids such as lysophosphatidylcholine and the platelet activating factor. These can activate macrophages and endothelial cells and serve as chemoattractants, thus promoting further LDL oxidation and the recruitment of immunocompetent cells. Such events may explain the strong, adaptive immune response to oxLDL.

Both cellular and humoral immune responses directed against LDL are elicited by oxidation. T cell clones derived from human plaques recognize oxidized LDL when presented by autologous monocytes in the context of HLA-DR [2]. This suggests that the atherosclerotic plaque is the site of an autoimmune reaction against oxidized LDL. Autoantibodies to oxLDL are frequent in patients with atherosclerosis [26]. Their titer may correlate to disease progression, although this is still controversial. Analyses of apoE knockout mice have shown that both IgM and IgG antibodies are formed against oxLDL [27] and that T cell help is involved in the production of IgG-antioxLDL (X. Zhou, S. Stemme and G.K. Hansson, unpublished observations). Interestingly, moderate hypercholesterolemia involves Th1 help to B cell-dependent antibody production. In contrast, the extreme hypercholesterolemia obtained when apoE knockout mice are fed a high-cholesterol diet results in a switch from Th1 to Th2 help, and the subsequent production of IgG1 antibodies to oxidized LDL. This suggests that cholesterol metabolism can modify immune responses, or that the concentration of the oxLDL antigen determines the type of T cell help to autoantibody production.

It is likely that macrophage-Th1 interactions elicit an inflammation in the atherosclerotic plaque. A cascade of mediators govern such responses, starting with the T cell and macrophage activating cytokines released upon immune activation. Thus, IFN-γ activates macrophages, leading to radical production, growth factor secretion, expression of procoagulant activity, enhanced antigen presenting capacity and expression of the proinflammatory cytokines, TNF-α and IL-1. Together with IFN-γ, these cytokines induce adhesion molecule expression and inhibit fibrinolytic activity on the endothelium, downregulate growth and collagen production by smooth muscle cells, and induce NO production in all these cells.

NO is an important regulator of vascular tone under normal conditions but also a mediator of inflammation. In the normal artery, small amounts of NO are produced continuously by an NO synthase constitutively expressed in the endothelium [28]. After diffusing to the smooth muscle cells of the arterial media, NO activates cGMP synthesis by nitrosylating the heme group of guanylyl cyclase. This induces a cascade that involves myosin kinase and results in relaxation of the smooth muscle. Proinflammatory cytokines induce the expression of a high-output NO synthase by smooth muscle cells themselves [8]. This results in the production of large amounts of NO with concomitant cGMP production, but also inhibition of mitochondrial respiration and eventually, apoptosis [8,29]. In vivo, cytokine-inducible NO production may be important to prevent thrombosis and vasospasm, but may also lead to cytotoxic changes in arterial cells [30,31].

To summarize, immune reactions are tightly linked to the initiation and development of atherosclerosis. Cellular immune responses involving macrophages, T cells and proinflammatory cytokines are particularly important and can account for many of the pathological phenomena associated with atherosclerosis. Recent animal experimental studies suggest that cell-mediated immune reactions aggravate atherosclerosis and also that immunization and immune-modulating strategies can inhibit the disease process.

Acknowledgements

Our work is supported by the Swedish Medical Research Council (prof. no 6816) and Heart-Lung Foundation.

References

1. Hansson GK. Cell-mediated immunity in atherosclerosis. Curr Opin Lipid 1997;8:301—311.
2. Stemme S, Faber B, Holm J, Wiklund O, Witztum JL, Hansson GK. T lymphocytes from human atherosclerotic plaques recognize oxidized LDL. Proc Natl Acad Sci USA 1995;92:3893—3897.
3. Geng YJ, Hansson GK. Interferon-γ inhibits scavenger receptor expression and foam cell formation in human monocyte-derived macrophages. J Clin Invest 1992;89:1322—1330.
4. Stemme S, Patarroyo M, Hansson GK. Adhesion of activated T lymphocytes to vascular smooth muscle cells and dermal fibroblasts is mediated by beta-1- and beta-2-integrin receptors. Scand J Immunol 1992;36:233—242.
5. Hansson GK, Hellstrand M, Rymo L, Rubbia L, Gabbiani G. Interferon-γ inhibits both proliferation and expression of differentiation-specific α-smooth muscle actin in arterial smooth muscle cells. J Exp Med 1989;170:1595—1608.
6. Amento EP, Ehsani N, Palmer H, Libby P. Cytokines and growth factors positively and negatively regulate interstitial collagen gene expression in human vascular smooth muscle cells. Arterioscl Thromb 1991;11:1223—1230.
7. Pober JS, Cotran RS. Cytokines and endothelial cell biology. Physiol Rev 1990;70:427—456.
8. Geng YJ, Hansson GK, Holme E. Interferon-γ and tumor necrosis factor synergize to induce nitric oxide production and inhibit mitochondrial respiration in vascular smooth muscle cells. Circ Res 1992;71:1268—1276.
9. Sarén P, Welgus HG, Kovanen PT. TNF-α and IL-1β selectively induce expression of 92-kDa gelatinase by human macrophages. J Immunol 1996;157:4159—4165.
10. Hansson GK, Holm J, Holm S, Fotev Z, Hedrich HJ, Fingerle J. T lymphocytes inhibit the vascular response to injury. Proc Natl Acad Sci USA 1991;88:10530—10534.
11. Hansson GK, Holm J. Interferon-γ inhibits arterial stenosis after injury. Circulation 1991;84: 1266—1272.
12. Adams DO. Molecular interactions in macrophage activation. Immunol Today 1989;10:33—35.
13. van der Wal AC, Becker AE, van der Loos CM, Das PK. Site of intimal rupture or erosion of thrombosed coronary atherosclerotic plaques is characterized by an inflammatory process irrespective of the dominant plaque morphology. Circulation 1994;89:36—44.
14. Zhou X, Stemme S, Hansson GK. Evidence for a local immune response in atherosclerosis. CD4+ T cells infiltrate lesions of apo E-deficient mice. Am J Pathol 1996;149:359—366.
15. Roselaar SE, Kakkanathu PX, Daugherty A. Lymphocyte populations in atherosclerotic lesions of apo E $-/-$ and LDL receptor $-/-$ mice. Decreasing density with disease progression. Arterioscl Thromb Vasc Biol 1996;16:1013—1018.
16. Smith JD, Trogan E, Ginsberg M, Grigaux C, Tian J, Miyata M. Decreased atherosclerosis in mice deficient in both macrophage colony-stimulating factor (op) and apolipoprotein E. Proc Natl Acad Sci USA 1995;92:8264—8268.
17. Dansky HM, Charlton SA, Harper MM, Smith JD. T and B lymphocytes play a minor role in atherosclerotic plaque formation in the apolipoprotein E-deficient mouse. Proc Natl Acad Sci USA 1997;94:4642—4646.
18. Gupta S, Pablo AM, Jiang X-C, Wang N, Tall AR, Schindler C. IFN-γ potentiates atherosclerosis in apoE knock-out mice. J Clin Invest 1997;99:2752—2561.
19. Puolakkainen M, Kuo CC, Shor A, Wang SP, Grayston JT, Campbell LA. Serological response to *Chlamydia pneumoniae* in adults with coronary arterial fatty streaks and fibrolipid plaques. J Clin Microbiol 1993;31:2212—2214.

20. Kuo CC, Gown AM, Benditt EP, Grayston JT. Detection of chlamydia pneumoniae in aortic lesions of atherosclerosis by immunocytochemical stain. Arterioscl Thromb 1993;13: 1501—1504.

21. Kaner RJ, Hajjar DP. Viral activation of thrombo-atherogenesis. In: Fuster V, Ross R, Topol EJ (eds) Atherosclerosis and Coronary Artery Disease, vol 1. Philadelphia: Lippincott-Raven, 1996;569—584.

22. Wick G, Schett G, Amberger A, Kleindienst R, Xu Q. Is atherosclerosis an immunologically mediated disease? Immunol Today 1995;16:27—33.

23. Xu Q, Dietrich H, Steiner HJ, Gown AM, Schoel B, Mikuz G, Kaufmann S, Wick G. Induction of arteriosclerosis in normocholesterolemic rabbits by immunization with heat shock protein 65. Arterioscl Thromb 1992;12:789—799.

24. Witztum JL, Steinberg D. Role of oxidized low-density lipoprotein in atherogenesis. J Clin Invest 1991;88:1785—1792.

25. Ylä-Herttuala S, Palinski W, Rosenfeld ME, Parthasarathy S, Carew TE, Butler S, Witztum JL, Steinberg D. Evidence for the presence of oxidatively modified low-density lipoprotein in atherosclerotic lesions of rabbit and man. J Clin Invest 1989;84:1086—1095.

26. Salonen JT, Ylä-Herttuala S, Yamamoto R, Butler S, Korpela H, Salonen R, Nyyssänen K, Palinski W, Witztum JL. Autoantibody against oxidised LDL and progression of carotid atherosclerosis. Lancet 1992;339:883—887.

27. Palinski W, Hörkkö S, Miller E, Steinbrecher UP, Powell HC, Curtiss LK, Witztum JL. Cloning of monoclonal autoantibodies to epitopes of oxidized lipoproteins from apolipoprotein E-deficient mice. Demonstration of epitopes of oxidized low-density lipoprotein in human plasma. J Clin Invest 1996;98:800—814.

28. Moncada S, Higgs A. The L-arginine-nitric oxide pathway. N Engl J Med 1993;329: 2002—2012.

29. Geng Y-J, Wu Q, Muszynski M, Hansson GK, Libby P. Apoptosis of vascular smooth muscle cells induced by in vitro stimulation with interferon-γ tumor necrosis factor-α and interleukin-1β. Arterioscl Thromb Vasc Biol 1996;16:19—27.

30. Hansson GK, Geng YJ, Holm J, Hårdhammar P, Wennmalm Å, Jennische E. Arterial smooth muscle cells express nitric oxide synthase in response to endothelial injury. J Exp Med 1994; 180:733—738.

31. Yan Z-Q, Yokota T, Hansson GK. Expression of inducible nitric oxide synthase inhibits platelet adhesion to the injured artery. Circ Res 1996;79:38—44.

Potential roles of mast cells in atherosclerosis: from fatty streaks to plaque rupture

Petri T. Kovanen
Wihuri Research Institute, Helsinki, Finland

Abstract. Recent immunohistochemical observations on atherosclerotic lesions in human aortas and coronary arteries have revealed that these lesions contain mast cells. The mast cells are filled with cytoplasmic secretory granules that contain histamine, heparin, the neutral proteases chymase and tryptase and a powerful proinflammatory cytokine, TNF-α. When activated, the mast cells degranulate and may in this way influence lipoprotein metabolism in their immediate environment. Indeed, experimental studies with rodent cells in culture have revealed that degranulation of mast cells induces binding of low-density lipoproteins (LDL) to the heparin proteoglycan component of the exocytosed granules. Granule chymase then degrades the apoB-100 component of the heparin-bound LDL particles and induces their fusion. Ultimately, the granule-bound fused LDL particles are carried into phagocytes (macrophages and smooth muscle cells), which then become foam cells. Chymase also degrades the apolipoprotein A component of high-density lipoprotein (HDL) and so blocks the high-affinity component of cholesterol efflux from the foam cells. As atherosclerotic lesions progress to more severe forms, the number of activated (degranulated) mast cells increases, especially in the vulnerable shoulder regions of coronary atheromas. In these areas, the activated mast cells may induce plaque rupture by stimulating other cells of the intima to secrete matrix metalloproteinases and through activating the secreted enzymes. Definition of the quantitative importance of mast cells in the pathogenesis of atherosclerosis and its complications remains an exciting challenge for the future.

Keywords: chymase, coronary heart disease, inflammation, macromolecular heparin, matrix metalloproteinases, tryptase.

Mast cells originate in the bone marrow. They develop from circulating multilineage c-kit$^+$, CD34$^+$, Ly$^-$, CD14$^-$ and CD17$^-$ hemopoietic progenitors, and accordingly, are different from circulating monocytes (CD14$^+$) and blood basophils (CD17$^+$) [1]. The morphologically indeterminate circulating progenitor cells then migrate into various tissues, notably the various mucosal surfaces and the skin. The chemokine responsible for the migration of the mast-cell precursors into peripheral tissues is thought to be the stem-cell factor, which is secreted by the stromal cells of the tissues. In the tissues, the precursors are then converted into mature mast cells, the hallmark of which is their very high content of cytoplasmic granules [2]. The granules have three main components: histamine, neutral proteases and proteoglycans.

Address for correspondence: Petri Kovanen MD, Wihuri Research Institute, Kalliolinnantie 4, 00140 Helsinki, Finland. Tel.: +358-9-636-494. Fax: +358-9-637-476.
E-mail: petri.kovanen@wihuri.fimnet.fi

Once activated, the mast cells degranulate and expel some of their granules into the extracellular fluid, where histamine is released from the proteoglycans, diffuses away and exerts its various functions (e.g., by increasing the vascular permeability to plasma proteins and plasma lipoproteins, such as the low-density lipoprotein (LDL) particles) [3]. A variable fraction of the proteoglycans is also released in soluble form. Another fraction of the proteoglycans, however, remains bound to the neutral proteases in the form of protease-proteoglycan complexes. These residual complexes are called granule remnants [4].

Mast cells in aortic and coronary fatty streaks

Human mast cells can be divided phenotypically into two types according to their content of neutral proteases: those containing tryptase and those containing both tryptase and chymase [5]. Since all mast cells and only mast cells contain tryptase, staining for this enzyme is the best method for detecting mast cells in human tissues. Therefore, to identify mast cells in arterial tissues, we routinely stain the tissue sections with monoclonal antibodies directed against tryptase. To define the phenotype of the mast cells, chymase is stained. Our studies have revealed that in the human arterial intima (whether normal or atherosclerotic), a highly variable fraction of the cells contain chymase, in addition to tryptase. Thus, in some subjects all of the mast cells contain chymase, in some subjects no mast cells contain chymase, and in yet other subjects a fraction of the mast cells contain chymase.

In a systematic study on the density of mast cells in human atherosclerosis, we first examined aortic intimas for their content of mast cells [6]. In normal aortic intimas and fatty streaks, the mast cells had an average density of $15/mm^2$ and amounted to 3% of all nucleated cells. The ratios of mast cells to T lymphocytes in normal intimas and in fatty streaks were 2:1 and 1:3, and to macrophages, correspondingly 1:4 and 1:10. In normal coronary intimas and fatty streaks, the mast cells had average densities of 1 and $5/mm^2$, and amounted to 0.1 and 0.9% of all nucleated cells, respectively [7]. Thus, in the coronary arteries the density of mast cells was 5-fold higher in the areas where foam cells were also present, as compared with areas without foam cells. To investigate whether the coronary mast cells were activated, electron microscopy was used to identify signs of degranulation. Degranulated mast cells were found to be more numerous in the intimal areas in which the atherosclerotic process was advancing. Thus, in the normal coronary intima about every fifth and in the fatty streaks about every other mast cell showed signs of degranulation. Similar figures have also been found in the aortic fatty streaks.

Mast cells in aortic and coronary atheromas

In aortic atheromas we made the surprising observation that mast cells are distributed unevenly in a typical way: $8/mm^2$ in the shoulder region, $1/mm^2$ in the fibrous cap, and a few or none in the lipid core region [7]. In coronary atheromas, the distribution of mast cells was also uneven: $6/mm^2$ in the shoulder region, and $2/mm^2$ in both the cap and the core regions. Notably, the increase in the number of degranulated mast cells was especially pronounced in the shoulder region of atheromas, the predilection site for atheromatous rupture. In this region, the proportion of degranulated mast cells was 85%, but in the normal intima only 18%. Moreover, in the shoulder region, the ratios of mast cells to T lymphocytes and macrophages were, on average, 1:4 (26%) and 1:8 (12%), respectively. Both T lymphocytes and macrophages are known to secrete histamine-releasing factors, and so may have activated the mast cells and triggered their degranulation. Another potentially important local activator of mast cells in the inflamed coronary atheromas is activated complement.

Mast cells in eroded or ruptured coronary atheromas

More recently, we identified the site of atheromatous erosion or rupture in patients who had died of acute myocardial infarction [8]. At the immediate site of erosion or rupture, mast cells amounted to 6% of all nucleated cells, in the adjacent atheromatous area to 1%, and in the unaffected intimal area to 0.1%. The proportions of the mast cells that were activated (degranulated) were 86% at the site of erosion or rupture, 63% in the adjacent atheromatous area, and 27% in the unaffected intima. From these figures, we could calculate that the density of degranulated mast cells was 200-fold higher at the eroded or ruptured site than in the unaffected intimal area. At the site of erosion or rupture, the numbers of T lymphocytes and macrophages were also increased, and the number of smooth muscle cells was decreased.

Mechanisms of mast cell-induced foam cell formation

To gain insight into the mechanisms by which mast cells might participate in the formation of foam cells, we used cell-culture methods employing mast cells derived from the rat peritoneal cavity [9]. These studies defined a tightly regulated sequence of events leading to foam-cell formation. When the mast cells were cocultured with rat or mouse peritoneal macrophages in the presence of LDL, and then stimulated to degranulate, the apolipoprotein (apo)B-100 component of the LDL particles was bound by the heparin proteoglycan component of the exocytosed granules. The granule-bound LDL was then proteolyzed by the (also granule-bound) chymase. On being proteolyzed, the LDL particles became unstable and fused into larger lipid droplets; thus the capacity of each exocytosed granule to bind and carry LDL was increased on average, from a full load of 10,000 to a full load of 50,000 LDL particles. Finally, the LDL-coated granule remnants were scavenged by the cocultured macrophages, the result being massive uptake of LDL by these cells, with ultimate formation of foam cells. Cultured rat aortic smooth muscle cells of synthetic phenotype could also ingest such LDL-coated granule remnants, and so become filled with cholesterol [10]. With the aid of immunoelectron microscopic studies, we have found evidence that in the human arterial intima, exocytosed mast cell granules bind apoB-100-containing lipoproteins, and that such LDL-loaded granule remnants may be ingested by intimal phagocytes (either macrophages or smooth muscle cells) [11].

Chymase-containing rat serosal mast cells, when stimulated, also effectively block the removal of cholesterol from macrophage foam cells in vitro. The chymase of exocytosed granules proteolyzes HDL_3 particles, thereby reducing their ability to induce efflux of cholesterol from the foam cells [12]. More recently, we found that inhibition of the high-affinity component of cholesterol efflux from cultured macrophage foam cells is due to degradation of the apolipoprotein A-I-containing particles in human serum and aortic intimal fluid [13].

Taken together, the experiments carried out with rodent mast cells suggest the possibility that stimulated mast cells, both by promoting the uptake of LDL and by inhibiting the release of cellular cholesterol, are potentially powerful accelerators of foam-cell formation in the intimal areas in which mast cells, macrophages and smooth muscle cells coexist (Fig. 1).

Potential roles of mast cells in the rupture of coronary atheromas

Novel functions for intimal mast cells have recently emerged, which are not directly related to the formation of foam cells. These functions relate to the concept that coronary atheromas may rupture because of increased activity of the enzymes involved in extracellular matrix digestion [14]. Mast cells of the human arterial intima, when stimulated, release their neutral proteases (tryptase and chymase) into the surrounding microenvironment. Even though tryptase and chymase have limited activity against the various components of the extracellular matrix, they may effectively activate the zymogen forms of matrix metalloproteinases (MMPs). MMPs are synthesized and secreted by the macrophages and smooth muscle cells of atherosclerotic lesions as inactive proforms (proMMPs), and consequently, upon secretion, still have to be activated. One of these matrix-degrading enzymes is interstitial collagenase (MMP-1), also present in human atheromas. We found that human chymase effectively activates proMMP-1 by cleaving the proenzyme at the position Leu^{83}-Thr^{84} [15]. Moreover, studies in other laboratories have demonstrated that tryptase can activate prostromelysin (proMMP-3) [16], which again can activate other MMPs. Finally, granules of mast cells in rupture-prone areas of human coronary atheromas contain TNF-α, a potent proinflammatory cytokine [17]. Importantly, TNF-α can induce macrophages to synthesize MMP-9 (92-kDa gelatinase), another member of the MMP family present in the coronary atheromas [18]. These findings, together with the observations that degranulated mast cells are present at the actual site of the coronary rupture, point to the possibility of a completely new plaque-destabilizing factor, that is, release of chymase, tryptase and TNF-α from mast cells in the coronary plaques.

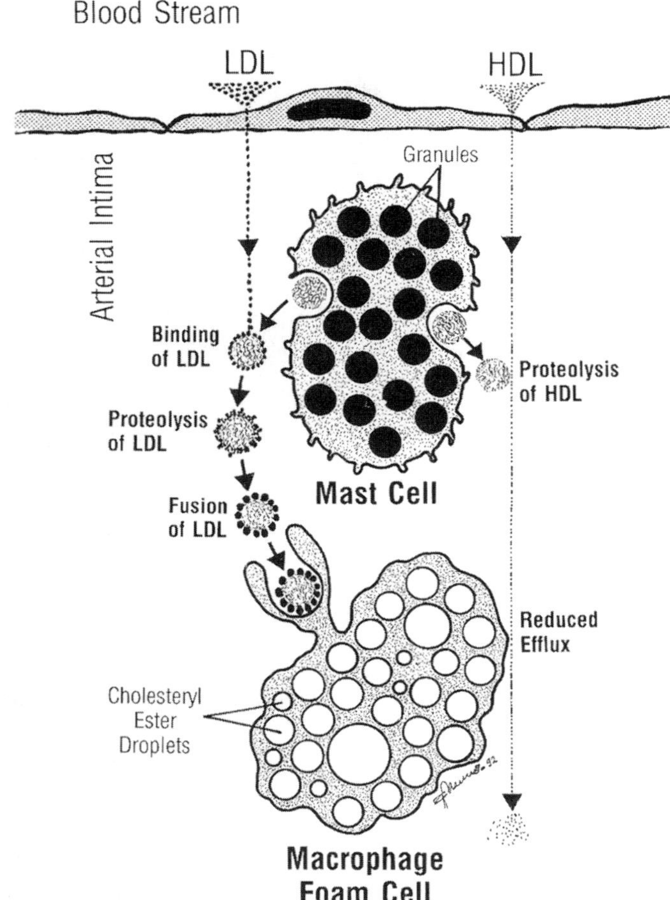

Fig. 1. The dual action of exocytosed mast cell granules on lipoprotein metabolism in the series of events by which a stimulated mast cell converts a macrophage into a foam cell. A degranulating mast cell is shown residing in the subendothelial space of the arterial intima. The exocytosed mast cell granules (i.e., granule remnants) bind and proteolyze LDL particles, so that the particles become unstable and fuse on the remnant surface (left). The granule remnants loaded with fused LDL are phagocytosed by the macrophage, and a macrophage foam cell is formed. Simultaneously, the remnants also proteolyze HDL particles and so block the high-affinity component of the HDL-dependent efflux of cholesterol from the macrophage foam cell (right). This dual action of granule remnants on lipoprotein metabolism facilitates the conversion of the macrophage into a foam cell (from [4] with permission).

References

1. Agis H et al. Monocytes do not make mast cells when cultured in the presence of SCF. Characterization of the circulating mast cell progenitor as c-kit$^+$, CD34$^+$, Ly$^-$, CD14$^-$, CD17$^-$, colony-forming cell. J Immunol 1993;151:4221—4227.

2. Schwartz LB, Austen KF. Structure and function of the chemical mediators of mast cells. Prog Allergy 1984;34:271—321.
3. Ma H, Kovanen PT. Degranulation of cutaneous mast cells induces transendothelial transport and local accumulation of plasma LDL in rat skin in vivo. J Lipid Res 1997;38:1877—1887.
4. Kovanen PT. The mast cell — a potential link between inflammation and cellular cholesterol deposition in atherogenesis. Eur Heart J 1993;14(Suppl K):105—117.
5. Irani AA et al. Two types of human mast cells that have distinct neutral protease compositions. Proc Natl Acad Sci USA 1986;83:4464—4468.
6. Kaartinen M, Penttilä A, Kovanen PT. Mast cells of two types differing in neutral protease composition in the human aortic intima: demonstration of tryptase- and tryptase/chymase-containing mast cells in normal intimas, fatty streaks, and the shoulder region of atheromas. Arterioscl Thromb 1994;14:966—972.
7. Kaartinen M, Penttilä A, Kovanen PT. Accumulation of activated mast cells in the shoulder region of human coronary atheroma, the predilection site of atheromatous rupture. Circulation 1994;90:1669—1678.
8. Kovanen PT, Kaartinen M, Paavonen T. Infiltrates of activated mast cells at the site of coronary atheromatous erosion or rupture in myocardial infarction. Circulation 1995;92:1084—1088.
9. Kovanen PT. Mast cells in human fatty streaks and atheromas: implications for intimal lipid accumulation. Curr Opin Lipid 1996;7:281—286.
10. Wang Y, Lindstedt KA, Kovanen PT. Mast cell granule remnants carry LDL into smooth muscle cells of the synthetic phenotype and induce their conversion into foam cells. Arterioscl Thromb Vasc Biol 1995;15:801—810.
11. Kaartinen M, Penttilä A, Kovanen PT. Extracellular mast cell granules carry apolipoprotein B-100-containing lipoproteins into phagocytes in human arterial intima: functional coupling of exocytosis and phagocytosis in neighboring cells. Arterioscl Thromb Vasc Biol 1995;15:2047—2054.
12. Lee M, Lindstedt LK, Kovanen PT. Mast cell-mediated inhibition of reverse cholesterol transport. Arterioscl Thromb 1992;12:1329—1335.
13. Lindstedt L et al. Chymase in exocytosed rat mast cell granules effectively proteolyzes apolipoprotein AI-containing lipoproteins, so reducing the cholesterol efflux-inducing ability of serum and aortic intimal fluid. J Clin Invest 1996;97:2174—2182.
14. Libby P. Molecular bases of the acute coronary syndromes. Circulation 1991;2844—2850.
15. Saarinen J et al. Activation of human interstitial procollagenase through direct cleavage of the Leu[83]-Thr[84] bond by mast cell chymase. J Biol Chem 1994;269:18134—18140.
16. Gruber BL et al. Synovial procollagenase activation by human mast cell tryptase: dependence upon matrix metalloproteinase 3 activation. J Clin Invest 1989;84:1657—1662.
17. Kaartinen M, Penttilä A, Kovanen PT. Mast cells in rupture-prone areas of human coronary atheromas produce and store TNF-α. Circulation 1996;94:2787—2792.
18. Sarén P, Welgus HG, Kovanen PT. TNF-α and IL-1β selectively induce expression of 92-kDa gelatinase by human macrophages. J Immunol 1996;157:4159—4165.

Autoimmunity to heat shock proteins in atherosclerosis

Georg Wick[1,2] and Qingbo Xu[2]

[1]*Institute for General and Experimental Pathology, University of Innsbruck Medical School; and* [2]*Institute for Biomedical Aging Research of the Austrian Academy of Sciences, Innsbruck, Austria*

Abstract. Based on data obtained from animal experiments and investigations in man, we have developed a new "immunological" hypothesis for the development of atherosclerosis. This concept proposes that the first stage of this disease is of an inflammatory, immunological type. Humoral and cellular immune reactions against certain types of stress proteins, the so-called heat shock proteins (hsp) 65/60 seem to play an important initiating role in atherogenesis. Stress proteins are phylogenetically highly conserved. Thus, a homology at the DNA and protein level of over 50% exists between hsp 65 of *Mycobacterium tuberculosis*, hsp 60 of *Escherichia coli* (GroEl) and the mammalian homologue hsp 60. Immune reactions against bacterial hsp 60 are essential to protect an organism from infection. This protection has, however, to be "paid for" with the risk of cross-reactions to autologous hsp 60. Hsp 60 and adhesion molecules are expressed by endothelial cells at those sites of the arterial vascular tree that are subject to major haemodynamic stress (e.g., the aortic arch and the branching of larger vessels). Pre-existing hsp 65/60-reactive T cells and antibodies, respectively, are able to react with these stressed endothelial cells and mediate the initial lesion. Protracted influence of these risk factors, especially high blood pressure and chemically modified (e.g., oxidized) low-density lipoproteins then lead to the development of classical atherosclerotic lesions, ranging from fatty streaks to fully blown plaques. Immunization of normocholesterolemic rabbits with recombinant hsp 65 leads to mononuclear cell infiltration at these predilection sites that can progress to classical atherosclerotic lesions (including foam cells) if the animals receive, in addition, a cholesterol-rich diet.

Keywords: atherosclerosis, autoimmunity, heat shock proteins.

Introduction

Observations in many laboratories have for a long time supported the idea that the immune system plays a primary or secondary role in the pathogenesis of atherosclerosis [1—3]. In the past decade we have developed a new "immunologic" hypothesis that postulates an autoimmune reaction against a stress protein, heat shock protein 60 (hsp 60), to be the initiating event in atherogenesis [3—5]. This concept is based on the results of studies in experimental animals and men that were triggered by our long-standing interest in two areas of research that are of relevance in this context; autoimmune disease [6], and the role of an altered lipid metabolism for the declining immune response in the elderly [7].

Hsp are the group of proteins that are classified into different families accord-

Address for correspondence: G. Wick MD, Professor and Chairman, Institute for Biomedical Aging Research of the Austrian Academy of Sciences, Rennweg 10, 6020 Innsbruck, Austria. Tel.: +43-512-583919. Fax: +43-512-5839198. E-mail: iba@oeaw.ac.at

ing to their molecular weight [8]. The 60 kD family comprises proteins that have important physiological functions, especially with regard to protein assembly and folding. Furthermore, they also act as chaperons and protect other proteins from the effects of mild stress. Hsp in general, and the hsp 60 family in particular are phylogenetically highly conserved. They constitute important antigenic components of all bacteria and a high degree of homology can be observed between these and eukaryontic hsp [9]. Thus, mycobacterial hsp 65 and human hsp 60 have a homology over 50% on the DNA and protein level. Even higher homologies exist between, for example, mycobacterial hsp 60, hsp 60 of *Chlamydiae* and *GroEl* of *E. coli*. Most human beings possess strong cellular and humoral protective immune responses against bacterial hsp 60. This protection has to be "paid for" by the danger of cross-reactivity with autologous hsp 60 leading to autoimmune damage of the cells expressing these [10,11]. Hsp 60 is a mitochondrial protein, but it is now clear that it is also transported to the cell surface and becomes accessible to T cells in an MHC-restricted fashion or to antibodies [12,13].

Immunization-induced arteriosclerosis in rabbits

Aiming at establishing an experimental autoimmune animal model for atherosclerosis in normocholesterolemic rabbits, we made the lucky observation that immunization with mycobacterial hsp 65 leads to the development of inflammatory, T lymphocyte-dominated, macrophage-containing lesions in the arterial intima of these animals, at those sites that are known to be subjected to increased haemodynamic stress. These are notorious predilection sites for atherosclerotic changes, for example, after feeding a high-cholesterol diet [14]. The lesions in hsp 65 immunized normocholesterolemic rabbits contained T cells that were mostly of the CD4$^+$. The majority of these cells expressed major histocompatibility complex (MHC) class II antigens [15]. In addition to these immunologic-inflammatory cellular elements, smooth muscle cell immigration from the media as well as the occurrence of fibrous caps was also observed, but foam cells were absent. In recombinant mycobacterial hsp 65-immunized rabbits, a cholesterol-rich diet entailed the development of fully blown atherosclerotic lesions that completely paralleled the human situation including foam cells. In addition to the production of antihsp 65 antibodies, the immunized rabbits also showed the expected high number of hsp 65-reactive T cells in the peripheral blood [15]. However, the frequency of the latter was significantly increased in lesion-derived T cell lines. Interestingly, T cells derived from lesions of rabbits that were not immunized but only fed a high-cholesterol diet also showed an increased frequency of hsp 65 responders as compared to the peripheral blood [15].

We were able to demonstrate that in rabbits the first inflammatory stage is still reversible, but fully blown lesions in animals that were concomitantly fed a high-cholesterol diet are not reversible [16]. T-cell depletion of rabbits by treatment with an anti-CD3 monoclonal antibody plus prednisolone prevented development of hsp 65-induced atherosclerosis (Metzler et al., unpublished observations).

Immunization with hsp 65 in rabbits led to atherosclerosis, but arthritis was not observed. Conversely, immunization of rats with hsp 65 entails the development of adjuvant arthritis, but not atherosclerosis. These differences may rely either on the recognition of different hsp 65 epitopes (atherosclerosis-conferring vs. arthritis-conferring epitopes) that cross-react with their mammalian counterparts expressed in different types of cells or tissues, or target cell-dependent influences on organ-specific expression of cross-reactive mammalian hsp 60 epitopes. These issues are now under investigation in our laboratory.

Vascular associated lymphoid tissues

Immunohistological studies in arterial human specimens also showed activated, mostly CD4$^+$, HLA-DR$^+$, Interleukin-2 receptor (IL-2R)$^+$ T cells to be among the first to accumulate in the intima at predilection sites for atherosclerosis [17]. In the earliest stages their number clearly exceed that of macrophages. As a matter of fact, such T cell accumulations together with macrophages and dendritic cells (but without granulocytes, K/NK cells and B cells) could already be observed in the arterial intima of children at the above-mentioned predilection sites, well before the development of fatty streaks [18].

We have tentatively denoted these so far unknown intimae accumulations of lymphoid cells, macrophages and dendritic cells, "vascular associated lymphoid tissue (VALT)" in analogy to the "mucosa associated lymphoid tissue (MALT)". We hypothesize that the VALT serves a similar function as the MALT, i.e., monitors the internal vascular surface for potentially dangerous autologous or heterologous antigenic material.

Subsequent immunohistological analyses revealed an unexpectedly high percentage of the lesion-infiltrating T cells in early human atherosclerotic lesions to express the T cell receptor (TCR) γ/δ . Since this type of T cell is known to have a high propensity for a non-MHC restricted reaction with hsp, this observation further supported our concept of a possible involvement of stress proteins in this initial inflammatory stage of atherosclerosis [19]. In addition, we showed that adhesion molecules (P-selectin and intercellular adhesion molecule-1, ICAM-1) were expressed by endothelial cells at the very same sites that were decorated with an antihsp 60 antibody (i.e., at regions of major haemodynamic stress) such as the aortic arch and arterial bifurcations [20]. Application of various stress factors (temperature, H_2O_2, cytokines, oxidized low-density lipoproteins, etc.) to monolayers of human venous and arterial endothelial cells led to the simultaneous expression of hsp 60 and ICAM-1, P-selectin and vascular adhesion molecule-1 (VCAM-1) in a coordinated fashion [21]. Thus, the prerequisites for interaction of hsp 65/60 specific T cells and also of antibodies with stressed endothelial cells were fulfilled.

Humoral immunity to HSP 60

An investigation of over 800 clinically healthy volunteers with concomitant sonographic assessment of their carotid arteries afforded significantly increased antihsp 65 serum antibody titers in those affected with atherosclerotic lesions as compared to the group without such changes [22]. These antibodies cross-react with recombinant human hsp 60 [23] as well as with *GroEl* and *Chlamydia* hsp 60 and vice versa (Mayr et al., submitted). These antibodies are not only of diagnostic relevance but also seem to play a pathogenetic role, since they were able to lyse stressed, but not unstressed endothelial cells in a complement-mediated fashion or via antibody-dependent cellular cytotoxicity (ADCC) [24].

Such antibodies have recently also been demonstrated in patients with coronary atherosclerosis. Interestingly, immediately after myocardial infarction, these patients showed a drop in antihsp 65 antibody titers, probably due to the release of hsp 60 by the infarcted tissue and subsequent immune complex formation [25].

It is important to note that arterial endothelial cells that have been subjected to higher blood pressure, and thus more pronounced mechanical stress throughout life, seem to have a lower threshold for the adhesion molecule- and hsp-inducing activity of other stressors. Thus, oxidized LDL acts as a potent stressor only on arterial but not venous human endothelial cells.

So far, we have identified three linear epitopes with which human antihsp 65 antibodies react, i.e., two N-terminal sequences (AA 97-109 and AA 197-187) and one C-terminal sequence (AA 504-512) [26], and we are now in the process of defining the most probably more important conformational epitopes.

Interestingly, we were able to demonstrate that cyclosporin A is a potent inducer of the expression of adhesion molecules and hsp 60 by itself, an observation that provides a molecular basis for the known increased frequency of atherosclerosis in patients treated with this immunosuppressive drug (Amberger et al., unpublished results).

Conclusion

We postulate that the earliest stage of arteriosclerosis consists in an immunologic inflammatory reaction against hsp 60, expressed by stressed endothelial cells. Due to the higher arterial blood pressure, the threshold of arterial endothelial cells for stressors that lead to the coordinated expression of adhesion molecules and hsp 60 is lower than in venous endothelial cells. Since nearly everybody possesses cellular and humoral immune reactivity against bacterial hsp 65 it depends not only on the immunological recognition of atherogenic hsp 60 epitopes but also on "how we treat" our endothelial cells, if a potentially dangerous cross-reactivity comes into effect. We, of course, do not dispute the well-proven role of classical risk factors, such as high blood pressure, high serum cholesterol and altered lipoprotein levels, tobacco-derived toxins, infections etc., but we assign a different initial role to these as stressors of endothelial cells entailing damage by

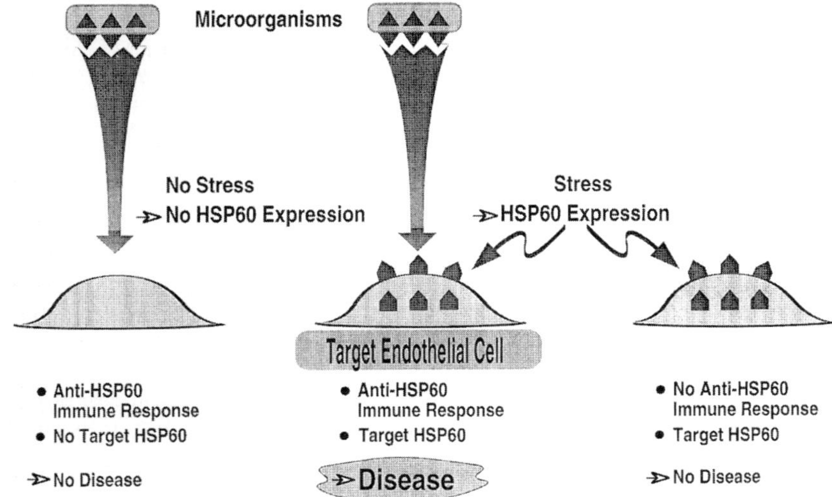

Fig. 1. Cellular and humoral response to hsp 60.

cross-reactive cellular and humoral immunity against hsp 60. In a second stage of atherogenesis (characterized by the appearance of foam cells) these risk factors play a different role, i.e., act as stimulators of cytokines and growth factors as well as chemoattractants. At present, we do not know if humoral or cellular antihsp 65/60 reactivity is the initiating factor for the disease, nor can we differentiate between a cross-reaction of antibacterial hsp 60 immunity with human hsp 60 or the emergence of a bona fide outreactivity (Fig. 1).

Acknowledgements

The original work by the authors was supported by the Austrian Research Fund (GW projects no 10677 and 12213, QX project no. 11615), the Jubiliäumsfonds of the Austrian National Bank (GW project no 5651), the Sandoz Foundation for Gerontological Research (GW) and the State of Tyrol (GW).

References

1. Hansson GK, Jonasson L, Seifert PS, Stemme S. Immune mechanisms in atherosclerosis. Arteriosclerosis 1989;9:567–578.
2. Libby P, Hansson GK. Involvement of the immune system in human atherogenesis: current knowledge and unanswered questions. Lab Invest 1991;64:5–15.
3. Wick G, Kleindienst R, Dietrich H, Xu Q. Is atherosclerosis an autoimmune disease? Trends Food Sci Technol 1992;3:114–119.
4. Wick G, Schett G, Amberger A, Kleindienst R, Xu Q. Is atherosclerosis an immunologically mediated disease? Immunol Today 1995;16:27–33.
5. Xu Q, Wick G. The role of heat shock proteins in protection and pathophysiology of the arterial

wall. Molec Med Today 1996;2:372—379.

6. Wick G, Brezinschek HP, Hála K, Dietrich H,Wolf H, Kroemer G. The obese strain of chickens: an animal model with spontaneous autoimmune thyroiditis. Adv Immunol 1989;47:433—500.

7. Wick G, Huber LA, Xu Q, Jarosch E, Schönitzer D, Jürgens G. The decline of the immune response during aging: the role of an altered lipid metabolism. Ann NY Acad Sci 1991;621: 277—290.

8. Morimoto RI. Cells in stress: transcriptional activation of heat shock genes. Science 1993;259: 1409—1410.

9. Young RA, Elliott TJ. Stress proteins, infection, and immune surveillance. Cell 1989;59:5—8.

10. Kaufmann SHE. Heat shock proteins and the immune response. Immunol Today 1990;11: 129—136.

11. Xu Q, Schett G, Seitz CS, Hu Y, Gupta RS,Wick G. Surface staining and cytotoxic activity of heat-shock protein 60 antibody in stressed aortic endothelial cells. Circ Res 1994;75: 1078—1085.

12. Wurttenberg AW, Shoel B, Ivanyi J, Kaufmann SHE. Surface expression by mononuclear phagocytes of an epitope shared with mycobacterial heat shock protein 60. Eur J Immunol 1991;21:1089—1096.

13. Cesare SD, Poccia F, Mastino A, Colizzi V. Surface expressed heat-shock proteins by stressed or human immunodeficiency virus (HIV)-infected lymphoid cells represent the target for antibody-dependent cellular cytotoxicity. Immunology 1992;76:341—343.

14. Xu Q, Dietrich H, Steiner HJ, Gown AM, Schoel B, Mikuz G, Kaufmann SHE,Wick G. Induction of arteriosclerosis in normocholesterolemic rabbits by immunization with heat shock protein 65. Arterioscl Thromb 1992;12:789—799.

15. Xu Q, Kleindienst R,Waitz W, Dietrich H,Wick G. Increased expression of heat shock protein 65 coincides with a population of infiltrating T lymphocytes in atherosclerotic lesions of rabbits specifically responding to heat shock protein 65. J Clin Invest 1993;91:2693—2702.

16. Xu Q, Kleindienst R, Schett G,Waitz W, Jindal S, Gupta RS, Dietrich H,Wick G. Regression of arteriosclerotic lesions induced by immunization with heat shock protein 65-containing material in normocholesterolemic, but not hypercholesterolemic, rabbits. Atherosclerosis 1996;123: 145—155.

17. Xu Q, Oberhuber G, Gruschwitz M,Wick G. Immunology of atherosclerosis: Cellular composition and major histocompatibility complex class II antigen expression in aortic intima, fatty streaks, and atherosclerotic plaques in young and aged human specimens. Clin Immunol Immunopathol 1990;56:344—359.

18. Wick G, Romen M, Amberger A, Metzler B, Mayr M, Falkensamer G, Xu Q. Atherosclerosis, autoimmunity and the vascular associated lymphoid tissue. FASEB J (In press).

19. Kleindienst R, Xu Q,Willeit J,Waldenberger F, Weimann S, Wick G. Immunology of atherosclerosis: demonstration of heat shock protein 60 expression and T-lymphocytes bearing $\alpha\beta$ or $\gamma\delta$ receptor in human atherosclerotic lesions. Am J Pathol 1993;142:1927—1937.

20. Seitz CS, Kleindienst R, Xu Q,Wick G. Coexpression of intercellular adhesion molecule-1 and heat shock protein 60 is related to increased adherent monocytes and T cells on aortic endothelium of rats in response to endotoxin. Lab Invest 1996;74:241—252.

21. Amberger A, Maczek C, Jürgens G, Michaelis D, Schett G, Xu Q, Wick G. Coexpression of ICAM-1,VCAM-1, ELAM-1 and Hsp 60 in human arterial venous endothelial cells in response to cytokines and oxidized low-density lipoproteins. Cell Stress Chaperons 1997;2:94—103.

22. Xu Q,Willeit J, Marosi M, Kleindienst R, Oberhollenzer F, Kiechl S, Stulnig T, Luef G,Wick G. Association of serum antibodies to heat shock protein 65 with carotid atherosclerosis. Lancet 1993;341:255—259.

23. Xu Q, Luef G,Weimann S, Gupta RS,Wolf H,Wick G. Staining of endothelial cells and macrophages in atherosclerotic lesions with human heat-shock protein reactive antisera. Arterioscl Thromb 1993;13:1763—1769.

24. Schett G, Xu Q, Amberger A, van der Zee R, Recheis H, Willeit J,Wick G. Autoantibodies

against heat shock protein 60 mediate endothelial cytotoxicity. J Clin Invest 1995;96: 2569—2577.
25. Hoppichler F, Lechleitner M, Tragweger C, Schett G, Dzien A, Sturm W, Xu Q. Changes of serum antibodies to heat-shock protein 65 in coronary heart disease and acute myocardial infarction. Atherosclerosis 1996;126:333—338.
26. Metzler B, Schett G, Kleindienst R, van der Zee R, Ottenhoff T, Hajeer A, Bernstein R, Xu Q, Wick G. Epitope specificity of antiheat shock protein 65/60 serum antibodies in atherosclerosis. Arterioscl Thromb Vasc Biol 1997;17:536—541.

New developments in animal models for atherosclerosis

Effect of multiple gene transfer in mouse models

Sandrine Séguret-Macé, Patrick Benoit, Florence Emmanuel, Jean Michel Caillaud, Laurent Bassinet, Isabelle Viry, Pierre Gallix, Didier Branellec, Patrice Denèfle and Nicolas Duverger
Rhône-Poulenc Rorer-Gencell Division, Centre de recherche de Vitry-Alfortville, Vitry-sur-Seine, France

Abstract. Low levels of high-density lipoproteins (HDL) account for 36% of patients with coronary heart disease (CHD). The concentration of HDL is inversely correlated with the risk of CHD indicating that HDL have antiatherogenic properties. Apolipoprotein A-I (apoA-I) is the major protein component of HDL. Lecithin cholesterol acyltransferase (LCAT) catalyzes the esterification of free cholesterol present in HDL. The potentials of these two genes in gene therapy for atherosclerosis were investigated. First, the roles of apoA-I and LCAT have been evaluated in relevant transgenic animal models. In transgenic apoA-I of mice and rabbits, the HDL levels were 2-fold increased and animals were protected against atherosclerogenesis. Human LCAT expression in transgenic mice also lead to an increase of HDL levels. Secondly, adenovirus-mediated transfer of human apoA-I and LCAT genes have been investigated. Mice infected with 3×10^9 pfu of a recombinant adenovirus encoding human apoA-I demonstrated a 300% increase in both levels of apoA-I and HDL 7 days after injection, indicating that transient expression of apoA-I produces elevation of HDL cholesterol of a magnitude correlated with important physiological effects. Similar data were obtained with a recombinant adenovirus encoding human LCAT. Plasma levels of HDL and apoA-I were increased by 600 and 250%, respectively, 7 days after infection (1×10^9 pfu). Overall, these studies show that adenovirus-mediated gene transfer of apoA-I and LCAT genes have therapeutic potential for the treatment of patients with low levels of HDL-cholesterol.

Introduction

More than half of patients with angiographically confirmed coronary heart disease before the age of 60 years have a familial lipoprotein disorder [1]. Reduced high-density lipoprotein (HDL) cholesterol is the most common lipoprotein abnormality (39% of cases) [1]. Epidemiological studies have consistently demonstrated a strong inverse correlation between plasma levels of HDL cholesterol and the incidence of coronary heart disease (CHD) [2,3]. HDL and its major apolipoprotein (apo) A-I are thought to directly limit the development of atherosclerosis.

In humans, apoA-I is synthesized by both liver and intestine [4]. ApoA-I represents 70% of the protein component of HDL and its concentration is directly correlated with HDL-cholesterol levels. ApoA-I plays a predominant role in the

---

Address for correspondence: Nicolas Duverger, Rhône-Poulenc Rorer-Gencell Division, Cardiovascular Department, Centre de recherche de Vitry-Alfortville, 13 Quai Jules Guesde-BP 14, 94403 Vitry-sur-Seine Cedex, France. Tel: +33-1-55-71-38-91. Fax: +33-1-55-71-24-22.
E-mail: nicolas.duverger@rhone-poulenc.com

molecular architecture of HDL [5]. ApoA-I-containing lipoproteins are heterogeneous in hydrated densities and sizes. In addition to the epidemiological data, several animal studies have shown that apoA-I prevents atherosclerosis development. Infusion of apoA-I-containing lipoproteins in rabbits inhibits lesion formation [6,7]. Overexpression of human apoA-I in specific inbred strains of animals (natural cholesterol-fed C57BL/6 mice [8] and New Zealand White rabbits [9]), or in genetically engineered strains of animals (apoE-deficient mice [10,11] and human apo(a) transgenic mice [12]) protects against atherosclerosis. ApoA-I-containing lipoproteins appear to exert their antiatherogenic effect by facilitating reverse cholesterol transport, during which cholesterol excess is transported away from cells of extrahepatic tissues and carried back to the liver, where it can be eliminated or reused [13].

Lecithin cholesterol acyltransferase (LCAT) is an enzyme primarily associated with HDL which uses the free cholesterol of HDL as substrate [14]. ApoA-I is the principal cofactor of the enzyme. LCAT catalyses the synthesis of cholesteryl esters and lysolecithin from lecithin and unesterified cholesterol present in the plasma. HDL particles are the main acceptors of cholesterol that desorbs from lipid interfaces. By maintaining a free cholesterol concentration gradient between peripheral cells and HDL and by participating in the maturation of HDL, LCAT plays a major role in reverse cholesterol transport.

LCAT is an important enzyme in the metabolic pathways of HDL. Subjects with partial or complete LCAT deficiency are characterized by low concentrations of HDL-cholesterol.

In this article, we showed the use of adenovirus-mediated gene delivery in human apoA-I transgenic mice, and we observed that transient human LCAT and apoA-I expression increased plasma levels of HDL-cholesterol as well as human apoA-I. Overall, these studies show that adenovirus-mediated gene transfer of apoA-I and LCAT genes have therapeutic potential for the treatment of patients with low levels of HDL cholesterol.

Experimental procedures

Recombinant adenoviruses preparation

Recombinant adenoviruses encoding human LCAT (AV CMV LCAT), apoA-I (AV RSV apoA-I) or β-galactosidase genes were prepared, purified and titered using standard techniques, as described previously [15]. The coding regions from apoA-I and LCAT cDNA are cloned under the control of the RSV-LTR (Rous sarcoma virus long terminal repeat) and CMV (cytomegalovirus) promoter, respectively.

Animal experiments

The study protocol was approved by the Animal Use Committee of Rhône-Poulenc Rorer. Human apoA-I transgenic mice [16] have been described previously (C57BL/6 background). Mice, 8—10 weeks old, were treated by tail-vein injection of purified recombinant adenovirus stocks. Blood was taken from the retro-orbital plexus of mice fasted for 3 h. Plasma was separated by centrifugation at 2,800 g for 20 min at 4°C.

Protein and lipoprotein analysis

Plasma-lipoprotein distribution was assayed by analytical gel filtration chromatography, with a Superose 6 HR 10/30 column (Pharmacia, Sweden). Plasma levels of human apoA-I were determined by rocket immunoelectrophoresis (SEBIA). There was no cross-reactivity between human and mouse apoA-I in this assay. LCAT activity was assayed by using an exogenous proteoliposome substrate as described by Chen and Albers [17]. We considered the level of LCAT to be directly proportional to its activity. Plasma cholesterol esterification rate (CER) was measured as previously described [18]. Total cholesterol (TC) and free cholesterol (FC) were measured with commercially available kits (Boehringer Mannheim, Germany). Cholesteryl ester (CE) values were calculated by subtracting FC from plasma TC concentrations.

In vitro cellular cholesterol efflux

Cellular cholesterol efflux studies were performed as described previously [19] with the rat Fu5AH hepatoma cells incubated with 2.5% diluted serum.

Statistical analysis

All data are expressed as mean ± SEM. Data were evaluated with ANOVA.

Results

Adenovirus-mediated human apoA-I gene transfer in human apoA-I transgenic mice

In order to avoid the effect of the immune reaction against the human protein, transgenic mice for human apoA-I were used for human apoA-I gene transfer. Basal levels of human apoA-I were 143 ± 5 mg/ml whereas endogenous mouse apoA-I was undetectable. Transgenic mice were injected with 3×10^9 pfu of the AV RSV apoA-I (n = 10) or with PBS (n = 5). Plasma levels of human apoA-I, triglycerides and HDL cholesterol were measured on a weekly basis (Fig. 1). Seven days after adenovirus administration, plasma level of human apoA-I increased from basal level to 425 ± 58 mg/dl (300% increase). These high levels of the transgene were still significantly higher (p < 0.0001) in AV RSV apoA-I treated mice than in mock-treated mice after 6 weeks. HDL-cholesterol levels (Fig. 1) were also increased in a parallel manner and rose from 97 ± 8 mg/dl to

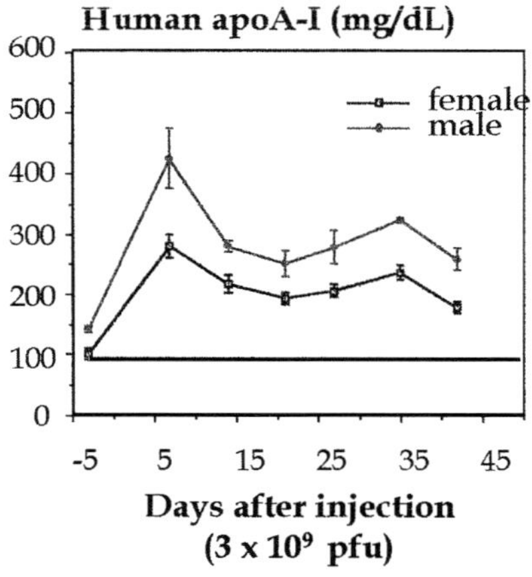

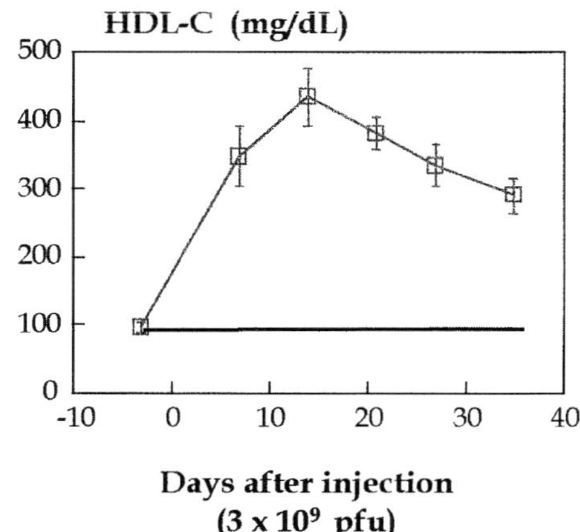

Fig. 1. Effects of adenovirus-mediated gene transfer on the transgene expression in human apoA-I transgenic mice. Mice were injected with 3×10^9 pfu of AV RSV apoA-I ($\bullet$, $\blacksquare$) or with PBS (basal line). Plasma levels of human apoA-I and HDL-cholesterol increased at day 7 and remained significantly elevated during the 6 weeks of the experiment ($p < 0.001$ and $p < 0.001$ for human apoA-I and HDL-cholesterol levels, respectively). Human apoA-I transgenic mice injected with PBS showed no variation in the human apoA-I levels.

346 ± 44 mg/dl (360% increase) at 7 days. After 5 weeks, the HDL-cholesterol levels were still significantly increased at 289 ± 26 mg/dl (297% of the basal level, $p < 0.0001$). Human apoA-I levels were still higher in AV RSV apoA-I treated mice than in mock-treated mice after 10 weeks (data not shown). No variation of triglycerides concentrations (mean levels: 138 ± 13 mg/dl) was observed following human gene transfer.

In order to get insights in the molecular mechanism of the protective effect mediated by human apoA-I, the promotion of cholesterol efflux from cells was investigated. Cholesterol efflux (Fig. 2) promoted from cholesterol preloaded Fu5AH cells was 1.55-fold greater ($p < 0.0008$) with the incubation of sera (14 days postinjection) from the AV RSV apoA-I treated mice than that from PBS-treated mice.

Adenovirus-mediated human LCAT gene transfer in human apoA-I transgenic mice

LCAT activities and cholesterol esterification rates were determined in the serum of human apoA-I transgenic mice after adenovirus-mediated human LCAT gene transfer. All parameters measured for this study were determined 3 days before and 6 days after injection, which corresponded to the time point for the peak of expression of human LCAT as well as for the major lipoprotein metabolism alterations observed. No variation in LCAT activities and lipoprotein metabolism were observed in mice infected with adenovirus encoding β-galactosidase gene. Six days after injection of the recombinant adenovirus encoding human LCAT,

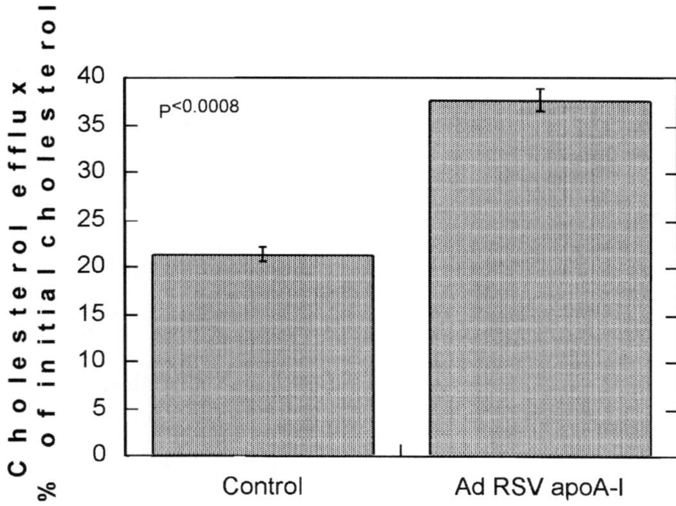

Fig. 2. Cholesterol efflux studies. 2.5% diluted sera from mice infected (14 days postinfection) with AV RSV apoA-I or PBS (control) were incubated with radiolabeled cholesterol preloaded Fu5AH cells for 4 h at 37°C. Values are expressed as percentage of initial cholesterol present in the cells that was found in the medium after incubation.

both plasma CER and LCAT activities levels were increased in human apoA-I transgenic mice (Table 1).

Plasma levels of lipid and lipoprotein in transgenic mice are presented in Table 2. When human apoA-I transgenic mice were infected with the recombinant adenovirus (1×10^9 pfu), TC and HDL-cholesterol levels were 12- and 13-fold increased, respectively. The CE/TC ratios in the plasma and in HDL increased after infection, indicating a CE accumulation in HDL.

To determine whether overexpression of LCAT would alter the ability of apoA-I-containing lipoproteins to promote cholesterol efflux (Fig. 3), Fu5AH hepatoma cells were incubated with 2.5% diluted serum from human apoA-I transgenic mice before and after infection with 5×10^8 pfu and 1×10^9 pfu of AV CMV

Table 1. Plasma LCAT activities and cholesteryl esterification rate in human apoA-I transgenic mice before and after infection with AV CMV LCAT.

	Human apoA-I transgenic mice J-73 (n = 6)	Human apoA-I transgenic infected mice (1×10^9 pfu) J + 6 (n = 6)
LCAT activity (nmol/ml/h)	38 ± 2	13253 ± 660[a]
CER (nmol/ml/h)	54 ± 5	318 ± 15[a]

[a]Different from corresponding noninfected mice ($p < 0.05$).

Table 2. Plasma levels (mg/dl) of lipid and lipoprotein in human apo A-I transgenic mice before and after infection with AV CMV LCAT.

	Human apoA-I transgenic mice J-3 (n = 6)	Human apoA-I transgenic infected mice (1×10^9 pfu) J+6 (n = 6)
Total cholesterol (TC)	93 ± 9	1177 ± 40^a
Cholesteryl ester (CE)	67 ± 9	991 ± 35^a
Free cholesterol	26 ± 3	186 ± 6^a
CE/TC	0.72 ± 0.04	0.84 ± 0.01^a
Non-HDL-cholesterol	11 ± 1	80 ± 7^a
Triglycerides	62 ± 21	653 ± 75^a
Phospholipids	292 ± 20	1280 ± 33^a
HDL-cholesterol	82 ± 10	1091 ± 36^a
HDL-cholesteryl ester	62 ± 9	932 ± 31^a
HDL-free cholesterol	21 ± 3	159 ± 5^a
CE/TC in HDL	0.74 ± 0.04	0.84 ± 0.01^a

[a]Different from corresponding noninfected mice (p < 0.05).

LCAT (6 days after injection). Overexpression of LCAT altered HDL metabolism of transgenic mice and increased the capacity of serum to produce cholesterol efflux. After infection, cholesterol efflux increased significantly with the incubation of serum from human apoA-I transgenic mice.

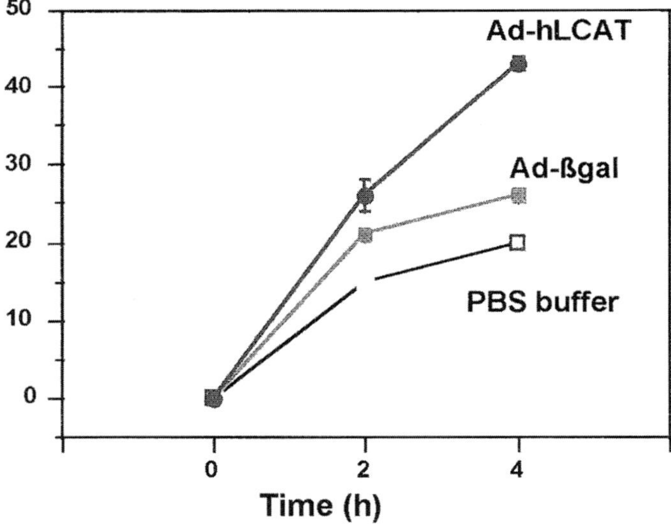

Fig. 3. Cholesterol efflux studies. 2.5% diluted sera from mice infected (14 days postinfection) with AV CMV LCAT, AV CMV βGal or PBS (control) were incubated with radiolabeled cholesterol preloaded Fu5AH cells for 4 h at 37°C. Values are expressed as percentage of initial cholesterol present in the cells that was found in the medium after incubation.

The rates of esterification of cholesterol effluxed from cells after incubation with sera obtained before human LCAT expression were 0.81 ± 0.06 nmol/ml/h in human apoA-I. The rates of esterification of cholesterol effluxed from cells after incubation with sera obtained during human LCAT expression were 1.35 ± 0.19 nmol/ml/h in human apoA-I transgenic mice.

Discussion

This study described the effects of administration of recombinant adenovirus encoding human apoA-I or human LCAT in the mouse model. The use of adenoviral vector permitted a high level of transgene expression which was associated with increased apoA-I and HDL-cholesterol concentrations. In addition, the utilization of the RSV-LTR promoter to control the apoA-I expression as well as transgenic mice as recipient mice allowed a long-term duration of human apoA-I expression.

Adenovirus-mediated gene delivery of human apoA-I demonstrated that it is possible to increase the levels of apoA-I and HDL-cholesterol in the plasma of human apoA-I transgenic mice by nearly 300%, whereas only moderate increases of these parameters were observed in normal mice. The dramatic difference in the level of transgene expression between transgenic and nontransgenic mice [20] reflected the lack of a reaction against the protein of foreign origin. The levels of human apoA-I expression obtained in transgenic animals were higher than those in the nontransgenic models, and the duration of expression was also increased from weeks to months. Nevertheless, immune reaction against viral proteins was still present with this first-generation adenoviral vector and contributed to the extinction of transgene expression by elimination of virus-tranduced cells. Recently, several groups have reported solutions to this problem, such as transient immunosupression, neonatal administration of the vector or modification of the viral vector. We showed here that immune response against the foreign protein is the major hurdle in obtaining stable expression (for few months) and producing data in the study of lipoprotein metabolism and atherogenesis. In addition, the use of RSV-LTR promoter, which may appear weaker at directing transgene expression at the peak level when compared with that of a CMV (cytomegalovirus) promoter, allowed a constant expression for a longer period of time without side effects such the hypertriglyceridemia which was observed by Kopfler et al. [20].

HDL and apoA-I-containing lipoproteins have been proposed as protecting against atherogenesis by removing cholesterol excess in peripheral cells and transporting it back to the liver [13]. Although other mechanisms have been proposed for the antiatherogenic role of HDL, the present in vitro cellular cholesterol efflux study strongly supports this hypothesis. In the cell-culture system for evaluation of cholesterol efflux efficiency [19], serum from AV RSV apoA-I infected mice promoted significantly higher cholesterol efflux than that of control mice.

The vast majority of hypoalphalipoproteinemic patients having some residual apoA-I levels in the circulation develops premature CHD 1. Data emerging from large epidemiological surveys have suggested that each percentage increase in HDL-cholesterol plasma concentration results in a 3—4% decrease in coronary heart disease risk [21]. In addition, overproduction of human apoA-I has been found in some subjects, and was associated with high HDL-cholesterol levels, an absence of CHD and longevity [22]. Therefore, overexpression of apoA-I to higher levels than normal concentrations can be considered as potential therapy in order to increase HDL concentration and induce inhibition or regression of atherosclerotic lesions in a large population.

LCAT occupies a central role in HDL metabolism, esterifying cholesterol at the surface of HDL and participating in the reverse cholesterol transport process. It has been suggested that LCAT may be antiatherogenic based on several lines of evidence. First, LCAT overexpression in transgenic mice led to an increase of HDL-cholesterol concentrations [23,24]. Secondly, human LCAT transgenic rabbits fed with an atherogenic diet have a decrease of apoB-containing lipoprotein levels as well as an increase of apoA-I-containing lipoprotein levels and are protected against atherogenesis [25]. Finally, in a small epidemiological study, it has been shown that LCAT activity correlated with HDL cholesterol and with a lower risk for developing cardiovascular diseases [26]. Here, we reported another potential therapy for hypoalphalipoproteinemic patients with adenovirus-mediated transfer of human lecithin cholesterol acyltransferase (LCAT) gene. Human LCAT gene transfer in human apoA-I transgenic mice led to an increase of HDL-cholesterol and human apoA-I plasma levels, probably due to a delay in apoA-I-containing lipoprotein catabolism.

The present studies demonstrate the potential of gene-transfer strategy in the appropriate animal model to get insight into the role of apoA-I and LCAT in lipoprotein metabolism. Similar constructs and animal models will be required to compare these two genes. In addition, new vectors should be designed to evaluate their possible synergistic effect.

References

1. Genest JJ, Martin-Munley S, McNamara J, Ordovas J, Jenner J, Myers R, Silberman S, Wilson P, Salem D, Schaefer E. Familial lipoprotein disorders in patients with premature coronary artery disease. Circulation 1992;85(6):2025—2033.
2. Miller G, Miller N. Plasma high-density lipoprotein concentration and development of ischaemic heart disease. Lancet 1975;1(7897):16—19.
3. Gordon D, Rifkind B. High-density lipoprotein — the clinical implications of recent studies. N Engl J Med 1989;321(19):1311—1316.
4. Higuchi K, Law S, Hoeg J, Schumacher U, Meglin N, Brewer HJ. Tissue-specific expression of apolipoprotein A-I (ApoA-I) is regulated by the 5′-flanking region of the human ApoA-I gene. J Biol Chem 1988;263(34):18530—18536.
5. Duverger N, Rader D, Duchateau P, Fruchart J, Castro G, Brewer HJ. Biochemical characterization of the three major subclasses of lipoprotein A-I preparatively isolated from human plasma. Biochemistry 1993;32(46):12372—12379.

6. Badimon J, Badimon L, Fuster V. Regression of atherosclerotic lesions by high-density lipoprotein plasma fraction in the cholesterol-fed rabbit. J Clin Invest 1990;85(4):1234—1241.

7. Miyazaki A, Sakuma S, Morikawa W, Takiue T, Miake F, Terano T, Sakai M, Hakamata H, Sakamoto Y, Natio M et al. Intravenous injection of rabbit apolipoprotein A-I inhibits the progression of atherosclerosis in cholesterol-fed rabbits. Arterioscl Thromb Vasc Biol 1995;15(11): 1882—1888.

8. Rubin E, Krauss R, Spangler E, Verstuyft J, Clift S. Inhibition of early atherogenesis in transgenic mice by human apolipoprotein AI. Nature 1991;353(6341):265—267.

9. Duverger N, Kruth H, Emmanuel F, Caillaud J, Viglietta C, Castro G, Tailleux A, Fievet C, Fruchart J, Houdebine L, Denefle P. Inhibition of atherosclerosis development in cholesterol-fed human apolipoprotein A-I-transgenic rabbits. Circulation 1996;94(4):713—717.

10. Paszty C, Maeda N, Verstuyft J, Rubin E. Apolipoprotein AI transgene corrects apolipoprotein E deficiency-induced atherosclerosis in mice. J Clin Invest 1994;94(2):899—903.

11. Plump A, Scott C, Breslow J. Human apolipoprotein A-I gene expression increases high-density lipoprotein and suppresses atherosclerosis in the apolipoprotein E-deficient mouse. Proc Natl Acad Sci USA 1994;91(20):9607—9611.

12. Liu A, Lawn R, Verstuyft J, Rubin E. Human apolipoprotein A-I prevents atherosclerosis associated with apolipoprotein(a) in transgenic mice. J Lipid Res 1994;35(12):2263—2267.

13. Fielding C, Fielding P. Molecular physiology of reverse cholesterol transport. J Lipid Res 1995; 36(2):211—228.

14. Jonas A. Lecithin-cholesterol acyltransferase in the metabolism of high-density lipoproteins. Biochim Biophys Acta 1991;1084:205—220.

15. Stratford-Perricaudet L, Makeh I, Perricaudet M, Briand P. Widespread long-term gene transfer to mouse skeletal muscles and heart. J Clin Invest 1992;90(2):626—630.

16. Rubin E, Ishida B, Clift S, Krauss R. Expression of human apolipoprotein A-I in transgenic mice results in reduced plasma levels of murine apolipoprotein A-I and the appearance of two new high-density lipoprotein size subclasses. Proc Natl Acad Sci USA 1991;88(2):434—438.

17. Chen CH, Albers JJ. Characterization of proteoliposomes containing apoprotein A-I: a new substrate for measurement of lecithin:cholesterol acyltransferase activity. J Lipid Res 1982;23: 680—691.

18. Stokke KT, Norum KR. Determination of lecithin:cholesterol acyltransfer in human blood plasma. Scand J Clin Lab Invest 1971;27:21—27.

19. de la Llera Moya M, Atger V, Paul J, Fournier N, Moatti N, Giral P, Friday K, Rothblat G. A cell culture system for screening human serum for ability to promote cellular cholesterol efflux. Relations between serum components and efflux, esterification, and transfer. Arterioscl Thromb 1994;14(7):1056—1065.

20. Kopfler W, Willard M, Betz T, Willard T, Gerard R, Meidell R. Adenovirus-mediated transfer of a gene encoding human apolipoprotein A-I into normal mice increases circulating high-density lipoprotein cholesterol. Circulation 1994;90(3):1319—1327.

21. Wilson P. High-density lipoprotein, low-density lipoprotein and coronary artery disease. Am J Cardiol 1990;66(6):7A—10A.

22. Rader D, Schaefer J, Lohse P, Ikewaki K, Thomas F, Harris W, Zech L, Dujovne C, Brewer HJ. Increased production of apolipoprotein A-I associated with elevated plasma levels of high-density lipoproteins, apolipoprotein A-I, and lipoprotein A-I in a patient with familial hyperalphalipoproteinemia. Metabolism 1993;42(11):1429—1434.

23. Mehlum A, Staels B, Duverger N, Tailleux N, Castro G, Fievet C, Luc G, Fruchart J, Olivecrona G, Skretting G et al. Tissue-specific expression of the human gene for lecithin: cholesterol acyltransferase in transgenic mice alters blood lipids, lipoproteins and lipases towards a less atherogenic profile. Eur J Biochem 1991;230(2):567—575.

24. Francone O, Gong E, Ng D, Fielding C, Rubin E. Expression of human lecithin-cholesterol acyltransferase in transgenic mice. Effect of human apolipoprotein AI and human apolipoprotein aII on plasma lipoprotein cholesterol metabolism. J Clin Invest 1995;96(3):1440—1448.

25. Hoeg J, Santamarina-Fojo S, Berard A, Cornhill J, Herderick E, Feldman S, Haudenschild C, Vaisman B, Hoyt RJ, Demosky SJ, Kauffman R, Hazel R, Marcovina S, Brewer HJ. Overexpression of lecithin:cholesterol acyltransferase in transgenic rabbits prevents diet-induced atherosclerosis. Proc Natl Acad Sci USA 1996;93(21):11448−11453.
26. Albers JJ, Bergelin RO, Adolphson JL, Wahl PW. Population-based reference values for lecithin-cholesterol acyltransferase (LCAT). Atherosclerosis 1982;43:369−379.

Overexpression of human apoC1 in transgenic mice inhibits binding of VLDL to LRP and the VLDL receptor

Miek C. Jong[1], Ko Willems van Dijk[2], Bart J.M. van Vlijmen[1], Marten H. Hofker[2] and Louis M. Havekes[1,3]

[1]*TNO-Prevention and Health, Gaubius Laboratory;* [2]*MGC-Department of Human Genetics, Leiden University; and* [3]*Departments of Cardiology and Internal Medicine, University Hospital, Leiden, The Netherlands*

Keywords: apolipoprotein E, hyperlipidemia, LDL receptor, lipoprotein lipase, triglycerides.

Introduction

Since increased plasma levels of very low density lipoprotein (VLDL) remnant lipoproteins predispose to atherosclerosis, it is of great importance that these lipoproteins are efficiently cleared from the circulation. Previous in vitro studies have suggested that the clearance of VLDL is effectively regulated by a balance between the amounts of apoC1 and apoE on the particle. Whereas apoE promotes VLDL remnant clearance, apoC1 has been reported to inhibit the apoE-mediated interaction of lipoproteins with LRP and the LDL receptor (LDLR) in vitro [1,2]. This inhibitory action of apoC1 on lipoprotein binding can easily be explained by the observation that apoC1 displaces apoE from the remnant particle [3]. However, recent in vivo studies with our transgenic mouse models lacking or overexpressing the apoC1 protein, reveal that apoC1 plays a more complex role in lipoprotein metabolism than previously thought.

Results

VLDL metabolism in apoC1-knockout mice

In an attempt to understand the role of apoC1 in lipoprotein metabolism in vivo, mice were generated that were deficient in apoC1 [4]. Suprisingly, mice with total apoC1-deficiency exhibit no overt changes in serum lipid levels when maintained on a sucrose-rich diet, but develop hypercholesterolemia on a high-fat/high-cholesterol diet (Table 1). These elevated levels of serum cholesterol on a high-fat diet were mainly due to an accumulation of VLDL particles in the circulation. Binding competition studies in vitro revealed that VLDL isolated from apoC1-deficient mice is a poor competitor for LDL in binding to the LDL receptor on

---

Address for correspondence: Miek C. Jong, Departments of Cardiology and Internal Medicine, University Hospital, P.O. Box 2215, 2301 CE Leiden, The Netherlands.

Table 1. Serum lipid levels and VLDL fractional catabolic rates in apoC1-deficient mice.

Mice	Diet	TC (mmol/l)	TG (mmol/l)	FCR (pool apoB/h)
Control	LFC	2.5 ± 0.4	0.4 ± 0.1	2.1 ± 0.1
apoC1-deficient	LFC	2.2 ± 0.4	0.4 ± 0.1	1.1 ± 0.3[a]
Control	HFC	5.0 ± 0.5	nd	1.4 ± 0.4
apoC1-deficient	HFC	7.8 ± 0.7[a]	nd	0.4 ± 0.1[a]

Total serum cholesterol (TC) and triglyceride (TG) levels were measured in fasted mice fed the sucrose-rich low-fat/low-cholesterol (LFC) diet or high-fat/high-cholesterol (HFC) diet for a period of 3 weeks. The fractional catabolic rate (FCR) was measured by following the disappearance of autologous (^{125}I)-apoB-labeled VLDL protein in the circulation. The values are the mean $\pm$ SD of at least six mice per group. nd: not detectable. [a]$p < 0.05$, indicating the difference between control and apoC1-deficient mice using nonparametric Mann-Whitney U tests.

HepG2 cells. In line with these findings, apoB-VLDL turnover studies showed a reduced VLDL-apoB FCR in apoC1-deficient mice to approximately half the rate of control mice (Table 1). Since no effect on VLDL-TG (TG) production and lipolysis was found [5], the absence of apoC1 solely seems to impair the uptake of lipoprotein particles by the liver.

VLDL metabolism in apoE*3Leiden transgenic mice coexpressing human apoC1

To investigate the influence of apoC1 on VLDL metabolism under conditions of hyperlipidemia, we examined the phenotypic expression in apoE*3Leiden transgenic mice overexpressing the human apoC1 gene (E*3L-C1) in relation to apoE*3Leiden transgenic mice without the apoC1 gene (E*3L) [6]. As presented in Table 2, both E*3L-C1 and E*3L mice exhibited elevated levels of serum cholesterol and TG as compared to control mice on a sucrose-rich diet. Elevated se-

Table 2. Serum lipid levels and VLDL fractional catabolic rates in apoE*3Leiden-C1 transgenic mice.

Mice	TC (mmol/l)	TG (mmol/l)	FCR (pool TG/h)	LR (pool TG/h)
Control	2.1 ± 0.4	0.2 ± 0.2	20.4 ± 0.1	6.3 ± 2.1
E*3L	4.3 ± 0.6[a]	0.6 ± 0.2[a]	11.0 ± 1.7[a]	1.8 ± 1.1[a]
E*3L-C1	4.3 ± 0.9[ab]	4.4 ± 1.1[ab]	3.5 ± 0.3[ab]	1.5 ± 0.9[a]

Total serum cholesterol (TC) and triglyceride (TG) levels were measured in fasted control, apoE*3-Leiden (E*3L) and apoE*3Leiden-apoC1 (E*3L-C1) transgenic mice fed the sucrose-rich diet for a period of three weeks. The fractional catabolic rate (FCR) was measured by following the disappearance of autologous (^{3}H)-TG-labeled VLDL in the circulation. The lipolytic rate (LR) was calculated from in vivo clearance of labeled VLDL in hepatectomized mice. The values are the mean $\pm$ SD of at least six mice per group. [a]$p < 0.05$, indicating the difference between control and APOE*3Leiden transgenic mice; [b]$p < 0.05$, indicating the difference between E*3L and E*3L-C1 mice, using nonparametric Mann-Whitney U tests.

rum lipid levels were mainly in the VLDL-sized lipoproteins. However, the increase in serum TG was much more pronounced in E*3L-C1 mice as compared to the E*3L mice (Table 2). To investigate the mechanisms underlying the pronounced hypertriglyceridemia in E*3L-C1 mice, VLDL-TG turnover studies were performed. The VLDL-TG FCR was strongly reduced in E*3L-C1 mice when compared with the respective FCR in E*3L and control mice (Table 2), whereas the production rate of VLDL was not significantly different in these mice. If similar turnover experiments were performed in hepatectomized mice, we found that the lipolysis of labeled VLDL-TG was not affected by overexpression of apoC1. However, both E*3L-C1 and E*3L mice showed a decreased lipolytic rate of VLDL-TG compared to control mice (Table 2). Thus, excess of apoC1 leads to a defect in the hepatic clearance of VLDL particles, whereas overexpression of the apoE*3Leiden gene influences the extrahepatic lipolysis of VLDL-TG.

VLDL metabolism in transgenic mice overexpressing human apoC1

Further experimental evidence that excess of apoC1 on the lipoprotein particle inhibits VLDL clearance was obtained from studies with transgenic mice that overexpress only the human apoC1 gene, thus without coexpression of the apoE*3Leiden gene [7]. On a sucrose-rich diet, apoC1 transgenic mice exhibit elevated levels of serum cholesterol and TG (Table 3), which was positively correlated with the level of transgene expression in the liver. In vivo VLDL-TG turnover studies revealed a reduced VLDL FCR in apoC1 transgenic mice as compared to control mice (Table 3). No differences were observed in the hepatic production and extrahepatic lipolysis of VLDL-TG. Furthermore, VLDL (as isolated from apoC1 transgenic and control mice) were found to be equally good substrates for lipoprotein lipase in vitro. Thus, these data indicate that an impaired hepatic uptake of VLDL particles is the major metabolic defect in human apoC1 transgenic mice.

Table 3. Serum lipid levels and VLDL fractional catabolic rates in apoC1 transgenic mice.

Mice	TC (mmol/l)	TG (mmol/l)	FCR (pool TG/h)
Control	1.8 ± 0.2	0.3 ± 0.2	13.7 ± 2.9
Low expressor	3.6 ± 0.7^a	1.5 ± 0.6^a	3.2 ± 1.8^a
High expressor	5.2 ± 1.0^{ab}	4.6 ± 1.7^{ab}	nd

Total serum cholesterol (TC) and triglyceride (TG) levels were measured in fasted control and apoC1 transgenic (low- and high-expressor) mice fed a regular chow diet. The fractional catabolic rate (FCR) was measured by following the disappearance of autologous (^{3}H)-TG-labeled VLDL in the circulation. The values are the mean $\pm$ SD of at least six mice per group. nd: not determined. ^{a}p < 0.05, indicating the difference between control and apoC1 transgenic mice; ^{b}p < 0.05, indicating the difference between low- and high-expressor apoC1 transgenic mice, using nonparametric Mann-Whitney U tests.

ApoC1 expression and LDL receptor deficiency

To investigate whether apoC1-enriched VLDL shows impaired binding to hepatic receptors other than the LDLR, apoC1 transgenic mice were crossbred with LDLR-deficient mice [7]. As shown in Table 4, mice heterozygous for the LDLR defect (LDLR$^{+/-}$) overexpressing human apoC1 have elevated levels of cholesterol and TG when compared with apoC1 transgenic mice having both functional alleles for the LDLR. Mice homozygous for the LDLR defect showed increased levels of cholesterol but not of TG. Overexpression of apoC1 in these mice caused a dramatic increase of both serum cholesterol and TG, which was confined to the VLDL/IDL-sized fractions (Table 4). Thus, in the absence of the LDLR, overexpression of apoC1 has a pronounced inhibiting effect on the clearance of VLDL-sized lipoproteins via an alternative clearance pathway.

The interaction of apoC1 with the remnant receptor (LRP)

To determine whether apoC1-enriched VLDL shows impaired binding to a receptor-associated protein (RAP)-sensitive pathway, RAP was overexpressed in apoC1/LDLR$^{-/-}$ mice via injection of recombinant adenovirus containing RAP cDNA (Ad-RAP). Five days after Ad-RAP transduction, control mice showed slightly elevated levels of serum cholesterol and TG (Table 4). Transfection of apoC1 transgenic mice with Ad-RAP further increased serum cholesterol and TG levels. Treatment of LDLR$^{-/-}$ mice with Ad-RAP strongly increased both serum cholesterol and TG, whereas in the extremely hyperlipidemic apoC1/LDLR$^{-/-}$ mice Ad-RAP did not significantly alter serum lipid levels (Table 4). These data indicate that RAP and apoC1 overexpression act on the same pathway in inhibiting the clearance of VLDL remnants by the liver. Since under these conditions of RAP transduction the clearance of α_2-macroglobulin, as a ligand for LRP, was completely inhibited [7], most probably apoC1 inhibition acts on the LRP pathway.

Table 4. Serum lipid levels in apoC1/LDLR-deficient mice and adenovirus-RAP injection.

Mice	Before Ad-RAP transduction		After Ad-RAP transduction	
	TC (mmol/l)	TG (mmol/l)	TC (mmol/l)	TG (mmol/l)
Control	2.2 ± 0.1	0.4 ± 0.2	3.1 ± 0.6	2.2 ± 0.3
ApoC1	3.6 ± 0.4	1.7 ± 0.4	7.1 ± 3.7	11 ± 9
LDLR$^{+/-}$	4.6 ± 0.8	0.2 ± 0.1	nd	nd
ApoC1/LDLR$^{+/-}$	10 ± 4	3.0 ± 2.2	nd	nd
LDLR$^{-/-}$	8.4 ± 0.9	0.5 ± 0.2	39 ± 8	17 ± 8
ApoC1/LDLR$^{-/-}$	52 ± 19	36 ± 19	60 ± 10	38 ± 7

Total serum cholesterol (TC) and triglyceride (TG) levels in fasted mice fed the Chow diet were measured before and 5 days after Ad-RAP (3×10^9 pfu) injection. Values represent the mean $\pm$ SD of at least five mice per group.

The interaction of apoC1 with the VLDL receptor

Apart from the inhibitory action of apoC1 on lipoprotein binding to the alternative remnant receptor, presumably LRP, we also investigated whether apoC1 modulates the binding of TG-rich lipoproteins to the VLDL receptor (VLDLR) [8]. Therefore, the VLDLR was overexpressed in the liver of apoC1 transgenic mice through injection of recombinant adenovirus containing VLDLR cDNA. Transduction with Ad-LacZ was used as a control. As shown in Table 5, Ad-VLDLR transductions reduced serum-cholesterol levels in $LDLR^{-/-}$ mice to approximately 60% (4.3 ± 0.5 vs. 10.4 ± 1.2 mmol/l). This reduction in serum cholesterol was reflected by a decrease in the IDL/LDL-sized particles in the circulation of transduced $LDLR^{-/-}$ mice. Serum TG levels were not affected upon Ad-VLDLR transduction. Remarkably, overexpression of the VLDLR in the liver of apoC1/$LDLR^{-/-}$ mice did not alter serum cholesterol levels in these mice (43.5 ± 19.5 vs. 36.5 ± 17.3 mmol/l) (Table 5), indicating that apoC1-rich lipoproteins are defective in binding to the VLDLR in vivo. In addition, overexpression of the VLDLR did not affect serum lipid levels in low and high expressor apoC1 transgenic mice as well (Table 5).

Overexpression of human apoC1 in transgenic mice has been reported to decrease the amount of apoE on the VLDL particle [7]. To investigate whether the reduced amounts of apoE on apoC1 transgenic VLDL was responsible for the defective binding of lipoproteins to the VLDLR, apoC1 transgenic VLDL was enriched with increasing amounts of human apoE, and in vitro binding studies were performed. Binding experiments at 4°C with CHO-cells overexpressing the VLDLR (CHO-VLDLR) revealed that VLDL as isolated from control mice bound considerably better than VLDL isolated from apoC1 transgenic mice (132 ± 1.9 vs. 78.2 ± 10.3 ng VLDL protein/mg cell protein) (Fig. 1). Furthermore, enrichment of control VLDL with apoE, strongly enhanced its uptake by CHO-VLDLR cells in a concentration-dependent manner. Remarkably, enrichment of apoC1 transgenic VLDL with apoE did not stimulate its binding to CHO-VLDLR cells (Fig. 1). These results indicate that apoC1 inhibits the

Table 5. Serum lipid levels in adenovirus-VLDLR transducted apoC1 transgenic mice.

Mice	Ad-β-Gal transduction		Ad-VLDLR transduction	
	TC (mmol/l)	TG (mmol/l)	TC (mmol/l)	TG (mmol/l)
$LDLR^{-/-}$	10.4 ± 1.2	1.2 ± 0.3	4.3 ± 0.5	1.1 ± 0.2
ApoC1/$LDLR^{-/-}$	36.5 ± 17.3	18.3 ± 13.1	43.5 ± 19.5	21.3 ± 15.1
Low expressor	4.9 ± 0.7	1.3 ± 0.6	4.8 ± 0.6	2.5 ± 1.6
High expressor	8.7 ± 3.4	7.5 ± 3.0	8.7 ± 1.5	9.5 ± 2.8

Total serum cholesterol (TC) and triglyceride (TG) levels in fasted mice fed the Chow diet were measured 5 days after Ad-β-Gal and Ad-VLDLR (3×10^9 pfu) injection. Values represent the mean ± SD of at least four mice per group.

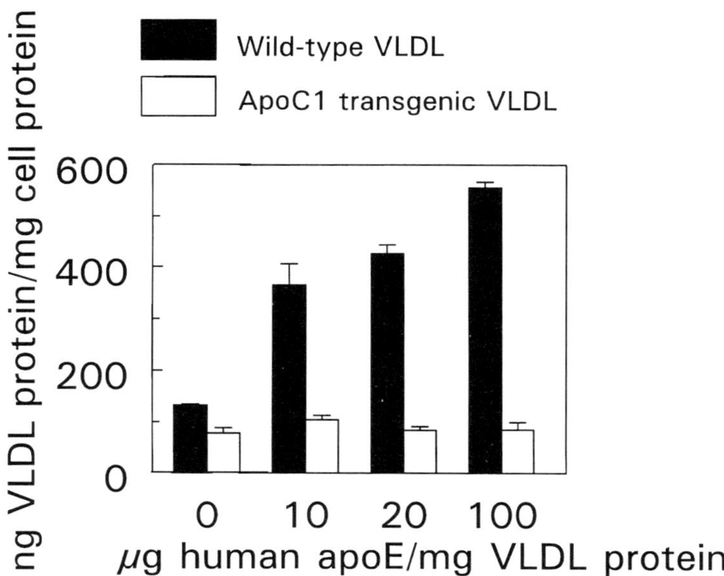

Fig. 1. Binding of VLDL to LDLR-negative CHO cells overexpressing the VLDR. The binding of VLDL isolated from control and apoC1 transgenic mice to CHO cells overexpressing the VLDR was measured upon incubation of the cells with 10 µg/ml of the respective ^{125}I-labeled VLDL fraction at 4°C for 3 h. Control and apoC1 transgenic VLDL were enriched with the amounts of human apoE as indicated. Values represent the specific binding and are the mean ± SD of four measurements.

apoE-mediated binding of TG-rich lipoproteins to the VLDLR in an irreversible manner.

Conclusions

Transgenic mice overexpressing human apoC1 develop hyperlipidemia due to an impaired clearance of VLDL particles from their circulation. Further in vivo studies revealed that apoC1 inhibits the binding of VLDL to hepatic receptors, in particular LRP. In addition, we also found that apoC1 impairs the recognition of lipoprotein particles by the VLDLR, independent of the amount of apoE on the particle. However, such a role for apoC1 could not be deduced from the results we obtained with apoC1-deficient mice. In the total absence of apoC1, VLDL clearance was hampered as well. These findings suggest that apoC1 influences VLDL metabolism in a discontinuous way. The variability in affinities of apoC1-enriched and apoC1-deficient TG-rich particles for the specific lipoprotein receptors points to a complex regulatory role for apoC1 in hyperlipidemia and in the delivery of lipoprotein constituents to different tissues. The recent findings that transgenic mice with high levels of apoC1 expression develop several abnormalities (including lack of hair, atrophic sebaceous glands, reduced amounts of sebum and adipose tissue) sustains this hypothesis (Jong et al., unpublished results).

References

1. Weisgraber KH, Mahley RW, Kowal RC, Herz J, Goldstein JL, Brown MS. Apolipoprotein C-I modulates the interaction of apolipoprotein E with β-migrating very low density lipoproteins (β-VLDL) and inhibits binding of β-VLDL to low-density lipoprotein receptor-related protein. J Biol Chem 1990;265:22453—22459.
2. Sehayek E, Eisenberg S. Mechanisms of inhibition by apolipoprotein C of apolipoprotein E-dependent cellular metabolism of human TG-rich lipoproteins through the low-density lipoprotein receptor. J Biol Chem 1991;266:18259—18267.
3. Swaney JB, Weisgraber KH. Effect of apolipoprotein C-1 peptides on the apolipoprotein E content and receptor-binding properties of beta-migrating very low-density lipoproteins. J Lipid Res 1994;35:134—142.
4. van Ree JH, Hofker MH, van den Broek WJAA, van Deursen JMA, van der Boom H, Frants RR, Wieringa B, Havekes LM. Increased response to cholesterol feeding in apolipoprotein C-1 deficient mice. Biochem J 1995;305:905—911.
5. Jong MC, van Ree JH, Dahlmans VEH, Frants RR, Hofker MH, Havekes LM. Decreased very low density lipoprotein fractional catabolic rate in apolipoprotein C1 deficient mice. Biochem J 1997;321:445—450.
6. Jong MC, Dahlmans VEH, van Gorp PJJ, Breuer ML, Mol MJMT, van der Zee A, Frants RR, Hofker MH, Havekes LM. Both lipolysis and hepatic uptake of VLDL are impaired in transgenic mice coexpressing human apolipoprotein E*3Leiden and human apolipoprotein C1. Arterioscl Thromb Vasc Biol 1996;16:934—940.
7. Jong MC, Dahlmans VEH, van Gorp PJJ, Willems van Dijk K, Breuer ML, Hofker MH, Havekes LM. In the absence of the low-density lipoprotein receptor, overexpression of apolipoprotein C1 in transgenic mice inhibits the hepatic uptake of very low density lipoproteins that is mediated via a receptor associated protein (RAP)-sensitive pathway. J Clin Invest 1996;98:2259—2267.
8. Jong MC, Dahlmans VEH, van Gorp PJJ, Willems van Dijk K, Koopman SJ, Chan L, Hofker MH, Havekes LM. The binding of VLDL to the VLDL receptor is inhibited by an excess of apoC1. Circulation 1996;94(Suppl):4081.

Analysis of chylomicron remnant metabolism by tissue-specific gene inactivation

Astrid Rohlmann[1], Michael Gotthardt[3], Robert E. Hammer[2] and Joachim Herz[1]

Departments of [1] Molecular Genetics and [2] Biochemistry, Howard Hughes Medical Institute, University of Texas Southwestern Medical Center, Dallas, Texas, USA; and [3] Max-Delbrueck-Center Berlin, Germany

Abstract. LDL receptor-related protein (LRP) is a multifunctional receptor participating in a diversity of physiological processes, i.e., regulation of plasminogen activation, clearance of α_2-macroglobulin/proteinase complexes and cellular uptake of toxins of microbial and plant origin. LRP is predominantly expressed in liver and brain. It was shown before that the complete knock out of the LRP by conventional gene inactivation is lethal, the embryos die early during gestation. This study uses the cre/loxP recombination system to knock out LRP in the liver and to analyze its role in lipid metabolism.

Two apoE-specific receptors are known to be expressed in the liver. One is the low-density lipoprotein (LDL) receptor, the other is the structurally similar LRP. The LDL receptor mediates endocytosis of apoE and apoB100 containing lipoproteins (LDL, intermediate density and remnant lipoproteins), and LRP has been postulated to mediate uptake of apoE/apoB48 containing chylomicron remnants (CR) into hepatocytes. The latter is supported by two lines of experiments.

The clearance of intravenously injected small chylomicrons in rodents and their endocytosis was analyzed in wild-type, LDL receptor deficient and receptor-associated protein (RAP) preinjected animals [1]. RAP is a molecular chaperon with high affinity to LRP and inhibits binding of the receptor to all of its known ligands, serving as a dominant negative regulator of LRP. The results of this study showed that the rapid endocytosis of CR was mainly mediated by the LDL receptor, however, in RAP preinjected animals CR endocytosis was diminished.

Another approach by Willnow et al. [2] used recombinant adenovirus for gene transfer of RAP into mice livers. In control experiments they observed a mild hepatocellular inflammation but ruled out changes in the metabolism of lipoproteins due to wild-type adenovirus injection. Overexpression of RAP in intact mice (wild-type and LDL receptor knock out) led to changes in the lipoprotein profiles: virus-injected wild-type mice showed total plasma cholesterol concentrations increased by 50%, whereas in LDL receptor knock out animals plasma cholesterol was elevated up to 300%, primarily because of apoB48/apoE-containing particles. This suggested a function for LRP as a backup receptor of CR clearance.

The experiments mentioned above used RAP to block LRP in the liver and elucidate its function in the absence of the LDL receptor. In the present study we used the cre/loxP technique to induce a tissue-specific knock out of LRP in the liver. The hepatic LRP knock out excludes any possible RAP mediated interactions to other receptors or proteins which may have affected the previous studies. In the following experiments we address the effect of LRP on metabolism of lipoproteins in vivo.

The first step of the cre/loxP technique requires the LRP gene to be "floxed", which means insertion of loxP sites that later serve as recognition sites for recombination. This is mediated by the cre-recombinase which has to be targeted to the floxed LRP gene. For this purpose we used two different strategies: 1) cre-recombinase expressing adenovirus was injected into the external jugular vein and is subsequently taken up by the liver; or 2) MX1 cre inducible transgenic mice were bred to the floxed LRP mice [3]. To induce the otherwise silent promoter, we injected polyinosinic:polycytidylic ribonucleic (pI:pC) acid, an inducer for macrophages to produce interferon which in turn stimulates the MX1 promoter.

Both approaches for the delivery of the cre-recombinase were carried out in adult mice, and animals were analyzed about 3 weeks after injections.

Four genotypes of mice were injected, and liver membrane proteins studied by immunoblotting with antibodies against LRP and LDL receptor. Wild-type mice still show expression of LRP and LDL receptor, excluding any side effects of the injections, as do injected LDL receptor knock-out animals that still express LRP. LRP expression in animals homozygous for the floxed LRP allele is greatly reduced after cre adenovirus injection, and hardly detectable using induction of the MX1 cre promoter. This also applies for the double-mutant mice where LRP is knocked out in the absence of the LDL receptor.

Studies of plasma lipoprotein homeostasis

Serum of injected animals was immunoblotted with antibodies against apolipoproteins B100, B48, E and A1. Results of the cre adenovirus injections are similar to the MX1 cre inducible system.

While apolipoprotein A1 remains unchanged among all four genotypes before and after injections, LDL receptor deficient mice show elevated levels of apolipoprotein E that are further enhanced after injections in double-mutant animals. ApoB100 and apoB48 levels are also increased in LDL receptor knock out animals. However, additional knock out of LRP by the cre recombinase in these mice dramatically increases apoB48 levels. The accumulation of apoB48/apoE containing lipoproteins in LDL receptor/hepatic LRP knock-out animals is consistent with the previous findings.

Studies of plasma cholesterol profiles and triglycerides

Serum of mice before and after LRP inactivation was subjected to FPLC fractionation to separate the lipoproteins by size. Wild-type mice and mice with floxed LRP alleles only show an HDL peak that was unchanged before and after cre induction. LDL receptor knock-out and LDL receptor knock out/LRP flox animals reveal an HDL and LDL peak in their plasma cholesterol profiles. In contrast, mice lacking both LDLR and LRP in the liver show an additional accumulation of plasma lipoproteins in the chylomicron remnant/VLDL size range. Triglyceride concentrations are increased approximately 2-fold compared to mice lacking only the LDL receptor.

Liver-specific LRP inactivation, as used in this study, suggests that the LDL receptor and LRP together are involved in the clearance of apoE-containing remnants.

Acknowledgements

We are indebted to Martina Anton and Frank Graham for sharing the cre-expressing adenovirus and to Wen-Ling Niu and Scott Clark for outstanding technical assistance. This work was supported by grants from the NIH (HL20948), the Keck Foundation, the Howard Hughes Medical Institute and the Perot Family Foundation. A.R. was supported by a fellowship from the Deutsche Forschungsgemeinschaft and M.G. by the Boehringer Ingelheim Fonds. J.H. is an Established Investigator of the American Heart Association and Parke-Davis Company.

References

1. Herz J, Qiu SQ, Oesterle A, DeSilva HV, Shafi S, Havel RJ. Initial hepatic removal of chylomicron remnants is unaffected but endocytosis is delayed in mice lacking the low density lipoprotein receptor. Proc Natl Acad Sci USA 1995;92:4611–4615.
2. Willnow TE, Sheng Z, Ishibashi S, Herz J. Inhibition of hepatic chylomicron remnant uptake by gene transfer of a receptor antagonist. Science 1994;264:1471–1474.
3. Rohlmann A, Gotthardt M, Hammer RE, Herz J. Inducible inactivation of hepatic LRP gene by Cre-mediated recombination confirms role of LRP in clearance of chylomicron remnants. J Clin Invest 1998;101:689–695.

Atherosclerosis XI.
B. Jacotot, D. Mathé and J.-C. Fruchart, editors.

Transgenic dissection of atherogenic profiles of plasma lipoproteins and arterial wall metabolism

Shun Ishibashi, Masako Shimada, Jun-ichi Osuga, Hiroaki Yagyu, Zhong Chen, Ken Ohashi, Kenji Harada, Yoshio Yazaki and Nobuhiro Yamda
The Third Department of Internal Medicine, Faculty of Medicine, University of Tokyo, Tokyo, Japan

Abstract. Genetically mutant mice produced using transgenic technology have emerged as valuable tools for investigating the pathological processes and for the development of new therapeutics of atherosclerosis. Currently, mice lacking low-density lipoprotein receptor (LDLRKO) or apolipoprotein E (APOEKO) are being widely used as animal models of atherosclerosis. Mice lacking both LDLR and apo E develop more severe atherosclerosis compared with those lacking an individual gene, implicating the additive nature of each gene. Introduction of other knockout or transgenic genes into these models is a useful approach for determining the roles of these genes in atherosclerosis. To investigate the atherogenic potentials of lipoprotein lipase (LPL) or apo E, we have generated LDLRKO mice overexpressing LPL or apo E. It has been shown that both proteins are protective against diet-induced hypercholesterolemia and atherosclerosis even in the absence of LDL receptor. Mice lacking apo B mRNA editing activity have been generated to compare the atherogenic potentials between apo B-100- and apo B-48-containing lipoproteins. Other potential target molecules which are being investigated will shortly be discussed. In conclusion, LPL and apo E may be promising target molecules for the treatment of atherosclerosis.

Keywords: apolipoprotein B, apolipoprotein E, cholesterol ester, gene targeting, knockout mouse, low-density lipoprotein receptor.

The initial event of atherosclerosis is characterized by the intimal accumulation of lipid-laden foam cells which are mostly originated from circulating monocytes. It is widely accepted that atherogenic lipoproteins infiltrate into the arterial wall, reside in the extracellular matrices, undergo modification such as oxidation, trigger the recruitment of monocytes into the arterial wall by releasing chemoattractant mediators, and elicit foam cell formation in the recruited cells as well as other cellular reactions subsequent to the uptake of these lipoproteins. Theoretically, every step in the sequence of events is essential for atherogenesis and the molecules involved in each step are the potential targets for the investigational genetic manipulation.

Techniques for the genetic manipulation of mouse embryos have substantially enhanced our capability to explore the pathological processes underlying athero-

Address for correspondence: Shun Ishibashi MD, PhD, The Third Department of Internal Medicine, Faculty of Medicine, University of Tokyo, 7-3-1 Hongo, Bunkyo-ku, Tokyo 113, Japan. Tel.: +81-3-3815-5411 (ext. 3129). Fax: +81-3-5802-2955.

sclerosis and develop new therapeutics. The low density lipoprotein receptor knockout (LDLRKO) [1,2] or apo E knockout mice (APOEKO) are being widely used as excellent animal models of atherosclerosis [3,4].

In the present paper, we review our current status of the understanding of the atherogenic profiles of plasma lipoprotein and arterial wall metabolism, which have emerged as a result of the application of transgenic technology.

Atherogenic profiles of plasma lipoprotein metabolism

LDL receptor

LDLRKO mice are a model of a common monogenic disease, familial hypercholesterolemia (FH). Patients with homozygous FH develop severe hypercholesterolemia and fulminant atherosclerosis and rarely survive the third decade of life when not treated properly. The hypercholesterolemia and atherosclerosis in the LDLRKO mice appears milder than the human equivalent when fed a normal chow which contains little fat and cholesterol [1,2]. The milder phenotype in the mice may be attributable to the lower non-HDL cholesterol levels and higher HDL-cholesterol levels as compared to human FH. Interestingly, LDLRKO mice are highly sensitive to dietary fat and develop severe hypercholesterolemia and atherosclerosis when challenged with an atherogenic diet which contains high fats and cholesterol [2].

Apolipoprotein E

APOEKO mice are a model of a rare disease, apo E deficiency, which has been described only in three families in the world. Patients with apo E deficiency exhibit type III hyperlipoproteinemia and their atherosclerosis is reportedly milder than that in homozygous FH. However, the APOEKO mice develop a more severe form of hypercholesterolemia and atherosclerosis than LDLRKO mice when fed a normal chow [3,4]. How can this reciprocity be accounted for? We would hypothesize that the apo E-dependent pathway for the lipoprotein clearance is more dominant in mice compared to humans. In support of this, the liver of the mice produces substantial amounts of lipoproteins containing apo B-48 that is collinear with the amino-terminal half of apo B-100 and lacks a domain required for the LDL receptor binding activity. APOEKO mice show marked accumulation of apo B-48, but not apo B-100, in the plasma, supporting the notion that the lipoproteins containing apo B-48 obligatorily require apo E for their hepatic clearance [5].

Conversely, mice overexpressing apo E are resistant to diet-induced hypercholesterolemia [6]. The hepatic overproduction of apo E alleviate hypercholesterolemia and atherosclerosis even in the absence of the LDL receptor (J. Osuga et al., unpublished observations).

Apolipoprotein B subspecies

To determine whether hepatic production of apo B-48 is responsible for the dominance of apo E-dependent plasma clearance of apo B-containing lipoproteins, we have generated mice lacking apo B-48 by inactivating a catalytic component of the apo B mRNA editing enzyme, APOBEC-1 [7]. In these mice, both the liver and small intestine lack the apo B mRNA editing activity, apo B-48 is eliminated completely from the plasma. Their LDL-cholesterol levels are elevated slightly, but are still far less than those in humans (30 vs. 100 mg/dl), suggesting that the hepatic production of apo B-48 is not the sole reason for the low plasma levels of LDL-cholesterol in mice and for the postulated dominance of apo E-dependent plasma clearance of apo B-containing lipoproteins in the mice.

We introduced this APOBEC-1 KO mutation into APOEKO mice to determine how much the hypercholesterolemia of the APOEKO mice is alleviated by substituting apo B-48 for apo B-100, whose binding to the LDL receptor does not require apo E [7]. The mice lacking both APOBEC-1 and apo E had significantly lower plasma cholesterol levels than the APOEKO mice, but the reduction was partial, indicating that apo B-100 does not fully substitute apo E, even if both share the LDL binding activities in common. These observations can be explained by assuming that apo E is necessary for both the efficient lipolytic conversion of VLDL containing apo B-100 to denser IDL and/or LDL and their direct hepatic uptake.

Mice lacking both LDL receptor and apo E (LDLR/APOEKO) are used for a study addressing whether the effects of the deficiency of apo E and the LDL receptor on the lipoprotein profiles and atherosclerosis are additive [5]. VLDL-cholesterol and LDL-cholesterol were markedly increased in APOEKO and LDLRKO mice, respectively. On the other hand, LDLR/APOEKO mice had combined elevation of the two lipoproteins. In proportion to the changes in the lipoproteins, atherosclerosis in LDLR/APOEKO mice is more severe than in either LDLRKO or APOEKO mice (S. Ishibashi et al., unpublished observations).

Lipoprotein lipase

Until recently, the role of lipoprotein lipase (LPL) in atherosclerosis has been controversial, because LPL catalyses the formation of both atherogenic (chylomicron remnants, IDL and LDL) and antiatherogenic lipoproteins (HDL). Transgenic mice overexpressing LPL are useful for addressing this question [8]. We have reported that LDL knockout mice overexpressing LPL (LPLTg/LDLRKO) showed a 2-fold decrease in plasma cholesterol levels compared with LDLRKO mice irrespective of the diets [9]. The results of the lipoprotein kinetics studies favor the notion that the overexpressed LPL reduced the plasma cholesterol levels not by stimulating the plasma clearance of apo B-containing lipoproteins, but by reducing the cholesterol contents of each lipoprotein particle. The atherosclerosis in the LPLTg/LDLRKO mice was suppressed disproportionately compared to the changes in plasma cholesterol levels (20- vs. 2-fold). We speculate that the apo B-containing lipoproteins which are excessively acted on by LPL substantially lose their atherogenecity. These findings are consistent with the recent reports that patients heterozygous and homozygous for the mutation in LPL genes develop clinically relevant atherosclerosis. Intervention that increases LPL activity may be alternative to the gene transfer of LDL receptor for the treatment of familial hypercholesterolemia.

Atherogenic profile of arterial wall metabolism

Cellular cholesterol ester cycle

Foam cells in the arterial walls exhibit a wide variety of cellular changes. In the lesions from the APOEKO mice, apoptotic cell death was observed, especially in the initial stage of atherosclerosis [10]. It is conceivable that the apoptotic cells are somehow involved in the further progression of atherosclerosis. The mechanisms behind the cell death are currently unknown. We speculate that oxidized cholesterol and/or cholesterol ester deposited in the cells, at least in part, play contributory roles in its progression.

We are currently investigating the role of cholesterol esterification and hydrolysis in the progression of atherosclerosis by using mice deficient in acyl CoA:cholesterol acyltransferase (ACAT) and neutral cholesterol ester hydrolase (NCEH) activity which have been generated by the disruption of ACAT and hormone-sensitive lipase (HSL) genes, respectively.

Acknowledgements

We are grateful to M. Okazaki (Tokyo Medical and Dental University) for HPLC analysis.

References

1. Ishibashi S, Brown MS, Goldstein JL, Gerard RD, Hammer RE, Herz J. Hypercholesterolemia in low density lipoprotein receptor knockout mice and its reversal by adenovirus-mediated gene delivery. J Clin Invest 1993;92:883–893.
2. Ishibashi S, Goldstein JL, Brown MS, Herz J, Burns DK. Massive xanthomatosis and atherosclerosis in cholesterol-fed low density lipoprotein receptor-negative mice. J Clin Invest 1994;93:1885–1893.
3. Zhang SH, Reddick RL, Piedrahita JA, Maeda N. Spontaneous hypercholesterolemia and arterial lesions in mice lacking apolipoprotein E. Science (Washington DC) 1992;258:468–471.
4. Plump AS, Smith JD, Hayek T, Aalto-Setälä K, Walsh A, Verstuyft JG, Rubin EM, Breslow JL. Severe hypercholesterolemia and atherosclerosis in apolipoprotein E deficient mice created by homologous recombination in ES cells. Cell 1992;71:343–353.

5. Ishibashi S, Herz J, Maeda N, Goldstein JL, Brown MS. The two-receptor model of lipoprotein clearance: tests of the hypothesis in "knockout" mice lacking the low density lipoprotein receptor, apolipoprotein E, or both proteins. Proc Natl Acad Sci USA 1994;91:4431—4435.
6. Shimano H, Yamada N, Katsuki M, Shimada M, Gotoda T, Harada K, Murase T, Fukazawa F, Takaku F, Yazaki Y. Overexpression of apolipoprotein E in transgenic mice: a marked reduction in plasma lipoproteins except high density lipoprotein, and resistance against diet-induced hypercholesterolemia. Proc Natl Acad Sci USA 1992;89:1750—1754.
7. Osuga J, Yagyu H, Ohashi K, Harada K, Yazaki Y, Yamada M, Ishibashi S. Effects of apo E deficiency on plasma lipid levels in mice lacking APOBEC-1. Biochem Biophys Res Commun 1997;236:375—378.
8. Shimada M, Shimano H, Gotoda T, Yamamoto K, Kawamura M, Inaba T, Yazaki Y, Yamada N. Overexpression of human lipoprotein lipase in transgenic mice. J Biol Chem 1993;268:17924—17929.
9. Shimada M, Ishibashi S, Inaba T, Yagyu H, Harada K, Osuga J, Ohashi K, Yazaki Y, Yamada N. Suppression of diet-induced atherosclerosis in low density lipoprotein receptor knockout mice overexpressing lipoprotein lipase. Proc Natl Acad Sci USA 1996;93:7242—7246.
10. Harada K, Chen Z, Ishibashi S, Osuga J, Yagyu H, Ohashi K, Yahagi N, Shionoiri F, Sun L, Yazaki Y, Yamada Y. Apoptotic cell death in atherosclerotic plaques of hyperlipidemic knockout mice. Atherosclerosis 1997;135:235—239.

Atherosclerosis XI.
B. Jacotot, D. Mathé and J.-C. Fruchart, editors.

Strategies for altering the mouse genome and their application in the study of atherogenesis

M.E. Hinsdale, H. Mezdour, P. Sullivan, L. Toth and N. Maeda
Department of Pathology and Laboratory Medicine, University of North Carolina, Chapel Hill, North Carolina, USA

Abstract. Three different strategies were used to model human dyslipidemias and atherosclerosis. The "in-out" two-step method was used to generate mice producing a truncated apolipoprotein (apo) B protein and an apoB100 protein with the putative LDL receptor binding sites replaced with unrelated sequence. These models, respectively, will allow us to study human hypobetalipoproteinemia and familial defective apoB100. Targeted gene duplication of the *Apob* gene at its endogenous chromosomal locus allowed us to increase circulating atherogenic apoB-containing particles. Targeted gene replacement of mouse *Apoe* with the human *APOE* alleles resulted in mice which produce human apoE2, E3, or E4 isoforms at physiological levels. These replacement models allow us to study the APOE isoform-specific effects in type III hyperlipidemia, hypercholesterolemia, atherosclerosis and Alzheimer's disease.

Keywords: dyslipidemia, hypobetalipoproteinemia, targeted gene duplication, targeted gene replacement.

Introduction

The method to introduce specific alterations at desired loci in the mouse genome by gene targeting in embryonic stem (ES) cells has evolved very quickly over the last 10 years, and has aided many areas of research in the biological sciences. Gene targeting in ES cells has been most commonly used to disrupt genes resulting in a null allele. These so-called "knock-out" mice have been useful as models for atherosclerosis [1—4]. However, the mutations that cause human diseases are not always null mutations but those leading to changes in the level of gene expression or in the function of the protein produced. Gene targeting can be used to generate mutations that alter the function (e.g., in-out/hit and run), the expression (e.g., gene-targeted duplication), and form (e.g., gene-targeted replacement) of a gene.

In-out two-step (or hit and run) strategy

This approach allows the introduction of a small mutation without disruption of the gene [5,6]. It is a two-step approach using an insertion (O-type) type construct which contains a selector for positive and negative gene(s), e.g., hypox-

---

Address for correspondence: N. Maeda, Department of Pathology and Laboratory Medicine, University of North Carolina, Chapel Hill, NC 27599-7525, USA.

1030

anthine phosphoribosyl transferase (*hprt*) gene, and regions of homology having the desired mutation (Fig. 1). The "in-step" is an insertion of the construct and results in partial gene duplication. The "in-step" recombinants are screened for a functional *hprt* gene. The gene which is selective for *hprt* can be used for both positive and negative selection, but must be used in an *hprt*-deficient ES cell line. The "out-step" is a spontaneous intrachromosomal recombination or unequal sister chromatid exchange within the duplicated sequences. This step removes the gene that is selective for *hprt*, plasmid sequence and duplicated sequences, and results in a gene which may or may not contain the desired mutation depending on the position of the recombination crossover. The "out-step" recombinants are screened for the loss of the *hprt* gene.

We used the "in-out" strategy on the *Apob* gene to generate two different alleles (Fig. 1) [7]. The "in-step" introduced a stop codon resulting in a truncated apoB protein (apoB81) 81% of the full length. The resulting homozygous mice were hypobetalipoproteinemic which is characterized by dramatically decreased plasma levels of apoB-containing proteins and total cholesterol (TC). Therefore, these mice model human hypobetalipoproteinemia resulting from apoB truncations [8]. The "out-step" resulted in an apoB100 protein with the putative LDLr binding sites replaced with human betaglobin sequence. This change models mutations which disrupt LDLr binding in humans causing familial defective apoB100 [9].

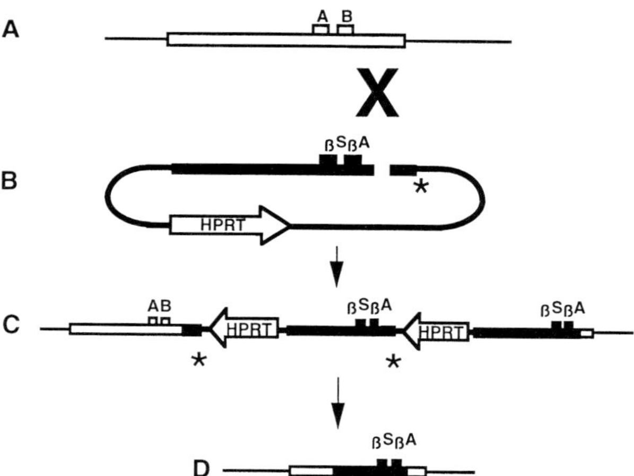

Fig. 1. Apob "in-out" strategy. A crossover "X" between exon 26 of the *Apob* locus (white box) (**A**) and the altered exon 26 homology of the targeting construct (thick black box) (**B**). The putative LDLr binding domains, A and B, in the targeting construct homology were replaced with human β-globin sequence, $\beta^S \beta^A$. The termination codon (*) produces the truncated apoB81 protein. The thin black line represents the plasmid sequence which contains the *hprt* selectable gene. The "in-step" (**C**) resulted in an integration of multiple copies of the construct. After the "out-step" (**D**), the targeted locus retained the desired mutation and had regained its normal structure due to loss of the duplicated homology, selectable marker *hprt*, and multiple construct copies.

Surprisingly, the resulting homozygous mice had normal plasma levels of apoB100-containing particles and TC. This suggests that a lack of the putative LDLr binding sites is not sufficient to increase circulating apoB100-containing particles in the mouse.

Targeted gene duplication

Targeted gene duplication increases the copy number of a gene at its endogenous locus and causes a quantitative change in gene expression [10]. This strategy uses an insertion (O-type) targeting construct that contains regions of homology flanking the locus (Fig. 2). The gap between the regions of homology in the construct is repaired during recombination using the endogenous locus as a template. The final result is a tandem duplication of the entire locus. The design of the construct must ensure that the basal promoter elements are duplicated, otherwise precise knowledge of the gene's regulatory elements is not needed for correct tissue and developmental expression of the duplicated gene. The fold increase in mRNA allows for a quantitative analysis of gene expression and phenotype.

Elevated plasma apoB-containing particles are associated with atherosclerosis [11]. Therefore, we planned to increase circulating apoB levels by duplicating the *Apob* locus (Fig. 2). An approximately 50 kb gap repair was accomplished with a total duplication of approximately 60 kb. Duplication of the *Apob* locus was quite efficient, being present in one out of 75 G418-resistant recombinants. The lipid profile of the heterozygote mice (three copy) on normal chow was not different from that of wild-type controls (two copy). In addition, the plasma apoB100

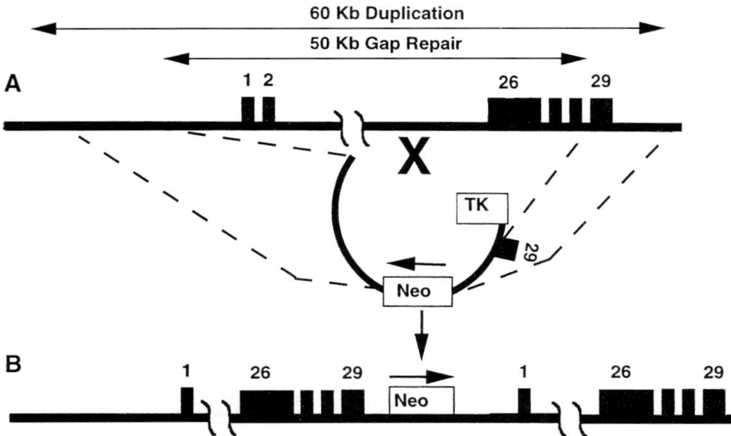

Fig. 2. Apob gene targeted duplication strategy. 5′ and 3′ ends of mouse *Apob* locus with exons (black boxes) are shown (**A**). Dashed lines indicate alignment of the targeting vector homology. With recombination, the gap between the areas of homology in the construct is repaired resulting in duplication of the locus (**B**).

level in heterozygotes, as measured by ELISA, was not different from that of controls. However, when challenged with a Western-style diet, the plasma TC increase was higher in the heterozygous males as compared to controls. Currently, heterozygotes are being crossed to generate homozygous (four copy) animals for further studies of dyslipidemia due to a higher production of apoB protein.

Targeted gene replacement

This strategy allows us to replace an endogenous gene with a modified form while preserving normal gene regulation [12]. The advantages of this strategy include simplified phenotype assessment due to the absence of the endogenous gene product, physiological levels of the modified protein since all endogenous controlling elements remain intact, and direct comparison of different structural mutants originating from allelic differences.

Our laboratory replaced the mouse *Apoe* gene with the three human alleles of apolipoprotein E, (*APOE*2*, *APOE*3*, *APOE*4*) (Fig. 3). The *APOE*3* allele is the most common in the human population. The second most common allele, *APOE*4*, is associated with elevated plasma LDL [13] and early onset of Alzheimer's disease [14]. Individuals homozygous for *APOE*2* are generally hypolipemic, but 5—10% develop type III hyperlipidemia [15].

The *APOE*3*-targeted replacement resulted in a mouse which only produces human APOE3 [12]. The tissue distribution and levels of human apoE3 mRNA expression in homozygous mutant mice (3/3) was similar to mouse apoE mRNA in wild-type controls. The plasma concentration of human apoE3 in the 3/3 mice was similar to mouse apoE in wild-type mice (1.30 ± 0.47 mg/dl vs. 1.13 ± 0.23 mg/dl, respectively). On normal chow, the 3/3 mice are normolipidemic; however, they had decreased plasma levels of β-migrating lipoproteins and a slower fractional catabolic rate as compared to controls (0.02 vs. 0.12%

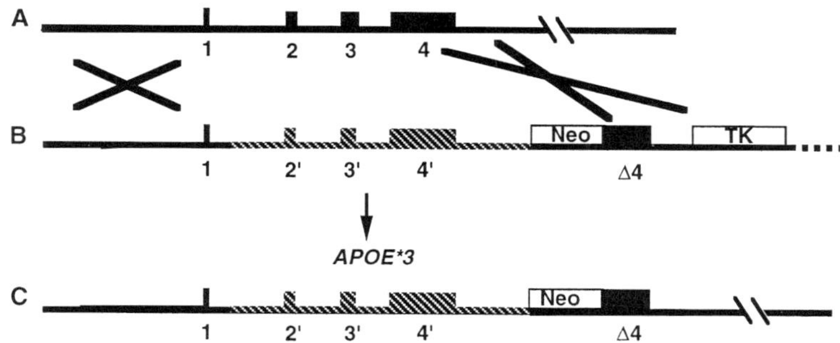

Fig. 3. Targeted gene replacement strategy. The endogenous *Apoe* locus contains 4 exons (black boxes) of which exon 1 is noncoding (**A**). Recombination with targeting construct (**B**) resulted in replacement of mouse exons 2—4 with human *APOE*3* sequence (hatched). The mouse fusion gene (**C**) produced mRNA encoding human apoE3.

change of injected dose/min, respectively). Furthermore, the 3/3 mice on a high-fat diet had a 3.5-fold higher plasma TC and at least 13-fold larger atherosclerotic plaques as compared to controls on the same diet. Thus, structural differences between mouse apoE and human apoE3 are sufficient to induce significant changes in lipid metabolism and atherogenesis.

In summary, gene targeting in ES cells allows us to introduce subtle mutations, duplications, and gene replacements in the mouse genome. These alterations result in physiologic changes in protein levels and/or function that alone or in combination with other mutations can model the complex genetics of atherosclerosis and dyslipidemia in humans.

Acknowledgements

We thank Dr Steven Young for the hybridoma cell lines which we used to obtain mouse apoB monoclonal antibody for the apoB100 ELISA. This work was supported by ARCOL fellowship (HM), NSF fellowship (LT), and NIH grants RR0011 (MEH) and HL42630 (NM).

References

1. Maeda N. Gene targeting in mice as a strategy for understanding lipid metabolism and atherogenesis. Curr Opin Lipid 1993;4:90—94.
2. Rubin EM, Smith DJ. Atherosclerosis in mice: getting to the heart of a polygenic disorder. TIG 1994;10:199—203.
3. Smithies O, Maeda N. Gene targeting approaches to complex genetic diseases: atherosclerosis and essential hypertension. Proc Natl Acad Sci USA 1995;92:5266—5272.
4. Breslow JL. Mouse models of atherosclerosis. Science 1996;272:685—688.
5. Valancius V, Smithies O. Testing an "in-out" targeting procedure for making subtle genomic modifications in mouse embryonic stem cells. Molec Cell Biol 1991;11:1402—1408.
6. Hasty P, Ramirez-Solis R, Krumlauf R, Bradley A. Introduction of a subtle mutation into the Hox-2.6 locus in embryonic stem cells. Nature 1991;350:243—246.
7. Toth LR, Smith TJ, Jones C, de Silva HV, Smithies O, Maeda N. Two distinct apolipoprotein B alleles in mice generated by a single "in-out" targeting. Gene 1996;178:161—168.
8. Linton MF, Farese RV Jr, Young SG. Familial hypobetalipoproteinemia. J Lipid Res 1993;34:521—541.
9. Innerarity TL, Weisgraber KH, Arnold KS, Mahley RW, Krauss RM, Vega GL, Grundy SM. Familial defective apolipoprotein B-100: low density lipoproteins with abnormal receptor binding. Proc Natl Acad Sci USA 1987;84:6919—6923.
10. Smithies O, Kim HS. Targeted gene duplication and disruption for analyzing quantitative genetic traits in mice. Proc Natl Acad Sci USA 1994;91:3612—3615.
11. Breslow JL. The genetic basis of lipoprotein disorders. J Int Med 1992;231:627—631.
12. Sullivan PM, Mezdour H, Aratani Y, Knouff C, Najib J, Reddick RL, Quarfordt SH, Maeda N. Targeted replacement of the mouse apolipoprotein E gene with the common human APOE3 allele enhances diet-induced hypercholesterolemia and atherosclerosis. J Biol Chem 1997;272:17972—17980.
13. Davignon J, Gregg RE, Sing CF. Apolipoprotein E polymorphism and atherosclerosis. Arteriosclerosis 1988;8:1—21.
14. Corder EH, Saunders AM, Strittmatter WJ, Schmechal DE, Gaskell PC, Small GW, Roses AD,

Haines JL, Pericak-Vance MA. Gene dose of apolipoprotein E type 4 allele and the risk of Alzheimer's disease in late onset families. Science 1993;261:921–923.

15. Mahley RW, Rall CR Jr. Type III hyperlipoproteinemia (dysbetalipoproteinemia): the role of apolipoprotein E in normal and abnormal lipid metabolism. In: Scriver SR, Beaudet AL, Sly WS, Valle D (eds) Metabolism and Molecular Basis of Inherited Disease, 7th edn, vol II. New York: McGraw-Hill, 1995;1953–1980.

Genetic epidemiology of CHD and its risk factors

Genetic susceptibility factors for restenosis after coronary angioplasty

Philippe Amouyel[1,2] and Christophe Bauters[1]
[1]*University and Centre Hospitalier Régional Universitaire de Lille, Lille; and* [2]*INSERM CJF 95-05, Institut Pasteur de Lille, Lille, France*

Abstract. *Background.* Percutaneous transluminal coronary angioplasty (PTCA) has become an established treatment for patients with atherosclerotic coronary artery lesions. However, the extent of this procedure is weakened by restenosis that occurs within 6 months after PTCA. Recently, intra-coronary stent implantation has been shown to significantly reduce angiographic restenosis. Not all subjects develop restenosis, suggesting that predisposing factors may underlie this phenomenon. Based on a candidate gene research strategy, we sought associations between restenosis after PTCA and various genetic polymorphisms.

Patients and Methods. More than 200 patients with PTCA and 200 patients with PTCA and coronary stenting were enrolled. Quantitative angiographic variables from computer-assisted coronary angiography were measured before and 6 months after angioplasty, in patients with and without stent implantation. DNA samples were recovered from each patient and genetic polymorphisms were characterised.

Results. We demonstrated that the deletion (D) allele of the angiotensin-I converting enzyme (ACE) gene, associated with increased levels of circulating and cellular enzyme, was not a risk factor for restenosis after PTCA. We reported that this polymorphism was associated with an increased risk of coronary artery occlusion after PTCA. Conversely, the *ACE* D allele was a major risk factor for restenosis after stent implantation, suggesting a possible association with neointimal hyperplasia, a predominant mechanism of restenosis after stenting.

Conclusions. The *ACE* D allele is a major risk factor for restenosis after coronary stenting and thus may be proposed to trace subjects at risk. ACE inhibitors may also be tested to reduce restenosis after coronary stenting particularly in D allele bearer subjects.

Keywords: genetic polymorphism, renin angiotensin system, restenosis, stent.

Introduction

Percutaneous transluminal coronary angioplasty (PTCA) constitutes a major treatment for patients with atherosclerotic coronary artery lesions. However, the benefit of this coronary balloon angioplasty is limited by the restenosis of the treated segment observed in 30—50% of the patients [1]. Several mechanisms underlie restenosis after PTCA: elastic recoil of the dilated segment, platelet-mediated thrombus formation, neointimal proliferation of smooth muscle cells, and vascular remodeling [2]. Restenosis requires other revascularisation procedures to avoid reoccurrence of myocardial infarctions or coronary heart dis-

---

Address for correspondence: Prof Philippe Amouyel, INSERM CJF 95-05, Institut Pasteur de Lille, 1 rue Albert Calmette, 59019 Lille Cedex, France. Tel.: +33-320-87-77-10. Fax: +33-320-87-78-94.
E-mail: Philippe.Amouyel@pasteur-lille.fr

eases. To fight against restenosis, various approaches have been proposed. Among these, intracoronary stent implantation has been shown to significantly reduce angiographic restenosis in humans [3,4]. The better long-term angiographic prognosis of this procedure is due to an improved acute result that decreases elastic recoil and the abolition of chronic remodeling. However, 20—30% of patients still develop restenosis, mainly due to an increase in neointimal thickening.

Several risk factors of restenosis have been described as diabetes, unstable angina and previous myocardial infarction; however, the observation that restenosis is by itself a risk factor for restenosis suggests that some patients are prone to restenosis after PTCA and may have an increased individual susceptibility underlain by a genetic predisposition. To explore genetic risk factors expressing after such a therapeutic procedure, family studies and genomic screening are difficult to achieve. The fastest and most convenient way to hunt for these risk factors seems to develop association studies comparing subjects with or without restenosis according to the genotype distribution of polymorphisms detected in candidate genes. The choice of these candidate genes is inferred from the knowledge of the mechanisms leading to restenosis. Thus, all the genes coding for proteins implicated in restenosis may be tested: coagulation factors, growth factors, oncogenes, extracellular matrix components and renin angiotensin system proteins. We will focus on a candidate gene from the renin angiotensin system, the angiotensin-I converting enzyme (ACE) gene. The locus of this gene contains a deletion (D)/insertion (I) polymorphism associated with part of the variability of the circulating and cellular levels of the enzyme: subjects with the DD genotype have higher levels of *ACE* than either ID or II genotype bearers [5]. Thus, we explored the influence of this polymorphism on restenosis after PTCA.

Patients and Methods

Between 1993 and 1996, 320 patients undergoing a PTCA without stenting and 257 patients undergoing a PTCA with stenting were recruited and had a systematic coronary angiography control 6 months after the procedure. Quantitative computer-assisted angiographic measurements were performed on end-diastolic frames with use of the computer-assisted evaluation of stenosis and restenosis (CAESAR) system (Fig. 1). A detailed description of this system has been reported previously [6]. This method allowed us to measure various parameters: the acute gain was defined as the difference between the minimal lumen diameter (MLD) immediately after the procedure and the MLD before the procedure; the late loss during the follow-up period was defined as the difference between the MLD immediately after the procedure and the MLD at follow-up; the net gain was defined as the difference between the acute gain and the late loss; the loss index is the ratio late loss to acute gain. To define restenosis, we also used a categorical approach with the classic criterion of > 50% diameter stenosis at follow-up.

Genomic DNA was extracted from white blood cells and the *ACE* fragment

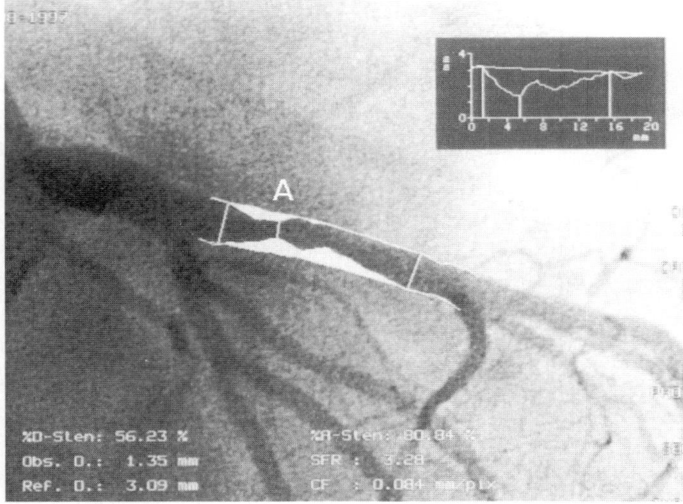

Fig. 1. Example of a quantitative computer-assisted measurement of a stenosis of the left anterior descending coronary artery. "A" corresponds to the minimal lumen diameter measured in mm.

containing the insertion/deletion was detected by polymerase chain reaction as described elsewhere [7].

Statistical analyses were performed with SAS software, version 6.10 (SAS Institute Inc., Cary, North Carolina). Mean and standard deviation (SD) values of quantitative data were calculated. Quantitative data were compared with a general linear model according to the *ACE* genotypes. Subjects were categorised into three classes according to their genotype (i.e., DD, ID and II). The tests were performed assuming an allele-dose effect. Qualitative data were tested with the use of Pearson's χ^2 test and Mantel-Haenszel linear test. Adjusted odds ratios were computed from a multivariate logistic regression model to provide an estimate of the relative risk of restenosis.

Results

In the sample of patients with PTCA without stenting, the results did not show any difference among *ACE* genotype groups in minimal lumen diameter (MLD) before PTCA, immediately after PTCA and at follow-up (Fig. 2). No other difference within the three genotypes could be detected in acute gain, late loss, loss index and restenosis qualitative estimation [8].

In this sample, we analysed the genotype distribution of the *ACE* polymorphism in patients with an occlusion at follow-up (Fig. 3). In subjects with the DD genotype, the odds ratio (an approximation of the relative risk in case-control studies) to develop an occlusion at follow-up after PTCA without stenting was 3.17 (95% confidence interval (1.11—8.99)) compared to patients bearing the

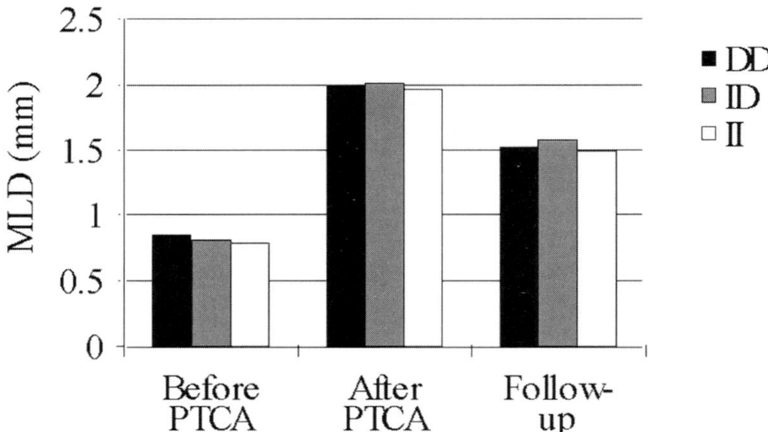

Fig. 2. Minimal lumen diameter (MLD) of patients with a PTCA without coronary stenting.

ID or II genotype [9].

Finally, we explored the impact of the *ACE* polymorphism on restenosis after PTCA with coronary stenting [10]. The MLD before and after the procedure and the acute gain did not differ significantly among the three genotype groups. At follow-up, the MLD had an inverse relationship to the number of D alleles. Late loss was more than 2-fold greater in the DD (0.89 ± 0.61 mm) than in the II group (0.40 ± 0.53 mm), the ID group being intermediate (0.60 ± 0.52 mm) (p < 0.0001). All these results were homogeneous across covariates (smoking,

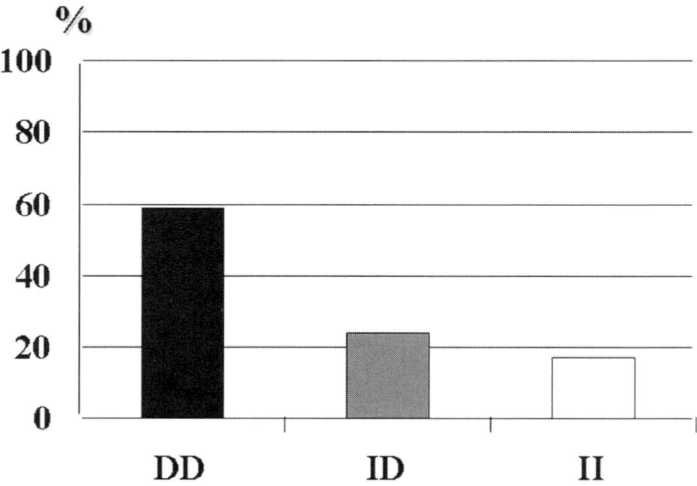

Fig. 3. Distribution of the ACE polymorphism genotype frequencies in patients with occlusion after PTCA without stenting.

diabetes, hypertension, unstable angina, previous myocardial infarction, ACE-inhibitor treatment, indication for stenting). The quantitative angiographic variables adjusted for diabetes, unstable angina, previous myocardial infarction, ACE inhibitor treatment, reference diameter, MLD after PTCA, indication for stenting and number of stents are presented in Fig. 4. The odds ratio of restenosis (defined as a $> 50\%$ diameter stenosis at follow-up) was 2.00 per number of D alleles (95% confidence interval = (1.03−3.88), p < 0.04).

Discussion

In two series of patients with PTCA with or without stenting, we observed that the deletion allele of *ACE* was a risk factor for post-PTCA occlusion and in-stent restenosis but not for restenosis after balloon angioplasty without stenting.

Contrary to the observation of Ohishi et al. [11] reporting that *ACE* polymorphism was a risk factor for restenosis after PTCA, we were unable to detect any association of the quantitative variables studied and *ACE* genotypes. A similar lack of association was also described by Samani et al. [12] in a series similar to ours. The series reported by Ohishi et al. [11], was composed of patients treated by emergency PTCA for acute myocardial infarction. Because this type of procedure in such patients is associated with a higher rate of restenosis due to the frequent occurrence of complete vessel occlusion [13], we investigated whether the *ACE* D allele might be a risk factor for total occlusion after PTCA without stenting. We reported that the risk of occlusion was increased in DD patients,

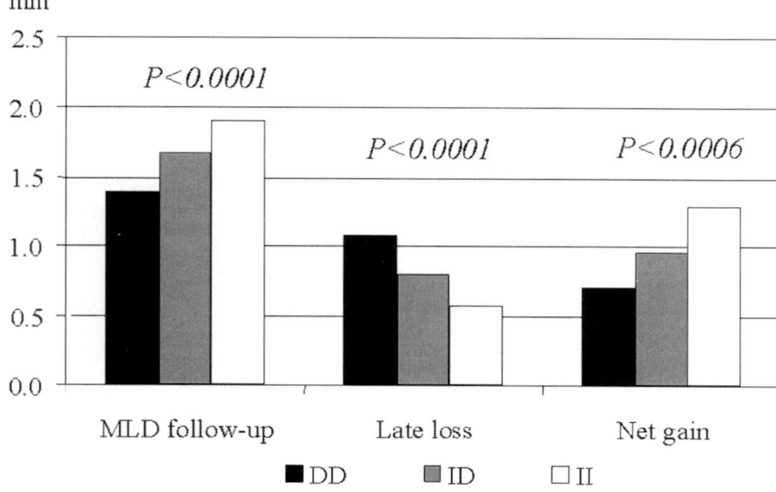

Fig. 4. Effect of the ACE genotypes on restenosis quantitative estimations after PTCA with stent implantation. Values are adjusted means for diabetes, unstable angina, previous myocardial infarction, ACE inhibitor treatment, reference diameter, MLD after PTCA, indication for stenting and number of stents.

and consequently might explain the discrepancies in the studies [9]. Indeed, the DD genotype is associated with increased levels of circulating ACE implicated in angiotensin II production. Angiotensin II is a potent vasoconstrictor and promotes increased plasma plasminogen activator-inhibitor 1 levels in humans [14]. This observation may constitute a possible link between ACE increased activity in DD subjects, and an increased risk of thrombosis implicated in the occurrence of acute myocardial infarction and occlusion after successful PTCA.

We reported that the *ACE* I/D was an independent predictor of late luminal narrowing after PTCA with coronary stenting [10]. Recent studies suggest that the contribution of neointimal hyperplasia to restenosis after balloon angioplasty is relatively limited and that lumen narrowing is in fact mostly related to vessel remodeling [15]. As the stent prevents the remodeling process, restenosis after coronary stenting is mainly the consequence of neointimal hyperplasia within the stent [16]. Various factors have been associated with neointimal hyperplasia [17]. Among these the components of the renin-angiotensin system are of major interest. Thus, factors such as *ACE* polymorphism, suspected to affect the degree of neointimal hyperplasia, will be more likely to influence restenosis after coronary stenting than restenosis after balloon angioplasty. The ACE influence on neointimal hyperplasia may be related to the role of this enzyme in the production of angiotensin II, a potent growth factor for smooth muscle cells.

The potential effect of the *ACE* polymorphism on restenosis lacking in balloon angioplasty but revealed after coronary stenting constitutes an example of gene-environment interaction [18]. The proliferation stimulus of neointimal growth due to the stent may be considered as the environmental factor. The neointimal proliferation, that does not seem to be pre-eminent in restenosis observed after PTCA without stent implantation, may be a major cause of restenosis after stent implantation, according to the number of D alleles in the genotype of a patient. If confirmed, this may be an example of an interaction between a therapeutic procedure and the genetic profile of a subject related to the concept of pharmacogenetics in the field of cardiovascular diseases. This observation may provide a way to assess the risk of a patient to develop a restenosis after a PTCA with coronary stenting and to plan a more intensive follow-up. This finding may also help to define a population in which the effects of medical drugs, such as ACE inhibitors, or of advanced gene therapy techniques should be tested.

Acknowledgements

This work was supported by the Centre Hospitalier et Universitaire de Lille, the Institut National de la Santé et de la Recherche Médicale (INSERM) and the Institut Pasteur de Lille.

References

1. McBride W, Lange RA, Hillis LD. Restenosis after successfull coronary angioplasty. Patho-

physiology and prevention. N Engl J Med 1988;318:1734—1737.

2. Waller BF. Crackers, breakers, stretchers, drillers, scrapers, shavers, burners, welders and melters — the future treatment of atherosclerotic coronary artery disease? A clinical-morphologic assessment. J Am Coll Cardiol 1989;13:969—987.

3. Serruys PW, de Jaegere P, Kiemeneij F, Macaya C, Rutsch W, Heyndrickx G, Emanuelsson H, Marco J, Legrand V, Materne P, Belardi J, Sigwart U, Colombo A, Goy JJ, van den Heuvel P, Delcan J, Morel MA, for the Benestent Study Group. A comparison of balloon-expandable-stent implantation with balloon angioplasty in patients with coronary artery disease. N Engl J Med 1994;331:489—495.

4. Fischman DL, Leon MB, Baim DS, Schatz RA, Savage MP, Penn I, Detre K, Veltri L, Ricci D, Nobuyoshi M, Cleman M, Heuser R, Almond D, Teirstein PS, Fish RD, Colombo A, Brinker J, Moses J, Shaknovich A, Hirshfeld J, Bailey S, Ellis S, Rake R, Goldberg S, for the Stent Restenosis Study Investigators. A randomized comparison of coronary-stent placement and balloon angioplasty in the treatment of coronary artery disease. N Engl J Med 1994;331:496—501.

5. Rigat B, Hubert C, Alhenc-Gelas F, Cambien F, Corvol P, Soubrier F. An insertion/deletion polymorphism in the angiotensin-converting enzyme gene accounting for half the variance of serum enzyme levels. J Clin Invest 1990;86:1343—1346.

6. Bertrand ME, Lablanche JM, Bauters C, Leroy F, McFadden EP. Discordant results of visual and quantitative estimates of stenosis severity before and after coronary angioplasty. Cathet Cardiovasc Diagn 1993;28:1—6.

7. Fogarty DG, Maxwell AP, Doherty CC, Hugues AE, Nevin NC. ACE gene typing. Lancet 1994; 343:851.

8. Hamon M, Bauters C, Amant C, McFadden EP, Helbecque N, Lablanche JM, Bertrand ME, Amouyel P. Relation between the deletion polymorphism of the angiotensin-converting enzyme gene and late luminal narrowing after coronary angioplasty. Circulation 1995;92:296—299.

9. Hamon M, Amant C, Bauters C, Lablanche JM, Bertrand M, Amouyel P. ACE polymorphism, a genetic predictor of occlusion after coronary angioplasty. Am J Cardiol 1996;78:679—681.

10. Amant C, Bauters C, Bodart JC, Lablanche JM, Grollier G, Danchin N, Hamon M, Richard F, Helbecque N, McFadden E, Amouyel P, Bertrand M. The D allele of the angiotensin I-converting enzyme is a major risk factor for restenosis after coronary stenting. Circulation 1997;96: 56—60.

11. Ohishi M, Fujii K, Minamino T, Higaki J, Katimani A, Rakugi H, Zhao Y, Mikami H, Miki T, Ogihara T. A potent genetic risk factor for restenosis. Nat Genet 1993;5:324—325.

12. Samani NJ, Martin DS, Brack M, Cullen J, Chauhan A, Lodwick D, Harley A, Swales JD, de Borno DP, Gershlick AH. Insertion/deletion polymorphism in the angiotensin-converting enzyme gene and risk of restenosis after coronary angioplasty. Lancet 1995;345:1013—1016.

13. Bauters C, Khanoyan P, McFadden E, Quandalle P, Lablanche JM, Bertrand M. Restenosis after delayed coronary angioplsty of the culprit vessel in patients with a recent myocardial infarction. Circulation 1995;91:1410—1418.

14. Ridker PM, Gaboury CL, Conlin PR, Seely EW, Williams GH, Vaughan DE. Stimulation of plasminogen activator inhibitor in vivo by infusion of angiotensin II. Circulation 1993;87: 1969—1973.

15. Mintz GS, Popma JJ, Pichard AD, Kent KM, Satler LF, Wong SC, Hong MK, Kovach JA, Leon MB. Arterial remodeling after coronary angioplasty. A serial intravascular ultrasound study. Circulation 1996;75:299—306.

16. Hoffmann R, Mintz GS, Dussaillant GR, Popma JJ, Pichard AD, Satler LF, Kent KM, Griffin J, Leon M. Patterns and mechanisms of in-stent restenosis: a serial intravascular ultrasound study. Circulation 1996;94:1247—1254.

17. Schwartz SM, deBlois D, O'Brien ERM. The intima. Soil for atherosclerosis and restenosis. Circ Res 1995;77:445—465.

18. Lindpainter K. Genetics of interventional cardiology, old principles, new frontiers. Circulation 1997;96:12—14.

Genetics, lipoproteins disorders and premature coronary artery disease

Jacques Genest Jr and Michel Marcil
Cardiovascular Genetics Laboratory, Clinical Research Institute of Montréal and the Cardiology Services, Centre Hospitalier de l'Université de Montréal (CHUM), Montréal, Québec, Canada

Abstract. Familial segregation of coronary artery disease (CAD) can be explained partly by shared environment, with risk factors such as cigarette smoking, social stress, diet and physical inactivity. A family history of premature CAD is an important, independent risk factor for the development of CAD. Familial hypercholesterolemia due to mutations of the LDL-receptor gene is seen in 3–5% of premature CAD cases. Other monogenic disorders such as defective apo B_{100}, type III dyslipidemia, familial HDL deficiency or Tangier disease are rare. Genetic factors strongly influence cardiovascular risk factors (hypertension, diabetes, obesity and dyslipoproteinemia). Lp(a) excess is predominantly genetically determined and may be the sole metabolic risk factor in some subjects with CAD. Familial lipoprotein disorders are seen in more than half of subjects with premature CAD. Most of these familial syndromes, including familial combined hyperlipidemia (seen in ~ 15% of premature CAD kindred), hypertriglyceridemia with low HDL (11%) and most cases of "isolated" reduced HDL-C (4%) are associated with increased plasma apo B levels and may reflect polygenic lipoprotein disorders often associated with other risk factors (visceral obesity, hypertension and insulin resistance). The search for genes causing lipoprotein disorders has followed the candidate gene approach, genomic scanning and transgenic models and, more recently, synteny with rodent genome and mRNA differential display. To understand the molecular genetics of CAD, one must carefully characterize the phenotype, perform large family studies or sib-pair analysis. Although multiple gene defects have been identified in candidate genes, the strength of association is often weak, reflecting the difficulty in defining quantitative genetic traits. The biochemistry and physiology determine cardiovascular risk and few genetic markers (if any) have proven to be clinically useful. Nevertheless, teasing gene-environment interactions will lead to a better understanding of genetic predisposition to developing CAD.

Keywords: coronary heart disease, genetics, lipoproteins.

Introduction

In the Western world, and in many developing countries, coronary artery disease (CAD), is the major cause of death. The direct costs to society in terms of health care, paramedical care and rehabilitation as well as the indirect costs of lost productivity are estimated at US$137 billion in the USA alone [1]. Worldwide, ischemic heart disease represents the principal cause of death in 1990. Projections made by Murray and Lopez [2] show that ischemic heart disease and

---

Address for correspondence: Jacques Genest Jr MD, Cardiovascular Genetics Laboratory, Clinical Research Institute of Montreal, 110 avenue des Pins Ouest, Montréal, Québec, Canada H2W 1R7. Tel.: +1-514-987-5715. Fax: +1-514-987-5767. E-mail: genestj@ircm.umontreal.ca

strokes will remain the principal causes of death by the year 2020. Epidemiological studies performed since the late 1950s have shown the importance of risk factors (male gender, age, heredity, smoking, high blood pressure, elevated cholesterol (C) level, reduced level of high density lipoprotein cholesterol (HDL-C) and diabetes) in determining cardiovascular risk [3]. Our ability to predict cardiovascular risk is based on mathematical models that take into account the traditional risk factors of increasing age, male gender, family history of premature CAD, cigarette smoking, blood pressure, elevated plasma cholesterol levels (especially low density lipoprotein cholesterol (LDL-C)), reduced HDL-C and the presence of diabetes mellitus as well as the presence of left ventricular hypertrophy [3]. This probabilistic analysis is, however, inaccurate. Recent trials for primary prevention of cardiovascular disease have shown that a large number of healthy men with elevated plasma cholesterol must be treated to prevent a handful of deaths.

In a study of families of probands with premature CAD, approximately 55% have a familial lipoprotein disorder [4]. The precise genetic defect(s) for the majority of these familial disorders remains unknown. It is hoped that a better understanding of the genes involved in CAD may allow for earlier detection and early treatment of affected subjects. The identification of genes involved in pathogenic mechanisms of atherosclerosis has been one of the successful endeavors of the application of molecular biology and molecular genetics. Despite this, molecular testing in young patients is unlikely to add predictive value to our ability to evaluate cardiovascular risk in healthy individuals. In the not so distant future, however, computer chip technology with silicone wafers imprinted with arrays of short DNA fragments will allow the rapid detection of mutations for virtually any gene [5]. Although promising from the technological point of view, the clinical applications of this technology in screening for genetic predisposition to chronic disease states such as cancer, cardiovascular disease, arthritis, neurological disorders are in the distant future. The major interest in searching for genes involved in premature CAD (defined here as occurring in subjects <60 years) lies predominantly in a better understanding of the effects of various genes on basic pathophysiological mechanisms of atherogenesis. The use of transgenic animal models and gene "knockout" animals has greatly helped to understand the contribution of single genes in complex pathological processes such as atherosclerosis. In the clinical setting, the characterization of these disorders may pave the way for selective gene therapy for affected individuals. For reasons of space limitation, this review will deal principally with the molecular genetics of lipoproteins associated with premature CAD.

Over a decade ago, association studies using bi-allelic markers such as restriction fragment-length polymorphisms (RFLP) attempted to associate variability at candidate genes (expressed as the presence or absence of an allele bearing a polymorphism) with the presence of CAD in case-control type of studies. Although this approach is still used, many such studies tend to be population-specific, are of small scale and do not have sufficient power to show the unequivocal association of specific genetic markers with CAD.

There are several strategies for the identification of genetic disorders associated with CAD. First, the candidate gene approach involves the study of polymorphisms or physiologically significant mutations of known genes and their association with a defined phenotype. Second, an approach using candidate loci derived from research on animal models such as atherosclerosis-susceptible strains of mice, and third, genome scanning in which random genetic markers on all 23 chromosomes are examined and associated with a clinical phenotype [6]. These techniques use bi- or multi-allelic polymorphisms in case-control type of studies. There are two major problems with these approaches. The first is the difficulty in assessing coronary artery disease noninvasively in family members other than in the proband and therefore in phenotype assignment. It is well appreciated that CAD represents a large spectrum of clinical manifestation and new techniques such as intracoronary ultrasound, which allows the detection of significant luminal narrowing in asymptomatic individuals. The second problem lies in the unknown mode of transmission of disease susceptibility genes (in terms of penetrance, age of expression and gender effects). This makes the use of the traditional family study with use of the LOD score problematic. Other methods, notably sib pair analysis may shed more light than traditional LOD-score based family studies.

There are several genetic lipoprotein disorders associated with premature CAD [7] (Table 1). These are either single cases or account for a relatively small proportion of subjects with premature CAD (with the exception of familial hypercholesterolemia that accounts for 3—5% of premature CAD cases) [4,8]. Our current state of knowledge is incomplete as new monogenic disorders are being characterized and the effects of genetic variability on plasma biochemical variables, the effects of gene-environment and gene-gene interactions are being better understood. Some monogenic disorders, especially familial hypercholesterolemia (FH), have such a profound impact on the development of CAD that the association between a genetic defect and CAD is easy to make. For most genetic disorders, we must accept the concept of a "middle distance reality" where genetic variability or specific mutations at a single gene are shown to alter the function of a protein or its product in plasma and this may influence cardiovascular risk [9].

Table 1. Genetic lipoprotein disorders and CAD [5].

	Gene involved	Plasma variable	Prevalence in premature CAD
Familial hypercholesterolemia	LDL receptor	LDL-C ↑↑↑	3—5%
Familial defective apo B	Apo B	LDL-C ↑↑↑	<1/500
Apo AI deficiency	Apo AI-CIII-AIV	HDL-C ↓↓↓	Very rare
Apo E deficiency, type III HLP	Apo E	Tg ↑↑ HDL ↓↓	<1%
Lp(a) excess	Apo (a)	Lp(a) ↑↑	Frequent

Familial hypercholesterolemia

Familial hypercholesterolemia is a lipoprotein disorder characterized by elevated LDL-C levels ($>$ 95th percentile of age- and gender-matched subjects), cutaneous manifestations in adults (tendinous xanthomas, xanthelasmas) and premature CAD in family members. Multiple defects in the LDL receptor (LDL-R) have been identified in subjects with FH. The prevalence of FH in the general population is approximately 1/500 (based on a study of familial lipoprotein disorders in survivors of myocardial infarction) [7,10]. In regions where genetic disorders are known to cluster because of a founder effect, the prevalence of FH may be as high as 1/270. The presence of homozygous FH (either due to the presence of identical alleles or compound heterozygotes), the affected subject dies usually before 30 years of age of coronary artery disease and severe atherosclerosis. With newer techniques of selective LDL filtration or extracorporeal precipitation, survival can be markedly prolonged and the rate of development of atherosclerosis can be decreased. Over 150 mutations have so far been characterized at the molecular and cellular levels. Many types of mutation have been characterized at the cellular physiology level: point mutations within the promoter region affecting the binding of nuclear factors that facilitate the transcription of the gene by RNA polymerase, point mutations (missense) changing a critical domain of the protein, nonsense mutations leading to truncated forms of the protein and large deletions leading to a null allele phenotype. Individual mutations may explain, in part, the phenotypic variability seen in FH subjects. Within specific populations, molecular diagnosis is available and may help in the diagnosis of difficult cases. Current DNA diagnostic methods rely on PCR-based techniques (or, in rare cases, Southern blotting analysis), and are performed only in specialized research centers.

The FH phenotype can also be caused by abnormalities in the ligand for the LDL-R, apolipoprotein B (apo B). To date, two mutations of apo B, in the region of the postulated LDL-R binding region have been identified. These mutations, known as apo $B_{Arg3500 \rightarrow Gln}$ and apo $B_{Arg3531 \rightarrow Cys}$ have been shown to have decreased affinity for the LDL-R and to accumulate in the plasma of affected individuals, giving a clinical phenotype indistinguishable from FH.

Familial apo E disorders

The apo E gene is located on chromosome 19 and codes for a 299 amino acid protein. Apo E is involved in receptor-mediated endocytosis of triglyceride-rich lipoproteins (IDL) and chylomicrons remnant lipoproteins. A rare disorder of the apo E gene leads to a lack of detectable apo E in plasma, severe dyslipoproteinemia and premature CAD [10]. The defect in apo E absence has been characterized as a mutation within the third intron of the apo E gene, causing a splicing defect and unstable mRNA for apo E and a lack of protein being secreted. Apo E gene defects are very rare. Two common polymorphisms of the apo E gene, apo E2 and apo E4, have a small but significant effect in plasma levels of LDL-cholesterol (3–5%) and triglycerides. Subjects carrying two copies of the apo E2 allele are at risk of developing a severe lipoprotein disorder (type III dyslipidemia) characterized by accumulation of apo E containing remnant lipoproteins and clinically by premature (often) vascular disease. Only approximately 1% of subjects with the apo E2/E2 genotype will develop type III dyslipoproteinemia; it is postulated that another defect (e.g., diabetes, familial combined hyperlipidemia/hyperapo B, hypertriglyceridemia) must be present for genetically predisposed subjects to develop the disease. In some studies, but not all, variability at the apo E locus has been associated with coronary artery disease.

Familial HDL deficiency syndromes

Rare disorders of apolipoprotein AI, the major apolipoprotein of high-density lipoprotein (HDL) particles, have been associated with premature CAD [11]. There are now 10 kindred characterized with apo AI deficiency due to defects at the apo AI gene locus. In four of these, there is an association with premature CAD but in others of various ethnic descent (German, Japanese, Turkish and Italian) no association with CAD was found. Although age at presentation may be a confounding factor in these various reports, it suggests that severe disorders of apo AI are not necessarily associated with premature CAD. Other genetic disorders associated with severe HDL deficiency include lipoprotein lipase deficiency or its activator, apo CII. These disorders are characterized by severe hypertriglyceridemia and the decreased HDL-cholesterol levels are considered to be secondary to severe hypertriglyceridemia. A deficiency of the enzyme LCAT is also associated with severe HDL-cholesterol deficiency. This disorder is very rare and does not appear to confer increased CAD risk. Tangier disease [7] is a disorder of unknown etiology characterized by severe HDL and apo AI deficiency, lymphoid tissue infiltration by lipid-laden macrophages, peripheral neuropathy and, in half the cases reported to date, premature CAD.

Lipoprotein (a) (Lp(a))

Lipoprotein (a) is a lipoprotein composed of a cholesterol ester core, one molecule of apo B which is covalently linked to one molecule of apo (a), a protein that shares homology to plasminogen and is composed of multiple repeats of a kringle domain homologous to those of plasminogen. The molecular size diversity of apo (a) is due to the number of kringle domains present on the protein. Variations in the apo (a) gene account for approximately 90% of plasma Lp(a) levels, with apo (a) size polymorphisms accounting for the major portion of this variability. Elevated plasma levels of Lp(a) have been associated in several studies with the presence of CAD but other studies failed to find such an association [7].

Familial lipoprotein lipase (LPL) deficiency (hyperchylomicronemia)

Subjects homozygous for functional LPL mutations have severe chylomicronemia, with recurrent pancreatitis that may be life threatening. Such patients have very low LDL-C levels and were considered to be protected from atherosclerosis. A recent report casts doubts on the protective effect of LDL deficiency and suggests that massive accumulation of chylomicrons (or the secondary severe HDL deficiency that results) can cause CAD [12]. The heterozygous state for LPL mutations may predispose to CAD by raising plasma triglyceride levels and lowering HDL-C levels [9].

Familial lipoprotein disorders

There are several familial disorders of lipoproteins that are associated with premature CAD [4]; these are summarized in Table 2. One of the most common is familial combined hyperlipoproteinemia (FCH), a disorder characterized by increases in plasma levels of total cholesterol, apo B, increase in the number of circulating LDL particles (that are usually small and dense) and increased plasma triglyceride levels within a family. The genetic etiology is unknown, although several genetic associations have been proposed. The diagnostic criteria for FCH rely on age and gender-specific cut-points for plasma lipids and lipoprotein lipid levels. There is, therefore, a considerable overlap between FCH and familial hypertriglyceridemia, familial hypoalphalipoproteinemia, the metabolic syndrome, hyperapo B and familial dyslipidemic hypertension [13]. We [14] and others [15,16] have recently described a novel lipoprotein disorder, familial HDL deficiency (FHD) in which probands have isolated hypoalphalipoproteinemia (all known causes having been excluded). These patients have marked hypercatabolism of HDL particles. This disorder may be a form of Tangier disease [17,18] but without the clinical manifestations seen in true Tangier disease subjects. Tangier disease and FHD may represent a novel class of lipoprotein disorders in which there is abnormal intracellular transport and efflux of cholesterol [19,20].

Table 2. Familial lipoprotein disorders associated with CAD.

	Gene(s) involved	Biochemical variables
Familial combined hyperlipidemia[a]	Unknown	Tg↑ LDL-C ↑ Apo B↑ HDL↓
Hyperapo B[a]	Unknown	Apo B ↑
Metabolic syndrome[a]	Unknown	Tg↑ Gluc ↑ Apo B↑ HDL↓ Insulin↑
Familial HDL deficiency	Unknown	HDL-C ↓↓ Apo AI↓↓
Familial dyslipidemic hypertension[a]	Unknown	Tg↑ LDL-C↑ BP↑
Elevated Lp(a)	Apo(a)	Lp(a) ↑
Tangier disease	Unknown	HDL-C ↓↓↓ Apo AI ↓↓↓
Small, dense LDL[a]	Unknown	Tg↑ HDL-C ↓ Apo B↑

[a]Overlapping disorders.

Potential genes of interest

As our understanding of lipoprotein metabolism continues to advance, genes that code for proteins involved in many aspects of lipoprotein assembly, secretion, metabolism and uptake are characterized [10,21]. These hold the key to many disorders of (yet) unknown etiology and may provide novel therapeutic paths. In some of these genes, specific mutations have been identified that lead to clinical syndromes that are associated with premature CAD (Table 1). Genetic mutations at several loci have yielded inconsistent or no associations with CAD despite perturbed lipoprotein metabolism.

Clinical relevance

Single gene disorders associated with premature CAD are, in general, rare and have little impact on the epidemiology of CAD within a population. The most prevalent defect seen in premature CAD is familial hypercholesterolemia due to mutations within the LDL-R gene. Other genetic defects account for less than 1% of premature CAD. These include type III dysbetalipoproteinemia, apo E absence, apo AI mutations (usually leading to apo AI absence from plasma), Tangier disease, or apo B_{3500}.

The screening of specific mutations for disorders identified in Table 1 is fraught with complex ethical issues as well as significant costs. Even in populations with a high prevalence of FH subjects known to have a small number of specific mutations of the LDL-R gene, genetic screening may not be cost-effective nor have sufficient predictive value in a clinical or health care policy setting. Furthermore, the plasma concentration of the biochemical variable (i.e., total or LDL-cholesterol in the case of FH) is necessary and, in most cases, sufficient to determine cardiovascular risk. An argument can be made that genetic screening in asymptomatic children of parents with premature CAD may help to detect a strong genetic predisposition to CAD. Experience with FH in children reveals that even young children with specific LDL-R mutations have very high LDL-C levels compared to age- and gender-matched children. Thus, for clinical purposes, the identification of a specific mutation in subjects with FH usually does not change the management of individual patients. In general, the therapeutic approach is based on the biochemical variable of the physiological process that is altered.

Genetic variability at candidate gene loci associations with CAD or altered plasma variables (especially plasma lipoprotein-lipid levels) has yielded inconsistent results and have little, if any, positive predictive value. From the point of view of health care expenditure, at the current time, genetic screening should be performed in highly specialized and experienced laboratories. Reimbursement for such tests remains problematic.

Nevertheless, research must be vigorously pursued in characterizing the effects of individual genes and specific mutations in cellular models and in transgenic and gene knockout animals. Gene therapy for familial hypercholesterolemia has already been attempted albeit with relatively modest results. The future of gene therapy will be oriented at correcting the basic defect (i.e., inserting a functional copy of the LDL-R in the liver of subjects with homozygous FH) or by enhancing the body's clearance of cholesterol by increasing the efficiency of the HDL-mediated cholesterol efflux.

Acknowledgements

The authors are supported by grants from the Medical Research Council of Canada, the Heart and Stroke Foundation of Canada and the Fonds de la Recherche en santé du Québec.

References

1. American Heart Association. Heart and Stroke Facts: 1995 Statistical Supplement. AHA publication 1995.
2. Murray CJL, Lopez AD. Mortality by cause for eight regions of the world: Global Burden of Disease Study. Lancet 1997;349:1269—1276 and: Alternative projections of mortality and disability by cause 1990—2020: global burden of disease study. Lancet 1997;349:1498—1504.
3. The Expert Panel. Summary of the second report of the National Cholesterol Education Program (NCEP) expert panel on detection, evaluation, and treatment of high blood cholesterol in adults (adult treatment panel II). J Am Med Assoc 1993;269:3015—3023.
4. Genest J Jr, Martin-Munley SS, McNamara JR, Ordovas JM, Jenner JL, Meyers RH, Silberman SR, Wilson PWF, Salem DN, Schaefer EJ. Familial lipoprotein disorders in patients with premature coronary artery disease. Circulation 1992;85:2025—2033.
5. Editorial. Chipping away at the human genome. Science 1996;272:1737.
6. Genome DataBase. Http://gdbwww.gdb.org/
7. Dammerman M, Breslow JL. Genetic basis of lipoprotein disorders. Circulation 1995;91:505—511.
8. Weber M, McNicoll S, Lussier-Cacan S, Marcil M, Connelly P, Rondeau C, Latour Y, Connelly P, Davignon J, Genest J Jr. Plasma lipoproteins, apolipoprotein B, apolipoprotein E phenotypes and metabolic factors in premature CAD in French Canadians. Can J Cardiol 1997;13:253—260.
9. Wittrup HH, Tybjaerg-Hansen A, Abidgaard S, Steffensen R, Schnohr P, Nordestgaard BG. A common substitution (Asn291Ser) in lipoprotein lipase is associated with increased risk of ischemic heart disease. J Clin Invest 1997;99:1606—1613.
10. Online Mendelian Inheritance in Man (OMIM©). Center for Medical Denetics, Johns Hopkins University, Baltimore, MD, and the National Center for Biotechnology Information, National Library of Medicine, Bethesda, MD; 1996. Smith M, McKusick VA (eds) Http://www3.ncbi.nih.gov/omim/.
11. Breslow JL. Familial disorders of high density lipoprotein metabolism. In: Scriver CR, Beaudet AL, Sly WS, Valle D (eds) The Metabolic and Molecular Basis of Inherited Disease, 7th edn. New York: McGraw-Hill, 1995;2031—2052.
12. Benlian P, DeGennes JL, Foubert L, Zhang H, Gagne SE, Hayden M. Premature atherosclerosis in patients with familial chylomicronemia caused by mutations in the lipoprotein lipase gene. N Engl J Med 1996;335:848—854.
13. Genest J Jr, Bard J-M, Fruchart J-C, Ordovas JM, Schaefer EJ. Familial hypoalphalipoproteinemia in premature coronary artery disease. Arterioscler Thromb 1993;13:1728—1737.
14. Marcil M, Boucher B, Frohlich J, Davignon J, Solymoss BC, Genest J Jr. Severe familial HDL

deficiency in French Canadian kindred: biochemical and molecular characterization. Arterioscl Thromb Vasc Biol 1995;15:1015–1024.

15. Emmerich J, Verges B, Tauveron I, Rader D, Sammaritano-Fojo S, Schaefer J, Ayrault-Jarrier M, Thieblot P, Brewer B Jr. Familial HDL deficiency due to marked hypercatabolism of normal apo AI. Arterioscl Thromb 1993;13:1299–1306.

16. Cheung MC, Mendez AJ, Wolf AC, Knopp RH. Characterization of apolipoprotein A-I and A-II-containing lipoproteins in a new case of high density lipoprotein deficiency resembling Tangier disease and their effects on intracellular cholesterol efflux. J Clin Invest 1993;19:522–529.

17. Serfaty-Lacrosniere C, Civiera F, Lanzberg A et al. Homozygous Tangier disease and cardiovascular disease. Atherosclerosis 1994;107:85–98.

18. Assman G, von Eckardstein A, Brewer HB Jr. Familial high density lipoprotein deficiency: Tangier disease. In: Scriver CR, Beaudet AL, Sly WS, Valle D (eds) The Metabolic and Molecular Basis of Inherited Disease, 7th edn. New York: McGraw-Hill, 1995;2053–2072.

19. Francis GA, Knopp RH, Oram JF. Defective removal of cellular cholesterol and phospholipids by apolipoprotein AI in Tangier disease. J Clin Invest 1995;96:78–87.

20. Rogler G, Trumbach B, Klima B, Lackner KJ, Schmitz G. HDL-mediated efflux of intracellular cholesterol is impaired in fibroblasts from Tangier disease patients. Arterioscl Thromb Vasc Biol 1995;15:693–690.

21. Havel RJ, Kane JP. Structure and metabolism of plasma lipoproteins. In: Scriver CR, Beaudet AL, Sly WS, Valle D (eds) The Metabolic and Molecular Basis of Inherited Disease, 7th edn. New York: McGraw-Hill, 1995;1841–1851.

Predisposing genes, high-risk environments and coronary artery disease: LPL and MMP-3 as examples

Steve E. Humphries[1], Rachel M. Fisher[1], George Miller[2], Shu Ye[3], Adriano Henney[3] and Philippa J. Talmud[1]

[1]*Department of Medicine, Centre for Cardiovascular Genetics, UCLMS, The Rayne Institute, London;* [2]*Wolfson Institute, St Bartholomew's Hospital, London; and* [3]*Wellcome Trust Centre for Human Genetics, Oxford, UK (current address)*

Abstract. Two examples of the modifying effects of environment on genotype on the development of coronary artery disease (CAD) will be presented. Two mutations in the LPL gene (D9N and N291S) have been identified that occur at a combined frequency of 4—6% in the general population resulting in a moderate reduction in the LPL activity/mass in vitro. Carriers have slightly elevated plasma TG and lower HDL-C levels, and when compounded by obesity show increased levels of plasma lipid increasing CAD risk. Abnormal matrix metalloproteinase (MMP) activity has been implicated in the pathogenesis of coronary atherosclerosis. A common sequence variant, 6As or 5As in the MMP-3 gene promoter, was identified. In patients with lipid levels lowered by treatment, the 5A/6A genotype had no effect on disease progression, but in 6A homozygous individuals whose lipid levels remained high, a significant progression of angiographic stenosis was observed. In vitro, compared to the 5A allele, the 6A promoter had a 2-fold lower strength. Low levels of stromelysin may thus predispose to matrix accumulation and progression of disease, but this may only be clinically important when the individual is also in a high-risk environment such as hyperlipidaemia.

Keywords: gene-environment interaction/plaque, lipoprotein lipase, stromelysin (MMP-3), triglycerides.

Introduction

Coronary artery disease (CAD) is a multifactorial disorder, with both genetic and environmental factors being involved to varying extents. Epidemiological studies have identified a number of these factors including high blood pressure, smoking, high dietary fat intake, obesity and the development of diabetes. These studies have also identified a number of plasma risk factors such as elevated levels of cholesterol and high levels of the clotting factor fibrinogen. However, details at the level of genotype may give added information, such as:

1. When a genotype predicts a level of a measurable risk factor at some future time such as the change in plasma lipid levels with the development of obesity, diabetes, and increasing age.
2. A genotype may give extra predictive information over classical risk factor

---

Address for correspondence: Prof Humphries, Department of Medicine, Centre for Cardiovascular Genetics, UCLMS, The Rayne Institute, University Street, London WC1E 6JJ, UK.
E-mail: shumphri@medicine.ucl.ac.uk

traits where the gene codes for a protein not easily measurable, e.g., heart muscle, the intestine and the liver or cells in the vessel wall.
In this review, examples of both of these types of genotype information will be presented.

Plasma triglycerides, lipoprotein lipase variants and obesity

A growing body of evidence supports the hypothesis that elevated plasma triglycerides may increase the risk of CAD. LPL is a key enzyme in the metabolism of triglyceride-rich lipoproteins by hydrolysing triglycerides in large TG-rich lipoproteins (chylomicrons and VLDLs). To date, two common missense mutations have been identified in the LPL gene [1], an aspartic acid to asparagine change in exon 2 (D9N) and an asparagine to serine change (N291S) in exon 6. In vitro D9N causes a 20—30% decrease in mass and activity, with retention in the cells suggesting a secretion defect [2]. In vitro S291 demonstrated reduced dimer stability with overall 30—50% reduced activity.

We examined the effect of the mutations on plasma lipid levels in 628 healthy individuals participating in the Northwick Park Heart Study II; 27 N9 and 24 S291 carriers were identified [3,4] with plasma TG levels 24 and 14% higher, respectively, than individuals with neither mutation. The relationship of BMI (divided according to tertiles) with plasma TG concentration in carriers and noncarriers is shown in Fig. 1. In the noncarriers, the expected graded increase in plasma TG across the BMI tertiles was seen. In carriers of either mutations, the increase in plasma TG concentration was much larger in the upper two BMI ter-

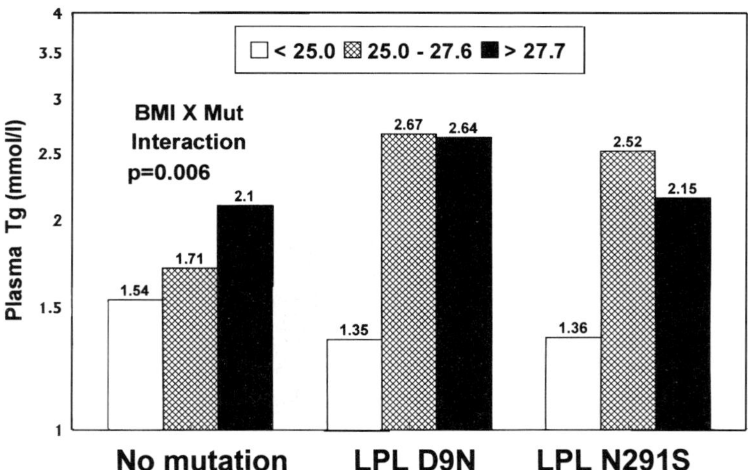

Fig. 1. Mean plasma triglyceride concentration according to tertiles of BMI in healthy noncarriers and carriers of the N9 (n = 26) or S291 (n = 24) LPL mutations. For carriers of either mutation the test for interaction between carriers/noncarriers and tertiles of BMI was p = 0.006. To test differences in triglyceride levels, values were log-transformed prior to statistical analysis.

tile groups compared to the lowest BMI tertile group. Thus both variants are implicated in causing elevated plasma TG concentrations, exaggerated at higher BMI. Obesity may promote overproduction of TG-rich lipoproteins from the liver, which overwhelms the partially deficient LPL in the adipose and muscle. Thus, carriers of these LPL mutations who are also moderately obese would be at increased risk of CAD.

Stromelysin genotype and progression of atherosclerosis

The acute event precipitating an MI is usually the rupture of an advanced foam-cell and lipid-laden atherosclerotic plaque, with the resulting thrombosis causing occlusion of the artery [5]. Thus the variability of expression of proteinases that could weaken and destroy the plaque is a process that is likely to be critical. Since the level of expression of these enzymes in the plaque is essentially impossible to measure, this is a second area of cardiovascular disease where a specific genotype, if it predicted high enzyme levels, may add information to measurable plasma risk factors for estimating CAD risk.

Members of the matrix metalloproteinase (MMP) family have been implicated in connective tissue remodelling during atherogenesis. By in situ mRNA hybridization, we originally demonstrated the presence of stromelysin-1 in coronary atherosclerotic plaques [6]. Stromelysin-1 is an MMP with a broad substrate specificity, degrading types II, IV and IX collagen, proteoglycans, laminin, fibronectin, gelatins and elastin. Expression of stromelysin-1 is primarily regulated at the level of transcription, where the promoter of the gene responds to various stimuli, including growth factors and cytokines (see [7] and references therein) mediated through a number of cis-elements located in the stromelysin-1 promo-

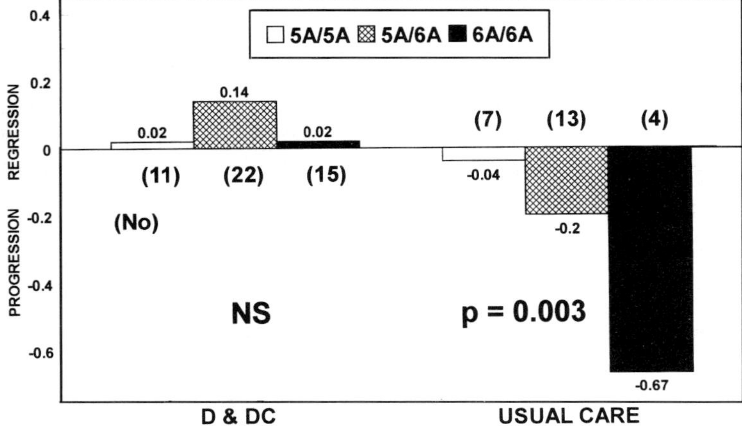

Fig. 2. Bar graph showing changes in mean width of coronary artery segments between baseline and 3-year follow-up angiography in men with different stromelysin genotypes, divided according to usual care or lipid-lowering regime.

ter, shown in Fig. 2. We identified a common polymorphism in the stromelysin gene promoter [7], located roughly 600 bp upstream from the start of transcription, where one allele has a run of six adenosines (6A) and another has five (5A). To investigate the relationship between this polymorphism and the progression of the disease, we genotyped men with CAD who participated in the St Thomas' Atherosclerosis Regression Study (STARS) randomised to receive usual care (UC), dietary intervention (D), or diet plus cholestyramine (DC), with angiography at baseline and at 39 months. Paired measurements were made using a computerized method on 489 segments, with a mean (SD) of 6.4 (2.0) segments analysed per patient. The study endpoints were the overall change (per patient) in mean and minimum absolute width of coronary segments (MAWS and MinAWS, respectively). Overall, the DC group showed regression of disease and the U group showed progression of disease, with the D group being intermediate. However, a strong association between the polymorphism and change in luminal diameter was seen in the UC group in which the decrease in MinAWS in patients homozygous for the 6A allele was 4.8-fold greater than that in those with other genotypes ($p < 0.01$). The findings were similar in measures of the change in MAWS, with a decrease 3.7-fold greater in individuals with the genotype 6A6A than in those with other genotypes ($p < 0.05$, Fig. 2B). No significant associations were observed in patients in the D or DC treatment groups. These results provide the first evidence of a link between genetic variation in stromelysin and progression of coronary atherosclerosis and support the hypothesis that connective tissue remodelling mediated by metalloproteinases contributes to the pathogenesis of atherosclerosis.

In vitro studies of promoter strength showed the 5A-allele expressed higher activity than the 6A allele in both cultured human foetal foreskin fibroblasts (HFFF2), and vascular smooth muscle cells [8]. Bandshift assays showed that a nuclear protein bound more strongly to the 6A than the 5A suggesting that this protein may be a repressor of transcriptional activity. Compared to other genotypes, individuals homozygous for the 6A allele would have lower stromelysin-1 levels in their arterial walls because of reduced gene transcription which would favour deposition of extracellular matrix in the atherosclerotic lesions. This would lead to the development of an atherosclerotic plaque with a thick cap, and result in a more rapid progression of angiographically defined stenosis.

Conclusions

We have described two genetic predictors for an individual's CAD risk, which may be useful over and above measures of classical risk factors. For the LPL variants, the modest reduction of lipolytic action appears likely to be important, particularly when individuals are also overweight. The clinical implications for obese carriers of these variants, is that they may experience a large and clinically useful reduction in TG concentration for a moderate loss of weight. For the stromelysin promoter we show that the 6A/5A polymorphism affects binding of nuclear proteins and thus influences the rate of transcription, resulting in changes in the levels of the protein and thus progression of plaque size, but this may only be clinically important in the presence of other factors (such as hyperlipidaemia) which promote plaque growth. A better understanding of the detailed molecular mechanisms of these effects, should allow the development of novel therapeutic strategies, where levels of transcription may be modulated by specific antagonists of such nuclear protein binding.

Acknowledgements

This work was supported by the British Heart Foundation (PG007 and 86-77) and the MRC (GJM)

References

1. Fisher RM, Humphries SE, Talmud PJ. Common variation in the lipoprotein lipase gene: effects on plasma lipids and risk of atherosclerosis. Atherosclerosis 1997;(In press).
2. Zhang H, Henderson H, Gagne SE, Clee SM, Miao L, Liu G, Hayden MR. Common sequence variants of lipoprotein lipase: standardized studies of in vitro expression and catalytic function. Biochim Biophys Acta 1996;1302:159—166.
3. Mailly F, Tugrul Y, Reymer PWA, Bruin T, Seed M, Groenemeyer BF, Asplund-Carlson A, Vallance D, Winder AF, Miller GJ, Kastelein JJP, Hamsten A, Olivecrona G, Humphries SE, Talmud P. A common variant in the gene for lipoprotein lipase (Asp9→Asn): functional implications and prevalence in normal and hyperlipidemic subjects. Arterioscler Thromb Vasc Biol 1995;15:468—478.
4. Fisher RM, Mailly F, Peacock RE, Hamsten A, Seed M, Yudkin JS, Beisiegel U, Feussner G, Miller G, Humphries SE, Talmud PJ. Interaction of the lipoprotein lipase asparagine 291→serine mutation with body mass index determines elevated plasma triacylglycerol concentrations: a study in hyperlipidaemic subjects, myocardial infarction survivors and healthy adults. J Lipid Res 1995;36:2104—2112.
5. Davies MJ, Richardson PD, Woolf N, Katz DR, Mann J. Risk of thrombosis in human atherosclerotic plaques: role of extracellular lipid, macrophage, and smooth muscle cell content. Br Heart J 1993;69:377—381.
6. Henney AM, Wakeley P, Davies MJ, Foster K, Hembry R, Murphy G, Humphries SE. Localization of stromelysin gene expression in atherosclerotic plaques by in situ hybridization. Proc Natl Acad Sci USA 1991;88:8154—8158.
7. Ye S, Watts GF, Mandalia S, Humphries SE, Henney AM. Preliminary report: genetic variation in the human stromelysin promoter is associated with progression of coronary atherosclerosis. Br Heart J 1995;73:209—215.
8. Ye S, Eriksson P, Hamsten A, Kirkinen M, Humphries SE, Henney AM. Progression of coronary atherosclerosis is associated with a common genetic variant of the human stromelysin-1 promoter which results in reduced gene expression. J Biol Chem 1996;271:13055—13060.

A quantitative genetic analysis of the angiotensin-1 converting enzyme (ACE) gene

Bernard Keavney, Colin A. McKenzie, John M.C. Connell, Cecile Julier, Peter J. Ratcliffe, Mark Lathorp and Martin Farrall
The Wellcome Trust Centre for Human Genetics, University of Oxford, Oxford, UK

The analysis of multiple polymorphisms in a candidate gene or region and the definition of their relationship to an underlying susceptibility or quantitative trait represents a major theoretical and practical bottleneck in the identification of variants for complex inherited disease and traits. Circulating angiotensin-I converting enzyme (ACE) levels are influenced by one or more major quantitative trait loci (QTL) that maps within or close to the ACE gene. ACE represents an important and experimentally tractable model trait for the development of strategies for variant identification.

We have undertaken a haplotype analysis of 10 polymorphisms spanning 26 kb at the ACE locus in a series of white British families that revealed a limited number of common haplotypes due to strong linkage disequilibrium operating over the whole region. A haplotype tree (cladogram) is proposed with three branches which account for the majority of the observed haplotypes. One branch is most likely derived following an ancestral recombination event. This evolutionary information was then used to direct a series of nested, measured haplotype analyses which exclude upstream sequences of the ACE promoter from harbouring the major ACE-linked variant. The importance of unlinked genetic influences was reinforced in this analysis. A combined cladistic/measured haplotype approach provides a powerful method to analyse polymorphisms within a gene in a search to identify variants that directly influence a quantitative trait.

Address for correspondence: Martin Farrall, The Wellcome Trust Centre for Human Genetics, University of Oxford, Windmill Road, Oxford, OX3 7BN, UK. Tel.: +44-1865-740-012. Fax: +44-1865-742-196.

Insulin resistance and lipoprotein metabolism

Abnormal reverse cholesterol transport in type II diabetes mellitus

F.D. Brites[1], J.-C. Fruchart[2], G.R. Castro[2], R.L. Wikinski[1]

[1] Laboratory of Lipids and Lipoproteins, Department of Clinical Biochemistry, School of Pharmacy and Biochemistry, University of Buenos Aires, Buenos Aires, Argentina; and [2] Service d'Etude et de Recherche sur les Lipoprotéines et l'Atherosclérose, Institut Pasteur de Lille, INSERM Unité 325, Lille, France

Abstract. Type II diabetes mellitus is generally preceded by hyperinsulinemia and the insulin-resistance syndrome, the latter being characterised by a clustering of atherogenic factors. The metabolic consequences of low HDL-cholesterol levels, frequently observed in these patients, are not fully understood. In moderate hypertriglyceridemic type II diabetic patients and in healthy normolipemic subjects, we tested the first step of reverse cholesterol transport (RCT), cellular cholesterol efflux, by incubating Fu5AH rat hepatoma cells with sera, obtained in fasting and postprandial (PP) states. We found significantly decreased cholesterol efflux promotion only in PP samples from diabetic patients. In HDL from patients the known triglyceride enrichment and cholesteryl ester depletion were further amplified in the PP state. The distribution of apo A-I-containing lipoproteins, analysed by two-dimensional electrophoresis, revealed that samples from patients exhibited an additional particle with pre-β mobility and low molecular weight (40 kDa). In the fasting condition decreased concentrations of HDL subfractions only containing apo A-I (LpA-I) were found in diabetic patients. This finding led us to study the metabolic role of LpA-I particles, isolated by immunoaffinity chromatography. Fasting and postprandial LpA-I particles from patients were less efficient in promoting cholesterol efflux from Ob1771 mouse adipose cells than control particles. Lecithin:cholesterol acyltransferase activity within LpA-I particles showed a 54% increase and an 18% decrease postprandially for control subjects and patients, respectively. The abnormal RCT described in these studies, reflects disturbances in the antiatherogenic function of HDL and their subfractions, thus contributing to the atherogenic clustering of factors in type II diabetes.

Keywords: cholesterol efflux, LpA-I, postprandial, pre-β-HDL.

In type II diabetes mellitus, cardiovascular atherosclerotic disease is the most frequent cause of mortality. It is generally preceded by hyperinsulinemia and by the insulin resistance syndrome, the latter being characterised by a clustering of atherogenic factors [1]. Among them, some lipoprotein abnormalities and their metabolic consequences are better known than others. The presence of fasting and postprandial hypertriglyceridemia is typical in type II diabetic patients, even under exhaustive glycaemic control [2]. Moreover, the appearance of abnormal triglyceride-rich lipoproteins contributes to atherogenesis in diabetic patients. Although LDL-C concentration is generally below the upper desirable

---

Address for correspondence: Fernando Brites, Laboratory of Lipids and Lipoproteins, Department of Clinical Biochemistry, School of Pharmacy and Biochemistry, Junin 956, Buenos Aires (1113), Argentina.

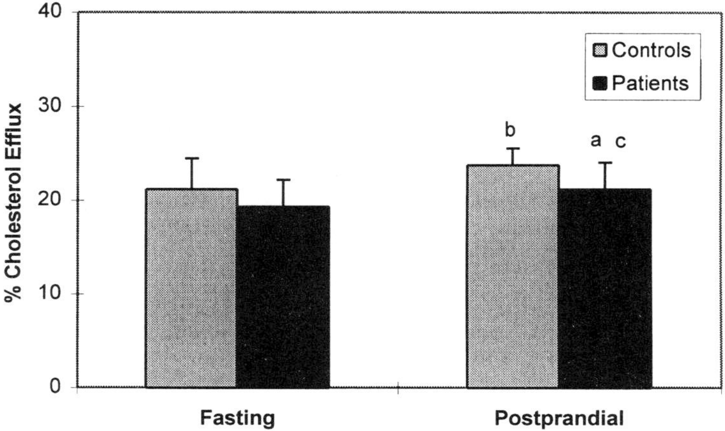

Fig. 1. Cholesterol efflux from Fu5AH rat hepatoma cells induced by serum samples from control subjects (n = 12) and diabetic patients (n = 31) in fasting and postprandial states. [a]p = 0.012 vs. control subjects in the same dietary condition by Mann-Whitney U test; [b]p < 0.01 and p < 0.001 vs. the fasting value for control subjects and diabetic patients, respectively, by Wilcoxon test. Results are expressed as mean ± SD.

value, there may be a preponderance of highly atherogenic small and dense LDL particles [3]. Finally, another dominant feature in these patients is a significant reduction in HDL-C concentrations [4].

The biological effects of low HDL-C levels are not fully understood. HDL plays

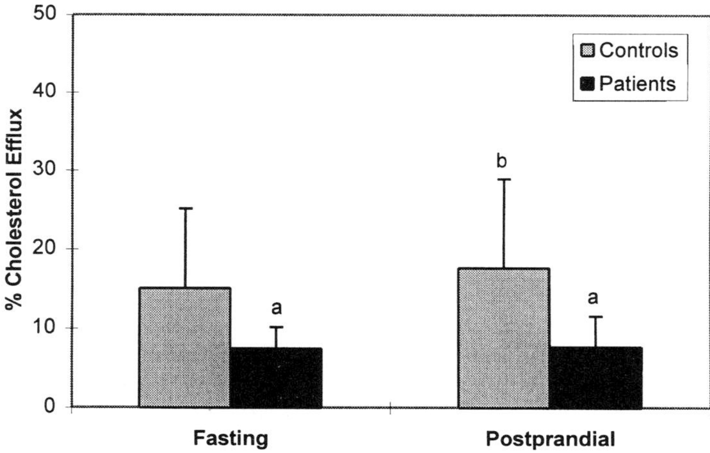

Fig. 2. Cholesterol efflux from Ob1771 adipose cells induced by LpA-I particles from control subjects (n = 10) and diabetic patients (n = 14) in fasting and postprandial states. [a]p < 0.05 vs. control subjects in the same dietary condition by Mann-Whitney U test; [b]p = 0.02 vs. the fasting value by Wilcoxon test. Results are expressed as mean ± SD.

its main role in reverse cholesterol transport by which excess cholesterol in peripheral tissues is transported to the liver for excretion [5]. This metabolic pathway consists of four main steps:

1. Free cholesterol efflux from peripheral cells and its uptake by pre-β_1-HDL fraction [6].
2. Free cholesterol esterification by the enzyme lecithin:cholesterol acyltransferase (LCAT).
3. Cholesteryl ester transfer from HDL to apo B-containing lipoproteins by the cholesteryl ester transfer protein (CETP).
4. Hepatic clearance of cholesteryl esters.

We have recently found (F. Brites, E. Cavallero, B. Jacotot, J.-C. Fruchart, R. Wikinski, G. Castro, unpublished data) that serum samples from moderate hypertriglyceridemic type II diabetic patients were less efficient to promote free cholesterol efflux from Fu5AH rat hepatoma cells than samples from healthy controls. This difference between both groups was only statistically significant in the postprandial state, though the higher cholesterol efflux induction in postprandial samples was evidenced for both diabetic patients and controls (Fig. 1).

Cholesterol efflux experiments carried out with whole serum or plasma provide useful information about the interaction of diverse parameters which participate in this complex process [7]. The reduced capacity of serum samples from diabetic patients to promote cellular cholesterol efflux might result from the low plasma levels of HDL-C, apo A-I and LpA-I particles (lipoprotein particles which only contain apo A-I but no apo A-II). Other factors such as the presence of triglyceride-enriched and cholesteryl ester depleted HDL particles, the increase in fasting and postprandial triglyceride concentrations and in LpC-III particle levels (lipoprotein particles which contain apo C-III) could also contribute to the less efficient release of free cholesterol from cellular membranes.

When the distribution of apo A-I-containing lipoproteins was analysed by two-dimensional electrophoresis, samples from patients and controls exhibited the pre-β_1, pre-β_2 and α-HDL subpopulations. Furthermore, an additional particle with pre-β electrophoretic mobility and low molecular weight (ca. 40 kDa), was only detected in all the samples from diabetic patients. We have proposed the term of pre-β_0 for this small particle. Pre-β_0 could be transformed into pre-β_1 after fusion with surface components coming from triglyceride-rich lipoproteins hydrolysed by lipoprotein lipase. Detection of this very small particle in type II diabetic patients could be due to a higher rate of production by an increased hepatic lipase activity on the triglyceride-enriched HDL and a diminished activity of lipoprotein lipase, the latter due to the insulin resistance syndrome and to higher LpC-III levels. The presence of this small particle might be, therefore, associated to an altered capacity of these serum samples to promote cellular cholesterol release.

When patients and controls were evaluated as a whole, a weak positive correlation was found between cholesterol efflux and LpA-I levels, whereas no correlation was seen with LpA-I:A-II (lipoprotein particles which contain both apo A-I

1068

and apo A-II). When divided in groups, the correlation with LpA-I:A-II became negative for controls and significantly positive for patients. The contrasting behaviour seen in patients and controls suggests that LpA-I:A-II play different roles in both groups. This is in line with the report of Marja-Riitta Taskinen in type II diabetic patients with or without coronary artery disease [8].

As regards the role played by LpA-I in reverse cholesterol transport, we found [9] that particles isolated by immunoaffinity chromatography from diabetic plasma exhibited a decreased capacity to induce cholesterol efflux from Ob1771 adipose cells both in fasting and postprandial states, whereas only control particles showed a significantly higher ability to promote cholesterol efflux after the test meal (Fig. 2). It is noteworthy that LCAT activity within LpA-I particles showed a 54% increase postprandially for control subjects, but an 18% decrease for type II diabetic patients. The alterations found in LpA-I metabolic functions in diabetic patients could be attributed to different factors. It must be noted that LpA-I particles from patients appeared depleted in cholesterol and phospholipids and relatively enriched in apolipoproteins as compared with LpA-I particles from control subjects. In addition, these particles showed an abnormal distribution of their subpopulations as separated on the basis of their size with a preponderance of smaller ones.

In conclusion, all the modifications found in samples from type II diabetic patients, whole serum and isolated LpA-I particles, could be responsible for an abnormal reverse cholesterol transport, specially in the postprandial condition. Therefore, the association between type II diabetes mellitus and atherosclerosis would be due, among several factors, to an ineffective antiatherogenic pathway.

Acknowledgements

F. Brites is a Research Fellow from the University of Buenos Aires. This study was performed as part of the INSERM-CONICET scientific exchange program.

References

1. Syvänne M, Taskinen MJ. Lipids and lipoproteins as coronary risk factors in non-insulin-dependent diabetes mellitus. Lancet 1997;350(Suppl I):20–23.
2. Cavallero E, Dachet C, Neufcour D, Wirquin E, Mathé D, Jacotot B. Postprandial amplification of lipoprotein abnormalities in controlled type II diabetic subjects: relationship to postprandial lipemia and C-peptide/glucagon levels. Metabolism 1994;43:270–278.
3. Austin MA, Edwards KL. Small, dense low density lipoproteins, the insulin resistance syndrome and non-insulin-dependent diabetes. Curr Opin Lipid 1996;7:167–171.
4. Berthezene F. Non-insulin dependent diabetes and reverse cholesterol transport. Atherosclerosis 1996;124:S39–S42.
5. Glomset JA. The plasma lecithin:cholesterol acyltransferase reaction. J Lipid Res 1968;9:155–167.
6. Castro GR, Fielding CJ. Early incorporation of cell-derived cholesterol into pre-β-migrating high density lipoprotein. Biochemistry 1988;27:25–29.
7. De la Llera Moya M, Atger V, Paul JL, Fournier N, Moatti N, Giral P, Friday KE, Rothblat G. A

cell culture system for screening human serum for ability to promote cellular cholesterol efflux. Arterioscler Thromb 1994;14:1056—1065.

8. Syvänne M, Castro G, Dengremont C, De Geitere C, Jauhiainen M, Ehnholm C, Michelagnoli S, Franceschini G, Kahri J, Taskinen MR. Cholesterol efflux from Fu5AH hepatoma cells induced by plasma of subjects with or without coronary artery disease and non-insulin-dependent diabetes: importance of LpA-I:A-II particles and phospholipid transfer protein. Atherosclerosis 1996;127:245—253.
9. Cavallero E, Brites F, Delfly B, Nicolaïew N, Decossin C, De Geitere C, Fruchart JC, Wikinski R, Jacotot B, Castro G. Abnormal reverse cholesterol transport in controlled type II diabetic patients. Studies on fasting and postprandial LpA-I particles. Arterioscler Thromb Vasc Biol 1995;15:2130—2135.

Atherosclerosis XI.
B. Jacotot, D. Mathé and J.-C. Fruchart, editors.

The insulin-resistant dyslipidemic syndrome of visceral obesity: an atherogenic cluster

Jean-Pierre Després
Lipid Research Center, Laval University, Sainte-Foy, Québec, Canada

Abstract. Considerable metabolic heterogeneity is found amongst obese patients. Numerous studies published over the last 15 years have emphasized the role of body-fat distribution, especially of visceral adipose tissue accumulation as a critical correlate of metabolic abnormalities, that have been in the past associated with excess fatness per se. Recent findings of the prospective Québec Cardiovascular Study have emphasized that the cluster of metabolic abnormalities found in visceral obese patients (hyperinsulinemia, hyperapo B, small dense LDL particles) is associated with a substantial increase in the risk of ischemic heart disease (IHD). These metabolic complications are even found in the prediabetic state, suggesting that the time for preventive endocrinology may have come.

Introduction

Clinicians are familiar with the considerable metabolic heterogeneity which can be found amongst obese patients. This metabolic heterogeneity raises the important problem of defining obesity from a medical standpoint. Obesity has been traditionally defined by a high accumulation of body fat. However, a substantial number of individuals who are not markedly overweight will eventually develop premature coronary heart disease and diabetes, whereas some obese patients will remain free from these common metabolic complications. In this regard, the development of imaging techniques such as magnetic resonance imaging or computed tomography [1] has allowed measurement (with good precision) of the amount of body fat, but also its distribution. In particular, the amount of adipose tissue located in the abdominal cavity can be measured, the so-called intra-abdominal or visceral adipose tissue. Studies that have been conducted in our laboratory have emphasized the importance of visceral adipose tissue as a critical correlate of the metabolic complications that have been in the past associated with excess fatness per se (for reviews, [2—4]). Thus, excess visceral adipose tissue accumulation has been associated with hyperinsulinemia resulting from an insulin-resistant state, glucose intolerance which may convert to non-insulin-dependent diabetes mellitus (NIDDM) among genetically susceptible individuals, hypertriglyceridemia, elevated LDL particle concentration, increased proportion of small dense LDL particles and reduced plasma HDL-cholesterol concentrations. These metabolic abnormalities have been reported to cluster among

Address for correspondence: Jean-Pierre Després PhD, Lipid Research Center, CHUL Research Center, 2705 Laurier Blvd, TR-93 Sainte-Foy, Québec, Canada G1V 4G2. Tel.: +1-418-654-2133. Fax: +1-418-654-2145. E-mail: jean-pierre.despres@crchul.ulaval.ca

1072

individuals with an excess accumulation of visceral adipose tissue, irrespective of the amount of total body fat.

The insulin-resistant dyslipidemic syndrome: the need to go beyond body weight and conventional plasma lipid management

Thus, some insulin-resistant dyslipidemic patients who would not be considered as being overweight from the current weight/height standards could benefit from a reduction in atherogenic visceral adipose tissue mass. Irrespective of the patient's body weight, excess visceral adipose tissue accumulation is associated with a cluster of metabolic complications which may contribute to increase the risk of NIDDM and cardiovascular disease.

These features of visceral obesity are reminiscent of the characteristics of the insulin-resistance syndrome which was described by Reaven at the end of the 1980s [5]. It is also important to emphasize that the insulin-resistant dyslipidemic state of visceral obesity is not frequently associated with marked elevations in plasma cholesterol and LDL-cholesterol levels [2–4]. Studies conducted in our laboratory have indicated that the clinician should not be misled by these apparently normal plasma cholesterol and LDL-cholesterol levels. Additional techniques such as gradient gel electrophoresis and the measurement of plasma apo B levels have revealed that visceral obese patients are characterized by a substantial increase in apo B concentrations as well as in the proportion of small, dense LDL particles [6].

The atherogenic metabolic complications of visceral obesity: the new metabolic triad

The risk of ischemic heart disease associated with the cluster of metabolic abnormalities found in visceral obesity has been examined in the Québec Cardiovascular Study, a prospective study in which 2,103 middle-aged male subjects were followed over a period of 5 years. This study indicated that fasting hyperinsulinemia was, among nondiabetic men, an independent risk factor for ischemic heart disease (IHD) [7,8]. Furthermore, an elevated apolipoprotein (apo) B concentration (which is another common complication of visceral obesity) was found to be a much better predictor of IHD risk than raised cholesterol or LDL-cholesterol levels [9]. Furthermore, this study indicated that fasting hyperinsulinemia associated with increased apo B levels (the synergic combination found in visceral obese patients) was associated with more than a 10-fold increase in the risk of ischemic heart disease, emphasizing the atherogenic nature of this cluster of metabolic abnormalities [8]. We also recently reported that the presence of small dense LDL particles was associated with an approximately 3-fold increase in IHD risk [10]. The IHD risk was further increased in the presence of elevated apo B levels [10]. As hyperinsulinemia, elevated apo B and an increased proportion of small dense LDL particles are abnormalities which are simultaneously found in visceral obese patients, we have examined the atherogenic potential of this triad of new metabolic complications in the sample of men in the Québec Cardiovascular Study. Unpublished results from our laboratory indicate that hyperinsulinemia combined with elevated apo B was associated with a 20-fold increase in the risk of ischemic heart disease when these metabolic alterations were accompanied by a high proportion of small dense LDL particles (Lamarche et al., unpublished observations). Thus, this "new triad" of metabolic alterations found in visceral obesity substantially increases the risk of ischemic heart disease, even in prediabetic individuals. Considering the high prevalence of visceral obesity in sedentary adult men (about 25%) [4], this cluster of related metabolic abnormalities may represent the most prevalent cause of coronary heart disease in our affluent societies.

The atherogenic metabolic cluster of visceral obesity: therapeutic implications

Therefore, it appears relevant to prevent visceral adipose tissue accumulation observed with age [11]. From a clinical standpoint, therefore, it would be important to target our intervention towards high-risk overweight patients, and to focus on obese patients with excess visceral adipose tissue and metabolic complications [4]. From a practical standpoint, we have shown that a simple anthropometric measurement such as the waist circumference is a crude but better correlate of the absolute amount of visceral fat than the waist-to-hip ratio which has been commonly used in epidemiological studies [12,13]. Recent observations from our laboratory have suggested that waist circumference values of 1 m and above among individuals below 40 years of age and of 90 cm and above among individuals between 40–60 years of age were associated with an increased likelihood of finding the cluster of metabolic abnormalities of visceral obesity [13]. Therefore, emphasis should be placed on the management of body waist rather than weight, and the objective of normalizing body fatness and weight is not always justified from a medical standpoint. Finally, whether the reduction in visceral adipose tissue mass which can be achieved by diet, exercise and pharmacotherapy reduces the incidence of diabetes and cardiovascular disease remains an unresolved issue. Answering this simple question would have tremendous public health implications. The costs of such a study would obviously be considerable but our inaction probably has a much greater impact on our health care expenses.

References

1. Després JP, Ross R, Lemieux S. Imaging techniques applied to the measurement of human body composition. In: Roche AF, Heymsfield SB, Lohman TG (eds) Human Body Composition. Champaign, IL: Human Kinetics 1996;149–166.
2. Després, JP, Moorjani S, Lupien PJ, Tremblay A, Nadeau A, Bouchard C. Regional distribution of body fat, plasma lipoproteins and cardiovascular disease. Arteriosclerosis 1990;10:497–511.
3. Després JP. Visceral obesity: a component of the insulin resistance-dyslipidemic syndrome. Can J Cardiol 1994;10(Suppl B):17B–22B.

4. Després JP. Dyslipidaemia and obesity. Baillière's Clin Endocrin Metab 1994;8:629–660.

5. Reaven GM. Role of insulin resistance in human disease. Diabetes 1988;37:1595–1607.

6. Tchernof A, Lamarche B, Prud'homme, Nadeau A, Moorjani S, Labrie F, Lupien PJ, Després JP. The dense LDL phenotype: association with plasma lipoprotein levels, visceral obesity, and hyperinsulinemia in men. Diabetes Care 1996;19:629–637.

7. Després JP, Lamarche B, Mauriège P, Cantin B, Lupien PJ, Dagenais GR. Risk factors for ischaemic heart disease: is it time to measure insulin? Eur Heart J 1996;17:1453–1454.

8. Després JP, Lamarche B, Mauriège P, Cantin B, Dagenais GR, Moorjani S, Lupien PJ. Hyperinsulinemia as an independent risk factor for ischemic heart disease. N Engl J Med 1996;334:952–957.

9. Lamarche B, Moorjani S, Lupien PJ, Cantin B, Bernard PM, Dagenais GR, Després JP. Apolipoprotein A-I and B levels and the risk of ischemic heart disease during a five-year follow-up of men in the Québec Cardiovascular Study. Circulation 1996;94:273–278.

10. Lamarche B, Tchernof A, Moorjani S, Cantin B, Dagenais GR, Lupien PJ, Després JP. Small, dense low-density lipoprotein particles as a predictor of the risk of ischemic heart disease in men. Circulation 1997;95:69–75.

11. Lemieux S, Prud'homme D, Moorjani S, Tremblay A, Bouchard C, Lupien PJ, Després JP. Do elevated levels of abdominal visceral adipose tissue contribute to age-related differences in plasma lipoprotein concentrations in men? Atherosclerosis 1995;118:155–164.

12. Pouliot MC, Després JP, Lemieux S, Moorjani S, Bouchard C, Tremblay A, Nadeau A, Lupien PJ. Waist circumference and abdominal sagittal diameter as indexes of abdominal visceral adipose tissue accumulation and related cardiovascular risk in men and women. Am J Cardiol 1994;73:460–468.

13. Lemieux S, Prud'homme D, Bouchard C, Tremblay A, Després JP. A single threshold value of waist girth identifies normal-weight and overweight subjects with excess visceral adipose tissue. Am J Clin Nutr 1996;64:685–693.

Insulin resistance, atherosclerosis and CHD

Steven M. Haffner

University of Texas Health Science Center at San Antonio, San Antonio, Texas, USA

Introduction

Non-insulin-dependent diabetes mellitus (NIDDM) is associated with a markedly increased risk of coronary heart disease (CHD) [1,2] which is generally greater in women (approximately 4-fold) than in men (approximately 2-fold) compared to nondiabetic subjects. Although the degree and duration of hyperglycemia are major risk factors for microvascular complications [3,4], in several studies, the duration of diabetes and the severity of hyperglycemia are not related or only weakly related to CHD in subjects with NIDDM [5—8]. In some recent Finnish studies, glycemia has been related to CHD in NIDDM subjects [9,10]. The absence of a strong relation between duration of diabetes and glycemia to CHD in NIDDM subjects suggests that events in the prediabetic state may increase the risk of both CHD and NIDDM. One likely candidate is hyperinsulinemia or insulin resistance [11]. Hyperinsulinemia and/or insulin resistance has been associated with increased CHD [12] although it has been questioned whether insulin itself has a direct atherogenic effect [13]. Clearly, both insulin resistance [14,15] and hyperinsulinemia [16,17] are strong predictors of NIDDM. Increased cardiovascular risk factors have also been found prior to the onset of NIDDM [18—21]. In one study [20], the increased atherogenicity in prediabetic subjects was no longer statistically significant after adjustment for insulin concentrations. Although, interestingly, no study has been done on whether prediabetic subjects have an increased risk of CHD. Since prediabetic subjects have increased cardiovascular risk factors, it seems logical that increased insulin levels in nondiabetics should also be associated with increased cardiovascular risk factors and disease.

The insulin-resistance syndrome

In 1988, Reaven suggested that insulin resistance may underlie a number of disorders including hypertension, dyslipidemia (especially high triglyceride and low high-density lipoprotein levels), impaired glucose tolerance, and CHD (Table 1) [11]. Reaven used the term "syndrome X" to describe these related disorders. We

---

Address for correspondence: Steven M. Haffner MD, Prof Med, University of Texas Health Science Center at San Antonio, 7703 Floyd Curl Drive, San Antonio, TX 78284-7873, USA. Tel.: +1-210-567-4737. Fax: +1-210-567-6955.

have proposed the name insulin-resistance syndrome (IRS), since this highlights the presumed etiology of the syndrome [22]. Although Reaven formulated his concept in terms of the harmful effects of insulin resistance ("low insulin-mediated glucose disposal"), many studies have used increased insulin concentrations as a surrogate for directly measured insulin resistance because the measurement of insulin resistance by the hyperinsulinemic euglycemic clamp insulin suppression test or the frequently sampled intravenous glucose tolerance test (FSIGT) is expensive and has limited patient acceptance. In nondiabetic subjects, increased insulin concentrations generally reflect insulin resistance [23]. In type II diabetes subjects, the fasting insulin level may be a reasonable surrogate for insulin resistance [23]. This is not true of the postglucose insulin level, however, because first-phase insulin secretion is decreased and thus insulin levels may be decreased following oral ingestion of glucose. There is, however, an additional problem with using insulin levels as surrogates for insulin resistance because most conventional insulin assays measure immunoreactive insulin which cross-reacts with proinsulin, and proinsulin is selectively increased in type II diabetes subjects [24]. The increasing use of "specific" or "true" insulin assays that do not cross-react with proinsulin may be helping to resolve this problem.

Insulin levels and cardiovascular risk factors

A number of reports have confirmed that elevated insulin levels are associated, "cross-sectionally", with increased triglyceride levels, decreased high-density lipoprotein levels and hypertension [25]. There are relatively few data, however, to help determine whether insulin concentrations predict the development of metabolic disorders. In the San Antonio Heart Study [22], increased fasting insulin levels significantly predicted the development of type II diabetes, low high-density lipoprotein (HDL) levels, high triglyceride levels, and hypertension over an 8-year follow-up. Moreover, subjects were more likely to develop multiple metabolic disorders than would be predicted from calculating the joint probabil-

Table 1. Syndrome X ("the insulin-resistance syndrome").

A. Original formulation (Reaven 1988)
   1. Hyperinsulinemia
   2. Impaired glucose tolerance
   3. Hypertension
   4. Increased triglyceride
   5. Decreased high-density lipoprotein cholesterol
B. Extensions
   1. Visceral adiposity
   2. Small dense LDL
   3. Increased PAI-1
   4. Decreased sex hormone binding globulin
   5. Postprandial lipemia

ity of developing each single disorder, suggesting that these metabolic disorders do indeed cluster; subjects who developed multiple metabolic disorders had higher insulin concentrations than those who developed only a single disorder.

Small dense LDL, insulin resistance and type II diabetes

A preponderance of smaller denser LDL (LDL subclass pattern B) has been identified as a risk factor for CHD in the general population [26] although this relationship has not been studied in diabetic subjects. Furthermore, LDL size has not been shown to be independent of triglyceride levels in nondiabetic subjects (however, it would be difficult to show statistical independence of LDL size given the strong correlation between these two variables.) Austin et al. [26] have suggested that most individuals can be assigned to one of two LDL subclass patterns (A or B). Smaller denser LDL (type B) is associated with increased triglyceride and decreased HDL cholesterol levels, male gender, hyperinsulinemia and insulin resistance [27–31]. Among these factors the concentrations of triglyceride and HDL cholesterol are most important suggesting that perturbations of these lipoproteins would be most important in changing LDL subclass pattern B to A. A number of studies have suggested that a preponderance of small dense LDL occurs in type II diabetes [27,29,32,33]. In normotriglyceridemic (i.e., triglyceride < 200 mg/dl) type II diabetic subjects, small dense LDL is also found [32] and even after adjustment for the higher triglyceride and lower HDL concentrations in a population-based study, smaller denser LDL was found in type II diabetic subjects relative to normoglycemic subjects [33]. In type II diabetic subjects, the composition of LDL was more abnormal (by preparative ultracentrifugation) in diabetic women than in diabetic men [34]. After intensive control of glycemia, the LDL composition normalized in this study. Thus, diabetic subjects have qualitative changes in LDL that may increase their risk of atherosclerosis even if their overall LDL levels are not different than in male diabetic subjects.

Hyperinsulinemia and the incidence of CHD

Hyperinsulinemia has been identified as a risk factor for CHD in several [35–38], but not in all, studies [39–41] (Table 2). The study of Welborn et al. [35], of both men and women, found a significant relationship between insulin and cardiovascular disease (CHD) only in men. The studies of Pyörälä et al. [36] and Eschwege et al. [12] showed that insulin concentrations were significantly related to CHD in men. Interestingly, the study of Folsom et al. [38] found a significant relation between insulin and CHD in women but not in men. The study by Després et al. [37] provides the strongest evidence that hyperinsulinemia is associated prospectively with the development of CHD. These authors did a nested case-control study in 91 male cases and 105 matched controls from the Quebec Cardiovascular Study. This study had more comprehensive lipid and lipoprotein measurements, including HDL cholesterol and apoprotein B (apo B), at

Table 2. Prospective studies of insulin in relation to cardiovascular disease.

Author	Journal	Year	Reference	Men	Women
Pyörälä	Acta Med Scand	1985	[36]	Y	—
Welborn	Diabet Care	1979	[35]	Y	N
Eschwège	Horm Metab Res	1985	[12]	Y	—
Welin	Diabetologia	1992	[40]	N	—
Orchard	Ann Epidemiol	1994	[39]	N[a]	—
Ferrara	Am J Epidemiol	1994	[41]	N	N
Després	N Engl J Med	1996	[37]	Y	—
Folsom	Diabet Care	1997	[38]	N	Y

Y = significant; N = not significant; — = not studied. [a]Significant interaction with apo E.

baseline, than previous studies (Table 3). In earlier studies [12,35,36], HDL cholesterol was not measured at baseline. Furthermore, the investigators in the Quebec study used an insulin assay that did not cross-react with proinsulin. The authors found that adjustment for other risk factors did not diminish the predictive power of insulin for CHD and that increased levels of both fasting insulin and apo B predicted CHD strongly.

The negative studies by Welin et al. [40] and Ferrara et al. [41] were performed in elderly subjects and thus could have represented a survival bias in that subjects who might have had CHD due to increased insulin resistance might have already died. The negative study by Orchard et al. [39] was done in high-risk subjects (Multiple Risk Factor Intervention Trial) and thus its study population might have been enriched in subjects with insulin resistance. Furthermore, there was an interaction of Apo E phenotype with insulin concentration in relation to CHD incidence in the MRFIT study [39]. Thus far, no study has prospectively shown an association between insulin concentrations and CHD in women. Furthermore, no prospective studies have examined the relationship of insulin resistance (as distinguished from insulin concentration) to CHD.

Insulin resistance and atherosclerosis

Only a few cross-sectional studies have found an association of insulin resistance

Table 3. Relation between fasting insulin at baseline and incident coronary heart disease.

Variable	Model 1 OR (95% C.I.) (univariate)	Model 7 OR (95% C.I.) (multivariate)
Insulin	1.7 (1.3—2.4)[b]	1.6 (1.1—2.3)[a]
Triglyceride	—	1.0 (0.7—1.5)
HDLC	—	1.0 (0.7—1.5)
Apo B	—	1.9 (1.3—2.9)[b]

[a]$p < 0.01$; [b]$p \leqslant 0.001$. Adapted from [37].

(as determined by the hyperinsulinemic euglycemic clamp) with atherosclerosis as measured by carotid ultrasound [42] or coronary angiography [43]. These studies [42,43], however, were small. The relationship between insulin resistance (as measured by the frequently sampled intravenous glucose tolerance test (FSIGT)) and atherosclerosis (as measured by β-mode ultrasound of the carotid) was recently reported in a large multiethnic population (398 Blacks, 457 Hispanics and 542 non-Hispanic Whites) [44]. In the Insulin Resistance Atherosclerosis Study (IRAS) there was a positive association between insulin resistance and the intimal medial thickness (IMT) of the carotid artery both in Hispanics and in non-Hispanic Whites. This effect was reduced but not totally explained by adjustment for traditional cardiovascular disease risk factors, glucose tolerance, measures of adiposity, and fasting insulin levels. However, there was no significant association between insulin resistance and intimal medial thickness in Blacks. The reasons for the lack of association between atherosclerosis and insulin resistance in Blacks are not well-understood but could relate partly to the increased insulin resistance observed in Blacks [45]; there may be a plateau effect below which only weak relations between insulin sensitivity and atherosclerosis are seen.

Conclusion

Type II diabetes is associated with a 2- to 4-fold excess of CHD, compared to nondiabetic populations. In most studies of type II diabetes, degree of hyperglycemia and duration of clinical diabetes have been found to be only weak risk factors for CHD development, while conventional CHD risk factors such as dyslipidemia and hypertension have consistently been identified as strong risk factors for CHD development. Hyperinsulinemia and insulin resistance, which are predictive of the development of type II diabetes, in some studies have been shown to be predictive of CHD development.

In order to prevent the excess risk of CHD in subjects with type II diabetes, a multifactorial approach will be necessary. Improved glycemic control is likely to have a beneficial, although probably minor, effect. Attention should be paid to the avoidance of weight gain. Aggressive treatment of cardiovascular risk factors will be necessary. As shown in the 4S study, for example, aggressive lowering of LDL levels in subjects with a prior myocardial infarction is at least as effective in reducing the reinfarction rate in type II diabetes subjects as in nondiabetic subjects [46]. Glucose lowering agents which do not raise concentrations (such as metformin, acarbose, and troglitazone), may lead to improvement in CHD risk factors relative to glucose lowering agents that raise insulin concentrations (sulfonylureas). Finally, primary prevention of type II diabetes is also important. At the 1996 American Diabetes Association meetings, the start of a major NIH funded project to prevent diabetes was announced. This study (Diabetes Prevention Project) will enroll 4,000 subjects with baseline IGT and follow them for 3—6 years. The four treatment arms are:

1) usual care;
2) intensive weight loss and increased physical activity;
3) metformin; and
4) troglitazone.

The primary endpoint will be the prevention of type II diabetes mellitus. The study will also test whether interventions reduce the progression of atherosclerosis using β-mode ultrasound of the carotids. This trial will help to assess how closely changes in insulin sensitivity are related to atherosclerosis and whether they are indeed mediated by changes in other CHD risk factors. This is critical because several studies have shown increased CHD risk factors prior to the onset of type II diabetes [18—21].

References

1. Kannel WB, McGee DL. Diabetes and glucose tolerance as risk factors for cardiovascular disease: the Framingham Study. JAMA 1979;241:2035—2038.
2. Wingard DL, Barrett-Connor E. Heart disease and diabetes. In: Diabetes in America, 2nd edn. National Institute of Health, National Institute of Diabetes and Digestive and Kidney Diseases, National Diabetes Data Group, 1995;429—448.
3. Diabetes Drafting Group. Prevalence of small vessel and large vessel disease in diabetic patients from 14 centers: the World Health Organization Multinational Study of Vascular Disease in Diabetics. Diabetologia 1985;28:615—640.
4. Klein R, Klein BEK, Moss SE et al. Glycosylated hemoglobin of diabetic retinopathy. JAMA 1988;260:2864—2871.
5. Herman JB, Medalie JH, Goldbourt U. Differences in cardiovascular morbidity and mortality between previously known and newly diagnosed adult diabetics. Diabetologia 1977;13: 229—234.
6. West KM, Ahuja MMS, Bennett PH et al. The role of circulating glucose and triglyceride concentrations and their interactions with other "risk factors" as determinants of arterial disease in nine diabetic population samples from the WHO Multinational Study. Diabet Care 1983;6: 361—369.
7. Fuller JH, Shipley MJ, Rose G et al. Coronary heart disease and impaired glucose tolerance: The Whitehall Study. Lancet 1980;1:1373—1376.
8. Morrish NJ, Stevens LK, Head J et al. A prospective study of mortality among middle-aged diabetic patients (the London cohort of the WHO Multinational Study of Vascular Disease in Diabetics). II. Associated risk factors. Diabetologia 1990;33:542—548.
9. Kuusisto J, Mykkänen L, Pyörälä K, Laakso M. NIDDM and its metabolic control predict coronary heart disease in elderly subjects. Diabetes 1994;43:960—967.
10. Laakso M, Lehto S, Pentillä I, Pyörälä K. Lipids and lipoproteins predicting coronary heart disease mortality and morbidity in patients with non-insulin-dependent diabetes. Circulation 1993;88:1421—1430.
11. Reaven GM. Banting Lecture 1988. Role of insulin resistance in human disease. Diabetes 1988; 37:1596—1607.
12. Eschwège E, Richard JL, Thibult N et al. Coronary heart disease mortality in relation with diabetes, blood glucose and plasma insulin levels: The Paris Prospective Study, ten years later. Horm Metab Res 1985;15(Suppl):41.
13. Stern MP. Perspectives in diabetes. Diabetes and cardiovascular disease: the "common soil" hypothesis. Diabetes 1995;44:369—374.
14. Warram JH, Martin BD, Krolewski AS, Soeldner JS, Kahn CR. Slow glucose removal rate and

hyperinsulinemia precede the development of type II diabetes in the offspring of diabetic parents. Ann Intern Med 1990;113:909—915.

15. Lillioja S, Mott DM, Spraul M, Ferraro R, Foley JE, Ravussin E, Knowler WC, Bennett PH, Bogardus C. Insulin resistance and insulin secretory dysfunction as precursors of non-insulin-dependent diabetes mellitus. Prospective studies of Pima Indians. N Engl J Med 1993;329: 1988—1992.

16. Haffner SM, Miettinen H, Gaskill SP, Stern MP. Decreased insulin secretion and increased insulin secretion are independently related to the 7-year risk of non-insulin-dependent diabetes mellitus. Diabetes 1995;44:1386—1391.

17. Saad MF, Knowler WC, Pettitt DJ, Nelson RG, Mott DM, Bennett PH. Sequential changes in serum insulin concentration during development of non-insulin dependent diabetes. Lancet 1989;1:1356—1359.

18. McPhillips JB, Barrett-Connor E, Wingard DL. Cardiovascular disease risk factors prior to the diagnosis of impaired glucose tolerance and non-insulin-dependent diabetes mellitus in a community of older adults. Am J Epidemiol 1990;131:443—453.

19. Medalie JH, Papier CM, Goldbourt U, Herman JB. Major factors in the development of diabetes mellitus in 10,000 men. Arch Int Med 1975;135:811—817.

20. Haffner SM, Stern MP, Hazuda HP, Mitchell BD, Patterson JK. Cardiovascular risk factors in confirmed prediabetic individuals. Does the clock for coronary heart disease start ticking before the onset of clinical diabetes? JAMA 1990;263:2893—2898.

21. Mykkänen L, Kuusisto J, Pyörälä K, Laakso M. Cardiovascular disease risk factors as predictors of type II (non-insulin-dependent) diabetes mellitus in elderly subjects. Diabetologia 1993; 36:553—559.

22. Haffner SM, Valdez RA, Hazuda HP, Mitchell BD, Morales PA, Stern MP. Prospective analyses of the insulin resistance syndrome (Syndrome X). Diabetes 1992;41:715—722.

23. Laakso M. How good a marker is insulin level for insulin resistance? Am J Epidemiol 1993;137: 959—965.

24. Haffner SM, Bowsher RR, Mykkänen L, Hazuda HP, Mitchell BD, Valdez RA, Gingerich R, Monterossa A, Stern MP. Proinsulin and specific insulin concentrations in high and low risk populations for type II diabetes. Diabetes 1994;43:1490—1493.

25. Zavaroni I, Bonora E, Pagliara M, Dall'Aglio E, Luchetti L, Buonanno G, Bonati PA, Bergonzani M, Gnudi L, Passeri M, Reaven GM. Risk factors for coronary artery disease in healthy persons with hyperinsulinemia and normal glucose tolerance. N Engl J Med 1989;320:702—706.

26. Austin MA, Breslow JL, Hennekens CHD, Buring JE, Willett WC, Krauss RM. Low density lipoprotein subclass patterns and risk of myocardial infarction. JAMA 1988;260:1917—1921.

27. Barakat HA, Carpenter JW, McLendon VD, Khazanie P, Leggett N, Heath J, Marks R. Influence of obesity, impaired glucose tolerance and NIDDM on LDL structure and composition: possible link between hyperinsulinemia and atherosclerosis. Diabetes 1990;39:1527—1533.

28. Haffner SM, Mykkänen L, Valdez RA, Paidi M, Stern MP, Howard BV. LDL size and subclass pattern in a biethnic population. Arteriosclerosis 1993;13:1623—1630.

29. Selby JV, Austin MA, Newman B, Zhang D, Quesenberry CP, Mayer EJ, Krauss RM. LDL subclass phenotypes and the insulin resistance syndrome in women. Circulation 1993;85:381—387.

30. Reaven GM, Chen YD, Jeppesen J, Maheux P, Krauss RM. Insulin resistance in individuals with small, dense lipoprotein particles. J Clin Invest 1993;92:141—146.

31. McNamara JR, Campos H, Ordovas JM, Peterson RM, Wilson PW, Schaefer EJ. Effect of gender, age and lipid status on low density subfraction distribution: results of the Framingham Offspring Study. Arteriosclerosis 1987;7:483—490.

32. Feingold KR, Grunfeld C, Doerrler W, Krauss RM. LDL subclass phenotypes and triglyceride metabolism in non-insulin-dependent diabetes. Arterioscler Thromb 1992;12:1496—1502.

33. Haffner SM, Mykkänen L, Stern MP, Paidi M, Howard BV. Greater effect of diabetes on LDL size in women than in men. Diabet Care 1994;17:1164—1171.

34. Caixàs A, Ordóñmez-Llanos J, de Leiva A, Payés A, Homs R, Pérez A. Optimization of glyce-

mic control by insulin therapy decreases the proportion of small dense LDL patients in diabetic patients. Diabetes 1997;46:1207—1213.

35. Welborn TA, Wearne K. Coronary heart disease incidence and cardiovascular mortality in Busselton with reference to glucose and insulin concentrations. Diabet Care 1979;2:154—160.

36. Pyörälä K, Savolainen E, Kaukola S, Haapakoski J. Plasma insulin as coronary heart disease risk factor: Relationship to other risk factors and predictive during 9½ year follow-up of the Helsinki Policeman Study population. Acta Med Scand 1985;701(Suppl):38—52.

37. Després JP, Lamarche B, Mauriége P, Cantin B, Dagenais GR, Moorjani S, Lupien PJ. Hyperinsulinemia as an independent risk factor for ischemic heart disease. N Engl J Med 1996;334:952—957.

38. Folsom AR, Szklo M, Stevens J, Liao F, Smith R, Eckfeldt JH. A prospective study for coronary heart disease in relation to fasting insulin, glucose, and diabetes: The Atherosclerosis Risk in Communities (ARIC) Study. Diabet Care 1997;20:935—942.

39. Orchard TJ, Eichner J, Kuller LH, Becker DJ, McCallum LM, Grandits GA. Insulin as a predictor of coronary heart disease: Interaction with Apolipoprotein E phenotype. A report from the Multiple Risk Factor Intervention Trial. Ann Epidemiol 1994;4:40—45.

40. Welin L, Eriksson H, Larsson B, Ohlson LO, Svardsudd K, Tibblin G. Hyperinsulinemia is not a major coronary risk factor in elderly men. The study of men born in 1913. Diabetologia 1992;35:766—770.

41. Ferrara A, Barrett-Connor EL, Edelstein SL. Hyperinsulinemia does not increase the risk of fatal cardiovascular disease in elderly men or women without diabetes: the Rancho Bernardo Study, 1984—1991. Am J Epidemiol 1994;140:857—869.

42. Laakso M, Sarlund H, Salonen R, Suhonen M, Pyörälä K, Salonen JT, Karhapää P. Asymptomatic atherosclerosis and insulin resistance. Arterioscler Thromb 1991;11:1068—1076.

43. Bressler P, Bailey SR, Matsuda M, DeFronzo RA. Insulin resistance and coronary artery disease. Diabetologia 1996;39:1345—1350.

44. Howard G, O'Leary DH, Zaccaro D, Haffner SM, Rewers M, Hamman R, Selby JV, Saad MF, Savage P, Bergman R. Insulin sensitivity and atherosclerosis. Circulation 1996;93:1809—1817.

45. Haffner SM, D'Agostino R, Saad MF, Rewers M, Mykkänen L, Selby J, Howard G, Savage PJ, Hamman RF, Wagenknecht LE, Bergman RN. Increased insulin resistance and insulin secretion in non-diabetic African Americans and Hispanics compared with non-Hispanic whites: the Insulin Resistance Atherosclerosis Study. Diabetes 1996;45:742—748.

46. Pyörälä K, Pedersen JR, Kjekshus J, Faergerman O, Olsson AG, Thorgeirsson G. Cholesterol lowering with simvastatin improves prognosis of diabetic patients with coronary heart disease. A subgroup analyses of the Scandinavian Simvastatin Survival Study (4S). Diabet Care 1997;20:614—620.

Lipoprotein abnormalities and insulin resistance

Richard W. James

Clinical Diabetes Unit, Division of Endocrinology and Diabetology, University Hospital, Geneva, Switzerland

Introduction

Non-insulin-dependent diabetes (NIDDM) is characterised by multiple anomalies affecting the three principal lipoprotein classes VLDL, LDL and HDL [1,2]. Whilst the disturbances manifest quantitatively for VLDL (hypertriglyceridaemia) and HDL (low HDL-cholesterol) they are less evident for LDL. Here they are of a more qualitative nature, notably with an increased prevalence of small dense particles, especially in poorly controlled patients [3]. This is an important cardiovascular disease (CVD) risk factor [4]. Qualitative abnormalities are also evident for VLDL (which are larger in size) and HDL where there is a decrease in particle diameter. To what extent specific aspects of the diabetic state contribute to these aberrations, and ultimately, to the increased incidence of vascular disease in diabetes, is an important question. Of particular interest in this respect is insulin resistance. We have attempted to address the question of the role of insulin resistance in lipoprotein anomalies with studies of four groups of subjects with varying degrees of insulin resistance. The subjects were studied before and after a hyperinsulinaemic clamp.

Methods

Participants were recruited from the personnel of the University Hospital, Geneva or patients attending the outpatients clinic of the hospital. Informed consent was obtained from all participants and the study was conducted according to the requirements of the Ethical Commission of the Medical Faculty. Four groups of subjects were defined: controls (group 1), obese glucose tolerant patients (group 2), obese glucose intolerant patients (group 3) and NIDDM patients (group 4). Characteristics of the groups are given in Table 1. Plasma samples were obtained before and after 4 h of hyperinsulinaemic clamp. Subfractions of VLDL (VLDL-1, Sf 100–400; VLDL-2, Sf 60–100; VLDL-3, Sf 20–60) and LDL (LDL-1, Sf 12–20; LDL-2, Sf 6–12; LDL-3, Sf 3–6) were isolated by cumulative flotation ultracentrifugation, as described previously in detail [3]. Concentrations of total protein and individual lipid components (triglycerides,

Address for correspondence: Dr Richard W. James, Clinical Diabetes Unit, Division of Endocrinology and Diabetology, University Hospital, 24 rue Micheli-du-Crest, 1211 Geneva 14, Switzerland.

1084

Table 1. Characteristics of study groups.

	Group 1	Group 2	Group 3	Group 4	p
n (M/F)	10.00 (7/3)	12.00 (8/4)	7.00 (5/2)	14.00 (10/4)	ns
Age	37.50 (3.1)	49.00 (2.8)	49.00 (3.7)	55.20 (2.6)	0.002
Glucose disposal	6.23 (0.5)	3.38 (0.4)	2.27 (0.6)	1.52 (0.4)	0.001
Insulin during clamp	521.00 (73)	659.00 (70)	667.00 (87)	757.00 (62)	ns
Fasting glucose	4.90 (0.4)	5.10 (0.4)	5.50 (0.5)	7.40 (0.3)	0.001
Free fatty acids	0.65 (0.07)	0.73 (0.06)	0.80 (0.08)	0.90 (0.06)	0.05
Triglycerides	1.23 (0.21)	1.40 (0.19)	1.39 (0.25)	1.69 (0.18)	ns
Cholesterol	4.77 (0.30)	5.13 (0.28)	5.09 (0.37)	4.61 (0.25)	ns
HDL-cholesterol	1.11 (0.06)	0.81 (0.06)	0.82 (0.07)	0.82 (0.05)	0.002
BMI	23.10 (1.7)	30.90 (1.6)	35.00 (2.0)	36.60 (1.3)	0.001

Mean values (SEM) are given with age in years, glucose disposal as mg/kg fat free mass/min, insulin in pmol/l and all other values in mmol/l. BMI, weight(kg)/height (m^2). Comparisons were made by ANOVA.

phospholipids, free and esterified cholesterol) were determined [3,5] and summed to give the total subfraction concentration. Statistical analyses were performed with the JMP statistical package (SAS Institute Inc., Cary, NC). Triglyceride and VLDL subfraction concentrations were converted to log values prior to analysis.

Results

As shown in Table 1, the control group was younger and nonobese. HDL-cholesterol was higher in this group, but there were no significant differences between the four groups for cholesterol and triglycerides. Free fatty acids tended to be higher in the diabetic patients. A similar degree of hyperinsulinaemia was achieved during the clamp (Table 1) where there were important and highly significant decreases of plasma free fatty acid concentrations. These were of a similar magnitude in all four groups (0.59–0.63mm/l) representing a 70–90% decrease (Fig. 1A). A less consistent impact of hyperinsulinaemia was observed on large VLDL (VLDL-1). Plasma concentrations were significantly decreased in controls (p = 0.001) and obese glucose tolerant patients (p = 0.023). However, there were no changes in concentrations of VLDL-1 for groups 3 and 4 (Fig. 1B). Conversely, at the opposing end of the VLDL spectrum, small VLDL (VLDL-3) were unaffected by the hyperinsulinaemic clamp in groups 1 and 2, but there were decreased concentrations in obese glucose intolerant and NIDDM patients (results not shown). In univariate analysis, the percentage decrease of large VLDL was positively correlated with glucose disposal (r = 0.67, p < 0.0001), negatively correlated with insulin resistance and positively correlated with the percentage fall in free fatty acids (r = 0.63, p < 0.0001). In forward stepwise regression analysis (including glucose disposal (insulin resistance), percentage fall in free fatty acids, indices of body weight and fat distribution, plasma lipid levels, gender and age), only insulin resistance (p < 0.0001) and gender (p

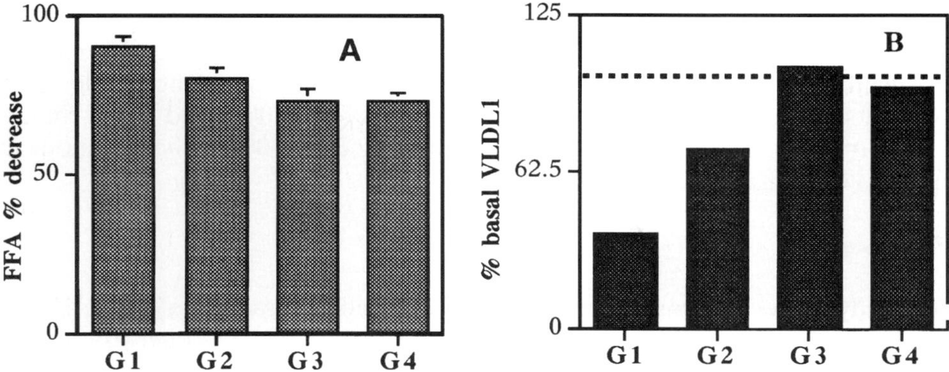

Fig. 1. Decreases in free fatty acids and VLDL-1 during the hyperinsulinaemic clamp. **A**: Percentage decrease in plasma free fatty acids during the hyperinsulinaemic clamp ($p < 0.0001$ for all groups). **B**: Plasma VLDL-1 concentrations after the hyperinsulinaemic clamp expressed as a percentage of basal, preclamp concentrations. G1 controls ($p = 0.001$); G2 obese glucose tolerant ($p = 0.02$); G3 obese glucose intolerant; and G4 NIDDM. The dotted line indicates the 100% value.

$= 0.007$) entered the model. This model accounted for 75% of the variations in the decrease of VLDL-1.

Subfractionation of LDL gives rise to three subfractions of which LDL-2 represents large particles and LDL-3 represents small dense LDL particles [3,6]. The ratio of the plasma concentrations of the two types of particle is thus an indication of the prevalence of small dense LDL particles. When analysed in plasma samples taken prior to installation of the hyperinsulinaemic clamp, a decrease in the ratio was observed when passing from the controls to the NIDDM patients: mean values (SEM); controls 3.53 (0.66), obese glucose tolerant 2.77 (0.56), obese glucose intolerant 2.40 (1.10), NIDDM 2.29 (0.42). Table 2 shows the univariate correlations between the ratio and various parameters. The strongest correlation was observed with fasting triglyceride concentrations, whilst HDL-cholesterol and glucose disposal were also significantly correlated with the

Table 2. Correlations between the LDL2/LDL3 concentration ratios and different parameters.

	Univariate correlation		Corrected for triglycerides	
	r	p	r	p
Triglycerides	− 0.57	0.0001	—	—
Glucose disposal	0.35	0.026	0.08	ns
HDL-cholesterol	0.50	0.001	0.36	0.022
% decrease FFA	0.20	ns	− 0.04	ns
Waist-to-hip ratio	− 0.30	0.063	− 0.16	ns
BMI	− 0.18	ns	− 0.02	ns
Cholesterol	− 0.07	ns	− 0.01	ns
Gender	0.19	ns	—	—

ratio. The waist-to-hip ratio was of borderline significance. When these univariate correlations were corrected for triglycerides, only HDL-cholesterol remained independently associated with the LDL2/LDL3 concentration ratio (Table 2). In forward stepwise regression analysis, triglycerides (p < 0.001) and HDL-cholesterol (p = 0.03) entered the model, which accounted for 40% of the variations in the ratio of LDL2/LDL3.

Discussion

The study shows that insulin modulates plasma concentrations of large VLDL, decreasing their levels in insulin-sensitive subjects. In contrast, concentrations of small VLDL were not altered, underlining the dichotomous action of insulin on triglyceride-rich lipoproteins. The action of insulin on large VLDL was impaired in glucose intolerant and NIDDM patients where no decrease was observed. This was very strongly associated with insulin resistance rather than a fall in plasma free fatty acid concentrations.

There is presently disagreement concerning the role of insulin in regulating VLDL levels. One hypothesis suggested a stimulatory effect of acute hyperinsulinaemia on VLDL production [7]. This has been strongly challenged with data indicating acute inhibition of VLDL production by insulin [8,9]. The latter would appear a logical action as it would limit hepatic release of VLDL during the post-prandial phase at a time when chylomicrons are available. This would minimise competition between the two types of triglyceride-rich lipoprotein for lipolytic and removal processes. In studies of obese patients, Lewis et al. [10] reported impaired action of insulin on plasma VLDL downregulation. The present data concur and demonstrate that it concerns only large VLDL. More importantly, the study suggests that in obesity the extent of impairment may depend on the degree of associated insulin resistance. The role of insulin in diabetic patients has been less clear. Cummings et al. [11] reported downregulation of VLDL synthesis in diabetic patients studied with stable isotope techniques indicating no impairment of insulin action. In contrast, a very recent study by Malmström et al. [12], employing a similar approach, did observe inhibition of synthesis of large VLDL during a hyperinsulinaemic clamp in NIDDM patients. The data from the NIDDM and obese glucose intolerant patients studied herein are consistent with the conclusions of impaired action of insulin on large VLDL synthesis and provide evidence of a graded effect depending on the degree of insulin sensitivity.

There was a worsening of the large to small LDL concentration ratio after the hyperinsulinaemic clamp in obese glucose intolerant and NIDDM patients. This is consistent with a more atherogenic profile given the role presently attributed to small dense LDL as a CVD risk factor. Whereas insulin can be directly implicated in qualitative modifications of VLDL, its involvement at the LDL level is less evident. The data suggest that triglycerides are the primary determinants of an increased prevalence of small dense LDL. No independent correlation with insulin resistance was apparent. However, insulin resistance could contribute to the production of small dense LDL by potentiating postprandial hypertriglyceridaemia. This would facilitate triglyceride and esterified cholesterol exchange between triglyceride-rich lipoproteins and LDL. The latter process is thought to predispose LDL to the formation of small dense LDL, probably due to the activity of hepatic lipase [13,14].

In conclusion, insulin action is impaired in glucose intolerant and NIDDM patients and this is related to the degree of insulin resistance. It would predispose such patients to a number of lipoprotein abnormalities, generating a more atherogenic profile. Specific aspects of the diabetic state (insulin resistance) can thus be directly implicated in pathological modifications to VLDL, but a direct role at the LDL level is less apparent. The data also illustrate metabolic dichotomy between large and small VLDL.

Acknowledgements

The study was supported by a grant from the Swiss National Research Foundation.

References

1. Pyörälä K, Laakso M, Uusitupa M. Diabetes and atherosclerosis: an epidemiological view. Diabet Metab Rev 1987;3:463—524.
2. Tomkin GH, Owens D. Insulin and lipoprotein metabolism with special reference to the diabetic state. Diabet Metab Rev 1994;10:225—252.
3. James RW, Pometta D. The distribution profiles of very low density and low-density lipoproteins in poorly controlled male, type 2 (non-insulin-dependent) diabetic patients. Diabetologia 1991; 34:246—252.
4. Austin MA, Breslow JL, Hennekens CH, Buring JE, Willett WC, Krauss RM. Low-density lipoprotein subclass patterns and risk of myocardial infarction. JAMA 1988;260:1917—1922.
5. James RW, Pometta D. Differences in lipoprotein subfraction composition and distribution between type 1 diabetic men and control subjects. Diabetes 1990;39:1158—1164.
6. Lindgren FT, Jensen LC, Hatch FT. The isolation and quantitative analysis of serum lipoproteins. In: Nelson GJ (ed) Blood Lipids and Lipoproteins; Quantitation, Composition, and Metabolism. New York: Wiley-Interscience, 1972;181—274.
7. Reaven GM, Chen Y-DI. The role of insulin in regulation of lipoprotein metabolism in diabetes. Diabet Metab Rev 1988;4:639—652.
8. Gibbons GF. Assembly and secretion of hepatic very low density lipoprotein. Biochem J 1990; 268:1—13.
9. Sparks JD, Sparks CE. Insulin regulation of triacylglycerol-rich lipoprotein synthesis and secretion. Biochim Biophys Acta 1994;1215:9—32.
10. Lewis GF, Uffelman KD, Szeto LW, Steiner G. Effects of acute hyperinsulinemia on VLDL triglyceride and VLDL apo B production in normal weight and obese individuals. Diabetes 1993;42:833—842.
11. Cummings MH, Watts GF, Umpleby AM, Hennessy TR, Kelly JM, Jackson NC, Sönksen PH. Acute hyperinsulinemia decreases the hepatic secretion of very low density lipoprotein apolipoprotein B-100 in NIDDM. Diabetes 1995;44:1059—1065.
12. Malmström R, Packard CJ, Caslake M, Bedford D, Stewart P, Yki-Järvinen H, Shepherd J, Tas-

kinen M-R. Defective regulation of triglyceride metabolism by insulin in the liver in NIDDM. Diabetologia 1997;40:454–462.

13. Zambon A, Austin MA, Brown BG, Hokanson JE, Brunzell JD. Effect of hepatic lipase on LDL in normal men and those with coronary artery disease. Arterioscl Thromb 1993;13:147–153.

14. Tan CE, Forster L, Caslake MJ, Bedford D, Watson TDG, McConnell M, Packard CJ, Shepherd J. Relations between plasma lipids and postheparin plasma lipases and VLDL and LDL subfraction patterns in normolipaemic men and women. Arterioscl Thromb Vasc Biol 1995;15:1839–1848.

Is insulin regulation of VLDL production defective in insulin resistance?

M.-R. Taskinen[1], R. Malmström[1], M. Caslake[2], D. Bedford[2], P. Stewart[2], J. Shepherd[2] and C. Packard[2]

[1]Department of Medicine, University of Helsinki, Helsinki, Finland; and [2]Royal Infirmary, Glasgow, UK

Keywords: apo B production, hyperinsulinism, type II diabetes.

Patients with type II diabetes are at greater risk of developing coronary heart disease (CHD) than the nondiabetic population [1–3]. Data from the Multiple Risk Factor Intervention Trial (MRFIT) highlights the excess risk of CHD in the presence of none or one to three traditional risk factors comprising smoking, hypertension and high cholesterol in diabetic populations as compared to non-diabetic population [3]. Data from the MRFIT study also shows that at any given cholesterol level the risk of cardiovascular mortality is higher in diabetic patients than in nondiabetic cohort. Thus, the traditional risk factors are operative but do not explain the excess CHD risk in diabetic cohorts. There is no shortage of potential candidates to explain the gap for the excess CHD risk between diabetic and nondiabetic populations. Diabetic dyslipidemia as an atherogenic condition has received particular attention in relation to the increased CHD risk [4]. In order to prevent premature vascular disease in type II diabetic patients we need to know the underlying mechanism of diabetic dyslipidemia.

Components of diabetic dyslipidemia

Diabetic dyslipidemia has a special profile. An elevated triglyceride level is the most common feature together with a low level of high-density lipoprotein (HDL) cholesterol. The concentration of serum and LDL cholesterol is similar or even lower than in a nondiabetic population matched for race, age and gender [5]. The presence of hypertriglyceridemia has a profound effect on the metabolic interaction of all other lipoproteins: VLDL, IDL, LDL and HDL subclasses. The metabolic consequences of an elevation of triglyceride-rich lipoproteins (TRLs) comprise exaggerated postprandial lipemia, preponderance of small dense LDL and compositional changes of HDL particles. We consider that the key abnormality in the sequence of events is a long-residence time of TRLs in cir-

Address for correspondence: Prof Marja-Riitta Taskinen, Department of Medicine, University of Helsinki, Haartmaninkatu 4, FIN-00290 Helsinki, Finland. Fax: +358-9-471-4694.

culation, due to the competition of both chylomicrons and endogenous VLDL particles for common removal pathways which become oversaturated [4]. In this scenario, the long-residency time allows excessive transfer of core lipids (triglycerides and cholesteryl esters) between TRLs and LDL and HDL particles. The end result of this transfer process is TG enrichment of both LDL and HDL particles. These TG-enriched particles are good substrates for hepatic lipase (HL) that produce small dense LDL particles and small dense HDL particles. The key issue is that even mild elevation of plasma triglycerides is associated with these potentially highly atherogenic changes in other lipoprotein subclasses.

New insights into pathogenesis of hypertriglyceridemia in type II diabetes

If the concept is acknowledged that the primary disturbance in diabetic dyslipidemia is the elevation of plasma triglycerides, the key question is "What are the underlying mechanisms behind the elevation of plasma triglycerides in type II diabetes?" The prevailing sequence of events has been as follows: insulin resistance results in compensatory hyperinsulinism that directly stimulates VLDL production in the liver, and the end result is the elevation of plasma triglycerides [6]. However, this concept is a topic of ongoing debate based on controversial data from both in vitro experiments and recent in vivo studies [7,8]. It has been reported that in studies using cultured hepatocytes insulin actually suppresses VLDL apo B production. In line with this, recent kinetic studies have shown that insulin acutely suppresses both VLDL apo and VLDL triglyceride production in man [8]. These pioneer studies have left several questions open to debate:
1. What is the actual site of insulin action on apo B production?
2. Are the acute and chronic effects of insulin similar or different?
3. What is the role of FFA flux in the regulation of metabolic pathways of apo B and triglycerides in the liver?
4. Most importantly, is the site of insulin action in the liver influenced by insulin resistance?

Consequently we have designed a series of experiments aimed to answer question 1. What is the major site of insulin action on VLDL apo B metabolism? Is the suppression of VLDL apo B production by insulin impaired in type II diabetic patients? To answer these questions we studied VLDL apo B metabolism using $3\text{-}^3\text{H}$ leucine during an 8.5-h infusion of saline (control), and during 8.5-h infusion of insulin and glucose (serum insulin ~ 540 pmol/l) in normal men (n = 7) and in type II diabetic men (n = 6). The kinetic analyses and multicompartmental modelling of the data were performed using a CONSAM modelling program, and a new non-steady-state multicompartmental model that allows us to take account of changes in apo B pool sizes during insulin infusion. The novel observation was that in normal men acute hyperinsulinemia suppresses VLDL1 apo B production, but has no effect on de novo VLDL2 apo B production [9]. The suppression of VLDL1 apo B production by insulin averaged 50% in normal men. It is worth noting that insulin had no effect on any kinetic parameters of apo B catabolic rates. In conclusion, we have uncovered an action of insulin on VLDL1 apo B production that was postulated to occur on the basis of cell-culture findings. Our data also provided evidence for the concept that VLDL1 and VLDL2 apo B metabolism are independently regulated, and that insulin only has a specific action on the flux of large buoyant VLDL1 particles.

The principal finding in type II diabetic men was in contrast to the observed 40—50% suppression seen in VLDL1 apo B release in normal men, insulin failed to suppress VLDL1 apo B production [10]. In fact, the actual VLDL1 apo B production rates were closely similar after saline and insulin infusions (701 ± 102 vs. 603 ± 145 mg/dl) in type II diabetic men. These data indicate that a component of insulin resistance is the failure of insulin in the liver to suppress the release of triglyceride-rich large VLDL1 particles. The impairment of this insulin action may be the root cause of elevation in plasma triglyceride-rich lipoproteins in type II diabetes and insulin resistance.

Conclusion

We envisage large VLDL1 particles as the liver's chylomicrons which should be released only in a fasting state when food is not available (Fig. 1). Postprandially, when abundant triglycerides are present in chylomicrons the physiological action of insulin would be to suppress the release of VLDL1 particles. This would also relieve postprandial competition between chylomicrons and VLDL1 particles and prevent fat intolerance. Thus the physiological role of insulin is to maintain the balance between intestine-derived and liver-derived triglyceride-rich particles. The failure to suppress VLDL1 particle release in type II diabetes contributes to postprandial lipemia, as well as to changes seen in other lipoprotein classes, and may be a potential link between diabetic dyslipidemia and CHD.

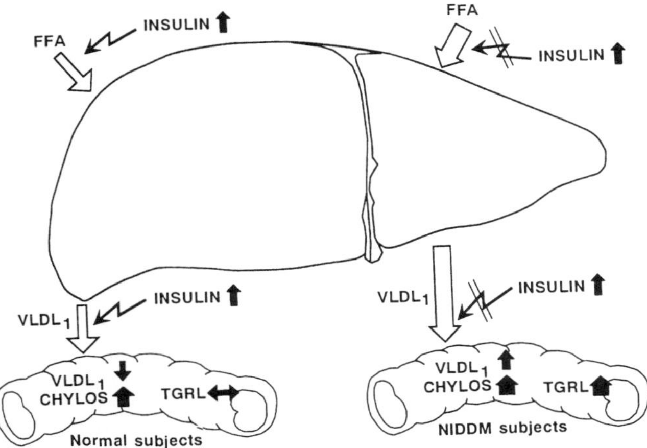

Fig. 1.

References

1. Pyörälä K, Laakso M, Uusitupa K. Diabetes and atherosclerosis: an epidemiologic view. Diabet Metab Rev 1987;3:464—524.
2. Bierman EL. Atherogenesis in diabetes. Arterioscl Thromb 1992;12:647—656.
3. Stamler J, Vaccaro O, Neaton JD, Wentworth D. Diabetes, other risk factors, and 12 year cardiovascular mortality for men screened in the multiple risk factor intervention trial. Diabetes Care 1993;16:434—444.
4. Syvänne M, Taskinen M-R. Lipids and lipoproteins as coronary risk factors in non-insulin-dependent diabetes mellitus. Lancet 1997;350(Suppl I):20—23.
5. Taskinen M-R. Quantitative and qualitative lipoprotein abnormalities in diabetes mellitus. Diabetes 1992;41(Suppl 2):12—17.
6. Reaven GM. Role of insulin resistance in human disease. Diabetes 1988;37:1595—1607.
7. Sparks JD, Sparks CE. Hormonal regulation of lipoprotein assembly and secretion. Curr Opin Lipid 1993;4:177—186.
8. Lewis GF. Fatty acid regulation of very low density lipoprotein production. Curr Opin Lipid 1997;8:146—153.
9. Malmström R, Packard CJ, Watson TDG et al. Metabolic basis of hypotriglyceridemic effects of insulin in normal men. Arterioscl Thromb Vasc Biol 1997;17:1454—1464.
10. Malmström R, Packard CJ, Caslake M et al. Defective regulation of triglyceride metabolism by insulin in the liver in non-insulin-dependent diabetes mellitus. Diabetologia 1997;40:454—462.

Platelets

Atherosclerosis XI.
B. Jacotot, D. Mathé and J.-C. Fruchart, editors.

Proteolytically activated receptors in the regulation of hemostasis

Wadie F. Bahou
Division of Hematology, State University of New York, New York, USA

Keywords: endothelium, G proteins, genetic mapping, serine proteases.

Introduction: serine proteases in cellular activation

Macromolecular assembly and generation of serine proteases on cellular surfaces is critically involved in the regulation of hemostatic, inflammatory or fibrinolytic pathways. This process, ultimately forming the fibrin gel, is further regulated by the recruitment of platelets and leukocytes to the activated endothelial cell surface, thereby functioning in an overlapping fashion to orchestrate physiological responses involving these pathways. In addition to participating in protease-generating pathways, proteases mediate a large number of cellular processes including migration and invasion, trophoblast implantation, embryomorphogenesis, tissue remodeling and angiogenesis [1]. The concept that serine proteases may display profound effects on cellular activation and proliferation is relatively new, and has evolved in parallel with a developing paradigm focusing on the molecular mechanisms of cellular/protease interactions. Thus, although α-thrombin functions as a critical regulator of the clotting cascade, it also initiates receptor-coupling responses, resulting in profound sequelae at the cellular level [2]. Recent observations have extended these cellular responses to other serine proteases. For example, both plasmin [3,4] and cathepsin G [5] modulate thrombin receptor responsiveness, although distinct cellular receptors for each of these two proteases have also been postulated based on known cellular activation sequelae. Likewise, accumulating evidence suggests that alternative thrombin receptors exist on rodent platelets [6], and that cell-surface receptors exist for a larger number of serine proteases regulating hemostatic and inflammatory pathways, including factor XIIa [7], Xa [8], VIIa [8], mast cell tryptases [9] and granzyme A [10] (Table 1). A recurring theme in these observations suggests that the active site is required for cellular activation, invoking a receptor proteolytic mechanism [2], thereby interdigitating with recent progress in the field of proteolytically activated receptors.

Address for correspondence: Wadie F. Bahou MD, Division of Hematology, HSC T15-040 State University of New York, Stony Brook, New York 11794-8151, USA. Tel.: +1-516-444-2059. Fax: +1-516-444-7530. E-mail: WBahou@mail.som.sunysb.edu

Table 1. Protease-cellular activation.

Protease	Cell	Effect
α-Thrombin	Platelets	Aggregation/proliferation
	Endothelial cells	
	Vascular smooth muscle cells	
	Fibroblasts	
Factor VIIa	Canine kidney	Calcium flux
Factor Xa	Canine kidney	Calcium flux
Plasmin	Endothelial	Arachidonic acid release
Granzyme A[a]	Neurons/astrocytes	Retraction
Cathepsin G	Platelets	Aggregation, calcium release
	Porcine aortic endothelial cells	
Tryptase	Smooth muscle cells	Mitogenicity
Factor XIIa[b]	HepG2 cell line	Mitogenicity

[a]May be mediated via PAR-1 activation; [b]not known to require proteolysis for cellular effect.

Proteolytically activated receptors (PARs)

PARs are members of a larger family of seven transmembrane cell-surface receptors that include the three β-adrenergic receptors, the two α2-adrenergic receptors, the five muscarinic receptors and the 5HT-1A serotonin receptor. Three PARs had been isolated to date, the thrombin receptor (PAR-1) [11], the proteinase activated receptor-2 (PAR-2) [12] and PAR-3 (a second "thrombin" receptor) [13]. Unlike the former class of receptors in which cellular activation events are initiated by standard receptor/ligand binding interactions, PARs are activated by cleavage at distinct sessile bonds located within the N-terminal extension (Table 2). The thrombin receptors PAR-1 and PAR-3 have evolved to contain

Table 2. Proteolytically activated receptors.

	PAR-1	PAR-2	PAR-3
Chromosome	5Q13	5Q13	5Q13
Gene structure	2 Exon	2 Exon	?
Function	Proliferation	Proliferation	?
	Aggregation		
Agonists	α-thrombin	Trypsin	α-thrombin
		Tryptase	
Peptide agonists	SFLLR(N)	SLIGKVD	—
(Ant)agonists	Cathepsin G	—	—
	Plasmin		
Expression			
Endothelial cells	Yes	Yes	Yes
Megakaryocytes/platelets	Yes	No	Yes

acidic hirudin-like domains, thereby serving to optimize interactions with their specific protease [11,13]. An irreversible cleavage within the extracellular domain of this receptor unmasks a new amino-terminus that presumably binds intramolecularly within other receptor domains to mediate downstream receptor coupling effects. Indeed, synthetic peptidomimetics representing the new N-terminus after receptor cleavage function as full receptor agonists irrespective of receptor cleavage, although their ability to recapitulate all thrombin's known cellular effects remains controversial. Structure/function determinants for proteolytically activated receptors have been extensively studied in the case of the thrombin receptor (PAR-1) and its activating peptides. A core pentapeptide sequence (TR$^{42-46}$, SFLLR) is sufficient for specifying receptor interactions, and site-directed mutagenesis studies have established that the peptide ligand "binding pocket" includes critical interactions involving Glu^{260} (extracellular loop 2) and Phe^{87} [14,15]. Like the thrombin receptor, PAR-2 is activated by proteolytic cleavage and by synthetic peptides corresponding to the newly generated N-terminus (SLIGKVD, human PAR$^{37-43}$ [16]). On vascular endothelial cells, PAR-2 is known to mediate proliferative responses, further highlighting functional similarities between PAR-2 and the TR on this cell type [17]. Recent reports suggest that PAR-2 is not expressed on platelets as evaluated by aggregometry using PAR-2-specific peptidomimetics [18]. While initial work identified trypsin as a PAR-2 activator, recent work from this [19] and other laboratories [20] have demonstrated that mast-cell tryptases can cleave, activate and recapitulate the mitogenic signal through PAR-2. Given evidence for functional coupling between PAR-1 and PAR-2 on this cell line, the identification of mast-cell tryptases as agonists for PAR-2 also suggests a previously unidentified link between hemostatic and inflammatory pathways mediated through endothelial cell activation [17]. Identified by "low-stringency PCR" using rat platelets, PAR-3 is clearly homologous to PAR-1 and PAR-2, and also appears to be a cleavable receptor [13]. To date, the only known protease agonist for PAR-3 is α-thrombin, as it appears to be specifically activated (and cleaved) by nanomolar concentrations of proteolytically active thrombin. However, the putative cleavage site K^{38}/T^{39} appears unusual for a thrombin substrate. Unexpectedly, unlike PAR-1 or PAR-2, PAR-3 does not appear to be able to be activated by synthetic peptidomimetics representing the new N-terminus after cleavage. The tissue distribution of murine PAR-3 is more limited than that of PAR-1, as Northern analysis and in situ hybridization detects expression primarily in spleen and splenic megakaryocytes. Although expression appeared to be evident in the bone marrow, the precise cells could not be delineated. Thus, although a more comprehensive analysis of cellular distribution is pending, composite evidence would suggest that PAR-3 is minimally expressed in megakaryocytes/platelets and vascular endothelial cells, as demonstrated in this laboratory (unpublished observations). Finally, although PAR-3 may represent the rodent platelet thrombin receptor, its role in human thrombin-mediated cellular activation events remains speculative at this time.

Molecular biology of PARs

Genomic characterization of both the human TR and PAR-2 genes has now been completed with evidence for relevant similarities [16,21]. Initial gene localization studies from this [22] and other laboratories [16] have confirmed that both TR and PAR-2 are present as single-copy genes in the region q13 of human chromosome 5. The coding regions of both genes are contained within two exons, with the presence in both genes of relatively small first exons each encoding less than 30 amino acids (Fig. 1). Likewise, the majority of the coding sequence of both genes is encoded by the larger second exon, which contains the enzymatic cleavage site. Both genes have a relatively large first intron separating the two exons. This remarkable similarity at the genetic level suggests that the PAR-1 and PAR-2 genes arose from a relatively recent gene-duplication event, and further intimated that additional PARs may be clustered within this region of the genome, a hypothesis that was subsequently confirmed with the isolation of PAR-3 (see below). Thus, although the molecular characterization of both PAR-1 and PAR-2

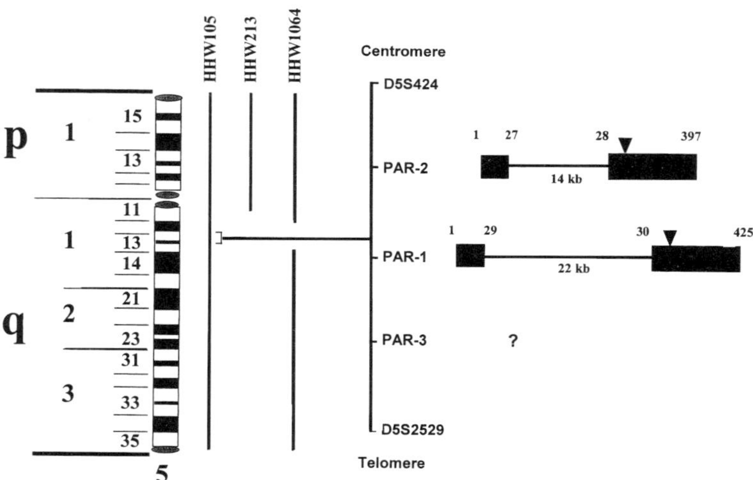

Fig. 1. Schema of human chromosome 5 summarizing the PAR gene cluster. The extent of the human chromosomal complements for the individual human:hamster somatic cell hybrids used for initial gene localization is indicated by the vertical lines [21]. HHW105 contains a monochromosomal 5 as its only human component, HHW213 contains a single human chromosome 5 lacking ~95% of the long arm of chromosome 5 with an intact 5p, and HHW1064 contains a single human chromosome 5 with a deletion spanning the region 5q11.2→5q13.3. Initial genomic analysis demonstrated cross-hybridizing signals only in genomic DNA from HHW105, confirming that the gene cluster is contained within the region 5q11.2→5q13.3 [21]. The centromeric/telomeric assignment with the flanking microsatellite markers D5S424 and D5S2529 represents a consensus from previous mapping data using the G3 radiation hybrid mapping panel [23]. Exons are represented by rectangles, introns by lines, and the proteolytic cleavage sites by arrows. Amino acid residues encoded by individual exons are detailed.

genes has been reported, the gene structure for PAR-3 is not complete, although a priori extrapolation would suggest a similar organization, based on the presumed evolution from a common ancestral gene. The 5'-untranslated region of the TR gene has been reported, although the molecular analysis of its promoter has not been characterized [21]. A region similar to an *Alu* J-subfamily of short interspersed repetitive sequences is present, and has been identified within the promoter regions for other genes (including transforming growth factor-α and the integrin β_3 subunit); a potential role in transcriptional gene regulation remains unestablished. Neither a TATA box nor CCAAT sequences are evident adjacent to the transcription initiation site. The thrombin receptor 5'-flanking region also contains putative sequence binding sites for the erythroid nuclear factor protein NF-E1 (WGATAMS). This activating protein is known to be expressed in megakaryocytes, suggesting that megakaryocyte-specific promoters may share overlapping regulatory elements with erythroid-specific genes. Octameric sequences similar to those found in enhancers modulating the expression of various megakaryocyte-specific genes are also identifiable, although their role (if any) in affecting TR expression remains speculative.

To further characterize the molecular genetics of these receptors, the genetic and physical mapping of all three PARs have now been completed. Two distinct radiation hybrid mapping panels of different resolution have been used to map and order the PAR genes within this region of the human genome [23]. Thus, all three PARs are tightly linked to the identical microsatellite marker D5S424 using a lower resolution mapping panel (G3) with an estimated resolution of ~ 500 kb. The interorder assignment of the genes has been preliminarily determined using a higher resolution mapping panel TNG3, and is displayed in Fig. 1. Within the gene cluster, PAR-2 would appear to be more centromeric and PAR-3 telomeric. All three PARs are contained within a single linked yeast artificial chromosome (YAC) contig WC5.7, known to contain the D5S424 microsatellite marker. Southern analysis and pulsed field gel electrophoresis have been completed as a means of more completely characterizing distances among these genes, using individual YACs known to encompass the PAR gene cluster. Thus, physical mapping by genomic analysis demonstrates that all three PARs are contained within identical restriction fragments of ~ 120 kb, confirming that the PAR gene cluster is maximally of this size. Based on the previously reported sizes of both PAR-1 (~ 27 kb [21] and PAR-2 (~ 19 kb [16]), it is not unreasonable to speculate that individual genes may be much closer, and that other PARs may be coclustered within this region of the genome. These observations appear to be especially relevant given data outlining the presence of other cellular PARs for known serine proteases (Table 1).

Attempts to elucidate molecular genetic defects in humans have followed from previous gene localization studies outlined above. The PAR gene cluster colocalizes to a region on human chromosome 5 that is contiguous to the proximal breakpoint in patients with the 5q-syndrome. This syndrome represents an unusual hematological disorder, and typically presents with thrombocytosis, refractory anemia and characteristic bone marrow features displaying dysmegakaryo-cytopoiesis with poorly lobulated nuclei. Although PAR-1 appears to be centro-meric (and not deleted) to the common proximal breakpoint as evaluated by fluorescent in situ hybridization (FISH) [24], potential deletions involving PAR-3 have not been studied. This analysis would appear appropriate given the evidence that PAR-3 is telomeric and abundantly expressed in megakaryocytes, making it a putative candidate gene involved in the dyspoietic maturation evident in these cells.

Acknowledgements

This work was supported by funding from the National Institutes of Health HL02431.

References

1. Liotta L, Steeg P, Stetler-Stevenson W. Cancer metastasis and angiogenesis: an imbalance of positive and negative regulation. Cell 1991;64:327–336.
2. Glenn KC et al. Thrombin active site regions are required for fibroblast receptor binding and initiation of cell division. J Biol Chem 1980;255:6609–6616.
3. Kimura M et al. Plasmin-platelet interaction involves cleavage of the functional thrombin receptor. Am J Physiol 1996;40:C54–C60.
4. Chang WC et al. Human plasmin induces a receptor-mediated arachidonate release coupled with G proteins in endothelial cells. Am J Physiol 1993;264:C271–C281.
5. Molino M et al. Proteolysis of the human platelet and endothelial cell thrombin receptor by neutrophil-derived cathepsin G. J Biol Chem 1995;270:11168–11175.
6. Kinlough-Rathbone RL, Rand ML, Packham MA. Rabbit and rat platelets do not respond to thrombin receptor peptides that activate human platelets. Blood 1993;82:103–106.
7. Schmeidler-Sapiro KT, Ratnoff OD, Gordon EM. Mitogenic effects of coagulation factor XII and factor XIIa on Hep G_2 cells. Proc Natl Acad Sci USA 1991;88:4382–4385.
8. Camerer E et al. Coagulation factors VII and X induce Ca^{2+} oscillations in madin-darby canine kidney cells only when proteolytically active. J Biol Chem 1996;271:29034–29042.
9. Brown JK et al. Tryptase-induced mitogenesis in airway smooth muscle cells. Potency, mechanisms and interactions with other mast cell mediators. Chest 1995;107:95S–96S.
10. Suidan HS et al. Granzyme A released upon stimulation of cytotoxic T lymphocytes activates the thrombin receptor on neuronal cells and astrocytes. Proc Natl Acad Sci USA 1994;91:8112–8116.
11. Vu T et al. Molecular cloning of a functional thrombin receptor reveals a novel proteolytic mechanism of receptor activation. Cell 1991;64:1057–1068.
12. Nystedt S et al. Molecular cloning of a potential proteinase activated receptor. Proc Natl Acad Sci USA 1994;91:9208–9212.
13. Ishihara H et al. Protease-activated receptor 3 is a second thrombin receptor in humans. Nature 1997;386:502–506.
14. Bahou W et al. Identification of a thrombin receptor sequence specifying activation-dependent responses. Blood 1994;84:4195–4202.
15. Gerstzen RE et al. Specificity of the thrombin receptor for agonist peptide is defined by its extracellular surface. Nature 1994;368:648–651.
16. Nystedt S et al. Molecular cloning and functional expression of the gene encoding the human proteinase-activated receptor 2. Eur J Biochem 1995;232:84–89.

17. Mirza H, Yatsula V, Bahou WF. The proteinase activated receptor-2 (PAR-2) mediates mitogenic responses in human vascular endothelial cells. J Clin Invest 1996;97:1705—1714.
18. Hwa JJ et al. Evidence for the presence of a proteinase-activated receptor distinct from the thrombin receptor in vascular endothelial cells. Circ Res 1996;71:581—588.
19. Mirza H et al. Mitogenic responses mediated through the proteinase activated receptor-α are induced by mast cell α- and β-tryptases. Blood 1997;(In press).
20. Molino M et al. Interactions of mast cell tryptase with thrombin receptors and PAR-2. J Biol Chem 1997;272:4043—4049.
21. Schmidt V, Vitale E, Bahou W. Genomic cloning and characterization of the human thrombin receptor gene: evidence for a novel gene family that includes PAR-2. J Biol Chem 1996;271:9307—9312.
22. Bahou WF et al. Chromosomal assignment of the human thrombin receptor gene: localization to region q13 of chromosome 5. Blood 1993;82:1532—1537.
23. Schmidt VA et al. The human thrombin receptor and proteinase activated receptor-2 genes are tightly linked on chromosome 5q13. Br J Haematol 1997;97:523—529.
24. Demetrick DJ et al. The thrombin receptor gene is centromeric to the common proximal breakpoint in patients with the 5q-syndrome: identification of a previously unrecognized chromosome 5 inversion. Br J Haematol 1996;92:339—343.

Integrin signalling kinases and their influence on the formation of lipid intermediates during platelet responses

Karine Missy, Muriel Laffargue, Sylvie Giuriato, Marie-Pierre Gratacap, Joël Tuech, Laurent Monnereau, Ashraf Ragab, Jeannie M.F. Ragab-Thomas, Patrick Raynal, Gérard Mauco, Monique Plantavid, Bernard Payrastre and Hugues Chap
Institut Fédératif de Recherche en Immunologie Cellulaire et Moléculaire, Université Paul Sabatier and Centre Hospitalo-Universitaire de Toulouse, INSERM Unité 326, Toulouse; Phospholipides Membranaires, Signalisation Cellulaire et Lipoprotéines, Hôpital Purpan, Toulouse, France

Abstract. Platelet activation results in a conformational change of integrin α_{IIb}/β_3, which upon fibrinogen binding allows aggregation to occur. This is accompanied by a number of integrin-dependent signalling events, including tyrosine phosphorylation of various proteins, as well as synthesis of phosphoinositides phosphorylated on the D-3 position of inositol ring (the most abundant being in this case phosphatidylinositol 3,4-bisphosphate or $PI(3,4)P_2$). We have reviewed our ongoing studies based mainly on the regulation of $PI(3,4)P_2$ synthesis, which might involve both a phosphoinositide 3-kinase (PI 3-kinase) and an inositol polyphosphate 5-phosphatase containing a Src-homology 2 domain called SHIP. Although many molecular details still remain to be identified, pharmacological evidence indicates that production of $PI(3,4)P_2$ might be required to maintain the organization of focal adhesions necessary for a stable aggregation to occur. Studies are in progress to identify potential targets of $PI(3,4)P_2$, among which are protein tyrosine kinases bearing pleckstrin homology (PH) domains (Tec kinase family).

Keywords: focal adhesion kinase, phosphatidylinositol 3,4-bisphosphate, phosphoinositide 3-kinase, SHIP (SH2 domain-containing inositol 5-phosphatase), wortmannin.

Introduction

It is now established that stimulation of platelets with various agonists such as thrombin results (among other responses) in a conformational change of integrin α_{IIb}/β_3, which is then able to bind fibrinogen, resulting in the onset of platelet aggregation [1]. However, fibrinogen binding to its membrane receptor is not simply a passive event allowing the formation of intercellular bridges between platelets, since a complex signalling pathway is triggered by integrin engagement. As recently reviewed [1], this involves various protein tyrosine kinases and lipid kinases. A number of them become associated with the submembranous cytoskeleton, where they form multiprotein signalling complexes participating in the organization of focal adhesions, similar to those observed in other nucleated

Address for correspondence: Prof Hugues Chap, INSERM Unité 326, Hôpital Purpan, F-31059 Toulouse Cedex, France. Tel.: +33-561-77-9400. Fax: +33-561-77-9401.

cells adhering to extracellular matrix. In particular, tyrosine kinases of the Src family have been identified in the cytoskeleton of activated platelets. This is also the case for focal adhesion kinase (FAK), which is concentrated in focal adhesions owing to its ability to interact with various integrins.

In these last years, our studies have been focused on the role and the regulation of phosphoinositide 3-kinase (PI 3-kinase), a "novel" lipid kinase participating in the formation of signaling complexes present in the submembrane cytoskeleton of activated platelets. This enzyme catalyzes the synthesis of the so-called D-3 phosphoinositides, which are not substrates of phospholipase C, and are increasingly considered as potential intracellular messengers. After briefly recalling the basis of the metabolism of these peculiar phospholipids, we will emphasize our current knowledge concerning both the regulation of PI 3-kinase and the possible role of the D-3 phosphoinositides synthesized in thrombin-stimulated platelets.

Phosphoinositide 3-kinases and their metabolic function

The structure of the two main D-3 phosphoinositides produced in activated cells,

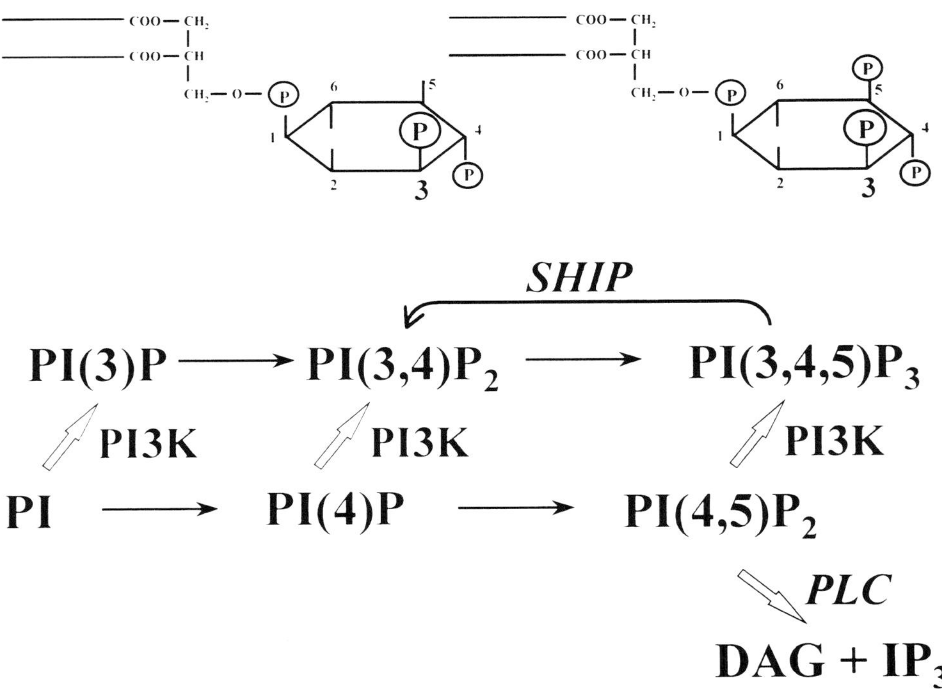

Fig. 1. Structure and biosynthetic pathways of D-3 phosphoinositides. The structures shown in the upper part of the scheme correspond to PI(3,4)P₂ (left) and to PIP₃ (right). Abbreviations not defined in the text: PI3K, PI3-kinase; PLC, phospholipase C; DAG, diacylglycerol.

including platelets, is presented in Fig. 1. In vitro phosphatidylinositol 3,4-bisphosphate (or PI(3,4)P$_2$) is obtained upon phosphorylation by PI 3-kinase of phosphatidylinositol 4-phosphate, whereas phosphatidylinositol 3,4,5-trisphosphate (PI(3,4,5)P$_3$ or PIP$_3$) is derived from phosphatidylinositol 4,5-bisphosphate, the main substrate of phospholipase C. Although phosphatidylinositol 3-phosphate can also be obtained in vitro, this phospholipid, which is constitutively present in low amounts, does not appear to vary significantly in relation to cell signalling. We and others [2—6] have found that PIP$_3$ is produced transiently in the first seconds of platelet stimulation with thrombin, whereas PI(3,4)P$_2$ accumulates more slowly. Moreover, the secondary accumulation of PI(3,4)P$_2$ is inhibited by the tetrapeptide RGDS (which competes for fibrinogen binding to integrin α_{IIb}/β_3), and it is hardly detected in thrombasthenic platelets, giving strong support to the view that its synthesis is a main signalling event occurring downstream of integrin α_{IIb}/β_3 [5].

As also indicated in Fig. 1, the synthesis of D-3 phosphoinositides involves PI 3-kinases, which now appear to form a large family of homologous enzymes [7,8]. Platelets contain at least two members of PI 3-kinase [9]: class IA contains a 110-kDa catalytic subunit associated to an 85-kDa regulatory subunit (p85α), which possesses various interacting motifs such as two Src-homology 2 (SH2) domains and one SH3 domain. This enzyme has been studied the most as yet, and its regulation implies specific association of p85α to phosphotyrosyl residues, resulting in a conformational change of the catalytic subunit, which then acquires its full activity. The other class of PI 3-kinase identified in platelets (class IB) is also heterodimeric, with a 110-kDa catalytic subunit and a putative p101 adaptor. In contrast to the former, class IB PI 3-kinase is directly activated by the $\beta\gamma$ dimer from heterotrimeric G-proteins [10]. Since activation of Gi occurs early in thrombin-stimulated platelets promoting, for instance, some specific protein phosphorylation steps [11,12], it is tempting to speculate that class IB PI 3-kinase might be responsible for the early and transient accumulation of PIP$_3$ in thrombin-stimulated platelets. In contrast, since integrin engagement has been shown in many instances to stimulate various protein tyrosine kinases [1], this led us to mainly focus our studies on class IA PI 3-kinase.

Behaviour of class IA PI 3-kinase in thrombin-stimulated platelets

A tight relationship between tyrosine kinases and PI 3-kinase is suggested by two types of data: in thrombin-stimulated platelets, tyrosine kinase inhibitors significantly decrease the production of PI(3,4)P$_2$ [13], and the p85α subunit of PI 3-kinase can be immunoprecipitated by an antibody specific for antiphosphotyrosine [13]. However, p85α is not tyrosine phosphorylated itself, suggesting that it is associated with other tyrosine phosphorylated proteins.

On the other hand, PI 3-kinase which is a cytosolic protein, becomes associated with the cytoskeleton as a consequence of platelet activation, together with a number of signalling proteins such as various protein tyrosine kinases,

1106

protein tyrosine phosphatases as well as other lipid kinases [6]. Translocation to
the cytoskeleton requires both integrin engagement and a full activity of protein
tyrosine kinases, since it is inhibited by RGDS and by tyrphostins. This suggested
that PI 3-kinase might undergo specific associations with other cytoskeletal proteins participating in the formation of signalling complexes. Although no binding
could be detected with pp60^{c-src}, the p85α subunit of PI 3-kinase could be immunoprecipitated with an antibody directed against FAK [6]. Additional experiments also indicated that p85α interacted at least via its SH3 domain with a pro-
line-rich sequence present in FAK, this specific event being responsible for an
activation of the catalytic subunit of PI 3-kinase [6].

As summarized in Fig. 2, these various data allowed us to suggest that integrin
engagement promotes two key events concerning PI 3-kinase: its association to
submembranous cytoskeleton allowing an appropriate positioning towards its
substrate present in the inner leaflet of the platelet membrane; a specific association with FAK, which results in an 8-fold increase of its specific activity. However,
it might well be that PI 3-kinase by itself is not sufficient to explain the relatively
large accumulation of PI(3,4)P$_2$ during platelet aggregation.

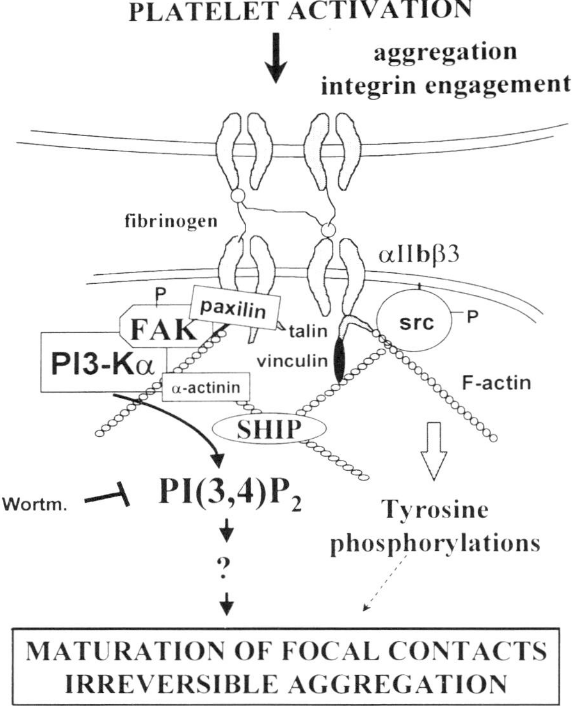

Fig. 2. Possible interactions of PI 3-kinase and of SHIP in the submembranous cytoskeleton of activated platelets. For the sake of clarity, PI 3-kinase is represented as a single entity, but is formed by
two subunits (p85α, regulatory subunit; p110, catalytic subunit).

Possible role of SHIP in the production of $PI(3,4)P_2$

The cDNA encoding a novel SH2 domain-containing inositol 5-phosphatase (SHIP) was recently cloned by three different groups [14—16]. SHIP is able to specifically dephosphorylate the 5-position of both inositol 1,3,4,5-tetrakisphosphate and PIP_3, producing inositol 1,3,4-trisphosphate and $PI(3,4)P_2$, respectively. The latter possibility is indicated in the metabolic scheme of Fig. 1. In a very recent study [17], we were able to show that SHIP is present in significant amounts in platelets as an active 5-phosphatase, and displays a behaviour very similar to that previously described for PI 3-kinase (upon thrombin stimulation, this cytosolic protein becomes tyrosine phosphorylated and is translocated to the cytoskeleton with a time course strictly parallel to the translocation of PI 3-kinase and to the synthesis of $PI(3,4)P_2$). Moreover, all these responses are simultaneously inhibited by the peptide RGDS or when platelets are incubated in the absence of shaking, which is required for aggregation to occur. Although this is only circumstantial evidence, these data suggest that SHIP also participates in multiprotein signalling complexes present in submembranous cytoskeleton and contributes to the production of $PI(3,4)P_2$ by hydrolyzing the PIP_3 produced by PI 3-kinase. This is also illustrated in Fig. 2.

A final question then concerns the mechanism by which accumulation of D-3 phosphoinositides (particularly $PI(3,4)P_2$) in focal-adhesion plaques might contribute to some platelet responses. Some pharmacological evidence is now available and will be briefly discussed.

Evidence for a role of D3 phosphoinositides in the stabilisation of platelet aggregates

Two relatively specific and unrelated inhibitors of PI 3-kinases (wortmannin and LY294002) are currently used to investigate the possible role of this enzyme in cell biology. In the case of platelets, Kovacsovics et al. [18] and ourselves (unpublished data) have observed that inhibition of PI 3-kinase is able to convert stable platelet aggregation induced by thrombin into a reversible process. The current interpretation of these data is to consider that PI 3-kinase is necessary to maintain a firm organisation of focal adhesion plaques to stabilize platelet aggregates. Although wortmannin or LY294002 themselves are not pharmacological agents to be used in vivo, this observation defines a potential target to design antithrombotic drugs, since a stable aggregation is certainly a very crucial step to allow the formation of a white thrombus able to resist the strong blood flow normally occurring in arterial vasculature.

Conclusion

Although all the molecular mechanisms regulating the synthesis of D-3 phosphoinositides in activated platelets are not yet elucidated, the main contribution of our laboratory was to define a paradigm where association of signalling proteins such as PI 3-kinase or SHIP to the submembranous cytoskeleton might allow an appropriate positioning of these enzymes towards their substrate. Further studies might allow a more specific dissection of their interactions with other signalling molecules also present on the cytoskeletal matrix. We have illustrated the example of a specific association between the p85α subunit of PI 3-kinase and FAK. There are certainly many more possibilities. For instance a major role of the small G-protein rhoA has been suggested in at least two studies [19,20], although the precise mechanism by which rhoA is necessary for the activation of PI 3-kinase is still unclear. We have also found a possible involvement of calpains in the control of the integrin-dependent accumulation of PI 3-kinase products in platelets [21].

Finally, a major challenge will be to understand how D-3 phosphoinositides in general, and $PI(3,4)P_2$ in particular, contribute to the stabilization of platelet aggregation via an effect on focal adhesion structures. This requires an identification of specific targets of D-3 phosphoinositides. Interesting candidates might be proteins carrying pleckstrin homology (PH) domains, among which are a group of tyrosine kinases such as Tec kinase or Bruton tyrosine kinase (Btk). In a recent study, Tec was identified in platelets and found to participate in the multi-protein signalling complexes adsorbed on the cystoskeletal matrix [22].

References

1. Clark EA, Brugge JS. Tyrosine phosphorylation in platelets. Potential roles in signal transduction. Trends Cardiovasc Med 1993;3:218—226.
2. Nola RD, Lapetina EG. Thrombin stimulates the production of a novel polyphosphoinositide in human platelets. J Biol Chem 1990;265:2441—2445.
3. Kucera GL, Rittenhouse SE. Human platelets form 3-phosphorylated phosphoinositides in response to α-thrombin, U46619, or GTPγS. J Biol Chem 1990;265:5345—5348.
4. Sultan C, Breton M, Mauco G, Grondin P, Plantavid M, Chap H. The novel inositol lipid phosphatidylinositol 3,4-bisphosphate is produced by human blood platelets upon thrombin stimulation. Biochem J 1990;269:831—834.
5. Sultan C, Plantavid M, Bachelot C, Grondin P, Breton M, Mauco G, Lévy-Toledano S, Caen JP, Chap H. Involvement of platelet glycoprotein IIb-IIIa (α_{IIb}-β_3 integrin) in thrombin-induced synthesis of phosphatidylinositol 3′,4′-bisphosphate. J Biol Chem 1991;266:23554—23557.
6. Guinebault C, Payrastre B, Racaud-Sultan C, Mazarguil H, Breton M, Mauco G, Plantavid M, Chap H. Integrin-dependent translocation of phosphoinositide 3-kinase to the cytoskeleton of thrombin-activated platelets involves specific interactions of p85α with actin filaments and focal adhesion kinase. J Cell Biol 1995;129:831—842.
7. Vanhaesebroek B, Leevers SJ, Panayotou G, Waterfield MD. Phosphoinositide 3-kinases: a conserved family of signal transducers. Trends Biochem Sci 1997;22:267—272.
8. Domin J, Waterfield M. Using structure to define the function of phosphoinositide kinase family members. FEBS Lett 1997;410:91—95.
9. Rittenhouse SE. Phosphoinositide 3-kinase activation and platelet function. Blood 1996;88:4401—4414.
10. Zhang J, Zhang WG, Benovic JL, Sugai M, Wetzker R, Gout I, Rittenhouse SE. Sequestration of a G-protein βγ subunit or ADP-ribosylation of rho can inhibit thrombin-induced activation of platelet phosphoinositide 3-kinases. J Biol Chem 1995;270:6589—6594.

11. Li RY, Gaits F, Ragab A, Ragab-Thomas JMF, Chap H. Tyrosine phosphorylation of an SH2-containing protein tyrosine phosphatase is coupled to platelet thrombin receptor via a pertussis toxin-sensitive heterotrimeric G-protein. EMBO J 1995;14:219—226.
12. Gaits F, Li RY, Bigay J, Ragab A, Ragab-Thomas JMF, Chap H. G-protein βγ subunits mediate specific phosphorylation of the protein tyrosine phosphatase SH-PTP1 induced by lysophosphatidic acid. J Biol Chem 1996;271:20151—20155.
13. Guinebault C, Payrastre B, Sultan C, Mauco G, Breton M, Lévy-Toledano S, Plantavid M, Chap H. Tyrosine kinases and phosphoinositide metabolism in thrombin-stimulated human platelets. Biochem J 1993;292:851—856.
14. Drayer LA, Pesesse X, De Smedt F, Woscholski R, Parker P, Erneux C. Cloning and expression of a human placenta inositol 1,3,4,5-tetrakisphosphate and phosphatidylinositol 3,4,5-trisphosphate 5-phosphatase. Biochem Biophys Res Commun 1996;225:243—249.
15. Ware MD, Rosten P, Damen JE, Liu L, Humphries K, Krystal G. Cloning and characterization of human SHIP, the 145-kD inositol 5-phosphatase that associates with SHC after cytokine stimulation. Blood 1996;88:2833—2840.
16. Kavanaugh WM, Pot DA, Chin SM, Deuter-Reinhard M, Jefferson AB, Norris FA, Masiarz FR, Cousens LS, Majerus PW, Williams LT. Multiple forms of an inositol 5-phosphatase form signaling complexes with Shc and Grb2. Curr Biol 1996;6:438—445.
17. Giuriato S, Payrastre B, Drayer LA, Plantavid M, Woscholski R, Parker P, Erneux C, Chap H. Tyrosine phosphorylation and relocation of SHIP are integrin-mediated in thrombin-stimulated human blood platelets. J Biol Chem 1997;272:26857—26863.
18. Kovacsovics TJ, Bachelot C, Toker A, Vlahos CJ, Duckworth B, Cantley LC, Hartwig JH. Phosphoinositide 3-kinase inhibition spares actin assembly in activating platelets but reverses platelet aggregation. J Biol Chem 1995;271:11358—11366.
19. Zhang J, King WG, Dillon S, Hall A, Feig L, Rittenhouse SE. Activation of platelet phosphatidylinositide kinase requires the small GTP-binding protein Rho. J Biol Chem 1993;268:22251—22254.
20. Gachet C, Payrastre B, Guinebault C, Trumel C, Ohlmann P, Mauco G, Cazenave JP, Plantavid M, Chap H. Reversible translocation of phosphoinositide 3-kinase to the cytoskeleton of ADP-aggregated human platelets occurs independently of RHO and without synthesis of phosphatidylinositol (3,4)-bisphosphate. J Biol Chem 1997;272:4850—4854.
21. Montsarrat N, Racaud-Sultan C, Mauco G, Plantavid M, Payrastre B, Breton-Douillon M, Chap H. Calpains are involved in phosphatidylinositol 3′,4′-*bis*phosphate synthesis dependent on the $\alpha_{IIb}\beta_3$ integrin engagement in thrombin-stimulated platelets. FEBS Lett 1997;404:23—26.
22. Laffargue M, Monnereau L, Tuech J, Ragab A, Ragab-Thomas JMF, Payrastre B, Raynal P, Chap H. Integrin-dependent tyrosine phosphorylation and cytoskeletal translocation of Tec in thrombin-activated platelets. Biochem Biophys Res Commun 1997;238:247—251.

The respective roles of GPIb and GPIIb-IIIa in blood platelet adhesion

Jan J. Sixma and Philip G. de Groot
Department of Haematology, University Hospital Utrecht, Utrecht, The Netherlands

Introduction

Blood platelet adhesion is an essential first step in formation of a haemostatic plug or thrombus. This process is mediated by adhesive proteins in the vessel wall and by adhesion receptors on the platelet membrane. In this respect, platelet adhesion is similar in general to the adhesion of cells to a connective tissue matrix. However, platelet adhesion occurs from flowing blood and this has several consequences that set it apart. The first consequence is that adhesive proteins do not necessarily have to be present in the vessel wall, but they can bind there when the vessel is breached and the subendothelial or perivascular connective tissue is exposed to the blood. Secondly, such adhesive proteins should not interact with the platelet in the circulation. A third consequence is that the interaction between the adhesive molecules and the respective receptors does occur under shear conditions, and this introduces special requirements. All these three special consequences of adhesion occurring from flowing blood are met by a single protein which is special to platelet adhesion: von Willebrand factor (vWF). VWF is a multimeric glycoprotein with a subunit of 270 kDa, which first dimerizes at the aminoterminus, then forms long multimers by the formation of disulfide bonds between the carboxytermini. The multimers have molecular weights up to 20 million kDa, which corresponds to a length of approximately 1 mm for the stretched out molecule [1,2]. VWF is synthesized by endothelial cells, deposited in part in the subendothelium and secreted in part towards the circulation. It is also synthesized by megakaryocytes, and this vWF is stored in the α-granule of the platelet from where it can be released upon activation of the platelet [3]. VWF binds to the subendothelium, and to perivascular collagen from plasma — this binding may precede platelet adhesion [4,5]. VWF may also be secreted from the platelet during adhesion, this vWF can also contribute to adhesion. In the circulation, vWF does not interact with the platelet unless the platelet is activated, or unless vWF is bound to a surface. The blood platelet has receptors for vWF: GPIb and GPIIb-IIIa. The question which will be the central theme of this review is how these two receptors function in platelet adhesion in flow, and in the subsequent aggregate formation under flow conditions. We will also see

---

Address for correspondence: Jan J. Sixma, Department of Haematology, Graduate School of Biomembranes, University Hospital Utrecht, P. O. Box 85500, 3508 GA, The Netherlands.

that although vWF may be the special adhesive molecule for platelet adhesion in flow, it is in no way the only adhesive molecule; adhesion as well as thrombus formation are complex mechanisms that are only partly understood today.

Role of GPIb in adhesion

The essential role of GPIb in platelet adhesion was established with the use of antibodies, mutated vWF molecules and by observations on a disease, the Bernard-Soulier syndrome in which GPIb is absent from the platelet [6]. In this disease, platelet adhesion is completely absent. The disease is characterized, however, by the presence of large platelets and by concomitant thrombocytopenia. Comparison of the adhesion in the Bernard-Soulier patients with results in other forms of macrothrombocytopenia showed that the adhesion defect was specific for the Bernard-Soulier syndrome (Nieuwenhuis HK, de Groot PhG, Sixma JJ unpublished). The studies with mutant vWF were performed with a recombinant product in which the A1-domain of vWF was deleted. Previous studies had shown that the A1-domain represents the interaction site with GPIb in the vWF molecule. The studies with the ΔA1-vWF showed no adhesion at all to surface-coated vWF (both under static and flow conditions), and little or no adhesion to collagen type I or III, or to fibrinogen and fibronectin at high shear rates [7—9]. The effect of antibodies on GPIb, or on the interaction site of GPIb on the platelet have demonstrated that platelet adhesion is abolished to the subendothelium and to surface-coated vWF at all shear rates and to collagen type I, III and IV at high shear rates [10—12]. The results of these studies show that GPIb is a receptor that is crucial to the interaction of the platelet with vWF. A first conclusion is that the interaction of GPIb with vWF is independent of the way in which vWF is bound to the surface. Up until now four different ways have been recognized in which vWF may bind to a surface. A specific binding site localized in the A3-domain of vWF has been found for binding to collagens type I and III [7,13]. A different binding site has been found for binding to subendothelium, a site which is probably identical to the binding site for collagen type VI, which is prominently present in subendothelium as microfibrils [14,15]. VWF binding in adhesion to collagen type IV, fibrinogen and to fibronectin is a special case. VWF does not bind to these proteins when they are coated to a surface, but adhesion at high shear rates is dependent on vWF (apart from the ligand receptor interaction responsible for the respective protein [8,9,12]). Morphological studies have demonstrated that vWF is present between the platelet and the surface and long threads of vWF have been found to anchor platelets. The exact binding characteristics of vWF under these conditions are unknown. The possibility cannot be excluded that platelets secrete a substance which binds to the surface to which vWF then binds. The last binding mode is the most nonspecific. VWF adsorbed to a surface works as an adhesive molecule regardless of the nature of the surface or the way of coating [16—18]. A second conclusion that can be drawn is that shear-rate effects on vWF may not be essential for the interaction of GPIb and vWF. Changes in conformation may occur when vWF is exposed to flow, but the observation that platelet adhesion to ΔA1-vWF is completely absent under static conditions indicates that this is not important for the interaction between GPIb and vWF.

VWF does not interact spontaneously with a blood platelet. In vitro such an interaction does occur in the presence of the snake-venom protein botrocetin or the carbohydrate substance ristocetin. Also bovine vWF shows spontaneous binding to human platelets and such binding may also occur when sialic acid residues are removed from vWF [19]. Spontaneous increased binding of vWF has been demonstrated in type IIB von Willebrand Disease (vWD) [20,21]. In this disease, specific point mutations in vWF have been found which are responsible for increased binding. Increased binding has also been found in platelet type vWD, a disease caused by specific mutations in GPIb responsible for spontaneous binding of vWF. Recent studies in our laboratory demonstrated that spontaneous binding of type IIB vWF at very low levels to platelets inhibited adhesion to collagen, whereas larger concentrations caused spontaneous platelet aggregation [22]. Taken together these results suggest that adsorption of vWF to any surface changes the conformation of the A1-domain of vWF in such a way that interaction with GPIb becomes possible [23].

Role of GPIIb-IIIa in adhesion

The first indication that GPIIb-IIIa is involved in adhesion to subendothelium came from studies in Glanzmann's thrombasthenia in which platelet spreading was diminished whereas adhesion by itself was not affected [24—26]. Later studies with antibodies confirmed these results. The ligand of GPIIb-IIIa involved in this spreading activity of GPIIb-IIIa has not been identified with certainty. Fibronectin, vWF or adsorbed fibrinogen could all play a role. In studies with isolated surface-coated proteins, GPIIb-IIIa was found to be the single primary receptor for fibrinogen at all shear rates. As mentioned above, this interaction was supported at high shear rates by a GPIb/vWF interaction [9]. On fibronectin, GPIIb-IIIa is also crucial. Both GPIc-IIa ($\alpha5\beta$) and GPIIb-IIIa are required for adhesion to occur [8]. On vWF, GPIb and GPIIb-IIIa are both necessary under flow conditions, whereas GPIb is sufficient under static conditions [18,27]. On collagens, laminin and thrombospondin, no function could be demonstrated for GPIIb-IIIa. For collagens this can be tricky to demonstrate. They induce also thrombus formation and this is obviously abolished when GPIIb-IIIa is blocked. An inhibition of platelet adhesion on subendothelium by RGD peptides was also reported, but as we recently discovered, this only occurs when citrate is used as anticoagulant and not under conditions where enough divalent cations are present. The interaction site for GPIIb-IIIa on fibronectin and vWF is the arginine-glycin-aspartic acid-(serine) (RGD(S)) sequence [28]. For fibrinogen, the situation is more complex. Two RGD sequences are present in the α-chain, but both these sequences are not essential for interaction with GPIIb-IIIa. Antibody studies but more convincingly studies with recombinant fibrinogen lacking the carboxyterminal amino acids of the γ-chain have indicated that this part of the molecule is critical for the interaction with GPIIb-IIIa [29]. Other sites have also been suggested but they are less firmly established. One of these sites is located at the β-chain (β15—42) [30] and another site may be present at residues 319 and 320 of the γ-chain. The way in which these sites interact is at present unknown.

GPIb and GpIIb-IIIa: how do they work?

The adhesion of leukocytes (the other cell type that adheres in flowing blood) has given important pointers how platelets may adhere. Leukoytes were found to adhere via a two step mechanism: firstly, interaction mediated by a rolling receptor for which the selectins appeared to be responsible, and then a second interaction leading to firm attachment mediated by an integrin [31]. This hypothesis has been firmly established by now and is supported by much evidence. For platelets, indications have been found that a similar sequence of events may operate. Adhesion on von Willebrand factor was shown to involve rolling, mediated by GPIb, and firm attachment, mediated by GPIIb-IIIa [32]. Interaction with fibrinogen was mediated directly by GPIIb-IIIa, and platelets were attached firmly at the moment they contacted the fibrinogen coated surface. However attractive this hypothesis is, and however convincing the data on surfaces coated with single proteins, not everything is yet explained about more complex surfaces such as the subendothelial matrix or on perivascular collagen. On these two surfaces, adhesion at high shear rates is dependent on at least three independent adhesion mechanisms, i.e., interaction between GPIa-IIa ($\alpha2\beta1$) and collagen [33], interaction between GPIb and vWF [25], and interaction between GPIc-IIa ($\alpha5\beta1$) and fibronectin [34]. GPIIb-IIIa, moreover, has been shown to be involved in platelet spreading, and as mentioned its ligand is currently unknown. Furthermore, GPVI a receptor for simple triple helical sequences in collagen is crucial for platelet activation and subsequent thrombus formation [35]. Whether GPIb works as a rolling receptor under these conditions is unknown. A possible reversal of roles should be kept in mind in which the interaction with the respective integrin comes first, before vWF can play a role. Such a sequence of events seems likely on surfaces to which vWF does not bind. What is also unknown, is the role of laminin and thrombospondin in the vessel wall in real life. Both are adhesive proteins for platelets, with GPIc'-IIa ($\alpha6\beta1$) as receptor for laminin, whereas the adhesion receptor for thrombospondin is not yet known [36,37]. Laminin is probably not very important since an inhibitory antibody had no major effect on the adhesion to subendothelium, but the role of thrombospondin is not clear.

Role of GPIb and GPIIb-IIIa in thrombus formation

The role of GPIIb-IIIa as a receptor essential to platelet-platelet interaction is firmly established. From the first finding of the lack of this receptor in Glanzmann's thrombasthenia (a disease showing complete lack of platelet-platelet interaction) until today when platelet aggregation in the clinic is inhibited by monoclonal antibodies against it, this contention has never been in doubt. Three problems remain: firstly, how is GPIIb-IIIa activated; secondly, what causes thrombus growth to stop; and thirdly, is GPIb involved in thrombus growth as well? Much work has been performed on signal response pathways leading to the activation of GPIIb-IIIa [38,39] and we will not dwell on it in this brief review. Instead, we will say a few words about the two other questions which have been and are the subject of our recent and current studies. When platelets adhere GPIIb-IIIa is activated and new platelets may interact via GPIIb-IIIa bound fibrinogen or other ligands. This would mean that platelet accumulation would continue until the thrombus would become occlusive, and transport of platelets to the thrombus would stop. Still, in practice, thrombus growth seems to be determined by the initial surface: collagen causing thrombus formation and subendothelium almost no growth, or by the simultaneous formation of thrombin via a tissue-factor-dependent pathway, or by the direct effect of very high shear rates at areas of stenosis [40]. We studied what happened at the surface of thrombus that does not grow any further. We found that GPIIb-IIIa on the platelets at the surface of thrombus is activated, but curiously enough it is not occupied by ligands [41]. What the reason is behind this is not known. It is evident, however, that this absence of ligands may serve as a mechanism to limit thrombus size. Further studies are required to find the basis for this phenomenon. That GPIb might play a role in platelet thrombus formation was suggested by observations showing a defect in it at high shear rates in vWD. VWF may serve as ligand for GPIIb-IIIa, however, and thus support platelet-platelet interaction. We recently were able to demonstrate that GPIb is the receptor for this vWF activity, and that GPIIb-IIIa interaction was inhibitory rather than supportive for platelet thrombus formation (Y.P. Wu, P.G. de Groot, J.J. Sixma, unpublished).

Conclusion

Platelet adhesion and thrombus formation are complex processes crucial to haemostasis. Many adhesive proteins and various receptors are involved. GPIb and GPIIb-IIIa are the two main receptors of the platelet and their respective roles are beginning to emerge. A precise definition of that role is not only of importance for understanding of the process but also as a background for rational drug design for antithrombotic agents.

References

1. Ruggeri ZM, Ware J. von Willebrand factor. FASEB J 1993;7:308—316.
2. Meyer D, Girma J-P. von Willebrand factor: structure and function. Thromb Haemost 1993;

70:99—104.

3. Wagner DD. Cell biology of von Willebrand factor. Ann Rev Cell Biol 1990;6:217—246.

4. Sakariassen KS, Bolhuis PA, Sixma JJ. Human blood platelet adhesion to artery subendothelium is mediated by factor VIII-von Willebrand factor bound to the subendothelium. Nature 1979;279:635—638.

5. Bolhuis PA, Sakariassen KS, Sander HJ, Bouma BN, Sixma JJ. Binding of factor VIII-von Willebrand factor to human arterial subendothelium precedes increased platelet adherence and enhances platelet spreading. J Lab Clin Med 1981;97:568—576.

6. Weiss HJ, Turitto VT, Baumgartner HR. Effect of shear rate on platelet interaction in von Willebrand's disease and Bernard-Soulier syndrome. J Lab Clin Med 1978;92:750—764.

7. Lankhof H, Van Hoeij M, Schiphorst ME, Bracke M, Wu YP, IJsseldijk MJW, Vink T, de Groot PG, Sixma JJ. A3 domain is essential for interaction of von Willebrand factor with collagen type III. Thromb Haemost 1996;75:950—958.

8. Beumer S, Heijnen HFG, IJsseldijk MJW, Orlando E, De Groot PG, Sixma JJ. Platelet adhesion to fibronectin in flow: the importance of von Willebrand Factor and GPIb. Blood 1995;86: 3452—3460.

9. Endenburg SC, Hantgan RR, Lindeboom-Blokzijl L, Lankhof H, Jerome WG, Lewis JC, Sixma JJ, de Groot PG. On the role of von Willebrand factor in promoting platelet adhesion to fibrin in flowing blood. Blood 1995;86:4158—4165.

10. Houdijk WPM, Sakariassen KS, Nievelstein PFEM, Sixma JJ. Role of factor VIII-von Willebrand factor and fibronectin in the interaction of platelets in flowing blood with monomeric and fibrillar collagen types I and III. J Clin Invest 1985;75:531—540.

11. Houdijk WPM, De Groot PG, Nievelstein PFEM, Sakariassen KS, Sixma JJ. Subendothelial proteins and platelet adhesion: von Willebrand factor and fibronectin, not thrombospondin, are involved in platelet adhesion to extracellular matrix of human vascular endothelial cells. Arteriosclerosis 1986;6:24—33.

12. van Zanten GH, Saelman EUM, Schut-Hese KM, Wu YP, Slootweg PJ, Nieuwenhuis HK, De Groot PG, Sixma JJ. Platelet adhesion to collagen type IV under flow conditions. Blood 1996; 88:3862—3871.

13. Cruz MA, Yuan H, Lee JR, Wise RJ, Handin RI. Interaction of the von Willebrand factor (vWF) with collagen. Localization of the primary collagen-binding site by analysis of recombinant vWF A domain polypeptides. J Biol Chem 1995;270:10822—10827.

14. De Groot PG, Ottenhof-Rovers M, Van Mourik JA, Sixma JJ. Evidence that the primary binding site of von Willebrand factor that mediates platelet adhesion to subendothelium is not collagen. J Clin Invest 1988;82:65—73.

15. Rand JH, Wu X-X, Potter BJ, Uson RR, Gordon RE. Colocalization of von Willebrand factor and type VI collagen in human vascular subendothelium. Am J Pathol 1993;142:843—850.

16. Olson JD, Zaleski A, Herrmann D, Flood PA. Adhesion of platelets to purified solid-phase von Willebrand factor: effects of wall shear rate, ADP, thrombin and ristocetin. J Lab Clin Med 1989;114:6—18.

17. Danton MC, Zaleski A, Nichols WL, Olson JD. Monoclonal antibodies to platelet glycoproteins Ib and Iib/IIIa inhibit adhesion of platelets to purified solid-phase von Willebrand factor. J Lab Clin Med 1994;124:274—282.

18. Wu YP, van Breugel HHFI, Lankhof H, Wise RJ, Handin RI, de Groot PhG, Sixma JJ. Platelet adhesion to multimeric and dimeric von Willebrand Factor and to collagen type III preincubated with von Willebrand Factor. Arterioscl Thromb Vasc Biol 1996;16:611—620.

19. Federici AB, de Romeuf C, De Groot PG, Samor B, Lombardi R, d'Alessio PA, Mazurier C, Mannucci PM, Sixma JJ. Adhesive properties of the carbohydrate-modified von Willebrand factor (CHO-vWF). Blood 1988;71:947—952.

20. de Marco L, Mazzuccato M, Del Ben MG, Budde U, Federici AB. Type IIB von Willebrand factor with normal sialic acid content induces platelet aggregation in the absence of ristocetin. JCI 1987;80:475—482.

21. de Marco L, Mazzucato M, De Roia D, Casonato A, Federici AB, Girolami A, Ruggeri ZM. Distinct abnormalities in the interaction of purified types IIA and IIB von Willebrand factor with the two platelet binding sites, glycoprotein complexes Ib-IX and IIb-IIIa. JCI 1990;86: 785−792.

22. Lankhof H, Damas C, Schiphorst ME, IJsseldijk MJW, Bracke M, Sixma JJ, Vink T, de Groot Ph G. Functional studies on platelet adhesion with recombinant von Willebrand Factor type 2B mutants R543Q and R543W under conditions of flow. Blood 1997;89:2766−2772.

23. Miyata S, Goto S, Federici AB, Ware J, Ruggeri ZM. Conformational changes in the A1 domain of von Willebrand factor modulating the interaction with platelet glycoprotein Iba. J Biol Chem 1996;271:9046−9053.

24. Weiss HJ, Turitto VT, Baumgartner HR. Platelet adhesion and thrombus formation on subendothelium in platelets deficient in glycoproteins IIb-IIIa and storage organelles. Blood 1986; 67:322−331.

25. Sakariassen KS, Nievelstein PFEM, Coller BS, Sixma JJ. The role of platelet membrane glycoproteins Ib and IIb-IIIa in platelet adherence to human artery subendothelium. Br J Haematol 1986;63:681−691.

26. Weiss HJ, Turitto VT, Baumgartner HR. Further evidence that glycoprotein IIb-IIIa mediates platelet spreading on subendothelium. Thromb Haemost 1991;65:202−205.

27. Hantgan RR, Endenburg SC, Sixma JJ, De Groot PG. Evidence that fibrin a-chain RGDX sequences are not required for platelet adhesion in flowing blood. Blood 1995;(In press).

28. Ginsberg MH, Loftus JC, D'Souza S, Plow EF. Ligand binding to integrins: common and ligand specific recognition mechanisms. Cell Diff Dev 1990;32:203−214.

29. Holmbäck K, Danton MJS, Suh TT, Daugherty CC, Degen JL. Impaired platelet aggregation and sustained bleeding in mice lacking the fibrinogen motif bound by integrin $a_{IIb}b_3$. EMBO J 1996;15(21):5760−5771.

30. Hamaguchi M, Bunce LA, Sporn LA, Francis CW. Spreading of platelets on fibrin is mediated by the aminoterminus of the b chain including peptide b15−42. Blood 1993;81:2348−2356.

31. Rosales C, Juliano RL. Signal transduction by cell adhesion receptors in leukocytes. J Leuk Biol 1995;57:189−198.

32. Savage B, Saldívar E, Ruggeri ZM. Initiation of platelet adhesion by arrest onto fibrinogen or translocation on von Willebrand factor. Cell 1996;84:289−297.

33. Saelman EUM, Nieuwenhuis HK, Hese KM, de Groot PG, Heijnen HFG, Sage EH, Williams S, McKeown L, Gralnick HR, Sixma JJ. Platelet adhesion to collagen types I through VIII under conditions of stasis and flow is mediated by GPIa/IIa (a_2b_1-integrin). Blood 1994;83: 1244−1250.

34. Beumer S, IJsseldijk MJW, De Groot PG, Sixma JJ. Platelet adhesion to fibronectin in flow: dependence on surface concentration and shear rate, role of membrane GP IIb/IIIa and VLA-5 and inhibition by heparin. Blood 1994;84:3724−3733.

35. Moroi M, Jung SM, Shinmyozu K, Tomiyama Y, Ordinas A, Diaz-Ricart M. Analysis of platelet adhesion to a collagen-coated surface under flow conditions: the involvement of glycoprotein VI in the platelet adhesion. Blood 1996;88:2081−2092.

36. Hindriks GA, IJsseldijk MJW, Sonnenberg A, Sixma JJ, De Groot PG. Platelet adhesion to laminin: role of Ca^{2+} and Mg^{2+} ions, shear rate, and platelet membrane glycoproteins. Blood 1992;79:928−935.

37. Agbanyo FR, Sixma JJ, De Groot PG, Languino LR, Plow EF. Thrombospondin-platelet interactions. Role of divalent cations, wall shear rate and platelet membrane glycoproteins. J Clin Invest 1993;92:288−996.

38. Faull RJ, Ginsberg MH. Inside-out signaling through integrins. J Am Soc Nephrol 1996;7(8): 1091−1097.

39. Leong L, Hughes PE, Schwartz MA, Ginsberg MH, Shattil SJ. Integrin signaling: roles for the cytoplasmic tails of $a_{IIb}b_3$ in the tyrosine phosphorylation of pp125[FAK]. J Cell Sci 1995;108: 3817−3825.

40. Barstad RM, Kierulf P, Sakariassen KS. Collagen-induced thrombus formation at the apex of eccentric stenoses — a time course study with non-anticoagulated human blood. Thromb Haemost 1996;75:685—692.
41. Heijnen HFG, Lozano Molero M, De Groot PG, Nieuwenhuis HK, Sixma JJ. Absence of ligands bound to glycoprotein IIb-IIIa on the exposed surface of a thrombus may limit thrombus growth in flowing blood. J Clin Invest 1994;94:1098—1112.

Molecular requirements for ligand recognition by β_3 integrins

Thomas J. Kunicki
Roon Research Center for Arteriosclerosis and Thrombosis, Division of Experimental Hemostasis and Thrombosis, Departments of Molecular and Experimental Medicine and Department of Vascular Biology, The Scripps Research Institute, La Jolla, California, USA

Abstract. With regard to the tripeptide motif arginine-glycine-aspartate (RGD), integrin specificity is modulated by the juxtaposition of the R and D side chains. The Fab molecules of the AP7 series contain the RGD sequence in CDR3 of their respective H chains (H3), and represent a valuable paradigm of natural RGD ligand behavior. The amino acid composition immediately adjacent to the RGD tripeptide can change the specificity of the ligand for β_3 integrins. AP7 (HPFYRGDGGN) binds exclusively to $\alpha_{IIb}\beta_3$, while AP7.4 (HPFYRGDGGA) binds solely to $\alpha_V\beta_3$. In comparison to $\alpha_V\beta_3$, $\alpha_{IIb}\beta_3$ is more selective with respect to the R and D side chain orientations that it will recognize. Affinity modulation, is also governed by differences in the immediate environment of the RGD sequence. We evaluated the binding of AP7.3, in which the H3 loop sequence of AP7 is replaced by that of the activation-dependent Fab molecule PAC1.1 (**RSPSYYRGDGAGP**). AP7 does not bind preferentially to activated $\alpha_{IIb}\beta_3$, while AP7.3 does. We conclude that very subtle changes in the position and/or orientation of the RGD sequence and its immediate flanking sequences are sufficient to modify integrin specificity and the dependence of ligand binding on the conformational state of the receptor.

The human integrins represent 22 different membrane glycoprotein heterodimers which result from the noncovalent pairing between 16 α and 8 β subunits [1—6]. These ubiquitous receptors mediate a wide range of cell adhesion events that are important to almost every fundamental area of human biology, including embryonal development, immunocompetence, wound healing and hemostasis.

As for their ligands, one commonly recognized binding site is the tripeptide sequence arginine-glycine-aspartate (RGD), present in numerous adhesive molecules, including fibrinogen or von Willebrand factor (vWF). This motif is recognized by $\alpha_{IIb}\beta_3$, $\alpha_V\beta_3$ and at least five other RGD-cognitive integrins [3,7—9]. Each of these "RGD-cognitive" integrins exhibits selective affinity for the variety of natural ligands that contain the RGD sequence.

Affinity modulation

Integrins undergo conformational transitions that can modulate ligand specificity and/or affinity. The single integrin that is most dramatically affected by cell stimulation is platelet $\alpha_{IIb}\beta_3$. In its "quiescent" or basal state, $\alpha_{IIb}\beta_3$ has a negli-

Address for correspondence: Thomas J. Kunicki PhD, Associate Professor, The Scripps Research Institute, 10550 North Torrey Pines Road, Maildrop SBR 13, La Jolla, CA 92037, USA. Tel.: +1-619-784-2668. Fax: +1-619-784-2174. E-mail: tomk@scripps.edu

gible affinity for its preferred ligands in soluble form but does retain the ability to mediate platelet attachment to one of these ligands, fibrinogen, when it is adsorbed to a surface [10]. Once the platelet is activated, however, the conformation and activity of $\alpha_{IIb}\beta_3$ changes such that it can engage fibrinogen, von Willebrand factor (vWF), fibronectin or vitronectin in soluble form and mediate attachment to any one of these proteins adsorbed to a surface [11,12]. We and others have accumulated evidence (some of which is presented below) that the structure of the RGD tract and its immediate environment markedly influence affinity modulation. However, the ultimate strength of the adhesive interaction between ligand and receptor in vivo is influenced by structural determinants in the ligand other than the RGD sequence [13−16], by post-ligand-binding events including outside-in signaling [17−19], by multiple contact points on the receptor [20−24] and by hemodynamic forces [25].

Molecular models of the RGD binding site

There are a number of natural or synthetic products that contain or mimic the RGD motif and bind differentially to $\alpha_{IIb}\beta_3$ vs. $\alpha_V\beta_3$ [18,26−36]. In an attempt to understand the behavior of such ligands better, Suehiro et al. [37] carefully compared the binding of various RGD ligands and peptides to the β_3 integrins as a function of divalent cation composition, and grouped ligands into four classes (Table 1). Class I, represented by RGD peptides and vitronectin, bind equivalently to $\alpha_{IIb}\beta_3$ and $\alpha_V\beta_3$. Class II, represented by the mimetic cHarGD, fibrinogen or fibrinogen γ-chain peptides, bind to both integrins in the presence of Mn^{2+}, but only with $\alpha_{IIb}\beta_3$ in the presence of Ca^{2+}. Class III, such as the disintegrin barbourin, bind exclusively to $\alpha_{IIb}\beta_3$ under any condition. Class IV,

Table 1. Classes of β_3 ligands (adapted from [37]).

Class	Ligands	Characteristicsa
I	Disintegrin Group A[a] (e.g., eristostatin), RGD peptides, vitronectin	Bind to both $\alpha IIb\beta_3$ and $\alpha V\beta_3$ in Ca^{2+} or Mn^{2+}
II	AP7, CHarGD, disintegrin group B[ab] (e.g., echistatin), fibrinogen, fibrinogen (γ-chain peptides)	Bind to $\alpha_V\beta_3$ in Mn^{2+} but not in Ca^{2+}; bind to $\alpha_{IIb}\beta_3$ in Ca^{2+} or Mn^{2+}
III	OPG2, barbourin	Bind only to $\alpha_{IIb}\beta_3$ and under all cation conditions
IV	AP7.4, osteopontin	Bind to $\alpha_V\beta_3$ in Mn^{2+} but not in Ca^{2+}; do not bind to $\alpha_{IIb}\beta_3$

[a]Disintegrin group A binds to resting or activated platelets with equivalent affinity [49,50]. Disintegrin group B binds to activated platelets with higher affinity [51]. [b]Cation-dependent reactivity of this group with $\alpha_V\beta_3$ remains to be determined.

represented by osteopontin, bind primarily to $\alpha_V\beta_3$. Two molecular vehicles provide valuable insight into RGD ligand behavior: the disintegrins [18,29–32] and the recombinant monoclonal Fab molecules of the AP7 series [34,35,38,39].

Disintegrins

Disintegrins are naturally occurring low molecular weight polypeptides that contain the sequence RGD, bind to any number of integrins (such as $\alpha_{IIb}\beta_3$ and $\alpha_V\beta_3$), and can be isolated from venom of vipers or pit vipers (for example, echistatin or trigramin) [18,29–31,40]. Barbourin, which is highly specific for $\alpha_{IIb}\beta_3$, is unique in that it contains the sequence KGD in place of RGD [41]. In the disintegrin molecule, a series of tightly packed and irregular loops form a rigid core that is constrained by multiple disulfide bonds (four in echistatin; six in kistrin), and the RGD sequence is located at the center of a flexible, hairpin loop that extends from this core [31,40,42–44]. Disintegrins that contain the tetrapeptide RGDW have about a 2-fold higher affinity for $\alpha_{IIb}\beta_3$ than for $\alpha_V\beta_3$ [32]. Conversely, RGDNP is about 5-fold more efficient in blocking $\alpha_V\beta_3$ than $\alpha_{IIb}\beta_3$, and about 10-fold more active than RGDW in inhibiting the activity of $\alpha_5\beta_1$. From these and earlier findings [27,34,45], one could argue that the RGD recognition site of $\alpha_{IIb}\beta_3$ prefers to bind to RGD in a locally hydrophobic environment and that efficacy of RGD peptides with respect to $\alpha_{IIb}\beta_3$ increases with increasing hydophobocity of the residue on the carboxy side of RGD. Thus, the peptide RGDW is about 200-fold more active in blocking $\alpha_{IIb}\beta_3$-mediated aggregation than is RGDS.

The AP7 Fab series

OPG2 is the parent molecule from which the members of the AP7 series were derived. Specificity of OPG2 (IgG1-κ isotype), which can bind to nonactivated platelets with high affinity (Kd = 25.4 nM), resides completely in the third heavy chain complementarity-determining region (H3) which contains the amino acid sequence arg-tyr-asp (RYD) contributed by the germline D-gene DSP 2.10 [34,35]. The binding of OPG2 to $\alpha_{IIb}\beta_3$ is completely inhibited by peptides that contain RYD or the substitution RGD at the same position [33,34]. Moreover, OPG2 fails to bind to mutant $\alpha_{IIb}\beta_3$ that includes CAM β_3 [34] which contains a single amino acid substitution at position 109 resulting in the complete absence of RGD recognition 21). Single amino acid substitutions within H3 alone (as described in detail below) result in complete loss of Fab binding to $\alpha_{IIb}\beta_3$ or any other integrin, significant changes in affinity for $\alpha_{IIb}\beta_3$ or dramatically altered specificy for other integrins.

Properties of RGD ligands that alter integrin specificity

In one series of comparisons, we were able to determine that the amino acid composition immediately adjacent to the RGD tripeptide can change the specificity of this Fab molecule for β_3 integrins. The sole difference in sequence between AP7 (which binds exclusively to $\alpha_{IIb}\beta_3$) and AP7.4 (which binds solely to $\alpha_v\beta_3$) is a single amino acid substitution within the H3 loop (HPFYRGDGGN in AP7 vs. HPFYRGDGGA in AP7.4) (Table 2). From X-ray crystallographic studies of OPG2 [46], the parent molecule of AP7 and AP7.4, we know that the Asn^{108} side chain can form a hydrogen bond with the side chain of Asp^{105}. Exchange of Asn^{108} with the nonionic residue, Ala, would eliminate that hydrogen bond, and the accomodation of this change by the mutated H3 loop probably leads to an altered orientation of the Arg^{103} and Asp^{105} side chains. Consequently, we would conclude that the Asn^{108}-Asp^{105} of OPG2 and AP7 maintains the Asn^{105} side chain in a particular orientation with respect to the Arg^{103} side chain such that the RGD tripeptide fits exclusively into the binding site of $\alpha_{IIb}\beta_3$.

Properties of RGD ligands that modulate relative affinity for different states of the integrin

Since affinity modulation is not governed by gross differences in molecular structure, more subtle differences in structure within the immediate environment of the RGD sequence may modulate ligand affinity. In another series of comparisons (Table 3), we exploited the binding properties of the AP7 Fab series and PAC1.1, the RGD-containing analog of the previously described RYD-containing antibody PAC1 [38,47,48]. AP7 Fab molecules bind with high affinity to either the nonactivated or the activated conformational states of $\alpha_{IIb}\beta_3$. On the other hand, recombinant PAC1.1 Fab molecules bind more avidly to the activated conformation of $\alpha_{IIb}\beta_3$, as reflected by an increase in affinity and number of sites. We compared the binding of AP7 to that of a newly engineered variant, AP7.3, in which the H3 loop sequence of AP7 was replaced by the H3 loop sequence of PAC1.1 [38]. Our findings clearly established that the amino acid environment within the immediate vicinity of the RGD tripeptide in macromolecular ligands is a major factor that regulates the sensitivity of ligand binding to the activation state of $\alpha_{IIb}\beta_3$.

Table 2. Comparative binding of recombinant fab molecules to β_3 integrins.

Fab	H3 sequence	Binds in the presence of							
		Ca^{2+} plus Mg^{2+}				Mn^{2+}			
		$\alpha_{IIb}\beta_3$	$\alpha_v\beta_3$	Platelets	M21	$\alpha_{IIb}\beta_3$	$\alpha_v\beta_3$	Platelets	M21
OPG2	HPFYRYDGGN	Yes	No	Yes	No	Yes	No	Yes	No
AP7	HPFYRGDGGN	Yes	No	Yes	No	Yes	Yes	Yes	Yes
AP7.4	HPFYRGDGGA	No	No	No	No	No	Yes	No	Yes
AP7.7	HPFYRYDGGA	No	No	No	No	No	No	No	No

From [39].

Table 3. Recombinant fab molecules employed to study affinity modulation of ligand binding to integrin $\alpha_{IIb}\beta_3$.

Fab	Framework	.......H3.......		
		V_H	D	J_H
OPG2	OPG2	.....Y C T R	H P F Y R Y D G G N	Y.....
AP7	OPG2	.....Y C T R	H P F Y R G D G G N	Y.....
AP7.1	OPG2	.....Y C T R	R S P S Y Y R G D G G N	Y.....
AP7.2	OPG2	.....Y C T R	H P F Y R G D G A G P	Y.....
AP7.3	OPPG2	.....Y C T R	R S P S Y Y R G D G A G P	Y.....
PAC1.1	PAC1	.....Y C T R	R S P S Y Y R G D G A G P	Y.....
PAC1	PAC1	.....Y C T R	R S P S Y Y R Y D G A G P	Y.....

From [38].

References

1. Hynes RO. Integrins: versatility, modulation and signaling in cell adhesion. Cell 1992;69: 11—25.
2. Hemler ME. VLA proteins in the integrin family: structures, functions, and their role on leukocytes. Ann Rev Immunol 1990;8:365—400.
3. Ruoslahti E. Integrins. J Clin Invest 1991;87:1—5.
4. Springer TA. Adhesion receptors of the immune system. Nature 1990;346:425—434.
5. Albelda SM, Buck CA. Integrins and other cell adhesion molecules. FASEB J 1990;4: 2868—2880.
6. Arnaout MA. Structure and function of the leukocyte adhesion molecules CD11/CD18. Blood 1990;75:1037—1050.
7. Cheng S, Craig WS, Mullen D et al. Design and synthesis of novel cyclic RGD-containing peptides as highly potent and selective integrin $\alpha_{IIb}\beta_3$ antagonists. J Med Chem 1994;37:1—8.
8. Busk M, Pytela R, Sheppard D. Characterization of the integrin alpha v beta 6 as a fibronectin-binding protein. J Biol Chem 1992;267:5790—5796.
9. Nishimura SL, Pytela R. Characterization of the integrin $\alpha_V\beta_8$. Molec Biol Cell 1993;4(Suppl): 285.
10. Savage B, Shattil SJ, Ruggeri ZM. Modulation of platelet function through adhesion receptors. A dual role for glycoprotein IIb-IIIa (integrin $\alpha_{IIb}\beta_3$) mediated by fibrinogen and glycoprotein Ib-von Willebrand factor. J Biol Chem 1992;267:11300—11306.
11. Haverstick DM, Cowan JF, Yamada KM et al. Inhibition of platelet adhesion to fibronectin, fibrinogen and von Willebrand factor substrates by a synthetic tetrapeptide derived from the cell-binding domain of fibronectin. Blood 1985;66:946—952.
12. Savage B, Ruggeri ZM. Selective recognition of adhesive sites in surface-bound fibrinogen by GP IIb-IIIa on nonactivated platelets. J Biol Chem 1991;266:11227—11233.
13. Charo IF, Nannizzi L, Phillips DR et al. Inhibition of fibrinogen binding to GPIIb-IIIa by a GP IIIa peptide. J Biol Chem 1991;266:1414—1421.
14. Kloczewiak M, Timmons S, Bednarek MA et al. Platelet receptor recognition domain on the gamma chain of human fibrinogen and its synthetic peptide analogues. Biochemistry 1989; 28:2915—2919.
15. Bowditch RD, Hariharan M, Tominna EF et al. Identification of a novel integrin binding site in fibronectin. Differential utilization by β_3 integrins. J Biol Chem 1994;269:10856—10863.
16. Bowditch RD, Halloran CE, Obara M et al. Integrin $\alpha_{IIb}\beta_3$ (Platelet GPIIb-IIIa) recognizes multiple sites in fibronectin. J Biol Chem 1991;266:23323—23328.

17. Chen Y-P, O'Toole TE, Shipley T et al. "Inside-out" signal transduction inhibited by isolated integrin cytoplasmic domains. J Biol Chem 1994;269:18307—18310.

18. Haung M, Lipfert L, Cunningham M et al. Adhesive ligand binding to integrin $\alpha_{IIb}\beta_3$ stimulates tyrosine phosphorylation of novel protein substrates before phosphorylation of pp125[FAK]. J Cell Biol 1993;12:473—483.

19. O'Toole TE, Katagiri Y, Tamura RN et al. Integrin cytoplasmic domains mediate inside-out signal transduction. J Cell Biol 1994;124:1047—1059.

20. D'Souza SE, Ginsberg MH, Burke TA et al. Localization of an Arg-Gly-Asp recognition site within an integrin adhesion receptor. Science 1988;242:91—93.

21. Loftus JC, O'Toole TE, Plow EF et al. A β_3 integrin mutation abolishes ligand binding and alters divalent cation-dependent conformation. Science 1990;249:915—918.

22. D'Souza SE, Ginsberg MH, Burke TA et al. The ligand binding site of the platelet integrin receptor GPIIb-IIIa is proximal to the second calcium binding domain of its alpha subunit. J Biol Chem 1990;265:3440—3446.

23. D'Souza SE, Ginsberg MH, Matsueda GR et al. A discrete sequence in a platelet integrin is involved in ligand recognition. Nature 1991;350:66—68.

24. Bajt ML, Loftus JC. Mutation of a ligand binding domain of β_3 integrin. Integral role of oxygenated residues in $\alpha_{IIb}\beta_3$ (GPIIb-IIIa) receptor function. J Biol Chem 1994;269:20913—20919.

25. Savage B, Saldivar E, Ruggeri ZM. Initiation of platelet adhesion by arrest onto fibrinogen or translocation on von Willebrand factor. Cell 1996;84:289—297.

26. Pierschbacher MD, Ruoslahti E. Cell attachment activity of fibronectin can be duplicated by small synthetic fragments of the molecule. Nature 1984;309:30—33.

27. Plow EF, Pierschbacher MD, Ruoslahti E et al. Arginyl-Glycyl-Aspartic acid sequences and fibronogen binding to platelets. Blood 1987;70:110—115.

28. Ruggeri ZM, Houghten RA, Russell SR et al. Inhibition of platelet function with synthetic peptides designed to be high-affinity antagonists of fibrinogen binding to platelets. Proc Natl Acad Sci USA 1986;83:5708—5712.

29. Huang T-F, Holt JC, Kirby EP et al. Trigramin: Primary structure and its inhibition of von Willebrand factor binding to glycoprotein IIb/IIIa complex on human platelets. Biochemistry 1989; 28:661—666.

30. Gan Z, Gould RJ, Jacobs JW et al. Echistatin. A potent platelet aggregation inhibitor from the venom of the viper, *Echis Carinatus*. J Biol Chem 1988;263:19827—19832.

31. Adler M, Lazarus RA, Dennis MS et al. Solution structure of Kistrin, a potent platelet aggregation inhibitor and GP IIb-IIIa antagonist. Science 1991;253:445—448.

32. Scarborough RM, Rose JW, Naughton MA et al. Characterization of the integrin specificities of disintegrins isolated from American pit viper venoms. J Biol Chem 1993;268:1058—1065.

33. Taub R, Gould RJ, Garsky VM et al. A monoclonal antibody against the platelet fibrinogen receptor contains a sequence that mimics a receptor recognition domain in fibrinogen. J Biol Chem 1989;264:259—265.

34. Tomiyama Y, Tsubakio T, Piotrowicz RS et al. The Arg-Gly-Asp (RGD) recognition site of platelet glycoprotein IIb-IIIa on nonactivated platelets is accessible to high-affinity macromolecules. Blood 1992;79:2303—2312.

35. Tomiyama Y, Brojer E, Ruggeri ZM et al. A molecular model of RGD ligands: antibody D gene segments that direct specificity for the integrin $\alpha_{IIb}\beta_3$. J Biol Chem 1992;267:18085—18092.

36. Niiya K, Hodson E, Bader R et al. Increased surface expression of the membrane glycoprotein IIb/IIIa complex induced by platelet activation. Relationship to the binding of fibrinogen and platelet aggregation. Blood 1987;70:475—483.

37. Suehiro K, Smith JW, Plow EF. The ligand recognition specificity of β_3 integrins. J Biol Chem 1996;271:10365—10371.

38. Kunicki TJ, Annis DS, Deng YJ et al. A molecular basis for affinity modulation of Fab ligand binding to integrin $\alpha_{IIb}\beta_3$. J Biol Chem 1996;271:20315—20321.

39. Kunicki TJ, Annis DS, Felding-Habermann B. Molecular determinants of RGD ligand specifi-

city for β3 integrins. J Biol Chem 1996;272:4103—4107.

40. Kunicki TJ, Orchekowski R, Annis D et al. Variability of integrin $\alpha_2\beta_1$ activity on human platelets. Blood 1993;82:2693—2703.

41. Scarborough RM, Rose JW, Hsu MA et al. Barbourin. A GPIIb-IIIa-specific integrin antagonist from the venom of *sistrurus M. Barbouri*. J Biol Chem 1991;266:9359—9362.

42. Senn H, Klaus W. The nuclear magnetic resonance solution structure of flavoridin, and antagonist of the platelet GP IIb-IIIa receptor. J Mol Biol 1993;232:907—925.

43. Calvete JJ, Schafer W, Soszka T et al. Identification of the disulfide bond pattern in albolabrin, an RGD-containing peptide from the venom of *Trimeresurus albolabris* significance for the expression of platelet aggregation inhibitory activity. Biochemistry 1991;30:5225—5229.

44. Calvete JJ, Wang Y, Mann K et al. The disulfide bridge pattern of snake venom disintegrins, flavoridin and echistatin. FEBS Lett 1992;309:316—320.

45. Plow EF, Pierschbacher MD, Ruoslahti E et al. The effect of Arg-Gly-Asp-containing peptides on fibrinogen and von Willebrand factor binding to platelets. Proc Natl Acad Sci USA 1985;82: 8057—8061.

46. Kodandapani R, Veerapandian B, Kunicki TJ et al. Crystal structure of the OPG2 Fab: an anti-receptor antibody that mimics an RGD cell adhesion site. J Biol Chem 1995;270:2268—2273.

47. Kunicki TJ, Ely KR, Kunicki TC et al. The exchange of Arg-Gly-Asp (RGD) and Arg-Tyr-Asp (RYD) binding sequences in a recombinant murine Fab fragment specific for the integrin $\alpha_{IIb}\beta_3$ does not alter integrin recognition. J Biol Chem 1995;270(28):16660—16665.

48. Abrams C, Deng Y-J, Steiner B et al. Determinants of specificity of a baculovirus-expressed antibody Fab fragment that binds selectively to the activated form of integrin $\alpha_{IIb}\beta_3$. J Biol Chem 1994;269:18781—18788.

49. McLane MA, Gabbeta J, Rao AK et al. A comparison of the effect of decorsin and two disintegrins, albolabrin and eristostatin, on platelet function. Thromb Haemost 1995;74(5): 1316—1322.

50. Lu X, Williams JA, Deadman J et al. Preferential antagonism of the interactions of the integrin $\alpha_{IIb}\beta_3$ with immovilized glycoprotein ligands by snake-venom RGD (Arg-Gly-Asp) proteins. Biochem J 1994;304:929—936.

51. Marcinkiewicz C, Rosenthal LA, Mosser DM et al. Immunological characterization of eristostatin and echistatin binding sites on α_{IIb} and $\alpha_v\beta_3$ integrins. Biochem J 1996;317:817—825.

Molecular insights into HDL and its properties

Structure-function relationships in apolipoprotein A-I: insights from the A-I$_{Milano}$ mutation

Guido Franceschini[1], Laura Calabresi[1], Cesare R. Sirtori[1], Franco Bernini[2], Ana Jonas[3], Donatella Taramelli[4] and Giuseppe Vecchio[5]

[1]*Center E. Grossi Paoletti, Institute of Pharmacological Sciences, University of Milano, Milan, Italy;* [2]*Institute of Pharmacology and Pharmacognosy, University of Parma, Parma, Italy;* [3]*Department of Biochemistry, University of Illinois at Urbana-Champaign, Urbana, Illinois, USA;* [4]*Institute of Medical Microbiology, University of Milano, Milan, Italy; and* [5]*Istituto di Chimica degli Ormoni, CNR, Milan, Italy*

Keywords: atherosclerosis, HDL, protein structure, reverse cholesterol transport.

Introduction

Apolipoprotein A-I (apoA-I) is the major protein constituent of human high-density lipoproteins (HDL) and seems to carry the major responsibility in the antiatherogenic activity of HDL. ApoA-I plays multiple roles in reverse cholesterol transport, the process by which excess cholesterol is removed from peripheral tissues (including the arterial wall), esterified in plasma and transported to the liver for excretion [1]. ApoA-I is the preferential acceptor of cell cholesterol, and acts as a cofactor for the lecithin cholesterol acyltransferase (LCAT) enzyme as well as a ligand for the putative HDL receptor. In addition, apoA-I displays unique properties that are not directly related to its major activities in reverse cholesterol transport, but possibly involved in HDL protection against vascular disease (i.e., prostacyclin stabilization, activation of fibrinolysis and modulation of complement function) [2].

The mature plasma apoA-I is a single polypeptide chain composed of 243 residues and lacks cysteine and isoleucine [3]. The most striking feature of the apoA-I sequence is the presence of internal repeat units of 11 or 22 amino acids, with the potential of forming amphipathic α-helices, interrupted by β-turns occurring at proline and glycine residues [4]. In the presence of phospholipids, apoA-I generates discoidal particles similar to nascent HDL (also known as reconstituted HDL (rHDL) [5]), in which the amphipathic helices run from side to side of the disk, with charged residues facing the aqueous phase and hydrophobic residues facing the acyl chains of the phospholipid bilayer [6]. Two relatively

Address for correspondence: Prof Guido Franceschini, Center E. Grossi Paoletti, Institute of Pharmacological Sciences, Via Balzaretti 9, 20133 Milano, Italy. Tel.: +39-2-6471690. Fax: +39-2-6470594. E-mail: Guido.Franceschini@unimi.it

distinct structural domains can be identified in apoA-I:
1) the amino-terminal end (residues 1–37), with very little α-helix potential and lipid-binding capacity; and
2) the central carboxy terminal fragment, which organizes in highly packed anti-parallel α-helices [6].

A hinged subdomain constituted by a pair of amphipathic helices, which could exist in two conformations, either bound to the lipoprotein surface or free in the aqueous milieu, has been identified within the central portion of apoA-I [7].

Apolipoprotein A-I$_{Milano}$ (A-I$_M$) is a molecular variant of apoA-I characterized by the Arg^{173}→Cys substitution [8], leading to the formation of a disulfide-linked homodimer (A-I$_M$/A-I$_M$). A-I$_M$/A-I$_M$ possesses molecular properties that are unique when compared to those of normal apoA-I: facilitated interhelix interactions, increased secondary structure and a more folded tertiary structure [9]. To evaluate the impact of the interchain disulfide bridge in A-I$_M$/A-I$_M$ on apoA-I functional properties, we prepared well-defined complexes of phosphatidylcholine (PC) and either apoA-I or A-I$_M$/A-I$_M$, and tested them for LCAT reactivity, promotion of cell cholesterol efflux and modulation of cell-cell interactions.

Generation of rHDL

The sizes and distributions of rHDL particles containing A-I$_M$/A-I$_M$ and apoA-I were examined by nondenaturing polyacrylamide gradient gel electrophoresis. The average size of rHDL generated with apoA-I increased from 7.8 to 17.6 nm with increasing PC:apolipoprotein weight ratio [10]. In contrast, the distribution of rHDL generated with A-I$_M$/A-I$_M$ changed with increasing PC:apolipoprotein ratio, but the same rHDL species with diameters of 8.2 and 12.5 nm, were present in all the preparations. Further incubation with LDL caused the disappearance of the 8.2 nm rHDL, with generation of a 7.8 nm rHDL particle and no changes in the 12.5 nm rHDL. The purified small (7.8 nm) and large (12.5 nm) rHDL species, containing one and two molecules of A-I$_M$/A-I$_M$ per particle, respectively, were compared with similarly sized apoA-I rHDL.

Investigations about the spectral properties of A-I$_M$/A-I$_M$ and apoA-I rHDL suggest that apoA-I possesses a remarkable degree of structural flexibility, manifested by drastic changes in secondary and tertiary structure in response to changes in particle size and composition. In contrast, A-I$_M$/A-I$_M$ adopts a similar, if not identical, conformation even when the lipid content and size of rHDL changes significantly [10]. Therefore, the introduction of the disulfide bridge in A-I$_M$/A-I$_M$ has two major effects on the generation of stable lipid/protein complexes, as follows:
1) it restricts particle size heterogeneity; and
2) limits the protein conformational flexibility.

Computer modeling of apoA-I and A-I$_M$/A-I$_M$ in rHDL is consistent with the experimental data in showing that apoA-I adopts different conformations, with the proposed hinged domain looping out of the rHDL surface in small particles and being in contact with lipids in the large rHDL. Instead, A-I$_M$/A-I$_M$ adopts identical conformations, with the C-terminal residues displaced with force out of the discs by the disulfide bridge and the hinged domain in the lipid-bound conformation.

Cholesterol efflux from cells

Facilitation of cholesterol efflux from peripheral cells is a major function of apoA-I in reverse cholesterol transport [1]. When incubated with lipid-laden mouse peritoneal macrophages, rHDL containing A-I$_M$/A-I$_M$ were significantly more efficient than those with apoA-I in promoting cholesterol efflux from the cell membrane, and inhibiting intracellular cholesterol esterification (Fig. 1). It is generally accepted that cholesterol efflux occurs in two steps: desorption from the cell membrane followed by diffusion into the extracellular fluid, where it is taken up by phospholipid-containing acceptor particles [11]. Acceptor-bound apolipoproteins can facilitate cholesterol efflux by interacting with specific lipid domains in the plasma membrane and substantially increasing the rate of choles- terol desorption; therefore, the more efficient efflux to the A-I$_M$/A-I$_M$ rHDL could be due to a preferential interaction with the membrane leading to higher rate of cholesterol desorption. It is intriguing that the C-terminal portion of apoA-I (which has a high affinity for lipid surfaces and has been involved in the initial binding of the apolipoprotein to the phospholipid bilayer [12]) is bound to the rHDL surface in the apoA-I-containing particles but loops out of the discs in A-I$_M$/A-I$_M$ rHDL. It thus appears that the hydrophobicity and the affinity for lipids of specific domains of apoA-I, which are able to dissociate from the HDL surface and interact with cell surfaces, can efficiently modulate cell cholesterol efflux to a apoA-I containing acceptors.

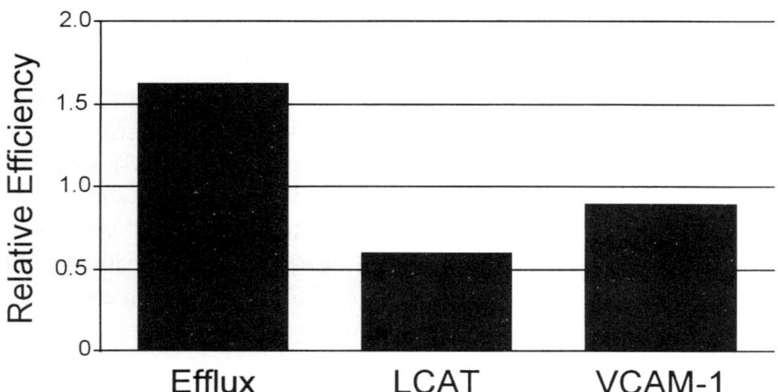

Fig. 1. Efficiency of 7.8 nm rHDL containing A-I$_M$/A-I$_M$, compared to apoA-I rHDL of similar size, in inhibiting cholesterol esterification in lipid-laden mouse peritoneal macrophages (Efflux), acting as substrates for LCAT and inhibiting cytokine-induced VCAM-1 expression in endothelial cells.

LCAT activation

Another major function of apoA-I in reverse cholesterol transport is the stimulation of cholesterol esterification through LCAT activation. As the reactivity of native and reconstituted HDL with LCAT is critically dependent on particle size, it is mandatory to compare protein/lipid complexes which are identical in size in studies comparing the LCAT activation capacity of different proteins. Two sets of cholesterol-containing apoA-I or $A-I_M/A-I_M$ rHDL with comparable diameters (7.8 and 12.5 nm) were incubated with purified enzyme. The large particles were more efficient substrates for LCAT than the smaller ones, independent of protein composition, but the $A-I_M/A-I_M$-containing particles were 40—70% less reactive with LCAT than their apoA-I size homologues (Fig. 1) [13]. Kinetic analyses showed that the constraints imposed by the disulfide bridge in $A-I_M/A-I_M$ result in a reduced ability to activate LCAT, but do not affect the binding of the enzyme to the substrate particles [13]. These results provide further support of the concept that LCAT activation by apoA-I is dependent on global protein conformation instead of specific amino acid sequences.

Cell-cell interactions

Evidence from a number of in vitro and in vivo studies suggests that HDL may also affect early stages of atherogenesis through mechanisms which are independent of their function in reverse cholesterol transport [14]. The onset of a vascular lesion involves adhesion of blood leukocytes to the dysfunctional endothelium, and subsequent transmigration of these cells into the intimal tissue. In cocultures of human aortic wall cells, HDL were able to inhibit LDL-induced binding of monocytes to target endothelial cells, and the subsequent transmigration and localization in the subendothelial space [15]. More recently, plasma-derived HDL have been shown to inhibit cytokine-induced expression of endothelial cell adhesion molecules in cultured endothelial cells [16]. By using a similar in vitro system, we could demonstrate that rHDL containing apoA-I or $A-I_M/A-I_M$ were similarly effective in inhibiting (by 50.4% and 44.8%, respectively) the TNFα-induced expression of the vascular cell adhesion molecule-1 (VCAM-1) (Fig. 1) [17]. How HDL inhibit cytokine-induced VCAM-1 expression is unknown. The results with apoA-I or $A-I_M/A-I_M$ rHDL suggest that the mechanism, which is likely to involve the modulation of adhesion molecule gene transcription [16] is rather unspecific, as two apolipoproteins with remarkably different secondary and tertiary structure display very similar activity.

Conclusions

The studies with synthetic HDL containing the disulfide-linked $A-I_M/A-I_M$ mutant indicate that changes in apoA-I primary sequence which affect protein conformation on the surface of HDL have distinct effects on major apoA-I functions. When compared to particles containing apoA-I, A-I$_M$/A-I$_M$ rHDL were more effective in promoting cell-cholesterol efflux, less efficient substrates in the LCAT reaction and equally potent in inhibiting cytokine-induced cell activation (Fig. 1). This suggests that these various functions depend on different structural features of apoA-I. The present results provide only indirect information on specific functional domains in apoA-I, which needs to be implemented with structure-function studies using recombinant apoA-I mutants [18]. The identification of specific domains involved in functions responsible for the antiatherogenic activity of apoA-I will provide the basis for the design of recombinant apoA-I molecules with improved antiatherogenic potential, that could become drugs with the objective of inhibiting initiation and fostering regression of atherosclerosis [19].

References

1. Franceschini G, Werba JP, Calabresi L. Drug control of reverse cholesterol transport. Pharmacol Ther 1994;61:289—324.
2. Franceschini G. Apolipoprotein function in health and disease: insights from natural mutations. Eur J Clin Invest 1996;26:733—746.
3. Brewer HB Jr, Fairwell T, Larue A, Ronan R, Houser A, Bronzert TJ. The amino acid sequence of human apoA-I, an apolipoprotein isolated from high-density lipoprotein. Biochem Biophys Res Commun 1978;80:623—630.
4. Segrest JP, Jones MK, De Loof H, Brouillette CG, Venkatachalapathi YV, Anantharamaiah GM. The amphipathic helix in the exchangeable apolipoproteins: a review of secondary structure and function. J Lipid Res 1992;33:141—166.
5. Jonas A. Reconstitution of high-density lipoproteins. Meth Enzymol 1986;128:553—582.
6. Brouillette CG, Anantharamaiah GM. Structural models of human apolipoprtoein A-I. Biochim Biophys Acta 1995;1256:103—129.
7. Calabresi L, Meng QH, Castro GR, Marcel YL. Apolipoprotein A-I conformation in discoidal particles: evidence for alternate structures. Biochemistry 1993;32:6477—6484.
8. Weisgraber KH, Rall SC Jr, Bersot TP, Mahley RW, Franceschini G, Sirtori CR. Apolipoprotein AI$_{Milano}$. Detection of normal AI in affected subjects and evidence for a cysteine for arginine substitution in the variant AI. J Biol Chem 1983;258:2508—2513.
9. Calabresi L, Vecchio G, Longhi R, Gianazza E, Palm G, Wadensten H, Hammarstrom A, Olsson A, Karlstrom A, Sejlitz T, Ageland H, Sirtori CR, Franceschini G. Molecular characterization of native and recombinant apolipoprotein A-I$_{Milano}$ dimer. The introduction of an interchain disulfide bridge remarkably alters the physicochemical properties of apolipoprotein A-I. J Biol Chem 1994;269:32168—32174.
10. Calabresi L, Vecchio G, Frigerio F, Vavassori L, Sirtori CR, Franceschini G. Reconstituted high-density lipoproteins with a disulfide-linked apolipoprotein A-I dimer: evidence for restricted particle size heterogeneity. Biochemistry 1998;(In press).
11. Johnson WJ, Mahlberg FH, Rothblat GH, Phillips MC. Cholesterol transport between cells and high-density lipoproteins. Biochim Biophys Acta 1991;1085:273—298.
12. Ji Y, Jonas A. Properties of an N-terminal proteolytic fragment of apolipoprotein AI in solution and in reconstituted high-density lipoproteins. J Biol Chem 1995;270:11290—11297.
13. Calabresi L, Franceschini G, Burkybile A, Jonas A. Activation of lecithin cholesterol acyltransferase by a disulfide-linked apolipoprotein A-I dimer. Biochem Biophys Res Commun 1997;232:345—349.
14. Soma MR, Donetti E, Parolini C, Sirtori CR, Fumagalli R, Franceschini G. Recombinant apo-

lipoprotein A-I$_{\text{Milano}}$ dimer inhibits carotid intimal thickening induced by perivascular manipulation in rabbits. Circ Res 1995;76:405−411.

15. Navab M, Imes SS, Hama SY, Hough GP, Ross LA, Bork RW, Valente AJ, Berliner JA, Drinkwater DC, Laks H, Fogelman AM. Monocyte transmigration induced by modification of low-density lipoprotein in cocultures of human aortic wall cells is due to induction of monocyte chemotactic protein 1 synthesis and is abolished by high-density lipoprotein. J Clin Invest 1991; 88:2039−2046.

16. Cockerill GW, Rye KA, Gamble JR, Vadas MA, Barter PJ. High-density lipoproteins inhibit cytokine-induced expression of endothelial cell adhesion molecules. Arterioscl Thromb Vasc Biol 1995;15:1987−1994.

17. Calabresi L, Franceschini G, Sirtori CR, de Palma A, Saresella M, Ferrante P, Taramelli D. Inhibition of VCAM-1 expression in endothelial cells by reconstituted high-density lipoproteins. Biochem Biophys Res Commun 1998;(In press).

18. Holvoet P, Zhao Z, Deridder E, Dhoest A, Collen D. Effects of deletion of the carboxyl-terminal domain of ApoA-I or of its substitution with helices of ApoA-II on in vitro and in vivo lipoprotein association. J Biol Chem 1996;271:19395−19401.

19. Sirtori CR. Recombinant apolipoproteins come of age. Nutr Metab Cardiovasc Dis 1995;5: 81−83.

Tryptophan residues stabilize the N-terminal domain of apolipoprotein A-I and promote its anchoring to lipid surfaces

W. Sean Davidson, Kirsten Arnvig McGuire and Ana Jonas

Department of Biochemistry, University of Illinois at Urbana-Champaign, Urbana, Illinois, USA

Abstract. *Background.* All the Trp residues of plasma apoA-I and recombinant proapoA-I are located in the N-terminal half of the proteins. Thus, these aromatic residues are useful probes of the N-terminal domain organization of apoA-I, its stability and its interaction with lipids.

Methods. Four Trp → Phe mutants of proapoA-I, with substitutions of two and four Trp residues, were prepared by PCR mutagenesis and expression in *Escherichia coli*. The purified proteins were studied by circular dichroism, fluorescence and absorbance methods in lipid-free and lipid-bound forms.

Results and Conclusions. The Trp → Phe mutants had very similar structures to wild-type pro-apoA-I, both in the lipid-free state and in reconstituted HDL. However, the lipid-free mutants with increasing contents of Phe residues had progressively lower free energies of unfolding, indicating that Trp side chains are important in stabilizing the N-terminal domain of apoA-I in solution. In addition, the Trp → Phe mutants cleared phospholipid liposomes at lower rates than proapoA-I, suggesting that Trp residues in the N-terminal domain participate in the initial anchoring of apoA-I to lipid surfaces.

Keywords: circular dichroism, fluorescence, phenylalanine, phospholipid, recombinant proapoA-I, reconstituted high-density lipoprotein.

Introduction

Several studies have suggested that apolipoprotein A-I (apoA-I) may be organized into distinct domains that roughly encompass the N- and C-terminal halves of the molecule. Fluorescence studies from our laboratory have shown that the Trp residues in the N-terminal half of the protein exist in nonpolar environments that are relatively protected from solvent [1,2]. Marcel and co-workers [3] have demonstrated the presence of discontinuous epitopes across the N-terminal and central regions of apoA-I suggesting substantial folding and contacts in these regions. Finally, in a recent study of apoA-I deletion mutants [4], we demonstrated that the N-terminal half of apoA-I is highly α-helical and is primarily responsible for the marginal stability of the protein in solution, whereas the C-terminal half is largely disorganized and unstable. Upon lipid-binding, the N-terminal half undergoes a rearrangement of α-helical segments without a major change in overall helicity. The C-terminal half, however, becomes highly helical and stabilizes the reconstituted HDL (rHDL) particles.

Address for correspondence: Prof Ana Jonas, Department of Biochemistry, University of Illinois at Urbana-Champaign, 506 South Mathews Avenue, Urbana, IL 61801, USA.

To determine in more detail the structural changes that occur throughout the N-terminal half of apoA-I, and to assess the role of Trp residues in apoA-I, we applied mutagenesis and spectroscopic techniques to probe the chemical environments of the five Trp residues that are present in the N-terminal half of recombinant proapoA-I [5]. In a recent publication we demonstrated that recombinant proapoA-I has essentially identical structural and functional properties to the mature apoA-I from human plasma [5]. Therefore, we feel justified in using Trp → Phe mutants of proapoA-I to study the N-terminal domain of apoA in this work.

Materials and Methods

Overexpression and purification of proapoA-I mutants

The four mutants of proapoA-I with two or four Trp → Phe substitutions, constructed in this study, are shown in Fig. 1. PCR-based mutagenesis techniques were used to modify the proapoA-I cDNA, inserted between NcoI and HindIII restriction sites of the pBluescript SK plasmid [5]. After the mutations were confirmed by DNA sequencing in the Biotechnology Center (University of Illinois, Urbana-Champaign), the mutant proapoA-I cDNAs were subcloned into the pET-28a, 5.8 kB expression plasmid, which was then transformed into BL-21 (DE3) *Escherichia coli* cells. The cells were induced with 2 mM IPTG and were grown for 5 h at 37°C, in the presence of 30 µg/ml of kanamycin.

Cells were lysed in 25 mM HEPES buffer containing 2% Triton X-100 and 50 µg/ml lysozyme, for 30 min at 4°C. After sonication and centrifugation, all of the proapoA-I mutant proteins were recovered in the supernatant fraction. The subsequent, general purification procedure is a modified version of the procedure we used previously to isolate recombinant proapA-I [5]. The first purification step exposed the supernatant proteins to 6 M guanidine hydrochloride (Gnd HCl). The following dialysis against 10 mM Tris buffer removed the denaturant and precipitated aggregated, denatured proteins, while the proapoA-I mutants refolded into soluble forms. Next, ammonium sulfate precipitation between 20 and 30% concentrations purified the proapoA-I mutants further and concentrated them for the subsequent phenyl sepharose chromatography step. The protein pellet from the ammonium sulfate precipitation step was dissolved in 20 mM Tris buffer, pH 8.0, and was passed through the phenyl sepharose column (Pharmacia, CL-4B; 1.5 × 20 cm). After extensive washing the proapoA-I mutants were eluted from the column with a gradient of Tris buffer from 0 to 60% ethylene glycol.

During the purification, 20% SDS-PAGE was used to follow proapoA-I mutant enrichment and isolation. Occasionally, to confirm the presence of apoA-I, polyclonal antiapoA-I antibodies were used in Western blots.

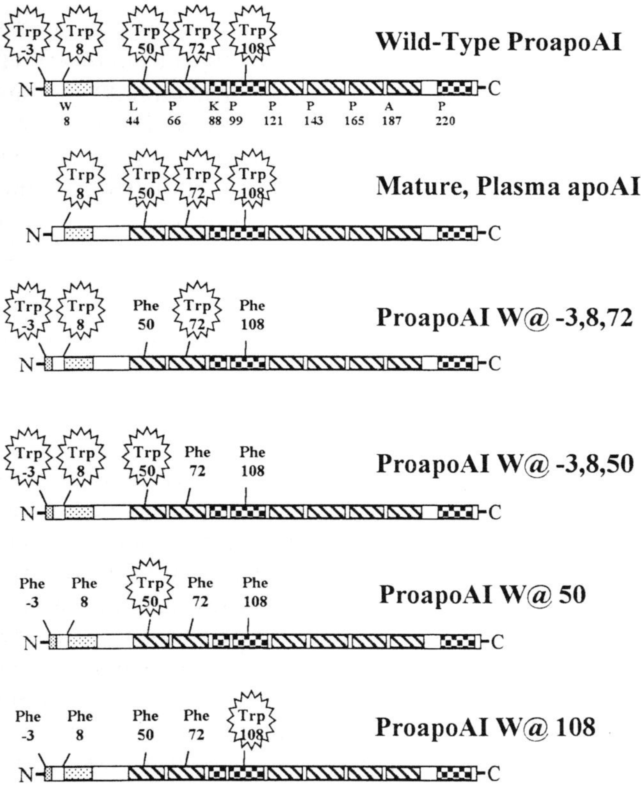

Fig. 1. ProapoA-I → Phe mutants constructed, expressed in *E. coli* and characterized in this study. The linear sequences of plasma apoA-I and recombinant proapoA-I and its Trp → Phe mutants show the location of the Trp residues and of the Phe substitutions. The cross-hatched segments in the sequences represent the putative amphipathic α-helical segments [17].

Spectroscopic analysis

The average α-helix contents of the proapoA-I mutants in lipid-free and lipid-bound states were determined by circular dichroism spectroscopy using a JASCO J-720 spectropolarimeter at the Laboratory for Fluorescence Dynamics (University of Illinois, Urbana-Champaign). Spectra were measured at 25°C in 0.1 cm cuvettes and the percent of α-helix content was determined from molar ellipticities at 222 nm by the method of Chen et al. [6]. The effect of Gnd HCl on the α-helix content of the mutant proteins and the free energy of unfolding were obtained as described by Aune and Tanford [7].

The wavelengths of maximum fluorescence of the Trp residues in the proapoA-I mutants were determined from uncorrected spectra using a Perkin-Elmer MPF-66 fluorescence spectrophotometer. The 0.1 mg/ml protein samples were excited at 295 nm, and the spectra were recorded from 305 to 375 nm using 4 nm excita-

1138

tion and emission slit widths.

To determine the kinetics of the lysis of dimyristroylphosphatidylcholine (DMPC) liposomes by the proapoA-I mutants, DMPC was dispersed in 10 mM Tris buffer, pH 8.0. An aliquot of the DMPC dispersion was added to a protein solution (total volume 0.8 ml) in a 2.5/1 mass ratio of DMPC to protein, and the absorbance of the samples was monitored at 325 nm for 2 h at 24.5°C in a Beckman DU-64 spectrophotometer.

Preparation and analysis of reconstituted HDL

Discoidal rHDL particles were prepared by the sodium-cholate method [8,9], using molar ratios of egg-phosphatidylcholine (egg PC): sodium cholate: protein of 100/100/1. The hydrodynamic diameters of the rHDL particles were estimated by native 8—25% polyacrylamide gradient gel electrophoresis (Pharmacia) by comparison with standard proteins.

Results

Figure 2 shows the SDS-PAGE gel of the purified proapoA-I mutants together with wild-type proapoA-I and a plasma apoA-I control. The recombinant proteins are at least 90% pure and migrate a little slower than plasma apoA-I due to the six additional amino acids of the prosegment.

Table 1 lists the α-helix contents, wavelengths of maximum fluorescence and

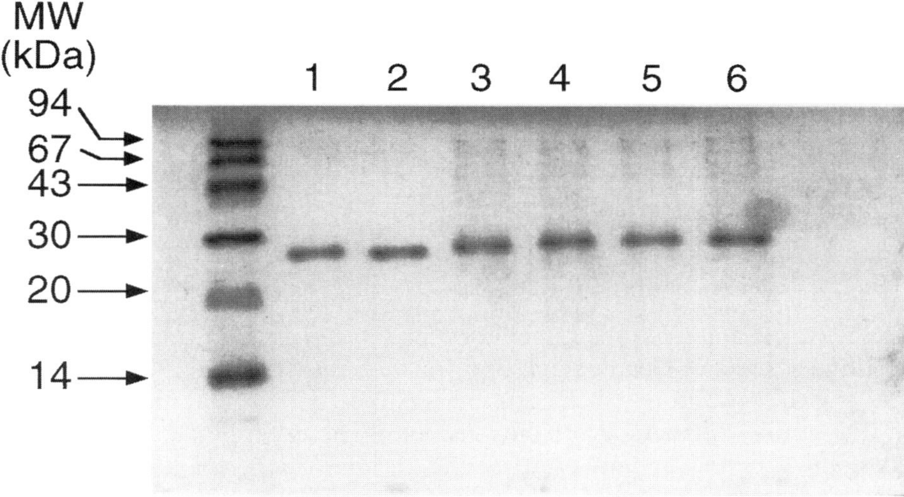

Fig. 2. SDS-PAGE (20%) gel of the proapoA-I Trp → Phe mutants after purification. Lane 1, wild-type proapoA-I; lane 2, plasma apoA-I; lane 3, proapoA-I Trp @ −3, 8, 72; lane 4, proapoA-I Trp @ −3, 8, 50; lane 5, proapoA-I Trp @ 50; and lane 6, proapoA-I Trp @ 108. The protein yields ranged from 1 to 5 mg of pure protein per liter of cell culture.

Table 1. Structural properties of the Trp → Phe mutants of proapoA-I in lipid-free form in solution.

Protein	α-helix[a] (%)	WMF[b] (nm)	ΔG_u[c] (kcal/mol)
Plasma apoA-I	56 ± 5	334 ± 1	2.7 ± 0.4
Wild-type proapoA-I	57 ± 8	336 ± 1	2.9 ± 0.4
Trp @ $-3, 8, 72$	58	335	1.8
Trp @ $-3, 8, 50$	58	336	1.7
Trp @ 50	53	338	1.3
Trp @ 108	60	332	1.4

[a]Calculated from CD spectra at 222 nm by the Chen et al. [6] method; [b]wavelength of maximum fluorescence (WMF) from uncorrected fluorescence spectra excited at 295 nm; [c]free energy of unfolding, (ΔG_u) calculated according to Aune and Tanford [7] from CD ellipticity values at 222 nm measured as a function of Gnd HCl concentration.

free energies of unfolding (ΔG_u) for the recombinant proteins in solution. The identical α-helix contents and similar blue shifted fluorescence maxima, indicate that by these criteria, the substitution of two or four Trp residues of proapoA-I with Phe residues does not affect the overall folding of apoA-I in solution, nor the chemical environments of the remaining Trp residues. In contrast, decreasing numbers of Trp residues in proapoA-I led to progressively lower ΔG_u values. This indicates that Trp residues stabilize the apoA-I N-terminal domain in solution.

Figure 3 depicts the kinetics of DMPC liposome disruption by apoA-I, proapoA-I and the Trp mutants of proapoA-I. Interestingly, the rates of liposome disruption by the proapoA-I mutants are slower than by the wild-type proapoA-I or by plasma apoA-I. Apparently, some of the hydrophobic Trp residues, and particularly Trp$_{50}$ may be involved in the initial anchoring of apoA-I to the DMPC bilayer.

In spite of the differences in the kinetics of spontaneous interaction with DMPC liposomes, all the mutant proapoA-Is were fully capable of forming discoidal rHDL particles with egg-PC by the sodium cholate method. The diameters

Table 2. Structural properties of the Trp → Phe mutants of proapoA-I in rHDL complexes with egg-PC.

Protein	Diameter[a] (nm)	α-helix[b] (%)	WMF[b] (nm)	ΔG_u[b] (kcal/mol)
Plasma apoA-I	98 ± 2	77 ± 8	333 ± 1	2.6 ± 0.5
Wild-type proapoA-I	100 ± 3	73 ± 5	335 ± 1	3.1
Trp @ $-3, 8, 72$	96	72	335	3.4
Trp @ $-3, 8, 50$	96	74	335	2.9
Trp @ 50	100	ND	336	ND
Trp @ 108	97	73	331	2.8

[a]Stokes diameters determined from native 8–25% polyacrylamide gradient gel electrophoresis by reference to standard proteins; [b]see the footnotes to Table 1. ND, not determined.

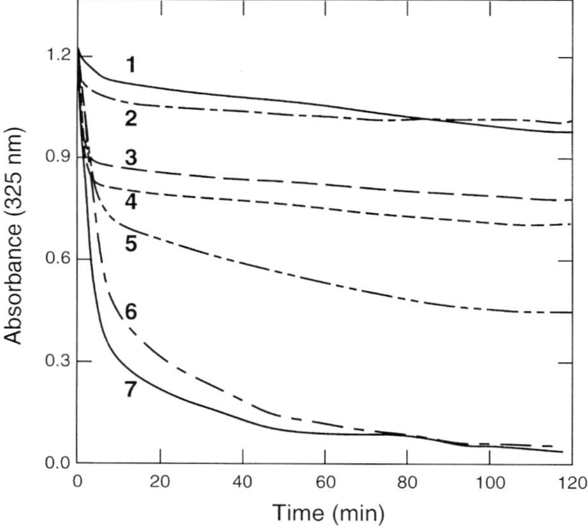

Fig. 3. Lysis of DMPC liposomes at 24.5°C by the Trp → Phe proapoA-I mutants. Absorbance at 325 nm is recorded as a function of time after addition of DMPC liposomes to the protein solutions at a mass ratio of 2.5/1, DMPC/protein. The curves correspond to: **1)** Trp @ −3, 8, 72; **2)** DMPC liposomes; **3)** Trp @ 108; **4)** Trp @ −3, 8, 50; **5)** Trp @ 50; **6)** plasma apoA-I; and **7)** wild-type proapoA-I.

of the rHDL, the α-helix contents, the wavelengths of maximum fluorescence and the ΔG_u values for the proteins in their lipid-bound state are given in Table 2. These parameters are almost identical for all the forms of lipid-bound proapoA-I indicating that the protein folding and stability are not affected by these point mutations, rather that the protein structure and stability are determined largely by the phospholipid.

Discussion

In recent work, we demonstrated that recombinant proapoA-I is essentially identical in its structural and functional properties to mature plasma apoA-I [5]. Therefore, the findings we present in this work on the Trp → Phe mutants of proapoA-I apply equally well to apoA-I.

Progressive substitution of the Trp residues in proapoA-I with two and four Phe residues yields proteins with very similar properties to the wild-type proapoA-I in terms of expression in and purification from *E. coli*, folding in solution and formation of discoidal complexes with egg-PC.

These results are not surprising because Trp → Phe substitutions are reasonably conservative [10,11]. However, the mutants did differ from proapoA-I and among each other in their stability in solution and rates of clearance of DMPC liposomes.

The properties of the Trp $\rightarrow$ Phe mutants in lipid-free form confirm our previous findings that the N-terminal half of apoA-I in solution is folded and the Trp residues are protected from solvent. In the mutants with single Trp residues, Trp @ 50 and Trp @ 108, small differences in chemical environment are revealed by a 6 nm difference in their wavelengths of maximum fluorescence. The difference decreases but does not disappear in the lipid-bound state (egg-PC rHDL), indicating that binding to lipid does not eliminate completely the effects of the protein environment on these two Trp residues.

Denaturation with Gnd HCl shows a progressive decrease in the stability of the mutants with fewer Trp residues (Table 1). Evidently Trp residues contribute significantly to the stabilization of the "molten globule" state of apoA-I in solution due to their highest relative hydrophobicity (3.4 kcal/mol for Trp vs. 2.5 kcal/mol for Phe) and largest volume [10] that contributes to van der Waals interactions, compared to other amino acid residues.

The most important and unexpected result from this study was the impaired ability of the Trp $\rightarrow$ Phe mutants to lyse DMPC liposomes. It is well-known from other work [12–14] that the C-terminus of apoA-I and several hydrophobic residues (Leu, Phe) within the C-terminus, are critical for the efficient, surfactant-like action of apoA-I in clearing DMPC liposomes. However, this study provides the first experimental evidence that the N-terminal half of intact apoA-I contains sequences and residues (e.g., Trp_{50}) that are also critical for this reaction. It appears that the initial interaction of apoA-I with DMPC bilayers at their phase transition temperature involves at least two anchoring sites in apoA-I: hydrophobic residues in the mostly unstructured C-terminus and the more exposed Trp residue (Trp_{50}) in the structured N-terminus of the molecule. Indeed, a very similar model for the interaction of apoA-I with phospholipid surfaces was proposed by Segrest and co-workers [15] based on the lipid affinities of synthetic, 22 mer peptides of apoA-I. They found that only the first (residues 44–65) and last (residues 220–241) amphipathic peptides were able to clear DMPC liposomes, and had the highest lipid affinities by several other experimental criteria. The results suggested that the two end helices of apoA-I are responsible for the initial interaction with phospholipid bilayers because they exhibit the greatest penetration into the bilayers. Our results confirm and expand this model by showing that a single amino acid substitution, Trp 50 $\rightarrow$ Phe, may affect the initial lipid-binding properties of apoA-I.

Finally, regardless of the number of Trp $\rightarrow$ Phe substitutions, the proapoA-I mutants are fully capable of forming discoidal rHDL complexes with egg-PC. Clearly the cooperative interactions with the phospholipids completely overcome the small structural and thermodynamic effects of conservative amino acid substitutions, as observed with a large number of natural [16] and engineered [14] conservative mutations in apoA-I that do not affect its properties in the lipid-bound state.

Acknowledgements

This work was supported by NIH grant HL-16059 and a postdoctoral fellowship of the American Heart Association, Illinois Affiliate to W. Sean Davidson (1995–1997).

References

1. Jonas A, Hefele-Wald J, Harms-Toohill KL, Krul ES, Kézdy KE. Apolipoprotein A-I structure and lipid properties in homogeneous, reconstituted spherical and discoidal high-density lipoproteins. J Biol Chem 1990;265:22123–22129.
2. Leroy A, Jonas A. Native-like structure and self-association behavior of apolipoprotein A-I in a water/n-propanol solution. Biochim Biophys Acta 1994;1212:285–294.
3. Marcel YL, Provost PR, Koa H, Raffai E, Dac NV, Fruchart J-C, Rassart E. The epitopes of apolipoprotein A-I define distinct structural domains including a mobile middle region. J Biol Chem 1991;266:3644–3653.
4. Davidson WS, Hazlett T, Mantulin WW, Jonas A. The role of apolipoprotein AI domains in lipid binding. Proc Natl Acad Sci USA 1996;93:13605–13610.
5. Arnvig-McGuire K, Davidson WS, Jonas A. High yield overexpression and characterization of human recombinant proapolipoprotein A-I. J Lipid Res 1996;37:1519–1528.
6. Chen Y-H, Yang JT, Martinez HM. Determination of the secondary structures of proteins by circular dichroism and optical rotatory dispersion. Biochemistry 1972;11:4120–4131.
7. Aune KC, Tanford C. Thermodynamics of the denaturation of lysozyme by guanidine hydrochloride. Biochemistry 1969;8:4586–4590.
8. Matz CE, Jonas A. Micellar complexes of human apolipoprotein A-I with phosphatidylcholines and cholesterol prepared from cholate-lipid dispersions. J Biol Chem 1982;257:4535–4540.
9. Jonas A. Reconstitution of high-density lipoproteins. Meth Enzymol 1986;128:553–582.
10. Creighton TE. Proteins. Structures and Molecular Principles. New York: W.H. Freeman Co., 1984.
11. Ladunga I, Smith RF. Amino acid substitutions preserve protein folding by conserving steric and hydrophobic properties. Protein (Eng) 1997;10:187–196.
12. Minnich A, Collet X, Roghani A, Cladaras C, Hamilton RL, Fielding CJ, Zannis V. Site-directed mutagenesis and structure-function analysis of human apolipoprotein A-I. J Biol Chem 1992;267:16553–16560.
13. Ji Y, Jonas A. Properties of an N-terminal proteolytic fragment of apolipoprotein AI in solution and in reconstituted high-density lipoproteins. J Biol Chem 1995;270:11290–11297.
14. Laccotripe M, Makrides SC, Jonas A, Zannis VI. The carboxyl-terminal hydrophobic residues of apolipoprotein A-I affect its rate of phospholipid binding and its association with high-density lipoprotein. J Biol Chem 1997;272:17511–17522.
15. Palgunachari MN, Mishra VK, Lund-Katz S, Phillips MC, Adeyeye SO, Alluri S, Anantharamaiah GM, Segrest JP. Only two end helixes of eight tandem amphipathic helical domains of human apoA-I have significant lipid affinity. Atherioscl Thromb Vasc Biol 1996;16:328–338.
16. Jonas A, von Eckardstein A, Kézdy KE, Steinmetz A, Assmann G. Structural and functional properties of reconstituted high-density lipoprotein discs prepared with six apolipoprotein A-I variants. J Lipid Res 1991;32:97–106.
17. Segrest JP, Jones MK, DeLoof H, Brouillette CG, Venkatachalapathi YV, Anantharamaiah GM. The amphipathic helix in the exchangeable apolipoproteins: A review of secondary structure and function. J Lipid Res 1992;33:141–166.

Interaction of the cholesteryl ester transfer protein with high-density lipoproteins from human and mouse plasmas

David Masson[1], Catherine Desrumaux[1], Florence Emmanuel[2], Nicolas Duverger[2] and Laurent Lagrost[1]

[1]*Laboratoire de Biochimie des Lipoprotéines, INSERM CJF 93-10, CHRU-Dijon, Faculté de Médicine, Dijon; and* [2]*Centre de Recherches de Vitry-Alfortville, Rhône-Poulenc Rorer, Gencell Division, Atherosclerosis Department, Vitry-sur-Seine, France*

Abstract. *Background.* Previous studies conducted with transgenic mice expressing the human cholesteryl ester transfer protein (CETP) together with human high-density lipoprotein (HDL) apolipoproteins (apo) provided new insights into the role of apolipoproteins in modulating plasma cholesteryl ester transfer activity in vivo. In particular, some studies in transgenic mice suggested that human CETP might interact preferentially with human apoAI when compared with mouse apoAI.

Methods. HDL were isolated from plasma samples from various sources; including normolipidemic human subjects, C57BL/6 control mice and transgenic mice that expressed either only human apoAI (HuAITg mice), only human apoAII (HuAIITg mice) or both human apoAI and human apoAII (HuAIAIITg mice). The distinct mouse lines did not express plasma cholesteryl ester transfer activity, and in all the experiments cholesteryl ester transfer activity was mediated by purified human CETP.

Results. In vitro studies revealed that human HDL, control mouse HDL and HuAIITg HDL contain a specific, heat-labile lipid transfer inhibitor activity that is absent from the HDL of HuAITg and HuAIAIITg mice. In complementary experiments, lipid transfer inhibitory activity was shown to be absent from the lipoprotein-deficient plasma fraction of HuAITg mice. Although affinity binding experiments indicated that the interaction of CETP with HDL from various sources is driven by electrostatic interactions, alterations in CETP-HDL binding did not account for differential lipid transfer inhibitory activity of plasma samples from various sources.

Conclusion. Lipid transfer inhibitory activity is present in human, control mouse and HuAIITg mouse plasmas, and it is carried by a heat-labile lipid transfer inhibitory protein (LTIP) that remains to be fully characterized. The observations of the present study suggest that the lack of lipid transfer inhibitory activity in HuAITg and HuAIAIITg mouse plasmas might relate to the displacement of endogenous LTIP by human apoAI.

Keywords: apolipoprotein A-I, apolipoprotein A-II, lipid transfer inhibitor protein, transgenic mouse.

Introduction

Peripheral cells can acquire some cholesterol through the endocytosis and hydrolysis of low-density lipoproteins (LDL). In turn, cholesterol excess can be removed from peripheral cells by the HDL that constitute the lipoprotein vehicle in the reverse cholesterol transport pathway. Cholesteryl ester transfer protein (CETP)

Address for correspondence: Laurent Lagrost, Laboratoire Central de Biochimie Médicale, Hôpital du Bocage, 21034 Dijon Cedex, France. Fax: +33-3-8029-3661.

is susceptible for playing an important role in determining the behaviour of plasma lipids, in particular by transferring cholesteryl esters from HDL towards the apoB-containing lipoproteins [1,2]. The proatherogenic or antiatherogenic properties of CETP are still largely debated today. In fact, the atherogenicity of CETP is probably dependent on the behaviour of the apoB-containing lipoproteins that can be taken up either by peripheral cells or hepatocytes [1]. The most recent in vivo studies in transgenic mice expressing human apolipoproteins AI and AII revealed that the apolipoprotein content of HDL can alter the efficacy of the CETP-mediated lipid transfer process. More precisely, previous studies suggested that human CETP might interact preferentially with human apoAI as compared with mouse apoAI [3–6]. The aim of the present study was to investigate further the role of human HDL apolipoproteins over mouse HDL apolipoproteins in determining the lipid transfer activity of human CETP.

Materials and Methods

HDL were isolated as the $1.070 < d < 1.210$ g/ml fraction of plasma samples from various sources, including normolipidemic human subjects, control mice and transgenic mice that expressed either only human apoAI (HuAITg) [7], only human apoAII (HuAIITg) [8] or both human apoAI and human apoAII [9]. All lipid assays were performed on a Cobas-Fara centrifugal analyzer using enzymatic methods. HDL apolipoproteins were analyzed by SDS electrophoresis in 80–250 g/l polyacrylamide gradient gels (Phastsystem, Pharmacia Biotech Inc.), and the distribution profile was obtained by image analysis of coomassie-stained gels on a BIO-RAD GS-670 imaging densitometer [10]. In some experiments, HDL were delipidated by using butanol-diisopropyl ether 40:60 (v/v) [11].

CETP was purified from citrated, normolipidemic human plasma using the sequential chromatographic procedure previously described [12]. No CETP activity was detected in isolated lipoprotein fractions or mouse plasma samples used throughout the study, and cholesteryl ester transfers were induced in all the experiments by the addition of purified human CETP.

Cholesteryl ester transfer activity was determined as the percentage of radio-labeled cholesteryl esters transferred from ^{3}H-CE-LDL to unlabeled acceptor HDL [10].

Results

Figure 1 shows the lipid and apolipoprotein composition of HDL that were ultra-centrifugally isolated from various plasma sources. Three main differences appeared when comparing the various HDL fractions. Firstly, human HDL contained higher amounts of triglycerides as compared with control and transgenic mouse HDL. Secondly, expression of human apolipoproteins in transgenic animals significantly increased the protein content of HDL. Lastly, the expression of human HDL apolipoproteins markedly modified the apoAI to apoAII ratio

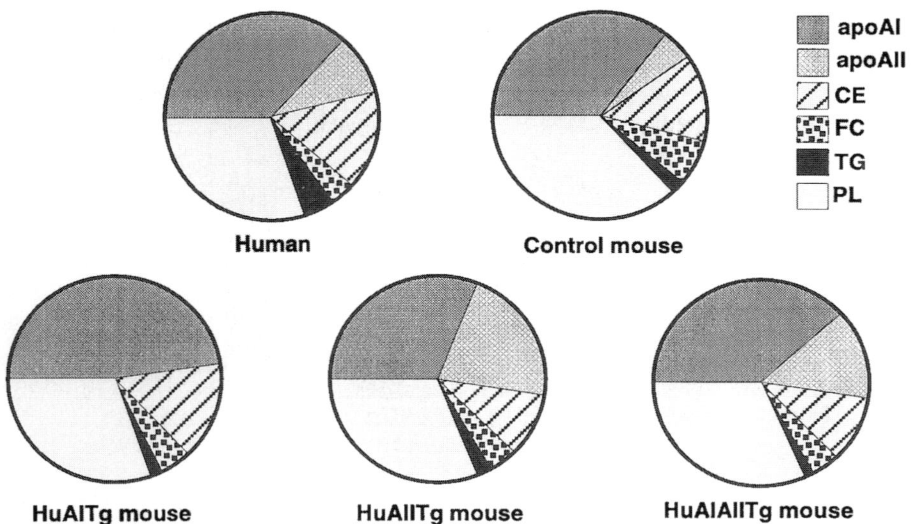

Fig. 1. Composition (mass percent) of HDL from human and mouse plasmas. CE = cholesteryl esters; FC = free cholesterol; TG = triglycerides; and PL = a phospholipids.

in transgenic mouse HDL. Indeed, the HuAITg mouse HDL contained mainly human apoAI, with only trace amounts of mouse apoAII being detectable. HuAIITg mouse HDL contained large amounts of mouse + human apoAII, while the coexpression of human apoAI and human apoAII in HuAIAIITg mice produced HDL particles with an apo AI to apoAII ratio similar to that of human HDL (Fig. 1).

With all the HDL fractions studied, cholesteryl ester transfer rates progressively increased until a maximal transfer value was obtained with an optimal HDL cholesterol concentration of 100 nmol/ml [10]. At the optimal concentration, cholesteryl ester transfer rates were significantly higher with control mouse HDL than with human HDL (p < 0.05). Raising the concentration of HuAITg HDL or HuAIAIITg HDL did not further modify the cholesteryl ester transfer rate, and similar transfer values were measured with HDL cholesterol concentrations of either 100 or 400 nmol/ml (Fig. 2). In contrast, raising the concentration of human HDL, control mouse HDL or HuAIITg mouse HDL from 100 nmol/ml up to 400 nmol/ml of cholesterol induced a significant inhibition of cholesteryl ester transfer activity (Fig. 2).

Whereas delipidated HDL apolipoproteins from control mice progressively reduced the cholesteryl ester transfer rate, the inhibition no longer appeared when HDL apolipoproteins were preheated for 1 h at 56°C [10]. In contrast, no significant inhibition of the CETP-mediated cholesteryl ester transfer reaction was observed when adding either heated or nonheated HDL apolipoproteins from HuAITg mice [10]. Although a good correspondence between the affinity of CETP for HDL and the electronegativity of the particles was observed among

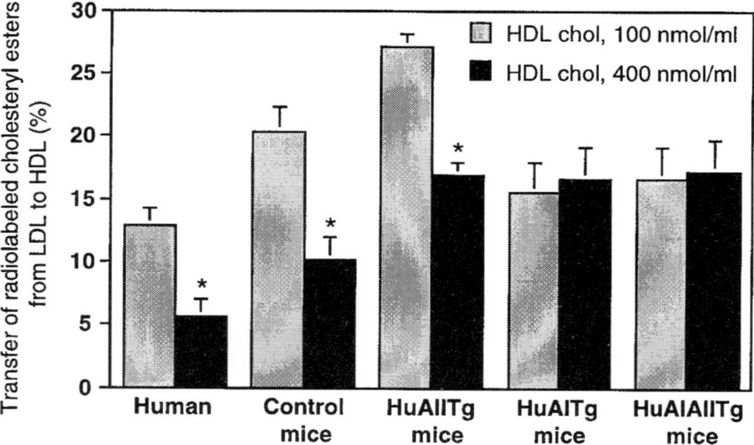

Fig. 2. Concentration-dependent effect of human, control mouse, HuAITg mouse, HuAIITg mouse and HuAIAIITg mouse HDL on CETP activity. Mixtures containing either 100 or 400 nmol/ml of HDL cholesterol, ^{3}H-CE-LDL (50 nmol of cholesterol/ml), and CETP (0.17 µg/ml) were incubated for 3 h at 37°C, and cholesteryl ester transfer rates were determined as described under "Materials and Methods". Each point represents the mean ± SD of triplicate determinations. [a]$p < 0.05$ vs. corresponding "100 nmol/ml" values.

studied samples, it is noteworthy that lipid transfer inhibitory activity was detectable only in control mouse HDL that displayed intermediate affinity and electronegativity values [10].

Discussion

The present study did not reveal a preferential interaction of human CETP with human apoAI vs. mouse apoAI, and higher cholesteryl ester transfer rates could be measured with control mouse HDL as compared with human HDL. Lipid transfer inhibitory activity was shown to be present in both control mouse and human plasmas, and it was shown to be carried by a heat-labile protein which might be identical to the lipid transfer inhibitor protein (LTIP) previously detected in plasma from various species [13—19]. Interestingly, the expression of human apoAI, but not the expression of human apoAII in transgenic mice is associated with the disappearance of plasma lipid transfer inhibitory activity from mouse plasma. The latter point might account for some of the variation in plasma cholesteryl ester transfer rates observed in transgenic animals expressing human HDL apolipoproteins in addition to CETP. Although we were not able to identify the mechanism of the inhibition of CETP activity, the variations in plasma lipid transfer inhibitory activity from one mouse line to another could not be explained by alterations in CETP-HDL binding. Although only speculative at this stage, lipid transfer inhibitory activity might relate to the ability of the putative LTIP to suppress the binding of neutral lipids to the neutral lipid

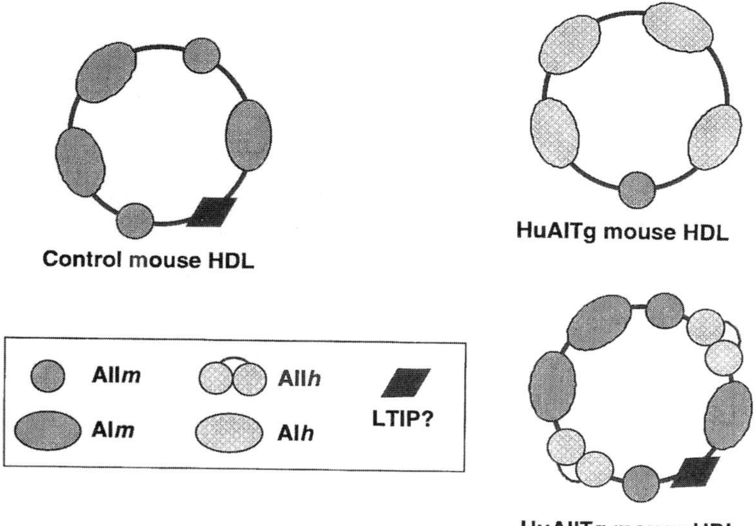

Fig. 3. Schematic representation of the protein content of HDL from control mouse, HuAITg mouse and HuAIITg mouse.

binding site of CETP, an hypothesis that deserves further investigation. Overall, the observations suggest that the lack of lipid transfer inhibitory activity in HuAITg mouse and in HuAIAIITg mouse plasmas might relate to the displacement of endogenous LTIP by human apoAI. As shown in Fig. 3, control mouse HDL contains mouse apoAI, as well as monomeric mouse apoAII in the surface, and our observations indicate that control HDL might also contain LTIP. In earlier studies with HuAITg mice, nearly all the mouse apoAI was shown to be replaced by human apoAI in plasma HDL, and a significant reduction in the mouse apoAII content was also reported [7,20]. As previously proposed for endogenous mouse apoAI, we postulate that LTIP might be also removed from the HuAITg HDL surface during assembly (Fig. 3). Unlike human apoAI, the expression of dimeric human apoAII in transgenic mice was not associated with marked changes in the levels of endogenous mouse apoAI and mouse apoAII [8]. Since we observed that lipid transfer inhibitory activity is present in HuAIITg mouse HDL, we suspect that LTIP might also be conserved in the HDL structure (Fig. 3). Thus, future comparative studies of the protein content of control mouse HDL and HuAITg mouse HDL might help with the identification and characterization of plasma LTIP.

References

1. Tall AR. Plasma lipid transfer proteins. J Lipid Res 1986;27:361—366.
2. Lagrost L. Regulation of cholesteryl ester transfer protein (CETP) activity: review of in vitro and

in vivo studies. Biochim Biophys Acta 1994;1215:209—236.

3. Hayek T, Chajek-Shaul T, Walsh A, Agellon LB, Moulin P, Tall AR, Breslow JL. An interaction between the human cholesterol ester transfer protein (CETP) and apolipoprotein A-I genes in transgenic mice results in a profound CETP-mediated depression of high-density lipoprotein cholesterol levels. J Clin Invest 1992;90:505—510.

4. Zhong S, Goldberg IJ, Bruce C, Rubin E, Breslow JL, Tall AR. Human apo A-II inhibits the hydrolysis of HDL triglyceride and the decrease of HDL size induced by hypertriglyceridemia and cholesteryl ester transfer protein in transgenic mice. J Clin Invest 1994;94:2457—2467.

5. Breslow JL. Transgenic mouse models of lipoprotein metabolism and atherosclerosis. Proc Natl Acad Sci USA 1993;90:8314—8318.

6. Tall AR. Plasma cholesteryl ester transfer protein and high-density lipoproteins: new insights from molecular genetic studies. J Int Med 1995;237:5—12.

7. Rubin EM, Ishida BY, Clift SM, Krauss RM. Expression of human apolipoprotein A-I in transgenic mice results in reduced plasma levels of murine apolipoprotein A-I and the appearance of two new high-density lipoprotein size subclasses. Proc Natl Acad Sci USA 1991;88:434—438.

8. Schultz JR, Gong EL, McCall MR, Nichols AV, Clift SM, Rubin EM. Expression of human apolipoprotein A-II and its effect on high-density lipoprotein in transgenic mice. J Biol Chem 1992;267:21630—21636.

9. Tremp GL, Duchange N, Branellec D, Cereghini S, Tailleux A, Berthou L, Fievet C, Touchet N, Schombert B, Fruchart JC, Zakin MM, Denèfle P. A 700-bp fragment of the human antithrombin III promoter is sufficient to confer high, tissue-specific expression on human apolipoprotein A-II in transgenic mice. Gene 1995;156:199—205.

10. Masson D, Duverger N, Emmanuel F, Lagrost L. Differential interaction of the human cholesteryl ester transfer protein with plasma high-density lipoproteins (HDLs) from humans, control mice and transgenic mice to human HDL apolipoproteins. Lack of lipid transfer inhibitory activity in transgenic mice expressing human apoAI. J Biol Chem 1997;272:24287—24293.

11. Cham BE, Knowles BR. A solvent system for delipidation of plasma or serum without protein precipitation. J Lipid Res 1976;17:176—181.

12. Lagrost L, Athias A, Gambert P, Lallemant C. Comparative study of phospholipid transfer activities mediated by cholesteryl ester transfer protein and phospholipid transfer protein. J Lipid Res 1994;35:825—835.

13. Morton RE, Zilversmit DB. A plasma inhibitor of triglyceride and cholesteryl ester transfer activities. J Biol Chem 1981;256:11992—11995.

14. Tollefson JH, Liu A, Albers JJ. Regulation of plasma lipid transfer by the high-density lipoproteins. Am J Physiol 1988;255:E894—E902.

15. Nishide T, Tollefson JH, Albers JJ. Inhibition of lipid transfer by a unique high-density lipoprotein subclass containing an inhibitor protein. J Lipid Res 1989;30:149—158.

16. Kushwaha RS, Hasan SQ, McGill HC Jr, Getz GS, Dunham RG, Kanda P. Characterization of cholesteryl ester transfer protein inhibitor from plasma of baboons (papio sp.). J Lipid Res 1993;34:1285—1297.

17. Morton RE, Steinbrunner JV. Determination of lipid transfer inhibitor protein activity in human lipoprotein-deficient plasma. Arterioscl Thromb 1993;13:1843—1851.

18. Morton RE, Greene DJ. Regulation of lipid transfer between lipoproteins by an endogenous plasma protein: selective inhibition among lipoprotein classes. J Lipid Res 1994;35:836—847.

19. Morton RE, Greene DJ. Enhanced detection of lipid transfer inhibitor protein activity by an assay involving only low-density lipoprotein. J Lipid Res 1994;35:2094—2099.

20. Chajek-Shaul T, Hayek T, Walsh A, Breslow JL. Expression of human apolipoprotein A-I gene in transgenic mice alters high-density lipoprotein (HDL) particle size distribution and diminishes selective uptake of HDL cholesteryl esters. Proc Natl Acad Sci USA 1991;88:6731—6735.

Definition of apolipoprotein A-I domains involved in reverse cholesterol transport

Yves L. Marcel and Philippe G. Frank
Lipoprotein and Atherosclerosis Group, University of Ottawa Heart Institute, Departments of Pathology and Laboratory Medicine, and Biochemistry, Ottawa, Ontario, Canada

Abstract. Four human apolipoprotein (apo) A-I mutants, including three with a deletion of two consecutive α-helices ($\Delta(100-143)$, $\Delta(122-165)$, $\Delta(144-186)$) and one with a C-terminal deletion $\Delta(187-243)$, have been expressed in *Escherichia coli*. The central deletion mutants were previously shown to exhibit a reduced phospholipid (PL)-binding capacity as well as reduced kinetics of association with PL for the two mutants $\Delta(122-165)$, and $\Delta(144-186)$. Also the deletion $100-143$ and within it the deletion of the helix between residues 100 and 121 decreases the stability of the protein, possibly due to the loss of helix interactions. To determine if these properties affect diffusional efflux of cellular cholesterol, discoidal complexes containing recombinant wild-type apoA-I (Rec.-apoA-I) or the mutant proteins and a constant PL/apoA-I molar ratio have been prepared and incubated with ^{3}H-cholesterol-labeled human skin fibroblasts. Central deletion mutants and Rec.-apoA-I had similar abilities to promote diffusional cholesterol efflux with comparable kinetics and saturating concentrations. Analysis of cholesterol efflux from cholesterol-loaded fibroblasts to lipid-free Rec.-apoA-I and each mutant including the C-terminal deletion also showed very little difference between these proteins. In contrast, efflux from cholesterol-loaded macrophages to the lipid-free apoA-I mutants demonstrated a different specificity with a much decreased cholesterol efflux to $\Delta(187-243)$, suggesting that the C-terminal domain of apoA-I is specifically important for macrophages. These results suggest that deletions of the central or C-terminal α-helices do not affect the ability of the resulting mutants to associate and to retain cellular cholesterol. However, specific cells require the presence of the C-terminal sequence and α-helices in a process, yet to be understood. Finally, the study of lecithin:cholesterol acyltransferase activation by the mutants with central deletions showed that helix $144-165$ is necessary for optimum esterification. These results provide a new mechanistic insight in the role of apoA-I domains in reverse cholesterol transport.

Keywords: cholesterol efflux, cholesterol esterification, HDL, lipid binding, protein structure.

Our current understanding of apolipoprotein (apo) A-I structure is largely derived from the recognition of multiple intragenic repeats coding for 22 amino acid sequences which form the amphipathic α-helices and the intervening random coil/turn sequences [1]. Computational analyses of these sequences have provided the basis for the models of apoA-I structure [2]. Model peptides and naturally occurring mutants of apoA-I have contributed further to the definition of the structure and function of apoA-I domains involved in lipid binding, cellular lipid efflux and LCAT activation [3,4]. To date, few informative mutagenesis

---

Address for correspondence: Yves L. Marcel, Lipoprotein and Atherosclerosis Group, University of Ottawa Heart Institute, 1053 Carling Avenue, Ottawa, Ontario, Canada K1Y 4E9.

studies of apoA-I have been done, owing, first to the difficulties of obtaining large amounts of purified protein [5—7], and second to the arbitrary nature of the selected mutations [8]. In the absence of solid data on the domain structure of apoA-I, unstable mutant proteins may be produced in which misfolding may interfere unpredictably with domains distal to the mutation. Informative mutagenesis with apoA-I is also complicated by the fact that most functions of apoA-I are interrelated. For example, mutant proteins must bind lipids before they can activate LCAT reaction. On the other hand, interaction of apoA-I with cells and efflux of lipids may or may not occur independently of an initial association with lipids.

Monoclonal antibodies against apoA-I have also been used to interact with specific domains and interfere with their function [9—11]. We have shown that antibodies reacting with apoA-I in different states of lipidation can exert different effects, as a result of either or both heterogeneous apoA-I structures in different lipid environments and different conformational modifications exerted by antibodies in these settings [12—14]. The different specificity and the inherent limitation of the two approaches using mutagenesis and specific antibodies have contributed to the conflicting results that currently form apoA-I domain characterization.

Here, we summarize results obtained with a series of deletion mutants of apoA-I designed to provide information on the role of central and C-terminal α-helices in lipid binding, cellular lipid efflux and LCAT activation. The strategy for mutagenesis aimed at minimal disruption of the predicted secondary structure and of the putative interhelix interactions. We deleted one at a time, a pair of adjacent amphipathic helices at the site of the proline punctuation that delineates the 22mer repeats [15]. This was postulated to represent a site of minimum disruption of the predicted secondary structure since it would not change the periodicity observed in the primary sequence. We hypothesized that these deletions would generate stably folded mutants and that the structure and function of each would reflect the importance of the deleted helix and the newly introduced interhelix interactions. The central deletion concerned residues 100—143, or 121—165, or 144—186, and the C-terminal deletion eliminated residues 187—243.

These initial assumptions were generally supported by the structural studies of the central deletion mutants whether in lipid-free or lipid-bound forms [15]. In the lipid-free form the stability of each central deletion mutant was similar and analogous to that of Rec. apoA-I. Also in the lipid-free form, the measured α-helix content of the mutants was similar to Rec. apoA-I with the exception of $\Delta(100—143)$ which had a significantly lower α-helicity [15].

When recombined with palmitoyl oleyl phosphatidylcholine (POPC) to form discoidal Lp2A-I of similar composition, a few significant changes appeared. While the deletions of residues 122—165 and 144—186 increased the stability of the mutants compared to Rec. apoA-I, $\Delta(100—143)$ had a lower stability. Similarly the α-helicity of mutants $\Delta(122—165)$ and $\Delta(144—186)$ was higher than that of Rec.apoA-I and in contrast with a slight decrease noted for mutant $\Delta(100-143)$. Assuming that on average 17 residues are required to form each apoA-I amphipathic α-helix, we could calculate that after deletion of two helices, mutant $\Delta(100-143)$ had the predicted remaining number of helices while mutants $\Delta(122-165)$ and $\Delta(144-186)$ still had eight helices, the same number as in Rec.apoA-I. This indicated that the last two mutants had formed two new helices presumably in the N-terminal domain. However, although these helices contributed to the increased stability of the protein in the lipoproteins formed, they could not substitute for the deleted helices and allow the mutant proteins to form Lp2A-I of a size and composition similar to the wild-type apoA-I. Moreover, whereas the size of Lp2A-I formed with plasma or Rec. apoA-I and different POPC levels could vary by about 1 nm, the size of Lp2A-I formed with each central deletion mutant remained nearly constant. This demonstrated the importance of the central helices in the formation of lipoproteins of different sizes and supported the theory that these helices form a hinge domain and associate with lipids only in large particles [15].

Having characterized the phospholipid-binding properties of the central deletion mutants and having established that they could form stable lipoproteins of similar size and composition, we then tested their ability to promote cellular cholesterol efflux. They were also compared to Rec.apoA-I and to a C-terminal deletion mutant, $\Delta(187-243)$. Using normal human skin fibroblasts labeled with ^{3}H-cholesterol we compared efflux to Lp2A-I of similar POPC content. Under these conditions the initial rates of efflux (between 0 and 2 h) mediated by each mutant were identical and equivalent to the rate of efflux to lipoproteins containing wild-type apoA-I. Fibroblasts loaded with cholesterol by preincubation with LDL and cholesterol/phospholipid liposomes were also used to study efflux to the lipid-free apolipoproteins. Again the rates were identical for all proteins independently of the deletion of a pair of central helices or the C-terminal helices.

These experiments were repeated with THP-1-derived macrophages. After differentiation in the presence of phorbol esters and cholesterol loading with acetylated-LDL, the cells were labeled with ^{3}H-cholesterol or with ^{3}H-choline. Efflux was studied between 0 and 24 h at the same molar concentration of lipid-free proteins. Whereas the central deletion mutants and Rec. apoA-I could mediate similar rates of efflux of either cholesterol or phospholipids, efflux to the C-terminal deletion mutant was significantly reduced for both lipids (70%). When we compared efflux to Lp2A-I containing similar ratio of POPC to apoA-I, the difference was much reduced but remained significantly lower to the C-terminal deletion mutant. These results show first that cholesterol efflux from fibroblasts does not require the presence of any particular sequence between residues 100 and the C-terminus, second, that within this sequence the deletion of any pair of amphipathic helices does not impair cholesterol efflux to the lipid-free or lipidated apoA-I proteins. On the other hand, the major decrease in lipid efflux from cholesterol-loaded macrophages to lipid-free $\Delta(187-243)$ suggests a requirement for the C-terminal sequence for interaction with macrophages. Alternatively, the

1152

larger lipid excess that can be accumulated in macrophages also yields a larger lipid efflux, and this may require the presence of the high lipid affinity helix present between residues 220 and 241 [4]. Further experiments will be needed to compare the binding properties of the various apoA-I mutants with macrophages and assess whether cell surface binding represents the limiting step.

Finally, we evaluated the effect of the different central deletions on the activation of LCAT reaction with discoidal Lp2A-I containing similar molar ratios of POPC and cholesterol to proteins. The initial rate of reaction was most decreased for the two mutants with deletion 122—165 and 144—186. Calculation of k_{cat} (V_{max}/ K_m) indicated that the activation of LCAT by these two mutants was significantly lower whereas deletion of residues 100—143 had no significant effect: Rec. apoA-I, 1.15; Δ(100—143), 0.83; Δ(122—165), 0.14; Δ(144—186), 0.09 nmol cholesterol esterified/h/μM apoA-I. Taken together with the results of Sorci-Thomas et al. [16] which showed significant decrease in LCAT activation upon deletion of residues 143—164 or 165—186, we conclude that the helix within 144—165 is the most important for LCAT activation. It is still unclear whether helix 165—186 is also directly involved in activation or its effects are related to the interactions with adjacent helices. Point-specific mutations should clarify this question.

In conclusion, multiple domains in apoA-I have been identified that are involved in the different steps of reverse cholesterol transport as well as in maintaining the stability of the protein in its lipid-free and lipid-bound forms.

References

1. Li W-H, Tanimura M, Luo C-C, Datta S, Chan L. The apolipoprotein multigene family: biosynthesis, structure-function relationships, and evolution. J Lipid Res 1988;245—271.
2. Brasseur R, Lins L, Vanloo B, Ruysschaert J-M, Rosseneu M. Molecular modeling of the amphipathic helices of the plasma apolipoproteins. Proteins 1992;13:246—257.
3. Anantharamaiah GM, Venkatachalapathi YV, Brouillette CG, Segrest JP. Use of synthetic peptide analogues to localize lecithin:cholesterol acyltransferase activating domain in apolipoprotein A-I. Arteriosclerosis 1990;10:95—105.
4. Palgunachari MN, Mishra VK, Lund-Katz S, Phillips MC, Adeyeye SO, Alluri S, Anantharamaiah GM, Segrest JP. Only the two end helixes of eight tandem amphipathic helical domains of human apo A-I have significant lipid affinity — Implications for HDL assembly. Arterioscler Thromb Vasc Biol 1996;16:328—338.
5. Brissette L, Cahuzac N, Desforges M, Bec J-L, Milne RW, Marcel YL, Rassart E. Expression and purification of recombinant human apolipoprotein A-I from Chinese hamster ovary cells or *E. coli*. Protein Exp Purif 1991;2:296—303.
6. Sorci-Thomas MG, Parks JS, Kearns MW, Pate GN, Zhang C, Thomas MJ. High level secretion of wild-type and mutant forms of human proapoA-I using baculovirus-mediated Sf-9 cell expression. J Lipid Res 1996;37:673—683.
7. Bergeron J, Frank PG, Emmanuel F, Latta M, Zhao YW, Sparks DL, Rassart E, Denèfle P, Marcel YL. Characterization of human apolipoprotein A-I expressed in *Escherichia coli*. Biochim Biophys Acta Lipids Lipid Metab 1997;1344:139—152.
8. Minnich A, Collet X, Roghani A, Cladaras C, Hamilton RL, Fielding CJ, Zannis VI. Site-directed mutagenesis and structure-function analysis of the human apolipoprotein A-I. Relation

between lecithin-cholesterol acyltransferase activation and lipid binding. J Biol Chem 1992;267: 16553—16560.

9. Banka CL, Bonnet DJ, Black AS, Smith RS, Curtiss LK. Localization of an apolipoprotein A-I epitope critical for activation of lecithin-cholesterol acyltransferase. J Biol Chem 1991;266: 23886—23892.

10. Fielding PE, Kawano M, Catapano AL, Zoppo A, Marcovina S, Fielding CJ. Unique epitope of apolipoprotein A-I expressed in pre-β-1 high-density lipoprotein and its role in the catalyzed efflux of cellular cholesterol. Biochemistry 1994;33:6981—6985.

11. Uboldi P, Spoladore M, Fantappiè S, Marcovina S, Catapano AL. Localization of apolipoprotein A-I epitopes involved in the activation of lecithin:cholesterol acyltransferase. J Lipid Res 1996;37:2557—2568.

12. Calabresi L, Meng Q-H, Castro GR, Marcel YL. Apolipoprotein A-I conformation in discoidal particles: evidence for alternate structures. Biochemistry 1993;32:6477—6484.

13. Bergeron J, Frank PG, Scales D, Meng QH, Castro G, Marcel YL. Apolipoprotein A-I conformation in reconstituted discoidal lipoproteins varying in phospholipid and cholesterol content. J Biol Chem 1995;270:27429—27438.

14. Meng Q-H, Calabresi L, Fruchart J-C, Marcel YL. Apolipoprotein A-I domains involved in the activation of lecithin:cholesterol acyltransferase. J Biol Chem 1993;268:16966—16973.

15. Frank PG, Bergeron J, Emmanuel F, Lavigne JP, Sparks DL, Denèfle P, Rassart E, Marcel YL. Deletion of central α-helices in human apolipoprotein A-I: effect on phospholipid association. Biochemistry 1997;36:1798—1806.

16. Sorci-Thomas M, Kearns MW, Lee JP. Apolipoprotein A-I domains involved in lecithin-cholesterol acyltransferase activation. Structure:function relationships. J Biol Chem 1993;268: 21403—21409.

Contribution of apo AII and LCAT oblique peptides to HDL metabolism

B. Vanloo[1], O. Perez-Mendez[1], G. Lambert[2], J. Tavernier[1], J. Vandekerckhove[1], R. Brasseur[3] and M. Rosseneu[1]

[1]*Department of Biochemistry, University of Gent, Gent, Belgium;* [2]*CJF INSERM 9508, Institut des Cordeliers, Paris, France; and* [3]*Centre de Biophysique Moleculaire Numérique, Faculty of Science and Agronomy, Gembloux, Belgium*

Abstract. Computer modeling of the apo AII 53—70 and the LCAT 56—68 segments suggests that these amphipathic helices are oriented at an angle of 30° at a lipid/water interface, due to the N-C hydrophobicity gradient along the helix. Mutant peptides were designed by computer modeling to be parallel (0°) or to retain the same orientation compared to a lipid bilayer. The capacity of the WT and variant peptides to induce fusion of pyrene-labeled PC/PE/chol vesicles was investigated. The excimer/monomer fluorescence ratio decreased under the addition of all oblique-orientated peptides, while the 0° peptide had no fusogenic activity. Release of calcein, entrapped inside the PC/PE/chol vesicles, was further demonstrated upon addition of the apo AII and LCAT oblique peptides. The apo AII 53—70 peptide and the oblique variant displaced up to 55% apo AI from HDL_3 as shown by gel filtration, whereas the 0° variant had no effect, thus suggesting that the C-terminal apo AII peptide is fusogenic and that it can displace apo AI from HDL_3. The insertion of the C-terminal hydrophobic end of the LCAT peptide into the lipid phase was demonstrated by moving the W61 residue of LCAT to position 57 and 68, respectively, and comparing the fluorescence properties of the variant peptides. The contribution of the 56—68 peptide to the enzymatic activity of LCAT was investigated by constructing and expressing LCAT deletion and substitution mutants. Results obtained both with the synthetic peptide and with the LCAT mutants suggest that in native LCAT, this domain might contribute to the interfacial substrate recognition of the enzyme. It might help further in destabilizing the lipoprotein lipid core and enhancing the diffusion of a phospholipid monomer into the active site of the enzyme.

Keywords: apoprotein, computer modeling, enzyme activity, fusogenic peptides.

Introduction

We identified a class of peptides that associate with lipids in membranes, commonly known as "oblique-orientated peptides". Due to an asymmetric distribution of hydrophobic residues along the axis of the α-helix, such peptides adopt an oblique orientation which can destabilize membranes or lipid cores, thereby facilitating remodeling of lipid cores and enhancing apoprotein transfer and lipid transport among lipoproteins [1]. Apolipoprotein AII and its C-terminal helix were shown to displace apo AI from high-density lipoproteins (HDL), thereby modulating the properties of HDL as a substrate for the lecithin cholesterol acyl

---

Address for correspondence: Berlinda Vanloo, Hospitaalstraat 13, B-9000 Gent, Belgium. Tel.: +32-9-224-0224 (ext. 220). Fax: +32-9-225-3489. E-mail: Berlinda.Vanloo @ rug.ac.be.

transferase (LCAT) enzyme [2]. The lipid-destabilizing properties of the apo AII C-terminal helical segment might contribute to this mechanism [2]. LCAT, which hydrolyses phospholipids and esterifies cholesterol in nascent and mature HDL, requires access to a monomeric phospholipid molecule from the substrate lipid core [3]. The first step of the enzymatic reaction, therefore, requires the destabilization of the organized lipoprotein core to enable diffusion of a lipid monomer into the active site of the enzyme. We identified a tilted core-destabilizing peptide at residues 56−68 in LCAT, which strongly resembles that of the lipases, and which might be involved in the interfacial recognition of the LCAT substrate [1]. In this paper we investigate the relationship between the fusogenic properties of the apo AII and LCAT peptides and their physiological activity.

Results

Fusogenic properties and apo AI displacement ability of the apo AII peptides

Lipid-destabilization properties of the apo AII 53−70 WT peptide and variants
The apo AII peptides were synthesized by solid-phase peptide synthesis and their sequence and properties are summarized in Table 1. Modeling of the peptides at a lipid/water interface was carried out as described by Brasseur [4]. In addition to the synthetic apo AII peptide spanning residues 53−70, we synthesized two variants: the AII 53−70 0°, orientated at an angle of 0° at a lipid/water interface, compared to 35° for the wild-type peptide, and another variant peptide AII 53−70 30° designed to retain an oblique orientation. Both sequences were modified by permutation of the wild-type peptide residues. The three peptides are predominantly hydrophobic and, moreover, they are amphipathic (Table 1).

The induction of intervesicular lipid mixing by peptides, as a measure of their fusogenic activity, was tested with PC/PE/Chol vesicles using a probe dilution assay [5]. The AII 53−70 WT and AII 53−70 30° peptides had fusogenic properties, as shown by the decrease of the E/M ratio after mixing unlabeled and labeled SUV's. The two oblique peptides induced lipid mixing in a concentration-dependent manner (Fig. 1A). The AII 53−70 0° peptide had no fusogenic activity, as predicted from computer modeling and the calculation of the peptide

Table 1. Properties of the synthetic apo AII 53−70 C terminal and the LCAT 56−68 peptides.

Peptide	Sequence	<Ho>	<µH>	Angle of insertion (°)
AII 53−70 WT	IKKAGTELVNFLSYFVEL	0.29	0.53	35
AII 53−70 0°	IKKAGLETVSFLNYFVEL	0.29	0.40	0
AII 53−70 30°	IKKAGLETVSFLNEFVYL	0.29	0.38	30
LCAT(56−68) WT	DFFTIWLDLNMFL	0.55	0.29	40
LCAT (56−68) W68	DFFNILLDLTMFW	0.55	0.37	38
LCAT (56−68) W57	DWTFIFLDLNMFL	0.55	0.20	50

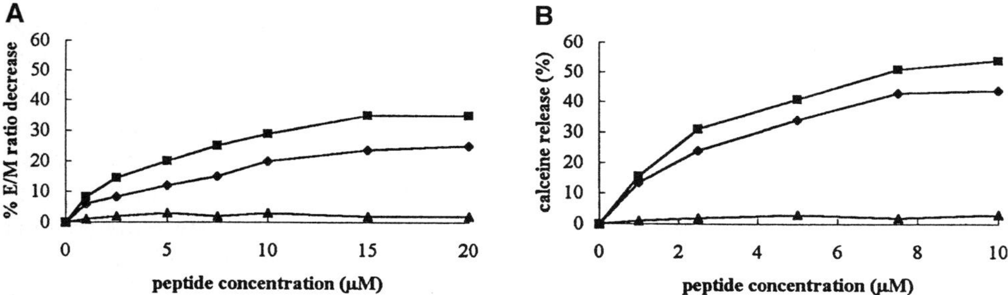

Fig. 1. **A**. Effect of the apo AII peptide concentration on the extent of lipid mixing of PC/PE/Chol SUV. Apo AII 53–70 WT peptide (■); apo AII 53–70 30° peptide (◆); apo AII 53–70 0° peptide (▲). **B**. Effect of the apo AII peptide concentration on the leakage of liposomal contents of PC/PE/Chol SUV. Apo AII 53–70 WT peptide (■); apo AII 53–70 30° peptide (◆); apo AII 53–70 0° peptide (▲).

orientation (Table 1). In order to test the membrane destabilization properties of the apo AII peptides, we monitored leakage of encapsulated calcein from PC/PE/Chol vesicles [5]. With the addition of 1–10 µM of the AII 53–70 WT, AII 53–70 30° peptides induced release of calcein from the vesicles (Fig. 1B), whereas the 0° variant had no effect.

Displacement of apo AI from native and reconstituted HDL

Mixtures of HDL$_3$ together with the apo AII C-terminal peptides were separated on a Superose 12 HR column, and Trp fluorescence measurement was used as a marker for apo AI. In agreement with the fusogenic activity on the peptides, the amount of apo AI released from HDL$_3$ increases with the amount of added peptide for both the AII 53–70 WT and the AII 53–70 30° variant (Fig. 2). The parallel-orientated variant was unable to displace apo AI from HDL (Fig.

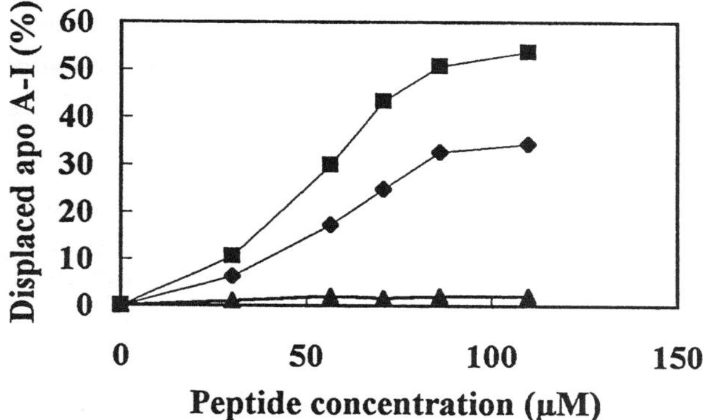

Fig. 2. Influence of the apo AII peptide amount on the displacement of apo AI from HDL$_3$. Apo AII 53–70 WT peptide (■); apo AII 53–70 30° peptide (◆); apo AII 53–70 0° peptide (▲).

2), thereby suggesting an association between apo AI displacement and orientation of the apo AII peptide.

Contribution of the LCAT 56—68 peptide to the activity of the LCAT enzyme

Lipid-mixing properties of the LCAT 56—68 peptide and variants

The sequence and properties of the LCAT 56—68 peptide and of two variants are summarized in Table 1. In order to probe the mode of insertion of this peptide into a lipid bilayer, we designed two mutants with an oblique orientation — but here Trp61 of the WT peptide was moved to position 57 and 68, at the N- and C-terminal end of the peptide, respectively (Table 1). In analogy with the apo AII peptides described above, the LCAT peptides are predominantly hydrophobic and are amphipathic.

The induction of intervesicular lipid mixing by peptides, as a measure of their fusogenic activity, was tested with PC/PE/Chol SUV, as for the apo AII peptides [5]. The three peptides had comparable fusogenic activity and decreased the E/M ratio after mixing unlabeled and labeled vesicles in a concentration-dependent manner (Fig. 3A). Leakage of encapsulated calcein from PC/PE/Chol vesicles was monitored upon addition of the peptides [5]. Addition of 1—10 μM of the LCAT peptides induced release of calcein from the vesicles (Fig. 3B) to a comparable extent.

Fluorescence emission spectra of the WT and variant peptides were recorded in the absence and presence of DMPC. Addition of DMPC vesicles to the WT and the W68 variant induced a significant blue shift of the maximal emission wavelength from 356 and 358 nm to 343 and 341 nm, respectively. In contrast, addition of lipids to the W57 variant shifted the maximal emission wavelength only slightly from 354 to 351 nm. These results, therefore, support the predicted orien-

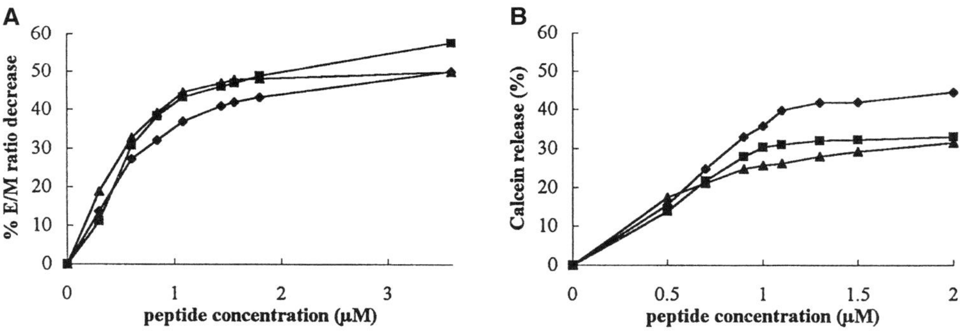

Fig. 3. **A**. Effect of the LCAT 56—68 peptide concentration on the extent of lipid mixing of PC/PE/Chol SUV. LCAT 56—68 WT peptide (■); LCAT 56—68 W68 peptide (◆); LCAT 56—68 W57 peptide (▲). **B**. Effect of the LCAT 56—68 peptide concentration on the leakage of liposomal contents of PC/PE/Chol SUV. LCAT 56—68 WT peptide (■); LCAT 56—68 W68 peptide (◆); LCAT 56—68 W57 peptide (▲).

Table 2. Mass and specific activity of mutant and WT LCAT transfectants (n = 3) in COS-1 cells.

Transfectant	Mass (μg/ml)	Specific activity	
		r-HDL (% of WT)	Monmeric (% of WT)
WT	2.3 ± 0.5	100	100
Δ56−68	1.6 ± 0.4	0	16 ± 5
W61-F	1.4 ± 0.3	105 ± 11	159 ± 12
W61-Y	1.6 ± 0.3	108 ± 13	172 ± 15
W61-L	1.1 ± 0.2	0	19 ± 5
W61-G	1.4 ± 0.2	0	18 ± 4

r-HDL: PLPC/cholesterol/apolipoprotein AI. Monomeric substrate: 1,2-bis-(1-pyrenebutanoyl)-*sn*-glycero-3-phosphocholine.

tation of the peptide and its insertion into the lipid through its C-terminal extremity, while the N-terminal residues remain in the aqueous phase, due to the oblique orientation of the peptide.

Expression and activity measurements of mutant recombinant LCAT
LCAT mutants were constructed by site-directed mutagenesis and expressed in COS-1 cells 6. Enzyme mass was measured by ELISA and activity was determined both on a monomeric substrate and on r-HDL consisting of discoidal apo AI/PLPC/Chol complexes [6] (Table 2). Deletion of the 56−68 segment in LCAT abolished activity on r-HDL, and strongly decreased activity on the monomeric substrate, supporting the role of this peptide in the interfacial activation of the enzyme. Mutations of W61 to an aromatic Phe or Tyr residue did not affect the activity of the LCAT mutant on r-HDL and even increased activity on the monomeric substrate. In contrast, substitution of the Trp by either Leu or Gly abolished activity on r-HDL and decreased the LCAT activity on the monomeric substrate.

Conclusion

These results support the hypothesis that oblique-orientated peptides are able to destabilize lipid bilayers and to induce vesicle fusion. Such peptides are probably involved in the physiological function of proteins, such as the displacement of apo AI from HDL by the apo AII C-terminal oblique peptide. In LCAT, the oblique peptide at residues 56−68 might participate in the interfacial substrate recognition, and in the destabilization of the lipid core of the phospholipid substrate, as suggested by the results obtained with the LCAT mutants.

References

1. Brasseur R, Pillot T, Lins L, Vandekerckhove J, Rosseneu M. Peptide in membranes: tipping the balance of membrane stability. Trends Biochem Sci 1997;22:167−217.

2. Benetollo C, Lambert G, Talussot C, Van Cauteren T, Rouy D, Dubois H, Baert J, Kalopissis A, Chambaz J, Denefle P, Brasseur R, Rosseneu M. Lipid-binding properties of synthetic peptide fragments of human apolipoprotein AII. Eur J Biochem 1996;242:657—664.
3. Jonas A. Lecithin-cholesterol acyltransferase in the metabolism of high-density lipoproteins. Biochim Biophys Acta 1991;1084:205—219.
4. Brasseur R. Differentation of lipid-associating helices by use of three-dimensional molecular hydrophobicity potential calculations. J Biol Chem 1991;266:16120—16127.
5. Pillot T, Goethals M, Vanloo B, Talussot C, Brasseur R, Rosseneu M, Vandekerckhove J, Lins L. Fusogenic properties of the C-terminal domain of the Alzheimer beta-amyloid peptide. J Biol Chem 1996;271:28757—28765.
6. Peelman F, Vinaimont N, Verhee A, Vanloo B, Verschelde JL, Labeur C, Séguret-Macé S, Duverger N, Hutchinson G, Vandekerckhove J, Tavernier J, Rosseneu M. A proposed architecture for Lecithin cholesterol acyl transferase. Identification of the catalytic triad and molecular modeling of LCAT. Protein Sci (Submitted).

Noninvasive assessment
of atherosclerosis

Common carotid artery intimal-medial thickness and risk of coronary heart disease

John R. Crouse III
Bowman Gray School of Medicine, Department of Internal Medicine, Winston-Salem, North Carolina, USA

Abstract. Several lines of evidence point to strong associations between extracranial carotid intimal-medial thickness (IMT) and risk of coronary heart disease. These include interassociations of cerebrovascular and coronary symptoms, interassociations of atherosclerosis of the two vascular beds and associations of indices of asymptomatic extracranial carotid atherosclerosis and stenosis with incident coronary events. However, although IMT, atherosclerosis and stenosis of the extracranial carotid arteries are associated with incident coronary events, these structural indices of disease do not precisely identify individuals at risk. Investigation of the composition of extracranial carotid plaques and of arterial function may provide new dimensions to identify arterial disease that may complement the currently used measures of arterial structure and help to identify individuals at risk more easily.

Keywords: clinical trial, endothelial function, plaque composition.

Interassociations of coronary artery and cerebrovascular disease have been known for some time and can be discussed in terms of interassociations of symptoms, interassociations of atherosclerosis of the two vascular beds (interassociations of structural manifestations of disease) and associations of asymptomatic structural manifestations of extracranial carotid disease (e.g., increased intimal-medial thickness (IMT), arterial stenosis) with incident fatal and nonfatal coronary events.

It is a common clinical observation that coronary events are responsible for most of the morbidity and mortality following transient ischemic attack and stroke [1] or carotid endarterectomy [2]. Heart-attack patients are also strongly predisposed to develop stroke [3].

Autopsy studies first identified associations of extracranial carotid atherosclerosis and coronary atherosclerosis [4,5]. We [6] and others [7,8] have also identified in vivo associations between increased IMT of the extracranial carotid arteries and CAD. These associations in general are graded so that increased extracranial carotid IMT is associated with increased extent and severity of CAD [9]. They are also robust, consistent and as strong as, if not stronger than, other risk factors. Rationale for these interassociations of structural manifesta-

---

Address for correspondence: John R. Crouse III MD, Bowman Gray School of Medicine, Department of Internal Medicine, Medical Center Boulevard, Winston-Salem, NC 27157, USA.

tions of arterial disease partly proceeds from shared risk factors for cerebrovascular and coronary artery disease [10], but the association of IMT and CAD often persists after control for common risk factors measured contemporaneously, suggesting that, because of its relative stability, IMT represents an index of the integrated impact of risk-factor exposure over long periods of time, or alternatively the role of additional "nontraditional" risk factors that might be of importance, but have not been measured such as elevated homocysteine [11], postprandial triglycerides [12] or chlamydia exposure [13].

Chambers and Norris showed many years ago that individuals with asymptomatic stenosis of the carotid arteries had a markedly increased risk of developing coronary heart disease (CHD) events [14]. More recently, Salonen and colleagues have noted a 6.7-fold increased risk of incident CHD associated with > 20% stenosis of the extracranial carotid arteries (Kuopio ischemic heart disease study (KIHD) [15]). However, although these studies identify an increased risk of CHD associated with extracranial carotid artery stenosis, approximately half the CHD events in the KIHD study (11/24) were associated with normal carotid arteries or wall thickening only, and although 412 individuals (32% of the population) had plaque or stenosis and experienced half the clinical CHD events, 96% of these remained free of CHD during the period of the study (Table 1). Thus, for the individual, there is only a loose association between stenotic carotid atherosclerosis (a structural manifestation of extracranial carotid disease) and clinical CHD events. It is similarly true that coronary artery stenosis only imperfectly predicts coronary events. This apparent paradox has been most eloquently elaborated by Brown et al., who first noted that small changes in progression and regression of stenosis of coronary arteries observed in clinical trials of cholesterol lowering were associated with a very dramatic reduction in clinical events [16].

At least six clinical trials have shown that cholesterol lowering retards progression of IMT of the extracranial carotid arteries (Table 2, [17–22]). In four of these trials, the authors observed net regression or 100% retardation of progression [17,18,20,22]. Qualitatively, therefore, this effect on atherosclerosis progression agrees with the clinical effects of HMGCoA reductase inhibitors to mark-

Table 1. Incident CHD odds ratios for levels of maximum stenosis: KIHD.

Stenosis	CHD		Odds ratio	95% C.I.
	No	Yes		
Normal	603	5	1.00	
Thickening	251	6	2.17	0.70–6.74
Plaque	375	11	4.15	1.51–11.47
Stenosis > 20%	37	2	6.71	1.33–33.91
Total	1266	24		

% CHD with "stenosis > 20%" = 8.3%

Table 2. Clinical trials with atherosclerosis outcome.

Clinical features							IMT progression rate difference (active drug vs. placebo)			
Trial [Ref]	No (F/ up,yr)	Symp- tom status	Rx[a]	Base LDL[b]	% Δ LDL	% Δ HDL[b]	Common[c] (Mm/yr)	Bif[c] (Mm/ yr)	Agg[c] (Mm/ yr)	% de- crease[d]
CLAS [17]	78(4)[e]	CABG	C+N	170	↓ 43%	↑ 37.0%	−0.035			REG
MARS [18]	30(2)[e]	CAD	L	155	↓ 45%	↑ 8.5%	−0.065			100%
PLAC-II [19]	151(3)	CAD	P	165	↓ 28%	↑ 3.9%	−0.016	−0.016	−0.008	30%
ACAPS[f] [20]	461(3)	None	L	157	↓ 28%	↑ 5.0%			−0.015	REG
KAPS [21]	447(3)[e]	None	P	186	↓ 27%	↑ 5.0%	−0.019	−0.012		40%
CAIUS[f] [22]	305(3)	None	P	178	↓ 22%	↑ 4.0%	−0.011	−0.027	−0.013	REG

[a]C = colestipol, N = niacin, L = lovastatin, P = pravastatin. [b]LDL, HDL: low-density lipoprotein, high-density lipoprotein, mg/dl. [c]Common, bif, agg common carotid IMT, bifurcation IMT, aggregate IMT. [d]% Decrease: REG = net regression. [e]Men only. [f]Multicenter.

edly reduce the risk of heart attack and stroke [16,23]. However, at least as regards recent studies of cholesterol lowering, clinical event reduction is often evident within 6 months of initiation of therapy [19], whereas the effects of risk-factor reduction on IMT progression (a structural manifestation of disease) become evident over 2–3 years.

These data suggest a loose association between effects of lipid-lowering agents to cause regression of stenosis and events, but a congruent relation of effects of lipid-lowering agents to cause regression of atherosclerosis and events. However, effects of cholesterol lowering on atherosclerosis regression are observed over a more prolonged period of time compared to effects on clinical events, and for the individual patient, atherosclerosis or even stenosis may not identify present and immediate danger of clinical events. This problem may partly derive from that aspect of arterial disease quantified by these structural manifestations: although they may represent the integrated effect of prolonged exposure to risk factors (as above), effects of interventions or changes in lifestyle that might in fact, rapidly reduce risk of incident clinical events might not be (in fact, are not) manifest as rapid change in atherosclerosis progression. Thus, other indices of arterial pathology that might be more rapidly responsive to risk-factor intervention could perhaps, add an additional dimension to studies of IMT with regard to identifying individuals at present risk (or with presently reduced risk) of incident events. In summary, to the extent that events may be conceptualized as relating to the processes of stenosis, progression of atherosclerosis, modification of plaque composition per se and plaque destabilization, the current measures of atherosclerosis quantitate only the first two.

For these reasons, investigators have used new technologies in an attempt to better quantify the characteristics of plaques, as well as to investigate the associations of nitric oxide mediated endothelial function with atherosclerosis/clinical events. As regards the former of these, several studies have used the ability of B-mode to quantify gray scale of extracranial carotid plaque as an index of plaque composition. These investigations have evaluated the association of these plaque characteristics with the development of clinical CHD events [24]. It is not altogether clear to what extent risk factors and/or prevalent vascular disease relate differently to plaque composition compared to IMT or stenosis per se. However, changes in plaque composition under the influence of risk-factor modification (e.g., cholesterol-lowering therapy) might well identify individuals at greater or lesser risk of developing clinical events. In the future it will be important to assess whether these changes occur in parallel with changes in IMT or provide unique information not available from studies of IMT. It will also be of interest to determine how rapidly change in these structural characteristics occurs. If change occurs over long periods of time it may be expected to reflect those elements now identified by IMT as regards associations with incident vascular events together with the attendant strengths and weaknesses.

Other investigators have focused attention on the associations of measures of arterial function rather than structure with atherosclerosis and with CAD. In these studies, individuals with and without CAD are evaluated for the ability of their brachial arteries to show a vasodilatory response to increases in blood flow induced by rapid deflation of a blood pressure cuff on the forearm. Research has identified associations between traditional cardiovascular disease risk factors and flow-mediated arterial dilation, and between flow-mediated arterial dilation and coronary artery disease. Furthermore, interventions that might be expected to improve cardiac outcome (e.g., lipid-lowering therapy [25], estrogen use [26], vitamin treatment [27]) improve arterial function over very short periods of time ranging from hours to months, and thus the time course for improvement in this functional manifestation of arterial disease may better reflect the change associated with risk-factor modification.

It is likely that in the future some combination of these measures of arterial structure and function will allow us to more precisely characterize those individuals at greatest risk for coronary artery disease; in addition, clinical trials using these indices as surrogate end points will provide evidence as regards mechanisms involved in reduction of coronary disease risk.

References

1. Crouse JR III. Assessment and management of carotid disease. Ann Rev Med 1992;43: 301–316.
2. Hertzer NR. Basic data concerning associated coronary disease in peripheral vascular patients.

Ann Vasc Surg 1978;1:616—620.

3. Komrad MS, Coffey CE, Coffey KS, McKinnis R, Massey EW, Califf RM. Myocardial infarction and stroke. Neurology 1984;34:1403—1409.

4. Solberg LA, Strong JP. Risk factors and atherosclerotic lesions. A review of autopsy studies. Arteriosclerosis 1983;3:187—198.

5. Holme I, Enger SC, Helgeland A, Hjermann I, Leren P, Lund-Larsen PG, Solberg LA, Strong JP. Risk factors and raised atherosclerotic lesions in coronary and cerebral arteries. Statistical analysis from the Oslo Study. Arteriosclerosis 1981;1:250—256.

6. Craven TE, Ryu JE, Espeland MA, Kahl FR, McKinney WM, Toole JF, McMahan MR, Thompson C, Heiss G, Crouse JR. Evaluation of the associations between carotid artery atherosclerosis and coronary artery stenosis: a case control study. Circulation 1990;82:1230—1242.

7. Geroulakos G, O'Gorman DJ, Kalodiki E, Sheridan DJ, Nicolaides AN. The carotid intima-media thickness as a marker of the presence of severe symptomatic coronary artery disease. Eur Heart J 1994;15:781—785.

8. Adams MR, Nakagomi A, Keech A, Robinson J, McCredie R, Bailey BP, Freedman SB, Celermajer DS. Carotid intima-media thickness is only weakly correlated with the extent and severity of coronary artery disease. Circulation 1995;92:2127—2134.

9. Wofford JL, Kahl FR, McKinney WM, Toole JF, Crouse JR. Relation of extent of extracranial carotid artery atherosclerosis as measured by B-mode ultrasound to the extent of coronary atherosclerosis. Arterioscl Thromb 1991;11:1786—1795.

10. Crouse JR. AWT and coronary heart disease. In: Touboul P-J, Crouse JR III (eds) Intima-Media Thickening and Atherosclerosis: Predicting the Risk. New York, London: Parthenon Publishing, 1996;105—115.

11. Selhub J, Jacques PF, Bostom AG, D'Agostino RB, Wilson PWF, Belanger AJ, O'Leary DH, Wolf PA, Schaefer EJ, Rosenberg IH. Association between plasma homocysteine concentrations and extracranial carotid-artery stenosis. N Engl J Med 1995;332:286—291.

12. Sharrett AR, Chambless LE, Heiss G, Paton CC, Patsch W. Association of postprandial triglyceride and retinyl palmitate responses with asymptomatic carotid artery atherosclerosis in middle-aged men and women. Arterioscl Thromb Vasc Biol 1995;15:2122—2129.

13. Melnick SL, Shahar E, Folsom AR. Past infection by *Chlamydia pneumoniae* strain TWAR and asymptomatic carotid atherosclerosis. Am J Med 1993;95:499—504.

14. Chambers BR, Norris JW. Outcome in patients with asymptomatic neck bruits. N Engl J Med 1986;315:860—865.

15. Salonen JT, Salonen R. Ultrasonographically assessed carotid morphology and the risk of coronary heart disease. Arterioscl Thromb 1991;11:1245—1249

16. Brown BG, Zhao X-Q, Sacco DE, Albers JJ. Lipid lowering and plaque regression, new insights into prevention of plaque disruption and clinical events in coronary disease. Circulation 1993;87:1781—1791.

17. Blankenhorn DH, Selzer RH, Crawford DW, Barth JD, Liu C, Liu C, Mack WJ, Alaupovic P. Beneficial effects of colestipol-niacin therapy on the common carotid artery. Circulation 1993;88:20—28.

18. Hodis HN, Mack WJ, LaBree L, Selzer RH, Liu C, Liu C, Alaupovic P, Kwong-Fu H, Azen SP. Reduction in carotid arterial wall thickness using lovastatin and dietary therapy. Ann Intern Med 1996;124:549—556.

19. Crouse JR III, Byington RP, Bond MG, Espeland MA, Craven TE, Sprinkle JW, McGovern ME, Furberg C. Pravastatin, lipids and atherosclerosis in the carotid arteries (PLAC-II). Am J Cardiol 1995;75:455—459.

20. Furberg CD, Adams HP, Applegate WB, Byington RP, Espeland MA, Hartwell T, Hunninghake DB, Lefkowitz DS, Probstfield J, Riley WA, Young B. Effect of lovastatin on early carotid atherosclerosis and cardiovascular events. Circulation 1994;90:1679—1687.

21. Salonen R, Nyyssonen K, Porkkala E, Rummukainen J, Belder R, Park J-S, Salonen JT. Kuopio Atherosclerosis Prevention Study (KAPS). Circulation 1995;92:1758—1764.

1168

22. Mercuri M, Bond MG, Sirtori CR, Veglia F, Crepaldi G, Feruglio FS, Descovich G, Ricci G, Rubba P, Mancini M, Gallus G Bianchi G, D'Alo G, Ventura A. Pravastatin reduces carotid intima-media thickness progression in an asymptomatic hypercholesterolemic Mediterranean population: the Carotid Atherosclerosis Italian Ultrasound Study. Am J Med 1996;101:627—634.

23. Crouse JR III, Byington RP, Hoen HM, Furberg C. Reductase inhibitor monotherapy and stroke prevention. Arch Int Med 1997;157:1305—1310.

24. Belcaro G, Nicolaides AN, Laurora G, Cesarone MR, De Sanctis M, Incandela L, Barsotti A. Ultrasound morphology classification of the arterial wall and cardiovascular events in a 6-year follow-up study. Arterioscl Thromb Vasc Biol 1996;16:851—856.

25. O'Driscoll G, Green D, Taylor RR. Simvastatin, an HMG-coenzyme A reductase inhibitor, improves endothelial function within 1 month. Circulation 1997;95:1126—1131.

26. Kieberman EH, Gerhard MD, Uehata A, Walsh BW, Selwyn AP, Ganz P, Yeung AC, Creager MA. Estrogen improves endothelium-dependent, flow-mediated vasodilation in postmenopausal women. Ann Intern Med 1994;121:936—941.

27. Levine, GN, Frei B, Koulouris SN, Gerhard MD, Keaney JF, Vita JA. Ascorbic acid reverses endothelial vasomotor dysfunction in patients with coronary artery disease. Circulation 1996;93:1107—1113.

Magnetic resonance imaging and angiography of atherosclerosis

Robert R. Edelman
Magnetic Resonance Imaging, Beth Israel-Deaconess Medical Center, Harvard Medical School, Boston, Massachusetts, USA

Atheromatous plaque can be directly imaged by magnetic resonance imaging (MRI), and work is underway to characterize plaque based on relaxation properties and spectroscopic features. Additionally, flowing blood has an appearance in MR images that is distinct from that of stationary tissue. This property can be used to generate magnetic resonance angiograms (MRA). The gold standard for imaging vascular disease is X-ray angiography, an invasive, costly and potentially hazardous procedure. Already MRA has supplanted a substantial portion of the X-ray angiograms carried out for extracranial carotid artery disease, and is increasingly being applied to imaging of the aorta and its major branches. Progress is also being made towards making coronary MRA a clinical reality.

The various features of plaque (e.g., lipid, collagen, calcium) show distinct signal intensities on T2-weighted spin-echo images. The atheromatous core, which is composed of cholesterol and cholesterol esters, has a shorter T2 relaxation time than the collagenous cap [1]. This method may eventually provide a means for discriminating between stable fibrous plaques and ones that are prone to hemorrhage.

Depending on the imaging technique used, blood may appear bright or dark. On spin-echo or fast spin-echo images, blood vessels usually appear dark. In order to create bright blood images, gradient-echo pulse sequences are used. In a gradient-echo sequence, only a single RF pulse is applied during each sequence repetition, so no signal is lost due to wash-out effects as occurs with spin-echo. Data for images on which blood is bright can be acquired as a series of overlapping thin sections (sequential two-dimensional) or as one or more thick volumes (three-dimensional). Each sequence has advantages, as discussed further on. Bright-blood techniques can be subcategorized into time of flight [2] and phase contrast [3]. The basis of time-of-flight techniques is that positive flow contrast is generated by inflow effects, whereas the background is saturated by the rapid repeated application of RF pulses. The basis for phase contrast is that the flow of blood along a magnetic-field gradient causes a shift in the phase of the MR signal. With phase contrast, pairs of images are acquired that have different sensitivities to flow. These are then subtracted to cancel background signal, leaving only the signal from flowing blood. Phase contrast also permits flow quantification [4], since the phase shift is proportional to the velocity.

Nowadays, the method of choice for MRA involves the combination of breath-hold three-dimensional gradient-echo sequences with short TR/TE and adminis-

1170

tration of a gadolinium chelate, typically in a double dose [5,6]. The contrast agent shortens the T1 to a low value (e.g., < 50 ms), so that the blood appears bright irrespective of flow patterns or velocities. The three-dimensional acquisition is advantageous in displaying detailed vessel anatomy and in reducing artifacts.

The heart of MR angiography is the ability to portray blood vessels in a projective format similar to that of X-ray angiography. Currently, projection images are created by postprocessing images acquired by a two- or three-dimensional gradient-echo sequence. Although image processing can be postponed until after the patient has left the MR suite, it is best done while the patient is still within the magnet so that additional scans can be obtained if needed. Most commonly, the images are processed by using a maximum intensity projection algorithm [7,8]. With this algorithm, the brightest pixels along a user-defined direction are extracted to create a projection image. Areas with poor flow contrast, including the edges of blood vessels and small vessels with slow flow, may be obscured by overlap with brighter stationary tissue [9].

A variety of artifacts, caused by phase or magnitude variations in the MR signal, afflict MRA. Within a voxel, blood protons flowing at different velocities accumulate a range or dispersion of phase shifts. Complex flow can produce signal loss due to intraview phase dispersion (i.e., it occurs during each repetition of the pulse sequence), ghost artifacts from view-to-view signal variations (i.e., occurring over multiple sequence repetitions) and flow displacement errors relating to the time delay between radiofrequency excitation and frequency encoding, or between phase and frequency encoding. These effects tend to falsely exaggerate the severity of a stenosis and are worst with two-dimensional MRA. Contrast-enhanced three-dimensional MRA using short TE has eliminated most of these artifacts.

Neurovascular applications

MR angiography is best established for the diagnosis of extracranial carotid bifurcation disease. A major incentive for developing a noninvasive means for evaluating the carotid bifurcation came from the North American symptomatic carotid endarterectomy trial, which showed that carotid endarterectomy significantly reduces the prevalence of stroke in symptomatic patients with stenosis, in which the diameter of the affected vessel is narrowed 70% or more [10]. The prevalence of major morbidity associated with conventional angiography is 0.5—3.0%. Duplex sonography is accurate but operator-dependent, and a minority of surgeons are willing to operate solely on the basis of a sonographic study. Occlusions cannot always be differentiated from critical stenoses. Moreover, tandem intracranial stenoses, which may preclude endarterectomy, are not accessible without the additional use of transcranial Doppler sonography or other noninvasive tests.

From a technical standpoint, MRA of the carotid bifurcation is aided by the paucity of motion artifacts and the availability of surface coils for the neck. Dedicated head and neck MRA coils are becoming available that permit efficient imaging of the aortic arch through the circle of Willis without the need for multiple coil placements (Fig. 1). Recent studies, in which three-dimensional sequences with short echo times were used to evaluate extracranial carotid stenoses found highly significant correlations (r values ranging >0.9) for diameters of stenoses measured using MRA and X-ray angiography [11,12]. The combination of duplex sonography and MRA, with X-ray angiography reserved for discordant cases, has been shown to be the most cost-effective approach for presurgical evaluation of extracranial carotid bifurcation disease [13]. As yet, the accuracy of MRA for evaluating the carotid and vertebral origins off the aortic arch is not known.

Body MRA

Stenosis of the renal artery afflicts a small percentage of patients with systemic hypertension. Neither duplex sonography nor radionuclide renography has been entirely satisfactory as a screening test, so that digital subtraction angiography remains the gold standard [14—16]. Excellent results are obtained noninvasively using contrast-enhanced three-dimensional MRA (Fig. 2) [17]. We use a breath-hold three-dimensional MRA sequence (e.g., TR/TE/flip angle = 5 ms/2 ms/

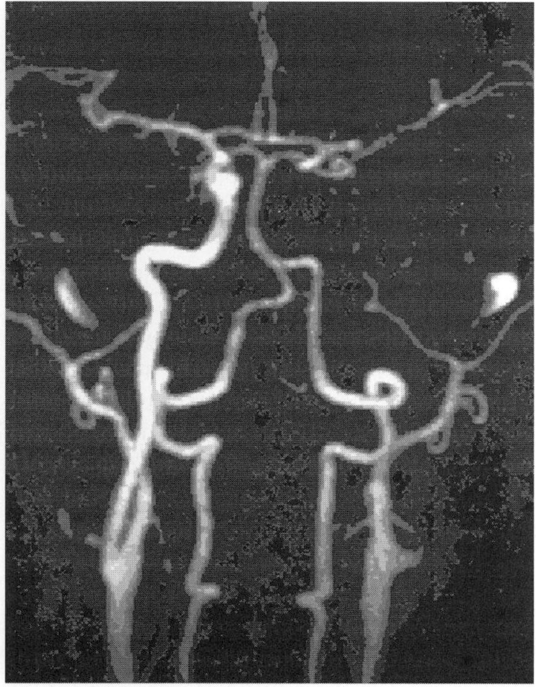

Fig. 1. Contrast-enhanced three-dimensional MRA of the head and neck showing occlusion of the left internal carotid artery due to dissection.

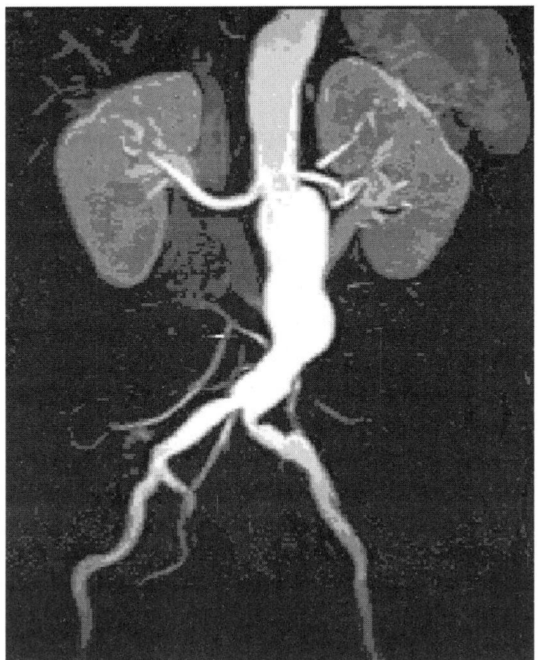

Fig. 2. Contrast-enhanced three-dimensional MRA of an abdominal aortic aneurysm.

40°) during the double-dose infusion of a gadolinium chelate. Because of its speed and insensitivity to flow artifacts, contrast-enhanced spiral CT is an alternative to MRA, but should not be used in patients with impaired renal function. MRA offers the advantage of a larger field of view, so that the entire abdominal aorta and iliac vessels can be encompassed in a single scan. It is also possible to measure blood flow and tissue perfusion by MR.

Although the peripheral arteries were the first vascular system in which the feasibility of MRA was demonstrated, only recently has its initial promise in this area become fulfilled [18]. Owen et al. showed that MR angiography depicts significantly more distal runoff vessels than X-ray angiography does; the finding of a patent run-off vessel may alter the choice between surgical revascularization and amputation [19].

Coronary artery MRA

Cardiovascular disease remains the leading cause of death in the USA with an estimated 1.2 million myocardial infarctions and 600,000 deaths per year attributed to coronary artery disease [20]. Minimally invasive tests for myocardial ischemia include single photon emission tomography (SPECT) [21,22] and positron emission tomography (PET) [23,24]. These tests reveal perfusion abnormalities, but do not depict the coronary artery stenoses that cause them nor do they provide direct measurements of coronary artery blood flow. The "gold standard" for evaluation of the coronary arteries is contrast angiography with over 500,000 diagnostic cardiac catheterizations performed annually in the USA. Despite the development of multiple noninvasive tests for the detection of myocardial ischemia, up to 20% of these coronary angiograms reveal insignificant coronary artery disease [25]. Information derived from such angiograms, however, is the standard by which mechanical interventions and many medical therapies are planned. In addition, prognostic information is also gained from data regarding coronary artery patency.

Hospital charges alone for cardiac catheterizations have been estimated at over US \$1.8 billion annually. In addition, coronary angiography carries with it a low, though finite major complication rate (death 0.12—0.20%, cerebrovascular accident 0.03—0.20%, myocardial infarction 0.0—0.25%) and minor complication rate (vascular complication, local infection 0.57—1.6%, or arrhythmias 0.30—0.63%) [26—28]. The high cost and associated risk make routine coronary angiography inappropriate for use as a screening test. Furthermore, while semiquantitative techniques exist for estimating the flow restriction caused by a coronary artery stenosis based on the conventional angiogram [29], they do not provide a quantitative measure of coronary artery blood flow.

The ability to perform noninvasive coronary angiography would represent a major improvement in patient care. Information regarding coronary anatomy could then be acquired with minimal risk, as well as in patients in whom coronary angiography is relatively contraindicated [30] due to severe allergic history to radiographic contrast agents, fever with documented infection, bleeding diatheses or recent gastrointestinal bleeding or cerebrovascular accident. Follow-up angiographic information in patients undergoing revascularization procedures could also be more readily obtained.

Human coronary arteries are small in caliber. The left main coronary artery is typically 4—6 mm in diameter [31] while the left anterior descending and left circumflex coronary arteries are generally 3—4 mm at their origins and taper distally. The right coronary artery, supplying less myocardium is smaller than the left main, and is typically 3—4 mm proximally. ECG-gated spin-echo and gradient-echo cine images only occasionally show portions of the coronary arteries, and these images are not adequate for detailed evaluation [32].

With standard gradient-echo acquisitions, an image cannot be obtained in less than a few hundred ms. This is obviously too long to freeze cardiac motion and avoid motion artifacts. Instead, the acquisition can be "segmented" into blocks of phase-encoding steps which are then interleaved to create an image, a method called "segmented turboFLASH". Segmentation can reduce the time for data acquisition within each cardiac cycle to 100 ms or less, which is adequate to minimize cardiac motion artifacts if imaging is done during diastole. The entire data collection is finished within 10—20 s, short enough to permit breath holding.

Using segmented turboFLASH, one consistently obtains good quality images of the proximal coronary arteries [33]. Sensitivity and specificity for coronary artery disease are in the 80—90% range [34], which is comparable to thallium scintigraphy. One problem has been poor flow contrast resulting from slow flow distal to a severe stenosis, making it difficult to distinguish from an occlusion. This problem might be ameliorated by the use of contrast agents. Blood pool contrast agents are currently under development that could greatly improve the quality of coronary artery images. Flow velocity measurements can be done pre- and postadministration of a vasodilator such as adenosine to obtain a measure of flow reserve, and help to determine the physiological significance of a coronary stenosis [35].

An important recent development is the introduction of navigator gating and correction to eliminate the need for breath holding. For navigator gating, MR data are only accumulated for image reconstruction when the navigator echo indicates that the interface of interest is within a certain operator-defined range. In this respect, navigator echoes perform a similar function to the bellows used for respiratory gating, but provide more consistent results. Because many data are rejected, acquisition times are typically increased by a factor of four or more, depending on breathing patterns. However, if a fast-imaging sequence such as segmented turboFLASH is used, scan times are still reasonable, in the order of a few minutes at most. Image sharpness is as good as with breath holding. Since navigator echoes permit signal averaging, signal-to-noise is increased and higher in-plane spatial resolution can be obtained (e.g., 0.5 mm). Moreover, navigator echoes ensure a consistent cardiac position from image to image, thereby minimizing misregistration artifact if one wishes to process a projection image.

Although most work to date has focused on two-dimensional acquisitions, three-dimensional acquisitions may offer certain advantages [36]. The slices (or partitions) are truly contiguous, residual motion artifacts tend to be averaged with the acquisition of multiple acquisitions as they would using multiple signal averages, and very thin sections (e.g., 1—2 mm) are readily obtained. Navigator gating permits the acquisition of artifact-free three-dimensional volumes within a reasonable acquisition period (e.g., 5—15 min, depending on breathing patterns).

References

1. Toussaint J-F, Southern JF, Fuster V, Kantor HL. T2-weighted contrast for NMR characterization of human atherosclerosis. Arterioscl Thromb Vasc Biol 1995;15:1533—1542.
2. Keller P. Time-of-flight magnetic resonance angiography. Neuroimag Clin N Am 1992;4:639—656.
3. Dumoulin CL. Phase contrast MR angiography techniques. Magn Reson Imag Clin N Am 1995;3:399—411
4. Walker MF, Souza SP, Dumoulin CL. Quantitative flow measurement in phase contrast MR angiography. J Comput Assist Tomogr 1988;12:304—313.
5. Prince MR. Gadolinium-enhanced MR aortography. Radiology 1994;191:155—164.

6. Prince MR. Body MR angiography with gadolinium contrast agents. MRI Clin N Am 1996; 4(1):11—24.

7. Saloner D. MRA: principles and display. In: Higgins CB, Hricak H, Helms CA (eds) Magnetic Resonance Imaging of the Body. Philadelphia: Lippencott-Raven Publishers, 1997;1345—1368.

8. Laub G. Displays for MR angiography. Magn Reson Med 1990;14:222—229.

9. Anderson C, Saloner D, Tsuruda J, Shapeero L, Lee R. Artifacts in maximum intensity projection display of MR angiograms. AJR 1990;154:623—629.

10. Collaborators NASCET. Beneficial effect of carotid endarterectomy in symptomatic patients with high-grade carotid stenosis. N Engl J Med 1991;325:445—453.

11. Anderson CM, Saloner D, Lee RE et al. Assessment of carotid artery stenosis by MR angiography: comparison with X-ray angiography and color-coded Doppler ultrasound. AJNR 1992; 13:989—1003.

12. Patel MR, Kuntz KM, Klufas RA et al. Preoperative assessment of the carotid bifurcation: can magnetic resonance angiography and duplex ultrasonography replace contrast arteriography? Stroke 1995;26:1753—1758.

13. Kent C, Kuntz KM, Patel MR et al. Perioperative imaging strategies for carotid endarterectomy: an analysis of morbidity and cost-effectiveness in symptomatic patients. JAMA 1995;274: 888—893.

14. Nally JV, Olin JW, Lammert GK. Advances in noninvasive screening for renovascular disease. Cleveland Clin J Med 1994;61:328—336.

15. Nally JV, Black HR. State-of-the-art review: captopril renography, pathophysiological considerations and clinical observations. Sem Nucl Med 1992;22(2):85—97.

16. Galanski M, Prokop M, Chavan A, Schaefer CM et al. Renal arterial stenoses: spiral CT angiography. Radiology 1993;189:185—192.

17. Holland GA, Dougherty L, Carpenter JP, Golden MA, Gilfeather M, Slossman F, Schnall MD, Axel L. Breath-hold ultrafast three-dimensional gadolinium-enhanced MR angiography of the aorta and the renal and other visceral abdominal arteries. AJR 1996;166:971—981.

18. Baum RA, Rutter CM, Sunshine JH et al. Multicenter trial to evaluate vascular magnetic resonance angiography of the lower extremity. JAMA 1995;274:875—880.

19. Owen RS, Carpenter JP, Baum RA, Perloff LJ, Cope C. Magnetic resonance imaging of angiographically occult runoff vessels in peripheral arterial occlusive disease. N Engl J Med 1992; 326:1577—1581.

20. Davis FA. Assessment of coronary artery disease. In: Yang SS, Bentivoglio LG, Maranhao V, Goldberg H (eds) Cardiac Catheterization Data to Hemodynamic Parameters, 3rd edn. Philadelphia, 1988;256.

21. Holman BL, Moore SC, Shulkin PM et al. Quantitation of perfused myocardial mass using Tl-201 and emission computed tomography. Invest Radiol 1983;18:322.

22. Cladwell JH, Williams DL, Harp GD et al. Quantitation of size of relative myocardial perfusion defect by single-photon emission computed tomography. Circulation 1984;70:1048—1056.

23. Marshall RC, Tillisch JH, Phelps ME et al. Identification and differentiation of resting myocardial ischemia and infarction in man with positron computed tomography, F-18 labeled fluorodeoxyglucose and N-13 ammonia. Circulation 1983;67:766—778.

24. Brunken R, Tillisch JH, Scwaiger M et al. Regional perfusion, glucose metabolism and wall motion in patients with chronic electrocardiographic Q-wave infarctions: evidence of persistence of viable tissue in some infarct regions by positron emission tomography. Circulation 1986;73:951—962.

25. Johnson LW, Lozner EC, Johnson D et al. Coronary arteriography 1984—1987: a report of the registry of the Society for Cardiac Angiography and Interventions. I. Results and complications. CCD 1989;17:5—10.

26. Davis K, Kennedy JW, Kemp HG et al. Complications of coronary arteriography from the collaborative study of Coronary Artery Surgery (CASS). Circulation 1979;59:1105.

27. Kennedy JW, and the Registry Committee of the Society for Cardiac Angiography. Complica-

tions associated with cardiac catheterization and angiography. Cath Cardiov Diag 1982;8:5.
28. Wyman RM, Safian RD, Portway V et al. Current complications of diagnostic and therapeutic cardiac catheterization. J Am Coll Cardiol 1988;12:1400.
29. Gould KL. Detecting and assessing severity of coronary artery disease in humans. Cardiovasc Inter Radiol 1990;13:5—13.
30. Guidelines for coronary angiography. A report of the American College of Cardiology/American Heart Association Task Force on assessment of diagnostic and therapeutic cardiovascular procedures (Subcommittee on Coronary Angiography). Circulation 1987;76:963A.
31. Paulin S. Coronary angiography. A technical, anatomic and clinical study. Acta Radiologica 1964;(Supp):125—137.
32. Paulin S, von Schulthess GK, Fossel E, Krayenbuehl HP. MR imaging of the aortic root and proximal coronary arteries. Am J Radiol 1987;148:665—670.
33. Edelman RR, Manning WJ, Burstein D, Paulin S. Coronary arteries: breath-hold MR angiography. Radiology 1991;181:641—643.
34. Manning WJ, Li W, Edelman RR. A preliminary report comparing magnetic resonance coronary angiography with conventional angiography. N Engl J Med 1993;328:828—832.
35. Edelman RR, Manning WJ, Gervino E, Li W. Flow velocity quantification in human coronary arteries with fast, breath-hold MR angiography. Magn Reson Imag 1993;3:699—703.
36. Li D, Kaushikkar S, Haacke EM, Woodard PK, Dhawale PJ, Kroeker RM, Laub G, Kuginuki Y, Gutierrez FR. Coronary arteries: three-dimensional MR imaging with retrospective respiratory gating. Radiology 1996;201(3):857—863.

Coronary calcification as a marker of arterial disease

Alain Simon, Jean Louis Megnien, Nicolas Denarie and Jaime Levenson
Centre de Médecine Préventive Cardiovasculaire, Hôpital Broussais, Paris, France

Abstract. Coronary calcium deposit is an anatomic marker of atheroma, but it has not yet been proven that it is an accurate marker of coronary stenosis. Coronary calcification can be detected noninvasively by X-ray imaging techniques, in particular, through electron beam computed tomography (EBCT). Although calcifications of coronary walls are associated with most traditional cardiovascular risk factors and globally reflect the multifactorial coronary-risk profile, their prognostic significance with regard to subsequent clinical outcomes has not yet been established in symptom-free subjects. The quantification of coronary calcium deposits by new X-ray techniques such as EBCT opens up a promising way for monitoring the progression of coronary atherosclerosis, in particular when under treatment. Finally, the detection of coronary calcification in symptom-free high-risk people should allow a better evaluation of coronary risk and better justification for decisions to vigorously treat cardiovascular risk factors.

Keywords: atherosclerosis, calcium, cardiovascular risk factors, computed tomography.

Introduction

Prevention of coronary heart disease, a major cause of morbidity and mortality, is of prime importance, and is traditionally based on the screening and treatment of established cardiovascular risk factors [1]. Increasing evidence indicates that prevention of coronary heart disease may be considerably enhanced by detecting early preclinical atherosclerosis, especially in coronary vessels [2]. The possibility of noninvasively detecting the presence of calcium deposits in coronary artery walls by radiographic techniques has opened up a promising way for the early detection of preclinical coronary atherosclerosis in subjects at high risk for coronary heart disease, but still free of clinical complications [3]. Coronary calcifications can be detected thanks to X-ray imaging (including digital fluoroscopy and X-ray computed tomography) [4]. Amongst these techniques, electron beam computed tomography (EBCT) has the ability to visualize the calcifications of large epicardial coronary vessels with high precision, and to totally quantify coronary artery calcium deposits [5].

Relation with atherosclerosis

Coronary calcium is an anatomic marker for significant coronary atheroma [3],

---

Address for correspondence: Prof Alain Simon, Centre de Médecine Préventive Cardiovasculaire, Hôpital Broussais, 96 rue Didot, 75674 Paris Cedex 14, France. Tel.: +33-1-4395-9392. Fax: +33-1-4539-1193.

but it has not yet been proven that even in the case of extended deposit, it is an accurate marker for coronary stenosis [4]. Evaluation studies of coronary calcification detected by EBCT as an indicator of significant angiographic stenosis have shown that the sensitivity of the presence of calcification varies from 85 to 100%, whereas its specificity varies from 41 to 76%, and its positive predictive value varies from 55–84%. Conversely, the absence of coronary calcification attested by EBCT has a negative predictive value for significant angiographic stenosis which ranges from 70 to 100% [4]. However, it must be emphasized that the absence of coronary calcium does not exclude at all the possibility of noncalcified atherosclerotic plaque which may even be subject to rupture. Also, coronary calcifications have been shown to be associated to extracoronary atherosclerosis detected echographically in peripheral large arteries (carotid, abdominal aorta, femoral) in an asymptomatic population at risk [6].

Relation with cardiovascular risk factors

Aging and male gender are two major risk factors for coronary calcification [4]. Other established risk factors for coronary calcifications are high blood cholesterol, low HDL-cholesterol, current smoking, high blood pressure, being overweight, diabetes mellitus and elevation of triglycerides [4,7]. In the presence of hypertension, the risk of coronary calcification is increased 2-fold and the risk of extended coronary calcium deposit (high EBCT-derived calcium score) is increased 5-fold [8]. Also, the extent of coronary calcium deposit reflects the multifactorial coronary risk profile estimated with the Framingham model in asymptomatic men [7]. The mechanisms by which cardiovascular risk factors are associated to coronary calcium deposit are not yet elucidated. It seems, however, that coronary calcification is an active process involving proteins of mineralization such as osteopontin, and their genetic expression induced by biological or mechanical injuries to the arterial wall.

Relation with clinical outcomes

A few preliminary prospective studies have given some arguments in favour of the prognostic significance of coronary calcifications in asymptomatic people. It has been shown in asymptomatic high-risk men that the presence of coronary calcification detected by fluoroscopy increases the 1-year risk of coronary event (angor, infarction, revascularization, death) by 3-fold [9]. Another study has also shown that extended deposit of coronary calcium considerably increases (by a factor of > 20) the short-term risk of acute cardiovascular complication (death, myocardial infarction, stroke) [10]. However, these studies are too limited in the number of subjects and the duration of follow-up. Further investigations are required to definitely confirm the relationship of coronary calcification and cardiac events in asymptomatic populations. Among the reasons for which coronary calcium (especially if the calcium deposit is important) may be predictive of future cardiac events, a major link may be that coronary calcification is a marker for overall atherosclerotic plaque burden, therefore; the higher the diffuseness of coronary atherosclerosis, the higher is the likelihood of potentially unstable lesions as a source of acute complications.

Relation with progression of atherosclerosis

The capability of new X-ray techniques, such as EBCT, to quantify coronary artery calcifications opens up a promising way for the noninvasive follow-up of coronary atherosclerosis, in particular under lipid-lowering or antihypertensive drugs therapy. To date, however, the reproducibility of coronary calcium quantification between two different EBCT scans is still too low [4,7] for accurately monitoring the progression of coronary calcium over time. Another limitation of using coronary detection by EBCT for monitoring progression of atherosclerosis is that EBCT usually measures calcium area and not volume.

Clinical perspectives

The detection of coronary calcium deposit should allow a better evaluation of coronary risk, and a better justification for decisions made about treatment of asymptomatic high-risk patients with preventive drug therapy (lipid-lowering agents, antioxidants, antihypertensive drugs or others) [2]. If the absence of coronary calcifications does not exclude noncalcified plaque (including unstable plaque) it makes the presence of significant coronary stenosis highly unlikely and can be considered as a condition of low risk of cardiovascular event in the next 2—5 years. Conversely, the presence of coronary calcification establishes the existence of coronary atherosclerosis, and the higher the deposit of calcium, the higher the likelihood of a cardiovascular event in the next 2—5 years [4]. Therefore, it follows that the evidence of coronary calcification in asymptomatic subjects is a major argument in favour of the decision to aggressively treat the modifiable risk associated with calcifications.

References

1. Oliver MF. Prevention of coronary heart disease-propaganda, promises, problems and prospects. Circulation 1986;73:1—9.
2. Simon A, Megnien JL, Levenson J. Coronary risk estimation and treatment of hypercholesterolemia. Circulation 1997;96:2449—2452.
3. Ultrafast CT for coronary calcification. Lancet 1991;337:1449—1450.
4. Wexler L, Brundage B, Crouse J, Detrano R, Fuster V, Maddahi J, Rumberger J, Stanford W, White R, Taubert K. Coronary artery calcification: pathophysiology, epidemiology, imaging methods and clinical implications. A statement for health profesionals from the American Heart Association. Circulation 1996;94:1175—1192.
5. Agaston A, Janowitz W, Hildner F, Zusmer N, Viamonte M, Detrano R. Quantification of coronary artery calcium using ultrafast computer tomography. J Am Coll Cardiol 1990;15: 827—832.

6. Mégnien JL, Séné V, Jeannin S, Hernigou A, Plainfossé MC, Merli I, Atger V, Moatti N, Levenson J, Simon A, PCV METRA Group. Coronary calcification and its relation to extracoronary atherosclerosis in asymptomatic men. Circulation 1992;85:1799—1807.

7. Simon A, Giral P, Levenson J. Extracoronary atherosclerotic plaque at multiple sites and total coronary calcification deposit in asymptomatic men. Association with coronary risk profile. Circulation 1995;92:1414—1421.

8. Mégnien JL, Simon A, Lemariey M, Plainfossé MC, Levenson J. Hypertension promotes coronary calcium deposit in asymptomatic men. Hypertension 1996;27:949—954.

9. Detrano RC, Wang ND, Tang W, French WJ, Georgiou D, Young E, Brezden OS, Doherty TM, Narahara KA, Brundage BH. Pronostic significance of cardiac cinefluoroscopy calcific deposits in asymptomatic high-risk subjects. J Am Coll Cardiol 1994;24:354—358.

10. Arad Y, Spadars LA, Goodman K, Lledo-Pereg A, Sherman S, Lerner G, Guerci AD. Predictive value of electron beam CT of the coronary arteries. 19-months follow-up of 1173 asymptomatic subjects. Circulation 1996;93:1951—1953.

Vascular endpoints for quantitating atherosclerosis for human gene therapy clinical trials

Jeffrey M. Hoeg[1], Mun K. Hong[2], Jafar Vossoughi[3], Gary S. Mintz[2], Ronald M. Summers[4], Robert F. Hoyt[1], Steven D. Wolff[1] and Martin B. Leon[2]

[1]*The National Heart, Lung and Blood Institute, National Institutes of Health, Bethesda, Maryland;*
[2]*Cardiology Research Foundation/Washington Cardiology Center, Washington, District of Columbia;*
[3]*Department of Biomedical Engineering, University of the District of Columbia, Washington, District of Columbia; and* [4]*Department of Radiology, National Institutes of Health, Bethesda, Maryland, USA*

Abstract. *Background.* Gene therapy for atherosclerosis requires new, more sensitive and specific vascular wall endpoints. Using normal, mutant and transgenic rabbits, as well as patients homozygous for familial hypercholesterolemia, an array of candidate methods for use in gene therapy studies have been systematically investigated.

Methods. Angiographic, intravascular ultrasound (IVUS), magnetic resonance imaging (MRI) and ultrafast computerized tomography (UFCT) studies were conducted in rabbits (WHHL) and patients homozygous for low-density lipoprotein receptor deficiency (FH).

Results. Angiography cannot detect types I—V atherosclerosis in WHHL rabbits. However, type II—V lesions are detected and quantitated by intravascular ultrasound (IVUS) and are associated with marked changes in the vascular compliance; these changes were correlated with the mural cholesterol content (r = −0.94; p < 0.001). Homozygous FH patients had substantial, diffuse, calcific coronary atherosclerosis detected by UFCT and IVUS. As in the rabbit models, nonobstructing lesions defined by angiography were associated with both structural and functional changes defined by both MRI and IVUS.

Conclusions. Direct quantitation of arterial wall thickness by IVUS, MRI and UFCT (as well as the quantitation of vascular compliance by MRI and US) provide more sensitive and specific methods for the evaluation of the efficacy of gene therapy to prevent and reverse atherosclerosis.

Keywords: familial hypercholesterolemia, intravascular ultrasound, low-density lipoproteins, magnetic resonance imaging, ultrafast computerized tomography, vascular compliance.

Introduction

As with many chronic diseases, atherosclerosis is the result of the interactions of a number of environmental and genetic factors. Recent studies in transgenic mice [1] and transgenic rabbits [2] have established that specific candidate genes can attenuate and even abolish diet-induced atherosclerosis. These results indicate that gene therapy to prevent atherosclerosis is feasible in man [3].

However, conventional clinical endpoints are inadequate for the purposes of

Address for correspondence: Jeffrey M. Hoeg MD, Chief of Section of Cell Biology, Molecular Disease Branch, National Heart, Lung and Blood Institutes, National Institutes of Health, Building 10, Room 7N115, 10 Center DR MSC 1666, Bethesda, MD 20892-1666, USA. Tel.: +1-301-496-5095. Fax: +1-301-402-0190. E-mail: jeff@mdb.nhlbi.nih.gov

phase II and phase III gene-therapy trials [4]. Cardiovascular morbidity and mortality trials with lipid-lowering drugs have required nearly 4,000 patients with 5—7 years of study to demonstrate efficacy. Although clinical trials focused upon angiography endpoints require as few as 200 patients with study durations as short as 1 year, clinical trials using therapeutic genes will be initiated on patients with inborn errors of metabolism. This is likely include as few as 10—20 patients. Therefore, new methods must be developed and validated in order to extend gene therapy to phase II and III clinical trials in man.

Table 1 summarizes the methods that can be considered for phase II and III gene therapy clinical trials. Epidemiologic and intervention studies have utilized morbidity and mortality as primary endpoints, and carotid artery ultrasound and coronary artery angiography have been used as surrogate endpoints for cardiovascular clinical events. We have initiated a series of studies in rabbits and man to evaluate the utility of ultrafast computerized tomography (UFCT), intravascular ultrasound (IVUS) and magnetic resonance imaging (MRI) in the detection and quantitation of atherosclerosis.

Materials and Methods

Male rabbits homozygous for the 12 base pair deletion in the low-density lipoprotein (LDL) receptor gene [5] and age-matched rabbits with normal LDL receptor function were studied. These rabbits develop severe aortic atherosclerosis that highly resemble the complex atherosclerosis in man [6]. The severity and extent of aortic atherosclerosis was assessed in these animals by aortography, intravascu-

Table 1. Techniques to detect and quantitate atherosclerosis.

Method	Quantitation[a]	Reproducibility	Advantages	Disadvantages
Angiography	++	++	Current "gold standard"	Lumenogram; doses not reflect mural processed
Carotid	+++	++	Noninvasive, quantitates atheroma	Does not assess coronary arteries
Trans-esophageal echo (TE echo)	+	+	Detects aortic lesions	Semiquantiative not reproducible
Magnetic resonance imaging (MRI)	?	?	Noninvasive, structural and rheologic	Not established
Ultrafast computerized tomography (UFCT)	?	++	Fast and relatively inexpensive	Detects only calcific atherosclerosis
Intravascula ultrasound (IVUS)	?	?	Sensitive and probes coronary artery wall	Expensive, invasive

[a]The semiquantitative scale is based upon 0 to a maximum of ++++ and reflects both sensitivity and specificity.

lar ultrasound, histopathologic evaluation and quantitation of the lipids in the arterial wall.

The investigation in patients homozygous for familial hypercholesterolemia was conducted within a study protocol approved by the Institutional Review Board of the National Heart, Lung and Blood Institute for patients 18 years or older. Consecutive patients referred to the Clinical Center of the National Institutes of Health with the diagnosis of homozygous familial hypercholesterolemia were evaluated. Initial evaluation included biochemical characterization (including plasma lipoprotein and apolipoprotein analyses), skin fibroblast assays for low-density lipoprotein receptor activity, and the evaluation of plasma lipoproteins in family members. After patients had given informed consent for participation, the extent of their atherosclerosis was evaluated by echocardiography, ultrafast computerized tomography (UFCT), coronary angiography, intravascular ultrasound and magnetic resonance imaging (MRI). The MRI scanning was performed using two separate strategies on two different 1.5 Tesla MRI scanners. One strategy optimized the resolution of the ascending aortic root image. This was accomplished by gating the pulse sequences to both heart and respiratory cycles. The scanning led to refined data acquisition permitting high-resolution images in both two- and three-dimensional renderings. The second strategy was designed to obtain rheologic information.

Results

Although it is not widely appreciated, the WHHL rabbits develop coronary artery disease. More than 20% of WHHL rabbits living more than 3 years experience sudden death. At postmortem evaluation, the hearts are engorged with blood secondary to the acute congestive heart failure the rabbits experienced (Fig. 1A). The coronary arteries are thickened and calcified reflecting atherosclerotic plaque (Fig. 1B). This coronary artery disease leads to recurrent myocardial infarction as reflected by the myocardial scarring (Fig. 1C) associated with the pulmonary congestion observed in acute congestive heart failure (Fig. 1D). These findings reinforce the utility of the WHHL rabbit as a model to investigate human atherogenesis and its sequelae.

The stiffness of the vascular wall was determined on control and WHHL aortae both before and after euthanasia. Prior to euthanasia, aortography and intravascular ultrasound were performed. After sodium pentobarbital euthanasia, the residual strain, a reflection of mural stiffness [7] was determined by obtaining 1–2 mm arterial rings using two parallel sections perpendicular to the axis of the vessel (Fig. 2). The ring was then cut on the dorsum of the vessel which permitted the ring to spring open due to the residual strain in the wall. Arteriography did not disclose any aortic lesions. However, intravascular ultrasound and histopathologic studies disclosed diffuse aortic disease. The cholesterol content in the aortae directly correlated with the compliance of the aorta determined by intravascular ultrasound as well as by the aortic residual strain. These findings

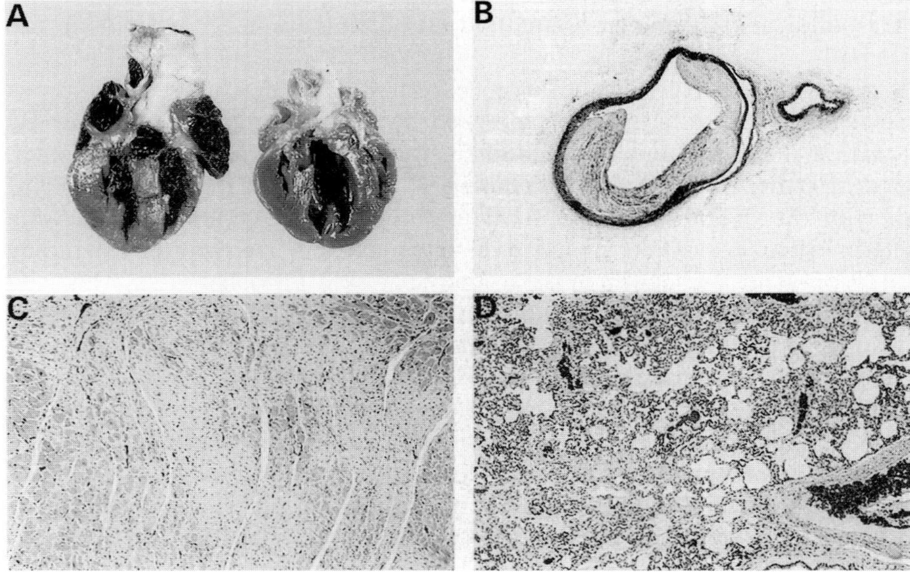

Fig. 1. Characterization of myocardial infarction in LDL-receptor deficient rabbits. The heart of a rabbit lacking functional LDL-receptors was harvested after a spontaneous death (**A**, left heart) and compared to a heart of a control rabbit of the same age, gender and size (**A**, right heart). The calcific coronary arteries and evidence of congestive heart failure is present in the LDL-receptor deficient heart. The coronary arteries demonstrated fibrocalcific plaque (**B**), while evidence of prior myocardial damage is evident from the fibrosis observed in the myocardium (**C**). Fluid indicative of congestive heart failure is evident in the lungs (**D**).

indicate that the biomechanical properties in human-like atherosclerosis precede changes that can be detected by conventional methods.

The parallel studies in homozygous familial hypercholesterolemic patients also indicated that angiography did not detect atherosclerosis in the coronary arteries. Intravascular ultrasound presented a sensitive means of identifying both calcific and noncalcific lesions. The calcific lesions can be quantitated by UFCT and highly correlates with the cumulative exposure to vasculotoxic low-density lipoproteins reflected in the cholesterol-year score [8]. In addition, MRI was useful in detecting plaque conformation and composition, as well as in quantitating altered vascular compliance-related properties.

These combined results indicate that different means of assessing the vascular consequences of hypercholesterolemia provide complementary means of characterizing atherosclerosis in vivo. Arteriography detects in the disease only late in the overall disease pathogenesis. In addition, arteriography is not a sensitive means of quantitating the extent of disease. Early detection of subtle changes in vascular compliance by MRI as well as the presence of calcific atherosclerosis by UFCT may become useful in risk-stratifying patients for interventional stud-

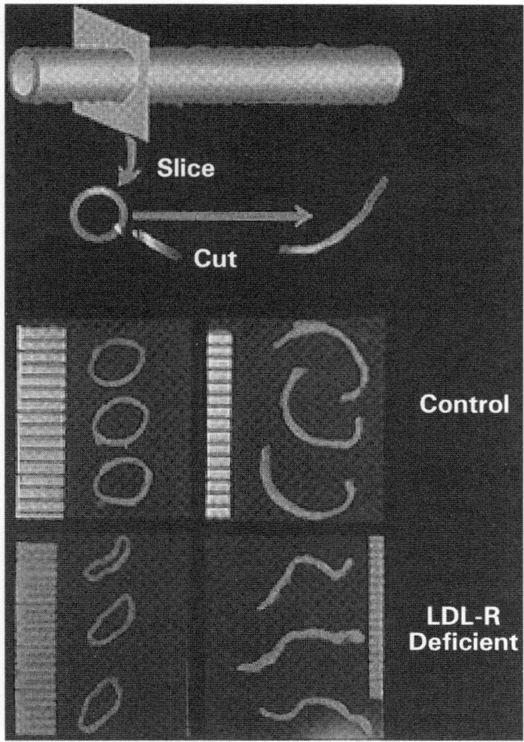

Fig. 2. The determination of residual strain. After harvestion, aortae from control and LDL-receptor deficient rabbits, the vessels were sliced perpendicular to the longitudinal axis. A cut in the ring released the residual strain that had accumulated in these vessels. In contrast to control, the LDL-receptor deficient rings sprang into a linear or even convex conformation, reflecting markedly increased vascular wall stiffness.

ies. These newer methods, particularly intravascular ultrasound and MRI rheological techniques, hold promise for quantitating early atherosclerosis and the impact of therapy on the underlying disease process.

References

1. Rubin EM, Smith DJ. Atherosclerosis in mice: getting to the heart of a polygenic disorder. Trends Genet 1994;10:199—203.
2. Hoeg JM, Santamarina-Fojo S, Berard AM, Cornhill JF, Herderick EE, Feldman SJ, Haudens-child CC, Vaisman BL, Hoyt RF Jr, Demosky SJ Jr, Kauffman RD, Hazel CM, Marcovina SM, Brewer HB Jr. Overexpression of lecithin:cholesterol acyltransferase in transgenic rabbits prevents diet-induced atherosclerosis. Proc Natl Acad Sci USA 1996;93:11448—11453.
3. Hoeg JM. Can genes prevent atherosclerosis? JAMA 1996;276:989—992.
4. Hoeg JM. Evaluating coronary heart disease risk: tiles in the mosaic. JAMA 1997;277:1387—1390.

5. Yamamoto T, Bishop RW, Brown MS, Goldstein JL, Russell DW. Deletion in cysteine-rich region of LDL receptor impedes transport to cell surface in WHHL rabbit. Science 1986;232:1230—1237.
6. Watanabe Y. Serial inbreeding of rabbits with hereditary hyperlipidemia (WHHL-rabbit): incidence and development of atherosclerosis and xanthoma. Atherosclerosis 1980;36:261—268.
7. Vaishnav RN, Vossoughi J. Residual stress and strain in aortic segments. J Biomech 1987;20:235—239.
8. Schmidt HH-J, Hill S, Makariou EF, Feuerstein IM, Dugi KA, Hoeg JM. Relation of cholesterol-year score to severity of calcific atherosclerosis and tissue deposition in homozygous familial hypercholesterolemia. Am J Cardiol 1996;77:575—580.

The clinical evaluation, development and regulation of new drugs, agents, substances affecting atherosclerosis cardiovascular diseases by lipoprotein related mechanisms

What guidelines are necessary to demonstrate efficacy and safety in "special" groups: women as a paradigm

John C. LaRosa
Tulane University Medical Center, New Orleans, Louisiana, USA

Abstract. Most studies of drugs effective in cardiovascular disease have been performed in middle-aged white men. Concern over coronary disease in men and women has increased over the past 10 years. FDA and NIH guidelines address the inclusion of women in trials including those of drug tolerance and efficacy. They indicate that enough women must be included to reassure clinicians that no gross differences exist in the safety or efficacy of test drugs. Generally, they do not require samples of sufficient size to demonstrate statistical significance in each subgroup unless there is preliminary evidence of differences in responses or clinical side effects. In general, some questions to answer in deciding when a separate clinical trial should be considered for a special group are:
1. Are there differences in the risk factor being modified compared with the "main" group?
2. Does evidence exist of a difference between or among groups in pharmacokinetics or pharmacodynamics of the drug being tested?
3. Do differences exist in the risk of a clinical event?
4. Is there evidence for a difference in the underlying disease process?
No common answer can be prescribed for each case, but the above considerations allow the development of a rationale for the creation of clinical trials in "special" groups.

Keywords: cholesterol lowering, clinical trials, coronary disease, FDA, NIH, women.

Most clinical trials in cardiovascular disease have concentrated on middle-aged white men [1]. This has been in part due to the extent of death and disability from coronary disease in men and the perception, at least in Western countries, of coronary disease as a major medical problem. In the USA and Northern Europe, women die almost as frequently of coronary disease as men do. Clinical disease presents itself 5–10 years later in women than in men. In the past the health concerns of women and their doctors, however, have focused on "female" diseases, such as breast and ovarian cancer, despite the fact that coronary disease causes 5–6 times the death and disability caused by reproductive cancers. In the last 10 years, it has become increasingly clear in the US and in Northern Europe that coronary disease is a cause for concern in both men and women. This, in turn, has led to serious discussion about the need to find ways of including more women in clinical trials.

In the US, two sets of guidelines, one developed by the Food and Drug Admin-

Address for correspondence: John C. LaRosa MD, Chancellor, Tulane University Medical Center, 1430 Tulane Avenue, SL76 New Orleans, LA 70112, USA. Tel.: +1-504-588-5295. Fax: +1-504-587-7357. E-mail: vpachec@mailhost.tcs.tulane.edu

1190

istration (FDA) [1], the other by the National Institutes of Health (NIH) [2], have specifically addressed the inclusion of women in clinical studies of cardiovascular disease interventions.

The FDA guidelines are specifically tailored to the issue of testing of new drugs and represent a sharp departure from previous FDA guidelines. The latter had been geared to minimal testing, particularly of women of childbearing age, in order to avoid potential problems of fetal toxicity.

New FDA guidelines include the following recommendations for the inclusion of women in new drug trials:

1. Women of all ages, including women of childbearing ages, should be eligible for inclusion in clinical trials of all phases.
2. There is, on the other hand, no requirement that women of childbearing age must be included in the early phase trials.
3. "Reasonable" numbers of women should be included in clinical trials to allow the detection of "significant" differences (these are not meant to be a statistical terms).
4. Specific pharmacokinetic studies that account for: a) the effects of the menstrual cycle and menopause status; b) the effect of exogenous hormones, such as in hormone replacement therapy or oral contraception; and c) the effect of the test drug on oral contraceptives (i.e., "b" is an attempt to examine the effects of exogenous hormones on drug pharmacokinetics, and "c" is an attempt to ascertain the effect of the drug on oral contraception).

With reference to clinical trials, the NIH guidelines apply particularly to the inclusion of women (and minorities) in Phase III clinical trials, i.e., trials to evaluate the efficacy of an experimental intervention. These guidelines may be summarized as follows:

1. If evidence of a "significant" (again, the word is not meant to have a statistical meaning) difference exists in the responses of men and women in early studies, sufficient numbers of women must be included in the trials to address the questions in the study separately for each gender.
2. If no data exist that imply differences in drug handling or drug effects then only enough women need be included to develop a "valid" analysis.
3. If there are data that definitively demonstrate that no difference exists in gender responses then there is no requirement that women be included in the studies, although it is nevertheless still encouraged.

The exclusion of strict statistical criteria in both of these sets of guidelines is deliberate and reflects the political as well as the scientific stimuli for their development. In essence, what they say is that enough women must be included to reassure investigators and practitioners that no gross differences exist either in the safety or efficacy of drugs being tested. Obviously, the guidelines were constructed in this way to side-step the potential for crippling statistical requirements that would have made the clinical trial testing too expensive because of the need to include groups at a relatively low risk of events.

For statistical purists, it is probably reasonable to assume that these guidelines represent a source of frustration and perhaps even disappointment. In a larger sense, what these guidelines represent is an attempt to answer, however incompletely, a very specific question, i.e., how much evidence is "enough" for a specific gender, race or age group, particularly when compelling evidence exists in a reference group, such as in the case of coronary atherosclerosis in white middle-aged men. A corollary question is how narrowly to define a "group". For example, is a study in white, elderly men applicable to white middle-aged men, black middle-aged men, black elderly men, etc.

There are, of course, no definitive answers to such questions. There is, however, widespread agreement that the gold standard for any group is a clinical trial specifically devoted to the study of the effects of the drug in that particular group (i.e., a specific clinical trial in white women over 65 of European extraction is the hard evidence of efficacy in that group).

The next step down the ladder of proof is a trial that includes members of the "special" group in sufficient numbers for researchers to be reasonably confident that the trends of the effects are in the same direction as in the major trial group. It is at this level that both the FDA and NIH guidelines operate.

A lower level of confidence is that defined by the state in which there is no inclusion of members of the "special" group in a clinical trial, but there is evidence either that the disease process is the same and/or that the effect of the agent on immediate surrogate risk factor being studied is the same. For example, it is assumed in the US that, despite the fact that there is no "substantial" inclusion of African-Americans in any of the clinical trials on the effect of cholesterol lowering on coronary disease, extrapolation is permitted. To the extent to which they have been studied, drugs appear to have the same effect in whites and blacks. In addition, atherosclerosis appears to be essentially the same process in both groups. It seems reasonable, therefore, to assume that the effects of cholesterol lowering will be the same.

The questions that must be addressed when looking at the adequacy of data on "special" groups might be summarized as follows:
1) has any of the group been included in clinical trials of relevance;
2) do the clinical trial data demonstrate trends in the same direction as in the "main" group;
3) is the underlying disease process the same in the "special" group as in the "main" group; and
4) is the risk factor being tested the same in its apparent effects on the disease process in the "special" group as in the "main" group?

Methods for making the most of small numbers of individuals of a particular group included in a clinical trial are also of value. These include; prerandomization stratification to ensure that participants in the trial are properly distributed and accounted for in the treated or control groups; poststudy subgroup analyses (although subject to concern that they may not preserve randomization) that can provide important information about trends in the "special" group; and meta-analyses of subgroups (i.e., examining effects in the same "special" group from a number of studies and statistically combining them to obtain a sufficient sample size to provide statistical significance).

As an example, how does all this play out in data addressing the issue of cholesterol lowering in women in available clinical trials? Reviews of this issue have already been published [3]. In general it may be said that, although included in clinical trials only in small numbers, women with established coronary disease appear in both subgroup analyses and meta-analyses to have at least the same degree of benefit as do men. In fact, there are indications in a number of studies, utilizing both angiographic as well as disease endpoints, that the response of women to LDL-cholesterol lowering may actually be greater [4—6]. This is a bit puzzling given the fact that human observational studies and some animal experiments indicate the arterial wall LDL uptake is not as pronounced in women as it is in men. These discrepancies may result from a failure to account for the degree of estrogenization of the women involved in these studies. Or they may indicate that once a woman has developed atherosclerosis, however, that process may have been affected by the presence of estrogen, she is at as much or more risk from elevated LDL compared with a man with similar disease.

Studies of primary prevention of coronary disease by cholesterol lowering in women are simply not adequate in number or size to draw any conclusions [3]. Given the high prevalence of coronary disease in women in Western society, however, it is prudent to regard women, particularly postmenopausal women, as at sufficient risk of developing coronary disease to be targets for at least routine hygienic interventions such as dietary change as well as exercise and weight control.

If the questions posed above are systematically answered for women, it is reasonable to conclude that there are probably sufficient numbers of women in clinical trials of secondary prevention (but not of primary prevention) to feel comfortable that the effects of cholesterol lowering are important and in the same direction as those found in men.

Given that, should a specific clinical trial of cholesterol lowering in women be mounted? The scientific community appears to have answered with a qualified yes. The antihypertensive and lipid-lowering treatment to prevent heart attack trial (ALLHAT), which is currently enrolling study subjects over 65 years of age for inclusion in a clinical trial of both blood pressure and cholesterol lowering, anticipates recruiting about 40% women [7].

Specific guidelines to define when a separate trial should be considered in a "special" group are not clearly defined. Some considerations that should be helpful in making that decision, however, include the following: are there significant differences in the risk factor (i.e., HDL, triglyceride, or diabetes in women), compared with the "main" group; is there evidence of a significant difference in the pharmacokinetics or pharmacodynamics of the drug being tested (i.e., the slower metabolism of alcohol in women); are there significant differences in the risk of the clinical event (i.e., the greatly increased risk of coronary artery disease in diabetic compared with nondiabetic women); and is there evidence of any significant difference in the underlying disease process (i.e., the effect of estrogen in ameliorating the activity of atherosclerotic plaques)?

These considerations at least allow the development for a rationale for the development of clinical trials in a "special" group. Such guidelines highlight the wisdom of both the FDA and NIH guidelines in requiring inclusion of the "special" groups without requiring the statistical straightjacketing that would preclude the completion of meaningful clinical trials to answer the major hypotheses being tested.

Acknowledgements

The author would like to thank Ann Morcos MA ELS, for excellent editorial assistance.

References

1. Merkatz RB, Temple R, Subel S, Feiden K, Kessler DA. Women in clinical trials of new drugs. A change in food and drug administration policy. The working group on women in clinical trials. N Engl J Med 1993;329:292–296.
2. Department of Health and Human Services. National Institutes of Health. RIN 0905-ZA18. NIH guidelines on the inclusion of women and minorities as subjects in clinical research. Federal Register 1994;59:14508–14513.
3. Walsh J, Grady D. Treatment of hyperlipidemia in women. JAMA 1995;274:1152–1158.
4. Kane JP, Malloy MJ, Ports TA, Phillips NI, Diehl JC, Havel RJ. Regression of coronary atherosclerosis during treatment of familial hypercholesterolemia and with combined drug regimens. JAMA 1990;264:3007–3012.
5. Waters D, Higginson L, Gladstone P, Kimball B, Le May M, Boccuzzi SJ, Lesperance J, CCAIT Study Group. Effects on monotherapy with an HMG-CoA reductase inhibitor on the progression of coronary atherosclerosis as assessed by serial quantitative arteriography. The Canadian Coronary Atherosclerosis Intervention Trial. Circulation 1994;89:959–968.
6. Sacks FM, Pfeffer MA, Moye LA et al. The effect of pravastatin on coronary events after myocardial infarction in patients with average cholesterol levels. N Engl J Med 1996;335: 1001–1009.
7. Davis BR, Cutler JA, Gordon DJ et al. Rationale and design for the Antihypertensive and Lipid Lowering Treatment to Prevent Heart Attack Trial (ALLHAT). Am J Hypertens 1996;9: 342–360.

Index of authors

Keyword index